THE WASHINGTON MANUAL™ OF SURGICAL PATHOLOGY

The Lauren V. Ackerman Laboratory of Surgical Pathology
Barnes-Jewish and St. Louis Children's Hospitals
Washington University Medical Center
Department of Pathology and Immunology
Washington University School of Medicine
St. Louis, Missouri

Editors

Peter A. Humphrey, MD, PhD
Louis P. Dehner, MD
John D. Pfeifer, MD, PhD

Wolters Kluwer | Lippincott Williams & Wilkins
Health

Philadelphia · Baltimore · New York · London
Buenos Aires · Hong Kong · Sydney · Tokyo

Senior Executive Editor: Jonathan W. Pine Jr.
Associate Managing Editor: Jean McGough
Project Manager: Karla Schroeder
Manufacturing Manager: Kathleen Brown
Senior Marketing Manager: Angela Panetta
Design Coordinator: Teresa Mallon
Cover Designer: Becky Baxendell
Production Services: Aptara, Inc.

Library of Congress Cataloging-in-Publication Data

The Washington manual of surgical pathology / editors, Peter A. Humphrey, Louis P. Dehner, John D. Pfeifer.
    p.   cm.
  Includes bibliographical references and index.
  ISBN-13: 978-0-7817-6527-5
  ISBN-10: 0-7817-6527-7
  1.   Pathology, Surgical—Handbooks, manuals, etc.   I. Humphrey, Peter A.
II.   Dehner, Louis P., 1940-   III. Pfeifer, John D.
  RD57.W37 2008
  617′.07—dc22

                                                            2008012371

The Washington Manual™ is an intent-to-use mark belonging to Washington University in St. Louis to which international legal protection applies. The mark is used in this publication by LWW under license from Washington University.

Care has been taken to confirm the accuracy of the information presented and to describe generally accepted practices. However, the authors, editors, and publisher are not responsible for errors or omissions or for any consequences from application of the information in this book and make no warranty, expressed or implied, with respect to the currency, completeness, or accuracy of the contents of the publication. Application of this information in a particular situation remains the professional responsibility of the practitioner.

The authors, editors, and publisher have exerted every effort to ensure that drug selection and dosage set forth in this text are in accordance with current recommendations and practice at the time of publication. However, in view of ongoing research, changes in government regulations, and the constant flow of information relating to drug therapy and drug reactions, the reader is urged to check the package insert for each drug for any change in indications and dosage and for added warnings and precautions. This is particularly important when the recommended agent is a new or infrequently employed drug.

Some drugs and medical devices presented in this publication have Food and Drug Administration (FDA) clearance for limited use in restricted research settings. It is the responsibility of health care providers to ascertain the FDA status of each drug or device planned for use in their clinical practice.

The publishers have made every effort to trace copyright holders for borrowed material. If they have inadvertently overlooked any, they will be pleased to make the necessary arrangements at the first opportunity.

To purchase additional copies of this book, call our customer service department at (800) 638-3030 or fax orders to (301) 223-2320. International customers should call (301) 223-2300.

Visit Lippincott Williams & Wilkins on the Internet: at LWW.com. Lippincott Williams & Wilkins customer service representatives are available from 8:30 am to 6 pm, EST.

10 9 8 7 6 5 4 3 2 1

THIS BOOK IS DEDICATED TO:

MY WIFE KAY, AND CHILDREN TOM AND JENNIFER
—P.A.H.

BECKY AND ALL MY CHILDREN
—L.P.D.

MY WIFE ANDREA, AND CHILDREN ETHAN AND CLAIRE
—J.D.P.

CONTENTS

III: GI TRACT

IV: BREAST

V: URINARY TRACT

VIII: SKIN

IX: NERVOUS SYSTEM

X: HEMATOPOIETIC SYSTEM

Gustavo Alvarez, MD
Surgical Pathology Fellow
Department of Pathology and Immunology
Washington University School of Medicine
St. Louis, Missouri

Emily A. Bantle, MD
Resident
Department of Pathology and Immunology
Washington University School of Medicine
St. Louis, Missouri

Dengfeng Cao, MD, PhD
Assistant Professor
Department of Pathology and Immunology
Washington University School of Medicine
St. Louis, Missouri

Zong-Ming E. Chen, MD, PhD
Surgical Pathology Fellow
Department of Pathology and Immunology
Washington University School of Medicine
St. Louis, Missouri

Rebecca D. Chernock, MD
Resident
Department of Pathology and Immunology
Washington University School of Medicine
St. Louis, Missouri

Kimberley G. Crone, MD
Dermatopathology Fellow
Department of Pathology and Immunology
Washington University School of Medicine
St. Louis, Missouri

Erika C. Crouch, MD, PhD
Professor
Department of Pathology and Immunology
Washington University School of Medicine
St. Louis, Missouri

Rosa M. Dávila, MD
Associate Professor
Department of Pathology and Immunology
Washington University School of Medicine
St. Louis, Missouri

Louis P. Dehner, MD
Professor
Department of Pathology and Immunology
Washington University School of Medicine
St. Louis, Missouri

Jamie K. Donnelly, MD
Surgical Pathology Fellow
Department of Pathology and Immunology
Washington University School of Medicine
St. Louis, Missouri

Samir K. El-Mofty, DMD, PhD
Professor of Oral and Maxillofacial
   Pathology
Associate Professor of Otolaryngology and
   Head and Neck Surgery
Associate Professor of Pathology
Department of Pathology and Immunology
Washington University School of Medicine
St. Louis, Missouri

John L. Frater, MD
Assistant Professor
Department of Pathology and Immunology
Washington University School of Medicine
St. Louis, Missouri

Omar Hameed, MD
Assistant Professor
Department of Pathology
University of Alabama School of Medicine
Birmingham, Alabama

Anjum Hassan, MD
Assistant Professor
Department of Pathology and Immunology
Washington University School of Medicine
St. Louis, Missouri

Phyllis C. Huettner, MD
Associate Professor
Department of Pathology and Immunology
Washington University School of Medicine
St. Louis, Missouri

Michael Hull, MD
Cytopathology Fellow
Department of Pathology and Immunology
Washington University School of Medicine
St. Louis, Missouri

Peter A. Humphrey, MD, PhD
Ladenson Professor
Department of Pathology and Immunology
Chief, Division of Anatomic and Molecular
   Pathology
Washington University School of Medicine
St. Louis, Missouri

Jason A. Jarzembowski, MD, PhD
Pediatric Pathology Fellow
Department of Pathology and Immunology
Washington University School of Medicine
St. Louis, Missouri

Michael J. Klein, MD
Professor
Department of Pathology
Director, Section of Surgical Pathology
University of Alabama School of Medicine
Birmingham, Alabama

Friederike Kreisel, MD
Assistant Professor
Department of Pathology and Immunology
Washington University
St. Louis, Missouri

Elise L. Krejci, MD
Surgical Pathology Fellow
Department of Pathology and Immunology
Washington University School of Medicine
St. Louis, Missouri

Hannah R. Krigman, MD
Assistant Professor
Department of Pathology and Immunology
Washington University School of Medicine
St. Louis, Missouri

Shashikant Kulkarni, MD
Assistant Professor
Departments of Pathology and Immunology,
   and Pediatrics
Director of Cytogenetics
Washington University School of Medicine
St. Louis, Missouri

Jochen K. M. Lennerz, MD, PhD
Resident
Department of Pathology and Immunology
Washington University School of Medicine
St. Louis, Missouri

James S. Lewis Jr., MD
Assistant Professor
Department of Pathology and Immunology
Washington University School of Medicine
St. Louis, Missouri

Helen Liapis, MD
Professor
Department of Pathology and Immunology
Washington University School of Medicine
St. Louis, Missouri

Anne C. Lind, MD
Assistant Professor
Department of Pathology and Immunology
Washington University School of Medicine
St. Louis, Missouri

Dongsi Lu, MD, PhD
Assistant Professor
Department of Pathology and Immunology
Washington University School of Medicine
St. Louis, Missouri

Deborah Novack, MD, PhD
Assistant Professor
Departments of Pathology and Immunology,
   and Internal Medicine
Washington University School of Medicine
St. Louis, Missouri

Anahit Nowrouzi, MD
Hematopathology Fellow
Department of Pathology and Immunology
Washington University School of Medicine
St. Louis, Missouri

Sushama Patil, MD
Neuropathology Fellow
Department of Pathology and Immunology
Washington University School of Medicine
St. Louis, Missouri

Arie Perry, MD
Professor
Department of Pathology and Immunology
Washington University School of Medicine
St. Louis, Missouri

John D. Pfeifer, MD, PhD
Associate Professor
Department of Pathology and Immunology
Associate Chief, Division of Anatomic and
  Molecular Pathology
Washington University School of Medicine
St. Louis, Missouri

Michelle L. E. Powers, MD
Hematopathology Fellow
Department of Pathology and Immunology
Washington University School of Medicine
St. Louis, Missouri

Jon H. Ritter, MD
Associate Professor
Department of Pathology and Immunology
Washington University School of Medicine
St. Louis, Missouri

Souzan Sanati, MD
Instructor
Department of Pathology and Immunology
Washington University School of Medicine
St. Louis, Missouri

Robert E. Schmidt, MD, PhD
Professor
Department of Pathology and Immunology
Chief, Division of Neuropathology
Washington University School of Medicine
St. Louis, Missouri

Kevin D. Selle, MT, HTL (ASCP)
Supervisor
Histology & Immunohistochemistry
  Laboratory
Barnes-Jewish Hospital
St. Louis, Missouri

Maria F. Serrano, MD
Surgical Pathology Fellow
Department of Pathology and Immunology
Washington University School of Medicine
St. Louis, Missouri

Morton E. Smith, MD
Professor Emeritus of Ophthalmology
Professor of Pathology
Washington University School of Medicine
St. Louis, Missouri

David E. Spence, MD
Resident
Department of Pathology and Immunology
Washington University School of Medicine
St. Louis, Missouri

Namsoo Suh, MD
Resident
Department of Pathology and Immunology
Washington University School of Medicine
St. Louis, Missouri

Kiran R. Vij, MD
Surgical Pathology Fellow
Department of Pathology and Immunology
Washington University School of Medicine
St. Louis, Missouri

Nathan C. Walk, MD
Dermatopathology Fellow
Department of Pathology and Immunology
Washington University School of Medicine
St. Louis, Missouri

Hanlin L. Wang, MD, PhD
Director, Gastrointestinal Pathology
Cedars-Sinai Medical Center
Los Angeles, California

Mark A. Watson, MD, PhD
Associate Professor
Department of Pathology and Immunology
Washington University School of Medicine
St. Louis, Missouri

Frances V. White, MD
Associate Professor
Department of Pathology and Immunology
Washington University School of Medicine
St. Louis, Missouri

Lourdes R. Ylagan, MD
Assistant Professor
Department of Pathology and Immunology
Washington University School of Medicine
St. Louis, Missouri

Barbara A. Zehnbauer, PhD
Professor
Department of Pathology and Immunology
Washington University School of Medicine
St. Louis, Missouri

Jing Zhai, MD, PhD
Assistant Professor
Department of Pathology and Immunology
Washington University School of Medicine
St. Louis, Missouri

PREFACE

"Welcome to the 32nd edition of the *Washington Manual of Medical Therapeutics*" is the opening salutation to the most recent edition of a publication that began as a handout to senior medical students, interns, and residents on the Ward Medical Service, as it was known at Barnes Hospital. This first edition of the *Washington Manual of Surgical Pathology* cannot make any claims about its immediate history, but it can harken back to the traditions that are the heritage of surgical pathology at Barnes Hospital, now Barnes-Jewish Hospital, which began with Lauren V. Ackerman, MD. When he came to this institution in 1948 as Director of Surgical Pathology, he was the first trained and board-certified pathologist to occupy a position previously held by surgeons. It was not until the early 1960s that surgical pathology was transferred to the Department of Pathology from the Department of Surgery. Dr. Ackerman initiated the paradigm of diagnostic excellence with the central focus on the patient, and advanced the vital role of the surgical pathologist as a consultant to clinicians. However, Dr. Ackerman was also keenly aware of the surgical pathologist as an educator and investigator of diseases from the observational perspective, and of the central role of the pathologist in correlating those findings with the clinical behavior of the disease process.

The systematic collection of those pathologic observations resulted in the first edition of *Surgical Pathology* in 1953 and lives on in the ninth edition of Rosai and Ackerman's *Surgical Pathology* in 2004. Although multivolume textbooks as well as subspecialty texts continue to have a central role in education and everyday clinical practice, this book is our attempt to respond to the immediate needs of an ever-accelerating world that defines the existence of pathology residents who never have enough time to "get it all done," pathologists in practice who can never sign out cases quickly enough to satisfy clinicians, and clinicians who need a ready and available reference in surgical pathology when the pathologist is not immediately available. For all of these individuals, it is our goal that this latest Washington Manual, written in the fast-access Washington Manual outline format, will fill a niche in our hectic world. In addition to this book, a companion Web site will offer the fully searchable text and an online-only image bank of over 1850 full-color images. (See the inside front cover for Web site access information.)

Most of the individuals who have contributed to this work have had their surgical pathology training in the Lauren V. Ackerman Laboratory of Surgical Pathology at Barnes-Jewish Hospital or are members of the faculty. In the tradition of all Washington Manuals, residents and fellows have likewise contributed to many of the chapters. We hope that the Ackerman tradition is appropriately served in this volume.

Peter A. Humphrey, MD, PhD
Louis P. Dehner, MD
John D. Pfeifer, MD, PhD

ACKNOWLEDGMENTS

The Washington Manual of Surgical Pathology would not have been possible without the participation of our colleagues who so willingly and generously provided their time and expertise to the project. All but one of the authors (special thanks to Dr. Michael Klein) are, or were, faculty or house staff in the Department of Pathology and Immunology at Washington University School of Medicine, which emphasizes the fact that academic surgical pathology at Washington University has always been a collaborative venture between faculty and trainees. Our current and previous chairmen, Dr. Herbert (Skip) Virgin and Dr. Emil Unanue, respectively, have not hesitated to provide the support required to maintain the tradition of diagnostic excellence, academic productivity, and education that forms the foundation of surgical pathology at Washington University School of Medicine.

We extend special thanks to our administrative assistants and secretaries, including Robyn Anderson, Elease Barnes, Margaret Chesney, Jeannie Doerr, Shari Jackson, and Mary Madden, who together typed virtually the entire book. We also acknowledge the artistic expertise of the staff at MedPic (the medical illustration service of Washington University School of Medicine), especially Vicki Friedman, Marcy Hartstein, and Lauren Rohde, who drew the figures for the book. Walter Clermont expertly and patiently edited all the electronic figures found at the associated Web site.

We are lucky to have had the opportunity to work with several wonderful people at Lippincott Williams & Wilkins. Jonathan W. Pine Jr., Senior Executive Editor, was receptive to the idea of a novel format in which the traditional Washington University Manual was combined with a Web site. Jean McGough, Associate Managing Editor, was a constant source of encouragement and support.

Most importantly, we need to thank our spouses and families for their patience and good humor (usually) when we were preoccupied with the writing and editing of the Manual. Over the past two years we have too often taken their support for granted.

Peter A. Humphrey
Louis P. Dehner
John D. Pfeifer

ORAL CAVITY AND OROPHARYNX
James S. Lewis Jr. and Rebecca D. Chernock

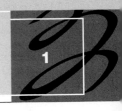

I. NORMAL ANATOMY

A. Oral cavity. The anterior aspect of the oral cavity extends from the mucocutaneous junction (vermillion border) of the lips to include the buccal mucosa (inside of cheek), maxillary and mandibular arches (teeth), retromolar trigone, anterior two thirds of the tongue (oral tongue), floor of mouth, and hard palate. Posteriorly, the oral cavity freely communicates with the oropharynx; the border between the two is marked by the junction of the hard and soft palate superiorly and the line of circumvallate papillae on the dorsal tongue (border between the anterior two thirds and posterior one third of the tongue) inferiorly.

The oral tongue is freely mobile and composed mainly of skeletal muscle. It has a dorsal (exposed) surface, ventral surface, and tip. The dorsal surface contains numerous papillae that have specialized taste receptors. The floor of the mouth lies beneath the tongue and is divided into sides by the midline frenulum (mucosal fold) of the tongue. It contains ostia of the submandibular and sublingual salivary glands, whereas the main duct of the parotid gland (Stenson's duct) enters the oral cavity through the buccal mucosa. The hard palate forms the roof of the oral cavity and consists of portions of the maxillary and palatine bones.

The oral cavity is lined by stratified squamous mucosa with prominent mucoserous glands in the submucosa. Most of the mucosa is nonkeratinizing with the exception of the hard palate, gingiva, and dorsal tongue, which become keratinized due to the friction of mastication.

B. Oropharynx. The oropharynx is the space posterior to the oral cavity that communicates with the nasopharynx superiorly and the larynx and hypopharynx inferiorly. The soft palate (posterior one third of the palate) marks the superior aspect of the oropharynx and is suspended from the posterior aspect of the hard palate. In contrast to the hard palate, the soft palate is fibromuscular without a bony skeleton. Whereas the oral aspect is covered with nonkeratinizing stratified squamous epithelium, the nasal surface is covered by pseudostratified ciliated columnar (respiratory-type) epithelium. Numerous mucoserous glands lie in its submucosa. The posterior one third of the tongue is rich in lymphoid tissue (known as the lingual tonsil); the palatine and lingual tonsils, together with the pharyngeal tonsil in the nasopharynx, are collectively known as Waldeyer's ring.

II. GROSS EXAMINATION, TISSUE SAMPLING, AND HISTOLOGIC SLIDE PREPARATION

A. Open and endoscopic biopsies. The majority of specimens from the oral cavity and oropharynx consist of open biopsies of lesions that can be visualized by the naked eye. The small biopsy pieces should be placed immediately into 10% buffered formalin or other appropriate fixative. Processing of the biopsies should include gross description of the tissue fragments with documentation of the number of pieces present; the biopsies should be entirely submitted, with three levels cut from each paraffin block for hematoxylin and eosin (H&E) examination.

B. Resections

1. Open procedure specimens are widely variable depending on the location of the tumor. Because many lesions encroach upon or invade the bone of the mandible or maxilla, composite resections with bone and soft tissue are common. As a generalization, all specimens need to be oriented appropriately, the soft tissue margins inked, and mucosal and soft tissue margins evaluated followed by sectioning of the tumor relative to cartilage/bone and tissue margins. Margins should be evaluated by either shave or radial sections, depending on the nature of the specimen. If the tumor is relatively distant from a margin, 1- to 2-mm shave sections are preferred. If the tumor approximates a margin to <1 to 2 mm, radial sections should be taken.

2. **Partial resections** with a CO_2 laser under an operating microscope are becoming more common. Because the inherent approach of this procedure is to excise the tumor piece by piece, the surgeon inks the individual pieces as he/she alone knows what constitutes the true margin. In the gross room all that is therefore required is to measure the pieces provided, describe them, and submit them entirely in sections perpendicular to the ink.

C. **Frozen sections** are a critical element of surgical therapy for tumors of the head and neck region. Although practices vary, at most institutions shave margins are submitted, taken by the surgeon from the periphery of the surgical defect after the tumor has been removed. In other cases, the surgeon may sample the tumor or suspicious sites to confirm and/or map the lesion, with additional samples from areas where the tumor is felt to be closest to the surgical margin.

For frozen sections, the tissue is submitted in saline to the pathology lab and then frozen in its entirety, with two H&E slides generated at representative levels well into the tissue. The tissue pieces should be evaluated grossly for mucosa (typically the shiny and pink-tan surface of the tissue) and, if mucosa is present, the specimen should be oriented in the frozen section block to demonstrate this surface on edge. It is critical to cut deeply into the block to obtain sections that represent the entire tissue submitted so that small foci of tumor are not missed by inadequate sampling.

The tissue that remains after frozen section is submitted for evaluation by permanent sections, which helps assure adequate sampling. Permanent sections can help resolve a number of issues from frozen section including freezing and cautery artifact, volume of tumor, and orientation (note that the margins of the main resection specimen should also be evaluated throughout their entirety because the separate frozen section specimens almost never cover the entire margins of a resection specimen). The final margin status is then a conglomerate of three sources: frozen section slides, permanent slides of the frozen tissue, and margins of the specimen itself.

III. DIAGNOSTIC FEATURES OF COMMON BENIGN DISEASES

A. **Inflammation.** Lichen planus, pemphigus vulgaris, and cicatricial pemphigoid are autoimmune disorders that predominately affect middle-aged adults and occur more frequently in women than men. They are diseases that affect mucosal sites as well as skin, so the oral cavity is sometimes involved as well.

1. **Lichen planus.** This disorder commonly affects the oral mucosa. Whereas skin involvement is usually self-limited, oral lichen planus follows a more protracted waxing and waning course. The oral lesions are typically asymptomatic unless ulceration occurs.

Any oral mucosal surface may be involved, and several patterns can be seen. The classic pattern is reticular with intersecting white keratotic streaks (Wickham's striae); the lesions are ill-defined, and the background may be erythematous due to mucosal atrophy. Some lesions may be mostly erythematous with minimal keratotic streaks, whereas others may show extensive keratinization and/or ulceration or form bullae. Microscopically, a dense submucosal band of lymphocytes is present, which may be less distinct in ulcerated lesions. The rete ridges may be hyperplastic (saw-toothed) or flattened. There is loosening of the basal layer of the epithelium, with degeneration of individual keratinocytes that may form eosinophilic colloid (cytoid or Civatte) bodies. The surface may show hyper- or parakeratosis. Although the histologic findings of lichen planus have been well defined, they are nonetheless not specific; for example, some oral lesions with a similar histologic picture may be due to a contact hypersensitivity reaction.

Asymptomatic patients require no treatment, but steroids (particularly topical) are often used for erosive or erythematous lesions. Some data suggest that there is an increased risk of malignant transformation in the erythematous, ulcerative, and bullous forms of oral lichen planus. Although this proposed risk of malignancy is controversial, these lesions at least require closer clinical follow-up.

2. **Pemphigus vulgaris.** This is an uncommon disorder that causes superficial ulceration of the skin and mucous membranes. Involvement of the oral mucosa may precede the development of skin lesions. The disease is caused by autoantibodies to desmogleins 1 and 3, cellular transmembrane proteins involved in the assembly of desmosomes. Cell-to-cell adhesion is impaired in the suprabasal epithelium, leading to clefting and ulceration. Flaccid bullae that easily rupture to form painful erosions can be seen on any oral mucosal surface. The lesions heal without scarring. Microscopically, intraepithelial separation with edema and acantholysis, which imparts a 'tombstone' appearance to the remaining attached basal cell layer (e-**Fig. 1.1**),* is seen at the edge of the ulcer. Acute and chronic inflammation are frequently present in the submucosa. Direct immunofluorescence is positive for immunoglobulin G (IgG) along cell membranes throughout the epidermis.

   Paraneoplastic pemphigus, which is associated with an underlying malignancy, may be distinguished from pemphigus vulgaris by the identification of a different pattern of antibody staining by direct immunofluorescence.

3. **Cicatricial or mucous membrane pemphigold.** This is a rare disease caused by various antibodies that target the basement membrane of mucous membranes and occasionally the skin. The oral mucosa is almost always involved, most commonly the gingiva. In contrast to pemphigus vulgaris, the variably sized bullae are not flaccid, and ruptured bullae heal with scarring. Microscopically, there is clefting between the epithelium and basement membrane, and the space may be filled with serous fluid containing sparse inflammatory cells. Direct immunofluorescence shows a linear band of IgG and C3 on the basement membrane. Treatment is with immunosuppression, but the disease is often progressive despite therapy.

B. **Infections.** Only a few of the numerous infections that may involve the oral cavity are discussed here.

1. **Fungal.** *Candida* species cause most of the fungal infections of the oral cavity. Other fungal infections that occur less frequently in the oral cavity include histoplasmosis, blastomycosis, and coccidiomycosis. *Candida* species are a part of the normal oral flora. Infections occur due to overgrowth, usually in the setting of a predisposing factor. *Candida albicans* is the most frequently isolated species. Local and systemic factors that favor overgrowth include immunosuppression, use of steroids or antibiotics, radiation therapy, xerostomia, use of dentures, and anemia. The extremes of ages are more often affected as well, and infection may be acute or chronic. Symptoms include a burning sensation or foul odor, although the infection may be asymptomatic.

   Several clinical patterns of oral candidiasis are seen. White plaques that are easily scraped off underlying erythematous mucosa are called pseudomembranous candidiasis (oral thrush); this is the most common type of oral candidiasis. Erythematous candidiasis appears as a red patch due to atrophy of the mucosa. Median rhomboid glossitis is a type of erythematous candidiasis that occurs in a specific location, namely a rhomboid-shaped area on the midline dorsal tongue, which over time may develop a nodular appearance. Angular cheilitis causes red fissuring and scaling at the labial commissures; predisposing factors include drooling and ill-fitting dentures. Chronic hyperplastic candidiasis presents as asymptomatic, white patches (due to the thickened, hyperplastic mucosa) that cannot be removed by scraping. This pattern is more common in immunocompetent individuals and may predispose to the development of carcinoma, although a causal relationship between the two has not been clearly demonstrated.

   Microscopically, an intraepithelial infiltrate of neutrophils is seen in all types of candidal infection. The epithelium may be ulcerated, although in chronic hyperplastic candidiasis it is thickened and hyperkeratotic (e-**Fig. 1.2**). Fungal pseudohyphae may be difficult to identify on routine H&E-stained slides. However, methenamine silver or periodic acid–Schiff (PAS) stains will highlight

*All e-figures are available online via the Solution Site Image Bank.

the fungal elements within the keratin and in the superficial squamous epithelium (e-**Fig. 1.2**, insetA).

2. **Viral.** Oral viral infections are highly prevalent, although frequently asymptomatic.

   a. **Human papillomavirus (HPV)** does not cause specific clinically symptomatic infection but is associated with several benign and malignant neoplasms in the oral cavity and oropharynx including squamous papillomas and squamous cell carcinoma (see respective sections to follow).

   b. **Herpes simplex virus (HSV)** causes a common oral viral infection with seroprevalence rates of up to 80% of the population. There are two common serotypes (HSV-1 and HSV-2), and HSV-1 is primarily associated with oral lesions. Gingivostomatitis occurs in 10% of initial infections, predominately in children, and is characterized by fever and a vesicular rash. The virus then latently infects sensory ganglia and may be reactivated periodically throughout life. Recurrent disease is manifested by clusters of vesicles that may cause a burning sensation at the mucocutaneous junction of the lip or nose. Intraoral lesions can also occur.

   Microscopically, the lesional mucosa is often ulcerated and acantholytic, with marked acute and chronic inflammation. There are typically individual necrotic squamous cells. Identification of the classic intranuclear eosinophilic inclusions within squamous epithelial cells is diagnostic of herpes virus infection; the inclusion-harboring cells are often single, detached, and multinucleated (e-**Fig. 1.3**). Immunohistochemical stains may be useful to confirm the diagnosis.

   c. **Epstein–Barr virus (EBV).** Acute EBV infection, although frequently asymptomatic, may cause pharyngitis and tonsillitis. The virus enters the host through oral epithelial cells, where it then gains access to and infects B lymphocytes. Acute EBV infection may produce reactive changes in the tonsils and lymph nodes that can mimic a hematopoietic malignancy.

   Latent EBV infection is virtually universal in adults and is usually asymptomatic. However, an EBV-driven proliferation of tongue epithelial cells, known as **hairy leukoplakia**, occurs in a high percentage of acquired immunodeficiency syndrome (AIDS) patients (approximately 80%); the lesions are asymptomatic unless superinfection with *Candida* occurs. Grossly, hairy leukoplakia appears as a flat, white, shaggy plaque on the lateral tongue. Microscopically, the epithelium is acanthotic with hyper- and parakeratosis. Perinuclear clearing with koilocytic-type change of individual cells is characteristic, and viral inclusions may give nuclei a smudged appearance. Inflammation is typically sparse. Definitive diagnosis relies on detection of EBV within the lesion by immunohistochemistry or in situ hybridization. Hairy leukoplakia is self-limited with no propensity for malignant transformation. Latent EBV infection has been implicated in the development of a variety of hematopoietic and non-hematopoietic malignancies as well (see Chaps. 3 and 43).

3. **Bacterial. Cervicofacial actinomycosis ("lumpy jaw").** *Actinomyces* are gram positive, saprophytic anaerobes that are part of the normal oral flora. The organisms are often incidentally found in sections of the tonsillar crypts. Occasionally, they are introduced into the soft tissues through trauma, particularly from dental manipulations, where an acute or chronic infection may ensue. *Actinomyces israeli* is the most common pathogenic species.

   Acute infections are suppurative, creating a nontender fluctuant mass. In the chronic phase, infections may form a more extensive firm fibrous mass mimicking a neoplasm. Sinus tracts may exit either the skin or mucosa (e-**Fig. 1.4**) and often discharge yellow clusters of tightly adherent *Actinomyces* bacteria that have the appearance of sulfur granules. Osteomyelitis may develop in adjacent bone. Microscopically, collections of radiating, filamentous organisms are seen in a background of neutrophils with surrounding granulation tissue and/or fibrosis. Cultures are often negative due to overgrowth of other organisms. Treatment with prolonged antibiotics is usually successful, although incision and drainage may be necessary.

C. Other non-neoplastic lesions
   1. Fibrous lesions. A number of different types of fibrous lesions occur in and around the oral cavity.
      a. Irritation fibroma. These are the most common oral mucosal mass lesions. They are painless reactive proliferations of fibrous tissue that develop in response to trauma from teeth or dentures. The lateral tongue and buccal mucosa along the bite line are the most common sites. Multiple fibromas may be seen in inherited syndromes including Cowden's syndrome and tuberous sclerosis. Linear, grooved fibromas occurring in the mucosa opposing the teeth or sulcus of the alveolar ridge are called epulis fissuratum and are denture-related.
      Grossly, irritation fibroma is usually pink to white, dome-shaped, and only a few millimeters in maximal diameter. Microscopically, there is a nodular deposition of dense collagen with associated chronic inflammation and overlying thinned mucosa (e-Fig. 1.5). Trauma-related changes such as hyperkeratosis and ulceration may be seen. The fibroblasts are spindled and indistinct; if larger, stellate fibroblasts are present, the lesion is called a **giant cell fibroma**, which, in contrast to irritation fibromas, is not associated with trauma and occurs at a younger age. Whereas typical irritation fibromas do not recur after simple resection, giant cell fibromas may.
      b. Gingival fibromatosis. This is generalized, but not necessarily symmetrical, enlargement of the gingiva which may be hereditary, drug-induced, related to poor oral hygiene, or idiopathic. When it is drug-induced, it is called **fibrous gingival hyperplasia** and frequently regresses with cessation of the inciting drug.
      Grossly, the gums are enlarged, smooth-surfaced, and firm. Microscopically, the submucosa shows dense eosinophilic to slightly basophilic fibrous tissue with associated mild chronic inflammation (e-Fig. 1.6). The surface squamous epithelium may have chronic inflammation or extreme elongation of the rete, but is otherwise unremarkable.
   2. Inflammatory papillary hyperplasia is a denture-associated lesion and is typically located beneath a denture base in the hard palate and alveolar ridges. Occasionally, it is seen in patients without dentures and may be associated with poor oral hygiene.
      Clinically, the mucosa looks "pebbly" with numerous, small, papular projections. Microscopically, the mucosa may be atrophic or demonstrate pseudoepitheliomatous hyperplasia. The underlying submucosa may vary from edematous to fibrotic, with mild chronic inflammation. Individual nodules may resemble an irritation fibroma or pyogenic granuloma. The condition is not premalignant, may subside with less denture wear, or may require surgical excision.
   3. Torus palatinus, torus mandibularis, and buccal exostosis are common developmental anomalies that continue to grow throughout life and typically present in adulthood. They are site-specific. Torus palatinus occurs in the midline of the hard palate, torus mandibularis occurs on the lingual surface of the mandible near the bicuspid teeth, and buccal exostosis is found on the facial surface of the alveolar bone. Any identical appearing bony proliferations at other oral sites are generically termed "bony exostosis" or "osteoma" and are not developmental, but rather trauma-related or true neoplasms that can be associated with Gardner's syndrome.
      Grossly, these lesions are broad-based, single, or lobulated masses with smooth surfaces (e-Fig. 1.7). Microscopically, they are composed of dense lamellar bone with scattered osteocytes and variable amounts of marrow. Ischemic changes with marrow fibrosis and loss of osteocytes from lacunae may be seen. Resection is not necessary except for cosmetic reasons or if the lesions become large. There is little risk of recurrence, and the lesions have no malignant potential.
   4. Fordyce granules. Sebaceous glands are normally found in the skin associated with hair follicles. When they are ectopically present in the oral mucosa, they are called Fordyce granules. They are common (present in up to 80% of adults) and can occur on any oral mucosal surface, although the buccal mucosa is most common. Most appear as scattered, 1 to 3 mm, white to yellow papules.

Microscopically, normal sebaceous glands are present in the submucosa without associated hair follicles. No treatment is necessary unless for cosmetic reasons (biopsies are rarely performed as the diagnosis is usually clinically apparent). Occasionally, Fordyce granules can coalesce to form the larger, cauliflowerlike lesion termed sebaceous hyperplasia.

5. **Cysts.** Included here are several of the more common soft tissue true cysts that have an epithelial lining. Odontogenic cysts, bone cysts, and salivary gland–derived pseudocysts (lacking a true epithelial lining) are discussed in Chapter 4.

   a. **Epidermoid cyst.** Intraoral epidermoid cysts are much less common than their counterparts in the skin and are thought to represent inclusions of surface epithelium or cystic change in odontogenic rests. They often present in teenagers and young adults. The most common site is the gingiva. Clinically, they are small (<1 cm) superficial nodules. When they occur in the midline floor of mouth, however, they can become much larger (>5 cm) and interfere with swallowing. Microscopically, they are lined by thin stratified squamous epithelium, with or without a granular cell layer, and are often filled with keratinous debris. Rupture with spillage of keratinous debris may elicit a granulomatous inflammatory reaction. Treatment is by simple surgical excision.

   b. **Dermoid cysts.** These are similar to epidermoid cysts but contain adnexal structures, such as sebaceous glands or hair follicles, in the cyst wall. If other tissue types are present, the lesion is termed a teratoid cyst.

   c. **Nasolabial cysts.** These rare cysts occur at the base of the nostril or at the superior aspect of the upper lip. They are thought to be derived from remnants of the embryonic nasolacrimal duct. Seventy-five percent of cases occur in women. More than 10% are bilateral. They present as slow growing masses, usually <1.5 cm, and they may have irregular contours. Soft tissue swelling with loss of the nasolabial fold or elevation of the nasal ala or floor may occasionally cause nasal obstruction. Pressure erosion of underlying bone is possible.

   Microscopically, the cysts may be lined by respiratory type, cuboidal, and/or stratified squamous epithelium with scattered mucus-filled goblet cells, with surrounding chronic inflammation. A fibrous or epithelial connection to the nasal mucosa is almost always present. Simple surgical excision is curative.

   d. **Lymphoepithelial cyst.** These cysts are thought to develop from invaginations of crypt epithelium within accessory tonsillar tissue. Clinically, they are painless submucosal nodules that are almost always <6 mm in diameter and typically occur in teenagers or young adults. Half of cases occur in the floor of the mouth; the lateral and ventral tongue, as well as the soft palate, are also common sites. They do not occur in the alveolar soft tissue.

   Microscopically, the cyst lining is an attenuated squamous epithelium with a poorly formed granular layer. The cyst is filled with orthokeratin and surrounded tightly by lymphoid aggregates with variable numbers of germinal centers. The cysts may become dissociated from the epithelium or remain connected, often with keratin plugging. Microscopically, the prominent lymphoid aggregates distinguish this cyst from an epidermoid cyst. Similar appearing cysts can be seen within the tonsils themselves from blockage of the crypt connection with the surface.

6. **Pseudoepitheliomatous hyperplasia** is a generic term for benign, downward proliferation of the epithelium that is important to distinguish from invasive, well-differentiated squamous cell carcinoma (SCC). Pseudoepitheliomatous hyperplasia is characteristically seen in association with specific lesions including inflammatory papillary hyperplasia, submucosal granular cell tumors, and fungal infections. It can also be seen adjacent to ulcers or be seen associated with myriad other lesions. Microscopically, irregular and pseudoinfiltrative nests of keratinizing squamous epithelium are sometimes seen beneath a markedly thickened surface epithelium; the papillae of the squamous epithelium may be markedly elongated and extend deeply into the submucosa (e-**Fig. 1.8**). However, in contrast to squamous dysplasia and carcinoma, cytologic atypia is absent.

7. **Amalgam tattoo.** Amalgam is a material used for dental fillings that is composed of a combination of metals. It can be inadvertently implanted into oral mucosa during a dental procedure, creating a tattoo that may be mistaken clinically for melanoma. The lesions present as painless, blue-gray pigmented macules that are variable in size and location. Microscopically, pigmented particles are seen scattered in the submucosa around vessels and along reticulin fibers. There is typically no tissue reaction.

IV. **NEOPLASTIC LESIONS.** The World Health Organization (WHO) classification of tumors of the oral cavity and oropharynx is listed in Table 1.1.

A. **Epithelial**

1. **Benign**

a. **Squamous papilloma.** Squamous papillomas are benign squamous proliferations caused by HPV. They are most common in the larynx but also occur as solitary lesions in the oral cavity and oropharynx.

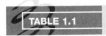

TABLE 1.1   **WHO Histological Classification of Tumors of the Oral Cavity and Oropharynx**

Malignant epithelial tumors
Squamous cell carcinoma
  Verrucous carcinoma
  Basaloid squamous cell carcinoma
  Papillary squamous cell carcinoma
Spindle cell carcinoma
Acantholytic squamous cell carcinoma
  Adenosquamous carcinoma
  Carcinoma cuniculatum
Lymphoepithelial carcinoma

Epithelial precursor lesions

Benign epithelial tumors
Papillomas
  Squamous cell papilloma and verruca
    vulgaris
  Condyloma acuminatum
  Focal epithelial hyperplasia
Granular cell tumor
Keratoacanthoma

Salivary gland tumors
Salivary gland carcinomas
  Acinic cell carcinoma
  Mucoepidermoid carcinoma
Adenoid cystic carcinoma
Polymorphous low-grade adenocarcinoma
Basal cell adenocarcinoma
Epithelial–myoepithelial carcinoma
Clear cell carcinoma, not otherwise
  specified
Cystadenocarcinoma
Mucinous adenocarcinoma
Oncocytic carcinoma
Salivary duct carcinoma

Myoepithelial carcinoma
Carcinoma ex pleomorphic adenoma

Benign epithelial tumors
Pleomorphic adenoma
Myoepithelioma
Basal cell adenoma
Canalicular adenoma
Ductal papilloma
Cystadenoma

Soft tissue tumors
Kaposi's sarcoma
Lymphangioma
Ectomesenchymal chondromyxoid tumor
Focal oral mucinosis
Congenital granular cell epulis

Hematolymphoid tumors
Diffuse large B-cell lymphoma (DLBCL)
Mantle cell lymphoma
Follicular lymphoma
Extranodal marginal zone B-cell lymphoma
  of mucosa-associated lymphoid tissue
  (MALT) type
Burkitt lymphoma
T-cell lymphoma (including anaplastic large
  cell lymphoma)
Extramedullary plasmacytoma
Langerhans cell histiocytosis
Extramedullary myeloid sarcoma
Follicular dendritic cell sarcoma/tumor

Mucosal malignant melanoma

Secondary tumors

Squamous papillomas are strongly associated with the nononcogenic HPV types 6 and 11, but have a very low infectivity so do not appear contagious. In the oral cavity and oropharynx, they occur in adults between 30 and 50 years of age, most commonly on the hard and soft palate and uvula.

Squamous papillomas have a characteristic morphology. Grossly, they are soft, exophytic, granular, and pink-red or tan. Microscopically, they consist of arborizing, papillary fronds of thickened but maturing squamous epithelium with nuclei that are slightly enlarged and irregular but not overtly dysplastic. Mitotic activity is usually present but is modest. Sometimes there is slight hyperplasia of the basal layer. Cells in the mid-layer often have cytoplasmic clearing, but frank koilocytosis is not regularly observed. Characteristically, there is no significant surface keratinization (e-**Fig. 1.9**).

Squamous papillomas are cured by simple excision. They have limited growth potential, rarely recur, and have essentially no risk of malignant transformation.

b. Condyloma acuminatum and verruca vulgaris. Both of these lesions, although much more common on the skin, can also occur in the oral cavity. Condylomas are considered a sexually transmitted disease and usually occur in young adults on the lips and soft palate as clusters of pink nodules that coalesce into more exophytic masses. They have more blunted, papillary fronds and more hyperkeratosis than squamous papillomas.

Verrucae also can occur intraorally, particularly in children, commonly on the lips and anterior tongue. They have a morphology identical to that of verruca of the skin with a broad base, marked papillomatosis, and hyperkeratosis with parakeratosis.

c. Verruciform xanthoma. This is a peculiar lesion of the oral cavity which has no relation to HPV and may be reactive in nature. It occurs in middle-aged to older adults and is most common on the alveolar ridges. Clinically and grossly, it is a well-demarcated, painless, and soft, slightly elevated mass. It may have a yellow or white color with a roughened surface. Microscopically, it consists of broad papillae with intervening cleftlike spaces covered by a slightly thickened, nondysplastic squamous epithelium with hyperkeratosis and parakeratosis. The diagnostic cells, which lie in the superficial submucosa, are foamy macrophages with abundant pale, flocculent cytoplasm and round to oval, bland nuclei (e-**Fig. 1.10**); these cells are filled with lipid and should be distinguished from the eosinophilic granular cells of granular cell tumor (see section E to follow).

Verruciform xanthoma is treated by conservative excision and has no risk of malignant transformation. Recurrences are rare.

2. Precursor (premalignant) squamous lesions. Precursor lesions are defined as altered squamous epithelium with an increased risk of progression to SCC, and are strongly associated with smoking and alcohol use. They may present as leukoplakia (white, thickened epithelium; see e-**Fig. 1.11**), erythroplakia (thin, erythematous, and red epithelium), or speckled erythroplakia (a mixture of both erythroplakia and leukoplakia).

The terms dysplasia or intraepithelial neoplasia should be used for these lesions. The likelihood of malignant change relates to the severity of dysplasia, although carcinoma can develop from any grade of dysplasia (as well as from normal epithelium). Atypia, on the other hand, is not considered synonymous with dysplasia and is used in a more general sense because the term may also describe changes seen in reactive epithelium. There are a number of changes that occur in dysplasia including nuclear abnormalities, architectural/organizational abnormalities, and abnormal keratinization. Unfortunately, there is poor agreement among pathologists about the minimum histopathologic changes that constitute dysplasia, and about the grading of dysplasia (several grading systems that have been proposed are shown in Table 1.2).

3. Malignant. SCC is the overwhelmingly most common malignant tumor of the oral cavity and oropharynx. It has a high male to female preponderance (3:1)

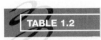

TABLE 1.2	Precursor Lesion Classification Schemes	

Ljubljana classification squamous intraepithelial lesions (SIL)	Squamous intraepithelial neoplasia (SIN)	2005 WHO classification
Squamous cell (simple) hyperplasia	Not applicable	Squamous cell hyperplasia
Basal/parabasal cell hyperplasia	SIN 1	Mild dysplasia
Atypical hyperplasia	SIN 2	Moderate dysplasia
Atypical hyperplasia	SIN 3	Severe dysplasia
Carcinoma in situ	SIN 3	Carcinoma in situ

and a strong relationship to tobacco smoking and alcohol consumption, with a multiplicative rather than additive relative risk. Although not as extreme, the risk of SCC is also increased with the use of snuff and chewing tobacco. Betel quid, commonly used in some parts of the world, is also a major risk factor. Finally, HPV, particularly type 16, has a major causative role in oropharyngeal SCC, leading to carcinomas that usually show a distinct nonkeratinizing morphology and less aggressive behavior.

   a. **Conventional or keratinizing-type SCC.** The gross appearance of keratinizing-type SCC is quite variable, ranging from fungating, exophytic tumors to endophytic, ulcerated tumors with raised edges. Most tumors elicit stromal fibrosis, so have firm and tan-white cut surfaces. Microscopically, these tumors consist of nests and sheets of cells with squamous differentiation. The cells typically have abundant eosinophilic cytoplasm and round to oval nuclei, often with prominent nucleoli. Well-differentiated tumors retain abundant pink or clear cytoplasm and often show keratin 'pearl' formation (e-**Fig. 1.12**). Moderately differentiated tumors (the majority of cases) have cells with more pleomorphism and a higher nucleus to cytoplasm ratio while still retaining a moderate amount of eosinophilic cytoplasm (e-**Fig. 1.13**). Poorly differentiated tumors often have single cells or small nests of cells with more mitotic activity and less cytoplasm (e-**Fig. 1.14**). Grading should be performed but has not been shown to predict clinical behavior. Perineural, lymphatic, and vascular space invasion are commonly seen.

      Treatment for oral cavity and oropharyngeal SCC typically consists of surgery followed by postoperative radiotherapy, the latter depending somewhat on the stage of disease. Small primary lesions without neck lymph node metastases, or with small lymph node metastases without extracapsular extension, may be treated by surgery alone. Radiotherapy, sometimes with chemotherapy and/or epidermal growth factor receptor (EGFR)-targeted drugs, is sometimes used, particularly for large tumors that are not surgically resectable. The overall survival for conventional SCC of the oral cavity is approximately 50%–55% at 5 years but varies greatly by tumor stage. For oropharyngeal carcinomas, the prognosis is slightly worse.

   b. **Nonkeratinizing SCC.** This entity is slowly gaining recognition as a specific subtype of head and neck SCC. Tumors with this morphology are only seen in the palatine tonsils and base of tongue and are virtually always HPV-associated (HPV16 in >95% of cases). Patients with nonkeratinizing SCC are, on average, 5 years younger than those with conventional SCC, and are less likely to be smokers. The most common clinical presentation is as an asymptomatic neck mass. Nonkeratinizing SCC arises in the crypts of the tonsillar tissue, so the tumors tend to be subsurface and thus clinically subtle. This feature, combined with the tumor's strong propensity for early metastasis to cervical lymph nodes, explains why the most common presentation is as a painless neck mass; better recognition of this tumor type has led to more intensive scrutiny of the tonsils and base of tongue in this clinical setting.

Grossly, nonkeratinizing SCC is endophytic, firm, and tan in most cases. However, because the tumors are often small and do not elicit much desmoplasia in the surrounding stroma, they can be quite difficult to identify grossly. Microscopically, they consist of ribbons of tumor cells lining the crypt epithelium and of nests and sheets of cells with smooth borders in the submucosa. The overlying surface epithelium is typically intact without dysplasia (e-Fig. 1.15). The cells are basal in appearance, with round to oval to spindled nuclei, relatively homogeneous chromatin without nucleoli, minimal cytoplasm, and very brisk mitotic activity with abundant apoptosis (e-Fig. 1.16). Central (comedo) necrosis is common in the tumor cell nests.

Immunohistochemistry is positive for cytokeratins, and for p16, a tumor suppressor protein that is aberrantly overexpressed in cells infected by HPV. In situ hybridization and polymerase chain reaction (PCR) are both positive for HPV16 or other high risk HPV types in almost all cases.

Treatment is most often by surgical resection with neck dissection followed by postoperative radiation therapy. Numerous studies have shown that the prognosis for HPV-related SCC of the oropharynx is better than for keratinizing type SCC, despite the fact that tumors commonly present with lymph node metastases and thus at high stage.

c. **Verrucous carcinoma** (VC) is a specific, well-differentiated and nonmetastasizing variant of SCC. It has also been called Ackerman's tumor *clinical*. It occurs in the larynx and oral cavity and grossly appears as a well-circumscribed, warty and exophytic, broad-based, white or tan mass (e-Fig. 1.17). It can become very large and dramatically invade soft tissues and bone. Microscopically, VC consists of very thick surface squamous epithelium with club-shaped papillae that have a broad pushing base; these blunt and downward-pushing projections have sometimes been likened to elephant's feet. There is usually prominent surface hyperkeratosis, and the sheets of tumor are composed of bland cells with abundant eosinophilic to clear cytoplasm, sometimes described as glassy in appearance. There is no cytologic atypia. The stroma directly beneath the tumor typically demonstrates prominent chronic inflammation, often with abundant plasma cells (e-Fig. 1.18).

The prognosis for pure VC is excellent. Although the tumor can be large and locally destructive, complete surgical resection is often curative. Radiation is also an acceptable treatment, particularly in poor surgical candidates. Conventional invasive SCC often arises from VC; when this occurs, the prognosis and behavior is the same as for conventional SCC. The lesion must be thoroughly sampled histologically before a diagnosis of pure VC is made.

d. **Spindle cell carcinoma** (SpCC) is the head and neck mucosal form of sarcomatoid carcinoma, a variant of SCC consisting of spindled or pleomorphic tumor cells that simulate a true sarcoma. It is clear from ultrastructural, immunohistochemical, and molecular studies that the sarcomatoid cells represent a clone of poorly differentiated, or divergently differentiated, carcinoma cells. SpCC has demographics similar to those of conventional SCC, occurring in the 5th to 6th decade, showing a strong association with smoking and alcohol use, and having a very high male to female ratio. It occurs most commonly in the larynx (particularly the glottis) followed by the oral cavity, hypopharynx, and nasal cavity. Up to 20% of patients have a history of previous radiation to the originating site, which is higher than that for conventional SCC.

Grossly, the vast majority of laryngeal and hypopharyngeal SpCC, and approximately 50% of oral SpCC, have a polypoid growth pattern resulting in an exophytic mass with a smooth and extensively ulcerated surface. Up to 75% of SpCC are biphasic tumors with areas of conventional SCC admixed with areas of spindled and/or pleomorphic tumor cells (e-Fig. 1.19); the spindled component usually predominates. The conventional squamous component may take the form of squamous dysplasia, carcinoma in situ, or invasive carcinoma; because the tumors are usually exophytic with extensive surface ulceration, the noninvasive component may be only a focal finding or may be effaced altogether. There may be a wide variety of architectural patterns including fascicular (e-**Fig. 1.20**), storiform, lacelike, or myxoid areas of growth. On occasion, the tumor cells may be widely spaced in an edematous stroma mimicking granulation tissue with cytologic atypia, a diagnostic pitfall. ✱ Approximately 5% of tumors will have definable heterologous sarcomatous differentiation, either osteo- or chondrosarcomatous. Immunohistochemistry in the spindle cell component is positive for cytokeratins and/or epithelial membrane antigen in approximately two thirds of cases, and for p63 in a similar percentage; vimentin is always positive, and a significant minority of tumors will be positive for smooth muscle actin.

Although any malignant spindle cell lesion of the mucosa of the upper aerodigestive tract should be considered an SpCC until proven otherwise, the differential diagnosis includes a true sarcoma, spindle cell melanoma, nodular fasciitis, and ulcers and granulation tissue with reactive atypia (particularly after radiation). When a conventional squamous carcinoma component is present intermingled with the spindle cells, the diagnosis of SpCC is confirmed without the need for additional studies.

Because SpCC is inherently a carcinoma, current treatment recommendations are essentially identical to those for conventional SCC, and taking all patients together, the prognosis does not appear different from conventional SCC. However, the prognosis is worse for oral cavity SpCC, although patients with exophytic tumors do better than those with any significant tissue invasion.

   e. **Papillary SCC** is a rare variant of SCC that has an exophytic, papillary growth pattern and a better prognosis. It is more common in the larynx than in the oral cavity and oropharynx.

   f. **Adenosquamous carcinoma** is another rare variant consisting of a mixture of SCC and adenocarcinoma with true gland formation, often with mucin production. The oral cavity and oropharynx are less common sites than the larynx. These tumors are typically more aggressive than conventional SCC.

B. **Melanocytic.** Melanoma is not uncommon in the oral cavity. It occurs in adults with an average age of approximately 60 years, but a very even incidence from age 20 to 80 years. Unlike cutaneous melanoma, in which sun damage underlies the development of most cases, no major etiology has been identified for oral lesions. There is a slight male preponderance and, also unlike cutaneous melanoma, oral lesions occur relatively equally among several races. Oral melanomas present as incidental pigmented lesions identified by a dentist or physician, as masses arising in a preexisting pigmented lesion, or simply as a new mass growing over a few months. The most common oral site is the hard palate (~40%), followed by the maxillary gingiva (~25%) (e-**Fig. 1.21**), the buccal mucosa, mandibular gingiva, and lip. Melanomas of the oropharynx are rare.

Grossly, most tumors are heavily pigmented and heterogeneous, with a brown, gray, or black color. There are sometimes satellite lesions without intervening pigmentation. Microscopically, most melanomas are deeply invasive, but two thirds retain a surface in situ component as well. Architecturally, the tumors consist of single cells and ill-defined sheets and nests of either epithelioid cells, spindle cells, or both. The large epithelioid cells have abundant cytoplasm (which can be eosinophilic to gray) and round to oval nuclei with a characteristic single, large, cherry red nucleolus (e-**Fig. 1.22**). Melanin pigment is commonly present. Spindle cells are less common and have cigar-shaped nuclei and moderate clear to eosinophilic cytoplasm. Plasmacytoid and rhabdoid cells can also be seen. Intranuclear cytoplasmic inclusions that are typical of melanomas at other sites are uncommon in oral melanomas. By immunohistochemistry, oral melanomas express the same proteins as other melanomas, namely MelanA, MART-1, HMB-45, S-100, and tyrosinase.

Treatment consists of radical resection with radiation, with or without chemotherapy. Neck dissection is performed only for clinically detected disease. The prognosis is poor; numerous studies have demonstrated a collective 5-year survival between 15 and 25%. Breslow thickness, unlike cutaneous lesions, is of very limited prognostic utility. Approximately 40% of patients will develop cervical lymph node metastases, and common distant metastatic sites include the lung, liver, and brain.

C. Neuroendocrine carcinomas are uncommon tumors in the head and neck region in general, and are very uncommon in the oral cavity and oropharynx. They are essentially all high grade with a small cell morphology, composed of cells with scant cytoplasm, crush artifact, granular chromatin without nucleoli, and extensive necrosis with brisk mitotic activity (i.e., morphologically identical to small cell carcinomas of the lung and other organs). Some are mixed with a component of SCC. Carcinoid tumors (low-grade neuroendocrine carcinomas) almost never occur in the oral cavity and oropharynx.

The prognosis for high-grade neuroendocrine carcinoma is very poor, with rapid progression of disease including the development of cervical lymph node metastases and distant metastatic disease.

D. Vascular

1. Pyogenic granulomas are benign lesions of the oral cavity that are better referred to as lobular capillary hemangiomas because this term more accurately reflects their origin. They occur in patients of all ages, are usually solitary, and are most common on the lips, tongue, and gingival and buccal mucosa. When they occur during pregnancy, they are usually on the gingiva, and they often grow rapidly. They usually present as small (a few centimeters or less) exophytic masses that bleed easily.

Grossly, they are polypoid or pedunculated; pink, red, or tan; and have a smooth surface. Microscopically, they consist of lobules of small capillaries with plump endothelial cells that have round to oval nuclei and occasional mitoses (e-**Fig. 1.23**), with larger central "feeder" vessels. Extensive surface ulceration with associated fibrin is usually present. The cells are positive for endothelial immunohistochemical markers such as CD34, CD31, and factor VIII–related antigen.

Pyogenic granulomas are benign neoplasms that are cured by simple excision. A small percentage may recur. Pregnancy-related lesions usually regress postpartum.

2. Hemangioma and **lymphangioma** are benign tumors composed of abundant blood or lymphatic vessels, respectively. Hemangiomas of the oral cavity usually occur in adults. They occur most commonly on the lip, buccal mucosa, and lateral tongue borders and present as painless, nodular or well-circumscribed, red or blue masses (e-**Fig. 1.24**) measuring <2 cm in maximal dimension. Microscopically, they consist of blood vessels ranging from small capillaries to large cavernous spaces. The endothelial lining cells can be plump and may have mitotic activity, a feature more common in children. There are a number of named histologic variants, most of which have no clinical significance.

Lymphangiomas (or cystic hygromas) are composed of dilated lymphatic channels. About 75% occur in the head and neck and, when presenting in the oral cavity, they are almost always found in children younger than 3 years. Histologically, they typically consist of very dilated lymphatic channels lined by bland, inconspicuous endothelial cells, with intraluminal eosinophilic material, lymphocytes, and occasional red blood cells. There often are interstitial aggregates of lymphocytes.

Both hemangioma and lymphangioma are benign lesions cured by conservative excision. Both lesions can be sclerosed as well. Large lymphangiomas are often debulked, often via serial resections to avoid major morbidity.

3. Kaposi's sarcoma (KS) is a locally aggressive tumor uniformly associated with human herpesvirus 8 (HHV-8) that predominantly involves the skin but can also involve mucosal sites. When KS involves the oral cavity, usually as a complication of AIDS, it is most commonly found in the palate, followed by the gingiva and dorsal tongue. Clinically, KS appears as purple, red-blue, or brown macules or plaques. Later in the disease course, the lesions become nodular and may ulcerate. The three histologic stages of KS (patch, plaque, and modular; all discussed in more detail in Chap. 39) can all be associated with oral KS (e-**Fig. 1.25**).

There are frequently associated collections of extravasated red blood cells and hemosiderin-laden macrophages. A characteristic feature that is sometimes seen is the pale, eosinophilic hyaline globule, which probably represents degenerating red blood cells. Immunohistochemistry is positive for the common endothelial markers CD34 and CD31.

The behavior of oral KS is variable. It is generally indolent in nonimmuno-compromised patients but is more aggressive in patients with AIDS. However, the mortality related to KS is highly dependent on other comorbidities such as opportunistic infections and systemic symptoms.

E. Neural/neuroectodermal. Granular cell tumors are benign, slow growing tumors of neural origin that occur at many anatomic sites. Approximately 50% occur in the head and neck region, and half of these occur in the tongue. They also occur in the buccal mucosa, floor of mouth, and palate, and are twice as common in women as men; approximately 10%–20% are multiple. Grossly, they are smooth, sessile, and firm with a pink or tan-white color. Microscopically, they consist of infiltrative nonencapsulated sheets and cords of bland cells with abundant eosinophilic granular cytoplasm and indistinct cell borders (e-Fig. 1.26). There is usually no significant stromal reaction. The nuclei are small, oval, and hyperchromatic with minimal atypia and no mitotic activity. A common feature is pseudoepitheliomatous hyperplasia of the overlying squamous epithelium, which can closely mimic SCC. Conservative excision is the treatment of choice, with a risk of recurrence of <10%. Malignant granular cell tumors are very rare but do occur.

F. Mesenchymal

1. **Peripheral ossifying fibroma** is a reactive proliferation of fibrous tissue on the gingiva which shows focal bone formation. It occurs over a broad age range, but young adults are most commonly affected. The lesions range from a few millimeters up to 2 cm in maximal dimension. They are essentially exclusive to the gingiva, particularly along the incisors, and present as sessile pink nodules, usually with surface ulceration. Microscopically, they consist of randomly distributed plump, but not atypical, fibroblasts with foci of mineralization ranging from dystrophic calcification, to cementum-like material, to well-formed bone (e-Fig. 1.27). Rare giant cells can be seen. The lesions should be excised down to the periosteum but will recur in 15%–20% of cases.

2. **Peripheral giant cell granuloma** is another reactive proliferation of the gingiva, particularly along the incisors, caused by chronic irritation. It presents over a wide age range, particularly in middle-aged to older adults, as a solitary broad-based nodule that is reddish or blue and <2 cm in diameter. Microscopically, it consists of a mixture of multinucleated osteoclast-like giant cells and plump spindled to oval mononuclear cells (e-Fig. 1.28). Hemosiderin, chronic inflammation, and foci of metaplastic bone are frequent. The differential diagnosis includes brown tumor of hyperparathyroidism, cherubism, and central (intraosseous) giant cell granuloma. The lesion is treated by local excision down to the bone, with recurrence in approximately 10% of cases.

3. **Congenital granular cell epulis** is a rare benign mesenchymal tumor that classically arises from the anterior alveolar ridge of a newborn. Girls are more frequently affected than boys by a ratio of 9:1. The tumor presents as a smooth, nonulcerated mass about 1 cm in size arising from the gingiva over the lateral incisor/canine area of the maxilla, or less commonly, the mandible. Grossly, it is polypoid and has a homogeneous firm pink or tan cut surface. Microscopically, it consists of a sheet of large cells that have abundant, granular, eosinophilic cytoplasm and round to oval, bland nuclei. The surface squamous epithelium is intact and shows no hyperplasia. By immunohistochemistry, the cells are positive only for vimentin, and specifically are negative for S-100.

Congenital granular cell epulis is not the newborn equivalent of a granular cell tumor and shows no neural differentiation. The tumor stops growing at birth and regresses over time, but most cases still require surgical resection. There is no recurrence, even after incomplete removal.

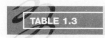

TABLE 1.3   2002 AJCC Staging Guidelines for Tumors of the Oral Cavity

PRIMARY TUMOR (T)
Primary tumor cannot be assessed (TX)
No evidence of primary tumor (T0)
Carcinoma in situ (Tis)
Tumor ≤2 cm in greatest dimension (T1)
Tumor >2 cm but not >4 cm in greatest dimension (T2)
Tumor >4 cm in greatest dimension (T3)
Tumor invades adjacent structures (i.e., through cortical bone*, into deep [extrinsic] muscle of
   tongue [genioglossus, hyoglossus, palatoglossus, and styloglossus], maxillary sinus, skin of
   face) (T4a)
Tumor invades masticator space, pterygoid plates, or skull base and/or encases internal carotid
   artery (T4b)
(Lip) Tumor invades through cortical bone, inferior alveolar nerve, floor of mouth, or skin of face,
   i.e., chin or nose (T4)

REGIONAL LYMPH NODES (N)
Regional lymph nodes cannot be assessed (NX)
No regional lymph node metastasis (N0)
Metastasis in a single ipsilateral lymph node, ≤3 cm in greatest dimension (N1)
Metastasis in a single ipsilateral lymph node, >3 cm but not >6 cm in greatest dimension (N2a)
Metastasis in multiple ipsilateral lymph nodes, none
>6 cm in greatest dimension (N2b)
Metastasis in bilateral or contralateral lymph nodes, none >6 cm in greatest dimension (N2c)
Metastasis in a lymph node >6 cm in greatest dimension (N3)

DISTANT METASTASIS (M)
Distant metastasis cannot be assessed (MX)
No distant metastasis (M0)
Distant metastases (M1)

STAGE GROUPING
The overall pathologic AJCC stage is
   Tis/N0/M0 (Stage 0)
   T1/N0/M0 (Stage I)
   T2/N0/M0 (Stage II)
   T3/N0/M0 (Stage III)
   T1/N1/M0 (Stage III)
   T2/N1/M0 (Stage III)
   T3/N1/M0 (Stage III)
   T4a/N0/M0 (Stage IVA)
   T4a/N1/M0 (Stage IVA)
   T1/N2/M0 (Stage IVA)
   T2/N2/M0 (Stage IVA)
   T3/N2/M0 (Stage IVA)
   T4a/N2/M0 (Stage IVA)
   T4b/Any N/M0 (Stage IVB)
   Any T/N3/M0 (Stage IVB)
   Any T/Any N/M1(Stage IVC)

*Superficial erosion alone of bone/tooth socket by gingival primary carcinoma is not sufficient to classify
a tumor as T4.
AJCC, American Joint Committee on Cancer.
From: Greene FL, Page DL, Fleming ID, Fritz AG, Balch CM, Haller DG, Morrow M, eds. AJCC Cancer
Staging Manual. 6th edition. New York: Springer; 2002. Used with permission. (A new AJCC TNM
staging system is scheduled for release in 2009; after its publication, the new staging scheme will appear
on the website for this book.)

V. PATHOLOGIC REPORTING OF ORAL CAVITY AND OROPHARYNGEAL MALIGNANCIES

A. Staging. The American Joint Committee on Cancer (AJCC) staging guidelines for oral cavity and oropharyngeal carcinomas are listed in Tables 1.3 and 1.4. Staging is extremely important for clinical management and establishing prognosis. Staging guidelines are applicable to all forms of carcinoma; any nonepithelial tumor type is

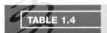

TABLE 1.4	**2002 AJCC Staging Guidelines for Tumors of the Oropharynx (Including Base of Tongue, Soft Palate, and Uvula)**

PRIMARY TUMOR (T)
Primary tumor cannot be assessed (TX)
No evidence of primary tumor (T0)
Carcinoma in situ (Tis)
Tumor ≤2 cm in greatest dimension (T1)
Tumor >2 cm but not >4 cm in greatest dimension (T2)
Tumor >4 cm in greatest dimension (T3)
Tumor invades the larynx, deep/extrinsic muscle of tongue, medial pterygoid, hard palate, or mandible (T4a)
Tumor invades lateral pterygoid muscle, pterygoid plates, lateral nasopharynx, or skull base or encases carotid artery (T4b)

REGIONAL LYMPH NODES (N)
Regional lymph nodes cannot be assessed (NX)
No regional lymph node metastasis (N0)
Metastasis in a single ipsilateral lymph node, ≤3 cm in greatest dimension (N1)
Metastasis in a single ipsilateral lymph node, >3 cm but not >6 cm in greatest dimension (N2a)
Metastasis in multiple ipsilateral lymph nodes, none >6 cm in greatest dimension (N2b)
Metastasis in bilateral or contralateral lymph nodes, none >6 cm in greatest dimension (N2c)
Metastasis in a lymph node >6 cm in greatest dimension (N3)

DISTANT METASTASIS (M)
Distant metastasis cannot be assessed (MX)
No distant metastasis (M0)
Distant metastases (M1)

STAGE GROUPING
The overall pathologic AJCC stage is
Tis/N0/M0 (Stage 0)
T1/N0/M0 (Stage I)
T2/N0/M0 (Stage II)
T3/N0/M0 (Stage III)
T1/N1/M0 (Stage III)
T2/N1/M0 (Stage III)
T3/N1/M0 (Stage III)
T4a/N0/M0 (Stage IVA)
T4a/N1/M0 (Stage IVA)
T1/N2/M0 (Stage IVA)
T2/N2/M0 (Stage IVA)
T3/N2/M0 (Stage IVA)
T4a/N2/M0 (Stage IVA)
T4b/Any N/M0 (Stage IVB)
Any T/N3/M0 (Stage IVB)
Any T/Any N/M1(Stage IVC)

AJCC, American Joint Committee on Cancer.
From: Greene FL, Page DL, Fleming ID, Fritz AG, Balch CM, Haller DG, Morrow M, eds. AJCC Cancer Staging Manual. 6th edition. New York: Springer, 2002. Used with permission. (A new AJCC TNM staging system is scheduled for release in 2009; after its publication, the new staging scheme will appear on the website for this book.)

excluded. A specific and very important point in staging involves bone involvement by tumor. To qualify as a T4 lesion, the tumor must erode through the bone cortex; superficial bone erosion is not sufficient for classification as T4.

B. Additional pertinent pathologic features. As with carcinomas at all upper aerodigestive tract sites, margin status, tumor differentiation, and the presence or absence of perineural or lymphvascular space invasion should be reported. Perineural invasion is particularly common in oral cavity carcinomas and is correlated with a poorer prognosis. The pattern of infiltration as well as the presence or absence of a host inflammatory response should also be reported, because both features have been correlated in many studies with a higher rate of local recurrence, a poorer prognosis, or both. Depth of invasion, particularly for T1 and T2 tumors, although not reflected in the staging system specifically, is important for clinical management and prognosis, and so should be reported.

Suggested Readings

Bouquot JE, Nikai H. Lesions of the oral cavity. In: Gnepp DR, ed. Diagnostic Surgical Pathology of the Head and Neck, 1st ed. Philadelphia: W.B. Saunders Publishers; 2001.

Slootweg P, Eveson JW. Tumours of the oral cavity and oropharynx. In: Barnes L, Eveson JW, Reichart P, Sidransky, eds. Pathology and Genetics Head and Neck Tumours. Lyon, France: IARC Press; 2005.

Thompson LDR, ed. Head and Neck Pathology, 1st ed. New York: Churchill Livingstone; 2006.

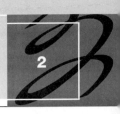

LARYNX

James S. Lewis Jr.

2

I. NORMAL ANATOMY

A. Macroscopic/gross. The larynx is a unique organ designed to produce phonation by modulation of the respiratory airstream. It is composed of several cartilaginous structures: the thyroid, cricoid, and arytenoid cartilages and the epiglottis. The hyoid bone sits above and is connected to the larynx by the thyrohyoid membrane (Fig. 2.1). The thyroid (and lesser so, cricoid cartilages) ossify in adults. In functional terms, the larynx is divided into three subsites. The glottis includes the true vocal folds or cords, below, and the false folds or cords, above. The space between them is called the ventricle, and its deeper recess the saccule. The true cords, with a hypocellular stroma called Reinke's space, are designed to vibrate for phonation, and the ventricle amplifies this further (e-Fig. 2.1).* The cords are manipulated by muscles that attach to and move the arytenoid cartilages, which sit at the posterior aspect of the vocal folds. The larynx can be divided into three compartments: the supraglottis, glottis, and subglottis, particularly for tumor management and staging purposes. The supraglottis includes the epiglottis, aryepiglottic folds, false cords, and ventricle. Glottis refers to the vocal cords from the edge of the ventricle to the free edge of the vocal cord. Subglottis refers to the area from the free edge of the vocal fold to the inferior border of the cricoid cartilage but has a slightly different definition for American Joint Committee on Cancer (AJCC) staging (see below).

B. Microscopic. The larynx is covered by a mixture of squamous and pseudostratified ciliated columnar (respiratory-type) epithelium. In smokers, however, often the entire endolarynx is covered by squamous epithelium. The true cords themselves are always covered by squamous epithelium. They contain a lamina propria area called Reinke's space, which lies between the epithelium and the vocal ligament and which consists of loose connective tissue with few capillaries, no lymphatics, and sparse seromucinous glands. It has been speculated that this is why very few T1 glottic carcinomas have lymph node metastases. The false cords and ventricle are typically lined by respiratory-type epithelium.

II. GROSS EXAMINATION, TISSUE SAMPLING, AND HISTOLOGIC SLIDE PREPARATION

A. Endoscopic biopsies. The majority of specimens from this region consist of endoscopic forcep biopsies. Appropriate management begins in the office or operating room when they are taken. The small pieces should be placed immediately into 10% buffered formalin or other appropriate fixative. These should undergo gross examination and description documenting the exact number of pieces present and then be entirely submitted with three levels cut from each paraffin block for hematoxylin and eosin (H&E) examination. For very small specimens or where few pieces are obtained from clinical masses, it is strongly recommended that one order unstained slides to be cut from the block on initial submission for potential use for immunohistochemistry or other special stains.

B. Resections

    1. Partial. These are widely variable specimens depending on the location of the tumor. Standard procedures include vertical hemilaryngectomy, and supraglottic or supracricoid laryngectomy. As a generalization, these need to be oriented

---

*All e-figures are available online via the Solutions Site Image Bank.

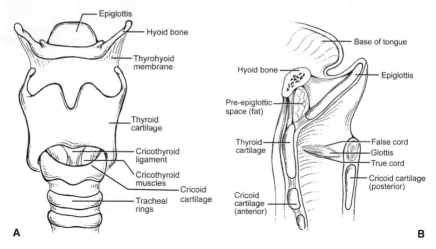

Figure 2.1. Larynx anatomy **(A)** anterior view, **(B)** sagittal cross section.

appropriately, the soft tissue margins inked, and margins demonstrated by shave or radial section followed by sectioning of the tumor relative to cartilage/bone and soft tissue margins. Margins should be evaluated by either shave or radial sections, depending on the nature of the specimen. If the tumor is relatively distant from a margin, 1- to 2-mm shave sections are preferred. If the tumor approximates a margin to <1 to 2 mm, radial sections are taken.

Partial resections with a CO_2 laser under an operating microscope are very common and becoming more so with time because of their low morbidity. Because an inherent part of this procedure is to cut into the tumor or to remove tumor in more than one piece, the surgeons ink the individual pieces themselves as they alone know what constitutes the true margin. In the pathology lab, the pieces are measured, described, and submitted entirely in sections perpendicular to the ink.

2. Total. For years, total laryngectomy has been the standard operation for malignancy. However, partial resections with preservation of function are increasingly common. Total laryngectomy is used most often now as salvage therapy for recurrences after partial surgery or definitive radiation and chemotherapy. Occasionally, patients present with such progressive disease that total laryngectomy is necessary as the initial surgery.

The usual approach to grossing a total laryngectomy is to initially ink the peripheral nonmucosal soft tissue margins and then open the larynx by a posterior vertical midline cut with scissors, propping it wide open with a small stick or portion of a wooden swab. After overnight formalin fixation, the specimen is ready for prosection. After orientation and measurement in three dimensions, any tumor is measured and described, specifically noting what structures are involved. The specimen typically includes the entire larynx and cartilages, small portions of hypopharyngeal mucosa bilaterally adjacent to the aryepiglottic folds, and the hyoid bone anterosuperiorly. Standard sections (Fig. 2.2) are taken as follows: (i) Margins: shaved inferior tracheal ring; shaved right and left hypopharyngeal mucosa; shaved postcricoid soft tissue; radial sections demonstrating anterior, anterolateral, and base of tongue inked soft tissue margins. (ii) Soft tissue/mucosa: bilateral vertical glottis (including both true and false cords); vertical anterior commissure; vertical midline epiglottis showing pre-epiglottic soft tissue space; bilateral aryepiglottic folds; four sections of tumor if not included in the previous sections. (iii) Cartilage/bone: vertical sections showing tumor and thyroid cartilage (at closest or at sites of gross invasion); sections of right and left wings of the hyoid bone (where closest to tumor or grossly involved by it.) Typically, all

Midline epiglottis showing pre-epiglottic soft tissue

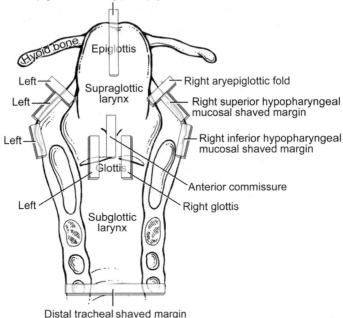

Distal tracheal shaved margin

Figure 2.2. Larynx grossing. Standard sections from a total laryngectomy are shown. Additional sections include sections of tumor (4–5 total), right and left postcricoid soft tissue shaved margins, and anterior soft tissue margins (either shaved or radial). Post decalcification, additional sections should include cartilage deep to the tumor showing involvement or nearest approach, any surrounding lymph nodes in neck soft tissue, of the hyoid bone (where closest to tumor or grossly involved by it). If necessary, sections of tracheostomy skin, thyroid lobe(s), and neck skin should also be submitted.

soft tissue and margin sections are taken first, and the entire specimen is bisected in the midline vertically and decalcified *in toto* overnight followed by cartilage and/or bone section acquisition.

C. **Frozen sections.** Frozen sections are a critical element of surgical therapy for tumors of the head and neck region. Although practices vary, most institutions have margins taken as small pieces by the surgeon from the periphery of the surgical defect after the tumor has been removed. Because laryngeal resections are quite variable, the sites where frozen sections are taken are not standard. For example, with total laryngectomies, sometimes no frozen sections are even felt to be clinically necessary. Otherwise, the surgeon may sample the tumor or suspicious sites to confirm and/or map the tumor and then margins taken from wherever the tumor is felt to be closest. These pieces are submitted individually to pathology in saline and frozen in their entirety with two H&E slides generated at representative levels well into the tissue. It is critical to obtain sections that represent the entire tissue submitted so that small foci of tumor are not missed by sampling error (i.e., missing significant but focal findings in the tissue at the time of frozen section by not sampling it well). The pieces should be evaluated grossly for mucosa—typically shiny and pink-tan on one surface of the tissue. If it is present, the specimen should be oriented to demonstrate this surface on one edge of the section with the submucosa below, just as a skin specimen would be. Additional sections should be cut if needed to assure that two quality sections are obtained.

The tissue that remains after frozen section is submitted for evaluation on permanent sections along with the remaining specimens to further assure adequate sampling of the tissue with quality paraffin embedding and sectioning. This process can help resolve a number of issues from frozen section including freezing and cautery artifact, amount of tumor represented, and orientation or embedding issues. The margins of the main resection specimen are also evaluated throughout its entirety because the separate frozen section specimens are small and almost never are able to cover the entire margin areas of a resection. The final margin status is then a conglomerate of all three sources: frozen section slides, permanent slides of the frozen tissue, and the margins of the specimen itself.

III. DIAGNOSTIC FEATURES OF COMMON DISEASES
  A. Inflammation and infection. Inflammation of the larynx (laryngitis) is quite commonly clinically, and can be divided into acute and chronic forms, which are variable by age. Most of the time, laryngitis will not necessitate the taking of specimens for pathologic evaluation. Infections can be caused by a myriad of agents including viruses, bacteria, fungi, and parasites. The pathologist must be alert to the possibility of infection, and a helpful reminder is the immune status of the patient, as many of these patients will be immunocompromised.

  Inflammation is essentially never present in the normal larynx, so the presence of inflammatory cells should be the first clue. Depending on the organism, the inflammation could take a number of different forms, almost all of which are typical for the type of organism when it presents in other locations. Examples of some of the major infections the pathologist might encounter include cytomegalovirus, herpes simplex virus, tuberculosis, rhinoscleroma (*Klebsiella rhinoscleromatis*), candidiasis, histoplasmosis, blastomycosis, cryptococcosis, coccidiomycosis, or rhinosporidiosis (*Rhinosporidium seeberi*). The resulting inflammation may cause mucosal ulceration, acute and chronic inflammation, necrosis, or granulomas. One should have a low threshold for ordering special stains [such as Gomori's methenamine silver (GMS), acid-fast bacillus (AFB), or periodic acid–Schiff (PAS)] to look for organisms.
  B. Nonneoplastic lesions
    1. Traumatic
      a. Vocal cord nodule. These are nonneoplastic degenerative stromal lesions of Reinke's space that are usually related to trauma due to misuse or vocal excess. As such, they have been referred to as singer's or screamer's nodules. They are more common in women and are commonly bilateral, characteristically occurring at the junction of the anterior and middle one third of the vocal cord as this is the point of maximal vibration during phonation. Macroscopically, they appear as gray or white broad-based nodules or polyps. Microscopically, they consist of squamous mucosa with or without hyperkeratosis, are only rarely ulcerated, and overlie a sparsely cellular myxoid, edematous, fibrous, fibrinous, or vascular stroma. In our experience, the myxoid appearance is most common and it may demonstrate small cystic spaces (e-**Fig. 2.2**).
      b. Contact ulcer. Also referred to clinically as *contact granulomas* or just *granulomas*, these are different from vocal cord nodules for they occur on the vocal process of the arytenoids as a result of forceful vocalization in people who must affect a low, deep, forceful voice (preachers, lawyers, salesmen). They are more common in men, can be unilateral or bilateral, and present as polypoid lesions. Microscopically, they are essentially granulation tissue polyps with an ulcerated mucosa and a stroma containing abundant small vessels in a haphazard configuration with plump endothelial cells. The stroma may be rich in lymphocytes, plasma cells, neutrophils, or histiocytes (sometimes including giant cells).
    2. Cysts. Laryngeal cysts may be divided into three categories: (i) ductal cysts, (ii) laryngoceles, and (iii) saccular cysts. All are cured by simple excision.
      a. Ductal cysts. These are the most common and result from obstruction of a minor salivary gland duct. With this obstruction, cystification occurs. Ductal cysts are typically small "bumps" on endoscopy and have a predilection for the cords, ventricle, aryepiglottic folds, and epiglottis. The lining may be squamous or oncocytic.
      b. Laryngocele. A laryngocele is the asymptomatic dilatation of the saccule (the deep aspect of the ventricle) by entrapped air. It may stay internal and show

up as a supraglottic mucosal bulge or may herniate above the thyroid cartilage to project externally into the neck soft tissue and present as a neck mass. Microscopically, it is lined by respiratory-type mucosa.

   c. Saccular cyst. This represents a mucin-filled dilatation of the saccule, either developmental or acquired. It is also typically lined by respiratory-type mucosa but it may be squamous or oncocytic on occasion. It is easily confused with a branchial cleft cyst.

3. Metabolic

   a. Amyloidosis is the term applied to the diverse collection of disorders with accumulation/deposition of amorphous extracellular material, all the types of which have been shown to be similar. The larynx is the most common site of localized amyloidosis, although this is still uncommon. It most commonly involves the false cord, followed by the true cord and ventricle. A subset of patients has multifocal disease, with approximately one-third having tracheal disease as well. The majority of patients have only localized disease, but systemic disease also occurs in a subset of patients. All patients should have a workup to rule out systemic amyloidosis with or without an associated plasma cell dyscrasia. The amyloid in localized laryngotracheal amyloidosis is always of the AL (or immunoglobulin type) type.

   b. Laryngeal amyloidosis usually macroscopically presents as a polypoid nodule covered by intact mucosa. Microscopically, it consists of sheets and nodular masses of amorphous, hypocellular eosinophilic material in the stroma (e-Fig. 2.3), in blood vessel walls, and in the basement membranes of mucoserous glands. It is confirmed by Congo Red special staining with "apple-green" birefringence on polarized microscopy. Thioflavin T staining with examination under fluorescence microscopy is also sometimes used.

C. Neoplastic lesions. The World Health Organization (WHO) classification of tumors of the larynx, hypopharynx, and trachea is listed in Table 2.1.

1. Benign

   a. Squamous papillomas are squamous proliferations caused by human papilloma virus (HPV) and are the most common benign tumors of the larynx. They are most common in the larynx but also occur in the trachea and bronchi in some cases. They also occur occasionally in the oral cavity and pharynx. There are two separate clinical settings: juvenile or juvenile-onset laryngeal papillomatosis (JOLP) and adult (or adult-onset) laryngeal papillomatosis (AOLP). Juvenile papillomas most often begin before age 5 and are much more likely than adult papillomas to be multifocal and to have an associated clinical impact. In a significant minority of patients, carpeting of the larynx occurs, requiring repeated laser excisions and occasionally tracheostomy or even laryngectomy for control and airway management. Papillomas tend to recur rapidly, but the disease severity usually regresses in early adulthood. In adult papillomas, the peak age is between 20 and 40 years, disease is usually unifocal or limited, and even when multifocal, it is less aggressive in nature. Only occasionally does it present as multifocal disease that recurs after excision.

     Squamous papillomas are strongly associated with HPV types 6 and 11, which are usually felt to be transmitted from the mother to the upper aerodigestive tract (UADT) of the neonate during vaginal delivery, thus explaining the occurrence in childhood. There is a very minimal risk of transformation to invasive carcinoma.

     Regardless of the clinical context, squamous papillomas have a typical morphology. Grossly, they appear as exophytic, granular, and friable pink, red, or tan lesions. Microscopically, they consist of arborizing, papillary fronds of thickened but maturing squamous epithelium with slight hyperplasia of the basal layer. Cells in the midlayer often have cytoplasmic clearing, but frank koilocytosis is not regularly observed. The nuclei are slightly enlarged and irregular but not overtly dysplastic-appearing, and mitotic activity is usually present but modest. Characteristically, there is minimal surface keratinization (e-Fig. 2.4). Frank dysplasia can be seen in some lesions and should be

TABLE 2.1 WHO Histological Classification of Tumors of the Hypopharynx, Larynx, and Trachea

Malignant epithelial tumors
Squamous cell carcinoma
   Verrucous carcinoma
   Papillary squamous cell carcinoma
   Basaloid squamous cell carcinoma
   Spindle cell carcinoma
   Adenosquamous carcinoma
   Acantholytic squamous cell carcinoma
Lymphoepithelial carcinoma
Giant cell carcinoma
Malignant salivary gland-type carcinomas
   Adenoid cystic carcinoma
   Mucoepidermoid carcinoma

Neuroendocrine tumors
Typical carcinoid
Atypical carcinoid
Small cell carcinoma, neuroendocrine type
Combined small cell carcinoma, neuroendocrine type

Benign epithelial tumors
Papilloma
Papillomatosis
Salivary gland-type adenomas
   Pleomorphic adenoma
   Oncocytic papillary cystadenoma

Soft tissue tumors
Malignant tumors
   Fibrosarcoma
   Malignant fibrous histiocytoma
   Liposarcoma
   Leiomyosarcoma
   Rhabdomyosarcoma
   Angiosarcoma
   Kaposi sarcoma
   Malignant peripheral nerve sheath tumor
   Synovial sarcoma
Borderline tumors/LMP
   Inflammatory myofibroblastic tumor
Benign tumors
   Schwannoma
   Neurofibroma
   Lipoma
   Leiomyoma
   Rhabdomyoma
   Hemangioma
   Lymphangioma
   Granular cell tumor

Hematolymphoid tumors

Tumors of bone and cartilage
Chondrosarcoma
Osteosarcoma
Chondroma
Giant cell tumor

Mucosal malignant melanoma

Secondary tumors

From Barnes L, Eveson J, Reichart P, Sidransky D, eds. *World Health Organization Classification of Tumours. Pathology and Genetics. Head and Neck Tumours.* Lyon: IARC Press; 2005. Used with permission.

reported. However, the correlation of overt dysplasia with the development of subsequent invasive carcinoma is not consistently reported in the literature.

b. **Granular cell tumors** are benign, slow growing tumors of neural origin that occur in a multitude of locations around the body. They are particularly common in the head and neck region with a minority occurring in the larynx. They are slightly more common in African Americans and typically present with hoarseness. Grossly, they are smooth, white polypoid tumors involving the posterior true cords, anterior commissure, false cords, or subglottis. Microscopically, they consist of infiltrative, nonencapsulated sheets and cords of bland appearing cells with abundant eosinophilic, granular cytoplasm, and indistinct cell borders. There is usually no significant stromal reaction. The nuclei are small, oval, and eccentric with minimal atypia and no mitotic activity. A common feature is pseudoepitheliomatous hyperplasia of the overlying squamous epithelium. This can be quite alarming and should prompt a search of the submucosa for granular cells (e-**Fig. 2.5**). Conservative endoscopic excision is the treatment of choice with a <10% risk of recurrence.

c. **Paragangliomas** are tumors recapitulating the paraganglia, specialized organs of the autonomic nervous system derived from neural crest. They occur in numerous locations throughout the body, and their behavior is largely dependent on site. Laryngeal paragangliomas are benign and are divided into two groups: superior and inferior. Superior paragangliomas are much more common and occur in the supraglottic larynx, from the false cord up into the aryepiglottic fold. They are polypoid submucosal lesions. Inferior paragangliomas occur along the cricoid cartilage in the subglottic region and often present as dumbbell-shaped lesions with both intra- and extralaryngeal components.

Microscopically, these tumors are identical to those arising elsewhere. They consist of polygonal to spindled cells with abundant eosinophilic to slightly basophilic cytoplasm and round to oval nuclei with a slightly granular chromatin. Nuclear pleomorphism may be striking, but there is minimal mitotic activity. They are arranged in nests (classically termed *zellballen*) and are highly vascular. By immunohistochemistry, they are strongly positive for synaptophysin and chromogranin A, virtually always negative for epithelial markers such as epithelial membrane antigen (EMA) and cytokeratin, and show the typical sustentacular (or supporting) cell staining for S-100 with the tumor cells themselves being negative.

2. **Precursor (premalignant) squamous lesions** are defined as altered squamous epithelium with an increased risk of progression to squamous cell carcinoma. The term dysplasia or intraepithelial neoplasia should be used for these lesions. Atypia, in contrast, is not considered synonymous with dysplasia or risk of squamous carcinoma, and is used in a more general sense. It may describe changes seen in reactive epithelium as well.

Unfortunately, there is poor agreement about the histopathologic changes that constitute dysplasia and about its grading. Also, there is poor correlation between the varying grades of dysplasia and subsequent risk of carcinoma. Several grading systems have been proposed (Table 2.2). Precursor lesions are strongly associated with smoking and alcohol use. Most precursor lesions present along the true cords, often bilateral, as opposed to other sites in the larynx. This presentation is likely a functional phenomenon as other laryngeal sites more often present as established invasive malignancy.

There are a number of changes that occur in dysplasia including nuclear abnormalities, architectural/organizational abnormalities, and abnormal keratinization. Hyperplasia manifests as thickening of the epithelium without any cytologic atypia. The changes of dysplasia, particularly mild dysplasia, are difficult to distinguish from hyperplasia or reactive change, and by the same token, the varying degrees of dysplasia are difficult to distinguish from each other. In broad terms, mild dysplasia shows nuclear enlargement, hyperchromasia, and increased nucleus to cytoplasm ratios limited to the lower third of the epithelium

| TABLE 2.2 | Precursor Lesion Classification Schemes |

Ljubljana classification Squamous Intraepithelial Lesions (SIL)	Squamous Intraepithelial Neoplasia (SIN)	2005 World Health Organization Classification
Squamous cell (simple) hyperplasia	N/A	Squamous cell hyperplasia
Basal/parabasal cell hyperplasia	SIN 1	Mild dysplasia
Atypical hyperplasia	SIN 2	Moderate dysplasia
Atypical hyperplasia	SIN 3	Severe dysplasia
Carcinoma in situ	SIN 3	Carcinoma in situ

N/A, not applicable.

(e-**Fig. 2.6**), moderate dysplasia into the middle third (e-**Fig. 2.7**), and severe dysplasia into the upper third or full thickness. However, severe dysplasia, in particular, may manifest as an expanded basal cell layer with maturation in the upper layers, particularly with bulbous or down-streaming tongues of basal epithelium toward the submucosa (e-**Fig. 2.8**). The epithelium is usually thickened but sometimes thinned, and hyperkeratosis may or may not be present.

3. **Malignant**

   a. **Squamous cell carcinoma** is the overwhelmingly most common malignant tumor of the larynx. It occurs with a peak in the sixth and seventh decades and, just as other UADT squamous cancers, has a high male-to-female ratio (5:1) and a strong relationship to tobacco use and alcohol consumption, with a multiplicative rather than additive relative risk when both are used. Most cases involve the glottis or supraglottic region. Glottic tumors present earliest and at the smallest size because of functional compromise and symptomology.

   The gross appearance of squamous cell carcinoma is quite variable, ranging from fungating, exophytic tumors to endophytic, ulcerated tumors with raised edges. Microscopically, it consists of nests and sheets of cells with abundant eosinophilic cytoplasm and round to oval nuclei, often with prominent nucleoli. Well-differentiated tumors retain abundant pink or clear cytoplasm and often show keratin "pearl" formation (e-**Fig. 2.9**). Moderately differentiated tumors have more pleomorphism and a higher nucleus to cytoplasm ratio in many of the cells while still retaining moderate eosinophilic cytoplasm (e-**Fig. 2.10**). Poorly differentiated tumors often have single cells or small nests of cells with more mitotic activity and less cytoplasm (e-**Fig. 2.11**). Grading should be performed but has not been shown to predict the clinical behavior of individual tumors. The majority of UADT squamous cell carcinomas are moderately differentiated. Although keratinization is commonly seen in well- and moderately differentiated carcinomas, its presence or absence does not have any clinical significance for laryngeal carcinoma.

      i. **Verrucous carcinoma** (VC) is a specific, well-differentiated, and non-metastasizing variant of squamous cell carcinoma. First described by Lauren Ackerman in the 1950s, this tumor has thus also been called "Ackerman's tumor." It occurs in the larynx and oral cavity and grossly appears as a well-circumscribed, warty and exophytic, broad-based white or tan mass. It can become very large. Microscopically, VC consists of very thick, club-shaped papillae with a broad pushing base. These blunt and downward-pushing projections have sometimes been likened to "elephant's feet." There is usually prominent surface hyperkeratosis, and the sheets of tumor have bland cells with abundant eosinophilic to clear cytoplasm, sometimes described as "glassy" in appearance. There is no cytologic atypia. The stroma directly beneath the tumor typically demonstrates prominent chronic inflammation, often with abundant plasma cells (e-**Fig. 2.12**).

The prognosis for pure VC is excellent. Although it can be large and locally destructive, complete surgical resection is often curative. Radiation is also an acceptable treatment, particularly in poor surgical candidates. However, routine invasive squamous cell carcinoma often arises from VC. When this occurs, the prognosis and behavior are the same as for typical squamous cell carcinoma.

ii. **Spindle cell carcinoma** (SpCC) is the term for a poorly differentiated carcinoma that adopts a sarcomatoid, spindled, or mesenchymal-appearing morphology but which is, nevertheless, of epithelial origin/differentiation. It is frequently biphasic with a spindled component and intermingled either in situ or invasive squamous cell carcinoma. It has the same demographics as routine squamous cell carcinoma.

Grossly, SpCC usually is polypoid with an ulcerated surface. The polypoid configuration is a classic feature. The glottis is the most common laryngeal site, and the surface is frequently extensively ulcerated. Microscopically, these tumors can be quite variable, but typically consist of sheets of spindle cells mimicking a fibrosarcoma or malignant fibrous histiocytoma (e-**Fig. 2.13**). There is usually brisk mitotic activity and necrosis. Foci of recognizable sarcomatous differentiation such as chondrosarcoma, osteosarcoma, or rhabdomyosarcoma sometimes occur. Most cases show some component of in situ or invasive squamous cell carcinoma, but it may take extensive sectioning to be seen.

If the tumor consists of spindle or pleomorphic cells only, immunohistochemistry for epithelial markers such as pancytokeratin, EMA, and p63 is usually very helpful. These are positive in anywhere from one fourth to one third of cases. With markedly extended cytokeratin panels, approximately three-quarters of tumors will demonstrate staining. These tumors do stain for certain mesenchymal markers as well, such as vimentin (every case), smooth muscle actin, and muscle specific actin. Whatever the case, a malignant spindle cell neoplasm involving/arising along the mucosa of the UADT should be considered a SpCC until proven otherwise, because sarcomas are distinctly uncommon at these sites. The differential diagnosis includes a granulation tissue polyp, true sarcoma, or inflammatory myofibroblastic tumor. The positive epithelial marker immunohistochemistry will distinguish SpCC from all of these other entities.

iii. **Basaloid squamous cell carcinoma** (BSCC) is an aggressive variant of squamous carcinoma composed almost entirely of basaloid cells. It has the same demographics as routine squamous cell carcinoma but has a predilection for the supraglottic larynx and for the hypopharynx, particularly the pyriform sinus region. It typically presents at high stage and, although this is somewhat controversial, is felt to be more aggressive than typical squamous cell carcinoma stage for stage.

Grossly, BSCC presents as a centrally ulcerated mass with thickening at the edges and commonly with extensive submucosal induration and spread at the periphery. Microscopically, there are two components. The first is basaloid cells with hyperchromatic round nuclei, inconspicuous nucleoli, and scant cytoplasm which grow in solid sheets or in rounded nests often with comedo-type central necrosis. The second is typical keratinizing type squamous cell carcinoma, either in situ or invasive which is always focal. The basaloid component of many tumors shows a characteristic hyalinized eosinophilic basement membrane material–like stroma in and around the tumor cells and forming small round nodules within tumor nests, akin to that seen in cylindromas of the skin (e-**Fig. 2.14**).

The differential diagnosis includes a neuroendocrine carcinoma or the solid variant of adenoid cystic carcinoma. The former expresses neuroendocrine markers in most cases and is also negative for high-molecular-weight keratins such as $34\beta E12$ and CK 5/6. Solid adenoid cystic carcinoma will show some evidence of myoepithelial differentiation so that with staining for p63, a marker of myoepithelial cells, adenoid cystic carcinoma will have staining only at the periphery of the nests. Squamous epithelium and squamous carcinomas also stain strongly for p63 so that BSCC will stain diffusely throughout the tumor. This differing staining pattern can thus help differentiate BSCC from solid adenoid cystic carcinoma (ACC).

    iv. Papillary squamous cell carcinoma (PSCC) is an uncommon variant of squamous cell carcinoma with the same demographics as typical squamous carcinoma. The larynx is among the most common sites of involvement, the supraglottis and glottis in particular, and only very rarely the subglottis. Grossly, it is a soft, polypoid and friable tumor. Microscopically, it is characterized by a predominantly papillary growth pattern with fibrovascular cores lined by full thickness markedly dysplastic squamous cells, which are most often very immature and basaloid appearing. There is usually minimal keratinization. Stromal invasion may or may not be present, but when it is, it has the appearance of typical squamous cell carcinoma. If frank invasion is not found, the lesion should be termed PSCC in situ.

    The differential diagnosis includes squamous papilloma, verrucous carcinoma, and typical squamous cell carcinoma with an exophytic growth pattern. The prognosis is believed to be better for this variant of squamous cell carcinoma, particularly when no invasive component is identified.

    v. Adenosquamous carcinoma. The larynx is the most common site for adenosquamous carcinoma (ASCC), followed by the oral cavity and sinonasal region. Again, it has the same demographics and clinical presentation as typical squamous cell carcinoma. Grossly, it is not unique, and is either exophytic or ulcerated with indurated edges. Microscopically, it consists of both true adenocarcinoma and squamous carcinoma. The two components are usually close to each other but still have a tendency to segregate. The squamous component can be either invasive or in situ carcinoma and has the same appearance as typical squamous carcinoma. This portion usually occupies the more superficial aspects, whereas the adenocarcinoma component, which may either be isolated glands or glandular structures within larger sheets of tumor, tends to occupy the deeper aspects of the mass. The glands usually show mucin production, which, although not strictly required for the diagnosis, is an important and common finding (e-**Fig. 2.15**). Mucicarmine or other mucin stains can be quite helpful to highlight it. Occasionally, signet ring type cells constitute the adenocarcinoma component.

    The differential diagnosis includes mucoepidermoid carcinoma, acantholytic or adenoid squamous cell carcinoma, and squamous cell carcinoma invading seromucinous minor salivary gland tissue. Mucoepidermoid carcinoma is the most important consideration (Table 2.3). Many ASCCs present at high stage and, although an uncommon tumor, reports strongly suggest that it has a worse prognosis than typical squamous cell carcinoma.

    b. Neuroendocrine tumors. Neuroendocrine carcinomas of the larynx are relatively uncommon and are divided into three major categories: well-differentiated (WDNEC or "carcinoid"), moderately differentiated (MDNEC or "atypical carcinoid"), and poorly differentiated (PDNEC). In the latter category, most tumors are essentially small cell carcinoma. However, more recently, some authors have defined a category of large cell neuroendocrine carcinoma similar to that seen in the lung. There is a clear spectrum of behavior among the subtypes, and MDNEC is the most common.

| TABLE 2.3 | Adenosquamous Carcinoma vs. Mucoepidermoid Carcinoma: Histologic Features |

Adenosquamous carcinoma	Mucoepidermoid carcinoma
Squamous carcinoma in situ	No squamous carcinoma in situ
Origin from squamous epithelium	Origin from seromucinous glands
Keratin pearls	Limited keratin pearls
Glands at lower invasive parts	Glands widely intermingled
No lobular arrangement	Lobular arrangement
No intermediate cells	Large, clear "intermediate cells"

Most neuroendocrine carcinomas of the larynx occur in the sixth to the eighth decade, and there is a strong male predominance. They occur most often in the supraglottis, and smoking is associated with MDNEC and PDNEC only. The histology of these tumors directly parallels that within the lung. WD-NEC is characterized by nests, trabeculae, and sheets of round, regular tumor cells with moderate eosinophilic to partially clear cytoplasm. Nuclei are round, regular, and show the typical "salt and pepper" or stippled chromatin. MD-NEC has a similar appearance but is less organized and shows more cellular pleomorphism, focal necrosis, and more prominent mitotic activity. Finally, PDNEC usually takes the form of small cell carcinoma with sheets of blue cells with nuclear molding, crush artifact, and delicate chromatin with indistinct nucleoli (e-**Fig. 2.16**). There is brisk mitotic activity and prominent necrosis. Large cell neuroendocrine carcinoma is high grade, akin to small cell carcinoma, but has larger cells with generous eosinophilic cytoplasm and frequently a more organized growth pattern with peripheral palisading, etc. All of these tumors will stain with neuroendocrine markers by immunohistochemistry (synaptophysin, chromogranin-A, CD56/N-CAM) but there tends to be less staining with the higher grade of the tumor. In particular, in PDNEC, the staining can become quite focal and sometimes only for one of the several neuroendocrine stains.

WDNEC has an excellent prognosis despite frequent local recurrence. Metastases are very uncommon. MDNEC has a worse prognosis with relatively frequent cervical lymph node metastases and occasional distant metastatic disease. Surgery is the treatment of choice for both of these. PDNEC has a dismal prognosis with frequent neck nodal and distant metastases. Patients are typically treated with radiation and chemotherapy rather than surgery.

c. **Mesenchymal tumors.** A great variety of mesenchymal tumors occur rarely in the larynx, the most common of which are the cartilaginous tumors chondroma and chondrosarcoma. Chondrosarcomas are the most common sarcoma of the larynx, occur in older adults, and are decidedly more common in men. They originate from the cricoid or thyroid lamina (3:1, cricoid to thyroid) and tend to present differently by site of origin with slowly progressive dyspnea for cricoid tumors or an anterior neck mass for thyroid tumors. Symptoms are usually present for a long period of time (often several years). Grossly, they consist of well-circumscribed, shiny white or gray lobulated masses with gritty areas of calcification and a glistening cut surface (e-**Fig. 2.17**). Microscopically, they consist of lobules of cartilage which, relative to normal, show increased cellularity and nuclear atypia with variability in size, more than one nucleus in individual lacunae, and binucleated cells (e-**Fig. 2.18**). The periphery is typically pushing and not infiltrative. The grading system is identical to that for chondrosarcomas elsewhere in the body, grades 1 to 3. As the grade progresses, the cells may show enlarged nuclei and nucleoli, but mitotic activity is only seen in high-grade tumors. It can be remarkably challenging to differentiate chondrosarcomas from chondromas, particularly on biopsy specimens.

TABLE 2.4 **2002 American Joint Committee on Cancer Staging Guidelines for Tumors of the Larynx**

PRIMARY TUMOR (T)

TX	Primary tumor cannot be assessed
T0	No evidence of primary tumor
Tis	Carcinoma in situ

Supraglottis

T1	Tumor limited to one subsite of supraglottis with normal vocal cord mobility
T2	Tumor invades mucosa of more than one adjacent subsite of supraglottis or glottis or region outside the supraglottis (e.g., mucosa of base of tongue, vallecula, medial wall of pyriform sinus) without fixation of the larynx
T3	Tumor limited to larynx with vocal cord fixation and/or invades any of the following: postcricoid area, pre-epiglottic tissues, paraglottic space, and/or minor thyroid cartilage erosion (e.g., inner cortex)
T4a	Tumor invades through the thyroid cartilage and/or invades tissues beyond the larynx (e.g., trachea, soft tissues of neck including deep extrinsic muscles of the tongue, strap muscles, thyroid, or esophagus)
T4b	Tumor invades prevertebral space, encases carotid artery, or invades mediastinal structures

Glottis

T1	Tumor limited to the vocal cord(s) (may involve anterior or posterior commissure) with normal mobility
T1a	Tumor limited to one vocal cord
T1b	Tumor involves both vocal cords
T2	Tumor extends to supraglottis and/or subglottis and/or with impaired vocal cord mobility
T3	Tumor limited to larynx with vocal cord fixation and/or invades the paraglottic space and/or minor thyroid cartilage erosion (e.g., inner cortex)
T4a	Tumor invades through the thyroid cartilage and/or invades tissues beyond the larynx (e.g., trachea, soft tissues of neck including deep extrinsic muscles of the tongue, strap muscles, thyroid, or esophagus)
T4b	Tumor invades prevertebral space, encases carotid artery, or invades mediastinal structures

Subglottis

T1	Tumor limited to subglottis
T2	Tumor extends to vocal cord(s) with normal or impaired mobility
T3	Tumor limited to larynx with vocal cord fixation
T4a	Tumor invades cricoid or thyroid cartilage and/or invades tissues beyond the larynx (e.g., trachea, soft tissues of neck including deep extrinsic muscles of the tongue, strap muscles, thyroid, or esophagus)
T4b	Tumor invades prevertebral space, encases carotid artery, or invades mediastinal structures

REGIONAL LYMPH NODES (N)

NX	Regional lymph nodes cannot be assessed
N0	No regional lymph node metastasis
N1	Metastasis in a single ipsilateral lymph node, ≤ 3 cm in greatest dimension
N2a	Metastasis in a single ipsilateral lymph node, >3 cm but <6 cm in greatest dimension
N2b	Metastasis in multiple ipsilateral lymph nodes, none >6 cm in greatest dimension
N2c	Metastasis in bilateral or contralateral lymph nodes, none >6 cm in greatest dimension
N3	Metastasis in a lymph node >6 cm in greatest dimension

DISTANT METASTASIS (M)

MX	Distant metastasis cannot be assessed
M0	No distant metastasis
M1	Distant metastasis

(*continued*)

TABLE 2.4	2002 American Joint Committee on Cancer Staging Guidelines for Tumors of the Larynx *(Continued)*		

STAGE GROUPING
The overall pathologic AJCC stage is

Stage 0	Tis	N0	M0
Stage I	T1	N0	M0
Stage II	T2	N0	M0
Stage III	T3	N0	M0
Stage III	T1	N1	M0
Stage III	T2	N1	M0
Stage III	T3	N1	M0
Stage IVA	T4a	N0	M0
Stage IVA	T4a	N1	M0
Stage IVA	T1	N2	M0
Stage IVA	T2	N2	M0
Stage IVA	T3	N2·	M0
Stage IVA	T4a	N2	M0
Stage IVB	T4b	Any N	M0
Stage IVB	Any T	N3	M0
Stage IVC	Any T	Any N	M1

From: Greene FL, Page DL, Fleming ID, Fritz AG, Balch CM, Haller DG, Morrow M, eds. AJCC Cancer Staging Manual. 6th edition. New York: Springer; 2002. Used with permission. (A new AJCC TNM staging system is scheduled for release in 2009; after its publication, the new staging scheme will appear on the website for this book.)

Chondrosarcomas display cytologic atypia with nucleoli in chondrocytes and will show at least some areas of more infiltrative growth at the periphery.

The vast majority of laryngeal chondrosarcomas are well-differentiated (Grade 1). However, interestingly, grade does not seem to affect prognosis. Surgery is directed at larynx-sparing complete excision, with total laryngectomy reserved for recurrence or uncontrolled local disease. Survival is >95% at 10 years.

IV. PATHOLOGIC REPORTING OF LARYNGEAL CARCINOMA

A. **Staging (AJCC).** Staging of laryngeal carcinomas is extremely important for clinical management and prognosis. For T-staging purposes, the larynx is divided into the supraglottis, glottis, and subglottis (Table 2.4). Although squamous cell carcinoma is the overwhelming type, staging guidelines are applicable to all forms of carcinoma. Any nonepithelial tumor type is excluded. The staging guidelines often require both clinical and pathologic input (for example, vocal cord fixation or not) for proper classification.

B. **Additional pertinent pathologic features.** As with carcinomas at all UADT sites, margin status, tumor differentiation, and the presence or absence of perineural or lymphvascular space invasion should be reported. In addition, the pattern of infiltration as well as the presence or absence of a host inflammatory response should be reported. All of these features have been correlated in many studies with a higher rate of local recurrence, a poorer prognosis, or both.

Suggested Readings

Barnes L, Tse LLY, Hunt JL, et al. Nonsquamous pathology of the larynx, hypopharynx, and trachea. In: Gnepp DR, ed. *Diagnostic Surgical Pathology of the Head and Neck,* Philadelphia: W.B. Saunders Publishers; 2001.

Gale N. Benign neoplasms of the larynx, hypopharynx, and trachea. In: Thompson LDR, ed. *Head and Neck Pathology,* New York: Churchill Livingstone; 2006.

Thompson LDR. Malignant neoplasms of the larynx, hypopharynx, and trachea. In: Thompson LDR, ed. *Head and Neck Pathology,* New York: Churchill Livingstone; 2006.

Thompson LDR. Non-neoplastic lesions of the larynx, hypopharynx, and trachea. In: Thompson LDR, ed. *Head and Neck Pathology,* New York: Churchill Livingstone; 2006.

Zidar N, Boffetta P. Tumours of the hypopharynx, larynx, and trachea. In: Barnes L, Eveson JW, Reichart P, Sidransky D, eds. *Pathology and Genetics Head and Neck Tumours,* Lyon, France: IARC Press; 2005.

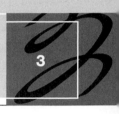
NASAL CAVITY, PARANASAL SINUSES, AND NASOPHARYNX

James S. Lewis Jr.

I. NORMAL ANATOMY

A. Nasal cavity. The normal sinonasal region consists of the central nasal cavity, paired bilateral paranasal sinuses, and the nasopharynx. The nasal cavity consists anteriorly of the nasal vestibule, the small hair-bearing region just inside the nasal ostia, with the remainder representing the nasal antrum. It has four walls, a central dividing septum, and paired bilateral turbinates: upper, middle, and lower. The nasal vestibule lining is an extension of the surrounding facial skin, and as such has a stratified, keratinizing squamous epithelium with associated skin-type appendages and hair. This extends for 1 to 2 cm into the nasal cavity. The nasal antrum is lined by pseudostratified ciliated columnar (respiratory-type) epithelium of ectodermal origin referred to as the Schneiderian membrane. The lamina propria beneath consists of minor-salivary gland-type mucoserous glands embedded in fibrovascular connective tissue with small ducts that convey their secretions to the surface. The turbinates have an even more richly vascular stroma. The roof of the nasal cavity contains the cribriform plate with olfactory mucosa, a modified respiratory-type epithelium with olfactory nerve cells and supporting cells.

B. Paranasal sinuses. The paranasal sinuses consist of the maxillary (largest), frontal, sphenoid, and ethmoid sinuses. They drain into the nasal cavity and are air-filled, intraosseous, and open. The ethmoid sinuses are small and complex (often referred to as the ethmoid labyrinth or air cells). All paranasal sinuses are in continuity with the nasal cavity so they have a similar mucosa. However, the mucosa of the sinuses is thinner, as is the lamina propria, which is also looser and less vascular. Seromucinous glands are also prominent in the lamina propria.

C. Nasopharynx. The nasopharynx is the most cephalad portion of the pharynx and is a cuboidal structure. Its roof is formed by the pharyngeal tonsil. The lateral walls are the most pathologically important because they contain the opening of the Eustachian tubes, and a depression posterior to the torus tubarius called the fossa of Rosenmüller. This is the most common site of origin for nasopharyngeal carcinoma (NPC). Because it is surrounded by bone and vital structures, the nasopharynx is poorly accessible for surgery on tumors arising there. The epithelial lining consists of a mixture of stratified squamous, intermediate (or transitional), and pseudostratified ciliated columnar epithelium.

II. GROSS EXAMINATION, TISSUE SAMPLING, AND HISTOLOGIC SLIDE PREPARATION

A. Endoscopic biopsies. The majority of specimens from this region consist of endoscopic forcep biopsies. Appropriate management begins in the office or operating room. The small pieces should be placed immediately into 10% buffered formalin or other appropriate fixative. If there is a suspicion of lymphoma, a minimum of three biopsy passes should be submitted in saline or RPMI medium and be directly given to the hematopathology service for triage and potential studies such as touch preparations and flow cytometry. Standard formalin-fixed specimens should undergo gross examination and description documenting the exact number of pieces present and then should be entirely submitted with three levels cut from each paraffin block for hematoxylin and eosin (H&E) examination. For very small specimens, or where few pieces are obtained from clinical masses, it is strongly recommended that additional unstained slides be cut from the block on initial submission for potential use in immunohistochemistry or special stains.

B. **Functional endoscopic sinus surgery (FESS; "sinus contents").** The tissue consists of fragments of ethmoid and maxillary ostium sinus bone and mucosa, resected inflammatory polyps, and nasal cavity and sinus tissue obtained by suction devices. These samples should be described, measured, and submitted for histologic examination. If firm or dense pieces are identified, they should be submitted as they may represent an unsuspected neoplasm. Otherwise, the pieces of intact tissue should be collected from the blood and fluid from the suction device, inspected grossly, and measured in aggregate; only one cassette of these fragments needs be submitted for histologic examination (one H&E level) with decalcification in EDTA or formic acid if gross pieces of bone are identified.

C. **Resections.** Surgical resections for sinonasal tumors are complex and varied, and are guided by tumor location, extent, and type. They always consist of soft tissue, mucosa, and bone. Margins are in very large part guided by frozen section. The main specimen should be oriented, the tumor identified, and mucosal, soft tissue, and bone margins identified. The specimen is described and measured. The soft tissue margins are inked and then mucosal and soft tissue margin sections taken first. Margins should be evaluated by either shave or radial sections, depending on the nature of the specimen. If the tumor is relatively distant from a margin, 1- to 2-mm shave sections are preferred. If the tumor approximates a margin to <1 to 2 mm, radial sections are taken. After this, the tumor is sectioned and sampled. Tumors should have four to five sections taken, or if small, should be entirely submitted for histologic examination. Often sectioning requires a saw to cut through bone to demonstrate the relationship of the lesion to the included structures. The bone is then decalcified, and shave sections from the bone margins are taken as well as sections demonstrating tumor involving bone.

D. **Frozen sections** are a critical element of surgical therapy for tumors of the head and neck region. Although practices vary, most institutions have margins taken as small pieces by the surgeon from the periphery of the surgical defect after the tumor has been removed. The pieces should be evaluated grossly for mucosa—typically shiny and pink-tan on one surface of the tissue. If it is present, the specimen should be oriented to demonstrate this mucosal surface on one edge of the section with the submucosa below. Two high quality sections should be obtained with the second level taken deep into the tissue to ensure adequate sampling at the time of frozen section.

  The tissue that remains after a frozen section is submitted for evaluation on permanent sections along with the remaining specimens. This is done to further assure adequate sampling of the tissue, and to help resolve a number of issues from frozen section including freezing and cautery artifact, amount of tumor represented, and orientation/embedding issues. The final margin status is therefore a conglomerate of three sources: frozen section slides, permanent slides of the frozen tissue, and the margins of the specimen itself.

III. **DIAGNOSTIC FEATURES OF COMMON DISEASES**
  A. **Inflammation and infection.** These processes are extremely common in the United States, necessitating a large amount of medical care, surgery, and also surgical specimens for evaluation. It has been estimated that up to 15% of the American population suffers from chronic sinusitis.
    1. **Acute rhinosinusitis.** Acute sinusitis is rarely seen by the pathologist because it is treated medically. However, typical histologic findings include neutrophils migrating through, and present in, the respiratory-type mucosa with luminal contents showing necrotic material with apoptotic neutrophil nuclear debris. Often, there are also abundant neutrophils in the luminal mucin.
    2. **Chronic rhinosinusitis.** Inflammation of the nasal cavity can result from allergy, upper respiratory tract infections, or cystic fibrosis. Sinusitis is thought to occur secondary to obstruction of the outflow of the paranasal sinuses by myriad etiologies such as edema and inflammation or anatomic abnormalities. Some of the most common obstructing agents are inflammatory polyps, a deviated septum, or

concha bullosa (air pocket in the middle turbinate). In children, developmental abnormalities may lead to chronic sinusitis from obstruction. Finally, rare genetic conditions such as immotile cilia syndrome (Kartagener's syndrome) cause chronic sinusitis. Complications include secondary bacterial infection and, in chronic allergic sinusitis, the development of inflammatory polyps (see section 4 below).

Specimens from FESS in chronic sinusitis typically show edema of the submucosa with a mixture of lymphocytes, plasma cells, and eosinophils. Sometimes, eosinophils are prominent. Their amount and distribution histologically do not have a clinical correlate other than suggesting that allergy is the underlying etiology for the sinusitis. When allergic mucin (see "Allergic fungal sinusitis") is present, eosinophils are usually very prominent in the intact sinus tissue.

3. **Wegener's granulomatosis** is a specific type of autoimmune disorder characterized by a necrotizing vasculitis that affects the nasal cavity and paranasal sinuses. It presents clinically with rhinorrhea, sinusitis, headache, nasal obstruction, anosmia, and sometimes middle ear and mastoid problems if inflammation obstructs the Eustachian tube. The majority of patients also have pulmonary and/or renal manifestations.

   Histologically, in biopsies of the sinonasal region, the diagnosis can be quite difficult. Features include mucosal ulceration, acute and chronic inflammation, necrosis, and granulomas. Wegener's granulomatosis causes a vasculitis which is often obscured by the inflammation, so elastic stains such as Vierhoff Von Gieser may be helpful to demonstrate the elastic fibers of inflamed vessels. The vasculitis involves arterioles, small arteries, and veins with changes ranging from fibrinoid necrosis with neutrophils and associated extravasated red blood cells and fibrin thrombi, to more granulomatous inflammation with multinucleated giant cells and histiocytes (e-Fig. 3.1).* It is very important to correlate the histologic findings with clinical information and laboratory investigation, which reveals cytoplasmic antineutrophil antibodies (cANCA) in approximately 90% of patients.

4. **Inflammatory polyps.** Sinonasal inflammatory polyps are nonneoplastic mucosal and submucosal projections that arise in longstanding chronic rhinitis, usually associated with allergy or asthma. They are seen most commonly in adults but can be seen in children as well, particularly in those with cystic fibrosis. Symptoms include headache, nasal obstruction, and rhinorrhea. They are multiple, often bilateral, and most commonly arise from the lateral nasal wall. Although nonneoplastic, they are capable of dramatic behavior including causing deviation of the septum, destruction of bone, and extension into the nasopharynx and rarely the orbit or cranial cavities.

   Grossly, inflammatory polyps can measure up to several centimeters and are boggy, gelatinous, and partially translucent. They often have a broad base. Microscopically, they consist predominantly of highly edematous or myxoid stroma with a mixed inflammatory infiltrate of lymphocytes, plasma cells, and variable eosinophils. There are few small vessels and minimal, bland spindled stromal cells. They typically are devoid of seromucinous glands, a feature that is particularly helpful in identifying them when they are in fragmented pieces with the remaining endoscopically resected tissue (e-Fig. 3.2). The surface is typically intact and lined by respiratory epithelium with a variably thickened basement membrane.

5. **Fungal infections** are relatively frequent and consist of several different pathologic entities that can involve any of the paranasal sinuses. They are best regarded broadly as "invasive" and "noninvasive" (Table 3.1).

   a. **Noninvasive.** Immunocompetent patients usually develop noninvasive fungal disease, either allergic fungal sinusitis or mycetoma ("fungus ball"). Clinically, these have similar presentations with typical symptoms of chronic sinusitis including headache, nasal discharge, stuffiness, and facial pressure.

   Allergic fungal sinusitis patients have asthma (present in >90% of cases), eosinophilia, atopy, and elevated total fungus-specific immunoglobulin E (IgE)

---

*All e-figures are available online via the Solution Site Image Bank.

TABLE 3.1	Fungal Sinusitis		

Entity	Clinical	Histology	Organism
Noninvasive: Allergic Fungal Sinusitis	Chronic sinusitis; inflammatory polyps; allergic symptoms; pan-sinusitis	Eosinophilic mucus; sheets of degenerating eosinophils; Charcot–Leyden crystals; sometimes fragmented hyphae in mucus	*Aspergillus;* dematiaceous fungi: *Bipolaris, Alternaria, Curvularia, Cladosporium*
Noninvasive: Mycetoma ("Fungus Ball")	Chronic sinusitis, mass lesion on imaging—usually one sinus cavity; usually nonallergic type presentation	Large intraluminal collections of fungal hyphae; minimal mucus; minimal inflammation	*Aspergillus;* dematiaceous fungi: *Bipolaris, Alternaria, Curvularia, Cladosporium*
Invasive: Acute Invasive Fungal Sinusitis	Severe acute sinusitis; fever; nasal discharge; ocular or neurologic deficits	Necrosis; thrombosis; hemorrhage; angioinvasive fungal hyphae in viable tissue; minimal inflammation	Common: Mucorales order—*Mucor, Rhizopus, Absidia, Cunninghamella;* Uncommon: *Aspergillus, Curvularia, Alternaria*
Invasive: Chronic Invasive Fungal Sinusitis	Slow, progressive onset; neurologic or orbital deficits; mass on imaging	Necrosis; angioinvasive fungal hyphae; granulomas	*Aspergillus*

concentrations. Endoscopy reveals thick, sticky, greenish or black to brown mucus, often described as the consistency of peanut butter. Microscopically, abundant brightly eosinophilic hypocellular mucin is present, distinct from the slightly basophilic staining of normal mucin. The mucin contains sheets of eosinophils that are degenerating and degranulating. These granules coalesce to form the classic Charcot–Leyden crystals also seen in the mucin (e-**Fig. 3.3**). The most common causative organisms are dematiaceous fungi such as *Curvularia* or *Alternaria,* and also *Aspergillus.* Fungal hyphae are fragmented and widely scattered in the mucin so they are rarely visible by H&E. Special stains such as Grocott's Methenamine Silver (GMS) are usually necessary for identification. If the typical histologic picture is present without identifying organisms, the term *allergic mucin* is used. If hyphae are identified, the term *allergic fungal sinusitis* is used.

Patients with mycetoma or fungus ball have typical chronic sinusitis but less often allergy-type symptoms. On endoscopy, the sinuses have mucopurulent, cheesy, or claylike material that microscopically consists of sheets of fungal hyphae with minimal mucin and inflammatory cells.

b. Invasive. The presence or absence of tissue invasion in fungal sinusitis is critical as patients with invasive disease are at great risk of morbidity and mortality. Patients with invasive fungal disease are usually immunocompromised, particularly due to diabetes mellitus, bone marrow or solid organ transplantation, or occasionally human immunodeficiency virus (HIV) infection.

Patients with invasive disease often are severely ill with fever, cough, nasal discharge, headache, and mental status changes. They sometimes have orbital and ophthalmologic symptoms due to eye involvement, or have neurologic deficits from cranial involvement. On endoscopy, there are dark ulcers of the mucosa and black, greasy necrotic tissue. The fungi are angioinvasive, so they cause extensive hemorrhage and necrosis. In the viable tissue, the microscopic findings include minimal inflammation with blood vessels filled with refractile fungal hyphae (e-Fig. 3.4). The order *Mucorales* is most common (e.g., *Mucor, Rhizopus, Absidia*), but other fungi including *Aspergillus* species are sometimes also causative. *Mucor* species have a unique morphology with bizarre, angulated hyphal fragments and elongated hyphae that are wide, irregular, and thick walled; typically there is a 90-degree angle branching without septation. Chronic invasive fungal disease sometimes occurs as a slowly progressive disease in patients with diabetes. They often have an orbital mass and functional deficits. Microscopically, there may be angioinvasive hyphae or granulomas

B. Nonneoplastic lesions. A number of lesions, developmental or mechanical, can occur in the sinonasal region and can be mass-like and simulate true neoplasms.

1. **Mucous impaction** is an uncommon lesion that occurs mostly in children and young adults with a long history of chronic sinusitis. It represents impaction of a large amount of mucus within the maxillary antrum. Grossly, it consists of translucent gray to pink material. Microscopically, it simply consists of slightly basophilic to eosinophilic extracellular mucin with a mixture of plasma cells, lymphocytes, and neutrophils with desquamated respiratory-type epithelium.

2. **Paranasal sinus mucoceles** are chronic, nonneoplastic cysts that form from obstruction of the sinus outlet by any of a number of processes. They occur most commonly in the ethmoid and frontal sinuses, and much less commonly in the maxillary and sphenoid sinuses. Grossly, they consist of a cyst filled with mucoid or gelatinous material. Microscopically, they consist of extracellular mucin as in mucous impaction but have a flattened respiratory-type epithelial lining that may have secondary squamous metaplasia.

3. **Respiratory epithelial adenomatoid hamartoma** (REAH) is a rare, benign lesion characterized by an adenomatoid proliferation of respiratory-type epithelium that occurs primarily on the posterior septum. Microscopically, it consists of a polypoid proliferation of variably sized, round to oval glands lined by ciliated respiratory-type epithelium with a markedly thickened basement membrane and no cytologic atypia or significant mitotic activity. The gland-like structures are often in direct continuity with the surface epithelium. The stroma is edematous and resembles that of an inflammatory polyp.

C. Neoplastic lesions. An extremely wide variety of neoplasms occur in the sinonasal region (Table 3.2).

1. **Benign**

   a. **Schneiderian papillomas.** The Schneiderian membrane is the ectodermally derived lining of the sinonasal tract. It gives rise to three different types of benign papillomas: exophytic, inverted, and oncocytic (Table 3.3). The distinction of these papillomas is important on clinical grounds due to the difference in behavior and risk of carcinoma development. For this reason, it is important to submit all papilloma tissue for microscopic examination.

      i. **Exophytic papilloma.** Also known as squamous or fungiform papilloma, the vast majority of these occur on the nasal septum, particularly anteriorly, in adults 20 to 50 years old. They are more common in men than women. Human papilloma virus (HPV; specifically the low risk types HPV 6 and 11) has been detected in a little over 50% of cases, so the virus may be important for pathogenesis. Exophytic papillomas are usually solitary and discrete, and patients present with epistaxis, unilateral nasal obstruction, or an asymptomatic mass.

         Clinically and grossly, these are warty gray-pink, nontranslucent growths with a broad base. Microscopically, they consist of exquisitely exophytic papillary fronds lined by a variably thickened epithelium that varies from squamous to ciliated pseudostratified columnar (respiratory-type) to a transitional form with features of both (e-Fig. 3.5). Scattered mucin-containing cells are sometimes seen, and the lining characteristically has abundant intraepithelial neutrophils, some in small collections simulating microabscesses. Surface keratinization is absent except in rare

| TABLE 3.2 | WHO Histological Classification of Tumors of the Nasal Cavity and Paranasal Sinuses |

Malignant epithelial tumors
Squamous cell carcinoma
  Verrucous carcinoma
  Papillary squamous cell carcinoma
  Basaloid squamous cell carcinoma
  Spindle cell carcinoma
  Adenosquamous carcinoma
  Acantholytic squamous cell carcinoma
Lymphoepithelial carcinoma
Sinonasal undifferentiated carcinoma
Adenocarcinoma
  Intestinal-type adenocarcinoma
  Nonintestinal-type adenocarcinoma
Salivary gland-type carcinomas
  Adenoid cystic carcinoma
  Acinic cell carcinoma
  Mucoepidermoid carcinoma
  Epithelial–myoepithelial carcinoma
  Clear cell carcinoma not otherwise specified
  Myoepithelial carcinoma
  Carcinoma ex pleomorphic adenoma
  Polymorphous low-grade adenocarcinoma
Neuroendocrine tumors
  Typical carcinoid
  Atypical carcinoid
  Small cell carcinoma, neuroendocrine type

Benign epithelial tumors
Sinonasal papillomas
  Inverted papilloma
  (Schneiderian papilloma, inverted type)
  Oncocytic papilloma
  (Schneiderian papilloma, oncocytic type)
  Exophytic papilloma
  (Schneiderian papilloma, exophytic type)
Salivary gland-type adenomas
  Pleomorphic adenoma
  Myoepithelioma
  Oncocytoma

Soft tissue tumors
Malignant tumors
  Fibrosarcoma
  Malignant fibrous histiocytoma
  Leiomyosarcoma
  Rhabdomyosarcoma
  Angiosarcoma
  Malignant peripheral nerve sheath tumor
Borderline and low malignant potential tumors
  Desmoid-type fibromatosis
  Inflammatory myofibroblastic tumor
  Glomangiopericytoma
    (Sinonasal-type hemangiopericytoma)
  Extrapleural solitary fibrous tumor

Benign tumors
  Myxoma
  Leiomyoma
  Haemangioma
  Schwannoma
  Neurofibroma
  Meningioma

Tumors of bone and cartilage
Malignant tumors
  Chondrosarcoma
  Mesenchymal chondrosarcoma
  Osteosarcoma
  Chordoma
Benign tumors
  Giant cell lesion
  Giant cell tumor
  Chondroma
  Osteoma
  Chondroblastoma
  Chondromyxoid fibroma
  Osteochondroma (exostosis)
  Osteoid osteoma
  Osteoblastoma
  Ameloblastoma
  Nasal chondromesenchymal hamartoma

Hematolymphoid tumors
  Extranodal natural killer (NK)/T-cell
    lymphoma
  Diffuse large B-cell lymphoma
  Extramedullary plasmacytoma
  Extramedullary myeloid sarcoma
  Histiocytic sarcoma
  Langerhans cell histiocytosis

Neuroectodermal
  Ewing sarcoma
  Primitive neuroectodermal tumor
  Olfactory neuroblastoma
  Melanotic neuroectodermal tumor of infancy
  Mucosal malignant melanoma

Germ cell tumors
  Immature teratoma
  Teratoma with malignant transformation
  Sinonasal yolk sac tumor (endodermal
    sinus tumor)
  Sinonasal teratocarcinosarcoma
  Mature teratoma
  Dermoid cyst

Secondary tumors

TABLE 3.3	Schneiderian Papillomas		
Type	**Common location**	**Pathology**	**Behavior**
Exophytic	Nasal septum	Exophytic fronds of bland epithelium—squamous, transitional, or respiratory-type; intraepithelial neutrophils and microcysts; thin basement membranes	Local recurrence; essentially no risk of invasive carcinoma
Inverted	Lateral nasal wall; paranasal sinuses	Pushing, endophytic nests of bland epithelium—squamous, transitional, or respiratory-type; lesser exophytic component at times; intraepithelial neutrophils and microcysts; thin basement membranes	Local recurrence; ~10% risk of invasive carcinoma
Oncocytic	Lateral nasal wall; paranasal sinuses	Exophytic and endophytic pushing nests of columnar, oncocytic cells with abundant, granular eosinophilic cytoplasm; intraepithelial neutrophils and microcysts	Local recurrence; ~5%–15% risk of invasive carcinoma

cases in which the lesion is near the vestibule and gets traumatized. There is minimal mitotic activity and no cytologic atypia.

After being completely removed, exophytic papillomas can recur locally in <25% of cases. However, there is no significant risk for developing carcinoma.

ii. **Inverted papilloma.** The most common type of Schneiderian papilloma, these are found primarily in adults between 40 and 70 years old. They characteristically arise from the lateral nasal wall in the region of the middle turbinate and ethmoid recesses, sometimes extending into the sinuses. In contrast to fungiform papillomas, only 8% of inverted papillomas arise from the nasal septum. They are only very rarely bilateral. HPV 6 and 11 have been reported to be present in widely variable numbers, but in a single large review, were detected in 38% of cases.

Microscopically, inverted papillomas are composed of numerous basement-membrane–enclosed, rounded ribbons of thickened epithelium identical to that seen in exophytic papillomas, again ranging from squamous to transitional to respiratory-type (e-**Fig. 3.6**). There is minimal mitotic activity, no significant cytologic atypia, and characteristically, there are abundant intraepithelial neutrophils singly and in clusters. The epithelium also contains numerous mucin-filled microcysts. An uncommonly mentioned feature is that some inverted papillomas can have an exophytic-appearing component. Any Schneiderian papilloma with a significant inverted and/or downward pushing component (more than a few nests) should be diagnosed as an inverted papilloma.

Uncommonly, there is surface keratinization and 5% to 20% show varying degrees of dysplasia. By itself, the dysplasia does not signify malignancy or a different clinical course for the patient. However, it is very important to thoroughly evaluate lesions that show dysplasia for carcinoma. In large series, approximately 10% to 15% of inverted papillomas were complicated by carcinoma, mostly squamous cell carcinoma, although a wide variety of carcinomas have been reported. In approximately 60% of cases associated with carcinoma, the malignancy was synchronous; in

40%, the malignancy was metachronous. A significant number of these papillomas will recur, particularly after conservative removal.

   iii. Oncocytic papillomas are the least common Schneiderian papillomas and have a variety of names including cylindrical cell papilloma and columnar cell papilloma. They occur in the same sites as inverted papillomas, namely, the lateral nasal wall and paranasal sinuses. Unlike the other Schneiderian papillomas, they have an equal male to female ratio, and studies have not identified an association with HPV.

   Grossly, they are fleshy, pink-tan, and papillary or polypoid. Microscopically, they typically have a mixture of exophytic and endophytic components and are lined by a unique two- to eight-cell layer of tall columnar oncocytic cells with abundant granular eosinophilic cytoplasm. The nuclei are slightly more atypical than in other Schneiderian papillomas with a wrinkled, dark to slightly vesicular appearance with small nucleoli. The epithelium also contains numerous mucin-filled microcysts and shows the typical intraepithelial neutrophils (**e-Fig. 3.7**).

   Oncocytic papillomas have a risk of carcinoma similar to inverted papillomas. A significant number will recur, particularly after conservative removal.

   b. Verruca vulgaris (nasal vestibule). As the nasal vestibule is essentially an extension of the surrounding nasal skin, verrucae occur here and have the same morphology as elsewhere (see Chapter 38).

2. Malignant

   a. Sinonasal undifferentiated carcinoma (SNUC). This tumor is an aggressive and clinicopathologically distinct form of sinonasal carcinoma. Patients are most commonly in their 50s or 60s and present with symptoms of short duration, including nasal obstruction and epistaxis, and often have orbital or cranial nerve deficits. The tumor most often arises in the nasal cavity, particularly anteriorly, or in the maxillary or ethmoid sinuses. It is usually bulky, often involving contiguous sites.

   There are no unique gross features. Tumors are usually >4 cm, poorly defined, and involve bone. Microscopically, there are a number of different growth patterns including nested, trabecular, or lobular. The tumor cells are small to moderate in size, have a small to moderate amount of cytoplasm with distinct cell borders, and have nuclei that range from hyperchromatic to vesicular, often with prominent nucleoli. There is abundant apoptosis, brisk mitotic activity, and often prominent necrosis (**e-Fig. 3.8**). By definition, there is a lack of definable differentiation.

   Immunohistochemistry is positive for pan-cytokeratin and epithelial membrane antigen. More specifically, simple keratins such as CK7, 8, and 19 are present, whereas more complex keratins such as CK5/6 are absent. Neuron-specific enolase (NSE) is positive in up to 50% of cases, but more specific neuroendocrine markers such as chromogranin A and synaptophysin are negative.

   SNNC is very aggressive with a mean survival of one to two years despite aggressive surgery, and radiation therapy.

   b. NPC. Although still relatively uncommon in the United States, NPC is important because of its relationship to Epstein–Barr Virus (EBV) and because of specific geographic predilections (the tumor is particularly common in the so-called "endemic" areas of Asia and North Africa). The latest World Health Organization (WHO) classification (2005) recognizes four major types: keratinizing, differentiated nonkeratinizing, undifferentiated, and basaloid (Table 3.4). NPC occurs in all age groups, with a peak incidence between 30 and 50 years of age. It is not uncommon in adolescents. Patients present with the typical sinonasal mass symptoms of nasal obstruction and epistaxis but also may have serous otitis media from Eustachian tube obstruction or, not infrequently, an asymptomatic neck mass from metastasis.

   The clinical and macroscopic appearance is nondescript. Microscopically, several different patterns are seen. The keratinizing type (WHO Type 1)

TABLE 3.4	2005 World Health Organization (WHO) Classification of Nasopharyngeal Carcinoma

Histology	Type
Keratinizing squamous cell carcinoma	1
Nonkeratinizing carcinoma, differentiated	2a
Nonkeratinizing carcinoma, undifferentiated	2b
Basaloid squamous cell carcinoma	3

has a morphology identical to that of keratinizing squamous cell carcinoma elsewhere in the head and neck. It is also graded the same from poorly to well differentiated. The differentiated nonkeratinizing type (WHO Type 2a) has stratified cells with an appearance similar to that of transitional cell carcinoma of the urinary bladder. The cells are moderately atypical with well-defined cell borders and a sharp interface of tumor nests with the surrounding stroma (e-**Fig. 3.9**). The undifferentiated nonkeratinizing type (WHO Type 2b) is the most common, most distinctive, and most challenging. It consists of syncytial aggregates/sheets of tumor cells with moderate eosinophilic cytoplasm; large, vesicular nuclei with prominent nucleoli; and a brisk lymphocytic infiltrate (e-**Fig. 3.10**). Occasionally, the cells are widely dispersed in small clusters or as single cells making the diagnosis of carcinoma difficult. Apoptosis and brisk mitotic activity are invariably present. Finally, basaloid squamous cell carcinoma (WHO Type 3) has a morphology identical to that seen in the same tumor in other regions of the head and neck. It is by far the least common type.

NPC has a number of interesting clinicopathologic features. First, given the location and anatomy of the nasopharynx, radiation therapy is the first-line treatment modality; surgery is uncommon and usually reserved for salvage therapy. Second, although EBV is strongly related to the tumorigenesis of nonkeratinizing NPC, in keratinizing NPC this relationship is tenuous at best. Third, nonkeratinizing NPC tends to metastasize to lymph nodes early in its course (60% to 85% overall), often to the posterior triangle (level V), and these tumors have a different staging system that reflects this (see AJCC staging below). Finally, despite advanced disease, nonkeratinizing NPC responds well to systemic therapy (5-year survival of approximately 65% in the United States); keratinizing NPC, although it much more often presents with localized disease, does not respond well to therapy (5-year survival of 20% to 40% in the United States).

c. **Squamous cell carcinoma/cylindric cell carcinoma.** Squamous cell carcinoma, although the overridingly most common carcinoma in most head and neck regions, constitutes only approximately 65% of carcinomas in the nasal cavity and paranasal sinuses. When it occurs in the nasopharynx, it is designated *keratinizing squamous cell carcinoma* (WHO Type 1; see section b. above and Table 3.4). Keratinizing, or typical, squamous cell carcinoma of the nasal cavity and paranasal sinuses has the same morphology as that occurring elsewhere in the upper aerodigestive tract. One particular issue related to squamous cell carcinoma of this region is the only modest association with smoking; tumors have been related to other exposures including nickel, chlorophenols, and textile dust, and some patients have had a prior Schneiderian papilloma.

A distinct variant of nonkeratinizating carcinoma occurs in this region, the so-called cylindrical cell carcinoma (Schneiderian or transitional carcinoma). The recent WHO classification simply terms it *nonkeratinizing carcinoma*. It has a papillary configuration with ribbons of invaginating tumor with pleomorphic cells without keratinization. These ribbons have a smooth border without clear stromal infiltration, which makes identification of invasion difficult (e-**Fig. 3.11**). This tumor type has been associated with HPV and is also reported by several authors to have a better prognosis, although the latter contention is still controversial.

  d. **Salivary gland–type tumors** constitute a small percentage of sinonasal tumors. They arise from submucosal seromucinous glands, and the most common are adenoid cystic carcinoma and pleomorphic adenoma, although almost all other types have been described. They are morphologically identical to their counterparts elsewhere.

  e. **Adenocarcinoma.** Primary nonsalivary gland–type adenocarcinomas of the sinonasal region are uncommon. A number of different classifications have been proposed. However, the most durable classification seems to be to divide them into intestinal and nonintestinal types.

   i. **Intestinal type.** Primary intestinal-type adenocarcinomas (ITACs) of the sinonasal region typically arise from the ethmoid sinuses or high in the nasal cavity. They have a strong association with occupational exposures, specifically wood dust (in carpenters), leather dust, nickel, or chromium compounds. Long exposures are necessary, and the latency period is several decades. Grossly, there are no characteristic features. Microscopically, these tumors can perfectly recapitulate gastrointestinal adenocarcinomas, including very well-differentiated tumors resembling colonic adenomas, typical "colonic-appearing" tumors with columnar glands with or without mucinous differentiation (e-**Fig. 3.12**), and high-grade tumors with a signet ring cell morphology.

   By immunohistochemistry, they stain very much like gastrointestinal adenocarcinomas, being positive for cytokeratin 20, CDX-2, MUC2, and villin. Cytokeratin 7 is variably positive, and carcinoembryogenic antigen (CEA) is usually positive. As such, it can be very difficult to separate these tumors from the rare metastasis to this region from a primary gastrointestinal adenocarcinoma.

   ITACs should be graded from poorly to well-differentiated, and the type (colonic, mucinous, papillary, signet ring cell, or solid) specified, as both have prognostic significance. The mortality is approximately 50% overall.

   ii. **Nonintestinal type.** These are uncommon tumors, most of which are low-grade. The low-grade tumors have a predilection for the ethmoid sinus and the high-grade tumors for the maxillary sinus. Low-grade tumors have a glandular or papillary growth pattern with numerous uniform, small glands arranged back-to-back and lined by a single layer of cuboidal to columnar cells with a moderate amount of eosinophilic cytoplasm and regular round nuclei. There is only mild nuclear pleomorphism, modest mitotic activity without atypical forms, and no necrosis. These tumors can have a papillary growth pattern and sometimes show clear cytoplasm. High-grade tumors have similar features, but also have solid areas and show moderate to severe nuclear pleomorphism with brisk mitotic activity and necrosis.

   By immunohistochemistry, nonintestinal type adenocarcinomas are positive for cytokeratin 7 and negative for the intestinal markers cytokeratin 20, CDX-2, and MUC2. Smooth muscle actin and p63 are negative; demonstration of the absence of a myoepithelial layer by these two markers is helpful in distinction from salivary gland-type adenocarcinomas. The prognosis for low-grade tumors is excellent, but for high-grade ones the prognosis is poor.

  f. **Neuroendocrine carcinomas** sometimes arise in the sinonasal region and are morphologically identical to those arising in the lung.

   i. **Low-grade neuroendocrine carcinoma** (i.e., carcinoid tumor) is extremely rare in this region.

   ii. **High-grade neuroendocrine carcinoma** (small cell carcinoma) is a rapidly proliferating, aggressive neoplasm that presents with epistaxis, nasal obstruction, and exophthalmos. It usually presents at an advanced stage with extensive local disease and lymph node or distant metastases. Microscopically, it consists of nests and sheets of small- to intermediate-sized blue cells with minimal cytoplasm, coarse chromatin, and frequent nuclear molding and crush artifact. Apoptosis is abundant, and there is brisk mitotic activity and necrosis. By immunohistochemistry, it is positive for pancytokeratin with a "dotlike" paranuclear staining pattern. It is variably positive for the neuroendocrine markers NSE, synaptophysin, and chromogranin A, but in most cases at least one of these markers is positive on careful inspection. The tumor is negative for S-100, CD99 (O13), and cytokeratin 20 (a feature sometimes helpful to exclude Merkel cell carcinoma).

g. Melanoma. Primary malignant melanoma of the sinonasal tract constitutes approximately 1% of all melanomas. It is more common in the nasal cavity than in the paranasal sinuses, and most patients are >50 years old, with tumors most often occurring on the middle or inferior turbinates or anterior septum. It has a variable macroscopic appearance, but usually is a sessile or polypoid lesion with mucosal ulceration. Most are heavily pigmented with a brown or black color. Microscopically, like melanomas elsewhere, it has a widely ranging appearance; although usually composed of high-grade epithelioid cells, some tumors are composed of a mixture of epithelioid and spindle cells. A junctional component with pagetoid spread of melanocytes in the intact mucosa is sometimes present.

Immunohistochemistry results are the same as for melanomas at other sites, with virtually all tumors expressing S-100, HMB-45, and melan-A. Cytokeratin reactivity, if present, is only focal. High-grade spindled melanomas tend to lose their melan-A and HMB-45 reactivity but will maintain S-100 reactivity.

Metastasis of melanoma to the sinonasal region from another primary site is not uncommon and should always be kept in mind in these cases. Metastases can almost perfectly recapitulate a primary lesion, although a junctional component at the surface mucosa essentially rules this out.

h. Olfactory neuroblastoma. This unique tumor arises almost exclusively in the upper nasal cavity from olfactory mucosa on the cribriform plate, upper lateral nasal wall, and superior turbinate. The presumed cell of origin is the reserve cell that gives rise to neuronal and sustentacular cells of olfactory mucosa. It occurs at any age but most commonly in the third and fourth decades, with the typical symptoms of nasal obstruction, epistaxis, and occasionally anosmia.

Macroscopically, the tumor usually is a unilateral, polypoid mass in the nasal cavity. Microscopically, it consists of small, round cells that are slightly larger than lymphocytes. The nuclei are round, with a uniform to delicately stippled chromatin without nucleoli. Many tumors have areas with fibrillary eosinophilic material reminiscent of neuropil (e-**Fig. 3.13**). Some tumors have a very lobulated and nested growth pattern, whereas others are diffuse. Homer–Wright rosettes (no central lumen) are relatively common. Mitotic activity is low, and there is only (uncommonly) necrosis or dystrophic calcification. Some tumors have been reported to show significant nuclear pleomorphism and high mitotic activity; however, this is very uncommon and merits strong consideration of another type of neoplasm, particularly, a high-grade neuroendocrine carcinoma. Rare findings include ganglion cells, melanin-containing cells, and divergent differentiation including glandular, squamous, and teratomatous features.

By immunohistochemistry, olfactory neuroblastoma shows strong cytoplasmic staining for synaptophysin, chromogranin A, and NSE. S-100 often highlights sustentacular cells at the periphery of nests and lobules, but is negative in tumor cells. A confusing finding is cytokeratin reactivity; this has been reported in up to 35% of cases, specifically for CAM 5.2, but less often for AE1/AE3. The staining is typically weaker and more focal than would be expected in a carcinoma.

Grading systems, most notably by Hyams, have been proposed, but their correlation with prognosis has not been consistently demonstrated.

TABLE 3.5	2002 American Joint Committee on Cancer (AJCC) Staging Guidelines for Tumors of the Nasal Cavity and Paranasal Sinuses

PRIMARY TUMOR (T)

Maxillary sinus

TX	Primary tumor cannot be assessed
T0	No evidence of primary tumor
Tis	Carcinoma in situ
T1	Tumor limited to maxillary sinus mucosa with no erosion or destruction of bone
T2	Tumor causing bone erosion or destruction including extension into the hard palate and/or middle nasal meatus, except extension to posterior wall of maxillary sinus and pterygoid plates
T3	Tumor invades any of the following: bone of the posterior wall of maxillary sinus, subcutaneous tissues, floor or medial wall of orbit, pterygoid fossa, or ethmoid sinuses
T4a	Tumor invades anterior orbital contents, skin of cheek, pterygoid plates, infratemporal fossa, cribriform plate, sphenoid or frontal sinuses
T4b	Tumor invades any of the following: orbital apex, dura, brain, middle cranial fossa, cranial nerves other than maxillary division of trigeminal nerve V2, nasopharynx, or clivus

Nasal cavity and ethmoid sinus

TX	Primary tumor cannot be assessed
T0	No evidence of primary tumor
Tis	Carcinoma in situ
T1	Tumor restricted to any one subsite, with or without bone invasion
T2	Tumor invading two subsites in a single region or extending to involve an adjacent region within the nasoethmoidal complex, with or without bony invasion
T3	Tumor extends to invade the medial wall or floor of the orbit, maxillary sinus, palate, or cribriform plate
T4a	Tumor invades any of the following: anterior orbital contents, skin of nose or cheek, minimal extension to anterior cranial fossa, pterygoid plates, sphenoid or frontal sinuses
T4b	Tumor invades any of the following: orbital apex, dura, brain, middle cranial fossa, cranial nerves other than V2, nasopharynx, or clivus

REGIONAL LYMPH NODES (N)

NX	Regional lymph nodes cannot be assessed
N0	No regional lymph node metastasis
N1	Metastasis in a single ipsilateral lymph node, 3 cm or less in greatest dimension
N2a	Metastasis in a single ipsilateral lymph node, >3 cm but not >6 cm in greatest dimension
N2b	Metastasis in multiple ipsilateral lymph nodes, none >6 cm in greatest dimension
N2c	Metastasis in bilateral or contralateral lymph nodes, none >6 cm in greatest dimension
N3	Metastasis in a lymph node >6 cm in greatest dimension

DISTANT METASTASIS (M)

MX	Distant metastasis cannot be assessed
M0	No distant metastasis
M1	Distant metastasis.

(continued)

TABLE 3.5 **2002 American Joint Committee on Cancer (AJCC) Staging Guidelines for Tumors of the Nasal Cavity and Paranasal Sinuses (*Continued*)**

STAGE GROUPING
The overall pathologic AJCC stage is

Stage 0	Tis	N0	M0
Stage I	T1	N0	M0
Stage II	T2	N0	M0
Stage III	T3	N0	M0
Stage III	T1	N1	M0
Stage III	T2	N1	M0
Stage III	T3	N1	M0
Stage IVA	T4a	N0	M0
Stage IVA	T4a	N1	M0
Stage IVA	T1	N2	M0
Stage IVA	T2	N2	M0
Stage IVA	T3	N2	M0
Stage IVA	T4a	N2	M0
Stage IVB	T4b	Any N	M0
Stage IVB	Any T	N3	M0
Stage IVC	Any T	Any N	M1

From: Greene FL, Page DL, Fleming ID, Fritz AG, Balch CM, Haller DG, Morrow M, eds. AJCC Cancer Staging Manual. 6th edition. New York: Springer, 2002. Used with permission. (A new AJCC TNM staging system is scheduled for release in 2009; after its publication, the new staging scheme will appear on the website for this book.)

i. Mesenchymal tumors

i. Angiofibroma. Also referred to as nasopharyngeal angiofibroma, this unique tumor is thought to arise from a fibrovascular nidus in the posterolateral nasal wall adjacent to the sphenopalatine foramen. It occurs virtually exclusively in boys aged 10 to 20 and presents with nasal obstruction, periodic epistaxis, and a nasopharyngeal mass. The reason it presents in the nasopharynx is because it is a pushing, well-circumscribed tumor, and it bulges posteriorly into the nasopharynx as it enlarges.

Grossly, the tumor is gray-white to tan, smooth, and lobulated, and it has a homogeneous cut surface. Microscopically, it consists of abundant vessels ranging from capillaries to large vessels, the latter often assuming a "staghorn" appearance (e-**Fig. 3.14**). These vessels are lined by a single layer of endothelial cells that can be flat to slightly plump without any cytologic atypia. The wall is typically devoid of smooth muscle and blends imperceptibly with the stromal component of the tumor, which has regularly distributed, plump, stellate spindle cells embedded in a dense collagenous stroma. The cells have vesicular chromatin, sometimes with small nucleoli, but no atypia and minimal mitotic activity. By immunohistochemistry, the stromal cells are positive for vimentin and negative for smooth muscle actin. The endothelial cells are positive for CD34. Otherwise, the tumors are negative for S-100, desmin, and cytokeratin.

This tumor is benign and grows as a pushing mass. However, it is capable of bone erosion from pressure. The virtually exclusive occurrence in adolescent boys, particularly the noted growth around puberty, has led investigators to demonstrate androgen receptors in most of the cases.

ii. Glomangiopericytoma. Also known as sinonasal-type hemangiopericytoma or hemangiopericytoma-like tumor, this is a somewhat uncommon tumor of perivascular myoid-type cells. All ages can be affected, but patients in their seventh decade predominate. Unilateral nasal cavity involvement

| TABLE 3.6 | 2002 American Joint Committee on Cancer (AJCC) Staging Guidelines for Tumors of the Nasopharynx |

PRIMARY TUMOR (T)

TX	Primary tumor cannot be assessed
T0	No evidence of primary tumor
Tis	Carcinoma in situ
T1	Tumor confined to the nasopharynx
T2	Tumor extends into the soft tissues
T2a	Tumor extends to the oropharynx and/or nasal cavity without parapharyngeal extension
T2b	Any tumor with parapharyngeal extension
T3	Tumor involves bony structures and/or paranasal sinuses
T4	Tumor with intracranial extension and/or involvement of cranial nerves, infratemporal fossa, hypopharynx, orbit, or masticator space

REGIONAL LYMPH NODES (N)

NX	Regional lymph nodes cannot be assessed
N0	No regional lymph node metastasis
N1	Unilateral metastasis in lymph node(s), 6 cm or less, above the supraclavicular fossa*
N2	Bilateral metastasis in lymph node(s), 6 cm or less, above the supraclavicular fossa*
N3*	Metastasis in a lymph node(s) >6 cm and/or to the supraclavicular fossa*
N3a	>6 cm
N3b	Extension to the supraclavicular fossa

DISTANT METASTASIS (M)

MX	Distant metastasis cannot be assessed
M0	No distant metastasis
M1	Distant metastasis

STAGE GROUPING
The overall pathologic AJCC stage is

Stage 0	Tis	N0	M0
Stage I	T1	N0	M0
Stage IIA	T2a	N0	M0
Stage IIB	T1	N1	M0
Stage IIB	T2a	N1	M0
Stage IIB	T2b	N0	M0
Stage IIB	T2b	N1	M0
Stage III	T1	N2	M0
Stage III	T2a	N2	M0
Stage III	T2b	N2	M0
Stage III	T3	N0	M0
Stage III	T3	N1	M0
Stage III	T3	N2	M0
Stage IVA	T4	N0	M0
Stage IVA	T4	N1	M0
Stage IVA	T4	N2	M0
Stage IVB	Any T	N3	M0
Stage IVC	Any T	Any N	M1

*Midline lymph nodes are considered ipsilateral.
From: Greene FL, Page DL, Fleming ID, Fritz AG, Balch CM, Haller DG, Morrow M, eds. AJCC Cancer Staging Manual. 6th edition. New York: Springer, 2002. Used with permission. (A new AJCC TNM staging system is scheduled for release in 2009; after its publication, the new staging scheme will appear on the website for this book.)

is most common, and the tumor is grossly polypoid, beefy-red to gray-pink, and soft. Microscopically, the tumor consists of numerous variably sized vascular channels that classically have a staghorn appearance. The intervascular stroma has a dense proliferation of closely packed cells with round to ovoid nuclei, and small amounts of eosinophilic cytoplasm. The tumor cells grow in short fascicles, sometimes with a storiform pattern. There is minimal nuclear pleomorphism, little mitotic activity, and no necrosis (e-**Fig. 3.15**). By immunohistochemistry, the cells are strongly and diffusely positive for CD34 and also for vimentin, smooth muscle actin, and factor XIIIa. The prognosis is excellent, with >90% survival at 5 years after surgery and a modest recurrence rate.

IV. PATHOLOGIC REPORTING OF SINONASAL MALIGNANCIES
   A. Staging (AJCC). Clinical staging of sinonasal cancers is important for prognosis and treatment, and differs by site. The 2002 Tumor, Node, and Metastasis (TNM) AJCC staging classification is given in Table 3.5 for the nasal cavity and paranasal sinuses and in Table 3.6 for the nasopharynx. Staging guidelines are applicable to all forms of carcinoma. Any nonepithelial tumor type is excluded.
   B. Additional pertinent pathologic features. A number of pathologic features not reflected in the AJCC staging have been proven important for head and neck squamous cell carcinomas, as well as for numerous other histologic types, including perineural invasion, lymphovascular space invasion, and positive margin status. All of these latter features have been demonstrated in numerous studies to correlate with a higher risk of local recurrence, a poorer prognosis, or both.

Suggested Readings
Barnes L, Tse LLY, Hunt JL, Brandwein-Gensler M, Curtin HD, Boffetta P. Tumours of the nasal cavity and paranasal sinuses. In: Barnes L, Eveson JW, Reichart P, Sidransky D, eds. *Pathology and Genetics Head and Neck Tumours.* Lyon, France: IARC Press; 2005.

Brandwein-Gensler M, Thompson LDR. Non-neoplastic lesions of the nasal cavity, paranasal sinuses, and nasopharynx. In: Thompson LDR, ed. *Head and Neck Pathology.* New York: Churchill Livingstone; 2006.

Chan JKC, Pilch BZ, Kuo TT, Wenig BM, Lee AWM. Tumours of the nasopharynx. In: Barnes L, Eveson JW, Reichart P, Sidransky D, eds. *Pathology and Genetics Head and Neck Tumours.* Lyon, France: IARC Press; 2005.

Perez-Ordonez B, Huvos AG. Nonsquamous lesions of the nasal cavity, paranasal sinuses, and nasopharynx. In: Gnepp DR, ed. *Diagnostic Surgical Pathology of the Head and Neck.* Philadelphia: W.B. Saunders Publishers; 2001.

Perez-Ordonez B, Thompson LDR. Benign neoplasms of the nasal cavity, paranasal sinuses, and nasopharynx. In: Thompson LDR, ed. *Head and Neck Pathology.* New York: Churchill Livingstone; 2006.

Thompson LDR. Malignant neoplasms of the nasal cavity, paranasal sinuses, and nasopharynx. In: Thompson LDR, ed. *Head and Neck Pathology.* New York: Churchill Livingstone; 2006.

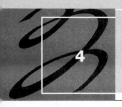

4 TUMORS AND CYSTS OF THE JAWS
David E. Spence and Samir K. El-Mofty

I. **NORMAL ANATOMY.** Of all the bones of the skeleton, the jaws are uniquely distinguished by harboring the odontogenic apparatus of the deciduous and permanent dentitions. The teeth germs are composed of three main components: the enamel organ, the dental papilla, and the tooth follicle. The enamel organ is composed of ectodermally derived epithelial cells, the ameloblasts, and is responsible for enamel formation. The dental papilla is of ectomesenchymal origin and produces the dentine. The tooth follicle is also ectomesenchymal; it surrounds the developing tooth and provides the supporting structures of the formed teeth, the periodontium. The odontogenic tissues may also be a source of a bewildering array of odontogenic cysts and tumors. Nonodontogenic cysts and tumors of the jaws will also be discussed in this chapter.

II. **ODONTOGENIC AND NONODONTOGENIC CYSTS.** Odontogenic cysts of the mandible and maxilla are relatively common and can present over a large age range. Accurate diagnosis is simplified by location, radiographic correlation, and microscopic examination (e-**Fig. 4.1**).* Odontogenic tumors by contrast are uncommon. They may be epithelial, mesenchymal, or mixed; they may be noncalcifying; or they may contain hard structures that mimic enamel, dentine, cementum, or bone. Although malignant odontogenic tumors are extremely rare, odontogenic carcinoma, sarcoma, and carcinosarcoma do occur.

A. **Odontogenic cysts.** With the exception of a few cysts that may develop along embryonic lines of fusion (known as nonodontogenic cysts), most jaw cysts are lined with epithelium that is derived from the odontogenic epithelium. Odontogenic cysts are classified as either developmental or inflammatory. Various types of odontogenic cysts are listed in Table 4.1.

1. **Developmental odontogenic cysts**

a. **A dentigerous cyst** (follicular cyst) is a unilocular cyst that forms in association with the crown of an impacted tooth, and is usually associated with a molar or canine tooth. Patients usually present with an asymptomatic, well-defined, expansive, radiolucent lesion. Microscopic examination shows a thin layer of cuboidal to slightly flattened epithelial cells. Focal keratinization, mucous cells, inflammation, and dystrophic calcification are possible. Enucleation and excision of the associated tooth are the treatment of choice. An eruption cyst is a subclass of dentigerous cyst associated with the erupting primary or permanent tooth.

b. **Keratocystic odontogenic tumors** (odontogenic keratocysts) usually present as asymptomatic unilocular cysts in the mandible or maxilla. Although more frequent in the 2nd to 4th decade, they may be seen at any age. Their incidence is higher in Caucasians and men, and roughly 5% of patients with odontogenic keratocysts have nevoid basal cell carcinoma (Gorlin) syndrome. Gross examination typically yields a cyst containing keratinous debris. Microscopic examination shows palisading basal cells covered by a few layers of squamous cells under a corrugated parakeratotic surface (e-**Fig. 4.2**). A key diagnostic feature is the lack of rete pegs. Satellite cysts and intramural epithelial cell proliferation are more commonly found in the syndrome-associated cases.

---

*All e-figures are available online via the Solution Site Image Bank.

TABLE 4.1	**Odontogenic Cysts**

Developmental
  Dentigerous cyst and eruption cyst
  Keratocystic odontogenic tumor (odontogenic keratocyst)
  Lateral periodontal cyst
  Gingival cyst of the adult
  Calcifying cystic odontogenic tumor (calcifying odontogenic cyst, Gorlin cyst)
  Glandular odontogenic cyst
Inflammatory
  Periapical (radicular) cyst
  Residual periapical (radicular) cyst

Exceptionally, dysplasia and carcinoma develop in the cyst. Treatment is surgical excision, and recurrence is common.

c. **Lateral periodontal cysts** generally present as well-demarcated radiolucent lesions in asymptomatic patients in their 5th to 7th decade. The typical locations are the lateral surface of the roots of the mandibular premolar teeth, although rare presentations in the maxilla may be encountered. Microscopic examination shows a thin layer of nonkeratinized epithelium with focal thickening and possible clear cells (e-Fig. 4.3). The adjacent soft tissue is not inflamed. A rare polycystic variant (botryoid odontogenic cyst) is characterized by rapid growth and an elevated probability of recurrence. Simple excision is typically curative.

d. **Gingival cysts** of the adult are infrequent lesions appearing on the buccal gingival of the mandible near the premolar and canine teeth. They represent the soft tissue counterparts of lateral periodontal cysts. Patients are typically in the 5th to 6th decade, and present with a pink to bluish overlying mucosal surface. Although usually unicystic, rare multicystic gingival cysts (gingival botryoid odontogenic cysts) may be seen. Microscopic examination shows a cyst lined by a thin layer of epithelium with rare focal thickening; the adjacent soft tissue is fibrotic and does not show inflammation. Treatment is simple excision.

e. **Calcifying cystic odontogenic tumors** (calcifying odontogenic cysts, Gorlin cysts) present as radiolucent asymptomatic lesions of the maxilla or mandible. The tumors can be unicystic, multicystic, and occasionally solid. Focal radio-opaque areas may be identified. The incidence peaks in the 2nd and 3rd decade, although cases occur in all age groups. Microscopic examination shows a proliferating layer of columnar palisaded basal cells similar to ameloblasts. The superficial layers frequently have larger ghost cells characterized by eosinophilic cytoplasm without nuclei (e-Fig. 4.4). Calcification of the tumor and adjacent soft tissue can be identified in some cases. Treatment is surgical excision, and recurrence is uncommon.

f. **Glandular odontogenic cysts** are recently defined lesions that have also been referred to as sialo-odontogenic cysts. The majority occur as radiolucent cysts in the anterior mandible or anterior maxilla. Patients typically present with pain and swelling, but some cases are asymptomatic. Microscopic examination demonstrates a unilocular/multilocular cyst with nonkeratinized epithelium, mucous-producing cells, and focal solid areas (e-Fig. 4.5). Hyaline bodies, ghost cells, and ciliated cuboidal eosinophilic cells may be present. Care should be taken to differentiate between a glandular odontogenic cyst and a central mucoepidermoid carcinoma. Surgical excision is the treatment of choice.

2. **Inflammatory odontogenic cysts.** Radicular (periapical) cysts are associated with nonviable carious teeth. The usual location is the apical third of the tooth root, with occasional cases involving the lateral root surface, and the cyst is more

common in the mandible. The typical age of patient is the 3rd to 6th decade. The most common presentation is pain and swelling, but presentation as an incidental finding on routine radiographic examination is not unusual. Microscopic examination reveals an inflamed, nonkeratinizing, stratified epithelium. Cholesterol crystals, foamy macrophages, dystrophic calcifications, and intraepithelial hyaline bodies (Rushton bodies) may be identified (e-Fig. 4.6). The *residual cyst* is a variant of radicular cyst that is seen at the site of an extracted tooth.

- **B. Nonodontogenic cysts.** This class of lesions includes a group of epithelium-lined cysts, as well as non–epithelium-lined bone cysts. The epithelium-lined cysts are believed to arise from epithelial remnants entrapped along embryonic lines of fusion and are referred to as "fissural cysts" (e-Fig. 4.7).
    - **1. Epithelial-lined nonodontogenic cysts "fissural cysts"**
        - **a. Nasopalatine duct cysts** (incisive canal cysts) are the most common of the fissural cysts. They are believed to arise from remnants of the nasopalatine duct. The cysts can develop almost at any age, but are most common in the 4th to 6th decades of life. Most studies show a slight male predilection. The most common presenting symptoms include swelling of the anterior palate, drainage, and pain.

            Radiographs usually demonstrate a well-circumscribed radiolucency, in or near the midline of the anterior maxilla, between and apical to the central incisor teeth. The lesion most often is round, oval, or pear-shaped. Microscopically, the epithelial lining of the cyst may be stratified squamous, pseudostratified columnar, simple columnar, or cuboidal. Commonly more than one epithelial type is present. Because the cyst arises within the incisive canal, moderately sized nerves and small muscular arteries and veins are usually found in the cyst wall (e-Fig. 4.8). Surgical enucleation is the treatment of choice.
        - **b. Globulomaxillary cysts** are believed to develop from epithelium entrapped during fusion of the globular portion of the medial nasal process with the maxillary process, although their origin continues to be a subject of debate.

            The cyst classically develops between the lateral incisor and cuspid teeth, although occasionally it has been reported between the central and lateral incisors. Radiographically, the cyst presents as well-circumscribed unilocular radiolucency between and apical to the teeth. The radiolucency is often pear-shaped. As the cyst expands, tilting of the adjacent teeth may occur. Microscopically, many of the cysts are lined with stratified squamous epithelium. Occasionally, however, the lining epithelium is of pseudostratified columnar ciliated type. Enucleation is the treatment of choice.
        - **c. Median palatal (palatine) cysts** are rare fissural cysts. They are believed to develop from epithelium entrapped along the embryonic line of fusion of the lateral palatal shelves of the maxilla. The cyst may be difficult to distinguish from the nasopalatine duct cysts, and some cases may actually represent a posteriorly placed nasopalatine duct cyst.

            Clinically, the cyst presents as a firm or fluctuant swelling in the midline of the hard palate, posterior to the incisive papilla. It is more frequent in young adults and is often asymptomatic. The average size of the cyst is 2 × 2 cm, but may become quite large. Radiographs demonstrate a well-circumscribed lucency in the midline of the hard palate. Microscopically, the cyst is commonly lined by stratified squamous epithelium, but areas of pseudostratified columnar epithelium may be seen. Surgical removal is the treatment of choice.
    - **2. Nonodontogenic non–epithelium-lined bone cysts** of the jaws
        - **a. Simple bone cysts** are known by multiple names: unicameral bone cyst, solitary bone cyst, progressive bony cavity, hemorrhagic cyst, traumatic bone cyst. The typical patient is younger than 20 years and has a well-demarcated osteolytic solitary lesion in the posterior mandible. Unusual cases have been seen in the maxilla. The cyst cavity is lined by fibrovascular tissue with hemosiderin-laden macrophages. Reactive bone and osteoclasts may be identified.
        - **b. Aneurysmal bone cysts** are rapidly enlarging blood-filled cystic lesions usually identified in the first three decades of life. The majority are

well-demarcated, unilateral pseudocysts located in the mandible (60%) and maxilla (40%). Aneurysmal bone cysts may be identified alone or in conjunction with another lesion (e.g., chondroblastoma, osteoblastoma). CT and MRI studies show characteristic layering of blood cells and serum. Microscopic examination shows a fibrotic stroma with giant cells, macrophages, and hemosiderin granules (e-**Fig. 4.9**). Areas of ossification may be present. Treatment is curettage and enucleation, and about 25% of the lesions recur.

III. **ODONTOGENIC TUMORS.** Odontogenic tumors are classified according to their composition into epithelial, mesenchymal, or mixed. Epithelial odontogenic tumors are composed only of odontogenic epithelium, whereas mesenchymal odontogenic tumors are composed principally of ectomesenchymal elements. Mixed odontogenic tumors contain epithelial and ectomesenchymal tissues. Inductive interactive action between the epithelial and ectomesenchymal elements may mimic normal odontogenesis, and thus dental hard tissues may, on occasion, be found in these tumors. As stated above, malignant odontogenic tumors are rare, but carcinomas, sarcomas, and carcinosarcomas do occur. Odontogenic tumors are listed in Table 4.2.

A. **Epithelial odontogenic tumors**

   1. **Ameloblastoma** is the most common clinically significant odontogenic tumor. Its relative frequency equals the combined frequency of all other odontogenic tumors, excluding odontoma. Ameloblastoma is a slow growing, locally invasive neoplasm. The tumor is encountered over a wide age range; it is rare in children and is most prevalent in the 3rd to 7th decade of life. There is no gender predilection. Some studies show an increased frequency in blacks.

   About 85% of ameloblastomas occur in the mandible, most often in the molar-ascending ramus area. About 15% of ameloblastomas occur in the maxilla, usually in the posterior region. Painless swelling or expansion of the jaw is the usual clinical presentation. If untreated, the lesion may grow slowly to massive or grotesque proportions. Pain and paresthesia are uncommon, even in large tumors. Radiographically, the most typical feature is that of a multilocular radiolucent lesion. Cortical expansion is frequently present. Microscopically, the lesion may present several patterns; these microscopic patterns have no bearing on the behavior of the tumor, and large tumors often show a combination of patterns.

   The follicular pattern is the most common and recognizable. It is composed of nests of epithelium that resemble the enamel organ of the developing teeth, dispersed in a mature fibrous connective tissue stroma. The core of the nests is composed of loosely arranged angular cells that resemble the stellate reticulum of the enamel organ. A single layer of tall columnar ameloblastlike cells surround the central core. The nuclei of these cells are placed away from the basement membrane (so-called reversed polarity) (e-**Fig. 4.10**). Cyst formation is common and may vary from microcysts forming within the follicles to large macroscopic cysts that may be several centimeters in diameter.

   The plexiform type of ameloblastoma consists of long anastomosing cords or large sheets of odontogenic epithelium bound by ameloblastic cells as seen in the follicular pattern, with similar stellate reticulumlike cores. Cyst formation is rare (e-**Fig. 4.11**).

   Unless removed in its entirety, ameloblastoma has a high recurrence rate. The tumor cells tend to infiltrate the surrounding marrow spaces, and the actual margin of the tumor often extends beyond its apparent radiographic or clinical margin. Marginal resection is therefore the most widely used treatment, but recurrence rates of up to 15% have still been reported. Many surgeons advocate that the margin of resection should be at least 1.0 cm past the radiographic limit of the tumor.

   2. **Calcifying epithelial odontogenic tumor** (Pindborg's tumor) is a rare tumor that presents as a slowly growing, painless, expansive lesion that favors the posterior mandible. The peak age of incidence is the 3rd to 7th decade, and the male-to-female ratio is equal. The radiographic appearance of the tumor changes over time. Early on, the tumor appears as a radiolucent lesion that can be

TABLE 4.2	WHO Histological Classification of Odontogenic Tumors*

BENIGN TUMORS
Odontogenic epithelium with mature fibrous stoma without odontogenic ectomesenchyme
Ameloblastoma, solid/multicystic type
Ameloblastoma, extraosseous/peripheral type
Ameloblastoma, desmoplastic type
Ameloblastoma, unicystic type
Squamous odontogenic tumor
Calcifying epithelial odontogenic tumor
Adenomatoid odontogenic tumor
Keratocystic odontogenic tumor

Odontogenic epithelium with odontogenic ectomesenchyme, with or without hard tissue formation
Ameloblastic fibroma
Ameloblastic fibrodentinoma
Ameloblastic fibro-odontoma
Odontoma
    Odontoma, complex type
    Odontoma, compound type
Odontoameloblastoma
Calcifying cystic odontogenic tumor
Dentinogenic ghost cell tumor

Mesenchyme and/or odontogenic ectomesenchyme with or without odontogenic epithelium
Odontogenic fibroma
Odontogenic myxoma/myxofibroma
Cementoblastoma

MALIGNANT TUMORS
Odontogenic carcinomas
Metastasizing (malignant) ameloblastoma
Ameloblastic carcinoma—primary type
Ameloblastic carcinoma—secondary type (dedifferentiated), intraosseous
Ameloblastic carcinoma—secondary type (dedifferentiated), peripheral
Primary intraosseous squamous cell carcinoma—solid type
Primary intraosseous squamous cell carcinoma derived from keratocystic odontogenic tumor
Primary intraosseous squamous cell carcinoma derived from odontogenic cysts
Clear cell odontogenic carcinoma
Ghost cell odontogenic carcinoma

Odontogenic sarcomas
Ameloblastic fibrosarcoma
Ameloblastic fibrodentino—and fibro-odontosarcoma

Modified from: Barnes L, Eveson J, Reichart P, Sidransky D, eds. *World Health Organization Classification of Tumours. Pathology and Genetics. Head and Neck Tumours.* Lyon: IARC Press; 2005. Used with permission.

mistaken for a cyst. As the lesion ages, it develops a poorly demarcated border and multiple radio-opaque foci. The lesion may be multilocular.

On microscopic examination, the tumor is characterized by clusters of pleomorphic polyhedral epithelial cells with a well-defined cell border and dense nuclear staining. The cells show mild-to-moderate nuclear pleomorphism and rare mitotic figures, and may contain multiple nuclei. Layered calcifications and amyloidlike globules are usually present (e-**Fig. 4.12**). Calcifying epithelial odontogenic tumors are generally treated surgically. Because the tumors tend to be infiltrating, treatment should include removal with a border of clinically and radiographically normal bone.

3. **Adenomatoid odontogenic tumors** (adenoameloblastomas) typically present as a slowly growing asymptomatic masses in the anterior portion of the maxilla or mandible in patients younger than 30 years. Women are affected twice as often as men. Radiographic examination demonstrates a radiolucent, well-defined lesion involving the crown of an unerupted or impacted tooth. Adjacent teeth may show root divergence without root resorption. Gross examination reveals a well-defined encapsulated mass of soft tissue with focal cystic and granular areas. Microscopic examination shows a well-defined fibrotic capsule surrounding a multinodular mass of eosinophilic spindle and polyhedral cells. Scattered among these cells are amphophilic globules with variable levels of calcification and lamination; these globules are periodic acid–Schiff positive and diastase resistant. In addition to the globules, small cystic spaces lined by a single layer of cuboidal to columnar cells with foamy cytoplasm and basally oriented nuclei are present (e-**Fig. 4.13**). Treatment is enucleation, and recurrence is extremely rare.

4. **Squamous odontogenic tumors** are benign lesions that present in patients over a wide age distribution. Patients generally present with tooth loosening in the absence of periodontal disease. Radiology demonstrates a radiolucent mass in the anterior maxilla or posterior mandible with tooth root involvement. Microscopic examination shows that the lesion is characterized by nodules of bland squamous cells with peripheral flattening of the basal cells, separated by a fibrous stroma (e-**Fig. 4.14**). Treatment is surgical excision with associated tooth removal.

5. **Malignant ameloblastoma and ameloblastic carcinoma.** Very rarely, ameloblastoma exhibits frank malignant behavior with development of metastasis. The frequency of such an event is difficult to determine but probably occurs in far less than 1% of all ameloblastomas.

   By definition, a tumor is malignant ameloblastoma when it shows histomorphologic features of a benign ameloblastoma, yet metastasizes. Metastasis, most often to the lungs, has been regarded as aspiration or implant metastasis. In such cases, the first evidence of metastasis is often discovered 1 to 30 years after surgical treatment of the primary lesion.

   The term ameloblastic carcinoma should be reserved for an ameloblastoma that has the cytologic features of malignancy in the primary tumor, in a recurrence, or in any metastatic deposit (e-**Fig. 4.15**). These lesions typically follow a markedly aggressive local course, but metastasis does not always occur.

B. **Mesenchymal odontogenic tumors**

1. **Odontogenic myxoma** is a benign tumor that has the potential for local infiltration, extensive bone destruction, and a relatively high recurrence rate. It is thought to be derived from the ectomesenchyme. Microscopically, it resembles the dental papilla of a developing tooth. Myxomas are most common in the 2nd and 3rd decade of life; although they occur in patients from 5 to 72 years old, they are uncommon in patients younger than 10 years or older than 50 years. Some studies show a female predilection. The lesion may be found at any location in the jaws, although some studies show a predominance of maxillary tumors.

   Myxomas vary in their radiographic appearance, from small and unilocular, to large and multilocular, with a 'soap bubble' appearance. Tooth displacement and cortical expansion are common in larger lesions. Maxillary tumors often extend into the maxillary sinus. Microscopic examination reveals a bland, monotonous, hypocellular proliferation of loose mesenchymal fibrous tissue. The cells are spindled or stellate, with long cytoplasmic processes. The nuclei are small and may be hyperchromatic. Mitoses are scarce. Small nests of odontogenic epithelium may be present but are not necessary for the diagnosis (e-**Fig. 4.16**).

   Because of their lack of encapsulation and infiltrative growth, myxomas tend to extend beyond their clinically anticipated boundaries. Recurrence rates as high as 25% are usually due to incomplete excision. Some recurrences occur years after excision.

2. **Benign cementoblastoma** (true cementoma) is a distinctive mesenchymal odontogenic tumor that is intimately associated with the roots of teeth. It is characterized by the formation of calcified cementumlike tissue deposited on the tooth root, most commonly mandibular molars. Although the tumor is detected in patients over a wide age range, it most commonly affects teenagers and young adults. Pain is a frequent symptom. The radiographic appearance of cementoblastoma is characteristic and is almost pathognomonic, namely, a radio-opaque mass that obliterates the radiographic details of the root of the affected tooth.

On microscopic examination, the peripheral part of the tumor resembles osteoblastoma. Central, thick trabeculae of cementum, which are strongly basophilic, are deposited on the intact or partially resorbed tooth root. Peripherally, bonelike trabeculae are rimmed with plump cementoblasts. The intervening fibrovascular tissue shows dilated vessels and occasional clusters of multinucleated osteoclastlike giant cells (e-**Fig. 4.17**).

Cementoblastoma is a slowly growing benign neoplasm, but it may attain a large size if not treated. The recommended treatment is surgical excision with extraction of the affected tooth. Recurrence is usually a result of incomplete removal.

3. **Cemento-ossifying fibroma** (COF) of the jaws is synonymous with ossifying fibroma and cementifying fibroma. It is a benign odontogenic neoplasm that is limited to the tooth-bearing areas of the jaws. COF is more often seen in the mandible (90%) and in women (83%). Most patients are in their 3rd to 4th decade, and present with a small, asymptomatic, expanding bone mass that does not erode the adjacent cortical bone. Larger lesions may present with facial deformation and pain. Radiographic examination demonstrates a well-circumscribed radiolucent lesion with patchy focal radio-opaque areas. Tooth displacement, resorption, and root divergence may be seen.

Microscopic examination shows a lesion characterized by a fibrous stroma with bone trabeculae and associated variable mineralized material that resembles dental cementum; either component may dominate in an individual lesion. The stroma is usually hypercellular; the bone trabeculae are usually woven, but lamellar bone may also be seen. Osteoblastic rimming may vary in extent (e-**Fig. 4.18**).

Most COFs are small tumors that can be shelled out or curetted out of the jaw bone with relative ease. Recurrence after adequate removal is seldom. Incompletely excised tumors continue to grow slowly, but may attain a large size.

C. **Mixed odontogenic tumors**

1. **Odontomas** represent the most highly differentiated of the mixed odontogenic tumors. They are considered by some pathologists to be hamartomas. Two types of odontomas are recognized: compound and complex. Compound odontoma is composed of many, sometimes even dozens of, small miniature teeth that are surrounded by a dental follicle, the same tissue that surrounds a normal developing tooth. This form of odontoma shows the highest degree histodifferentiation and morphodifferentiation (e-**Fig. 4.19**). In contrast, the complex odontoma is composed of a mass of intermixed enamel and dentine with no resemblance to normal or miniaturized teeth (e-**Fig. 4.20**).

The compound odontoma occurs most often in the anterior segment of the jaws, particularly the canine area in association with an impacted canine tooth. It is the most common odontogenic tumor. It is found most often in the 2nd decade of life and is more common in males than in females by a 3:2 ratio.

Complex odontomas occur most often in the posterior segment of the jaws, primarily in association with an impacted third molar tooth. They are the second most common odontogenic tumor and are usually discovered in the early 3rd decade of life. Like compound odontomas, there is a male gender predilection of 2:1.

Odontomas are typically discovered when radiographic examination is performed because of a delay in eruption of a tooth. They may be mostly radiolucent with areas of opacity, and may be associated with an odontogenic cyst (particularly dentigerous cyst) or with calcifying odontogenic cyst. They are treated by surgical excision.

2. **Ameloblastic fibroma** is a true neoplasm composed of both epithelial and mesenchymal types of tissues, but without calcified structures. The tumor is typically seen in adolescent patients. The average patient age is 14 years, and there is an equal male-to-female distribution. Patients usually present with a well-defined unilocular or multilocular lesion in the mandible (80%). Association with an unerupted tooth is common. Gross examination demonstrates a smooth, well-defined lesion with a tan-white cut surface. Microscopic examination demonstrates a lesion characterized by a background of immature connective tissue that resembles dental papilla with cords, strands, and nests of cuboidal to columnar epithelial cells. The epithelial nests are indistinguishable from those seen in follicular ameloblastoma, with a central stellate reticulumlike component and peripheral palisaded columnar cells showing reversed nuclear polarity. A prominent basement membrane separates the epithelial cells from the stroma (e-**Fig. 4.21**). Treatment is by enucleation and thorough curettage and, if necessary, extraction of the involved tooth. Recurrence is uncommon. Malignant transformation is extremely rare but has been documented.

3. **Ameloblastic fibrosarcoma and odontogenic carcinosarcoma.** Sarcomatous transformation of the mesenchymal component of ameloblastic fibroma, in association with benign epithelial elements, is designated ameloblastic fibrosarcoma. Tumors with both a sarcomatous and carcinomatous components are termed odontogenic carcinosarcoma.

   a. **Ameloblastic fibrosarcoma** typically presents as an expansive mandibular mass measuring 4 to 6 cm in maximum dimension in an adolescent or young adult. The tumor has a high propensity for recurrence if conservatively treated, and can occasionally metastasize. Death more frequently results from aggressive local growth.

      Microscopically, the architecture of ameloblastic fibrosarcoma resembles that of ameloblastic fibroma, albeit with a malignant connective tissue component. The epithelial cords and nests are widely separated by a hypercellular stroma. The fibroblast cells are round or fusiform and pleomorphic, with hyperchromatic nuclei and a high mitotic rate (e-**Fig. 4.22**). Ameloblastic fibrosarcoma can arise in an existing or recurrent ameloblastic fibroma. Multiple recurrences are usually associated with increasingly malignant cytologic features.

   b. **Odontogenic carcinosarcoma** is extremely rare. One case developed in a pre-existing ameloblastic fibroma in a 19-year-old pregnant woman, exhibited sudden growth, and was painful to palpation. The lesion was radiolucent and extended from the left body of the mandible into the ramus, reaching the condyle. Microscopically, areas of benign ameloblastic fibroma were associated with malignant epithelial and mesenchymal components. Interestingly, Ki67 labeling scores differed significantly between the two components of the tumor; the score of the carcinosarcoma score was much higher than that of the ameloblastic fibroma. The tumor was resected en bloc with no evidence of recurrence after 2 years of follow-up.

IV. **NONODONTOGENIC TUMORS.** The jaws, like other bones in the skeleton, can be a site of a wide variety of benign and malignant bone tumors. These entities are discussed in other parts of this manual. This chapter will mainly address tumors and tumorlike lesions that occur predominantly or exclusively in the jaws (Table 4.3).

   A. **Benign fibro-osseous lesions** are a group of lesions that share similar histomorphologic features although they have a differing clinical and radiographic presentation and behavior. Microscopically, fibro-osseous lesions are composed of fibrous connective tissue stroma containing mineralized structures that may be bone or cementum. Proper diagnosis requires correlation of history and clinical and radiographic findings. The more important types of fibro-osseous lesions of the jaws are discussed here.

      1. **Fibrous dysplasia** is a skeletal anomaly in which normal bone is replaced by poorly organized and inadequately mineralized, immature woven bone and

TABLE 4.3	Nonodontogenic Tumors

Benign Fibro-osseous Lesions
   Fibrous dysplasia
   Juvenile ossifying fibroma
      Trabecular
      Psammomatoid
   Cemento-osseous dysplasia
      Periapical
      Florid
Giant Cell Lesions
   Central (intra-osseous) giant cell granuloma
   Brown tumor of hyperparathyroidism
   Cherubism
   Aneurysmal bone cyst

fibrous connective tissue. Fibrous dysplasia is separated into two forms. The polyostotic form involves multiple bones, whereas the monostotic form is limited to a single site. Polyostotic fibrous dysplasia is less common, and a few of these cases may be associated with skin pigmentation and endocrine anomalies, a condition known as the McCune–Albright syndrome. The craniofacial skeleton, particularly the mandible and maxilla, is involved in 20%–25% of cases of monostotic fibrous dysplasia.

In craniofacial fibrous dysplasia, the condition is not strictly monostotic, but may extend by continuity to adjoining bones across suture lines. The maxilla is involved more often than the mandible. Most patients present in their 2nd to 3rd decade with a painless expanding bone mass. The mass does not involve the overlying bone cortex, and growth halts when the patient reaches skeletal maturity. The radiographic appearance can be variable, but the majority of patients present with a poorly defined lesion that is radiolucent when small, but becomes radio-opaque as it enlarges, often described as having a ground glass appearance. The lesion blends imperceptibly with the surrounding bone.

Microscopic examination demonstrates a bland fibrovascular stroma with numerous irregular trabeculae of woven bone merging to form complex shapes described as resembling Chinese letters. The bone trabeculae are not rimmed with osteoblasts, and lamellar bone is rarely identified (e-**Fig. 4.23**). Repair of the deformity is usually attempted after the cessation of growth with skeletal maturity. Radiation is contraindicated due to the elevated risk of radiation-induced sarcomas.

2. **Juvenile ossifying fibroma** (JOF), also known as juvenile active and juvenile aggressive ossifying fibroma, is used in the literature to describe two distinct clinicopathologic entities: trabecular JOF (TrJOF) and psammomatoid JOF (PsJOF).

   a. **TrJOF.** The great majority of the patients are children and adolescents with equal gender distribution. Clinically, the lesions are characterized by progressive and sometimes rapid expansion. The maxilla is more commonly affected than the mandible. Radiographically, the tumor is expansive and may be fairly well demarcated, with cortical thinning and perforation. Depending on the amount of calcification, the lesion may show varying degrees of radiodensity.

   Microscopically, TrJOF is composed of a cell-rich fibrous stroma containing bundles of cellular osteoid and bone trabeculae, without osteoblastic rimming. Aggregates of multinucleated giant cells are invariably present in the stroma (e-**Fig. 4.24**). Cystic degeneration and aneurysmal bone cyst formation may occur. The clinical course of TrJOF following conservative treatment is characterized by recurrence; eventual complete cure can be achieved by re-excision without resorting to radical surgery. Malignant transformation has not been reported.

b. PsJOF. Unlike TrJOF, PsJOF is a lesion that affects predominantly the extragnathic skull bones, particularly the periorbital bones. Occasional cases are encountered in the jaws, particularly the mandible. Affected patients tend to be older than those who have TrJOF. There is no sex predilection.

On radiographic examination, the tumor appears expansive with well-defined borders that may be corticated. Sclerotic changes within the lesion may impart a ground glass appearance. The tumors vary in size from 2 to 8 cm. Cystic changes are not uncommon and present as areas of low density in the CT scans.

Microscopically, the tumor is noteworthy for multiple, round, uniform, small ossicles that are basophilic and resemble psammoma bodies. The psammomatoid structures are embedded in relatively cellular stroma composed of stellate and spindle-shaped cells (e-Fig. **4.25**). Aneurysmal bone cyst formation is not uncommon. Surgical excision is the treatment of choice; multiple recurrences are not unusual. No malignant changes are observed.

3. Cemento-osseous dysplasia of the jaws is a nonneoplastic, presumably dysplastic, fibro-osseous lesion of the tooth-bearing areas of the jaws. Two types are recognized: periapical cemento-osseous dysplasia and florid cemento-osseous dysplasia.

a. Periapical cemento-osseous dysplasia, also known as periapical cementoma, is a relatively common condition, particularly in middle-aged black female patients. The anterior mandibular teeth are typically the site of this lesion. The condition is nonexpansive and asymptomatic, and is typically identified in routine dental radiographs as periapical radiolucencies, which become progressively mineralized in older lesions. Microscopic examination shows a poorly demarcated lesion consisting of fibrovascular stroma with trabeculae of bone and smooth globular masses of cementumlike material (e-Fig. **4.26**) The bone and cementum may merge with adjacent bone, but will not involve adjacent teeth. No treatment is required. It is of importance to distinguish the lesion from the periapical inflammatory disease.

b. Florid cemento-osseous dysplasia is uncommon. It usually presents in middle-aged or older black women, is usually asymptomatic, and may be incidentally discovered on routine radiographic examination. Radiographically, it is characterized by extensive sclerotic areas often involving the posterior quadrants of the mandible and maxilla bilaterally in the tooth-bearing areas, usually symmetrically (e-Fig. **4.27**). Microscopically, florid cemento-osseous dysplasia is analogous to periapical cemento-osseous dysplasia, although the former also shows large sclerotic masses that are hypocellular and extremely dense, and have small marrow spaces and Haversian systems. It is of importance to recognize the clinical radiographic features of the lesion so that the patient is not subject to surgical intervention. In fact, surgery is contraindicated because it may result in local infection, pain, and a complicated clinical course.

B. Giant cell lesions of the jaws. Giant cell lesions of the jaws are heterogeneous clinical entities that share similar microscopic features.

1. Central giant cell granuloma, or intra-osseous granuloma of the jaws, is also known as giant cell reparative granuloma. It is a localized osteolytic lesion of the mandible (66% of cases) and maxilla (33%). The majority of patients are younger than 30 years, and women outnumber men by a ratio of 2:1.

Giant cell granulomas are typically nonaggressive and present on routine dental radiographs as small, radiolucent, expansive masses that do not erode into the cortex. The majority occur in the anterior mandible, commonly crossing the midline. Microscopically, the lesions are unencapsulated and are composed of focal or evenly dispersed aggregates of multinucleated osteoclastlike giant cells in a richly vascular stroma with little collagen deposition (e-Fig. **4.28**). Two types of mononuclear stromal cells are identified: spindle-shaped fibroblastic cells and polygonal macrophagelike cells. Areas of ossification and hemosiderin granules may be present.

A rare aggressive variant characterized by pain, rapid growth, and cortical perforation with a marked tendency for recurrence may be an example of "true" giant cell tumor of bone. The lesion may show increased mitotic activity and evenly distributed larger giant cells that have an increased number of nuclei.

Central giant cell granuloma of the jaws is usually treated by curettage. Recurrent lesions often respond to further conservative surgery. A number of alternative nonsurgical approaches have been used in recent years, including intralesional corticosteroid injections, subcutaneous calcitonin injections, and interferon-a therapy.

2. **Brown tumor of hyperparathyroidism.** Brown tumor is an osseous lesion that develops in bones affected by primary or secondary hyperparathyroidism. It is currently less frequently encountered because the diagnosis of hyperparathyroidism is now often made on the basis of elevated serum calcium levels in asymptomatic adults.

   The lesions may be solitary or multifocal, and the mandible is a common site of involvement. Radiographically, Brown tumors are well-defined lytic lesions that are microscopically identical to central giant cell granuloma. Treatment is aimed at correction of the hyperparathyroid state; complete resolution usually occurs within 6 months after removal of a parathyroid adenoma.

3. **Cherubism** is a rare dominant genetic disease with complete male penetrance and a 50–70% penetrance in women. It typically presents in children 1 to 5 years old as painless bilateral symmetric jaw expansion that slowly increases in size until puberty; at puberty, the lesion undergoes variable regression. The lesions may be unilocular or multilocular with a 'soap bubble' appearance on radiographic examination.

   Microscopically, the lesions are essentially similar to those of central giant cell granuloma. However, the giant cells in cherubism tend to be less numerous and are placed in a less cellular stroma. The pathologic process in cherubism is self-limited, and treatment is dictated by cosmetic and functional needs. Curettage and contouring of bone are the treatments of choice.

Suggested Readings

Delair D, Bejarano P, Peleg M, El-Mofty SK. Ameloblastic carcinosarcoma arising in ameloblastic fibroma: a case report and review of literature. *Oral Surg Oral Med Oral Pathol Oral Radiol Endod.* 2007;103:516–520.

El-Mofty SK. Cemento-ossifying fibroma and benign cementoblastoma. *Semin Diag Pathol.* 1999;16:302–307.

El-Mofty SK. Psammomatoid and trabecular juvenile ossifying fibroma of the craniofacial skeleton: two distinct clinicopathologic entities. *Oral Surg Oral Med Oral Pathol Oral Radiol Endod.* 2002;93:269–304.

El-Mofty SK, Kyriakos M. Soft tissue and bone lesions. In: Gnepp DR, ed. *Diagnostic Surgical Pathology of the Head and Neck.* Philadelphia: WB Saunders; 2001:505–604.

Nevill BW, Damm DD, Allen CM, Bouquot JE, eds. Odontogenic cysts and tumors. In: *Oral and Maxillofacial Pathology*, 2nd ed. Philadelphia: WB Saunders; 2002:589–642.

Philipsen HP, Reichart PA, Slootweg PJ, Slater LJ. Odontogenic tumors. In: Barnes L, Eveson JW, Reichart P, Sidransky D, eds. *Pathology and Genetics of Head and Neck Tumours.* Lyon, France: IARC Press; 2005.

Slootweg PJ, El-Mofty SK. Ossifying fibroma. In: Barnes L, Eveson JW, Reichart P, Sidransky D, eds. *Pathology and Genetics of Head and Neck Tumours.* Lyon, France: IARC Press; 2005.

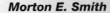

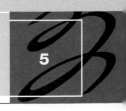

THE EYE
Morton E. Smith

5

I. DISEASES OF THE CONJUNCTIVA

A. Two benign conditions on the conjunctiva are the pterygium and the pingeculum. Histopathologic sections show only chronic inflammation, congested vessels, and elastotic (actinic) degeneration.

B. Neoplasms of the conjunctiva fall into one of three categories: squamous (surface epithelium), melanocytic, or lymphoid.

    1. Neoplasms arising from the surface epithelium range from benign papillomas (e-**Fig. 5.1**),* to CIN (conjunctival intraepithelial neoplasia) (e-**Fig. 5.2**), to invasive squamous cell carcinoma. The staging scheme for conjunctival carcinomas is given in Table 5.1.

    2. Melanocytic lesions of the conjunctiva range from nevi, to primary acquired melanosis (PAM) to melanoma (e-**Fig. 5.3**). Primary acquired melanosis itself is further divided into atypia, melanoma in situ, and melanoma arising from PAM. The staging scheme for melanomas of the conjunctiva is given in Table 5.2.

    3. Lymphomas of the conjunctiva can range from primary localized low-grade lymphomas, to high-grade lymphomas associated with systemic disease.

II. DISEASES OF THE CORNEA.
The host tissue from a corneal transplant procedure is traditionally referred to as the corneal "button," and the surgical procedure itself is often referred to as a penetrating keratoplasty (PKP). In the gross room, corneal buttons are merely bisected and each half is embedded with the cut side down. The most common reasons for a PKP to be performed are Fuchs dystrophy, pseudophakic bullous keratopathy, keratoconus, and graft failure.

A. Fuchs dystrophy is an aging process usually occurring in women older than 60 years. The corneal endothelial cells diminish in number and function, leading to chronic edema of the cornea. If conservative therapy is unsuccessful, PKP is necessary. Histopathologically, Fuchs dystrophy consists of loss of the endothelial cells, thickening of Descemet's membrane, and the presence of excrescences along Descemet's membrane (known as guttae). Often epithelial bullae (or blebs) are seen (e-**Fig. 5.4**).

B. Pseudophakic bullous keratopathy is the term used when endothelial cell decompensation follows cataract extraction (usually months later) with intraocular lens implantation. Histopathologically, endothelial cell loss is seen, but there are no guttae.

C. Keratoconus shows central thinning, stromal fibrosis, and breaks in Bowman's layer (e-**Fig. 5.5**). When a PKP fails (for example, due to immunologic rejection or a leaking wound), a regraft may be necessary. Peripheral scars are the key features on the "button" from the second procedure (e-**Fig. 5.6**). Often there is a retrocorneal membrane.

D. Ulcerative keratitis may or may not reveal the offending microorganism when special stains are performed (e.g., Gram for bacteria; Gomori's Methenamine Silver [GMS] and periodic acid-Schiff [PAS] for fungi; GMS and PAS for *Acanthamoeba*). Herpes simplex keratitis has a characteristic histopathologic appearance including loss of Bowman's layer, stromal fibrosis and vascularization, interstitial keratitis (consisting

---

*All e-figures are available online via the Solution Site Image Bank.

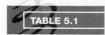

TABLE 5.1	Carcinoma of the Conjunctiva

Definition of TNM. These definitions apply to both clinical and pathologic staging.

PRIMARY TUMOR (T)

TX	Primary tumor cannot be assessed
T0	No evidence of primary tumor
Tis	Carcinoma in situ
T1	Tumor ≤5 mm in greatest dimension
T2	Tumor >5 mm in greatest dimension, without invasion of adjacent structures
T3	Tumor invades adjacent structures, excluding the orbit
T4	Tumor invades orbit with or without further extension
T4a	Tumor invades orbital soft tissues, without bone invasion
T4b	Tumor invades bone
T4c	Tumor invades adjacent paranasal sinuses
T4d	Tumor invades brain

REGIONAL LYMPH NODES (N)

NX	Regional lymph nodes cannot be assessed
N0	No regional lymph node metastasis
N1	Regional lymph node metastasis

DISTANT METASTASIS (M)

MX	Distant metastasis cannot be assessed
M0	No distant metastasis
M1	Distant metastasis

STAGE GROUPING
No stage grouping is presently recommended.

From: Greene FL, Page DL, Fleming ID, Fritz AG, Balch CM, Haller DG, Morrow M, eds. AJCC Cancer Staging Manual. 6th edition. New York: Springer, 2002. Used with permission. (A new AJCC TNM staging system is scheduled for release in 2009; after its publication, the new staging scheme will appear on the website for this book.)

of plasma cells and lymphocytes in the corneal stroma), and often granulomatous inflammation near Descemet's membrane (e-**Fig. 5.7**).

    E. Other rare entities for which a PKP is performed include hereditary stromal dystrophic diseases, for example, macular dystrophy (due to acid mucopolysaccharide abnormalities), granular dystrophy (due to hyaline degeneration), and lattice dystrophy (due to amyloid).

III. VASCULAR AND INFECTIOUS DISEASES AND TRAUMA. Eyes are often enucleated because they are "blind and painful." The reasons for an eye becoming blind and painful are numerous, but usually it is because of the development of secondary glaucoma. The antecedent event can range from previous accidental trauma or previous surgical trauma to specific disease entities such as retinal vascular disease (including diabetes or central retinal artery or vein occlusion), chronic inflammatory disease, or chronic retinal detachment.

    A. Secondary glaucoma. The key histopathologic finding in most cases of secondary glaucoma is a closed angle by peripheral anterior synechia. The term "closed angle" merely means that the anatomical angle formed by the cornea and iris, and occupied by the trabecular meshwork (the main outflow channel for aqueous humor), is occluded. The occlusion is caused by an adhesion of the iris against the trabecular meshwork (e-**Fig. 5.8**). Occasionally, in contrast to the closed angle appearance, there is a postcontusion angle recession. The retina in glaucoma exhibits atrophy of the nerve fiber layer and loss of ganglion cells; the optic nerve shows cupping of the disc (e-**Fig. 5.9**) and atrophy of the nerve.

    B. Retinal vascular diseases. The occluded angle may be due to neovascularization of the iris (e-**Fig. 5.10**). The two most common causes of neovascularization of the iris are diabetes and central retinal vascular occlusion (of the artery or vein).

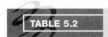

TABLE 5.2	Malignant Melanoma of the Conjunctiva

Definition of TNM

Clinical
PRIMARY TUMOR (T)

TX	Primary tumor cannot be assessed
T0	No evidence of primary tumor
T1	Tumor of the bulbar conjunctiva
T2	Tumor of the bulbar conjunctiva with corneal extension
T3	Tumor extending into the conjunctival fornix, palpebral conjunctiva, or caruncle
T4	Tumor invades the eyelid, globe, orbit, sinuses, or central nervous system

REGIONAL LYMPH NODES (N)

NX	Regional lymph nodes cannot be assessed
N0	No regional lymph node metastasis
N1	Regional lymph node metastasis

DISTANT METASTASIS (M)

MX	Distant metastasis cannot be assessed
M0	No distant metastasis
M1	Distant metastasis

Pathologic
PRIMARY TUMOR (T)

pTX	Primary tumor cannot be assessed
pT0	No evidence of primary tumor
pT1	Tumor of the bulbar conjunctiva confined to the epithelium
pT2	Tumor of the bulbar conjunctiva not >0.8 mm in thickness with invasion of the substantia propria
pT3	Tumor of the bulbar conjunctiva >0.8 mm in thickness with invasion of the substantia propria or tumors involving the palpebral or caruncular conjunctiva
pT4	Tumor invades the eyelid, globe, orbit, sinuses, or central nervous system

REGIONAL LYMPH NODES (N)

pNX	Regional lymph nodes cannot be assessed
pN0	No regional lymph node metastasis
pN1	Regional lymph node metastasis present

DISTANT METASTASIS (M)

pMX	Distant metastasis cannot be assessed
pM0	No distant metastasis
pM1	Distant metastasis

STAGE GROUPING
No stage grouping is presently recommended.

From: Greene FL, Page DL, Fleming ID, Fritz AG, Balch CM, Haller DG, Morrow M, eds. AJCC Cancer Staging Manual. 6th edition. New York: Springer, 2002. Used with permission. (A new AJCC TNM staging system is scheduled for release in 2009; after its publication, the new staging scheme will appear on the website for this book.)

Microscopic examination of the retina reveals the key features of diabetes: lipoproteinaceous exudates, intraretinal hemorrhages, neovascularization of the inner surface of the retina (proliferative diabetic retinopathy) (**e-Fig. 5.11**), and often hemorrhage into the vitreous. In cases of old central retinal vein or artery occlusion, the retina exhibits atrophy and cystoid degeneration of the inner two-thirds of the retina, lipoproteinaceous exudates, and often a persistence of hemorrhage due to venous occlusion.

C. Intraocular inflammation and infection. Severe inflammatory disease that can lead to a blind and painful eye includes diffuse uveitis of unknown etiology, diffuse granulomatous uveitis secondary to sympathetic ophthalmia (e-**Fig. 5.12**), sarcoidosis, toxoplasmosis, and necrotizing retinitis (often seen with cytomegalovirus [CMV] retinitis and Herpes retinitis).

D. Trauma. Many eyes are enucleated because of severe trauma. If there is no attempt by the ophthalmologist to repair a ruptured globe, the pathology specimen usually consists of a ruptured globe with massive intraocular hemorrhage (e-**Fig. 5.13**). Often there is loss of intraocular contents such as the lens or a portion of the retina. If an attempt has been made by the surgeon to salvage the ruptured globe and the eye is then enucleated days or weeks after the repair, the histopathologic description may be the same as described above (i.e., massive intraocular hemorrhage) or may show additional findings such as endophthalmitis (vitreous abscess).

E. Phthisis bulbi. When an eye undergoes a slow chronic degenerative process from such insults as a previous trauma, complications of surgery, chronic inflammation, or chronic retinal detachment, the eye becomes phthisical. Clinically, the eye has hypotony (very low intraocular pressure) and starts to shrink. The histopathologic appearance of such eyes is that of diffuse degeneration, atrophy, and architectural distortion of all layers of the eye. Often there is diffuse ossification (e-**Fig. 5.14**).

IV. INTRAOCULAR NEOPLASMS

A. Gross room processing of enucleated globes follows a standard protocol as shown in Figure 5.1. Larger cassettes are required for processing.

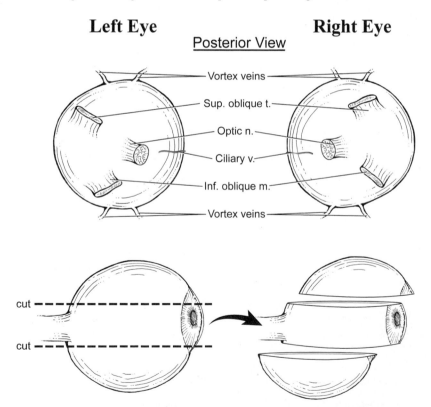

Figure 5.1. The globe is identified as to right eye or left eye using anatomic landmarks (*upper panel*). Two cuts (traditionally referred to as the p.o. sections) are then made in a transverse plane, passing in relation to the pupil and optic nerve as shown (*lower panel*). The superior cap (also known as the superior calotte) and inferior cap are usually not processed unless abnormalities are seen.

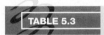

TABLE 5.3   Malignant Melanoma of the Uvea

Definition of TNM. These definitions apply to both clinical* and pathologic staging.

PRIMARY TUMOR (T)

All Uveal Melanomas

TX	Primary tumor cannot be assessed
T0	No evidence of primary tumor

Iris

T1	Tumor limited to the iris
T1a	Tumor limited to the iris not >3 clock hours in size
T1b	Tumor limited to the iris >3 clock hours in size
T1c	Tumor limited to the iris with melanomalytic glaucoma
T2	Tumor confluent with or extending into the ciliary body and/or choroid
T2a	Tumor confluent with or extending into the ciliary body and/or choroid with melanomalytic glaucoma
T3	Tumor confluent with or extending into the ciliary body and/or choroid with scleral extension
T3a	Tumor confluent with or extending into the ciliary body with scleral extension and melanomalytic glaucoma
T4	Tumor with extraocular extension

Ciliary Body and Choroid

T1*	Tumor ≤10 mm in greatest diameter and ≤2.5 mm in greatest height (thickness)
T1a	Tumor ≤10 mm in greatest diameter and ≤2.5 mm in greatest height (thickness) without microscopic extraocular extension
T1b	Tumor ≤10 mm in greatest diameter and ≤2.5 mm in greatest height (thickness) with microscopic extraocular extension
T1c	Tumor <10 mm in greatest diameter and ≤2.5 mm in greatest height (thickness) with macroscopic extraocular extension
T2*	Tumor 10–16 mm in greatest basal diameter and between 2.5 and 10 mm in maximum height (thickness)
T2a	Tumor 10–16 mm in greatest basal diameter and between 2.5 and 10 mm in maximum height (thickness) without microscopic extraocular extension
T2b	Tumor 10–16 mm in greatest basal diameter and between 2.5 and 10 mm in maximum height (thickness) with microscopic extraocular extension
T2c	Tumor 10–16 mm in greatest basal diameter and between 2.5 and 10 mm in maximum height (thickness) with macroscopic extraocular extension
T3*	Tumor >16 mm in greatest basal diameter and/or >10 mm in maximum height (thickness) with extraocular extension
T4	Tumor >16 mm in greatest diameter and/or >10 mm in maximum height (thickness) with extraocular extension

REGIONAL LYMPH NODES (N)

NX	Regional lymph nodes cannot be assessed
N0	No regional lymph node metastasis
N1	Regional lymph node metastasis

DISTANT METASTASIS (M)

MX	Distant metastasis cannot be assessed
M0	No distant metastasis
M1	Distant metastasis

Histopathologic Type. The histopathologic types are:
Spindle cell melanoma
Mixed cell melanoma
Epithelioid cell melanoma
Histopathologic Grade (G)

GX	Grade cannot be assessed

(Continued)

TABLE 5.3	(Continued)

STAGING GROUPING

Stage 1	T1	N0	M0
	T1a	N0	M0
	T1b	N0	M0
	T1c	N0	M0
Stage II	T2	N0	M0
	T2a	N0	M0
	T2b	N0	M0
	T2c	N0	M0
Stage III	T3	N0	M0
	T4	N0	M0
Stage IV	Any T	N1	M0
	Any T	any N	M1
GI	Spindle cell melanoma		
G2	Mixed cell melanoma		
G3	Epithelioid cell melanoma		

Note: When basal dimension and apical height do not fit this classification, the largest tumor diameter should be used for classification. In clinical practice, the tumor base may be estimated in optic disc diameters (dd) (average: 1 dd = 1.5 mm). The height may be estimated in diopters (average: 3 diopters = 1 mm). Techniques such as ultrasonography, visualization, and photography are frequently used to provide more accurate measurements.

From: Greene FL, Page DL, Fleming ID, Fritz AG, Balch CM, Haller DG, Morrow M, eds. AJCC Cancer Staging Manual. 6th edition. New York: Springer, 2002. Used with permission. (A new AJCC TNM staging system is scheduled for release in 2009; after its publication, the new staging scheme will appear on the website for this book.)

B. The most common primary intraocular neoplasm is melanoma of the uvea (iris, ciliary body, and choroid). Melanomas usually occur in light complexion adults, and melanomas of the iris have a better prognosis than do melanomas of the ciliary body and/or choroid. Although many intraocular melanomas can be treated by excision or brachytherapy, many patients do not seek medical attention until the melanoma has become so large that the only course of management is enucleation of the globe. The staging scheme for melanoma of the uvea is given in Table 5.3.

Primary intraocular melanoma usually arises from the ciliary body or choroid as an ellipse or "almond shape" (e-Figs. 5.15 and 5.16), which eventually breaks through Bruch's membrane and becomes mushroom shaped (e-Fig. 5.17). Microscopically, intraocular melanomas are composed of cells ranging from spindle to epithelioid, with the latter having a worse prognosis (e-Figs. 5.18 and 5.19). Other histopathologic features that predict prognosis are size (e-Fig. 5.20); extrascleral extension (e-Fig. 5–20); location (those arising from the iris have best prognosis, from the ciliary body [e-Fig. 5.21] and peripapillary have a poorer prognosis), necrosis; mitotic figures; and a spiral vascular pattern.

C. Retinoblastoma is the most common ocular neoplasm in children. The usual age for clinical presentation in nonfamilial cases is 1 year, and the usual clinical appearance is leukocoria. Histopathologically, retinoblastoma arises from the retina and is composed of small blue cells intermingled with anastomosing pools of pink necrosis, giving rise to the traditional description of "islands of blue tumor in a sea of pink necrosis" (e-Figs. 5.22 and 5.23). Scattered flecks of purple calcium are often seen. Cytologically, the tumor is composed of cells with hyperchromatic, oval-shaped blue nuclei with scant cytoplasm, densely packed together. There are many apoptotic bodies and numerous mitotic figures (e-Fig. 5.22). More differentiated retinoblastomas often exhibit Flexner–Wintersteiner rosettes (e-Fig. 5.24). Extension into the optic nerve, and especially presence of tumor at the surgical margin of the nerve, predicts a poor prognosis (e-Fig. 5.25). The staging scheme for retinoblastoma is given in Table 5.4.

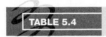

TABLE 5.4	Retinoblastoma

Definition of TNM

Clinical classification (cTNM)
PRIMARY TUMOR (T)

TX	Primary tumor cannot be assessed
T0	No evidence of primary tumor
T1	Tumor confined to the retina (no vitreous seeding or significant retinal detachment); no retinal detachment or subretinal fluid >5 mm from the base of the tumor
T1a	Any eye in which the largest tumor is ≤3 mm in height and no tumor; Is located closer than 1 disc diameter (dd) (1.5 mm) to the optic nerve or fovea
T1b	All other eyes in which the tumor(s) are confined to the retina regardless of location or size (up to half the volume of the eye). No vitreous seeding. No retinal detachment or subretinal fluid >5 mm from the base of the tumor
T2	Tumor with contiguous spread to adjacent tissues or spaces (vitreous or subretinal space)
T2a	Miminal tumor spread to vitreous and/or subretinal space. Fine local or diffuse vitreous seeding and/or serous retinal detachment up to total detachment may be present, but no clumps, lumps, snowballs, or avascular masses are allowed. The tumor may fill up to 2/3 the volume of the eye.
T2b	*Maximal tumor spread to the vitreous and/or subretinal space.* Vitreous seeding and/or subretinal implantation may consist of lumps, clumps, snowballs, or avascular tumor masses. Retinal detachment may be total. Tumor may fill up to 2/3 the volume of the eye
T2c	Unsalvageable intraocular disease. Tumor fills >2/3 the eye or there is no possibility of visual rehabilitation or one or more of the following are present:
	■ Tumor-associated glaucoma, either neovascular or angle closure
	■ Anterior segment extension of tumor
	■ Hyphema (significant)
	■ Massive vitreous hemorrhage
	■ Tumor in contact with lens
	■ Orbital cellulitislike clinical presentation (massive tumor necrosis)
T3	Invasion of the optic nerve and/or optic coats
T4	Extraocular tumor

REGIONAL LYMPH NODES (N)

NX	Regional lymph nodes cannot be assessed
N0	No regional lymph node involvement
N1	Regional lymph node involvement (preauricular, submandibular, or cervical)
N2	Distant lymph node involvement

DISTANT METASTASIS (M)

MX	Distant metastasis cannot be assessed
M0	No distant metastasis
M1	Metastasis to central nervous system and/or bone, bone marrow, or other sites

Pathologic classification (pTNM)
PRIMARY TUMOR (pT)

pTX	Primary tumor cannot be assessed
pT0	No evidence of primary tumor
pT1	Tumor confined to the retina, vitreous, or subretinal space. No optic nerve or choroidal invasion
PT2	Minimal invasion of the optic nerve and/or optic coats
pT2a	Tumor invades optic nerve up to, but not through, the level of the lamina cribrosa
pT2b	Tumor invades choroid focally

(Continued)

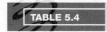

TABLE 5.4	**(Continued)**
pT2c	Tumor invades optic nerve to, but not through, the level of the lamina cribrosa and invades the choroid focally
pT3	Significant invasion of the optic nerve and/or optic coats
pT3a	Tumor invades optic nerve through the level of the lamina cribrosa but not to the line of resection
pT3b	Tumor massively invades the choroid
pT3c	Tumor invades the optic nerve through the level of the lamina cribrosa but not to the line of resection and massively invades the choroid
pT4	Extraocular tumor extension that includes:
	Invasion of optic nerve to the line of resection
	Invasion of orbit through the sclera
	Extension both anteriorly or posteriorly into the orbit
	Extension into the brain
	Extension into the subarachnoid space of the optic nerve
	Extension to the apex of the orbit
	Extension to, but not through, the chiasm
	Extension into the brain beyond the chiasm
Regional lymph nodes (pN)	
pNX	Regional lymph nodes cannot be assessed
pN0	No regional lymph node involvement
pN1	Regional lymph node metastasis
Distant metastasis (pM)	
pMX	Distant metastasis cannot be assessed
pM0	No distant metastasis
pM1	Distant metastasis
pM1a	Bone marrow
pM1b	Other sites

STAGE GROUPING
No stage grouping is presently recommended.

From: Greene FL, Page DL, Fleming ID, Fritz AG, Balch CM, Haller DG, Morrow M, eds. AJCC Cancer Staging Manual. 6th edition. New York: Springer, 2002. Used with permission. (A new AJCC TNM staging system is scheduled for release in 2009; after its publication, the new staging scheme will appear on the website for this book.)

V. DISEASES OF THE LACRIMAL GLAND AND LACRIMAL SAC

A. Lacrimal gland lesions are similar to lesions of the parotid gland. Infiltrative lesions include dacryoadenitis, sarcoidosis, benign lymphoid hyperplasia, and lymphoma. Intrinsic lesions of the lacrimal gland include pleomorphic adenoma, adenoid cystic carcinoma, and mucoepidermoid carcinoma. The staging scheme for lacrimal gland carcinoma is given in Table 5.5.

B. Lacrimal sac dacryolithiasis often contains *Actinomyces* organisms. Tumors of the lacrimal sac include papillomas, transitional cell carcinoma, and other rare entities such as plasmacytoma or lymphoma.

VI. DISEASES OF THE ORBIT.
Common lesions in the orbit include lymphoma, cavernous hemangioma in young adults, capillary (juvenile) hemangioma in children, idiopathic orbital inflammation (also known as inflammatory pseudotumor), schwannoma, infectious abscesses, dermoid cysts, and lymphangiomas. Less common lesions include rhabdomyosarcoma, granular cell tumor, optic nerve glioma, optic nerve sheath meningioma, alveolar soft part sarcoma, fibrous histiocytoma, melanoma, plasmacytoma, and metastatic carcinoma.

The morphologic features of all these lesions are the same as when they occur in other soft tissue sites. The staging scheme for sarcomas of the orbit is given in Table 5.6.

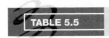

| TABLE 5.5 | Carcinoma of the Lacrimal Gland |

Definition of TNM
PRIMARY TUMOR (T)

TX	Primary tumor cannot be assessed
T0	No evidence of primary tumor
T1	Tumor ≤2.5 cm in greatest dimension, limited to the lacrimal gland
T2	Tumor >2.5 cm but not >5 cm in greatest dimension, limited to the lacrimal gland
T3	Tumor invades the periosteum
T3a	Tumor not >5 cm invades the periosteum of the lacrimal gland fossa
T3b	Tumor >5 cm in greatest dimension with periosteal invasion
T4	Tumor invades the orbital soft tissues, optic nerve, or globe with or without bone invasion; tumor extends beyond the orbit to adjacent structures, including brain

REGIONAL LYMPH NODES (N)

NX	Regional lymph nodes cannot be assessed
N0	No regional lymph node metastasis
N1	Regional lymph node metastasis

DISTANT METASTASIS (M)

MX	Distant metastasis cannot be assessed
M0	No distant metastasis
M1	Distant metastasis

STAGE GROUPING
No stage grouping is presently recommended.

From: Greene FL, Page DL, Fleming ID, Fritz AG, Balch CM, Haller DG, Morrow M, eds. AJCC Cancer Staging Manual. 6th edition. New York: Springer, 2002. Used with permission. (A new AJCC TNM staging system is scheduled for release in 2009; after its publication, the new staging scheme will appear on the website for this book.)

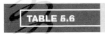

| TABLE 5.6 | Sarcoma of the Orbit |

Definition of TNM
PRIMARY TUMOR (T)

TX	Primary tumor cannot be assessed
T0	No evidence of primary tumor
T1	Tumor ≤15 mm in greatest dimension
T2	Tumor >15 mm in greatest dimension without invasion of globe or bony wall
T3	Tumor of any size with invasion of orbital tissues and/or bony walls
T4	Tumor invasion of globe or periorbital structure, such as eyelids, temporal fossa, nasal cavity and paranasal sinuses, and/or central nervous system

REGIONAL LYMPH NODES (N)

NX	Regional lymph nodes cannot be assessed
N0	No regional lymph node metastasis
N1	Regional lymph node metastasis

DISTANT METASTASIS (M)

MX	Distant metastasis cannot be assessed
M0	No distant metastasis
M1	Distant metastasis

STAGE GROUPING
No stage grouping is presently recommended.

From: Greene FL, Page DL, Fleming ID, Fritz AG, Balch CM, Haller DG, Morrow M, eds. AJCC Cancer Staging Manual. 6th edition. New York: Springer, 2002. Used with permission. (A new AJCC TNM staging system is scheduled for release in 2009; after its publication, the new staging scheme will appear on the website for this book.)

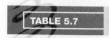

TABLE 5.7	Carcinoma of the Eyelid

Definition of TNM

PRIMARY TUMOR (T)

TX	Primary tumor cannot be assessed
T0	No evidence of primary tumor
Tis	Carcinoma in situ
T1	Tumor of any size, not invading the tarsal plate or, at the eyelid margin, ≤5 mm in greatest dimension
T2	Tumor invades tarsal plate or, at the eyelid margin, >5 mm but not >10 mm in greatest dimension
T3	Tumor involves full eyelid thickness or, at the eyelid margin, >10 mm in greatest dimension
T4	Tumor invades adjacent structures, which include bulbar conjunctiva, sclera and globe, soft tissues of the orbit, perineural space, bone and periosteum of the orbit, nasal cavity and paranasal sinuses, and central nervous system

REGIONAL LYMPH NODES (N)

NX	Regional lymph nodes cannot be assessed
N0	No regional lymph node metastasis
N1	Regional lymph node metastasis

DISTANT METASTASIS (M)

MX	Distant metastasis cannot be assessed
M0	No distant metastasis
M1	Distant metastasis

STAGE GROUPING
No stage grouping is presently recommended.

From: Greene FL, Page DL, Fleming ID, Fritz AG, Balch CM, Haller DG, Morrow M, eds. AJCC Cancer Staging Manual. 6th edition. New York: Springer, 2002. Used with permission. (A new AJCC TNM staging system is scheduled for release in 2009; after its publication, the new staging scheme will appear on the website for this book.)

VII. DISEASES OF THE EYELID. The common benign and malignant lesions of the eyelid are identical to those that occur at other cutaneous sites (see Chapters 38 and 39). The staging scheme for carcinoma of the eyelid is given in Table 5.7.

Suggested Readings

Eagle R. *Eye Pathology, an Atlas and Basic Text*. Philadelphia: W. B. Saunders; 1999.

Sassani J, ed. *Ophthalmic Pathology with Clinical Correlations*. Philadelphia: Lippincott-Raven; 1997.

Smith ME. Chapter 23. Pathology. In: Krachmer JH, ed. *The Requisites in Ophthalmology*. St. Louis, MO: Mosby; 2002.

Yanoff M, Fine B. *Ocular Pathology*, 5th ed. St. Louis, MO: Elsevier/Mosby; 2002.

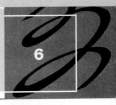

SALIVARY GLANDS

James S. Lewis Jr. and Elise L. Krejci

6

I. NORMAL ANATOMY

A. Macroscopic/gross. Salivary glands are exocrine organs that secrete components of saliva that both break down carbohydrates and lubricate the passage of food. There are three major paired salivary glands: the parotid, the submandibular, and the sublingual. There are also numerous minor salivary glands located in the submucosa of the entire upper aerodigestive tract, from the lips and nasal cavity to the major bronchi.

The paired parotid glands are each composed of a superficial lobe and a deeper smaller lobe; the facial nerve runs between the two lobes and is intimately associated with them. Each parotid gland normally contains an average of 20 intraglandular lymph nodes. The parotid glands secrete serous fluid, which passes through Stensen's duct to empty into the oral cavity near the second maxillary molar.

The submandibular glands (also referred to as the submaxillary glands) secrete a mixture of serous and mucous fluid. This fluid drains through Wharton's duct to empty at the floor of the mouth.

The sublingual glands secrete a mixture of serous and mucous fluid that travels through many small ducts, some of which empty into the floor of the mouth directly, and some of which coalesce into a larger (Bartholin's) duct to empty into Wharton's duct and then into the mouth.

B. Microscopic. The major salivary glands are enclosed by a connective tissue capsule and divided into lobules composed of ducts and acini; the minor salivary glands are unencapsulated. The acini are lined by epithelial cells (either serous or mucinous) surrounded by myoepithelial cells, the latter of which are specialized contractile (and possibly regenerative) cells that lie between the acinar cells and the basement membrane and contract to aid in the movement of glandular secretions. Myoepithelial cells are inconspicuous in normal salivary gland sections.

A single acinus may be composed of a mixture of serous and mucous cells. Serous cells are pyramidal in shape and contain periodic acid-Schiff (PAS)-positive granules within their cytoplasm. Mucous cells are rounder with basally oriented nuclei. The parotid gland is almost exclusively serous, the sublingual gland almost exclusively mucinous, and the submandibular gland is mixed serous and mucinous (e-**Figs. 6.1 to 6.3**).* The acini secrete fluid into the intercalated ducts, which are lined by a low simple cuboidal epithelium. Intercalated ducts are also the source of reserve cells that can repopulate the acinar system. The intercalated ducts join to form striated ducts, which merge to form interlobular ducts, which ultimately empty into the large named ducts.

II. GROSS EXAMINATION, TISSUE SAMPLING, AND HISTOLOGIC SLIDE PREPARATION

A. Biopsies of many salivary gland lesions are taken prior to surgery to characterize them and direct management.

   1. Fine needle aspiration (FNA) is the procedure of choice for initial characterization of salivary gland lesions for many reasons (see cytology section below).

---

*All e-figures are available online via the Solution Site Image Bank.

2. Core needle and incisional biopsies of the parotid gland can damage the facial nerve branches so are almost never performed.
B. Resections. Some salivary gland masses are removed in their entirety without a previous tissue diagnosis. Superficial parotidectomy remains the initial procedure of choice for benign (or benign-appearing) parotid gland tumors. Submandibular gland resections are usually performed without taking any significant periglandular soft tissue, although for more aggressive-appearing lesions or known malignancy, more tissue may be included with the specimen. The rare sublingual gland tumors necessitate a resection of the floor of mouth that is qualitatively similar to those performed for mucosal-based squamous carcinomas of the same area.

In general, salivary gland specimens are small enough to prosect the day of receipt. The gland should be described, and its dimensions recorded. The deep (covered by muscle and fascia) and superficial (covered by subcutaneous fat) surfaces of the parotid gland can sometimes be deciphered, and should then be differentially inked. Otherwise, the typical approach to the specimen is to ink the entire surface with only one color. The specimen is then serially sectioned, and any mass or focal lesions described with dimensions, color, texture, and distance to the margins. Four to five sections of the tumor, including representative areas of the closest inked margins, should be taken. At least one section of the normal surrounding gland should also be taken. For the parotid gland, the surrounding gland should be thoroughly searched for intraparenchymal lymph nodes, which should be separately submitted.

III. DIAGNOSTIC FEATURES OF COMMON DISEASES
A. Inflammation and infection. Sialadenitis, or inflammation of the salivary glands, can be divided into bacterial causes, viral causes, and autoimmune disease.
1. **Bacterial sialadenitis** is rare and is generally a result of obstruction by stones (sialolithiasis). The causative organism is usually *Staphylococcus aureus*, followed by *Streptococcus viridans* and gram-negative rods. Surgical specimens from bacterial sialadenitis are almost never seen; however, sialadenitis may lead to an abscess that requires surgical drainage. Gross specimens may show a purulent exudate or a relatively intact gland. Microscopic sections can show an abscess, cystic degeneration, and/or bacterial colonies.
2. **Viral sialadenitis** is most commonly caused by mumps (paramyxovirus), but can also be associated with Epstein–Barr, coxsackie, influenza A, and parainfluenza viruses. Surgical specimens are rarely encountered; however, grossly infected glands are boggy and edematous, and microscopically, chronic inflammation may be seen.
3. **Autoimmune sialadenitis** is relatively common, usually taking the form of Sjögren's syndrome (characterized by facial swelling, dry mouth, and dry eyes, which together are called "sicca" syndrome) with associated rheumatoid arthritis and hypergammaglobulinemia. On physical examination, bilateral, symmetric enlargement of the salivary and lacrimal glands is seen. An important specimen in this context is a minor salivary gland biopsy, typically taken from the inner lip as a diagnostic tool in the workup of a patient with suspected autoimmune disease.

Grossly, the major glands usually have a discrete, tan nodularity. Microscopically, in early disease, there is a lymphoplasmacytic septal inflammatory infiltrate with little to no abnormality of the parenchyma. The so-called "focus score," a nodular collection of >50 lymphocytes, is considered diagnostic of chronic sialadenitis. In larger glands or in more severe disease, there is typically an extensive lymphoid infiltrate with germinal centers (e-**Fig. 6.4**); the acini are often atrophic, and interstitial fibrosis may be seen. In late disease, acini may be completely absent with the only residual epithelium being ducts with an associated dense intraepithelial lymphocytosis (referred to as "epimyoepithelial islands"). In Sjögren's syndrome, the lymphocytic infiltrate is polyclonal, which can be used to exclude a Mucosa-Associated Lymphoid Tissue (MALT) lymphoma.

B. **Lymphoepithelial cystic lesions**
   1. **Acquired immune deficiency syndrome (AIDS)-related parotid cysts (ARPCs)** are benign lymphoepithelial cysts. Patients present with unilateral or bilateral, painless, slowly enlarging parotid masses. They sometimes have associated cervical lymphadenopathy and/or nasopharyngeal swelling. Grossly, these lesions have multiple cystic spaces usually containing serous fluid. Microscopically, ARPCs consist of cysts that most often have a mature squamous epithelial lining, although the lining is sometimes cuboidal or columnar with goblet cells. Below the epithelium, the cyst wall has dense lymphoid tissue with germinal centers (e-**Fig. 6.5**). Occasionally, lesions within the gland can lack cystic change and appear similar to epimyoepithelial islands.

   Unlike autoimmune sialadenitis, the vast majority of human immunodeficiency virus (HIV) patients with ARPC have no autoimmune symptoms, no sicca syndrome from glandular dysfunction, and no serum autoantibodies. The etiology of ARPC is thus unclear. Patients usually have bilateral disease by radiology, even if there are no symptoms and no clinical mass in the contralateral gland. If the diagnosis is established by radiology and cytology, surgery is not necessary for other than cosmetic reasons.
   2. **Benign lymphoepithelial cysts** are unifocal lesions that occur in patients in their 5th and 6th decades. They are usually unilateral, almost always involve the parotid gland, but sometimes can be seen in the oral cavity. There is no association with systemic or other disease. Grossly, they consist of well-circumscribed unilocular cysts with contents ranging from serous to mucoid to caseous; keratinous debris may be present. Microscopically, they consist of a cyst lined by benign mature squamous epithelium without papillary projections; in rare cases, the lining is cuboidal or columnar with goblet cells. Below the epithelium, the cyst wall has dense lymphoid tissue with germinal centers. Excision is curative, and the lesion does not recur.

C. **Nonneoplastic lesions**
   1. **Chronic sialadenitis** (or chronic sclerosing sialadenitis) is usually unilateral and clinically can mimic a true salivary gland neoplasm; when it occurs in the submandibular gland, it is known as Kuttner's tumor. Chronic sialadenitis most commonly results from sialolithiasis with obstruction, although some cases may be due to an autoimmune process, to radiation therapy, or to duct strictures. Grossly, it is characterized by a very hard, fibrotic gland. Histologic examination of the gland early in the disease process shows dilated ducts filled with secretions with an associated lymphoplasmacytic infiltrate occasionally with germinal center formation. As the disease progresses, fibrosis surrounds the ducts and results in lobulation of the gland (e-**Fig. 6.6**) with acinar atrophy. Surgical excision may be required.
   2. **Necrotizing sialometaplasia** is a rare inflammatory/destructive lesion that simulates malignancy that is thought to occur because of ischemic injury. Although it can occur anywhere along the UADT, the vast majority of cases occur in the hard palate. Men are slightly more commonly affected, and the average patient age is 46 years. Clinically, the lesion consists of a sharply defined and deep ulcer that develops rapidly (over a few days) and can persist for months. Grossly, the lesion consists of loose tissue with a surface ulcer without a distinguishing mass lesion. Microscopically, the most typical feature is coagulative necrosis of the minor salivary gland lobules with a prominent associated inflammatory response. There is extensive squamous metaplasia of the ducts (an alarming feature), but the lesion retains its overall lobular architecture (e-**Fig. 6.7**). The surface squamous mucosa may show pseudoepitheliomatous hyperplasia. The lack of peripheral infiltration and the retained lobular architecture are keys to the benign nature of the lesion. No specific therapy is indicated because the lesion is self-healing.
   3. **Lithiasis** results from concretions within the salivary gland duct system that coalesce to form a stone. Sialolithiasis most frequently involves the submandibular gland and may result in secondary chronic sclerosing sialadenitis. Distention of the duct system can result in swelling and pain of the affected gland. Sialoliths are

always visible on radiologic examination and are often seen in Wharton's duct of the submandibular gland. Treatment often requires removal of the stone and the affected portion of the gland.

4. **Mucoceles** are the most common nonneoplastic lesion of salivary gland tissue, and are defined as pooling of mucin in a cystic cavity. Two types of mucoceles are recognized. In the retention type, the mucin is within a dilated duct. In the extravasation type, the mucin accumulates in the soft tissue. The lower lip is the most common site of mucoceles, followed by the tongue, the floor of the mouth (where the lesion is termed a "ranula"), and the buccal mucosa. The peak incidence of mucoceles is in the 3rd decade. Grossly, a mucocele presents as a cystic cavity in the connective tissue that is filled with glistening fluid. Microscopically, the cyst wall may or may not have an epithelial lining, depending on the type; those of the retention type have a lining and usually no surrounding inflammation, whereas those of the extravasation type consist of mucin with surrounding inflammatory cells and no lining. Some late lesions consist only of a collection of foamy histiocytes containing mucin (e-Fig. 6.8), which can be confirmed by a PAS stain. Surgical excision is generally curative.

IV. **NEOPLASMS.** Neoplasms of the salivary gland can be roughly classified based on the component of normal salivary gland toward which they differentiate, namely acinar cells, myoepithelial cells, or ductal cells. However, most neoplasms have dual differentiation because almost all show some myoepithelial differentiation. Most benign neoplasms have a malignant counterpart. The World Health Organization (WHO) classification of tumors of the salivary gland is listed in Table 6.1.

A. **Benign neoplasms**

1. **Pleomorphic adenoma** (PA) is the most common neoplasm of the salivary glands. Ninety percent of PAs occur in the parotid gland (PAs represent 60% of parotid gland neoplasms); the remaining cases occur in the hard palate or submandibular gland. The tumor occurs in a wide age range of patients, but the peak incidence is in the 4th or 5th decade. The tumor presents as a slow-growing, painless mass that usually is between 2 and 5 cm in diameter. On gross examination, these tumors appear well-circumscribed and are not usually encapsulated; they are never encapsulated when occurring in minor salivary glands. Sectioning reveals a rubbery, myxoid, tan-white mass. The microscopic appearance, as the name suggests, is highly variable, but always shows an intimate admixture of epithelial and mesenchymal elements. The epithelial component consists of ductal structures with an associated myoepithelial layer, but also may contain collections of myoepithelial cells that may be spindled, clear, plasmacytoid, or basaloid. The mesenchymal, or stromal, component is typically myxoid, hyaline, or chondroid (e-Fig. 6.9). Although defined subcategories have no significant clinical importance, pleomorphic adenomas have been divided into a myxoid type (>80% mesenchymal-type tissue), cellular type (>80% epithelial-type tissue), and mixed or classic type (generally an equal mix of components).

   Treatment requires complete excision (with a rim of uninvolved tissue) as PAs are likely to recur if tumor is left behind or transected. Multinodular growth is very uncommon in primary tumors but is quite frequent in recurrent disease (yielding a so-called "buckshot" pattern), which makes therapy for recurrence difficult (e-Fig. 6.10).

2. **Warthin's tumor** (papillary cystadenoma lymphomatosum) is the second most common benign salivary gland tumor and is found exclusively in the parotid gland. It is the most common bilateral or multifocal salivary gland tumor, presents in the 6th or 7th decade, and is associated with smoking. Grossly, it presents as a soft, brown or yellow mass that is composed of cysts that are classically filled with viscous brown fluid. Microscopically, the lesion has a classic and highly reproducible morphology with a cystic and/or papillary epithelial lining composed of two layers of epithelial cells with oncocytic features (e-Fig. 6.11). The epithelium overlies a dense and closely applied, polyclonal lymphoid component that forms germinal centers. Warthin's tumors may show a giant cell reaction, fibrosis, or squamous metaplasia from trauma/cyst rupture or after FNA. Tumors are treated with surgical excision and rarely recur. Malignant

TABLE 6.1	WHO Histological Classification of Tumors of the Salivary Glands

Malignant epithelial tumors
Acinic cell carcinoma
Mucoepidermoid carcinoma
Adenoid cystic carcinoma
Polymorphous low-grade adenocarcinoma
Epithelial–myoepithelial carcinoma
Clear cell carcinoma, not otherwise specified
Basal cell adenocarcinoma
Sebaceous carcinoma
Sebaceous lymphadenocarcinoma
Cystadenocarcinoma
Low-grade cribriform cystadenocarcinoma
Mucinous adenocarcinoma
Oncocytic carcinoma
Salivary duct carcinoma
Adenocarcinoma, not otherwise specified
Myoepithelial carcinoma
Carcinoma ex pleomorphic adenoma
Carcinosarcoma
Metastasizing pleomorphic adenoma
Squamous cell carcinoma
Small cell carcinoma
Large cell carcinoma
Lymphoepithelial carcinoma
Sialoblastoma

Benign epithelial tumors
Pleomorphic adenoma
Myoepithelioma
Basal cell adenoma
Warthin's tumor
Oncocytoma
Canalicular adenoma
Sebaceous adenoma
Lymphadenoma
   Sebaceous
   Non-sebaceous
Ductal papillomas
   Inverted ductal papilloma
   Intraductal papilloma
   Sialadenoma papilliferum
Cystadenoma

Soft tissue tumors
Hemangioma

Hematolymphoid tumors
Hodgkin's lymphoma
Diffuse large B-cell lymphoma
Extranodal marginal zone B-cell lymphoma

Secondary tumors

From: Barnes L, Eveson J, Reichart P, Sidransky D, eds. *World Health Organization Classification of Tumours. Pathology and Genetics. Head and Neck Tumours.* Lyon: IARC Press: 2005. Used with permission.

TABLE 6.2	Four Major Patterns of Basal Cell Adenoma

Tubular
Solid
Trabecular
Membranous ("dermal anlage tumor")

transformation is very rare and takes the form of either squamous cell carcinoma or lymphoma.

3. **Basal cell adenomas** are benign tumors that are composed of small basaloid cells. They generally occur in adults, and 75% occur in the parotid gland. They usually present as an asymptomatic, slowly growing mass. The membranous subtype (dermal anlage tumor) may be multicentric and sometimes is associated with various adnexal tumors of the skin.

On gross examination, these tumors are usually solid, well-circumscribed, and pink to brown, although they can be cystic. Microscopically, there are four patterns (Table 6.2), but regardless of pattern, the tumor is composed of two cell types. Small cells with little cytoplasm typically lie at the neoplasm's edge, frequently show peripheral palisading, and give the tumor its basaloid appearance; more polygonal basaloid cells with slightly more cytoplasm and round to oval nuclei with more open chromatin usually lie in the tumor's center. The trabecular and membranous patterns have a "jig-saw puzzle" appearance with rounded nests of tumor shaped like puzzle pieces (e-**Fig. 6.12**), and the membranous pattern additionally shows hyalinized, eosinophilic, linear, or nodular basement membrane–like material around the nests. Basal cell adenomas are immunopositive for pan-cytokeratin S-100, smooth muscle actin, and muscle-specific actin, all evidencing myoepithelial differentiation.

The differential diagnosis for basal cell adenoma includes basal cell adenocarcinoma and adenoid cystic carcinoma, both of which, unlike basal cell adenoma, show infiltrative growth and/or perineural invasion. Simple excision of basal cell adenoma is usually curative and recurrence is rare, except in the membranous type, where the recurrence rate approaches 25%.

4. **Canalicular adenomas** are benign salivary tumors thought to arise from the excretory ducts, and are the second most common salivary gland lesion of the upper lip. These tumors almost always arise from the minor salivary glands, particularly of the upper lip, and are frequently multifocal. Women and African Americans are more commonly affected, and the peak incidence is in the 7th decade. Canalicular adenomas present clinically as an asymptomatic, fluctuant or firm 1- to 2-cm submucosal nodule that grows slowly.

On gross examination, these tumors are not encapsulated but are well circumscribed, and have a tan to pink, cystic or solid cut surface. Histologically, canalicular adenomas are composed of long strands or tubules of columnar epithelial cells with a loose, collagenous stroma. There are typically two rows of columnar cells which are situated opposite each other. These strands may take on a "beaded appearance" with tubules coming together and then separating. The epithelial cells lining the tubules have eosinophilic cytoplasm and range from cuboidal to basaloid. Pleomorphism is not present, and mitotic counts are low. The epithelial cells are immunopositive for cytokeratin and S-100.

The differential diagnosis for canalicular adenoma includes pleomorphic adenoma and basal cell adenoma. However, the pattern of growth of canalicular adenoma is virtually always distinctive enough to make the diagnosis. Simple local excision is performed with an attempt to obtain clear margins. Recurrence is rare.

5. **Myoepitheliomas** are benign tumors which, as the name implies, are composed almost exclusively of myoepithelial cells, although a small percentage (<10%) of

the tumor can be made up of ductal cells. In this regard, myoepitheliomas are sometimes considered to lie at one end of a biologic spectrum, with pleomorphic adenoma in the middle, and basal cell adenoma at the opposite end. Myoepitheliomas occur with approximately equal frequency in the parotid gland and minor salivary glands (specifically the hard and soft palate) and present as slowly growing, painless masses in adults. Men and women are affected equally.

Grossly, these neoplasms are well-circumscribed and encapsulated with a tan to white cut surface. Histologically, they consist of sheets and cords of tumor cells that can be classified into four major subtypes: spindle cell, hyaline, plasmacytoid, and clear cell, all of which usually have a collagenous or myxoid stroma. The spindle cell type can show an interlacing, fascicular pattern of growth (e-**Fig. 6.13**). Loosely cohesive myoepithelial cells with eosinophilic cytoplasm and eccentric round nuclei are present in the plasmacytoid variant. The clear cell type is composed of small tubules lined by a single layer of cuboidal cells surrounded by one or more layers of clear cells. Immunostains are often required for diagnosis; myoepithelial cells are strongly positive for S-100 and cytokeratin and are variably reactive to smooth muscle actin and glial fibrillary acid protein (GFAP).

Simple excision is generally the treatment of choice unless malignant features are encountered (consisting of infiltrative growth and/or perineural invasion). Myoepitheliomas have a similar, but slightly lower, recurrence rate than pleomorphic adenomas.

B. Malignant neoplasms

1. **Mucoepidermoid carcinoma** is a malignant glandular tumor composed of mucous, intermediate, and epidermoid (or squamoid) cells. These tumors are the most common salivary gland malignancy. They usually arise in the parotid gland (the major salivary glands account for more than half of all cases), but the tumors also arise from minor salivary glands in the oral cavity, particularly in the hard palate, buccal mucosa, lip, and retromolar trigone. Rarely, the tumor also arises intraosseously in the mandible and maxilla, but primary tumors of intraosseous sites are considered odontogenic in origin and have a different clinical behavior. Mucoepidermoid carcinomas are slightly more common in women, and the mean age of affected patients is approximately 45 years, although the tumor also occurs in children; in fact, mucoepidermoid carcinoma is the most common pediatric salivary gland carcinoma. Patients usually present with a painless, slowly growing mass. An intraoral tumor may mimic a mucocele or vascular lesion clinically if it presents as a blue-red superficial nodule.

Grossly, these tumors can have both solid and cystic components, often with mucinous material within the cysts. Microscopically, the hallmark of these tumors is the presence of the three different cell types. These three cell types can occur in sheets, nests, duct-like structures or cysts, in which the three cell types are in variable proportions. Intermediate cells frequently predominate, and range from small basal cells with minimal basophilic cytoplasm to larger oval cells with pale eosinophilic cytoplasm. The mucin-producing cells (mucocytes) occur singly or in clusters and have pale, foamy cytoplasm, distinct cell membranes, and eccentric small nuclei (e-**Fig. 6.14**); they frequently line cystic spaces and are positive with mucicarmine or PAS stains. Epidermoid or squamoid cells have abundant eosinophilic cytoplasm and vesicular nuclei with open chromatin; they are not truly squamous as they lack intercellular bridges, and only very rarely is there true keratinization. A population of clear cells is often scattered throughout the tumor; these cells usually have a high glycogen content, which can be demonstrated by PAS staining.

The differential diagnosis includes necrotizing sialometaplasia, which is discerned by its residual normal lobules of minor salivary gland tissue, presence of necrosis and an associated dense inflammatory infiltrate, and lack of cytologic atypia. Adenosquamous carcinoma and squamous cell carcinoma both have true squamous differentiation with some intercellular bridges or keratinization, often with associated surface squamous dysplasia or carcinoma in situ. Immunohistochemistry is of little utility in the diagnosis of mucoepidermoid carcinoma. Finally,

TABLE 6.3	Brandwein Grading System for Mucoepidermoid Carcinoma

Parameter	Point value
Cystic component <25%	+2
Tumor front invades in small nests and islands	+2
Pronounced nuclear atypia	+2
Lymphatic and/or vascular invasion	+3
Neural invasion	+3
Necrosis	+3
4+ mitoses/10 HPF	+3
Bony invasion	+3

Grade	Point score/mortality (%)
Low (I)	0
Intermediate (II)	2–3
High (III)	4 or more

Adapted from *Am J Surg Pathol* 2001;25:835.

many mucoepidermoid carcinomas possess a t(11;19)(q21;p13) translocation. Although the utility of testing for the translocation for diagnosis has not been established, tumors that carry the rearrangement are associated with a better clinical outcome.

Prognosis is highly dependent on the grade of the tumor, and the grade is in turn dependent on the relative amounts of the various tumor types. Low-grade lesions are markedly cystic, and have abundant well-differentiated mucous cells. High-grade lesions are more solid with squamous and intermediate cells predominating. Different grading systems have been proposed with inconsistent results, although the grading system presented in Table 6.3 has gained acceptance for its reproducibility.

Wide local excision is recommended. Radiation therapy has not been shown to be beneficial except for palliation of unresectable or recurrent disease. The prognosis for low-grade tumors is excellent (>90% survival at 5 years) but drops greatly for high-grade tumors (about 50% survival at 5 years).

2. **Polymorphous low-grade adenocarcinoma** (PLGA) arises exclusively from the minor salivary glands and accounts for 25% of all minor salivary gland tumors. The tumor's most common site is the palate, particularly at the junction of the hard and soft palate; less common sites include the upper lip, buccal mucosa, and posterior third of the tongue. PLGA arises more commonly in women and tends to present in the 4th to 6th decades, often as a very slow growing mass that may have been present for years.

On gross examination, PLGA is a circumscribed, nonencapsulated, and pale yellow or tan mass that generally ranges from 1 to 3 cm. Microscopically, the architectural features of this tumor are quite variable, as the name suggests. PLGA may consist of solid nests, lobules, cribriform glandlike structures, or duct-like arrangements; another common pattern is concentric whirling of the cellular nests in a single file arrangement in a pattern that has been termed "the eye of the storm." Stromal hyalinization is characteristic. Cytologically, the tumor cells are quite regular with moderate eosinophilic cytoplasm and characteristic round to oval nuclei with open chromatin. There is very little mitotic activity and no necrosis. The periphery of the tumor shows marked infiltrative growth, and perineural invasion is a very common finding (e-**Fig. 6.15**). The differential diagnosis includes pleomorphic adenoma (although the myxochondroid areas of pleomorphic adenoma are not seen in PLGA, and pleomorphic adenoma does not show an infiltrative growth pattern or perineural invasion) and adenoid cystic carcinoma (although adenoid cystic carcinoma has different cytologic features, consisting of basaloid cells with dark chromatin and little cytoplasm). Conservative resection is the treatment of choice. Recurrence occurs in 10% to 15% of patients. Neck dissection is only recommended for significant adenopathy or proven metastasis because lymph node metastases are distinctly uncommon. Distant metastases are even more uncommon. Patients have an excellent long-term prognosis even in the presence of recurrent/metastatic disease; deaths due to PLGA are extremely uncommon.

3. **Acinic cell carcinoma** accounts for only 1% to 3% of salivary gland tumors. It occurs in the pediatric to geriatric age groups, although most cases are evenly distributed in the 2nd through 7th decades. This tumor is the second most common childhood salivary gland malignancy (after mucoepidermoid carcinoma), and 80% arise in the parotid gland. Acinic cell carcinoma presents usually as a slow growing mass, which is occasionally painful.

Grossly, acinic cell carcinoma presents as a single, usually circumscribed, solid mass that can undergo cystic degeneration. Histologically, the tumor is highly variable. The architecture can be solid/lobular, microcystic, papillary-cystic, or follicular. Small tumors can be easily missed because the acinar cells are so well differentiated. The characteristic cell, the acinic cell, has the appearance of a salivary acinar cell with abundant granular, basophilic cytoplasm and a small, round, eccentrically placed nucleus (e-**Fig. 6.16**); PAS stains will highlight the cytoplasmic zymogen granules, which are resistant to diastase digestion. Despite the name, a number of other cell types can also be present including eosinophilic, clear, and vacuolated cells. Architecturally, acinic cell carcinomas often have a mixture of architectural patterns, and characteristically there is a dense associated lymphoid infiltrate. Although the periphery of the tumor may not be infiltrative, this should not be interpreted as a finding of benignancy. The differential diagnosis includes normal parotid gland, and, for the eosinophilic and clear cell types, tumors such as oncocytic carcinoma or clear cell carcinoma; the papillary variant of acinic cell carcinoma must be differentiated from cystadenocarcinoma.

Acinic cell carcinoma must be adequately resected because the tumor will recur in approximately one third of cases. Although classically regarded as a low-grade malignancy, 10% to 15% of these tumors will metastasize to regional lymph nodes or distantly, particularly to the lungs and bones. Survival is approximately 80% at 5 years and 70% at 10 years; tumor grade does not correlate well with behavior although dedifferentiation (in which typical acinic cell carcinoma is mixed with much higher grade carcinoma) has consistently been associated with a poor outcome.

4. **Adenoid cystic carcinoma** is one of the most recognizable salivary gland tumors. It comprises 10% of all salivary gland malignancies, and is the most common malignancy of the minor salivary glands. Although the tumor occurs in patients over a wide age range, the peak incidence is in patients between 40 and 60 years of age. The tumor is slowly growing, but nonetheless relentlessly progressive. Perineural invasion is extremely common, so cranial nerve involvement, including facial nerve palsy, may be the presenting symptom, with or without associated pain.

Grossly, the tumor is solid, light tan, firm, and well circumscribed. Histologically, several architectural patterns are found including cribriform, tubular, solid, and mixed. Tumors are graded based on the predominant pattern (Table 6.4). The tubular variant has double cell-lined ducts, and the solid variant has only lobules of tumor cells without defined architecture (e-**Fig. 6.17**). The classic and most easily recognized pattern, however, is cribriform (e-**Fig. 6.18**), which consists of nests of cells arranged around gland-like spaces filled with PAS-positive, granular basophilic material (the cribriform spaces are actually extracellular cavities containing reduplicated basal lamina as well as myxoid material produced by the tumor cells). The cells in adenoid cystic carcinoma, regardless of architectural type, are basaloid, with little cytoplasm, have round to oval nuclei that are dark and hyperchromatic without nucleoli, and are usually quite regular with little mitotic activity (except for the solid type, in which mitotic activity may be

| TABLE 6.4 | Grading of Adenoid Cystic Carcinoma |

Predominant pattern	Grade
Tubular	I
Cribriform	II
Solid	III

prominent). Perineural invasion is seen in the majority of cases, particularly at the tumor's periphery. As with most other salivary gland neoplasms, immunohistochemistry is of little utility in the diagnosis. The pseudocyst material will stain for collagen type IV and laminin; the neoplastic cells show strong immunoreactivity for cytokeratins and partial immunoreactivity for the myoepithelial markers S-100, smooth muscle actin, calponin, and p63.

The differential diagnosis for low-grade (tubular) tumors most importantly includes polymorphous low-grade adenocarcinoma, epithelial–myoepithelial carcinoma, and basal cell adenocarcinoma. None of these tumors, however, will show the basaloid and hyperchromatic nuclei characteristic of adenoid cystic carcinoma. High-grade neuroendocrine carcinomas and basaloid squamous cell carcinoma also enter into the differential diagnosis of solid-type adenoid cystic carcinoma. Although usually very bland-appearing microscopically, adenoid cystic carcinoma is highly malignant and progressive. Five- and ten-year survival rates are only 62% and 40%. Local recurrence is extremely common, particularly in the first 5 years after surgery, although late recurrences also occur. Involvement of bone, submandibular gland origin, and solid histologic type (grade III) all adversely affect prognosis; whether identification of perineural invasion also adversely affects prognosis is controversial.

5. **"Malignant mixed tumor"** is a broad term that is used to encompass true malignant mixed tumors, carcinoma ex pleomorphic adenoma, and metastasizing mixed tumor.

   a. **True salivary gland malignant mixed tumor** (or carcinosarcoma) is a malignant neoplasm that is composed of both carcinomatous and sarcomatous components, and is exceedingly rare. The mean age of individuals is 58 years, and one third of patients have evidence of a preexisting pleomorphic adenoma. Two-thirds of cases arise in the parotid gland, approximately 15% in the submandibular gland, and approximately 15% in the palate.

      Grossly, there is typically a firm, tan-white mass with hemorrhage, necrosis, and, on occasion, grittiness or calcification. Microscopically, there is an intimate admixture of the two components. The carcinomatous component typically takes the form of high-grade duct carcinoma or undifferentiated carcinoma (e-Fig. 6.19); the sarcomatous component is usually chondrosarcoma or osteosarcoma, but fibrosarcoma, leiomyosarcoma, and even liposarcoma occur. Treatment consists of wide local excision combined with radiotherapy. The tumors are very aggressive, with up to two-thirds of patients dying of disease, usually within 30 months.

   b. **Carcinoma ex pleomorphic adenoma** is defined as a mixed tumor in which carcinoma is present. This tumor accounts for >95% of malignant mixed tumors, and is most common in the parotid gland, followed by the minor salivary glands, the submandibular gland, and the sublingual gland. Most patients are in their 6th and 7th decades, which is approximately 1 decade older than the age of most patients who have pleomorphic adenomas. The classic history is a patient with a longstanding mass that undergoes rapid growth over a period of several months.

      Grossly, these tumors can reach up to 25 cm in diameter, and the average size is more than twice that of pleomorphic adenomas. The carcinomatous component is usually an infiltrative, hard, white to tan-gray mass with hemorrhage and necrosis. Microscopically, the proportions of the carcinoma and the pleomorphic adenoma are quite variable, and the pleomorphic adenoma component may be replaced by scarring or overgrown by the malignant component. The malignant component most often is a poorly differentiated adenocarcinoma not otherwise specified, salivary duct carcinoma, or undifferentiated carcinoma but low grade carcinomas like myoepithelial carcinoma sometimes occur.

Prognosis and management are highly dependent on the type of carcinoma and extent of invasion. The malignant component should be classified as noninvasive (intracapsular), minimally invasive ($\leq$1.5 mm in greatest extent), or invasive (>1.5 mm). Wide resection is the treatment of choice, with lymph node dissection and radiation therapy reserved for widely invasive tumors or tumors with obvious cervical lymph node metastases.

   c. **Metastasizing mixed tumor** is the least common form of malignant mixed tumor. These tumors have the same bland morphology of a pleomorphic adenoma, but metastasize either to local lymph nodes or distantly (usually to bone and lung). Often, there is a protracted clinical course with many recurrences at the primary site; overall mortality due to the tumor is 40%.

6. **Salivary duct carcinoma** is one of the most aggressive primary salivary gland tumors. This tumor simulates the appearance of high-grade ductal carcinoma of the breast, and accounts for <10% of salivary gland tumors. Men are more commonly affected in a ratio of 4:1, and patients generally present in the 6th decade with a rapidly growing parotid mass with facial nerve involvement and often skin ulceration.

   Grossly, these tumors are solid and white with hemorrhage, necrosis, and cystic areas. Infiltration of the surrounding tissue is usually apparent. Histologically, ductal carcinoma in situ with a cribriform pattern is present in a pattern similar to that of breast ductal carcinomas, often with comedo-type necrosis. The tumor's invasive component consists of large cells with abundant eosinophilic cytoplasm and large, round nuclei with vesicular chromatin and prominent nucleoli (e-**Fig. 6.20**). The neoplasm shows marked tissue infiltration with stromal desmoplasia and brisk mitotic activity, and vascular and perineural invasion are common. By immunohistochemistry, salivary duct carcinomas are positive for low- and high-molecular-weight cytokeratins, carcinoembryogenic antigen (CEA), androgen receptors, and human epidermal growth factor receptor 2 (HER2)/neu (in a distinct membrane-staining pattern). The differential diagnosis includes metastatic breast carcinoma, poorly differentiated squamous cell carcinoma, and mucoepidermoid carcinoma; in this regard, the presence of intraductal carcinoma is the most important finding because it argues for a diagnosis of a primary salivary duct carcinoma rather than metastasis.

   Salivary duct carcinoma is the most aggressive salivary gland tumor. One third of patients develop local recurrence, about one half distant metastases, and overall 65% of patients die of their disease, most within 4 years of diagnosis. Wide local excision with neck dissection and postoperative radiotherapy is the treatment of choice.

7. **Epithelial–myoepithelial carcinoma** is a low-grade tumor that accounts for 0.5% to 1% of salivary gland neoplasms. It occurs in older patients, predominantly in the parotid gland, and rarely in the larynx or paranasal sinuses.

   Grossly, the tumor is firm and well-demarcated, averaging 2 to 3 cm in diameter. Microscopically, the tumor is usually well-demarcated and partially encapsulated, with invasion by tumor into the adjacent parenchyma. The classic morphology is of ductal structures lined by eosinophilic cells with a prominent supporting layer of clear myoepithelial cells (e-**Fig. 6.21**), although the myoepithelial cell component may be present as large sheets of cells with only focal ductal differentiation. Classically, the stroma between the tumor nests is eosinophilic and hyalinized. Cytologically, the individual tumor cells are bland with minimal mitotic activity. Immunohistochemically, the duct-lining cells are positive for low-molecular-weight cytokeratins and the myoepithelial cells positive for calponin, smooth muscle actin, and p63. The differential diagnosis includes pleomorphic adenoma myoepithelioma/myoepithelial carcinoma and the tubular variant (Grade I) of adenoid cystic carcinoma.

Epithelial–myoepithelial carcinoma is a moderately aggressive tumor with a recurrence rate of 40%. Metastases to lymph nodes, lung, or liver occur in 15% of patients, and overall survival at 5 years is about 80%. Treatment is wide local excision with or without radiotherapy.

8. **Squamous cell carcinomas** are only rarely primary in the salivary gland. Metastases to the intraparotid lymph nodes from primary skin cancers of the head and neck, particularly of the scalp, ear, and face, are much more common. Most patients are in their 6th to 8th decade, and sometimes there is a history of prior radiation therapy. About 80% of tumors arise in the parotid gland and 20% in the submandibular gland, and the tumors typically are high stage at the time of diagnosis. By definition, the diagnosis of primary squamous cell carcinoma is restricted to the large salivary glands, because tumors arising in the minor salivary glands cannot be reliably distinguished from primary squamous carcinoma of the surrounding mucosa.

   Grossly, the neoplasm is a firm, white, infiltrative, and nonencapsulated mass. Histologically, it is identical to other typical squamous cell carcinoma of the UADT. Prominent desmoplasia is usually present, and perineural invasion and extension of the tumor into periglandular soft tissue are frequently also present.

   As noted above, the differential diagnosis most importantly includes metastatic squamous cell carcinoma. High-grade mucoepidermoid carcinoma can have a largely squamoid appearance but lacks keratinization, has a more heterogeneous cell population, and almost always demonstrates mucous cells.

   Primary squamous carcinomas are aggressive tumors, and the 5-year survival of patients is approximately 25%. Treatment involves radical surgery, neck dissection, and radiotherapy.

9. **Metastasis to the salivary glands** or, more commonly, to intra- or periglandular lymph nodes, is a frequent occurrence. Because the parotid gland has an average of 20 intraparenchymal lymph nodes whereas the submandibular gland does not contain any lymph nodes, the vast majority of metastases to the parotid gland are from primary tumors of the head and neck, whereas >85% of metastases to the submandibular gland are from non–head and neck sites.

   The parotid lymph nodes drain the scalp, face, ear skin, external auditory canal, and tympanic membrane, so skin tumors such as squamous cell carcinoma and melanoma account for approximately 80% of metastases to the gland. The remaining metastases are from non–head and neck primary tumors, most commonly lung, kidney, and breast carcinomas.

   The opposite distribution of metastases is seen for the submandibular gland. More than 85% of metastases arise from infraclavicular primary tumors, most commonly breast, kidney, and lung carcinomas (particularly small cell carcinoma of the lung).

10. **Pediatric tumors** are uncommon. Hemangioma is the most frequent, but as noted above, most salivary gland neoplasms that occur in adults can also occur in children. However, there are two congenital tumors that bear mentioning.

    a. **Sialoblastoma** is an extremely rare, potentially aggressive neoplasm that recapitulates the embryonic stage of salivary gland development and is thought to develop from retained blastematous cells. Clinically, it is seen in the perinatal to neonatal period, usually involving the parotid gland. This tumor may grow quickly and cause skin ulceration or airway compromise.

       Grossly, the mass is lobulated and partially circumscribed. Microscopically, it is composed of nests or nodules of basaloid cells with scanty cytoplasm, round to oval nuclei, and fine chromatin with small nucleoli. The mitotic rate is highly variable and can be quite high. Complete surgical excision with a rim of normal tissue is the treatment of choice. Although local recurrence is relatively common, occurring in up to 30% of cases, metastasis is extremely uncommon.

b. **Salivary anlage tumor**, also referred to as a congenital pleomorphic adenoma, occurs in male neonates in the first 2 weeks of life and is associated with respiratory obstruction or difficulty feeding. Sometimes the mass is spontaneously passed or inadvertently removed by airway suctioning. On examination, a mass attached by a thin stalk to the posterior nasal mucosa or nasopharynx is sometimes present.

Grossly, salivary anlage tumors are firm and tan-yellow with a smooth surface. Microscopically, the tumor's surface shows nonkeratinizing squamous epithelium, with a deeper stroma composed of bland spindled cells and intervening squamous islands, an overall histology that suggests a hamartoma rather than a true neoplasm. The treatment is simple excision of the mass. The lesion does not recur or spread.

V. PATHOLOGIC REPORTING OF MALIGNANT SALIVARY GLAND TUMORS
   A. **Staging: American Joint Committee on Cancer (AJCC).** Clinical staging of salivary gland cancers is important for prognosis and treatment decisions. The 2002 Tumor, Node, Metastasis (TNM) AJCC staging classification is provided in Table 6.5. Minor salivary gland carcinomas are staged according to the anatomic site of origin (e.g., oral cavity, sinus, larynx). Staging guidelines are applicable to all forms of carcinoma. Any nonepithelial tumor type is excluded.
   B. **Additional pertinent pathologic features.** Pathologic features such as tumor grade, positive resection margins, and skin or bone invasion have been demonstrated in numerous studies to correlate with a higher risk of local recurrence, a poorer prognosis, or both, and so should always be reported. Perineural and lymphovascular space invasion should also always be reported when observed, because they have been correlated with distant metastases in some studies even though they are not predictive of recurrence or poorer prognosis.

CYTOLOGY OF THE SALIVARY GLANDS
Rosa M. Dávila

FNA biopsy is a valuable tool in the evaluation of salivary gland masses. Most FNA biopsies are performed on major salivary glands; only 1% are from minor salivary gland masses (*Diagn Cytopathol* 2000;22:139). In the parotid gland, the sensitivity of FNA is reported to range from 66% to 92%, and the specificity from 86% to 100% (*Diagn Cytopathol* 2007;35:47); maximum utility requires correlation of the cytologic findings with clinical and radiologic information. The preoperative distinction between a benign and a malignant lesion makes it possible to avoid unnecessary surgery.

I. INFLAMMATORY PROCESSES
   A. **Acute sialadenitis** is usually caused by *Staphylococcus aureus*. It is not a common target of FNA biopsy because it is usually diagnosed based on the patient's clinical signs and symptoms. However, patients with atypical presentations may undergo FNA to determine the nature of the lesions. Samples from acute sialadenitis have numerous neutrophils and cellular debris intermixed with benign salivary gland elements (e-**Fig. 6.22**).
   B. **Chronic inflammation** is seen in various conditions such as chronic sialadenitis and lymphoepithelial lesion. Benign intraparenchymal lymph nodes and Warthin's tumor are also included in the cytologic differential diagnosis of chronic inflammation because they have an abundant lymphoid component (*Diagn Cytopathol* 1997;17:183). The lymphoid component is usually polymorphous and accompanied by histiocytes and scattered plasma cells. In the case of a lymphoepithelial lesion or Warthin's tumor, an epithelial component is also present. When a lymphoma is considered in the differential diagnosis, ancillary testing such as flow cytometry is usually useful.

II. BENIGN NEOPLASMS
   A. **Pleomorphic adenoma** is the most common benign neoplasm of the salivary gland. Aspirates from pleomorphic adenoma show stroma and epithelial and/or

TABLE 6.5 | **Tumor, Node, Metastasis (TNM) Staging Scheme for Tumors of the Major Salivary Glands**

PRIMARY TUMOR (T)

TX	Primary tumor cannot be assessed
T0	No evidence of primary tumor
T1	Tumor ≤2 cm in greatest dimension without extraparenchymal extension*
T2	Tumor >2 cm but not >4 cm in greatest dimension without extraparenchymal extension*
T3	Tumor >4 cm and/or tumor having extraparenchymal extension*
T4a	Tumor invades skin, mandible, ear canal, and/or facial nerve
T4b	Tumor invades skull base and/or pterygoid plates and/or encases carotid artery

REGIONAL LYMPH NODES (N)

NX	Regional lymph nodes cannot be assessed
N0	No regional lymph node metastasis
N1	Metastasis in a single ipsilateral lymph node, ≤3 cm in greatest dimension
N2a	Metastasis in a single ipsilateral lymph node, >3 cm but not >6 cm in greatest dimension
N2b	Metastasis in multiple ipsilateral lymph nodes, none more than 6 cm in greatest dimension
N2c	Metastasis in bilateral or contralateral lymph nodes, none >6 cm in greatest dimension
N3	Metastasis in a lymph node, >6 cm in greatest dimension

DISTANT METASTASIS (M)

MX	Distant metastasis cannot be assessed
M0	No distant metastasis
M1	Distant metastasis

STAGE GROUPING

The overall pathologic AJCC stage is

Stage I	T1	N0	M0
Stage II	T2	N0	M0
Stage III	T3	N0	M0
Stage III	T1	N1	M0
Stage III	T2	N1	M0
Stage III	T3	N1	M0
Stage IVA	T4a	N0	M0
Stage IVA	T4a	N1	M0
Stage IVA	T1	N2	M0
Stage IVA	T2	N2	M0
Stage IVA	T3	N2	M0
Stage IVA	T4a	N2	M0
Stage IVB	Tyb	Any N	M0
Stage IVB	Any T	N3	M0
Stage IVC	Any T	Any N	M1

AJCC, American Joint Committee on Cancer; TNM, tumor, node, metastasis.
*Note: Extraparenchymal extension is clinical or macroscopic evidence of invasion of soft tissues. Microscopic evidence alone does not constitute extraparenchymal extension for classification purposes. From: Greene FL, Page DL, Fleming ID, Fritz AG, Balch CM, Haller DG, Morrow M, eds. AJCC Cancer Staging Manual. 6th edition. New York: Springer; 2002. Used with permission. (A new AJCC TNM staging system is scheduled for release in 2009; after its publication, the new staging scheme will appear on the website for this book.)

myoepithelial elements (e-Fig. **6.23**). The stroma may have a fibrillar or myxoid appearance, with permeation by small myoepithelial cells. The epithelial component can be arranged in clusters or sheets and exhibit small nuclei with inconspicuous nucleoli and scant cytoplasm. The myoepithelial cells may acquire a plasmacytoid appearance and can be confused with plasma cells. Squamous and mucinous epithelial elements may be evident when metaplasia has occurred.

   B. **Warthin's tumor** usually yields an epithelial component, lymphoid component, and debris derived from the cystic space of the lesion (e-Fig. **6.24**). The epithelial cells have an oncocytic appearance with distinct cell borders, abundant granular and eosinophilic cytoplasm, round nuclei, and prominent nucleoli.

III. MALIGNANT NEOPLASMS

   A. **Mucoepidermoid carcinoma.** Smears from low-grade mucoepidermoid carcinoma have intermediate cells and scattered mucin-producing cells (e-Fig. **6.25**). The intermediate cells show minimal cellular and nuclear pleomorphism, scant to moderate cytoplasm, and inconspicuous nucleoli. Mucin-producing cells have abundant clear cytoplasm, small nuclei, and small nucleoli; the amount of extracellular mucin varies, and it is easier to assess in air-dried Romanowski-stained slides. Cellular debris, macrophages, and cholesterol crystals may also be present when the tumor has a cystic component.

   High-grade mucoepidermoid carcinoma displays marked nuclear pleomorphism, nuclear hyperchromasia, and irregularly clumped chromatin. Although its malignant appearance is evident, squamous or mucinous differentiation may be difficult to identify. Occasional keratinizing cells or vacuolated cells can be seen, and a necrotic component is often present (e-Fig. **6.26**).

   B. **Adenoid cystic carcinoma** is readily identified when well-defined cylinders and/or spheres of acellular stroma accompany the small epithelial cells. The stromal structures are colorless in Papanicolaou-stained slides but magenta in air-dried, Romanowski-stained slides (e-Fig. **6.27**). The epithelial cells lack significant nuclear and cellular pleomorphism and have scant cytoplasm, round nuclei, and small nucleoli. The lack of overtly malignant nuclear features may lead to a false-negative diagnosis (*Arch Pathol Lab Med* 2005;129:26). In poorly differentiated adenoid cystic carcinoma, the cells exhibit more nuclear abnormalities and the stromal cylinders or spheres are usually absent.

   C. **Acinic cell carcinoma** consists of cells that resemble normal acinar cells of the salivary gland. High cellularity, the absence of a ductal component, and the presence of single cells are usually helpful in reaching the correct diagnosis. The neoplastic cells have abundant lacelike, finely granular cytoplasm or finely vacuolated cytoplasm, round nuclei, and small but prominent nucleoli (e-Fig. **6.28**). It is not uncommon to find naked nuclei from the neoplastic cells in the background. When the tumor is poorly differentiated, it is easier to arrive at a malignant diagnosis, but the lack of resemblance to normal acinar cells often does not permit specific classification of acinic cell carcinoma by FNA.

Suggested Readings

Eveson JW. Malignant neoplasms of the salivary glands. In: Thompson LDR, ed. *Head and Neck Pathology.* New York: Churchill Livingstone; 2006.

Eveson JW, Auclair P, Gnepp DR, El-Naggar AK. Tumors of the salivary glands. In: Barnes L, Eveson JW, Reichart P, Sidransky D, eds. *Pathology and Genetics Head and Neck Tumors.* Lyon, France: IARC Press; 2005.

Gnepp DR, Brandwein MS, Henley JD. Salivary and lacrimal glands. In: Gnepp DR, ed. *Diagnostic Surgical Pathology of the Head and Neck.* Philadelphia: W.B. Saunders Publishers; 2001.

Richardson MS. Non-neoplastic lesions of the salivary glands. In: Thompson LDR, ed. *Head and Neck Pathology.* New York: Churchill Livingstone; 2006.

Torske K. Benign neoplasms of the salivary glands. In: Thompson LDR, ed. *Head and Neck Pathology.* New York: Churchill Livingstone; 2006.

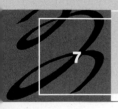

THE EAR
Peter A. Humphrey

I. NORMAL ANATOMY. The ear is composed of the external ear, the middle ear, and the inner ear. The external ear is made up of the auricle, which leads to the external auditory canal. The auricle has a supporting plate of elastic cartilage, which also helps to form the outer two thirds of the external auditory canal. Skin lines both the auricle and the canal; the main distinctive histological features of this skin are that the squamous lining of the inner half of the canal is thinned, and that modified apocrine glands called ceruminal glands are present in the outer third of the canal. The clustered ceruminal glands are lined by cuboidal epithelial cells that have an eosinophilic cytoplasm that often harbors a granular golden-yellow pigment (**e-Fig. 7.1**).*

The middle ear, or tympanic cavity, lies within the temporal bone. It is separated from the external auditory canal by the tympanic membrane, a thin fibrous sheet that has an external keratinizing squamous epithelial lining and an inner cuboidal cell lining. The middle ear contains the three auditory ossicles (malleus, incus, and stapes), ossicle ligaments, tendons of the ossicular muscles, auditory tube, the tympanic cavity itself, epitympanic recess, mastoid cavity, and chorda tympani of the facial nerve (cranial nerve VII). The auditory or eustachian tube connects the tympanic cavity with the nasopharynx. The tympanic cavity is lined by a single layer of flattened to cuboidal respiratory epithelium, whereas most of the auditory tube is lined by a low ciliated epithelium.

The inner ear is located within the petrous portion of the temporal bone and is composed of a membranous labyrinth surrounded by an osseous labyrinth. The membranous labyrinth houses the cochlea and the vestibular apparatus, both of which are supplied by cranial nerve VIII. There are several parts to the cochlea: the cochlear duct with the organ of Corti (the end organ of hearing), and the scala vestibuli and scala tympani, which hold perilymph. The organ of Corti has thousands of neurotransmitting hair cells. The vestibular apparatus, which functions in motion and position sensing, consists of three semicircular canals and the utricle and saccule. The ampullae of the canals have a sensory end organ, the crista ampullaris, with neurosensory hair cells. The utricle and saccule also possess a sensory end organ, the macula, which has neurosensory hair cells and otoliths. There is also a blind sac in the membranous labyrinth known as the endolymphatic sac, which is lined by tall columnar epithelium arranged on papillae.

II. GROSS EXAMINATION AND TISSUE SAMPLING

    A. External ear. Biopsy and excision specimens should be handled like skin specimens from other anatomic sites (see Chap. 38–40).

    B. Middle and inner ear. Samples from the middle ear are often obtained in cases of suspected cholesteatoma. For these cases, it should be noted whether bone fragments are present. Standard hematoxylin and eosin (H&E) slide preparation is sufficient. Ossicles from the middle ear can be described in a gross examination only. For middle ear and inner ear neoplasms, which are uncommon, use of ink to mark the peripheral margins is not usually necessary because these tissues are typically received as small fragments. In those rare cases in which the patient has a history of lymphoma or lymphoma is suspected clinically, fresh tissue should be processed according to the standard lymphoma work-up protocol. For all other middle ear samples, all tissue should be submitted for histological examination, with H&E slide generation.

---

*All e-figures are available online via the Solution Site Image Bank.

III. COMMON DISEASES OF THE EXTERNAL EAR

   A. Nonneoplastic diseases. The common diseases of skin that involve the pinna and external ear canal are covered in the chapters on skin (Chap. 38–40). Some diseases have a particular predilection for the skin of the ear, including gout, keloids (often secondary to ear piercing), angiolymphoid hyperplasia with eosinophilia (epithelioid or histiocytoid hermangioma), and chondrodermatitis nodularis (discussed below).

   1. Congenital anomalies of the ear that may be seen by the surgical pathologist include accessory tragi, branchial cleft abnormalities, congenital aural sinuses, and salivary gland ectopia.

   a. Accessory tragi are found at birth and clinically and macroscopically are most often solitary, sessile, or pedunculated polyps in the preauricular area. Microscopically, skin, hair follicles, and a central fibrofatty core with or without cartilage are observed (e-**Fig. 7.2**). They should not be misdiagnosed as a papilloma, fibroma, or chondroma.

   b. Anomalies of the first branchial cleft present near the ear as cysts, sinuses, and fistulas. The epithelial lining can be squamous or respiratory; Type I pure squamous cell–lined cysts can be confused with keratinous cysts. Lymphoid tissue can be found in the wall (e-**Fig. 7.3**). Type II defects can harbor skin including adnexal structures and cartilage (e-**Fig. 7.4**); associated salivary gland tissue may also be present when the process extends into or near the parotid gland.

   c. Congenital aural sinuses are distinguished from branchial cleft anomalies by location: Branchial cleft abnormalities are found in infra- or postauricular sites, whereas congenital aural sinuses are present in a preauricular location.

   2. Chondrodermatitis nodularis helicis is a condition of uncertain etiology that occurs on the skin of the external ear, usually on the upper part of the helix. Clinically, middle-aged or older, typically male, patients present with a small (<1 cm), painful nodule that can be ulcerated and can exhibit a crust. This appearance can clinically simulate actinic keratosis or squamous cell carcinoma. Microscopically, there is a somewhat funnel-shaped ulcer with associated dermal collagen edema and degeneration. There may be surrounding pseudoepitheliomatous squamous cell hyperplasia (e-**Fig. 7.5**), granulation tissue and fibrosis, and a predominantly lymphocytic inflammatory cell infiltrate, although the infiltrate can be mixed. A perichondritis with destruction of cartilage can be seen but is uncommon. Superficial or shave biopsies may show only a few of the above findings. Curettage and cautery are used for treatment, with recurrence in a minority of patients.

   3. Otitis externa is inflammation of the external auditory canal and/or pinna and is very common in clinical practice. Biopsy is generally not indicated.

   4. Necrotizing (malignant) otitis externa is usually caused by *Pseudomonas aeruginosa* infecting diabetic patients, but fungi can also be the causative agent. Microscopically, the response is one of necrotizing inflammation.

   B. Neoplasms of the external ear. The 2005 World Health Organization histological classification of tumors of the ear is given in Table 7.1. The most common neoplasms of the external ear are basal cell carcinoma and squamous cell carcinoma of the skin of the ear. Of the tumors of the external ear, only the rare ceruminous gland tumors are specific for this site.

   1. Benign ceruminous gland tumors include ceruminous adenoma, chondroid syringoma, and syringocystadenoma papilliferum. The latter two entities have the same histopathologic features as when they occur at other sites. Ceruminous adenomas are rare, and are seen in adult patients who present with a painless mass of the outer half of the external auditory canal (*Am J Surg Pathol.* 2004;28:308). Grossly, they are 0.4- to 4-cm polypoid growths. Microscopically, there are regular oxyphilic glands and small cysts lined by an inner ceruminous cell layer and an outer spindled to cuboidal myoepithelial cell layer (e-**Fig. 7.6**). Cerumen pigment, cytokeratin (CK)7 expression in ceruminal cells, and p63 and CK5/6 expression in the myoepithelial cells can be helpful in the distinction from

TABLE 7.1	2005 WHO Histological Classification of Tumors of the Ear

Tumors of the External Ear
Benign tumors of ceruminous glands
  Adenoma
  Chondroid syringoma
  Syringocystadenoma papilliferum
Cylindroma
Malignant tumors of ceruminous glands
  Adenocarcinoma
  Adenoid cystic carcinoma
  Mucoepidermoid carcinoma
Squamous cell carcinoma
Embryonal rhabdomyosarcoma
Osteoma and exostosis
Angiolymphoid hyperplasia with eosinophilia
Tumors of the Middle Ear
Adenoma of the middle ear
Papillary tumors
  Aggressive papillary tumor
  Schneiderian papilloma
  Inverted papilloma
Squamous cell carcinoma
Meningioma
Tumors of the Inner Ear
Vestibular schwannoma
Lipoma of the internal auditory canal
Hemangioma
Endolymphatic sac tumor
Hematolymphoid Tumors
B-cell chronic lymphocytic leukemia/small lymphocytic lymphoma
Langerhans cell histiocytosis
Secondary Tumors

From: Barnes L, Eveson J, Reichart P, Sidransky D, eds. *World Health Organization Classification of Tumours. Pathology and Genetics. Head and Neck Tumours.* Lyon: IARC Press: 2005. Used with permission.

adenocarcinoma and middle ear adenoma. There is about a 10% recurrence rate, which is associated with incomplete excision.

2. **Malignant tumors of ceruminous glands** include adenocarcinoma, adenoid cystic carcinoma, and mucoepidermoid carcinoma. The latter two are histologically identical to those arising in salivary glands. Ceruminous adenocarcinomas show infiltrative growth and range from cytologically bland to markedly atypical with an increase in mitotic activity. Perineural invasion is uncommon, but can be a useful diagnostic clue favoring adenocarcinoma when detected, especially in small biopsy samples. Ceruminous adenocarcinomas are locally aggressive.

3. **Other unusual neoplasms and tumorlike conditions of the external ear** include malignant melanoma, benign fibro-osseous lesion, osteoma and exostosis, and idiopathic pseudocystic chondromalacia (which is a nonneoplastic swelling of the pinna due to fluid accumulation within the cartilage of the ear).

IV. **COMMON DISEASES OF THE MIDDLE EAR**
  A. **Nonneoplastic middle ear diseases.** The common disorders include choristoma, inflammation, infection, cholesterol granuloma, and cholesteatoma.

1. **Choristomas** in the middle ear are composed of benign salivary gland, glial, or sebaceous gland tissue.
2. **Otitis media** is one of the most common diseases of childhood. Most acute purulent cases are due to bacterial infection by *Streptococcus pneumoniae* or *Haemophilus influenzae*. Tissue samples are not usually procured, but in chronic cases tissue may be removed. Microscopically, granulation tissue, scar tissue, chronic inflammation, calcific debris, and sclerotic or reactive bone can be seen. Occasionally, neutrophils and foreign body–type giant cells are present. There may be associated polypoid granulation tissue, cholesterol granulomas, cholesteatoma, or tympanosclerosis. Entrapped metaplastic glands should not be mistaken for neoplastic glands.
3. **Cholesterol granulomas** are found in a number of chronic ear diseases. Cholesterol clefts, a foreign body–type giant cell reaction, and hemosiderin deposition are characteristic.
4. **Cholesteatoma** may be congenital or acquired (*Eur Arch Otorhinolaryngol.* 2004;261:6). The congenital form is found in infants and young children, is defined as occurring in the presence of an intact tympanic membrane, and may result from an epidermoid cell rest (epidermoid formation). In the acquired form, seen mainly in older children and adults, there is an association with severe otitis media and a perforated tympanic membrane. Histologically, there are three major elements: keratin (e-Fig. 7.7), stratified squamous epithelium, and fibrous and/or granulation tissue. Downgrowth of the epithelium into underlying subepidermal connective tissue may be appreciated. Marked vascular congestion and abscess formation may also be found. Cholesteatoma is not a neoplasm, but can be locally destructive; ossicle(s) and the bony wall of the middle ear can be eroded. There is an increased cell proliferation index in the squamous epithelium of cholesteatoma (*Acta Otolaryngol.* 2003;123:377) and overexpression of cathepsin enzymes (*Laryngoscope.* 2003;113:808), abnormalities that may be related to the local growth but are not required for diagnosis.
B. **Neoplasms of the middle ear** include paraganglioma, adenoma of the middle ear, papillary tumors, meningioma, and squamous cell carcinoma (Table 7.1).
   1. **Paraganglioma** (also known as glomus tumor, glomus tympanicum, or chemodectoma) is the most common tumor of the middle ear (but still rare). It usually presents clinically with hearing loss or tinnitus in patients in the 5th and 6th decade of life. They can be solitary or part of a familial paraganglioma–pheochromocytoma syndrome caused by germline mutations in *SDHB, SDHC,* and *SDHD* genes (Nathanson K, Baysal BE, Drovdlic C, Komminoth P, Neumann HP in DeLellis RA, Lloyd RV, Heitz PU, and Eng C, eds. *Pathology and Genetics. Tumors of Endocrine Organs.* Lyon, France: IARC Press; 2004:238–242). The head and neck paragangliomas in this syndrome are bilateral/multicentric. Clinically, paraganglioma is bulging, red, pink, or bluish (and not white like a cholesteatoma). Biopsy may result in brisk bleeding.

   Microscopically, sections usually demonstrate the classical zellballen appearance with nests of small uniform epithelioid cells that have a peripheral layer of flattened cells. Sclerosis and vascularity can be pronounced in some tumors; in the former circumstance, the nested pattern may not be apparent (e-Fig. 7.8). Immunohistochemical stains can be confirmatory and particularly contributory in small biopsy samples, which may display significant crush artifact. Chromogranin A and synaptophysin immunostains are positive, whereas carcinoembryogenic antigen and keratin immunostains are negative. Only a few S-100–positive peripheral sustentacular cells may be visualized. These tumors are slow growing and can recur after surgery and/or radiation treatment. Intracranial extension develops in a small minority of patients, and about 1%–2% of patients suffer from metastatic spread. It is not possible to predict aggressive behavior based on histopathological features.
   2. **Adenoma of the middle ear** is a benign glandular neoplasm with variable neuroendocrine and mucin-secreting differentiation (*Arch Pathol Lab Med.* 2006;130:1067). The clinical presentation is an adult (mean age in the 40s)

with muffled hearing, tinnitus, and/or a sensation of pressure and/or fullness. The neoplasms are variably colored and only uncommonly penetrate through the tympanic membrane. Microscopic architectural patterns include closely packed small glands and solid and/or trabecular arrangements. The glands lack a myoepithelial layer. Cytologically, the cuboidal to columnar glandular cells are bland, with uniform small nuclei and rare nucleoli. Mitoses should not be identified. The immunoprofile includes positivity for cytokeratin and neuroendocrine markers such as chromogranin and synaptophysin. In the past, this immunophenotype was viewed as being indicative of a carcinoid tumor of the middle ear, but it is now recognized that expression of neuroendocrine markers is a characterized feature of most middle ear adenomas. Recurrence has been reported in a small minority of cases, usually after incomplete surgical excision.

3. **Papillary tumors of the middle ear** include aggressive papillary tumor, Schneiderian papilloma, and inverted papilloma types, although only a few cases of Schneiderian-type papilloma and inverted papilloma have been described. Aggressive papillary tumors are more common (*Adv Anat Pathol.* 2006;13:131), and are also known as low-grade papillary adenocarcinomas and endolymphatic sac tumors (Heffner tumor). Patients with a mean age in the 30s present with hearing difficulty and vertigo; 15% of patients have a family history of von Hippel–Lindau syndrome. Microscopically, there are complex interdigitating papillae with fibrous cores. The lining cells are cuboidal to columnar with bland nuclear cytology and eosinophilic cytoplasm. Mitoses are absent. Cystic spaces with a colloid-like material simulating thyroid follicles can be present. Immunostains show positivity for keratin, with variable S-100, glial fibrillary acid protein, and synaptophysin immunoreactivity, but thyroglobulin immunostaining is negative. Despite the bland histological appearance, the tumor is a slowly growing, locally aggressive, but nonmetastasizing neoplasm. Temporal bone invasion is common, and the tumor may extend into the cerebellum. Outcome is related to size of the tumor and adequacy of excision; radical surgical excision affords the best chance for cure. Recurrence is seen in about 20% of cases, with tumor-specific death in about 13% of patients.

4. **Meningioma in the middle ear** is a rare neoplasm that is more likely to represent secondary extension from an intracranial meningioma than from a primary middle ear meningioma. Patients with primary middle ear meningiomas present at a mean age of 50 years with hearing changes and sometimes otitis and pain (*Mod Pathol.* 2003;16:236). The histopathological features are similar to intracranial meningiomas, with meningothelial meningioma predominating (e-**Fig. 7.9**). Vimentin and epithelial membrane antigen immunostains are positive, and cytokeratin immunostains are negative. Meningiomas are slowly growing neoplasms and can recur following incomplete surgical excision. The 5-year survival is 83%.

5. **Squamous cell carcinoma in the middle ear** is uncommon and is typically advanced at presentation. Its development is not clearly related to chronic otitis media and is not related to cholesteatoma. Microscopically, the carcinoma is keratinizing and displays a variable degree of differentiation. Outcome is related to tumor extent and margin status at surgery, but not histologic grade. The 5-year survival is roughly 50% (*Int J Radiat Oncol Biol Phys.* 2007;68:1326).

6. **Other rare neoplasms of the middle ear** include embryonal rhabdomyosarcoma (e-**Fig. 7.10**), lipoma, hemangioma, osteoma, ossifying fibroma, and teratoma.

7. **Metastasis to the ear** is uncommon, accounting for only 2%–6% of all neoplasms of the ear. Most patients have known, widely disseminated cancer. The middle ear is the most common site for metastatic spread. Breast, lung, and prostate are, in order, the common primary sites of origin for the metastatic deposits.

V. NEOPLASMS OF THE INNER EAR. Vestibular schwannoma, lipoma, and hemangioma are the most common neoplasms of the inner ear. Endolymphatic sac tumors also arise in the inner ear (the aforementioned aggressive papillary tumor of the middle ear is thought to represent an endolymphatic sac tumor with extension into the middle ear).

A. Vestibular schwannoma (acoustic neuroma) is relatively common: Unilateral vestibular schwannoma accounts for 5%–10% of all intracranial tumors, and has been found in about 1% of autopsies. Bilateral vestibular schwannoma, found in 5% of all vestibular schwannoma cases, is characteristic of neurofibromatosis type 2 (an autosomal dominant condition with mutations in the NF2 gene on 22q12). Patients, who are often in their 40s or 50s, present with progressive hearing loss and tinnitus. Grossly, the size range is a few millimeters to 6 cm in maximal dimension. The smaller tumors are round to oval, whereas large tumors can assume a mushroom shape. The cut surfaces are yellow, and can exhibit hemorrhage and cystic change. Microscopically, the attributes are the same as in soft tissue schwannomas (**e-Fig. 7.11**), with Antoni A regions with Verocay bodies, and Antoni B areas. Mitotic figures should be rare. Degenerative nuclear atypia should not be taken as a sign of malignancy. S-100 immunoreactivity is strong.

B. Lipomas of the internal auditory canal resemble lipomas at other anatomic sites, except that cranial nerves VII or VIII or their branches may be present in the lipoma.

Suggested Readings

Barnes L. The eax. In: Silverberg SG, ed in chief, *Silverberg's Principles and Practices of Surgical Pathology and Cytopathology*, Philadelphia: Churchill Livingstone Elsevier; 2006:2268–2287.

Barnes L, Eveson JW, Reichart P, Sidransky D, eds. Tumors of the Ear, Chapter 7. In: *Pathology and Genetics Head and Neck Tumours*, Lyon, France: IARC Press; 2005.

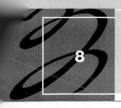

8 LUNG
Jon H. Ritter and Hannah R. Krigman

I. **NORMAL ANATOMY.** The lung is defined by airway branching, first into right and left lobes, then segments, and finally, the functional unit of the lung, the lobule. Arteries follow the airways, whereas veins and lymphatics flow toward lobular septa and finally to the hilum and main pulmonary veins. Bronchi are lined by a pseudostratified respiratory epithelium that includes goblet cells, which is separated by basement membrane from a delicate submucosa. Larger airways have a smooth muscle wall that contains minor salivary glands and a cartilaginous skeleton; bronchioles have lost the latter components. Each lobule has a central bronchovascular bundle; the interstitial space between the pulmonary artery branches and the bronchioles is eventually continuous with the alveolar interstitium. Lymph nodes occur within the lung and are discontinuous along the bronchi.

Progressive branching of the airways leads to the alveolar ducts, from which alveoli spring. Normal alveolar walls are very delicate and have a fine elastic tissue matrix. The barrier between the blood in capillaries and air in the alveolar space consists of the endothelial cell, the basement membrane, the wispy alveolar interstitium, epithelial cell basement membrane, and the flattened type 1 pneumocyte. Type 2 pneumocytes can proliferate to replace injured type 1 cells.

The visceral pleura consists of an inner vascular layer that abuts the alveolar tissue, a connective tissue layer, and an outer layer of mesothelium. The visceral pleura is reflected back at the hilum and becomes continuous with the parietal pleural layer that lines the chest cavity.

II. **SPECIMEN HANDLING AND REPORTING**
   A. **Samples.** Biopsies of lung tissue for diagnosis are obtained endoscopically (transbronchial or endobronchial biopsy), via radiologically guided procedures (usually needle core biopsies), or for peripheral disease, via wedge biopsies. Resections can involve a single lobe, two lobes, or an entire lung (pneumonectomy).
   B. **Gross examination and sampling**
      1. **Endoscopic biopsies are usually submitted in a single cassette.** The fragments are small; use of a nylon mesh bag or a filter paper wrap is preferable to submission on biopsy sponges because tissue can be compressed or lost in the pores of sponges. The number of fragments, range of size, and color should be recorded. Three hematoxylin and eosin (H&E)-stained levels should be examined. For smaller biopsies, additional unstained levels may be cut at the time of initial sectioning in case special stains are needed.

      Core biopsies of nodules presumed to represent neoplasms are performed under computed tomography (CT) guidance. They should be processed as for endoscopic biopsies.
      2. **Wedge resections are performed for either non-neoplastic or neoplastic processes.** The specimen should be measured in three dimensions and weighed. Assessment of alveolar architecture may be improved by gently inflating the specimen by injection of formalin at multiple sites. If the specimen is inflated, the gross description should include this fact. Wedge biopsies generally have multiple staple lines, which should be cut off as close to the staples as possible; ideally, sections are taken perpendicular to the staple line. The entire specimen should be submitted in non-neoplastic cases; levels are usually not necessary. If the specimen is obtained for diagnosis of a neoplasm, the presence and

dimensions of any masses should be described, as well as the distance to the staple line.

3. **Lung resections should be described as lobectomy, bilobectomy, or right or left pneumonectomy.** The specimen should be measured in three dimensions and weighed. Any additional designation by the surgeon (e.g., sutures) should be described. If a portion of chest wall is attached to the specimen, its size in three dimensions and the number of ribs or other attached structures should be noted. For lobectomy and pneumonectomy specimens, insufflation by injection of formalin into the bronchial orifices improves fixation and visualization of changes. Occasionally, obstruction of bronchi by tumor makes this technique ineffective, in which case the lung can be expanded by injection of formalin at multiple sites. The pleural surface should be described; areas of puckering, dullness, or adhesions should be noted, as should adhesions of lobes together in multilobe resections. Areas of pleural distortion over a mass should be marked with ink. The hilar area should be examined and the number and size of bronchial stumps noted. The lung can be sectioned in either parasagittal or in coronal planes; it is important to choose planes to highlight the extent of tumor, pleural invasion, invasion of adjacent structures, proximity to the hilum, and relationship to major airways and vessels. At least four sections of tumor should be taken, including one or two with the closest pleural surface (which may be at the hilum). If tumor is invading structures such as a rib, chest wall, or mediastinal soft tissue, a section that shows tumor in the lung in continuity with the involved structure should be taken. Other sections should include normal appearing lung, areas distal to the tumor that show obstructive pneumonia, and any additional nodules or lesions. The previously removed vascular and bronchial margins, hilar lymph nodes, and peribronchial lymph nodes should be submitted as well.

C. **Adjunct information.** For both non-neoplastic and neoplastic samples, the radiographic findings are an important adjunct to diagnosis. Either review the radiograph directly, or review its interpretation; old films may provide information on the pace of disease, and the distribution of abnormalities, the presence of lymphadenopathy, and the extent of disease all contribute to the final diagnosis. For non-neoplastic cases, a review of the clinical history, including the presence of systemic illnesses, medications, exposures, laboratory data including cultures, serologies, and pulmonary function tests, assists in understanding the non-neoplastic biopsy.

D. **Microscopic description**

1. A description of small biopsies includes the number of pieces and their constituent elements: alveolar tissue, bronchial wall, and superficial detached fragments of epithelium. The number of fragments is important; six fragments are considered to be representative of lung. The low-power impression of normal or abnormal alveolar architecture should be included. Expansion of the alveolar septa may be by inflammatory tissue, cellular tissue, or acellular fibrosis. Alveolar spaces may be empty, or filled with blood, histiocytes, or exudates. The vasculature may be unremarkable, thickened, show inflammation or vasculitis, or contain tumor or thromboemboli. The bronchial epithelium can be columnar, squamous, or dysplastic. The absence or presence and type of granulomas should be described. Inflammatory cells should be noted and characterized as to type and distribution, whether alveolar, septal, peribronchial, perivascular, or diffuse. The results of special stains for organisms or fibrosis should be reported.

   Biopsies for a neoplasm should include the same quantitation of the biopsy fragments as for non-neoplastic samples, as well as a description of the neoplasm. An in situ or dysplastic component should be described, if present. Detectable vascular space invasion should be noted.

2. The pathology report of wedge resections for non-neoplastic processes should contain the same information as for smaller biopsies, but should also include additional assessment of larger airways and vessels, and distribution of any non-neoplastic processes. Fibrosis, for example, can be diffuse, peripheral, or sparing the periphery. Similarly, inflammation or granulomas can be perivascular, peribronchial, or distributed along septa.

3. Definitive resections of neoplasms, from wedge resections to pneumonectomies, should provide as much information as possible. Prior sampling (endoscopic biopsy, mediastinoscopies, or previous wedge resections) and prior treatment (chemotherapy or irradiation) should be included in the pathology report. Margins should be evaluated, and the non-neoplastic lung should be described.

III. NON-NEOPLASTIC DISEASE

A. **Acute lung injury patterns.** When evaluating lung biopsies taken for medical diseases, identification of patterns of acute lung injury should be a major point of emphasis. These patterns represent the response of the lung to an acute injury, and immediately switch the diagnostic considerations away from the chronic fibrosing interstitial lung diseases. The commonly recognized patterns of acute lung injury include diffuse alveolar damage (DAD), bronchiolitis obliterans-organizing pneumonia (BOOP), and acute interstitial pneumonia (AIP). All three processes share key findings: They all feature fibrosis characterized by loose, fibroblast-rich, new fibrous tissue; they are temporally uniform; and they may be potentially reversible, at least before significant collagen fibrosis develops.

1. **DAD is the prototypical pattern of acute lung injury (e-Fig. 8.1).**[*] It is the pattern of histologic changes underlying the clinical syndrome of acute respiratory distress syndrome (ARDS), the clinical triad of diffuse lung infiltrates, hypoxemia, and decreased pulmonary compliance. DAD has myriad causes, as detailed in Table 8.1. DAD is caused by cellular injury to pulmonary epithelial and endothelial cells. The initial insult causes edema from leaky capillaries, and the sloughed cellular material and fibrinous exudate form hyaline membranes; there is often surprisingly little inflammation in this early phase, known as the exudative stage. By 5 to 6 days after the initializing event, the edema and hyaline membranes begin to disappear, and hyperplastic and regenerative type 2 pneumocytes are prominent. By 7 days, the process of organization is well underway, with interstitial and airspace fibroblastic proliferations; this stage is known as the proliferative or organizing phase. During organization, the alveolar exudates may be incorporated into the alveolar wall if proliferating type 2 pneumocytes grow on top of the exudate rather than along original alveolar basement membrane. Likewise, alveolar collapse may lead to further remodeling of prior airspaces. This process of organization and fibrosis may resolve at some point, or can continue along the path of fibrosis leading to the appearance of honeycomb lung within 3 to 4 weeks.

   The hallmark of biopsies with DAD is spatial and temporal uniformity; that is, the process is similar across all areas of the tissue because the inciting injury is diffuse. By the time most patients are sick enough to have a biopsy, this process has been present for at least several days, and hence is in the organizing phase. A search for such etiologic clues as viral inclusions, or fungus by silver stains is important, but the identification of the etiology for DAD is generally a clinicopathologic correlation exercise. When patients recover, they may essentially be normal, or may be left with some degree of lung impairment. Trichrome or similar stains may be helpful when reviewing these biopsies. Cases that show cellular fibrosis but in which trichrome stains do not show significant collagen deposition are thought to be reversible; however, after significant collagen is present in the areas of fibrosis, the process is not likely to resolve.

2. **AIP** is histologically similar to DAD, but has no definable cause and could thus also be considered as idiopathic DAD. The patients, often young adults, present with rapid onset of respiratory failure. There is often a history of a flu-like illness, and some studies have suggested that a herpes-like virus may be present in some cases. By the time patients have a biopsy, the lung almost always shows a picture identical to that of organizing phase DAD. Most patients die of disease within 2 months; this rapid form of interstitial lung disease was classically described as "Hamman–Rich syndrome."

---

[*]All e-figures are available online via the Solution Site Image Bank.

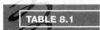

TABLE 8.1	Etiology of Diffuse Alveolar Damage

Category	Selected agents
Infections	Viruses
	Mycoplasma
	Other infections in immunocompromised patients
Inhaled toxins	Oxygen
	Smoke
Drugs	Chemotherapeutic agentss
	Amiodarone
	Nitrofurantoin
Shock	Traumatic
	Cardiogenic
	Other
Sepsis	Any organism
Miscellaneous	Radiation
	Burns
	Cardiopulmonary bypass
	Pancreatitis
	Lupus

3. **BOOP is another manifestation of acute lung injury (e-Fig. 8.2).** Some authors now advocate the substitution of the term cryptogenic organizing pneumonia (COP). Causes are detailed in Table 8.2. Idiopathic cases tend to present in older adults with fever, cough, and some dyspnea; there may be an antecedent respiratory infection. Radiographs show patchy, peripheral air-space filling opacities that may appear in different areas of the lung over time. Histologic sections show a very distinctive pattern of immature fibroblastic tissue within terminal bronchioles and alveolar ducts, which often has an elongated or "hook-like" configuration; these are often referred to as "Masson bodies" and can also be seen in peribronchiolar alveolar spaces. Because of the luminal filling of terminal bronchioles, there is often an associated localized obstructive pneumonia in the form of accumulation of lipid-filled macrophages. Because BOOP is centered on terminal airways, low-power views of wedge biopsies show a somewhat nodular configuration in contrast to the diffuse nature of injury in DAD. Thus, BOOP shares the temporal uniformity of DA, but not the homogeneous spatial appearance; nonetheless, the basic lesion of epithelial and endothelial cell injury is identical to that seen in DAD. It is important to emphasize that many, if not most,

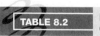

TABLE 8.2	Processes Associated with Bronchiolitis Obliterans-Organizing Pneumonia (BOOP) Response

1. Idiopathic BOOP
2. Collagen vascular diseases
3. Toxins
4. Organizing infection
5. Proximity to a variety of space-occupying lesions including neoplasms, granulomas, infarcts, and abscesses
6. Distal to bronchiectasiss
7. Acute infection
8. Immune mediated pneumonitides

cases of BOOP are secondary to some other process. Consequently, the finding of a pattern of BOOP on a biopsy should lead to a careful search of the tissue for lesions that can be associated with BOOP, such as granulomas, vasculitis, or viral inclusions indicative of viral infection.

Although the distinction between nodular versus diffuse involvement (and consequently, distinction between BOOP and DAD/AIP) may be obvious in wedge biopsies, transbronchial biopsies may show features such as organizing airspace fibrosis and type 2 pneumocyte hyperplasia without a clear indication of the spatial distribution of the process. In such cases, a more generic diagnosis of "organizing acute lung injury" may be used. This conveys the essential information for patient care—that is, the diagnosis defines the patient as having an acute injury, with attendant lung response, as opposed to a chronic idiopathic interstitial lung disease.

B. Idiopathic interstitial pneumonitis
 1. **Usual interstitial pneumonitis (UIP) is the prototypical chronic interstitial pneumonitis.** It is so named because it represents the underlying pathology in at least 80% of cases that fall under the clinical term of idiopathic pulmonary fibrosis. UIP is most often a disease of older adults, but has been reported in all age groups, including children. By the time of diagnosis, patients have often had several years of slowly developing shortness of breath. Pulmonary function tests show restrictive disease corresponding to the small lungs seen by chest x-ray examination. CT scans demonstrate honeycombing, most commonly at the lung bases and lung periphery, as well as traction bronchiectasis (e-**Fig. 8.3**). Gross examination shows coarse sponge-like lung corresponding to the honeycombing seen on radiograph. Microscopically, the disease is characterized by spatial and temporal heterogeneity. Temporal heterogeneity refers to the coexistence of old honeycomb scars (defined as cystic spaces lined by bronchiolar type epithelium) with areas of ongoing fibrosis (fibroblastic foci). The fibroblastic foci represent small areas of developing fibrosis, consistent with the insidious progression of this disease. Acute inflammation is often restricted to the honeycomb areas, which may contain mucoid debris. Spatial heterogeneity refers to the finding that the most severe fibrosis is in the subpleural areas and along lobular septa; more central parts of the pulmonary lobule typically show less severe disease. Chronic inflammation is mild and patchy within areas of fibrosis; autoimmune or connective tissue disorders (CTDs) should be considered in cases with more extensive chronic inflammation. Related changes in the lung include secondary pulmonary hypertension and type II pneumocyte hyperplasia. The clinical course both before and after diagnosis is variable; most patients die within 5 years of diagnosis, although some patients have a more protracted course. In the process known as acute exacerbation of UIP, histologic sections show DAD superimposed on a background of UIP; the precise etiology for acute exacerbation of UIP is not known (which parallels the fact that the etiology of UIP itself is generally unknown).

 2. **Nonspecific interstitial pneumonitis (NSIP) is the second most common form of idiopathic interstitial pneumonitis.** As with UIP, patients tend to be middle aged or older. Many patients have underlying CTDs such as rheumatoid arthritis or lupus. Pulmonary function tests show a restrictive pattern. CT scans disclose significant differences from those in UIP; honeycombing is rarely a prominent feature in NSIP, but ground glass opacities, linear opacities, and small nodular infiltrates are frequently present (e-**Fig. 8.4**).

 Microscopically, the process has a more homogeneous appearance than UIP. Biopsies usually lack subpleural accentuation, but instead show more uniform involvement of both central and peripheral parts of the lobule. The process is generally more cellular than UIP with a mixed interstitial acute and chronic inflammatory infiltrate. Cases may show features of organizing pneumonia or BOOP, and small nondescript granulomas may be seen in some cases. Honeycombing, if seen on microscopic sections, is usually more focal and should not be a dominant pattern. The foregoing findings are characteristic of the cellular or mixed patterns of NSIP; because they bear significant resemblance to processes such as chronic hypersensitivity pneumonia or unresolved or slowly resolving organizing pneumonia, it is not clear that cases labeled as NSIP do not represent some unusual variants of the latter groups. A third pattern of NSIP, namely the sclerotic variant, consists of hyaline-like interstitial fibrosis. Although the full characterization of NSIP is still evolving, the one unifying feature of NSIP is that the patients seem to survive longer, and with less disability, than do those patients whose biopsies show UIP.

3. **Desquamative interstitial pneumonia (DIP) and related lesions.** DIP is a rare form of interstitial pneumonia characterized by abundant macrophage exudates that fill the alveolar spaces. In most patients, this process is related to cigarette smoking, although rare examples have been reported in nonsmokers; most patients are middle aged or older. Radiographic studies are dominated by ground glass opacities reflective of the filling of alveolar spaces, and microscopic sections feature dramatic filling of the alveolar spaces by macrophages that tend to be light brown due to smoking-related pigment (e-**Fig. 8.5**). DIP is spatially homogeneous in that virtually any microscopic field from involved lung will show identical features. The alveolar walls may be thin and delicate, or may show some mild inactive hyaline fibrosis. Honeycomb changes are rare. DIP has an excellent prognosis; in cases related to cigarette use, the primary therapy is smoking cessation.

   Less dramatic findings along the same spectrum of smoking-related changes include respiratory bronchiolitis (RB) and RB–associated interstitial lung disease (RB-ILD). RB shows macrophages similar to those in DIP, but limited to the lumen of terminal airways; it is often most prominent in the upper lobes and is thought to be the precursor of centriacinar emphysema (e-**Fig. 8.6**). RB-ILD is similar with the addition of mild interstitial fibrosis surrounding the terminal bronchioles.

4. **Lymphoid interstitial pneumonitis (LIP) is another rare idiopathic form of interstitial pneumonitis.** LIP can occur in patients of any age. When LIP occurs in children, it is often a harbinger of human immunodeficiency virus (HIV) infection; similarly, LIP has been described in immunocompromised patients as a manifestation of Epstein–Barr virus (EBV) infection. Some cases of LIP are related to Sjogren's syndrome. Chest radiographs demonstrate infiltrates of a variety of patterns. Microscopically, there is diffuse expansion of the pulmonary interstitium by a mixed inflammatory cell infiltrate that includes small lymphocytes, plasma cells, germinal centers, and histiocytes. There may be some associated interstitial fibrosis. Many cases previously described as LIP likely represent examples of pulmonary mucosal associated lymphoid tissue lymphomas (MALTomas) or related neoplasms. Immunostains should show a mixed pattern of CD3-positive T cells and CD20-positive B cells. In cases of suspected LIP, flow cytometry or molecular studies to assess clonality are very useful to exclude lymphoma.

5. **Giant cell interstitial pneumonitis (GIP) is very rare.** Most cases are now known to represent a reaction to various heavy metals. Consequently, optimum diagnosis is made by the combination of accurate history and spectrophotometric analysis of lung tissue.

C. **Other noninfectious, non-neoplastic pulmonary processes**
   1. **Connective tissue diseases (CTDs).** Lung involvement in CTDs is extremely common and variable. Prominent patterns of involvement for selected disorders are summarized in Table 8.3. There is significant overlap among these entities, and assignment to a specific entity should not be made on the basis of pulmonary findings. Also, many of the lung findings in CTDs overlap with the "idiopathic" interstitial lung diseases.
   2. **Drug-induced pulmonary changes.** Prominent pathologic findings associated with drug reactions are listed in Table 8.4. It should be clear from this list that drug reactions can mimic virtually any non-neoplastic condition, which emphasizes the need for accurate history and correlation with the clinical setting.
      a. **Amiodarone.** Perhaps 5%–10% of patients experience a pulmonary complication related to amiodarone therapy. The drug inhibits phospholipase, so the hallmark of exposure is accumulation of phospholipids, which in the lung

TABLE 8.3	Pulmonary Manifestations of Connective Tissue Disorders	

Disease	Pleural changes	Pulmonary changes
Rheumatoid arthritis	Nonspecific pleuritis Necrobiotic nodules	Interstitial pneumonia and fibrosis Bronchiolitis Necrobiotic nodules Vasculitis Pulmonary hypertension Systemic amyloidosis
Systemic lupus erythematosus	Fibrinous pleuritis Effusions Pleural fibrosis	Chronic interstitial pneumonia Diffuse alveolar damage Intra-alveolar hemorrhage Vasculitis, both large vessel and capillaritis Pulmonary hypertension
Scleroderma		Interstitial fibrosis with UIP-like pattern Interstitial fibrosis with NSIP-like pattern Pulmonary hypertension
Polymyositis and dermatomyositis		Interstitial fibrosis Bronchiolitis obliterans-organizing pneumonia
Sjogren's syndrome		Lymphocytic inflammation of tracheobronchial glands, atrophy of glands Peribronchiolar lymphocytic inflammation Lymphoid hyperplasia/Lymphoid interstitial pneumonitis Lymphomas including mucosal associated lymphoid tissue lymphomas (MALTomas)

manifest as accumulations of foamy macrophages (e-**Fig. 8.7**); note that accumulation of foamy macrophages is seen in almost all patients on the drug to varying degrees, and does not by itself indicate toxicity. Toxicity occurs as early as 1 month after initiation of therapy, with an average of 10 to 12 months, and is associated with higher doses. Patients present with a variety of symptoms, such as cough, dyspnea, chest pain, fever, and myalgias. Radiographs can show a mixture of airspace infiltrates, interstitial disease, or even isolated collections. Microscopically, toxicity has several manifestations, including a cellular chronic interstitial pneumonitis, characterized by chronic inflammation in the interstitium, pneumocyte hyperplasia, and fibrosis, with foamy alveolar macrophages and lipids in cells within the interstitium and pneumocytes. Rarer cases show a dose-independent reaction that resembles hypersensitivity pneumonitis (HP). Still other cases show a pattern of DAD and/or BOOP-like injury.

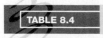

TABLE 8.4	Pulmonary Manifestations of Drug Reactions

- Chronic interstitial pneumonia
- Diffuse alveolar damage
- Bronchiolitis obliterans-organizing pneumonia
- Obliterative bronchiolitis
- Eosinophilic pneumonia
- Pulmonary hemorrhage
- Pulmonary edema
- Pulmonary veno-occlusive disease
- Large and small vessel vasculitis

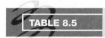 TABLE 8.5	Agents Implicated in Hypersensitivity Pneumonitis

1. Thermophilic *Actinomyces*
2. Molds
3. Animal proteins
4. Rarely, exposure to drugs (i.e., methotrexate, amiodarone)

   b. Methotrexate therapy is also commonly complicated by pulmonary toxicity (that does not seem to be related to total dose) in perhaps 5%–10% of patients. Radiographically, patients have diffuse infiltrates. Microscopically, there are multiple patterns of injury, including: (a) cellular interstitial pneumonitis, with nodular collections of lymphocytes, plasma cells, histiocytes, eosinophils, and poorly formed granulomas; (b) HP (many of these patients are on low-dose therapy); (c) BOOP (with the poorly formed granulomas); (d) DAD; and (e) severe pulmonary edema.

  3. Hypersensitivity pneumonitis (HP), also known as extrinsic allergic alveolitis (EAA), is a disease caused by exposure to organic antigens; classically the exposure is to thermophilic *Actinomyces,* but a variety of organic agents have been implicated (Table 8.5). Acute HP occurs with exposure to a large amount of antigen; within 4 to 6 hours dyspnea, cough, fever, and diffuse infiltrates develop. Pulmonary function tests show moderate to severe restriction and decreased carbon monoxide diffusing capacity (DLCO); severe hypoxemia is also present. Radiology studies show airspace disease, ground glass, and some small nodular opacities. Symptoms improve in 12 to 18 hours, and within 2 to 3 days the radiographic findings resolve. Microscopically, acute inflammation, edema, and exudates may be seen, but because of the rapid course of the disease, biopsies are rarely taken.

    Chronic HP is due to repeated or prolonged exposure to a small amount of antigen; it is typically due to episodic exposure to some organic antigen, but the offending antigen is eventually identified in only 1/3 to 1/2 of cases. Chronic HP has several histopathologic characteristic (e-Fig. 8.8), including chronic interstitial inflammation with many CD8+ T cells, vague granulomas or giant cells in the interstitium, and chronic bronchiolitis, sometimes with BOOP. Eosinophils are not part of the disease, despite the hypersensitivity label. Most patients respond to therapy (including steroids and/or removal of the offending antigen) or have stable disease, with a minority progressing to fibrosis and end-stage lung disease. There is overlap between chronic HP and some cases labeled as NSIP, and investigators have suggested that they may actually be the same process.

  4. Sarcoidosis is a systemic disease of uncertain etiology. Although some molecular genetic studies suggest that sarcoid represents a hypersensitivity-like reaction to mycobacterial infection, standard stains and cultures do not show organisms. There is frequent lung involvement, although it is usually mild, and as many as 2/3 of patients are asymptomatic. Most cases involve the hilar and mediastinal nodes, as well as the lung, but isolated involvement of either site can occur. In symptomatic patients, pulmonary function tests show mixed restriction and obstruction and decreased DLCO; lung volumes tend to be preserved.

    The basic histologic lesion of sarcoid is a noncaseating granuloma with enveloping fibrosis (e-Fig. 8.9). The individual granulomas can coalesce to form larger nodules. The granulomas follow the lymphatic routes, and so are present along airways; for this reason, transbronchial lung biopsies produce a diagnosis in up to 80% of cases. The giant cells in the granulomas may contain various structures, including Schaumann bodies, asteroid bodies, and oxalate crystals (the latter are produced endogenously by the giant cells, and thus polarizable material in the giant cells should not be taken as evidence of foreign body exposure). Sarcoid also includes varying degrees of interstitial lymphoid infiltrates. Stains for fungi and mycobacteria should be performed in all cases. Some cases otherwise typical for sarcoid show minimal central fibroinoid material in the granulomas; true caseation should raise concern that the diagnosis is not sarcoidosis.

Unusual clinicopathologic features of sarcoid include massive pleural effusions associated with chest pain, suggesting mesothelioma or pleural tumors, or one large nodule or multiple nodules with cavitation mimicking primary or metastatic tumor within the lung. Rare cases of sarcoidosis produce peripheral infiltrates that simulate eosinophilic pneumonia or granulomatous vascular impingement that can simulate veno-occlusive disease. End-stage cases often are dominated by the presence of apical bullous disease; the granulomas at this stage may be largely "burnt-out" and replaced by hyalinized fibrous tissue that tracks along the lymphatic routes.

The differential diagnosis of sarcoid is always granulomatous infection, and it is important to note that up to 10%–15% of biopsies with granulomas and negative special stains are culture-positive. Infection should always be suspected if the granulomas are necrotizing. The differential diagnosis also includes a drug reaction, berylliosis, aluminum exposure, HP, and granulomatous vasculitis.

5. **Pulmonary eosinophilic granuloma (EG; also called Langerhans cell histiocytosis or histiocytosis X) is a disease of adults, with most cases presenting in the 3rd and 4th decades of life.** There is a history of cigarette smoking in almost 90% of cases, indicating that this disease should be considered as another facet of smoking-induced lung disease. Patients with pulmonary EG usually have disease limited to lung; although some are asymptomatic, most complain of cough, dyspnea, fever, or weight loss. Pneumothorax is another documented presentation of EG. Radiologic studies show an upper lobe predominance; cysts and small stellate nodules can be seen by high-resolution CT scans. Because of the smoking history, there is often coexistent emphysema, DIP, RB, or RB-ILD.

The characteristic histologic picture of EG (e-**Fig. 8.10**) is a stellate interstitial collection, often near small airways, of eosinophils and Langerhans cells. Langerhans cells feature a unique convoluted nucleus, and a moderate amount of cytoplasm; some binucleated forms may also be present. An admixture of pigmented alveolar macrophages ("smoker's macrophages") is also often present. Langerhans cells can be easily demonstrated by immunostains for S-100 and CD1a; alveolar macrophages stain for CD68, but not S-100 or CD1a. In contrast to the cellular lesions just described, resolved or "burnt out" lesions in chronic disease may consist only of hyalinized stellate scars in the upper lung zones; immunostains may highlight a few Langerhans cells in these scars, or may be completely negative. About 10%–20% of cases progress to fibrosis, but most patients improve with cessation of smoking; rare patients develop severe pulmonary hypertension. Eosinophilic pneumonia is one important differential consideration in small biopsies, but can be easily dismissed by correlation with radiographic and clinical features; in addition, the macrophages in eosinophilic pneumonia will be negative for S-100 and CD1a. Eosinophilic pleuritis may develop after pneumothorax, and may raise concern for EG in the lung, but reactive mesothelial cells are negative for S-100 and CD1a.

6. **Lymphangioleiomyomatosis (LAM) is a disease that essentially occurs only in woman of reproductive age.** Although classified as an interstitial disease, it features preserved lung volumes, unlike most fibrosing diseases. CT scans show diffuse involvement of the lung by cysts of rather uniform size that feature some mural thickening around the cystic spaces, a finding that serves to distinguish LAM from processes such as emphysema; in fact, high-resolution CT images are so characteristic that the first pathologic specimen seen in patients is often the explanted lungs. Patients present with obstructive lung symptoms or spontaneous pneumothorax, and also may demonstrate large chylous pleural effusions. Microscopic sections of LAM (e-**Fig. 8.11**) show a proliferation of abnormal smooth muscle-like cells in the lung. In many cases these cells seem to swirl away from the native smooth muscle of airways and vessels. Vascular compromise is linked to microhemorrhages, so many cases show abundant hemosiderin within

the lung. Although LAM is centered in the lung, it also involves lymph nodes in the pulmonary hilum, mediastinum, and abdomen in many cases. The smooth muscle-like cells stain with vimentin, desmin, and smooth muscle actin, and also may express estrogen and progesterone receptor. LAM also shows cross-lineage staining with melanoma markers including HMB-45 and melan-A. In this regard, the cells of LAM share the staining attributes of the members of the perivascular epithelioid cell tumor (PEComa) family (including the sugar tumor of lung, renal angiomyolipomas, and some soft tissue tumors) (see Chap. 46). LAM also shows overlap with tuberous sclerosis (TS) in that some TS patients develop an identical cystic lung disease, and both LAM and TS share an association with angiomyolipomas in the kidney and elsewhere. The course of the disease is unpredictable; transplantation has been the only long-term option for those with severe disease.

7. **Alveolar proteinosis refers to a peculiar accumulation of intra-alveolar eosinophilic, granular periodic acid–Schiff (PAS)-positive protein and phospholipid.** It was initially reported as an idiopathic process, but a relation to immune deficiency, hematologic malignancies, infections, and various exposures is now recognized. Classic exposure-related cases are associated with massive acute silica exposure, which is believed to "poison" the alveolar macrophages and thus inhibit their ability to clear alveolar debris.

   Clinically, patients present with slowly progressive alveolar infiltrates and complain of dyspnea, cough, or sputum production with fever; CT scans show "crazy-paving" with alveolar infiltrates and septal line thickening. The diagnosis is often apparent from the milky appearance of lavage fluid; biopsies shows complete filling of the alveolar spaces by granular eosinophilic debris that is PAS-positive and diastase-resistant (e-Fig. 8.12). Findings often include cholesterol clefts (acicular clefts), globular eosinophilic debris, and macrophages. In most cases, the underlying alveolar structure appears normal, although some chronic cases may eventually show fibrosis. Secondary infection of the fluid by *Nocardia,* mycobacteria, and fungi has been reported. *Pneumocystis* infection can microscopically mimic alveolar proteinosis, although the material in alveolar proteinosis lacks the frothy appearance characteristic of *Pneumocystis* infection.

8. **Pulmonary amyloidosis occurs in several forms.**
   a. Tracheobronchial amyloidosis is rare, and features focal or diffuse amyloid deposition in the airway submucosa and around bronchial glands; the amyloid may show calcification or ossification. The patients may have symptoms of wheezing, lobar collapse, or recurrent infections, and the airways are prone to bleeding; this form does not usually feature systemic involvement.
   b. Nodular pulmonary amyloidosis is also typically confined to lung, with no systemic disease; patients are usually asymptomatic but have a well-circumscribed peripheral nodule or nodules that are evident on radiographic studies Grossly, the mass is often described as waxy or "lardaceous." Microscopic sections show nodules of amyloid with an associated foreign body reaction, lymphoplasmacytic infiltrate, and foci of calcification and metaplastic bone formation (e-Fig. 8.13).
   c. In contrast to the previous types of pulmonary amyloid, the diffuse septal form is most often seen with disseminated primary amyloidosis. Patients present with dyspnea, hypoxemia, and an increased A/a gradient. Chest x-rays show diffuse fine reticulonodular infiltrates. Microscopic sections show deposits in the alveolar interstitium, around vessels, and sometime in the airways and pleura (e-Fig. 8.14).

D. **"Allergic" diseases**
   1. **Eosinophilic pneumonia can be divided into acute and chronic forms.** The acute forms include the "simple form," also known as Loeffler's syndrome; this is an acute, self-limited process with fleeting infiltrates and peripheral blood eosinophilia, and is rarely biopsied. The tropical form is usually linked to filaria infection, and also presents as an acute illness. The chronic form is more likely to require biopsy for diagnosis.

Chronic eosinophilic pneumonia (CEP) has a variable presentation, from acute illness with fever, dyspnea, and weight loss, to vague respiratory complaints. Many patients have a history of asthma, and laboratory tests reveal elevated blood immunoglobulin E (IgE) and peripheral blood eosinophilia. Chest x-rays show patchy nonsegmental infiltrates, often peripheral, that may cross fissures, a pattern that is sometimes described as the "photographic negative of pulmonary edema." There are myriad underlying causes; major categories include drugs (antibiotics such as nitrofurantoin, sulfonamides, penicillins, anti-inflammatory agents, and chemotherapeutics), fungus (*Aspergillus* and *Candida*), parasites, nickel vapor, and idiopathic cases. Histologic sections of CEP (e-**Fig. 8.15**) show an alveolar filling process consisting of a mixture of eosinophils and macrophages. Necrosis of eosinophils may be present, forming an "eosinophilic abscess." Charcot–Leyden crystals will also be present, as well as interstitial and perivascular eosinophils, lymphocytes, plasma cells, and areas of BOOP.

2. **Mucoid impaction of bronchi (MIB) is the filling of bronchi by viscous mucus,** usually associated with another underlying disease such as asthma, cystic fibrosis, or chronic bronchitis. Patients present with evidence of lobar collapse or an irregular branching mass-like density. Histologic sections of the impacted material in most cases show "allergic mucin" that consists of laminated collections of eosinophils, eosinophil debris, and mucinous exudates. Fungal hyphae, most often *Aspergillus* (e-**Fig. 8.16**), may also be present on a pattern that overlaps with allergic bronchopulmonary aspergillosis (ABPA). A related process is plastic bronchitis, which is impaction of airways by neutrophilic debris.

3. **ABPA is a related form of hypersensitivity to fungal organisms, most often *Aspergillus*.** The disease almost always occurs in asthmatic patients, and is usually diagnosed by a combination of clinical features that include pulmonary infiltrates and proximal bronchiectasis, and skin testing that shows reaction to fungal antigens, precipitating antibodies to fungal antigen, elevated IgE levels, and peripheral blood eosinophilia. Tissue sections show a combination of eosinophilic pneumonia, MIB, and bronchocentric granulomatosis (granulomatous destruction of bronchioles).

E. **Vasculitis and related diseases** constitute an important collection of lung diseases, many of which have been historically included in the category of "angiitis and granulomatosis." Patients with vasculitis and related lesions often present with alveolar hemorrhage, the cause of which can be categorized (Table 8.6) based on the histologic finding of capillaritis (see below) and the immunofluorescence findings. Large pulmonary vessels may also be involved by vasculitis (e-**Fig. 8.17**); common etiologies of large vessel pulmonary artery vasculitis are presented in Table 8.7.

1. **Wegener's granulomatosis is the prototypical lung vasculitis.** It most often presents in middle age with pulmonary symptoms including cough, hemoptysis,

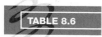

TABLE 8.6   **Pulmonary Hemorrhage Syndromes**

Syndrome	Capillaritis	Immunofluorescence
Goodpasture's	+/–	+, Linear staining
Idiopathic hemosiderosis	–	–
Wegener's	+	–
Microscopic polyarteritis	+	–
Collagen vascular disease (SLE)	+	–
Idiopathic rapidly progressive GN	+	+, Granular staining
Toxins	–	–

Abbreviations: SLE, systemic lupus erythematosus G.

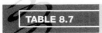

TABLE 8.7	Differential Diagnosis of Pulmonary Large Vessel Vasculitis
Involvement by systemic vasculitides	Polyarteritis nodosa, Behcet's, Takayasu's, giant cell arteritis
Classic causes	Wegener's, necrotizing sarcoid granulomatosis, Churg–Strauss syndrome
Other primary entities with large vessel vasculitis	Collagen vascular disease, malignancy, toxins and drugs
Secondary	Infection, pulmonary hypertension, others

and fever. Other patients present with upper respiratory complaints or renal failure, depending on the dominant sites of disease. Chest radiographs may show alveolar filling due to hemorrhage, multiple nodules with cavitation, or even a single massive nodule. Microscopic features in the lung reflect a classic triad of findings (e-**Fig. 8.17**): (a) Vasculitis which involves arteries, veins, and capillaries (capillaritis). Acute vascular lesions show fibrinoid necrosis; chronic lesions may show only vascular scarring or perivascular chronic inflammation. Capillaritis consists of neutrophils, nuclear dust, and fibrin microthrombi in lung capillaries, analogous to leukocytoclastic vasculitis in the skin. (b) Necrosis that is often described as geographic necrosis, and classically has an abscess-like appearance with a hematoxyphilic hue, surrounded by pallisaded histiocytes. (c) Granulomatous inflammation composed of palisades of histiocytes, scattered giant cells, and poorly formed granulomas.

Other microscopic features can include acute or chronic alveolar hemorrhage; airway disease including bronchocentric granulomatosis-like lesions, BOOP, chronic bronchitis and bronchiolitis; interstitial lesions including fibrosis and nonspecific chronic inflammation; DAD; and pleural lesions such as fibrinous pleuritis, granulomas, or chronic inflammation. Serology studies in most cases of Wegener's reveal anti-neutrophil cytoplasmic antibodies with a cytoplasmic staining pattern (c-ANCA) positivity; the anti-neutrophil antibodies will show a cytoplasmic pattern of staining, and PR3 is usually the antigen. Rarely, ANCA will be positive with a Perinuclear Pattern (PANCA).

2. **Microscopic polyarteritis (MPA) is the lung equivalent of leukocytoclastic vasculitis.** It is often associated with p-ANCA and has many other associations including drug-related cases, infection (hepatitis B, bacteria), Henoch–Schönlein purpura, collagen vascular disease, cryoglobulinemia, and idiopathic cases. The basic lesion is capillaritis, which has two main features: neutrophils in the alveolar septae and capillary walls with neutrophilic nuclear dust, and microscopic fibrin thrombi in capillaries (e-**Fig. 8.18**). Arteriolitis or venulitis are also often present. Because the differential diagnosis includes acute lung injury or acute pneumonia, MPA is a diagnosis of exclusion.

3. **Churg–Strauss syndrome (allergic angiitis and granulomatosis) is another ANCA-related vasculitis.** Nearly all patients have a history of asthma. Many patients also have skin lesions, neuropathy, central nervous system (CNS) disease, or heart failure; most cases have been diagnosed by biopsy of sites other than lung. The histopathologic findings are a combination of two features: (a) vasculitis that can affect both arteries and veins, with giant cell infiltration of vessel walls; there may also be transmural eosinophilia with fibrinoid necrosis and small pallisaded granulomas and (b) eosinophilic infiltrates that resemble eosinophilic pneumonia consisting of a combination of histiocytes and eosinophils that fill alveoli.

F. **Bronchiolitis**
   1. **Obliterative bronchiolitis (OB; constrictive bronchiolitis, bronchiolitis obliterans), although it has a name that is similar to BOOP, is a completely different disease that is characterized by the progressive narrowing and luminal compromise of small airways by subepithelial fibrosis.** Conditions

TABLE 8.8	Causes of Obliterative Bronchiolitis

- Idiopathic
- Chronic lung allograft rejection
- Graft-versus-host disease
- Immunodeficiency states
- Drugs (penicillamine)

- Rheumatoid arthritis
- Postinfection (viruses)
- "Pop-corn lung"
- Inhaled toxins

associated with this process, many of which have some immunologic basis, are listed in Table 8.8. Patients present with insidious onset of shortness of breath and obstructive pulmonary functions with air-trapping. Wedge biopsies are often required for diagnosis, and it is common to see a spectrum of small airway changes in such biopsies ranging from virtually normal, to partial scarring, to total luminal obliteration by fibrous tissue (e-Fig. 8.19). Inflammation is variable, and there will be mucus trapped distal to areas of severe luminal compromise. Although the disease may stabilize for some time, the changes are generally irreversible.

2. **Cellular bronchiolitis** is a descriptive name given to forms of bronchiolitis that feature marked acute and chronic bronchiolar inflammation. Conditions associated with this lesion are listed in Table 8.9.

IV. **INFECTIOUS PROCESSES**
   A. **Viral infections.** Typically, viral infections of the lung are self-limited and do not require biopsy for diagnosis. In contrast, in the setting of immunocompromise or severe pulmonary dysfunction from infection, an attempt to identify the etiology of pneumonia by tissue biopsy is often made. Viral cultures may require 1 to 4 weeks for growth, so in some instances a biopsy can provide a specific diagnosis in far less time. In addition to the findings in H&E-stained slides, immunostains, electron microscopy, and serology can be used to increase diagnostic sensitivity.
      1. **Cytomegalovirus (CMV)** typically affects immunocompromised patients; because most people are exposed to CMV in childhood, many cases represent re-activation of latent infection. Patients may develop fever, cough, or shortness of breath. Chest x-rays show diffuse infiltrates, and biopsies show interstitial pneumonitis as well as DAD or nodular inflammation. Enlarged cells with nuclear and/or cytoplasmic inclusions are pathognomic for CMV infection. In H&E-stained sections, nuclear inclusions have an eosinophilic core (6 μm) with a surrounding cleared zone, whereas the cytoplasmic deposits are basophilic (e-Fig. 8.20). Epithelial cells, vascular cells, and even stromal cells can exhibit inclusions. Immunohistochemistry for CMV will decorate the enlarged cells; electron microscopy demonstrates virions in the inclusions, whereas a PAS stain with diastase highlights the cytoplasmic deposits.
      2. **Herpesvirus (HSV).** Both HSV types I and II can induce pneumonitis, and immunocompromised hosts are more prone to Herpes viral pneumonia. Clinically, HSV pneumonia may result from extension of upper airway disease with primarily bronchiolar inflammation, or from systemic infection which presents as multiple small perivascular inflammatory nodules. Three findings are characteristic

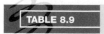

TABLE 8.9	Conditions Associated with Cellular Bronchiolitis

- Infections: bacteria, viral, mycoplasma
- Toxin/fume exposures
- Asthma
- Bronchiectasis
- Central obstruction

- Collagen vascular diseases (i.e., Sjogren's syndrome)
- Wegener's granulomatosis
- Transplant rejection/graft-versus-host disease
- Diffuse pan-bronchiolitis (Homa's disease)

of HSV: necrosis; individual cells with inclusions (e-**Fig. 8.21**) (featuring eosinophilic nuclear inclusions with perinuclear clearing; single cells with amphophilic nucleoplasm may represent early inclusions); Herpes viral giant cells (which contain two or more nuclei with ground glass central nuclear clearing and coarsely granular, sharply defined nuclear borders; the nuclei are often molded against one another). Immunohistochemistry using antibodies to HSV decorates the giant cells and the individual cells with inclusions.

3. **Varicella zoster (VZV)** is the causative agent for chicken pox and shingles. Primary infection in healthy adults and immunocompromised children can result in pneumonia. The underlying lung injury pattern can be either DAD with hyaline membranes and proteinaceous exudates, or nodular inflammation with central necrosis that calcify and persist on chest x-ray. Biopsies of VZV infections show giant cells similar to those of HSV.

4. **Adenovirus infection generally presents with symptoms typical of an upper respiratory infection;** pneumonia develops in a small percentage of healthy and immunocompromised children and adults. Two patterns of infection evolve. Some patients develop necrotizing bronchiolitis and pneumonia, whereas others respond with DAD with hyaline membranes and exudates. In adenoviral infections, both alveolar lining cells and bronchial epithelial cells may exhibit blurred and hyperchromatic nuclear chromatin (so-called smudge cells) (e-**Fig. 8.22**). The bronchial damage of adenovirus may result in fibrosing or constrictive bronchiolitis.

5. **Respiratory syncytial virus (RSV)** affects primarily small children and infants; premature infants and immunocompromised children are particularly prone to infection. RSV infection exhibits some seasonality, and is more common in fall and winter. RSV can induce bronchiolitis with symptoms of cough, wheezing, and respiratory distress. Biopsies show necrotizing bronchiolitis and/or interstitial pneumonia.

6. **Measles virus.** With the advent of vaccination, infection by measles virus is rare, and evolution to pneumonia rarer. Most patients are immunocompromised, and the characteristic skin rash is present. The underlying pathology is DAD, with associated individual and giant cells with viral inclusions; the alveolar spaces may contain exudates, and necrosis may be present. Both eosinophilic intranuclear and cytoplasmic inclusions develop in both alveolar and vascular lining cells. Measles pneumonia features a distinctive multinucleate giant cell thought to derive from coalescence of type II pneumocytes, the Warthin–Finkeldey giant cell, which contains up to 60 nuclei.

7. **Parainfluenza and influenza generate nonspecific patterns,** consisting of varying degrees of DAD, bronchial necrosis, and peribronchial inflammation.

B. **Bacterial infections**

1. **Mycoplasma** induces acute and chronic bronchiolitis, with necrosis and denudation of bronchial epithelium. The bronchial lumina may contain acute inflammatory cells admixed with denuded epithelium. Acute and chronic inflammatory cells often traverse the bronchial wall. Alveolar spaces may exhibit bronchopneumonia, with BOOP or DAD.

2. **Mycobacterial infections.** Infections with mycobacteria are typically grouped into tuberculosis (TB) and other (atypical) mycobacterial infections. The most common stain used to demonstrate organisms in tissue sections is the Ziehl–Neelsen stain; immunofluorescent (auramine–rhodamine) and immunohistochemical stains can also be used to identify mycobacteria. Polymerase chain reaction (PCR)-based genetic methods can also be used to detect (and speciate) the organism in tissue sections.

   a. **TB.** Multidrug resistance has emerged in this organism and, consequently, the pathologic spectrum of tubercular infection is expanding. The causative organism is *Mycobacterium tuberculosis*, which is transmitted via inhalation of organisms. Histologically, the tubercular granuloma is a classic pallisaded necrotizing granuloma. Granulomas may caseate and coalesce, creating nodules with central necrosis, or even cavitary masses. Organisms may be found in multinucleate giant cells or at the periphery of necrosis (e-**Fig. 8.23**). Lymph nodal involvement may be present. Miliary TB is unlikely to be sampled in biopsy or resection specimens.

b. Atypical mycobacterial infection. *Mycobacterium avium intracellulare* (MAI) is the most common of the atypical mycobacterial infections, and is more common among immunocompromised patients, in whom it presents with nonspecific fever and malaise. Radiographs show diffuse or patchy infiltrates. Histologic findings vary from more typical non-necrotizing punctuate granulomas, to bronchiolitis, to necrotizing granulomatous pneumonia, to diffuse pneumonitis (in which abundant pneumocytes in alveoli or interstitium are present and contain abundant organisms by acid-fast stains).

C. Fungal infections

1. *Candida* **infection arises in several contexts.** Mucocutaneous candidiasis can arise in immunocompetent adults, but arises more frequently in immunocompromised patients; the trachea or bronchial tree can have plaques of fungus admixed with desquamated cells and neutrophils. Impaired host defenses potentiate invasive disease; in the lungs, vascular invasion results in hemorrhagic necrosis. Direct inoculation into the bloodstream from iatrogenic sources (catheters, surgery) or other inoculation (drug abuse) results in disseminated disease. Lung transplant patients can develop infection at the sites of anastomosis. *C. albicans* is the most prevalent species; other species more often infect compromised hosts. All species exhibit the same basic morphology: nonbranching, aseptate pseudohyphae forming "box-car" like chains of cells; yeast forms bud from pseudohyphae (e-**Fig. 8.24**). Yeast forms are visible on H&E, PAS, or silver stains.

2. **Mucormycosis.** Infection by several members of the Phycomycetes class result in clinically and morphologically identical disease, including *Mucor, Absidia,* and *Rhizopus,* among others. Almost all cases occur in the setting of diabetic ketoacidosis (sinonasal or rhinocerebral disease) or immunosuppression from hematologic malignancies. Lung involvement may be the primary focus, or develop secondary to head and neck disease. Lung lesions are typified by hemorrhagic pneumonia; fungal thrombi with distal infarction are often present. The dual circulation of the lung (bronchial and pulmonary arterial systems) results in perfusion of infarcted areas with hemorrhagic necrosis, associated with varying amounts of inflammation. Keys to identification of these organisms include the finding of wide, ribbon-like nonseptate hyphae with irregular wide angle branching. The pseudohyphae are often described as "empty" and stain poorly with most special stains.

3. *Aspergillus* **species cause a wide spectrum of disease, dependent on both host immune status and site of growth.** Colonization with *Aspergillus* can induce an allergic response, including ABPA, sinusitis, and HP; *Aspergillus* can also colonize mucus or grow in a pre-existing cavity, and sinus or cavitary lung lesions both can harbor fungus balls. Transplant anastomoses are also prone to colonization by *Aspergillus* species (e-**Fig. 8.25**). The characteristic lung lesion is the target lesion with a sharply delineated hemorrhagic border, which reflects the fact that the fungus is frequently vasoinvasive and produces hemorrhagic infarcts. In well-preserved areas, organisms have relatively uniform septa that are thinner than those of *Mucor.* The hyphae branch at ~45 degrees; the reproductive form (fruiting body) is only rarely seen in tissues. Degenerate hyphae can be mistaken for *Mucor,* with empty or dilated forms; acute angle branching, occasional septa, and more intact forms indicate the correct diagnosis.

4. *Cryptococcus.* The most common pathogen of this germ is *C. neoformans,* which is usually an opportunistic infection but rarely also infects normal hosts after massive exposure. The common portal of entry is the lungs; patients remain virtually asymptomatic while the fungus spreads to other sites. The organism can be seen in the lung as "naked masses of organisms," as intracellular forms resembling those of histoplasmosis, or in granulomas with surrounding fibrosis (so-called "cryptococcomas") (e-**Fig. 8.26**). The organisms are larger than *Candida* or *Histoplasma,* with an average diameter of 4 to 10 μm; only yeast forms are found in tissue. The diameter of cryptococcal forms varies in large part with

capsule thickness, a function of host immune status, and mucicarmine stains the capsule strongly (generally considered a diagnostic feature). Capsule-deficient forms are common in cancer or acquired immunodeficiency syndrome (AIDS) patients, and may be much more difficult to diagnose definitively.

5. **Blastomycosis is generally seen in the middle of the United States.** Infection usually involves lungs and skin; spore inhalation is the mode of transmission for virtually all cases. Pulmonary blastomycosis takes several forms; the most common is a solitary focus of infection with variable associated lymph nodal disease, which usually heals and leaves a fibrous scar. Progressive disease is less common; infection spreads throughout the lung as miliary foci that range from neutrophil-rich abscesses to tubercle-like granulomas. The causative agent maintains a variably sized yeast form in tissue ranging from 5 to 25 μm, and has a thick, refractile, double-contoured wall; unlike *Cryptococcus*, this wall is negative or very weakly mucin-positive (e-**Fig. 8.27**).

6. **Histoplasmosis.** In the United States, infection is usually caused by *H. capsulatum* from bird or bat droppings. In tissue, the fungus reverts to a primitive yeast, 2 to 5 μm in diameter, with occasional unequal budding. Primary histoplasmosis produces a mild, self-limited febrile illness in most cases, with hyalinized granulomas (e-**Fig. 8.28**), but can result in a progressive, disseminated, fatal disease. Cases with active disease can also produce a granulation tissue-like pattern with vague granulomas. The organism can also induce secondary scarring forms of inflammation, such as sclerosing mediastinitis with calcified granulomas, in which organisms are often not identified. Rare cases manifest as diffuse growth within macrophages.

7. **Coccidiomycosis** is caused by *Coccidioides immitis*, a soil-borne saprophyte typically found in the southwestern United States. Patients typically have travel histories to that region, and present with an acute febrile illness (some infections are asymptomatic). Infection develops in both immunocompetent and immunocompromised individuals. The inhaled organisms transform into spherules, thick-walled sacs 60 to 80 μm in diameter containing multiple endospores (e-**Fig. 8.29**); reproduction in tissue results from rupture of the spherule with release of endospores. Microscopically, the organisms create a nodule, typically with noncaseating granuloma formation; cavitation may occur. Lymph node involvement may be present, and disseminated infection may result. The organisms can be demonstrated with Gomori's Methenamine Silver (GMS) or PAS stains.

8. **Pneumocystis carinii pneumonia (PCP).** *Pneumocystis carinii* was formerly considered a parasite, but genetic analysis suggests that it is best classified as a fungus. Infection is generally seen among immunocompromised patients. Chest x-ray classically shows diffuse infiltrates that correspond to the diffuse alveolar infiltrates that are almost diagnostic microscopically (e-**Fig. 8.30**). Cytologically, the infiltrate exfoliates in lavage specimens as alveolar casts. PCP can induce interstitial pneumonitis or granulomatous inflammation; these variant forms are often seen in chronic disease or, with partially treated disease, may progress to cavitating or cystic disease in the upper lobes, and are associated with extrapulmonary disseminated disease. The cysts stain well with GMS in most cases; in degenerate cases, immunostains may be of some help. The organism has a helmet or cup shape, often referred to as a "dented ping-pong ball."

D. **Parasite infections**

Dirofilariasis. *Dirofilaria* are nematodes, the most common pathogen of which is *D. immitis,* the common dog heartworm. Although this parasite does not have a life cycle in the human host, occasional infection can develop with adult nematodes via transmission by a mosquito bite. Infection can result in noncaseating granulomas presenting as a nodule in the lung (or other organ). Cross-sections of the organism's refractile cuticle 10 to 14 μm in greatest diameter may be seen in histologic sections. Endovascular thrombi with organisms have been reported as well.

V. **SELECTED PNEUMOCONIOSES**

A. **Asbestosis is an interstitial lung disease caused by asbestos.** It usually occurs in workers heavily exposed for a prolonged period of time. There is often a long latency period, usually at least 15 years, between exposure and the disease. Mild disease shows no symptoms; with increasing severity, patients complain of dyspnea, dry cough, weight loss, and chest pain. Radiographic findings are characterized by small irregular opacities, most prominent in the bases of the lung. The American Thoracic Society has defined six clinical criteria of a clinical diagnosis of asbestosis, including exposure, a latency period, rales, decreased lung volumes and DLCO by pulmonary function tests, and chest x-ray infiltrates. Thankfully, pathologic criteria include just two required findings: the presence of peribronchiolar fibrosis (*fibroelastosis*) and associated asbestos bodies (e-**Fig. 8.31**). Grading of asbestosis can be performed: grade 1 = fibrosis confined to respiratory bronchioles; grade 2 = fibrosis involves alveolar ducts or two tiers of alveoli; grade 3 = fibrosis involves all alveoli between two bronchioles; grade 4 = honeycombing. The lungs show a high fiber burden: 98%–99% of cases have at least 2000, and most have 10,000 to 100,000 or more asbestos bodies per gram of wet lung tissue, which correlates to at least several asbestos bodies per tissue slide in the majority of cases (iron stains often help to demonstrate asbestos bodies). If pathologic examination of biopsy or lung resections suggests asbestosis, or if there is clinical suspicion for asbestosis, it is prudent to set tissue aside for fiber analysis (fiber studies on either fresh lung tissue or formalin fixed and embedded tissue), although it is not required for diagnosis in most cases. Classically, asbestosis is required to attribute pulmonary carcinomas to asbestos exposure; asbestosis plus smoking increases the risk for lung carcinomas by a multiplicative factor, to perhaps 50X nonsmoking, nonasbestotic controls. Pleural plaques and mesothelioma, which are also asbestos-related pleuropulmonary lesions, are discussed in the chapter on serosal membranes (Chap. 11).

  B. Silicosis is produced by silica deposition in the lung. Occupations at risk include sand-blasting, grinding, mining, plastering, and masonry, among many others. Silicosis typically produces infiltrates in the mid-lung zones, in contrast to other types of pulmonary fibrosis. Lymph nodes in the chest will also show characteristic "egg-shell" calcifications on x-ray. The characteristic lung lesion is the silica nodule; nodules have a lymphangitic distribution, so are seen along the bronchovascular tree and in the pleura (e-**Fig. 8.32**). Early nodules are cellular and are composed of a swirling collection of fibrohistiocytic cells; birefringent particles can be seen in these nodules with polarized microscopy. Older lesions become progressively hyalinized; they may coalesce to form irregular masses that can mimic pulmonary neoplasms. The relationship of silicosis to the development of pulmonary neoplasms is debated, but appears to be a small risk, if present at all. Nodules may also include other material such as iron or carbon, in which case a diagnosis of mixed dust fibrosis is appropriate.

VI. PULMONARY TRANSPLANTATION

  A. Gross processing of transplant specimens. Pulmonary transplantation is now a well-established therapy for various end-stage lung diseases, including emphysema/chronic obstructive pulmonary disease, cystic fibrosis, lymphangioleiomyomatosis, pulmonary hypertension, and pulmonary fibrosis of various causes. Examination of the explanted, native lungs should include thorough documentation of the underlying disease process. A minimum of one section per lobe should be submitted for diffuse processes, as well as sections of the hilar lymph nodes. Cases of pulmonary hypertension may require additional sections to document plexiform lesions, and any mass or focal abnormality should be sampled thoroughly. Examination should be comprehensive enough to exclude foci of malignancy, or infections which may recur, due to the immunocompromised status of transplant recipients.

    The allograft is most often surveyed by transbronchial biopsy, and occasional wedge biopsies, both at scheduled protocol intervals as well as in response to changes in clinical condition. A minimum of five pieces of alveolar tissue is considered adequate for assessment in this setting. In general, three levels of H&E-stained sections are obtained; some authors advocate protocols with adjunct special stains for infectious organisms on all biopsies. We reserve such stains for cases with suggestive H&E findings.

B. **Microscopic features of transplant biopsies.**
   1. **Preservation injury is the first change seen in post-transplant biopsies.**
   This change reflects ischemic damage that develops in the lung in the interval
   between removal from the donor and re-implantation. Preservation injury produces a picture of classic lung injury that may exhibit features of DAD or BOOP
   (e-**Fig. 8.33**). The appearance sometimes suggests viral infection, but for biopsies
   taken in the first 1 to 2 weeks after transplant, it is generally too early for opportunistic infections to become manifest. One important differential diagnosis for
   early acute graft injury is humoral or hyperacute rejection (discussed below).
   2. **Opportunistic infections.** Biopsies after the first week or two must be surveyed
   for opportunistic infections, the most frequent of which is CMV, the features
   which are detailed above (IVA1.) (e-**Fig. 8.20**). Important clues of CMV infection include interstitial neutrophils and alveolar fibrin exudates, findings that
   warrant immunostains for CMV because transplant patients may not always
   develop classic inclusions. Importantly, CMV may produce perivascular inflammation, a finding that mimics acute rejection. Other viral infections often seen
   include HSV (e-**Fig. 8.21**) and adenovirus (e-**Fig. 8.22**); a variety of nonspecific pneumonitis patterns may represent other viruses without pathognomonic
   features. The results of culture, serologic, and molecular tests for infectious organisms must be integrated with biopsy data by the transplant clinician.
      Because most transplant patients currently receive prophylactic therapy
   against *Pneumocystis* infection, it is a rare complication. Fungal infections seen
   more commonly are *Aspergillus* or *Candida* colonization of the bronchial tissue
   in the region of the airway anastomosis, likely related to tissue ischemia (e-**Fig.
   8.25**); invasive growth within the lung is much less common. The presence of
   foamy macrophages in a transbronchial biopsy may be an indicator of fungal
   infection and should be followed with silver stains to exclude intrahistiocytic
   organisms such as *Histoplasma*.
   3. **Acute rejection is another primary concern in all follow-up biopsies.** The
   2007 revised lung allograft rejection scheme is provided in Table 8.10. The basic lesion of acute rejection is lymphocytic infiltration surrounding blood vessels and airways. The perivascular inflammation is reflected in the "A" scores
   (e-**Fig. 8.34**). T cells are the main cell type present in acute rejection; more severe
   rejections feature larger, more active cells, and will also show eosinophils and
   neutrophils; see Table 8.11 for more details.
      Airways are another target of rejection and are reflected in the "B" scores
   (e-**Fig. 8.35**, Table 8.11). Airway inflammation is less specific for rejection, and
   can be seen with chronic airway infections, obstruction, and preservation injury, among other causes. In general, A and B grades tend to follow each other,
   although they can be discordant, particularly if small biopsies are obtained.

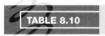

TABLE 8.10	Revised Scheme for Lung Allograft Rejection*
A: Acute rejection	**B:** Small airway inflammation/ lymphocytic bronchiolitis
A0: None	B0: None
A1: Minimal	B1R: low grade (previous B1, B2)
A2: Mild	B2R: high grade (previous B3, B4)
A3: Moderate	BX: ungradable
A4: Severe	
C: Chronic airway rejection - Bronchiolitis obliterans	
C0: absent	
C1: present	
D: Chronic vascular rejection	

*After: Stewart S, Fishbein MC, Snell GI, et al. Revision of the 1996 Working Formulation for the
standardization of nomenclature in the diagnosis of lung rejection. *J Heart Lung Transplant.* 2007;26:122.

TABLE 8.11   **Key Characteristics/Features in the Grading of Lung Allograft Cellular Rejection**

"A" lesions

Grade	Circumferential perivascular infiltrates	Cytologic features of infiltrate	Endothelialitis	Airway infiltrate
A0	None	N/A	N/A	Usually absent
A1	Rare, hard to see at scanning power 1- to 2-cell-thick cuffs	Small, "resting" lymphocytes	Usually absent	Often modest
A2	More vessels with infiltrate, easily seen at scanning power, 2- to 5-cell-thick cuffs	More "activated" lymphocytes, also eosinophils	Sometimes	Common
A3	Often many vessels, infiltrates into adjacent septa, "stellate"	More activated, many eosinophils, can be neutrophils	Almost always	Usually present
A4	May be confluent, Associated lung injury	Similar to A3	Almost always, vasculitis-like	Usually present, severe

"B" lesions

Grade	Severity	Epithelial damage
B0	None	N/A
B1R	Mild	No
B2R	Moderate to severe	Yes, individual cell apoptosis, to ulcers, or total denudation of epithelium

Humoral rejection is a form of acute rejection that has been recognized more recently. It often occurs in cases that show donor–recipient cross-match positivity in which the recipient has anti-donor antibodies, and is a similar process to hyperacute rejection. Clinically, there may be immediate graft dysfunction, noted even in the operating room, as a result of extensive vascular thrombosis and acute inflammation. Histologically, the features are still being defined, but findings include neutrophil infiltrates in the interstitium and small-vessel fibrinoid vasculitis that may lead to graft damage including necrosis and hemorrhage. In some cases of suspected humoral rejection seen outside of the immediate postoperative period, the changes may be much more subtle; it has been suggested that immunostains for C4d may be helpful to identify these cases of humoral rejection.

4. **Chronic airway rejection is a major problem in lung transplantation.** Bronchiolitis obliterans syndrome (BOS) is the clinical feature of chronic airway rejection, defined by a drop of forced expiratory volume (FEV) below 80% of the post-transplant maximum value. Chronic airway rejection is reflected in the "C" score. The pathologic lesion is subepithelial fibrosis of airways that leads to a picture of OB (e-**Fig. 8.36**). This subepithelial fibrosis pushes the mucosa toward the center of the lumen, with progressive luminal compromise; the findings in individual airways range from partial eccentric thickening, to complete obliteration of the airway resulting in a small fibrous scar next to an accompanying artery. Air-trapping and features of localized obstructive pneumonitis may also be seen due to bronchiolar dysfunction. The development of chronic rejection correlates with increasing episodes of acute rejection, and also with the severity of the lymphocytic infiltrate around airways, although the mechanisms of chronic rejection are still poorly understood.

5. **Post-transplant lymphoproliferative disorder (PTLD) is another serious post-transplant process;** changes in immunosuppressive regimens have resulted in a decreased incidence of the disease. In lung transplant patients, there is a propensity for PTLD to develop in the transplanted lung, although lymph nodes, the gastrointestinal tract, and tonsils appear to be other preferred sites. The vast majority of cases, in particular those that occur early in the transplant course, are EBV-positive, with a B cell phenotype. There should be a high index of suspicion for PTLD in any lung allograft biopsy that shows an intense infiltrate with cytologic atypia or necrosis, or where the clinical history suggests nodules or a mass. Cases usually fall into three general categories: plasma cell hyperplasia, consisting of cases that show low-grade findings; polymorphous PTLD, which is composed of a mixed population of atypical lymphoid cells; and monomorphous PTLD, consisting of cases that consist of a monotonous population of high grade, malignant-appearing cells (e-**Fig. 8.37**). Monomorphous cases are much less likely to regress following diminution of immunosuppression, as compared to the lower grade lesions; thus, higher grade cases are likely to require cytotoxic therapy. In allograft biopsies, if there is a question of PTLD versus a rejection-related infiltrate, a simple panel of CD3, CD20/CD79a, and EBV studies will provide dichotomous results: The infiltrate in severe rejection or infections is almost always a CD3-predominant infiltrate, whereas the infiltrate in PTLD is positive for CD20 and CD79a, as well as EBV, in the great majority of cases. Adjunctive studies to indicate clonality may also be of value in terms of diagnosis, classification, and prognosis. It is important to note that rare examples of PTLD may have the morphology of Hodgkin disease, and that late cases of EBV-negative lymphoid neoplasms (4 or 5 years after transplant) that resemble non-Hodgkin lymphomas can also develop.

6. **Recurrent disease.** With the exception of a few cases of sarcoid, recurrence of the native lung disease in allografts is not a significant problem. There are reports of occasional cases of carcinoma arising in transplanted lungs, as well as in the native lung in the setting of unilateral transplant; these patients fare poorly.

VII. **NEOPLASMS.** The World Health Organization (WHO) classification of lung neoplasms is presented in Table 8.12. Malignancies of the lung are the most common

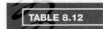

TABLE 8.12	WHO Histological Classification of Tumors of the Lung

Malignant epithelial tumors
Squamous cell carcinoma
   Papillary
   Clear cell
   Small cell
   Basaloid

Small cell carcinoma
   Combined small cell carcinoma

Adenocarcinoma
   Adenocarcinoma, mixed subtype
   Acinar adenocarcinoma
   Papillary adenocarcinoma
   Bronchioloalveolar carcinoma
      Nonmucinous
      Mucinous
      Mixed nonmucinous and mucinous or indeterminate
Solid adenocarcinoma with mucin production
   Fetal adenocarcinoma
   Mucinous ("colloid") carcinoma
   Mucinous cystadenocarcinoma
   Signet-ring adenocarcinoma
   Clear cell adenocarcinoma

Large cell carcinoma
   Large cell neuroendocrine carcinoma
   Combined large cell neuroendocrine carcinoma
   Basaloid carcinoma
   Lymphoepithelioma-like carcinoma
   Clear cell carcinoma
   Large cell carcinoma with rhabdoid phenotype

Adenosquamous carcinoma

Sarcomatoid carcinoma
   Pleomorphic carcinoma
   Spindle cell carcinoma
   Giant cell carcinoma
   Carcinosarcoma
   Pulmonary blastoma

Carcinoid tumor
   Typical carcinoid
   Atypical carcinoid

Salivary gland tumors
   Mucoepidermoid carcinoma
   Adenoid cystic carcinoma
   Epithelial-myoepithelial carcinoma

Preinvasive lesions
   Squamous carcinoma in situ
   Atypical adenomatous hyperplasia
   Diffuse idiopathic pulmonary neuroendocrine cell hyperplasia

(continued)

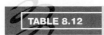 **TABLE 8.12** WHO Histological Classification of Tumors of the Lung *(Continued)*

Mesenchymal tumors
    Epithelioid hemangioendothelioma
    Angiosarcoma
    Pleuropulmonary blastoma
    Chondroma
    Congenial peribronchial myofibroblastic tumor
    Diffuse pulmonary lymphangiomatosis
    Inflammatory myofibroblastic tumor
    Lymphangioleiomyomatosis
    Synovial sarcoma
        Monophasic
        Biphasic
    Pulmonary artery sarcoma
    Pulmonary vein sarcoma

Benign epithelial tumors
Papillomas
    Squamous cell papilloma
    Exophytic
    Inverted
    Glandular papilloma
    Mixed squamous cell and glandular papilloma
Adenomas
    Alveolar adenoma
    Papillary adenoma
    Adenomas of the salivary gland type
    Mucous gland adenoma
    Pleomorphic adenoma
    Others
    Mucinous cystadenoma

Lymphoproliferative tumors
    Marginal zone B-cell lymphoma of the mucosal associated lymphoid tissue (MALT) type
    Diffuse large B-cell lymphoma
    Lymphomatoid granulomatosis
    Langerhans cell histiocytosis

Miscellaneous tumors
    Hamartoma
    Sclerosing hemangioma
    Clear cell tumor
    Germ cell tumors
    Teratoma, mature
    Immature
    Other germ cell tumors
    Intrapulmonary thymoma
    Melanoma

Metastatic tumors

From: Travis WD, Brambilla E, Müller-Hermelink HK, Harris CC, eds. *World Health Organization Classification of Tumours. Pathology and Genetics. Tumours of the Lung, Pleura, Thymus and Heart.* Lyon: IARC Press; 2004. Used with permission.

cause of cancer-related mortality in the United States. Despite decades of warnings, cigarette smoking remains the predominant risk factor for the development of pulmonary carcinoma. There has been speculation that a shift in location and cell type for pulmonary carcinomas is related to changes in cigarette usage. Some data suggest that filtered cigarettes, which remove larger tar particles, have allowed carcinogens to penetrate to more distal parts of the lung and produce peripheral adenocarcinomas instead of central squamous carcinomas or small cell carcinomas caused by larger particles. Changes in tobacco formulation over the years may also have played some role in these changes. Other risk factors for lung carcinoma, either proven or speculative, include asbestos exposure, radiation, various chemicals, heavy metals, viral infection, fibrosing lung diseases, immunosuppression, and genetic syndromes. Outside of these causes, there remain some cases of lung carcinomas for which there is no clear etiologic factor.

Up to 10% of patients with head and neck carcinomas may harbor a concurrent lung primary carcinoma; therefore, the finding of a lung nodule in a head and neck cancer patient should not automatically be assumed to represent metastatic disease. Similarly, 2%–5% of lung carcinoma patients present with apparent synchronous lung primary tumors (which may be due to the greatly improved resolution of CT techniques that can now detect additional small nodules in patients with a dominant lung masses); histologic sampling of these lesions often shows alveolar proliferations with varying degrees of atypia that may represent precursor lesions in the peripheral lung similar to squamous dysplasia in the more central airways.

A. Pathologic reporting. The important data to be included in a diagnostic report of a primary pulmonary neoplasm are summarized in Table 8.13. Generally, tumor size is assessed by gross examination, and this measurement suffices unless there is confounding fibrosis or peritumoral pneumonia. The extension of tumor through the pleura covering the lung (visceral pleura) or into the pleura lining the chest wall (parietal pleura) should be noted; an elastin stain can delineate these layers in some cases. Lymphatic and venous invasion should be noted separately. The status of the margins of resection should be listed, and any abnormalities in the adjacent lung should be described. The American Joint Committee on Cancer (AJCC) pathologic staging of lung carcinomas is provided in Table 8.14.

Currently, there is great interest in prognostic and predictive markers for lung carcinomas. Despite the extensive literature on this topic, the features that still remain most relevant to outcome are those described as important for reporting above. Outside of those ancillary tests required to identify if a specific patient qualifies for a specific therapy (e.g., for various epidermal growth factor receptor [EGFR] inhibiting drugs), no immunohistochemical or molecular tests are currently standard of care. There is hope that gene expression signatures, several of which are currently under study, may provide valuable information in terms of prognosis and response to therapy.

B. Non-small cell carcinomas

1. Adenocarcinoma is now the most common subtype of lung carcinoma, accounting for 40% or more of all primary lung carcinomas. This subtype is relatively more common in women. More than two thirds of cases arise in the

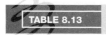

| TABLE 8.13 | Diagnostic Features to be Reported with Lung Carcinoma Resections |

▪ Tumor type	▪ Associated conditions in non-neoplastic lung
▪ Grade	▪ T stage
▪ Tumor size	▪ N stage
▪ Pleural involvement	▪ M data
▪ Lymphatic invasion	▪ Overall stage (American Joint Committee on Cancer [AJCC])
▪ Venous invasion	
▪ Margins	

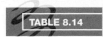

TABLE 8.14	Tumor, Node, Metastasis (TNM) Staging Scheme for Lung Cancer

PRIMARY TUMOR (T)

TX	Primary tumor cannot be assessed, or tumor proven by the presence of malignant cells in sputum or bronchial washings but not visualized by imaging or bronchoscopy
T0	No evidence of primary tumor
Tis	Carcinoma in situ
T1	Tumor 3 cm or less in greatest dimension, surrounded by lung or visceral pleura, without bronchoscopic evidence of invasion more proximal than the lobar bronchus (1)
T2	Tumor with any of the following features of size or extent: **1.** More than 3 cm in greatest dimension **2.** Involves main bronchus, 2 cm or more distal to the carina **3.** Invades visceral pleura **4.** Associated with atelectasis of obstructive pneumonitis that extends to the hilar region but does not involve the entire lung
T3	Tumor of any size that directly invades any of the following: chest wall, diaphragm, mediastinal pleura, parietal pericardium; or tumor in the main bronchus less than 2 cm distal to the carina but without involvement of the carina; or associated atelectasis or obstructive pneumonitis of the entire lung
T4	Tumor of any size that invades any of the following: mediastinum, heart, great vessels, trachea, esophagus, vertebral body, carina; separate tumor nodules(s) in the same lobe; tumor with malignant pleural effusion (2)
Notes:	**1.** The uncommon superficial spreading tumor of any size with its invasive component limited to the bronchial wall, which may extend proximal to the main bronchus, is also classified T1. **2.** Most pleural effusions with lung cancer are due to tumor. In a few patients, however, multiple cytopathologic examinations of pleural fluid are negative for tumor, and the fluid is non-bloody and is not related to the tumor; in these patients, the effusion should be excluded as a staging element and the patient should be classified as T1, T2, or T3.

REGIONAL LYMPH NODES (N)

NX	Regional lymph nodes cannot be assessed
N0	No regional lymph node metastasis
N1	Metastasis in ipsilateral peribronchial and/or ipsilateral hilar lymph nodes and intrapulmonary nodes, including involvement by direct extension
N2	Metastasis in ipsilateral mediastinal and/or subcarinal lymph node(s)
N3	Metastasis in contralateral mediastinal, contralateral hilar, ipsilateral or contralateral scalene, or supraclavicular lymph node(s)

DISTANT METASTASIS (M)

MX	Distant metastasis cannot be assessed
M0	No distant metastasis
M1	Distant metastasis, includes separate tumor nodule(s) in a different lobe (ipsilateral or contralateral)

(*continued*)

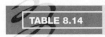

TABLE 8.14	Tumor, Node, Metastasis (TNM) Staging Scheme for Lung Cancer *(Continued)*		
STAGE GROUPING			
Occult Carcinoma	TX	N0	M0
Stage 0	Tis	N0	M0
Stage 1A	T1	N0	M0
Stage 1B	T2	N0	M0
Stage IIA	T1	N1	M0
Stage IIB	T2	N1	M0
	T3	N0	M0
Stage IIIA	T1	N2	M0
	T2	N2	M0
	T3	N1	M0
	T3	N2	M0
Stage IIIB	Any T	N3	M0
	T4	Any N	M0
Stage IV	Any T	Any N	M1

From: Greene FL, Page DL, Fleming ID, Fritz AG, Balch CM, Haller DG, Morrow M, eds. *AJCC Cancer Staging Manual.* 6th edition. New York: Springer; 2002. Used with permission. (A new AJCC TNM staging system is scheduled for release in 2009; after its publication, the new staging scheme will appear on the website for this book.)

periphery of the lung, often in a subpleural location, often with an associated scar (e-**Fig. 8.38**). Pulmonary acinar adenocarcinoma, sometimes designated as adenocarcinoma of no special type, represents the most common form of pulmonary adenocarcinoma. This variant of adenocarcinoma features a glandular, tubular, or solid growth pattern. The cytologic features range from very bland and well differentiated to highly anaplastic forms. Subtypes of adenocarcinoma include papillary, invasive micropapillary, mucinous, enteric-like, clear cell, glassy cell, and bronchioloalveolar carcinoma (BAC) (see below B1a.). Because of the peripheral location of most adenocarcinomas, they have a higher rate of resectability than do many other non-small cell carcinomas, and also tend to involve the visceral pleura. Finally, because lymphatic and vascular invasion, with consequent lymph node metastases, are quite common, relatively small peripheral adenocarcinomas may have mediastinal lymph node involvement.

Electron microscopic and immunostaining studies show that pulmonary adenocarcinomas can resemble many different respiratory cell types, including bronchial cells, goblet cells, Clara cells, and alveolar pneumocytes. Immunostains show consistent positivity for epithelial membrane antigen (EMA), various cytokeratins including cytokeratin 7, various surfactants and related proteins, and the nuclear marker thyroid transcription factor-1 (TTF-1) (e-**Fig. 8.39**). TTF-1 has been shown to be quite useful in differentiating primary pulmonary adenocarcinomas from lung metastases of adenocarcinomas from a variety of origins, and can also identify metastatic pulmonary adenocarcinomas in distant metastatic sites. Because very poorly differentiated adenocarcinomas, as well as some mucinous pulmonary carcinomas, do not express TTF-1, TTF-1 negativity does not provide definitive evidence that a tumor is not of pulmonary origin; such a determination must be based on all available clinical, radiographic, and pathologic information. In addition, TTF-1 is not specific for pulmonary adenocarcinoma and may be expressed by thyroid carcinomas and neuroendocrine carcinomas (NECs) arising at a variety of other anatomic sites. As expected in many adenocarcinomas, pulmonary adenocarcinoma also expresses many generic carcinoma markers including carcinoma embryonic antigen (CEA), the B72.3-related antigen, CD15, and MOC31.

a. **BAC is a specialized form of pulmonary adenocarcinoma.** With the relative and absolute increase of peripheral lung carcinomas, as discussed above, an increasing number of primary lung cancers present as ground glass opacities on chest imaging. Clinicians and radiologists often characterize these as BAC, but the morphologic diagnosis of BAC is somewhat rare because the restrictive WHO guidelines demand that BAC maintain an alveolar architecture. WHO criteria specify that BAC must grow primarily in a lepidic pattern; cases with any significant component of destructive invasion, as indicated by desmoplasia, should be classified as invasive adenocarcinomas. Pure BAC is therefore rare; it develops relatively more often in women and in nonsmokers. It is much more common as a peripheral component of an invasive adenocarcinoma, in which case it is best reported as adenocarcinoma with bronchioloalveolar features.

BAC may present as a solitary peripheral nodule or multiple nodules, with lobar consolidation that mimics pneumonia, or rarely with diffuse involvement of the entire lung. BACs are well-differentiated neoplasms. The tumor cell nuclei are often only modestly atypical, but are abnormal by their monotonous nature, and may be differentiated from reactive alveolar processes in part by this cellular uniformity. So-called sclerosing BAC may have some expansion of the alveolar interstitial by fibrosis without invasion, but many postulated examples of this tumor are actually invasive adenocarcinoma. Because BAC grows very slowly, there may be a central elastotic scar that is degenerative or involutional and so should not be labeled as invasive growth; these scars may feature calcification or even metaplastic bone. Some example of BAC can have extensive lymphocytic infiltrates, often with a nodular pattern. BAC has been classically divided into type I and type II.

i. Type I BAC are mucinous and may resemble pulmonary goblet cells, gastric mucous cells, or intestinal epithelium, both morphologically and in terms of mucin types (e-Fig. 8.40). Mucinous BAC is often multifocal, and may present with bronchorrhea. The cells grow along alveoli, often with a discontinuous appearance, and mucin and muciphages may fill the involved alveolar spaces. Invasive mucinous carcinomas, including signet-ring lesions, are often found in continuity with mucinous BAC. Another type of adenocarcinoma closely related to mucinous BAC, is so-called enteric type adenocarcinoma, which closely resembles colonic or other gut carcinomas. Finally, the so-called mucinous cystadenoma may be associated with mucinous BAC; this rare low-grade mucinous lung lesion resembles mucinous cystadenomas in other sites, and so is best considered as a lesion of low malignant potential. Metastatic adenocarcinoma of gastric, pancreatic, or intestinal origin is the most important differential consideration for mucinous BAC.

Mucinous BAC and related invasive adenocarcinomas of the lung often show immunostaining coexpression of cytokeratins 7 and 20 (e-Fig. 8.41), but may be negative for TTF-1. CDX2 staining may be of some utility, as most pulmonary mucinous neoplasms do not react with this immunostain. Adequate clinical history and correlation with the appearance and stage of the primary tumor is of great importance in this differential.

ii. Type II BAC cells can resemble several bronchial and alveolar cell types including type II pneumocytes and Clara cells (e-Fig. 8.42). Type II tumors, as compared to type I lesions, are more likely to present as solitary masses, although multiple type II tumors have occurred. Tumors with type II pneumocyte differentiation commonly have intranuclear pseudoinclusions, whereas Clara cell lesions may show PAS-positive apical granules.

b. **Atypical alveolar hyperplasia (AAH)** is a lesion closely related to BAC. In fact, molecular genetic studies show virtually identical abnormalities in cases

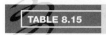

TABLE 8.15	Atypical Alveolar Hyperplasia versus Bronchioloalveolar Carcinoma	
	Atypical alveolar hyperplasia	**Bronchioloalveolar carcinoma**
Size	Small, usually <5 mm	>5 mm
Clinical presentation	Often unsuspected, may be found in sections of grossly "normal" lung or in or in sections of margins	Radiographic and gross lesion is present
Cytologic features	Mildly atypical, but polymorphous	Mildly atypical, monomorphous

of AAH and BAC. Key features in the separation of these lesions are presented in Table 8.15. In fact, AAH and BAC are best considered as the peripheral lung equivalents of dysplasia and carcinoma in situ, with a postulated role as precursors of invasive peripheral adenocarcinomas.

2. **Squamous cell carcinoma (SCC) is most frequently a central lesion arising in larger airways although peripheral lesions do occur; primarily endobronchial tumors are unusual.** Postobstructive pneumonia has been reported in up to one half of SCC. SCC is prone to central necrosis, and cavitation is a common radiologic finding. Squamous dysplasia and carcinoma in situ not infrequently accompany SCC and may be the only material retrieved by endoscopic biopsy. The histology of SCC does not differ significantly from that of SCC that occurs at other body sites; both keratinizing and nonkeratinizing variants occur, as well as basaloid and clear cell forms (e-**Fig. 8.43**). Unlike pulmonary adenocarcinoma, SCC does not generally express TTF-1 or other markers of pulmonary differentiation; for this reason, immunophenotyping of SCC is not particularly useful.

   Poorly differentiated SCC should not be confused with small cell carcinoma; SCC lacks the individual cell necrosis, crush artifact, and nuclear molding seen in small cell carcinoma. The distinction between small cell carcinoma and SCC can be facilitated by immunostains for p63; SCC generally reacts with antibodies to p63 whereas small cell carcinoma does not. SCC also seems to be somewhat less prone to nodal metastasis, whereas small cell carcinomas can have extensive lymph nodal or distant spread with relatively small tumors, SCC can be quite large and confined to the lung.

3. **Large cell carcinoma is an undifferentiated epithelial neoplasm.** Neither squamous differentiation (keratin, cytoplasmic bridges) nor glandular features (mucin, acinar formation) are seen by light microscopy, although ultrastructural studies have shown both squamous and glandular elements. Exhaustive and expensive attempts to subclassify undifferentiated large cell carcinoma into a specific diagnostic category offer no clinical utility; the finding of a tumor so poorly differentiated that standard sampling and diagnostic techniques cannot demonstrate clear cut squamous or glandular differentiation provides prognostic information in itself. These tumors are generally aggressive. Large randomized clinical trials have shown that demonstration of neuroendocrine markers in non-small neoplasms in general and large cell neoplasms in particular (outside of the defined neuroendocrine tumor types delineated below) does not denote responsiveness to small-cell carcinoma–specific chemotherapeutic regimens.

4. **Giant cell carcinoma is a unique variant of large cell carcinoma.** The tumor grows as a large bulky peripheral mass, and often invades the pleura and chest wall. Giant cell carcinoma is composed of large epithelioid cells, many of which are multinucleated (e-**Fig. 8.44**). The cells grow in large sheets and are loosely cohesive. An intense acute and chronic inflammatory cell infiltrate almost always permeates giant cell carcinoma. A spindle cell component often mixes with the giant cell pattern, producing what has sometimes been designated as

pleomorphic carcinoma. Unique aspects of giant cell carcinoma include a propensity to metastasize to abdominal sites including the small bowel, and an association with leukemoid reaction. Reactivity for epithelial markers including cytokeratin and EMA is generally maintained; documentation of these markers in a giant cell carcinoma distinguishes this tumor from such possible mimics as malignant fibrous histiocytoma, anaplastic large cell lymphoma, or choriocarcinoma.

5. **Clear cell carcinoma does not represent a distinct primary form of pulmonary carcinoma;** rather, lung carcinomas with cytoplasmic clearing represent variants of other forms of non-small cell carcinoma. Clearing has been reported in 25% or more of all pulmonary adenocarcinomas, squamous carcinomas, and even large cell carcinomas (e-**Fig. 8.45**). Of course, a pulmonary clear cell neoplasm should raise concern for a metastatic clear cell carcinoma, typically of renal origin, as well as the rare pulmonary clear cell tumor (see below VIIJ2).

6. **Adenosquamous carcinoma is an uncommon variant of pulmonary carcinoma.** These tumors are generally associated with a smoking history. The diagnosis should be reserved for tumors in which there is clearly recognizable differentiation into squamous (intercellular bridges and possibly keratinization) and glandular elements (acını). Solid adenocarcinomas, with minimal squamoid differentiation or foci of cytoplasmic eosinophilia, should not be interpreted as adenosquamous carcinoma; similarly, SCCs that contain rare droplets of intracytoplasmic mucin are better classified as SCCs. Also, high-grade mucoepidermoid carcinomas in the lung may be better classified as adenosquamous carcinomas.

7. **Other rare types of lung carcinoma** include lymphoepithelial-like carcinoma (e-**Fig. 8.46**), non-small cell carcinoma with rhabdoid features, and invasive micropapillary carcinoma.

C. **Neuroendocrine neoplasms (see Table 8.16) constitute a spectrum of neoplasms, from lesions of little clinical significance to highly malignant tumors.** The exact origin of these neoplasms remains speculative. Although the airways contain neuroendocrine cells, known as Kulchitsky cells, the idea that all neuroendocrine tumors arise from pre-existing neuroendocrine cells is probably not true; neuroendocrine differentiation may simply be a reflection of the totipotential nature of malignant neoplasms. In general, better differentiated tumors show greater variety in secretory products, and have greater number of neuroendocrine granules on ultrastructural examination.

1. **Neuroendocrine cell hyperplasia is the simplest neuroendocrine lesion seen in the lungs.** As its name implies, this process consists of an increased number of neuroendocrine cells in the bronchial and bronchiolar epithelium. This

TABLE 8.16   Features of Pulmonary Neuroendocrine Neoplasms

WHO terminology	Alternative terminology	Cell size	Nuclear atypia	Mitoses	Necrosis	Malignant potential
Carcinoid	Grade 1 NEC	Medium to large	None	<2/hpf	None	Low
Atypical carcinoid	Grade 2 NEC	Medium to large	Mild	2–10/hpf	Focal	Intermediate
Large cell neuroendocrine carcinoma	Grade 3 NEC, large cell type	Large	Marked	>10/hpf	Extensive	High
Small cell neuroendocrine carcinoma	Grade 3 NEC, small cell type	Small	Marked	High	Extensive	High

Abbreviations: WHO, World Health Organization; NEC, neuroendocrine carcinoma; hpf, high power field.

lesion is often not apparent by standard histology and only visualized through the use of immunostains for neuroendocrine markers. The lesion likely represents a reactive process and may be associated with conditions that cause airway inflammation or injury, and is of little or no clinical significance. It is the one lung neuroendocrine lesion that can be safely thought of as benign in essentially all cases.

2. **Carcinoid tumors should be considered grade 1 NECs.** Carcinoids can be divided into central lesions, which have an association with cartilaginous airways (often designated as typical carcinoids), and peripheral types, which lack such an association. Carcinoid tumors tend to occur on average as much as one to two decades earlier than standard lung carcinomas. In addition, they do not show any convincing relationship to cigarette smoking (in contrast to higher grade neuroendocrine tumors). The clinical presentation of patients with carcinoid tumors varies based on the tumor's location. Central tumors, which are slowly growing, often present with airway-related symptoms including wheezing, recurrent pneumonias, and cough (e-Fig. 8.47). In contrast, peripheral carcinoids are often asymptomatic and are discovered incidentally as a pulmonary "coin lesions." Unlike small bowel carcinoids, they essentially will never be associated with the carcinoid syndrome, although cases of Cushing's syndrome have been reported due to adrenocorticotropic hormone (ACTH) release.

Grossly, central carcinoid tumors usually present as yellow-tan polypoid intraluminal masses covered by normal respiratory tract mucosa; they almost always measure <5 cm. Microscopic sections show a variety of architectural patterns including trabeculae, rosettes, papillary formations, and areas of solid growth (e-Fig. 8.48). The tumors have vascular stroma, which can also feature elements including amyloid and bone. The individual cells tend to have moderate to abundant cytoplasm, which is often granular and eosinophilic. The tumor cells have nuclei that are regular and round to oval; the chromatin is granular and is often referred to as having a "salt and pepper" character. Mitotic activity should be essentially absent; the most recent WHO standard is ≤2 mitoses per 10 high-power field (hpf). Necrosis should be absent. Peripheral carcinoid tumors are morphologically identical to central tumors, although peripheral carcinoid tumors often exhibit a spindled morphology. Tumors with a peripheral location and spindled pattern should not be designated automatically as atypical carcinoid tumors (see below VIIC3).

Well-differentiated NECs contain abundant neurosecretory granules and show strong expression of chromogranin and synaptophysin; they are also immunopositive for epithelial markers such as cytokeratin. Carcinoid tumors have low malignant potential. Only about 5% of patients present with lymph node metastases; <5% of cases show distant metastatic disease, with spread to the liver, brain, bones, and skin. Long-term survival is in excess of 95%.

a. **Carcinoid tumorlets are microscopic proliferations (≤4 mm in size) that are otherwise histologically and immunophenotypically identical to carcinoid tumors (e-Fig. 8.49);** distinction is based solely on size. Tumorlets tend to occur in distal airways, and may be single lesions incidentally discovered in resection specimens; rare patients may have hundreds of these lesions in their distal airways. Multiple carcinoid tumorlets have some association with chronic airway diseases. Tumorlets have little or no clinical significance.

b. **Paraganglioma** features nested cells, a fine fibrovascular stroma, cells with eosinophilic to granular cytoplasm and some spindling, and regular nuclei, so it can be difficult to distinguish from carcinoid tumor. Although paraganglioma shows immunopositivity for chromogranin and synaptophysin, it is not reactive with antibodies to cytokeratin; in addition, the tumor contains S-100–positive sustentacular cells that are not present in carcinoid tumors.

c. **Chemodectomas.** Multiple pulmonary chemodectomas were once considered a variant of paraganglioma, but now are known to have no relationship to paraganglioma. So-called chemodectomas consist of 1- to 2-mm stellate proliferations that fill the pulmonary interstitium and feature bland epithelioid cells in a whirling pattern. These tumors share immunoreactivity for EMA and vimentin, and have been labeled as "minute meningothelial-like nodules." They are of no clinical significance.

3. **Atypical carcinoid tumor, better designated as grade 2 NEC, is more rare than carcinoid tumor, and more evenly divided between central and peripheral locations (e-Fig. 8.50).** Because more tumors are peripheral, airway-related symptoms are less common. In addition, there is a closer relationship to cigarette smoking. These tumors tend to be slightly larger than grade 1 lesions at the time of diagnosis, but it is microscopic features that distinguish grade 2 NEC (atypical carcinoid) from grade 1 NEC (carcinoid). The tumor cells tend to be slightly smaller than those of classic carcinoid tumors, and some modest nuclear pleomorphism is also usually present. Spindling of the cells is also more common than with grade 1 cases, and mitotic activity is more frequent; up to 10 mitoses per 10 hpf is an accepted criterion. Necrosis may be present, but is usually limited. Because the cells are moderately differentiated, neuroendocrine immunostains tend to be relatively strongly positive.

Atypical carcinoids show significantly greater malignant potential than classic carcinoids. About 25% of patients with atypical carcinoid tumor have lymph nodal metastases at presentation, and approximately 25% of patients are dead of disease at 5 years after diagnosis.

4. **Large cell NEC (LCNEC) can also be designated grade 3 NEC.** It is an extremely lethal form of lung carcinoma, and is the most recent variant of NEC to be described. The demographics of LCNEC are similar to those of other lung carcinomas; almost all cases have been reported in cigarette smokers. The vast majority of the tumors are found in the periphery of the lung, and thus they tend to present with the same sort of nonspecific symptoms as do other lung carcinomas. The gross appearance of the tumor is similar to that of other lung carcinomas, and may include necrosis or cavitation (**e-Fig. 8.51**).

The microscopic features of LCNEC are quite distinctive. The tumor has an organoid appearance in which large solid nests of tumor are separated by scant fibrovascular stroma. In some cases, the tumor seems to fill up the pre-existing alveolar spaces. Tumors may show palisading of tumor cells at the periphery of the nests, and features such as spindling or rosettes may also be present. The dominant feature in most cases is extensive necrosis, which may make up the bulk of the tumor mass. The tumor cells themselves are generally polygonal, and have a significant amount of cytoplasm. LCNEC can be distinguished from small cell NEC based on several factors: At lower power microscopy, the nuclei of the tumor do not touch (as do the nuclei in small cell carcinomas, see below VIIC5); the nuclear/cytoplasmic ratio is significantly lower than that of small cell carcinoma; the nuclear chromatin may be vesicular and nucleoli are often prominent; and finally, crush artifact and nuclear molding are not usually prominent.

Mitotic activity is one of the key features of this tumor; the tumor should feature at least 10 mitoses per 10 hpf, although the actual rate is generally far higher. Combined with the extensive necrosis described above, it is generally relatively straightforward to separate this LCNEC from lower grade tumors such as atypical carcinoid. In fact, LCNEC probably has the greatest overlap with non-small cell carcinomas such as poorly differentiated squamous carcinomas. Thus, immunostains can be quite helpful in diagnosis. LCNEC shows reliable staining with pan-cytokeratin antibodies (because of the increased amount of cytoplasm in the tumor, cytokeratin stains do not show the dot-like pattern that is typical of small cell carcinoma, but rather show strong circumferential cytoplasmic staining). The majority of cases of LCNEC also show positive staining for chromogranin, synaptophysin, CD56, and CD57, although the more poorly differentiated nature of LCNEC is reflected in more focal reactivity for these neuroendocrine markers. LCNEC often also shows positive staining for p53.

The prognosis for LCNEC is quite poor. Although the great majority of patients present with node-negative lesions at diagnosis, most patients rapidly develop recurrent or metastatic disease. The overall survival at 5 and 10 years is poor, approximately 20% and 10%, respectively.

5. **Small cell lung carcinoma (SCLC) is classically described as high-grade NEC.** The incidence of SCLC is decreasing, but SCLC still accounts for at least 10% of all primary lung carcinomas. This tumor type has a very strong association with cigarette smoking. At least 95% of patients present with a central mass composed of hilar and/or mediastinal adenopathy; the adenopathy often is larger than any radiographically definable intrapulmonary mass (e-**Fig. 8.52**). The bulky tumor in the mediastinum leads to a variety of clinical presentations, including cough, hemoptysis, lobar collapse, shortness of breath from pleural effusions, chest pain, hoarseness from recurrent laryngeal nerve invasion, or superior vena cava syndrome. A significant number of patients also present with signs or symptoms referable to distant spread, such as neurologic symptoms (brain metastases), bone lesions, or symptoms due to abdominal organ involvement. Paraneoplastic syndromes are common, including the syndrome of inappropriate secretion of antidiuretic hormone, Eaton–Lambert syndrome, and Cushing's syndrome (related to ACTH production).

Because small cell carcinomas are rarely resected, the gross features of the tumor are seldom seen in the surgical pathology laboratory. These features include a large central mass that tends to spread along the bronchial tree, with involvement of hilar lymph nodes often in a contiguous fashion with the primary tumor. Some cases show an endobronchial lesion; <5% of cases present as a peripheral pulmonary nodule.

The microscopic appearance of small cell carcinoma varies with the method of sampling (e-**Fig. 8.53**). Endobronchial biopsies commonly have the so called "oat cell" appearance characterized by small cells (about twice the diameter of a resting lymphocyte) with dark hyperchromatic nuclei. There is scant to barely visible cytoplasm, and crush artifact and nuclear molding are prominent; nucleoli are not usually prominent. Individual apoptotic cells are often seen, and more extensive confluent necrosis may be present. Mitotic figures are frequent. The cells tend to stream through the tissue in irregular sheets, although some cases may show rosettes, palisades, or trabecular growth patterns. Small cell carcinoma often has a slightly different appearance in larger tissue samples, such as resected primary tumors or lymph node biopsies. The cells are oftentimes slightly larger (up to four times the diameter of a resting lymphocyte), but still feature dark hyperchromatic nuclei, often with nucleoli. Crush artifact and nuclear molding may be less prominent. Necrosis is often widespread; one well-known feature of small cell carcinoma with excessive necrosis is the so-called Azzopardi effect, which is the coating of a blood vessel walls by nucleic acid to produce dark blue ring-like structures in the midst of otherwise eosinophilic necrotic areas.

Immunostains can be helpful in the diagnosis of small cell carcinoma. Cytokeratin immunostains often produce a dot-like perinuclear pattern of positivity due to the small amount of cytoplasm and the condensation of cytoskeletal elements in the tumor cells; stains for CD45 can exclude lymphoma. In cases with classic morphology, this simple panel (cytokeratin and CD45) is sufficient for the diagnosis of small cell carcinoma. If additional stains are requested to confirm neuroendocrine differentiation, it should be noted that small cell carcinomas have very few neurosecretory granules, and hence, chromogranin stains are relatively insensitive. Similarly, synaptophysin and CD57 stains are positive in only approximately 50%–60% of cases. Stains for neural cell adhesion molecule (NCAM) (CD56) are more sensitive, and stains for TTF-1 are also positive in the majority of cases of pulmonary small cell carcinoma. The cells of small cell carcinoma may also express CD99, bcl2, p53, and CEA, although these stains generally are not obtained in a diagnostic context.

Because small cell carcinoma has spread extensively at the time of diagnosis in most cases, treatment is generally nonsurgical. Survival remains poor. Modern chemotherapy and radiation regimens produce significant disease remissions in the majority of patients, but relapse within a few months is common. Overall 5-year survival is in the range of 5%–10%.

NEC may also be mixed with non-small cell carcinoma. This combination is rarely if ever seen with low-grade lesions, but is seen in a small minority of cases of LCNEC and small cell carcinoma. Admixed non-small cell components are rarely seen in bronchial biopsy specimens, but are detected in up to 10% of resected small cell cancer cases; this discrepancy is probably related to sampling volume. When recurrences occur after treatment of small cell carcinoma, a dominant non-small cell component may be present; it is likely that this shift in phenotype represents selective survival of a previously minor admixed non-small cell component not targeted by treatment directed against small cell carcinoma.

D. **Sarcomatoid carcinoma and related neoplasms.** A subset of primary pulmonary carcinomas has sarcoma-like features. Although traditionally these tumors have been given a variety of names, including carcinosarcoma and spindle cell carcinoma, sarcomatoid carcinoma is our currently preferred designation for all carcinomas with sarcoma-like features. Patients with sarcomatoid carcinoma have a similar age and smoking history as those with other forms of pulmonary carcinoma. Sarcomatoid carcinoma, however, presents in two distinct patterns. Some cases present as a polypoid intraluminal mass within a large central airway; these tumors tend to be small, most likely because patients present with airway-related symptoms early in the course of the tumor's growth. In contrast, other patients present with a bulky peripheral mass, often with pleural and chest wall invasion. Microscopic sections show malignant spindled tumor cells (e-**Fig. 8.54**), which may transition from areas of non-small cell carcinoma. Various heterologous elements such as malignant cartilage or osteoid may also be seen.

The major differential is with "true" pulmonary sarcomas, and sarcomatoid mesotheliomas. To diagnose sarcomatoid carcinoma, the sarcoma-like tumor must be proven to show some evidence of an epithelial lineage. This can be accomplished by immunostaining; reactivity for cytokeratins, EMA, p63, or other generic carcinoma markers such as CEA, will be present in the majority of (although certainly not all) examples of sarcomatoid carcinoma. Electron microscopy, with identification of epithelial features such as cell junctions, may be quite useful in this context. In many cases, extensive sampling is enough to demonstrate an epithelial component by showing transition from sarcoma-like areas to classic areas of squamous carcinoma or adenocarcinoma; the finding of such a transition provides definitive evidence as to the nature of the neoplasm. Differentiation from mesothelioma may be difficult in that immunophenotypes may overlap; WT1 and calretinin expression would favor mesothelioma. Clinical presentation as a single intrapulmonary mass may also be a critical feature to appreciate for sarcomatoid carcinoma, because mesothelioma tends to present as a diffuse pleural neoplasm.

Behavior of sarcomatoid carcinomas varies with the clinical presentation. Cases presenting as a small intraluminal polypoid airway lesion have a fair prognosis. In contrast, those cases occurring as large bulky peripheral tumors have a poor outcome because high-stage disease at presentation is common.

E. **Fetal adenocarcinoma is also known as monophasic pulmonary blastoma.** It is a tumor of adults, although it occurs on average several decades earlier than other non-small cell carcinomas. Most patients are smokers. The tumors generally are found in the periphery of the lung, average 4 to 5 cm, and are usually well-circumscribed. Microscopically, the tumor is composed of closely packed glands and tubules with scant intervening stroma (e-**Fig. 8.55**). Cribriform and vaguely papillary patterns can also be seen. The constituent cells are cytologically bland columnar cells with cytoplasmic clearing that resembles secretory endometrium. The glandular lumina are often filled with solid morules; the cells of these morules have nuclear clearing. Ultrastructural and immunohistochemical studies of fetal adenocarcinomas show pneumocyte-like differentiation, including expression of surfactants and Clara cell antigens. In addition, the glandular and morular cells contain neurosecretory granules with immunoexpression of neuroendocrine markers. The prognosis for this tumor is excellent; more than 80% of patients are cured by surgical

TABLE 8.17	Blastoma-like Lung Neoplasms

Tumor type	Age at diagnosis	Smoking history	Size	Malignant glands	Malignant stroma	Prognosis
Monophasic pulmonary blastoma	3rd to 4th decade	Yes	Small	Yes	No	Excellent
Biphasic pulmonary blastoma	3rd to 4th decade	Yes	Large, fleshy	Yes	Yes	Poor
Pleuropulmonary blastoma	Children (rare adults)	No	Large, solid and/or cystic	No	Yes	Variable, dependent on type

resection, an outcome that contrasts markedly with the poor prognosis of biphasic pulmonary blastoma.

F. Biphasic pulmonary blastoma. Like sarcomatoid carcinoma, biphasic pulmonary blastoma features both a malignant glandular and malignant stromal component. Biphasic pulmonary blastoma must be distinguished from pleuropulmonary blastoma (PPB) (see Table 8.17 and below VIIG). Despite the designation as a blastoma, biphasic pulmonary blastoma occurs almost exclusively in adults, albeit at a younger age (third or fourth decade of life) than most non-SCLCs. Most patients are cigarette smokers and present with a large peripheral mass often accompanied by pleural effusions and/or adenopathy. On gross examination the tumors are fleshy and may show necrosis, cystic change, or hemorrhage. Microscopic examination shows a characteristic biphasic pattern with endometrioid-type glands similar to those of monophasic blastoma, although the epithelial component may also be more poorly differentiated and consist of ill-defined cords and sheets of cells without obvious differentiation (e-Fig. 8.56). The malignant stromal component may resemble the blastemal component of Wilms' tumor or can include ill-defined spindle cells as well as malignant elements such as chondrosarcoma, osteosarcoma, or myogenic sarcomas. In contrast to monophasic blastoma, the outcome is poor, with most patients dying within 2 years of presentation.

G. PPB arises almost exclusively in children, although very rare cases have been described in young adults. There is a familial component to many cases of PPB, and many patients have relatives with a variety of other childhood and adult neoplasms; Washington University is the home of a PPB registry (http://ppbstudy.wustl.edu). The tumors present in the lung, most often in the subpleural area. PPB is subclassified based on gross features: predominately cystic (type 1), solid and cystic (type 2), or solid (type 3) (e-Fig. 8.57). When cystic, the lesion is often confused with a variety of benign cystic conditions including cystic adenomatoid malformation; the misdiagnosis is often discovered when the lesion recurs. Microscopic sections of the cystic cases show that the cysts are lined by benign epithelium with an underlying stroma that can have a variety of appearances, ranging from mature fibroblastic cells to overtly malignant cells with a sarcomatous appearance. The more solid cases similarly show sarcomatous-like malignant cells; rhabdomyoblasts and malignant cartilage may be included. Unlike monophasic and biphasic pulmonary blastoma, PPB does not include a malignant epithelial component. The majority of patients with completely excised cystic lesions that are confined to the lung demonstrate long-term survival; the prognosis is much more guarded for predominantly solid lesions.

H. Salivary gland tumors. Minor salivary glands are present all along the tracheobronchial tree. The airway can be the site of any of the neoplasms that can occur in the minor salivary glands. Although rare examples of pleomorphic adenoma (e-Fig.8.58), acinic cell tumor (Fechner's tumor), and oncocytoma have been reported, two salivary gland type neoplasms occur with a high enough frequency to warrant further discussion.

1. **Mucoepidermoid carcinoma.** Low-grade forms of this tumor tend to present as a polypoid intraluminal mass, and cases have been described in both adults and children. Histologic sections show a mixture of mucus-producing cells, clear cells, and squamous cells (e-Fig. 8.58). There is minimal mitotic activity, and necrosis is lacking. Many cases have abundant, mucus-filled cystic areas. The tumor is generally indolent, with local invasion and local recurrence the primary concerns; local resection is often curative. The major differential diagnostic considerations include mucus gland adenoma (which lacks the locally invasive character of mucoepidermoid carcinoma), and squamous carcinoma (which tends to show more extensive keratinization and less mucus production). High-grade forms of mucoepidermoid carcinoma similar to those described in the salivary glands also occur in the lung; because such high-grade tumors have a prognosis similar to other forms of non-small cell carcinoma, by convention they are generally considered to represent adenosquamous carcinomas.

2. **Adenoid cystic carcinoma.** (ACC) also occurs in the tracheobronchial tree. It is more common in the trachea, but also arises in the larger bronchi. Most tumors are found in middle aged to older adults, and many patients present with a long history of airway symptoms such as wheezing; the long history reflects the indolent nature of these tumors. ACC is usually 2 to 5 cm at the time of diagnosis; the tumors may grossly appear well circumscribed, but microscopically most extend beyond the gross area of disease. The histology of the tumor in the lung is identical to the analogous tumor of the salivary glands, with uniform, modestly atypical polygonal cells arranged in nests, cribriform patterns, and solid sheets (e-Fig. 8.59). Many of the tumor nests contain characteristic eosinophilic matrix material. As in the salivary glands, perineural invasion is common. Immunostains are consistent with the proposed myoepithelial origin of this tumor, demonstrating immunopositivity for cytokeratin, vimentin, actin, and S-100. Many cases are CD117 positive (it is not clear whether this finding has any therapeutic implications). Positive resection margins are common because of the infiltrative growth pattern; postoperative radiation therapy may help to control incompletely resected tumors for extended periods of time. Intrapulmonary metastasis eventually occurs in many cases as a late complication; even these metastases tend to be slow growing, and many patients survive with metastatic disease for an extended period of time.

I. **Sarcomas.** Primary sarcomas of the lung are distinctly uncommon. Before concluding that a tumor is a primary pulmonary sarcoma, primary pulmonary sarcomatoid carcinoma and metastatic sarcomas to the lung must be excluded. It is therefore important to know details of the clinical history and radiologic findings before labeling a lung tumor as a primary sarcoma. Fibrohistiocytic, fibroblastic, smooth muscle, and vascular sarcomas have been reported as primary lung sarcomas, as have primary neurogenic, osteogenic, and cartilaginous sarcomas. "Small blue cell tumors" of the lung include members of the Ewing's sarcoma/primitive neuroectodermal tumor family and rhabdomyosarcoma. Lung sarcomas are essentially identical in appearance to their soft tissue counterparts.

1. **Synovial sarcoma is a tumor that has recently been recognized to occur in both the lung and pleural spaces;** it occurs in relatively younger adults than do primary lung carcinomas. The tumor may show calcifications on radiographs, but otherwise has few defining clinical or radiographic features (e-Fig. 8.60). Histologic sections show features identical to those of synovial sarcomas of the soft tissue (see Chap. 46). Immunostains are tremendously helpful for averting a misdiagnosis; synovial sarcomas of the lung demonstrate expression of cytokeratin and EMA staining in both the glandular and spindle cell areas, and the tumor cells may also be positive for CD34 and CD99. The differential diagnosis includes other biphasic pulmonary tumors such as sarcomatoid carcinoma and

biphasic mesothelioma. Molecular demonstration of a t(X:18) translocation can be a helpful aid in diagnosis. As with synovial sarcoma arising in other locations, recurrence or metastasis may take many years to develop, but the ultimate prognosis is poor, with the majority of patients eventually dying of the disease.

2. **Epithelioid hemangioendothelioma (EH) was originally termed "intravascular bronchioloalveolar tumor."** EH presents most commonly in women of young to middle age. Patients may be asymptomatic or present with cough or shortness of breath. Radiology typically shows multiple small pulmonary nodules. Histologic sections show nodules containing pale staining, hyaline to myxoid stroma in which the pre-existing alveolar structure is often still apparent. The neoplastic cells are present within this stoma; they are small and epithelioid and often contain an intracytoplasmic lumen that represents a primitive attempt at vessel formation (e-**Fig. 8.61**). Ultrastructural studies show endothelial cell features such as Weibel–Pallade bodies; the cells also react with antibodies for vascular markers, including CD31 and CD34. Although the tumor grows slowly, most patients eventually go on to develop progressive disease with respiratory failure.

3. **Kaposi's sarcoma (KS) is another vascular tumor that may involve the lung.** Pulmonary involvement occurs almost exclusively in the setting of immunocompromise, predominantly HIV/AIDS, and rarely in solid organ transplant recipients. Pulmonary KS most often coexists with cutaneous disease. Radiographic studies show nodular infiltrates, and a pleural effusion may be present; symptoms include cough, fever, and hemoptysis. KS spreads via lymphovascular routes and thus is seen along the bronchial tree, along pulmonary vessels, and along the pleural and lobular septa; histology shows typical lesions of KS, with spindled cells arranged to form slit-like vascular spaces, extravasated erythrocytes, and hemosiderin (e-**Fig. 8.62**). Patients who have pulmonary KS have a poor prognosis, determined not only by the response of KS to chemotherapy but also by the course of the underlying HIV infection.

4. **Pulmonary artery sarcoma is another rare but deadly lung sarcoma.** Patients tend to be middle aged or older, and typically present with shortness of breath or signs of right-sided heart failure. Imaging studies often show intravascular filling of the pulmonary artery trunk, which may be interpreted as thromboembolic disease. The tumor may be situated in the main pulmonary artery trunk or in one or both of the main right and left artery branches; the sarcoma may extend distally into progressively smaller branches within the lung. The histologic features of pulmonary artery sarcoma are variable, including smooth muscle, fibrohistiocytic, endothelial, and even chondroid or osteoid differentiation. The prognosis of pulmonary artery sarcoma is poor; even in cases with complete resection, distal recurrences within the ipsilateral lung are the rule. To date, radiation and chemotherapy have not been particularly effective in treating this sarcoma.

5. **Thoracopulmonary small cell tumor, also known as Askin tumor, is now known to be a member of the Ewing's sarcoma/primitive neuroectodermal tumor family of neoplasms.** This highly malignant tumor most often presents in children and young adults and is typically very large at presentation; it may literally fill an entire hemithorax (e-**Fig. 8.63**). The exact site of origin is often unclear, although most tumors probably originate from the chest wall with secondary invasion into the lung. The tumor consists of a classic small blue cell proliferation, growing in sheets or rosettes. Necrosis may be prominent. The tumor shows staining for CD99 as well as various neuroendocrine markers. Most cases demonstrate a characteristic t(11;22) translocation (see Chap. 46).

J. Miscellaneous neoplasms

1. **Pulmonary hamartoma (chondroid hamartoma) is a benign proliferation usually seen in adults.** The tumor usually occurs as a solitary peripheral mass with a radiographic appearance of a so-called "coin lesion." A minority of cases involve the more central airways or even the trachea. Chondroid hamartomas may be part of a heritable syndrome in some cases; Carney's triad consists of

pulmonary hamartomas, gastric stromal tumors, and extra-adrenal pheochromocytomas. Grossly, the tumor is a well circumscribed, nodular lesion (e-**Fig. 8.64**). Histologic sections disclose a mixture of benign mesenchymal components, including cartilage, mature adipose tissue, and smooth muscle. Bronchial type epithelium is usually present within the lesion, although this is thought to represent entrapped tissue rather than a true component of the proliferation. Radiographic diagnosis of this lesion can be confidently made based on the presence of adipose tissue and calcifications within the cartilaginous component; for this reason, hamartomas are often not resected.

2. **Pulmonary clear cell tumor, or sugar tumor, is a unique pulmonary tumor composed of cells with clear cytoplasm.** The tumor generally arises in adults and presents as a well circumscribed, nodular mass; most are found incidentally in asymptomatic patients. The tumor usually measures <5 mm in greatest dimension. Histologic sections show epithelioid cells with bland nuclei and abundant clear cytoplasm (e-**Fig. 8.65**). The cells grow either in nests separated by fine fibrovascular stroma or in a more sheet-like pattern. PAS stains are positive due to abundant intracellular glycogen, as confirmed by ultrastructural studies that may also show premelanosomes within the tumor cells. Immunostains show a unique pattern of vimentin positivity, as well as positivity with melanocyte markers such as HMB-45 or melan-A, with expression of actin and CD117 as well.

The histogenesis of this tumor has long been debated; most recently it has been suggested that it is a member of the family of tumors known as PEComas. The most important neoplasm in the differential diagnosis is metastatic renal cell carcinoma; in this regard, it is important to emphasize that pulmonary clear cell tumors uniformly lack expression of epithelial markers such as cytokeratin and EMA. The behavior of pulmonary clear cell tumor has generally been considered to be benign, although rare tumors show malignant behavior.

3. **Inflammatory myofibroblastic tumor (IMT) has traditionally been given a variety of names, including inflammatory pseudotumor and plasma cell granuloma.** IMT is the most common benign lung tumor in children, but occurs in adults as well. The most common presentation is a relatively small solitary peripheral module; IMT also occurs as an endobronchial lesion. Patients may be asymptomatic or may present with a variety of systemic signs and symptoms, including fever, anemia, and polyclonal hypergammaglobulinemia; systemic manifestations usually resolve with removal of the tumor. In most cases, the tumor is confined to the lung, although occasional cases may exhibit more aggressive local behavior, including invasion of mediastinal structures.

Microscopic sections show a proliferation of spindled myofibroblastic cells with a haphazard pattern of vague fascicles (see Chap. 46) (e-**Fig. 8.66**). The spindle cells are characteristically bland and mitotic figures are rare, without abnormal mitotic figures; necrosis is unusual. There is often a marked inflammatory cell infiltrate in the lesion that may include plasma cells, lymphocytes with lymphoid follicles, acute inflammation and eosinophils. The stroma varies from myxoid to densely collagenized and keloid-like. Immunohistochemical stains show that the spindle cells are positive for vimentin and smooth muscle actin, and are negative for cytokeratin, CD34, and desmin. ALK-1 is variably expressed in IMTs of the lung, in contrast to some other sites. The plasma cells are polyclonal by light chain studies. The immunophenotype of IMT can be used to rule out several tumors in the differential diagnosis such as spindle cell carcinoma, solitary fibrous tumor, and fibrohistiocytic neoplasms.

IMT of the lung is usually cured by surgery. Recurrence is rare, but more common if the lesion invaded adjacent structures at the time of resection. Extremely unusual cases of malignant transformation to a high-grade fibroblastic or round cell neoplasms have been reported.

It must be emphasized that non-neoplastic inflammatory processes occur in the lung that are also capable of producing a mass-like lesion, such as organizing pneumonia, infarcts, scars, and confluent granulomas. These processes must always be included in the differential diagnosis of IMT.

K. Hematolymphoid lesions. Hematolymphoid neoplasms and pseudoneoplasms can involve the lung, both primarily and as part of systemic disease. Fresh tissue should be set aside for flow cytometry whenever possible. In cases for which only fixed tissue is available, a variety of molecular studies including gene rearrangement analysis can also be used to evaluate clonality. By definition, primary pulmonary lymphomas should not have evidence of disease outside of the lung or hilar lymph nodes.

1. **MALTomas commonly arise in the lung and constitute the most common form of primary pulmonary lymphoma.** MALTomas for the most part correspond to marginal zone lymphoma, and many harbor a t(8;11) translocation, which may be relatively specific for lung MALTomas. Most cases occur in adults; there is no specific relationship to infection or autoimmune disorders. Pulmonary MALToma may have a nodular or diffuse appearance, with an infiltrate composed of small lymphocytes, monocytoid cells, and plasmacytoid cells (e-Fig. 8.67) that may replace or disrupt the appearance of pre-existing germinal centers. The cells also infiltrate the bronchial mucosa with production of "lymphoepithelial lesions" as are seen with MALToma in other sites. The infiltrating cells are positive for CD19, CD20, and bcl-2, but negative for CD5, CD10, CD23, and cyclin D1.

2. **Large cell lymphoma.** Pulmonary large cell lymphoma generally presents as a solitary mass lesion involving a single lobe of the lung. These masses may develop central necrosis. Pulmonary large cell lymphomas are usually either of diffuse large cell type or are immunoblastic, and are of B-cell lineage (e-Fig. 8.68).

3. **Lymphomatoid granulomatosis (LYG) is the name for a lung lesion now known to be a malignant lymphoma, now also known as angiocentric immunoproliferative lesion (AIL).** It is an EBV-related B-cell proliferation analogous to PTLD or AIDS-related lymphoma. In fact, patients with LYG often have some underlying immunodeficiency. LYG usually is seen in middle aged or older adults, and shows multiple nodules that may suggest metastatic disease; concomitant skin and CNS involvement is quite common. Patients have respiratory symptoms such as cough or dyspnea, or may have constitutional symptoms. Microscopically, vasculocentric and angiodestructive lymphoid infiltrates that involve all layers of the vessel are the hallmark of LYG (e-Fig. 8.69); this vascular infiltration is hypothesized to result in infarct-like necrosis of the lung seen in the higher grade cases. Grade 1 lesions have infiltrates composed mainly of small T cells, plasma cells, and histiocytes; CD20 and EBV stains show only rare atypical B cells (<5 per hpf). Grade 2 cases show a greater number of atypical B cells (5 to 20 per hpf). Grade 3 cases have abundant large, atypical B cells.

4. **Leukemic infiltrates.** The lung may be the site of acute leukemic infiltrates in cases of acute myelogenous leukemia (AML), representing a granulocytic sarcoma or extramedullary myeloid tumor. Infiltration of airways, interstitial infiltrates, or nodular parenchymal masses are possible manifestations. Histologic clues to a diagnosis of AML include blast-like cells and the presence of immature eosinophilic precursors. Many cases are initially thought to represent a large cell lymphoma; one of the first clues to the current diagnosis is the absence of expression of either B- or T-cell markers in the presumed lymphomatous cells.

   The lung may also show extensive involvement by chronic lymphocytic leukemia/small lymphocytic lymphoma. In this setting, the infiltrate presents as nodular expansions along lymphatic routes in the lung.

5. **Other hematolymphoid diseases.** The lung has been the reported primary site of a variety of hematolymphoid lesions, including Hodgkin disease, intravascular lymphomatosis, plasmacytomas (e-Fig. 8.70), and Castleman disease. However, it should be reiterated that secondary involvement of the lung in patients with advanced hematolymphoid disease is very common, can occur with essentially all entities, and so must always be excluded.

6. **Pseudolymphoma.** Small nodular lymphoid deposits in the lung have been called pseudolymphoma; however, with the advent of more specific diagnostic techniques, many of these lesions have been shown to be lymphomas, such as

MALTomas. For lesions that can be demonstrated to be polyclonal, the term lymphoid hyperplasia is more appropriate.

L. Metastatic tumors. It is prudent to include metastatic disease in the differential diagnosis of every lung tumor. Metastasis should be suspected when a tumor type is encountered that would be unusual as a lung primary tumor. Also, presentation as multiple nodules, the finding of a tumor that is predominantly within lymphatics or vessels, and a tumor that appears very well circumscribed without a host stromal and inflammatory reaction should also raise suspicion for a secondary lung tumor. Clinical history, liberal use of special stains, and radiologic consultation can all be used to evaluate the possibility of metastatic disease.

CYTOLOGY OF THE LUNG
Lourdes R. Ylagan

I. METHODS OF SPECIMEN PROCUREMENT AFFECT CYTOLOGIC EVALUATION.
Cytologic evaluation of lung masses is accomplished by the analysis of sputum, bronchial wash, bronchial brush, fine needle aspirates (FNA), or pleural effusion specimens. Detection of malignancy depends on the type of procurement technique used. Sputum specimens yield the lowest quantity of exfoliated carcinoma cells, FNA specimens yield the highest. Endobronchial and transthoracic FNA for central and peripheral lung masses, respectively, yield similarly cellular specimens.

II. SPECIMEN ADEQUACY
   A. Sputum specimens, bronchial wash, bronchioalveolar lavage, and bronchial brush specimens are generally submitted fresh in a clean vial or ThinPrep® vial, and then Papaniculaou stained in the lab. Direct smears produced from endobronchial brush specimens usually carry some degree of air-drying artifact, and are therefore not the reparation of choice. The presence of alveolar macrophages and bronchial epithelial cells render these specimen types adequate for evaluation (e-**Fig. 8.71**).
   B. Fine needle aspirates of lung masses, whether obtained via endoscopic or transthoracic approaches, are DiffQuik® and Papaniculaou stained.
   C. Pleural effusions are generally submitted fresh, in toto, from which a well mixed portion (generally 2–300 ml) is used to prepare both a cytospin DiffQuik® and ThinPrep® Papanicolaou stained slide preparation. Benign mesothelial cells are generally found in these specimens (e-**Fig. 8.72**), with or without inflammation.

III. DIAGNOSTIC CATEGORIES
   A. Negative for malignancy. This diagnosis is rendered when the specimen shows only alveolar macrophages, benign bronchial epithelial cells, and mixed inflammatory cells. This diagnosis is also used when fungal elements are identified, or when viral cytopathic changes are seen.
   B. Atypical cytology. This diagnosis is rendered when the specimen shows bronchial epithelial cells which can be interpreted as reactive, but in which there is the absence of evidence of an underlying lesion. A repeat aspirate or tissue biopsy is usually suggested. An aspirate which shows markedly reactive bronchial epithelial cells which maybe interpreted as positive for carcinoma should be repeated if the cells are adjacent to ciliated bronchial epithelium (e-**Fig. 8.73**).
   C. Suspicious for malignancy. This diagnosis is rendered when rare malignant cells are present, but the quantity is insufficient for a definitive diagnosis of malignancy. This diagnosis usually prompts a repeat diagnostic procedure before definitive surgical treatment.
   D. Positive for malignancy. This diagnosis is rendered when both the quality and quantity of malignant cells are sufficient for an unequivocal diagnosis of malignancy.

IV. COMMON LUNG LESIONS
   A. Squamous cell carcinoma, a type of non-small cell carcinoma, consists of cells with varying degrees of keratinization, inconsistent size and shape, polygonal to amphophilic cytoplasm, and dark pyknotic nuclei. The background usually shows so-called dirty necrosis with abundant keratinized cellular debris (e-**Fig. 8.74**).

B. Adenocarcinoma, another type of non-small cell carcinoma, shows cells with fine foamy to vacuolated cytoplasm, and vesicular nuclei with prominent nucleoli. There is typically no background necrosis unless the tumor is large (e-**Fig. 8.75**).

C. Small cell carcinoma or large cell neuroendocrine carcinoma must be distinguished from non-small cell carcinomas since they respond well to chemotherapy. Small cell carcinoma is composed of cells with only a small amount of cytoplasm; nuclei that show a molding pattern, fine granular chromatin, and streaming; apoptotic debris; and cellular necrosis (e-**Fig. 8.76**).

D. Mesothelioma is usually seen in association with a pleural effusion. Cytologically, the cells show variability in size, with those in clusters having scalloped edges. A cell-in-cell arrangement is often present. Enlarged and convoluted nuclei, with or without nucleoli, are typical (e-**Fig. 8.77**). Appropriate immunohistochemical stains to rule out an adenocarcinoma should be performed. Asbestos fibers (e-**Fig. 8.78**) may be seen in bronchioalveolar lavage specimens from these patients.

E. Metastases to the lung are common, and should be evaluated on the basis of the patient's clinical history. The diagnostic approach to tumors of unknown origin presenting as lung metastases is the same as for tumors of unknown origin presenting at other sites (*Semin Oncol* 1993;20:206).

Suggested Readings

Churg A, Green FYH, eds. *Pathology of Occupational Diseases.* New York: Igaku-Shoin; 1988.

Churg AM, Myers JL, Tazelaar HD, Wright JL. *Thurlbecks Pathology of the Lung,* 3rd ed. Thieme; 2005.

Colby TV, Koss MN, Travis WD. AFIP Atlas of Tumor Pathology. Series III. *Tumors of the Lower Respiratory Tract.* Washington, DC: Armed Forces Institute of Pathology; 1996.

Dail DH, Hammar SP, eds. *Pulmonary Pathology.* New York: Springer Verlag; 1994.

Katzenstein AA. *Katzenstein and Askin's Surgical Pathology of Non-Neoplastic Lung Disease,* 4th ed. : WB Saunders Company; 2006.

Roggli VL, Greenberg SD, Pratt PC, eds. *Pathology of Asbestos-Associated Diseases.* Boston: Little, Brown and Company 1992.

Stocker JT, Dehner LP, eds. *Pediatric Pathology.* Philadelphia: JB Lippincott Co.; 1992.

Tomashefski TF, Cagle PT, Farver CF, Fraire AE. *Dail and Hammar's Pulmonary Pathology. Vol. 1 Non-neoplastic Lung Disease.* 3rd ed. : Springer Verlag; 2008.

Travis WD, Brambilla E. Müller-Hermelink HK, Harris CC. *Pathology & Genetics of Tumours of the Lung, Thymus And Heart (World Health Organization Classification of Tumours).* : WHO Press; 2004.

Travis WD, Colby TV, Koss MN, Rosado-de-Christenson ML, Müller NL, King TE. *AFIP Atlas of Non-Tumor Pathology. Series I. Non-Neoplastic Disorders of the Lower Respiratory Tract.* Washington, DC: Armed Forces Institute of Pathology; 2002.

Wick MR, Leslie KG. *Practical Pulmonary Pathology: A Diagnostic Approach.* : Churchill Livingstone; 2005.

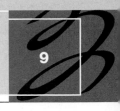

CARDIOVASCULAR SYSTEM

Jochen K. M. Lennerz

HEART

I. NORMAL ANATOMY. The normal weight of the adult heart is 300 to 350 g (men) and 250 to 300 g (women). Cardiomegaly above a critical weight of 500 g is associated with ischemic changes (**III.C.3**) and is termed *cor bovinum*. The normal ventricular thickness is 0.3 to 0.5 cm on the right and 1.2 to 1.5 cm on the left (**e-Fig. 9.1**),* measured at the base of the papillary muscles (Fig. 9.1). The heart is composed of three layers: the epicardium (including the serous or visceral pericardium, and the main branches of the coronary arteries), the muscular myocardium, and the endocardium (with an ill-defined subendocardial layer that contains many Purkinje fibers).

Microscopically, the normal myocardium is a syncytium of myocardial fibers (cardiac myocytes) that have centrally located nuclei (**e-Fig. 9.1**). Cardiac myocytes are a specialized form of striated muscle; faint dark eosinophilic intercalated discs between the myocytes form the mechanical and electrical couplings. Numerous capillaries with sparse interstitial tissue are found between the myocardial fibers (**e-Fig. 9.1**).

The atrioventricular valves (mitral and tricuspid) are composed of an annulus, leaflets, chordae tendinae, and papillary muscles. The semilunar valves (aortic and pulmonic) are composed of three cusps (each with a sinus), which meet at the three commissures (corpora arantii; **e-Fig. 9.2**). Valves are relatively avascular and are lined by endothelial cells on a thin layer of collagen and elastic tissue on the atrial/arterial side, a thicker layer of dense collagen on the ventricular side, and loose myxoid connective tissue (zona spongiosa) in between. The fibrous and spongiotic regions are normally of equal thickness (**e-Fig. 9.2**).

The conduction system is composed of specialized myocytes, with fewer intercalated disks and higher glycogen content. Masson trichrome, Verhoeff–van Giesen, and Alcian blue stains can be used to demonstrate the conduction system (**e-Fig. 9.3**). Exact knowledge of the topographic anatomy and correct sampling techniques are paramount (**e-Fig. 9.4**).

II. GROSS EXAMINATION AND TISSUE HANDLING

    A. Endomyocardial biopsies are usually taken via a right-sided cardiac catheter; the most common indications are monitoring of heart transplant rejection and grading of adriamycin toxicity. To avoid sampling errors, a minimum of three, preferably four, samples of myocardium are recommended (**e-Fig. 9.5**). The tissue fragments should be counted and measured during gross examination; their color and consistency should be noted. The tissue should be placed between foam pads or wrapped in filter paper for routine processing. Examination of at least three levels is recommended; some laboratories keep the intervening sections for additional stains if they are required to assess myocyte damage and fibrosis. Histologically, an adequate biopsy contains at least 50% myocardium, excluding previous biopsy sites (**e-Fig. 9.5**). Occasional cases require fresh frozen tissue or glutaraldehyde fixation for special techniques such as molecular diagnostics or electron microscopy (**III.C.2.e,g**), respectively. Adipose tissue between cardiomyocytes is a normal finding and does not indicate ventricular perforation (**e-Fig. 9.5**).

---

*All e-figures are available online via the Solution Site Image Bank.

Coronary Arteries - Bypasses - Sectioning

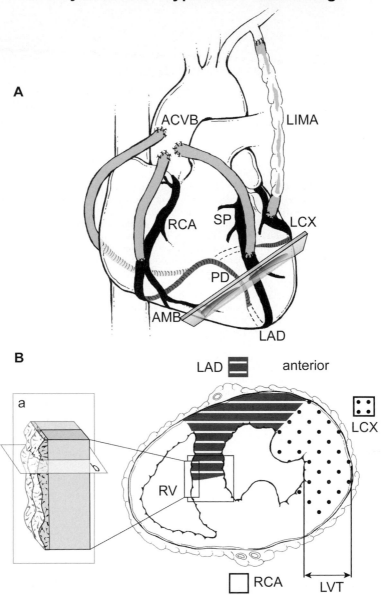

Figure 9.1. Coronary arteries, bypasses, sectioning of the ventricles. **A:** Left coronary artery branches into left circumflex (LCX) and left anterior descending (LAD), the latter supplies the anterior septum via septal perforators (SP). The right coronary artery (RCA) supplies the atrioventricular-node (not shown), branches into the acute marginal branch (AMB) and the posterior descending artery (PD). The origin of the PD determines the distribution type (right vs. left). Examples of aorto-coronary venous bypass (ACVB) and left internal mammary artery (LIMA) grafts are displayed in *gray*. **B:** Slice from plane illustrated in **a**. The myocardium displays the supplying arteries for mapping of myocardial infarctions. The ventricular thickness (LVT) is measured on the level of the anterior papillary muscle. The *large septal square* illustrates a section to determine myocyte disarray. The *small rectangle* close to the right ventricle (RV) illustrates a myomectomy specimen, which is sectioned perpendicular to the endocardial surface; preferred is horizontal (*a*) or vertical (*b*).

B. Cardiac valves are often removed because of calcific degeneration or perforation as sequelae of bacterial endocarditis (e-**Fig. 9.2**). Most valves are received in fragments; if possible, the description should include the distribution of vegetations (e-**Fig. 9.6**) and presence or absence of nonsurgery-related leaflet destruction. In cases of calcific degeneration, slow acid decalcification after fixation may be necessary. Sections are taken from the free edge to the annulus.

Prosthetic valves are typically removed because of thrombosis, anastomotic or valvular leakage, mechanical failure, or infection. Evaluation of the prosthetic valve ring attachment is therefore critical as infective endocarditis typically affects this region. For most mechanical heart valves, it is not possible to submit any tissue for histology, unless vegetations are present. For bioprosthetic valves, however, the valve cusp is submitted.

Valves from patients treated with the appetite-suppressant drug Fen-phen (a combination of fenfluramine and phentermine) show patterns of changes that resemble carcinoid valve disease with superficial layers of myofibroblastic proliferation on otherwise normal valve architecture.

C. Myomectomy specimens from ventricular aneurysm repair or septal myomectomy procedures should be measured, weighed, and sectioned at 3-mm intervals, perpendicular to the endocardial surface (Fig. 9.1). All layers of the heart should be described. For cardiac tumors, appropriate sections should assess the inked specimen resection margins (**IV.A.**).

D. Heart explant specimens should be weighed, described, and dissected as outlined (Fig. 9.2). In addition, the valves (circumference or diameter) and walls (Fig. 9.1) should be measured. The septal and ventricular configuration (concentric vs. dilatative ventricular hypertrophy) should be described.

III. DIAGNOSTIC FEATURES OF COMMON DISEASES OF THE HEART

A. Disorders of the endocardium

1. Infective endocarditis is characterized by bacterial colonization of the valve forming vegetations that are red, irregular (e-**Fig. 9.6**), and composed of granulation tissue and thrombus; their friability explains the propensity for associated septic embolization (e-**Fig. 9.2**). The myocardium is typically not involved. *Staphylococcus aureus* typically produces acute endocarditis, whereas *Streptococcus viridans* produces subacute endocarditis. Several organisms normally found in the oral cavity are also causative, and have been referred to as the Gram-negative HACEK organisms (*Hemophilus aphrophilus, Actinobacillus actinomycetemcomitans, Cardiobacterium hominis, Eikenella corrodens,* and *Kingella kingii*). *Staphylococcus epidermidis* also causes infective endocarditis, more common in the setting of prosthetic valves. Healed infective endocarditis leaves residual valve damage, often fenestrations, usually with a hemodynamic jet lesion and adjacent endocardial fibrosis.

2. Nonbacterial thrombotic endocarditis (*marantic endocarditis*) produces small (rarely >0.5 cm), pink, bland, and sterile vegetations attached to the valve surface at the lines of closure (e-**Fig. 9.6**). It is typically seen in cachectic patients with a hypercoagulable state (e.g., Trousseau syndrome).

3. Libman–Sacks endocarditis is seen in 4% of cases of systemic lupus erythematosis and is characterized by flat, pale tan, spreading bands of vegetations located on both surfaces of the valves or chordae tendinae (e-**Fig. 9.6**). Affected, in order of frequency, are the tricuspid, mitral, pulmonic, and aortic valves.

4. Rheumatic heart disease (RHD) is a sequela of rheumatic fever (RF) caused by *Streptococcus pyogenes* (group A or β-hemolytic streptococcus). Aschoff nodules (ANs) are a characteristic feature and appear as interstitial collections of plump mononuclear cells with occasional neurophils arranged in a granulomalike formation, although the presence or number of ANs does not correlate with clinical course or activity of the rheumatic process. The most characteristic cellular component of ANs is the Aschoff giant cell, which has two or more nuclei with prominent nucleoli; another characteristic feature is the presence of Anitschkow cells, which are mononuclear histiocytes that are often arranged in a palisade around the center of the granuloma. The macroscopic pattern is variable (e-**Fig. 9.6**).

Dissection Techniques of the Heart

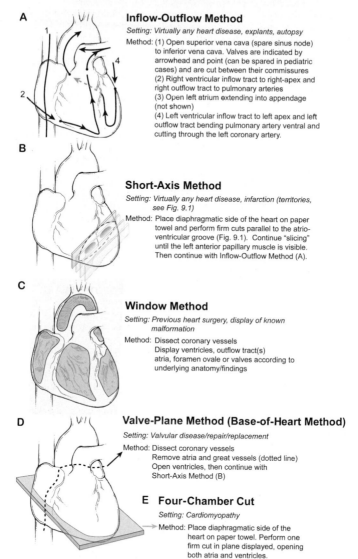

A

Inflow-Outflow Method

Setting: Virtually any heart disease, explants, autopsy

Method: (1) Open superior vena cava (spare sinus node) to inferior vena cava. Valves are indicated by arrowhead and point (can be spared in pediatric cases) and are cut between their commissures
(2) Right ventricular inflow tract to right-apex and right outflow tract to pulmonary arteries
(3) Open left atrium extending into appendage (not shown)
(4) Left ventricular inflow tract to left apex and left outflow tract bending pulmonary artery ventral and cutting through the left coronary artery.

B

Short-Axis Method

Setting: Virtually any heart disease, infarction (territories, see Fig. 9.1)

Method: Place diaphragmatic side of the heart on paper towel and perform firm cuts parallel to the atrio-ventricular groove (Fig. 9.1). Continue "slicing" until the left anterior papillary muscle is visible. Then continue with Inflow-Outflow Method (A).

C

Window Method

Setting: Previous heart surgery, display of known malformation

Method: Dissect coronary vessels
Display ventricles, outflow tract(s) atria, foramen ovale or valves according to underlying anatomy/findings

D

Valve-Plane Method (Base-of-Heart Method)

Setting: Valvular disease/repair/replacement

Method: Dissect coronary vessels
Remove atria and great vessels (dotted line)
Open ventricles, then continue with Short-Axis Method (B)

E Four-Chamber Cut

Setting: Cardiomyopathy

Method: Place diaphragmatic side of the heart on paper towel. Perform one firm cut in plane displayed, opening both atria and ventricles.

Figure 9.2. Dissection techniques of the heart.

The valvular disease characteristic of chronic RHD is usually the result of multiple recurrent episodes of acute RF, and typically develops many decades after the initial insult. RHD is the most common cause of mitral stenosis, and in up to 75% of cases the mitral valve is the only valve affected. In 25% of cases the mitral and aortic valve are affected. Progressive fibrosis leads to thickening of the valve and chordae that eventually leads to fusion of the mitral leaflets at the commissures, producing the classic "fish mouth" appearance.

5. Endocardial fibroelastosis is an uncommon condition that can result in restrictive cardiomyopathy. Pearly-white fibroelastic thickening, caused by accumulation of collagen and elastic fibers typically in the left ventricular endocardium (e-**Fig. 9.3**), is often associated with aortic valve obstruction. The disease occurs either focally or diffusely in children from birth to age 2.

6. Loeffler's endocarditis is also known as fibroelastic parietal endocarditis with blood eosinophilia. Classically, three stages (acute necrotic myocarditis, organizing thrombus, and endomyocardial fibrosis) are distinguished. The cardiac lesions are associated with dense eosinophilic infiltration of other organs, and the disease is usually rapidly fatal.

B. Disorders of the valves

1. Myxoid change is stromal accumulation of glycosaminoglycans as a sign of degeneration (e-**Fig. 9.2**). The layered architecture is preserved; if the architecture is absent or distorted, the differential diagnosis should include RHD. The chordae tendinae are thinned and elongated in myxomatous degeneration, whereas in RHD they are shortened and thickened.

2. Mitral valves are removed for acquired postinflammatory stenosis (e.g., RHD) and may show commissural fusion, cusp scarring, and dystrophic calcification (e-**Fig. 9.2**). RHD vegetations are composed mainly of fibrin and are usually no more than 2 mm in size. Cases of mitral insufficiency or myxomatous degeneration show a floppy valve with redundant and ballooned leaflets with abundant myxoid change.

3. Tricuspid valves are most commonly removed for insufficiency or infective endocarditis.

4. Aortic valves are removed for stenosis and are typically heavily calcified, sometimes with commissural fusion (senile calcific aortic stenosis), postinflammatory scarring, or calcification due to a congenitally bicuspid valve (present in 1% of the population).

5. Pulmonary valves are usually excised because of stenosis due to congenital heart disease (most commonly as a component of tetralogy of Fallot).

C. Disorders of the myocardium

1. Myocarditis is the underlying etiology in about 10% of patients with new-onset cardiac dysfunction. If not fatal, myocarditis often proceeds to dilated cardiomyopathy. Findings in subsequent biopsies, using the first specimen as a reference point, include: ongoing/persistent myocarditis, resolving/healing myocarditis (damage substantially reduced), or resolved/healed myocarditis (damage no longer present). The so-called Dallas criteria (*Hum Pathol.* 1987;18:619) are often used to categorize myocarditis mainly on histopathological findings, although it has been suggested that the criteria are no longer adequate (*Circulation.* 2006;113:593). The World Health Organization defines myocarditis as a minimum of 14 infiltrating leukocytes per square millimeter, preferably T cells, with as many as four macrophages (also known as the Marburg criteria; see *Circulation.* 1996;93:841). The diagnosis of *active myocarditis* classically requires the presence of an inflammatory infiltrate (usually lymphocytic) and myocyte necrosis/degeneration or damage not characteristic of an ischemic event; *borderline myocarditis* indicates the absence of necrosis and/or damage and can be applied to any form of inflammatory infiltrate.

a. Primary viral myocarditis accounts for most cases of myocarditis in developed countries. Cardiac involvement typically follows the primary viral infection by several days. The most commonly associated agents are enteroviruses (coxsackie A and B), adenovirus, echovirus, poliovirus, influenza viruses A and B, and human immunodeficiency virus (HIV). The infiltrate is composed mainly of lymphocytes with associated myocyte damage (e-**Fig. 9.7**). Eosinophils are typically not seen. Primary viral myocarditis includes four clinical pathological manifestations: fulminate, chronic active, eosinophilic, and giant cell myocarditis.

b. Fulminant myocarditis has a distinct onset within 2 weeks of presentation of profound left ventricular dysfunction without dilatation. Biopsy shows multiple foci of active inflammation and necrosis. Patients usually show complete histological and functional recovery or die within 2 weeks.

c. Chronic active myocarditis has an indistinct onset with moderate ventricular dysfunction and active or borderline myocarditis. Ongoing inflammation and fibrosis may result in the development of restrictive cardiomyopathy with 2 to 4 years after presentation.

d. Eosinophilic myocarditis can be attributed to eosinophilic syndromes or allergic reactions that result in left ventricular compromise. Eosinophils and myocyte damage are present in the biopsy (e-**Fig. 9.7**). This entity, sometimes referred to as *hypersensitivity myocarditis*, is linked to treatment with methyldopa, antibiotics (penicillin, sulfonamides, streptomycin), anticonvulsants, and antidepressants, and also shows eosinophils and occasional giant cells. The myocardium has little myocyte necrosis, and the inflammatory infiltrate is lymphohistiocytic and predominantly perivascular (e-**Fig. 9.7**). In some cases, the infiltrate is subendocardial or appears as poorly formed granulomas.

The differential diagnosis of eosinophilia in the myocardium includes parasitic infection, allergy, a hypereosinophilic syndrome, and hematologic malignancies. Cytomegalovirus infection should enter the differential diagnosis in an immunosuppressed patient.

e. Idiopathic giant cell myocarditis, also known as Fiedler's myocarditis, is associated with autoimmune diseases (e.g., inflammatory bowel disease, hypothyroidism) and is rapidly fatal if untreated. It typically occurs in young, healthy, white adults and presents as congestive heart failure. Diffuse, geographic myocardial necrosis with a mixed inflammatory infiltrate including eosinophils and multinucleated giant cells in the absence of granulomas is typical (e-**Fig. 9.8**). The giant cells have the immunohistochemical profile of histiocytes.

f. Other organisms associated with myocarditis include bacteria, fungi, spirochetes (especially *Borrelia burgdorferi*), *Rickettsiae*, *Chlamydia*, parasites (including *Toxoplasma gondii* in immunocompromised patients), and helminths (trichinosis).

g. Chagas disease, the most common form of protozoal myocarditis, is caused by the hemoflagellate *Trypanosoma cruzi* and is uncommon in the United States. However, in endemic regions of South and Central America it accounts for 25% of all deaths of 25- to 40-year-olds; up to 80% of patients with Chagas disease develop myocarditis. Histologically, myofibers contain parasites with an associated mild chronic inflammatory infiltrate. In the acute phase, dense inflammation with myocyte necrosis and trypanosome amastigotes in myocytes is characteristic, whereas the chronic phase shows interstitial and perivascular lymphoplasmacytic infiltrate without fibrosis.

h. Secondary myocarditis can occur in the setting of collagen vascular diseases, RF, drugs, heat stroke, and radiation.

i. Granulomatous myocarditis (e-**Fig. 9.9**) can be seen in tuberculosis or sarcoidosis.

j. Cardiac sarcoidosis shows non-necrotizing granulomas (e-**Fig. 9.9**) in a background of fibrosis and necrosis. Cardiac involvement, although present in 25% of systemic cases of sarcoidosis, is usually patchy; therefore, a single negative endomyocardial biopsy does not exclude the disease. The differential diagnosis in cases of suspected cardiac sarcoidosis includes idiopathic giant cell myocarditis, amyloid, Chagas disease, and Fabry disease.

2. Cardiomyopathy

a. Ischemic cardiomyopathy (**III.C.3.**) is usually secondary to severe coronary artery disease (e-**Fig. 9.10**).

b. Hypertrophic cardiomyopathy is typically seen in healthy individuals younger than 30 years, but can be seen at almost any age. Affected individuals suffer from angina, exertional dyspnea, or sudden cardiac death as a result of diastolic dysfunction due to ventricular thickening. In hypertrophic obstructive cardiomyopathy, there is classically asymmetric ventricular septal hypertrophy (with a wall thickness of 15 to 30 mm), with associated fibrous endocardial plaques and mitral valve thickening. Microscopically, disarray of myofibers (e-**Fig. 9.11**), myofiber hypertrophy, basophilic degeneration, and interstitial fibrosis are characteristic, although nonspecific. More than 400 disease-causing mutations in 11 genes encoding for myocardial contractile proteins have been implicated (*Neth Heart J.* 2007;15:184).

c. Dilated cardiomyopathy, also known as congestive cardiomyopathy, presents as cardiac failure due to progressive cardiac dilatation with systolic dysfunction. Hypertrophy (increased weight with normal or reduced wall thickness) and marked dilatation of all chambers is typical (e-Fig. 9.12). Histological examination shows nonspecific abnormalities; in about 50% of the cases, leukocytic infiltrates are present in endomyocardial biopsies. A significant number of cases are thought to be postviral or associated with alcohol use or chemotherapeutic agents. Pheochromocytoma is also associated with dilated cardiomyopathy. Dilated cardiomyopathy occurring in the peripartum period (up to 6 months after delivery) is known as peripartum cardiomyopathy. About 90% of familial cases show autosomal dominant inheritance, and 5–10% are X-linked. In addition to the genes affected by hypertrophic cardiomyopathy, additional mutations in cytoskeletal, nuclear envelope, and mitochondrial proteins have been found (*Circulation.* 2002;66:219).

d. Restrictive (obliterative) cardiomyopathy is uncommon in developed countries. The ventricles are normal or slightly enlarged but not dilated; in contrast, the atria exhibit relative bilateral dilatation. Patchy or interstitial fibrosis is found histologically (e-Fig. 9.13). The eosinophilic form shows an eosinophil-rich myocardial infiltrate, whereas the noneosinophilic form (more common in the United States) shows nonspecific findings. Restrictive cardiomyopathy is typically caused by endomyocardial fibrosis or hemochromatosis, but is often idiopathic.

e. Infiltrative cardiomyopathy is descriptive of a broad panel of metabolic diseases, and can be assigned to any disorder that restricts ventricular filling.

   i. Cardiac amyloidosis histologically shows amorphous, eosinophilic, extracellular material (e-Fig. 9.14). Cardiac amyloidosis is associated with restrictive features due to associated decreased ventricular compliance, and presents with diastolic dysfunction. Grossly, the myocardium appears stiff and rubbery or waxy. The diagnosis of amyloid is confirmed by demonstrating apple-green birefringence with polarized light using a Congo red stain and/or electron microscopy (e-Fig. 9.14).

   ii. Hereditary hemochromatosis is a homozygous autosomal recessive disorder resulting from *HFE* gene mutations. The mutation results in unregulated uptake of iron in the small intestine, leading to iron deposition in the liver (hepatomegaly), pancreas (diabetes mellitus), skin (hyperpigmentation), or heart (dilated or restrictive cardiomyopathy). In the heart, myocytes and interstitial macrophages contain abundant brown pigment (e-Fig. 9.15), which can be demonstrated to be iron by the Prussian blue stain, but there is little correlation between the amount of cardiac iron and systolic dysfunction. Increased cardiac iron must be distinguished from lipofuscin; the latter is more finely granular, derived from normal intracellular lipid peroxidation, and is not stained by Prussian blue (e-Fig. 9.15). Iron overload is not specific for hereditary hemochromatosis but can also be seen in the setting of thalassemia, multiple transfusions, hemosiderosis, or hemolytic anemia.

   iii. Other infiltrative cardiomyopathies include Loeffler's endocarditis, endocardial fibroelastosis, and mitochondrial myopathies.

f. Arrhythmogenic right ventricular cardiomyopathy is also known as right ventricular dysplasia, parchment right ventricle, and Uhl's anomaly. This uncommon variant of familial cardiomyopathy shows replacement of the myocardium by adipose and fibrous tissue, predominantly in the inferior and infundibular wall, without associated coronary artery sclerosis. The genetics of the disease have recently begun to be characterized (*J Cardiovasc Electrophysiol.* 2005;16:927).

g. Drug- and/or radiation-induced cardiomyopathy (*Cancer Treat Rev.* 2004; 30:181) is caused by drugs such as adriamycin and cyclophosphamide and shows primarily subcellular changes that are best seen by electron microscopy.

  i. Adriamycin (doxorubicin) toxicity is characterized by dose-dependent changes, predominately in the subendocardial region. It frequently occurs after lifetime doses >500 mg/m^2. Vacuolization of myocytes (mainly due to marked dilatation of the sarcoplasmic reticulum) is initially present (e-**Fig. 9.16**), followed by the appearance of typical "adria-cells" that show loss of cross-striations, myofilamentous bundles, and accompanying homogeneous basophilic staining (corresponding to ultrastructural fragmentation of sarcomeres). There is no accompanying inflammation. Because the microscopic features are not specific for adriamycin toxicity, clinical correlation is required (*Environ Health Perspect.* 1978;26:181, and *Int J Cardiol.* 2007;117:6).

  ii. Cyclophosphamide toxicity may produce hemorrhagic necrosis, interstitial hemorrhage, extensive capillary thrombosis, fibrin deposition, and necrosis of myocardial fibers.

  iii. Radiation enhances the changes seen with chemotherapy. Constrictive pericarditis, myocardial fibrosis, and coronary artery lesions are also associated with radiation therapy.

  3. Myocardial ischemia & ischemic heart disease

  a. The appearance of a myocardial infarct is dependent on its age (e-**Fig. 9.17**). Following acute ischemia, the histologic changes include waviness of fibers (after 1 to 3 hours), progressing to coagulative necrosis with contraction bands (after 4 to 12 hours), and infiltration by neutrophils (after 2 to 24 hours). In cases of reperfusion, contraction band necrosis can be seen after 18 to 24 hours as the cells begin to lose cross-striations and nuclear detail. Total coagulative necrosis can be seen by 24 to 72 hours.

  b. Chronic ischemic heart disease culminates in diffuse myocardial atrophy (brown atrophy) with patchy perivascular and interstitial fibrosis, with progressive ischemic necrosis. The heart is small with chocolate-colored myocardium that shows excessive lipofuscin deposition within the fibers.

  c. Microscopic arteriopathy is a term used to designate the changes in peripheral coronary arteries that undergo sclerotic changes (e-**Fig. 9.18**) resulting in a small lumen (>75% reduction in cross-sectional area). The disease is typically seen in chronic hypertension or with cocaine-induced cardiomyopathy, but will to some degree occur in chronic heart transplant rejection, where it becomes the rate-limiting step to long-term survival.

D. Disorders of the pericardium

  1. Acute pericarditis (e-**Fig. 9.19**) is idiopathic in 90% of cases, but can be caused by viruses (coxsackie B, echoviruses, influenza, mumps, Epstein–Barr virus [EBV]) or bacteria (*Staphylococcus aureus, Streptococci,* or *Haemophilus influenza*). Acute serous pericarditis can be secondary to acute RF, connective tissue disorders (e.g., systemic lupus erythematosus), uremia, metastatic malignancy, and renal transplantation. In contrast, acute fibrinous or serofibrinous pericarditis can be secondary to myocardial infarction (typically after 1 to 3 days), uremia, chest radiotherapy, RF, systemic lupus erythematosis, cardiac surgery, pneumonia, pleural infection, and cardiac trauma. Caseous pericarditis is usually due to *Mycobacterium tuberculosis* infection. Healed acute pericarditis usually results in a focal pearly thickened epicardial plaque, also known as a "soldier's plaque."

  2. Chronic pericarditis can lead to constrictive pericarditis where the heart is encased by a thick layer of fibrous tissue. Constrictive pericarditis can follow caseous pericarditis or radiotherapy, but is usually idiopathic.

  3. Neoplasms. Although primary neoplasms of the pericardium are very rare (including mesothelioma, germ cell tumors, and angiosarcoma), pericardial involvement is present in up to about 10% of patients with disseminated malignancy.

  4. Pericardial effusions. Effusions can be as large as 500 mL in some settings, such as congestive heart failure and hypoproteinemia. However, in acute cardiac tamponade, rapid accumulation of as little as 200 to 300 mL can cause cardiac compression and death.

IV. NEOPLASMS OF THE HEART. The four most common cardiac primary tumors (and tumorlike conditions) are all benign and account for 70% of cardiac neoplasms. Primary malignancies of the heart are very rare; involvement of the heart by a malignancy is far more likely to represent metastasis by lung carcinoma, breast carcinoma, melanoma, lymphoma, leukemia, renal cell carcinoma, and choriocarcinoma. In cases of metastatic spread to the heart, the pericardium is often involved.

A. Cardiac myxoma is the most common primary tumor of the heart. In the sporadic form, the tumor typically occurs in middle-aged women, and is grossly a spherical, soft gray-white, gelatinous, lobulated tumor 1 to 10 cm in maximal dimension, typically attached by a stalk to the left atrium near the fossa ovalis (e-**Fig. 9.20**). In familial cases (e.g., Carney complex, NAME syndrome (*n*evi, *a*trial myxoma, *m*yxoid neurofibroma, and *e*phelides), or LAMB syndrome (*l*entigines, *a*trial myxomas, *m*ucocutaneous myxomas, and *b*lue nevi), the mean age of patients is mid-20s, and the tumor is more often attached to the right atrium or is multicentric. Microscopically, myxomas consist of plump spindled or stellate cells in abundant loose myxoid stroma (e-**Fig. 9.20**). Heterologous elements including cartilage, foci of ossification (petrified myxoma), or gland formation (glandular myxoma) can be seen, but have no prognostic significance (e-**Fig. 9.20**).

B. Papillary fibroelastoma occurs typically on the ventricular surface of the semilunar valves or the atrial surface of the atrioventricular valves. The tumor accounts for 75% of all valvular tumors, and can be up to 7 cm in greatest dimension. In children, the right side is predominantly affected. The branching avascular papillae are composed of fibroelastic myxoid stroma and are lined by hyperplastic endothelium (e-**Fig. 9.20**).

C. Lipomas typically have a subendocardial location in the left ventricle.

D. Rhabdomyoma presents as a single (10% of cases) or multiple (90% of cases) well-circumscribed gray-white firm myocardial nodule up to 6 cm in size that often protrudes into the ventricle. The tumor is often discovered in the first year of life, and is the most common cardiac tumor in the pediatric age group. Patients usually present with heart failure or arrhythmias. Microscopically, the tumor is composed of mixtures of round and polygonal cells with glycogen-rich vacuoles (e-**Fig. 9.20**) that are separated by strands of cytoplasm radiating from the center of the cell (so-called "spider-cells"). Rhabdomyoma is mitotically inactive, noninvasive, and nonmetastasizing; some tumors even regress spontaneously after the first year of life. The tumor is thought to be hamartomatous and is associated with tuberous sclerosis. Rhabdomyoma cells are immunoreactive for vimentin, desmin, actin and myoglobin; focal HMB45-positive cells can be present.

E. Intramural cardiac fibroma usually occurs as a single, white, rubbery lesion (e-**Fig. 9.20**). The tumor cells are typically immunopositive for vimentin and smooth muscle actin, indicating myofibroblastic differentiation; immunoreactivity for the muscle-specific markers desmin and myoD1 is absent.

F. Other benign tumors include mesothelial/monocytic incidental cardiac excrescences (also known as cardiac MICE; e-**Fig. 9.19**), calcified amorphous tumor of the heart (also known as cardiac CAT), lipomatous hypertrophy of the atrial septum, mesothelioma of the atrioventricular node, adenomatoid tumor, epithelioid or histiocytoid hemangioma, paraganglioma (extra-adrenal pheochromocytoma), schwannoma, and granular cell tumor.

G. Angiosarcoma is the most common primary malignant tumor of the heart. It typically involves the right atrium as a large mass with intracavitary extension, and may also infiltrate the myocardium. Primary angiosarcoma of the heart is typically more poorly differentiated than elsewhere (e-**Fig. 9.20**). Other rare primary cardiac sarcomas include Kaposi's sarcoma, leiomyosarcoma, liposarcoma, and rhabdomyosarcoma.

H. Carcinoid heart disease, seen in ~50% of patients with carcinoid syndrome, typically affects the heart's right side, particularly the ventricular outflow tract and pulmonic valve. Gross findings include prominent hypertrophy and plaquelike thickening of

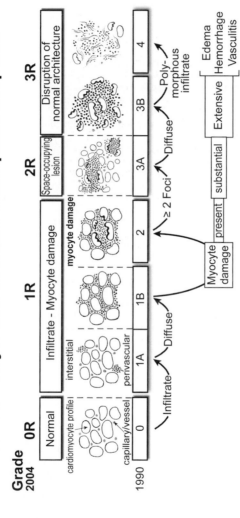

Figure 9.3. Grading of cellular rejection in heart transplant biopsies. The grading is illustrated from left to right, where the highest grade finding present determines the diagnosis. Comparison of original (1990) and revised grading (2004) schemes is schematically illustrated (see also **e-Fig. 9.21**). *Open circles* represent cardiomyocyte profiles; *small dots* represent vessels or inflammatory infiltrate. The main diagnostic feature of each grade is provided. The diagnostic features required for the 1990 grading are provided below the scheme. Based on *J Heart Transplant.* 1990;9:587; *J Heart Lung Transplant.* 2005;24:1710; and *Heart Transplant Pathol.* 2007;131:1169.

the endocardium. Microscopically, the valvular cusps show proliferation of smooth muscle and collagen deposition, without valve destruction. There are no carcinoid tumor cells in the lesion.

V. CARDIAC TRANSPLANTS. The most sensitive method for the evaluation of cellular rejection is microscopic examination of an adequate myocardial biopsy. Often the sample will be taken from a previous biopsy site and show healing foci of ischemic injury with varying degrees of inflammatory infiltrates, changes that should not be confused with acute rejection. The revised and original grading scheme for acute cellular rejection (Fig. 9.3) refers to the histologic findings (**e-Fig. 9.21**); however, the presence or absence of myocyte necrosis should always be documented (*J Heart Lung Transplant.* 2005;24:1710).

A. Quilty effect (**e-Fig. 9.22**) refers to the presence of a dense subendocardial lymphocyte infiltrate (*Am J Cardiovasc Pathol.* 1988;1:139), composed of predominately B lymphocytes. Quilty 'A' lesions are limited to the endo/subendocardium, whereas Quilty 'B' lesions extend into underlying myocardium, where there is often associated myocyte damage (*Curr Opin Cardiol.* 1997;12:146). There is no consensus as to the pathogenesis or clinical significance of Quilty 'B' lesions because up to 20% of posttransplant biopsies show this finding (also known as cyclosporine effect). Quilty lesions have no known adverse prognostic effect, and are not associated with EBV infection responsible for posttransplant lymphoproliferative disorders. Quilty effect is therefore classified as one of four nonrejection findings.

B. Ischemic injury is the second nonrejection finding. It presents either early (up to 6 weeks posttransplant) or late, and is related to allograft coronary disease.

C. Infection and lymphoproliferative disorders are the two other nonrejection findings in biopsies, characterized by diffuse infiltration by small to medium-sized lymphocytes in a pattern resembling rejection (*J Heart Lung Transplant.* 2005;24:1710).

D. So-called transplant arteriopathy or cardiac allograft vasculopathy is characteristic of chronic rejection. It features concentric luminal narrowing of small vessels by intimal thickening and medial proliferation with relative preservation of the internal elastic lamina, a pattern thought to represent an accelerated form of atherosclerosis. In cases with complete vascular obstruction ischemic damage can be found, although ischemic events are clinically silent due to the lack of cardiac reinnervation after transplantation.

VESSELS

I. NORMAL ANATOMY. The luminal endothelial cell layer defines vessels. Arteries have three layers (**e-Fig. 9.18**): the intima (composed of the endothelium, internal elastic lamella, and subendothelial connective tissue), media (smooth muscle), and adventitia (connective tissue). Venous vessels have the same three layers, but a thinner media and a thicker adventitia.

Endothelial cells are characterized by immunoreactivity for CD34, CD31, vimentin, endothelin, and von Willebrand factor. Endothelium also stains for Factor VIII–related antigen and *Ulex europaeus* I lectin, both stronger in blood vessels in comparison to lymphatic vessels. The smooth muscle cells of the media express desmin. Depending on the anatomic site, pericytes and smooth muscle or glomus cells are located along the outside of the vessel; these cells show immunoreactivity for actin, vimentin, and myosin.

The size of arterial vessels is typically defined in relation to vessels in the kidney. The aorta is categorized as a large artery, the renal and lobar arteries as medium-sized arteries, and the arcuate and interlobular arteries as small arteries (Fig. 9.4). The next smallest arterial vessels, arterioles, are defined by either a media that has two to five layers of smooth muscle cells or a luminal radius that equals the wall thickness.

II. GROSS EXAMINATION AND TISSUE HANDLING. Temporal artery biopsies are typically about 2 to 3 cm long. Because arteritis can have a patchy distribution with so-called skip areas (**III.A.1.**), proper tissue handling is essential to ensure a maximum diagnostic yield from the biopsy. The external aspect of the vessel should be inked (to ensure that the microscopic sections include the entire wall); the vessel should then be serially sectioned at 3-mm intervals. After processing, embedding of the vessel segments should

Vascular Tree and Distribution of Typical Vasculitides

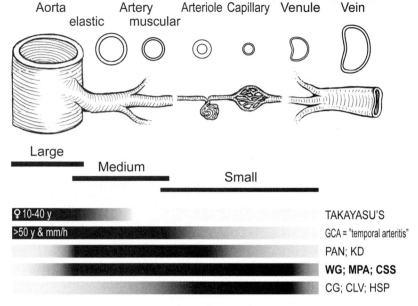

Figure 9.4. Overview of the vascular tree and typical vasculitides. TA = temporal arteritis; GCA = giant cell arteritis; PAN = panarteritis nodosa; KD = Kawasaki disease; WG = Wegener's granulomatosis; MPA = microscopic polyangiitis; CSS = Churg–Strauss syndrome; CG = cryoglobulemia; CLV = cutaneous leukocytoclastic vasculitis; HSP = Henoch–Schönlein purpura. **Bold**face type indicates ANCA-positive. See also **e-Fig. 9.18** and **e-Fig. 9.23**.

result in tissue sections with complete ringlike profiles that have an inked external surface. At least three levels should be examined. Orienting the vessel segments in agar prior to processing (*Ann Diagn Pathol.* 2001;5:107) is a simple way to ensure that proper orientation is achieved during embedding.

    Although embolectomy specimens are easy to gross, the submission of all tissue can have tremendous clinical impact, because the pathologist may ascertain the exact source of an embolus (e.g., endocarditis, atrial myxoma) in a minute piece of tissue.

III. DIAGNOSTIC FEATURES OF COMMON DISEASES. Vascular diseases affect all organs and contribute to the histopathological presentation of a variety of diseases.

  A. Vasculitides. Vasculitis is a noninfectious inflammatory disease of the vessel wall and surrounding tissue. The Chapel Hill classification system for vasculitis based on the size of the vessels (Fig. 9.4) is widely used (*Arthritis Rheum.* 1994;37:187).

    1. Large vessel vasculitides

      a. Giant cell arteritis is also known as temporal arteritis. Three of the following five diagnostic criteria by the American College of Rheumatology (ACR) are required for a diagnosis of giant cell arteritis: age >50 years, recent localized headache, temporal artery tenderness, erythrocyte sedimentation rate ≥50 mm/h, and a temporal artery biopsy demonstrating vasculitis (e-**Fig. 9.23**). It is worth noting that up to 60% of patients with clinical features of giant cell arteritis show no evidence of vasculitis by arterial biopsy (*Baillieres Clin Rheumatol.* 1991;5:387).

        There are four key diagnostic features of the vasculitis associated with giant cell arteritis: transmural inflammation, giant cells in close relation to disrupted elastic lamellae, intimal thickening, and marked intimal edema. Giant cells are not required for the diagnosis, but typically are present if a substantial or granulomatous inflammatory infiltrate is present. Noncontiguous foci of inflammation, so-called skip areas, are occasionally present; patches of arteritis can be <0.3 mm long, which emphasizes the importance of microscopic examination of multiple tissue levels (*Arch Ophthalmol.* 1976;94:2072). The diagnosis of 'healed' (e-**Fig. 9.**23) or subacute cranial arteritis is an indication for prolonged steroid therapy, and so is an important differential diagnosis. Focal aggregates of lymphocytes and/or macrophages in the media, irregular fibrosis and scarring of the media, breaks of the internal elastic lamella (involving up to 25% of the circumference), and irregular intimal fibrosis are the histologic hallmarks. Because the media does not contain blood vessels in normal arterial vessels, medial neovascularization is a useful indicator of previous inflammation.

Normal changes in the arteries of elderly persons can complicate diagnosis. However, arteriosclerosis typically does not include inflammation, and the associated intimal and medial fibrosis is concentric and not irregular. Although the internal elastic lamella may show fragmentation, long breaks are uncommon.

   b. Takayasu's arteritis. Clinical findings and vascular distribution are necessary to distinguish Takayasu's arteritis from giant cell arteritis because both diseases show identical morphologic features. In >80% of cases, Takayasu's arteritis affects women in the age range of 10 to 40 years. The aorta and typically the left mid- to proximal subclavian artery are affected, although in 50% of patients the pulmonary arteries and abdominal aorta are involved. In contrast, giant cell arteritis occurs in patients >50 years of age and typically involves the external carotid artery branches.

2. **Medium vessel vasculitides**
   a. Polyarteritis nodosa is a rare systemic, necrotizing vasculitis that is **not** associated with glomerulonephritis. The lesions are segmental, and may be only partially circumferential. The inflammation may cause weakening of the arterial wall, with subsequent aneurysmal dilatation and localized rupture.
   b. Kawasaki disease is febrile illness of childhood of unknown etiology that is characterized by a self-limited acute vasculitic syndrome. Microscopically, the vasculitis consists of an acute necrotizing arteritis similar to polyarteritis nodosa. Differentiation from polyarteritis nodosa is based on the distinctive clinical picture and age at presentation.

3. **Small vessel vasculitides.** This group of diseases is subclassified based on the presence or absence of anti-neutrophil cytoplasmic antibodies (ANCA). Because cytoplasmic ANCA (c-ANCA) mainly recognize proteinase 3 and perinuclear ANCA (p-ANCA) mainly recognize myeloperoxidase, the terms PR3-ANCA and MPO-ANCA, respectively, are now in common use (*Arch Intern Med.* 1996;156:440). ANCA-associated small-vessel vasculitides are the most common vasculitides in adults.
   a. ANCA-positive. There are four ANCA-positive small-vessel vasculitides: Wegener's granulomatosis, microscopic polyangiitis, Churg–Strauss syndrome, and drug-induced small-vessel vasculitis.
      The absence of granulomas defines microscopic polyangiitis. When granulomas are present, the distinction between Churg–Strauss syndrome and Wegener's granulomatosis is made based on the presence or absence of asthma and eosinophilia, respectively.
   b. ANCA-negative. There are three main ANCA-negative small-vessel vasculitides: Henoch–Schönlein purpura, cryoglobulinemia, and so-called non-ANCA small-vessel diseases.
      The presence of immunoglobulin A (IgA)-dominant immune deposits in small vessels (*N Engl J Med.* 1997;337:1512) is indicative of Henoch–Schönlein purpura, the most common vasculitis in children (e-**Fig.** 9.23). The absence of IgA deposits, together with the presence of serum cryoglobulins, is diagnostic of cryoglobulinemia. In the absence of both IgA and cryoglobulins, the differential diagnosis includes various non-ANCA small-vessel

vasculitides including paraneoplastic small-vessel vasculitis, inflammatory bowel disease vasculitis, and immune complex small-vessel vasculitis (a category which itself includes lupus vasculitis, rheumatoid arthritis, Goodpasture's syndrome, Sjögren disease, drug-induced immune complex vasculitis, Behçet disease, and infection-induced immune complex vasculitis). The diagnostic criteria for this group of vasculitides have been well described (*Am Fam Physician.* 2002;65:1615 and *N Engl J Med.* 1997;337:1512).

B. Amyloid angiopathy. The deposition of waxy, extracellular, amorphous, weakly eosinophilic material in the absence of an inflammatory reaction, without intimal myofibroblasts or collagen deposits, is the hallmark of amyloid angiopathy.

IV. NEOPLASMS OF THE VESSELS
   A. Benign
      1. Leiomyoma is the most common benign tumor of veins, and usually arises in the peripheral veins. Leiomyomas that arise in the inferior vena cava have a prominent luminal component and often represent extension of a uterine leiomyoma in the setting of intravascular leiomyomatosis.
      2. Rare benign neoplasms of the large arteries include inflammatory pseudotumor and benign fibrous histiocytoma. Paragangliomas occur within the aortic adventitia.
      3. Benign lesions of the endothelium are covered in the chapter on soft tissue tumors (Chapter 46).
   B. Malignant
      1. Leiomyosarcoma is the most common malignant neoplasm of veins, and differentiates toward smooth muscle cells of the media (e-**Fig. 9.24**). The tumor usually shows extension into the adjacent soft tissues; only rarely is the tumor confined to the vascular lumen. Most cases arise in the inferior vena cava, in women (the female to male ratio is >4:1) in their 6th decade. Microscopically, the tumor has the same morphologic features as leiomyosarcomas that occur at other sites.
      2. Aortic intimal sarcoma is the most common malignant neoplasm of large arteries, and is thought to arise from the pluripotent mesenchymal cells of the intima. By definition the tumor is luminal (e-**Fig. 9.24**), although some cases show focal extension into or through the media. Most cases arise within the abdominal aorta in patients in their 7th decade. Microscopically, the tumor is poorly differentiated and shows myofibroblastic or fibroblastic differentiation, although rare cases show specific histologic differentiation such as angiosarcoma or osteosarcoma. Cytologically, the tumor cells are usually spindle-shaped with marked atypia and pleomorphism.

      An analogous rare tumor, intimal pulmonary sarcoma, involves the pulmonary arteries, usually in patients in their 5th decade who present with symptoms suggestive of recurrent pulmonary emboli. As with aortic intimal sarcoma, a subset of cases has the morphology of a specific sarcoma type.

Suggested Readings
Anderson RH, Becker AE. *Cardiac Anatomy: An Integrated Text and Color Atlas.* New York: Raven Press; 1982.
Anderson RH, Becker AE. *Cardiac Anatomy: An Integrated Text and Color Atlas.* Gower Medical Publishing; 1980.
Bharati S, Lev M. *The Pathology of Congenital Heart Disease.* New York: Futura Publishing Company; 1996.
Bloom S, ed. *Diagnostic Criteria for Cardiovascular Pathology: Acquired Diseases.* Philadelphia: Lippincott-Raven Publishers; 1997.
Bowker TJ, Wood DA, Davies MJ, et al. Sudden, unexpected cardiac or unexplained death in England: a national survey *Q J Med.* 2003;96:269.
Fowles R, ed. *Cardiac Biopsy.* New York: Futura Publishing Company; 1992.

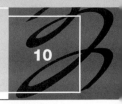
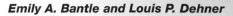

I. GROSS ANATOMY. The mediastinum is as much what it is as what it is not. It is located in the thoracic cavity and is generally divided into superior, anterior, middle, and posterior compartments and is bounded by the pleura laterally. Generally the first rib defines its superior limit and the diaphragm its inferior border. The sternum, ribs, and thoracic vertebrae (T1 through T11–12) constitute the skeletal confines of the mediastinum. The thymus, heart with its great vessels, lungs, and esophagus are among the most obvious organs that occupy the anterior (thymus), middle (heart), and posterior (esophagus and aorta) mediastinum. The aortic arch and the proximal segment of the aorta (ascending and proximal aorta) are located in the superior mediastinum, which is bounded by the manubrium sterni anteriorly and thoracic vertebrae 1 through 4. The embryological aspects of the mediastinum are basically those of the organs and structures that occupy this compartment.

One of the important considerations in the definition of the mediastinum relates to those structures and organs with observable pathology on imaging studies and the accompanying differential diagnosis. For instance, the anterior mediastinum is the site of the thymus with its varied associated pathology from Hodgkin lymphoma (HL) and non-Hodgkin lymphoma (NHL), to thymoma, to germ cell neoplasms. The pathology of the posterior mediastinum is dominated by a variety of neurogenic neoplasms and bronchoenteric developmental cysts.

II. GROSS EXAMINATION, TISSUE SAMPLING, AND HISTOLOGIC SLIDE PREPARATION

A. Fine needle aspiration biopsy (FNAB) is generally performed as an image-guided or endoscopically directed procedure on suspected pathology in the anterior or middle mediastinum. Given the broad range in pathologic processes in the anterior and middle mediastinum, an advanced level of experience is often required and even recommended. One of the more common specimens is the lymph node with a differential diagnosis of an infectious and/or granulomatous process, metastasis, or lymphoma. Metastasis, usually a carcinoma of the lung or elsewhere (squamous cell carcinoma of the head and neck, papillary thyroid carcinoma, or renal cell carcinoma) accounts for over 50% of diagnoses. NHL (lymphoblastic lymphoma and mediastinal large B-cell lymphoma) and HL presenting in the mediastinum are the most common primary malignant neoplasms in this site. A strong suspicion about an NHL can be voiced in the case of a lymphoblastic lymphoma, but both large B-cell lymphoma and HL of the nodular sclerosis subtype have a considerable fibrous component that may complicate the ability to obtain a diagnostically satisfactory cellular specimen.

B. Biopsy. Tissue samplings from the anterior mediastinum are generally small (<1 cm in maximal dimension) and often consist of multiple fragments that have been obtained via mediastinoscopy. These specimens, commonly intrathoracic lymph nodes, are submitted for intraoperative frozen section consultation to ascertain their metastatic status for purposes of operability of a non-small-cell carcinoma of the lung. In a minority of cases, the primary pulmonary tumor is an intermediate-grade neuroendocrine carcinoma and, less often, a small cell carcinoma. In addition to metastatic carcinoma, "negative" lymph nodes may contain granulomas in varying stages of activity and type (the so-called naked granulomas of sarcoidosis), or simply a carpet of pigmented macrophages. There is a false negative rate of 5%–6% at frozen section of metastatic carcinoma of the lung in mediastinal and peribronchial

141

lymph nodes; a small subcapsular metastatic focus the presence of which is only detected in deeper permanent sections is the usual source of the discrepancy.

Mediastinal biopsies in those cases with a clinical suspicion about a disease process other than metastatic carcinoma present the intraoperative dilemma of performing a frozen section because of the small amount of tissue; a discussion with the surgeon is helpful in these cases. As noted previously, these specimens are often quite small, and substantial tissue may be lost in the facing of the block, resulting in minimal remaining tissue for permanent sections and additional studies. When a lymphoma is suspected, tissue should be set aside for flow cytometry; when the lymphoma is a suspected HL, every fragment of tissue is critical in the search for Reed–Sternberg cells and their confirmation by immunohistochemistry.

Both benign and malignant processes in the mediastinum may be accompanied by a substantial fibroinflammatory reaction that encases the underlying pathology. It is necessary in some cases to recommend a rebiopsy when all efforts have been exhausted to establish the diagnosis, when the only findings are those of chronic inflammation and fibrosis or small fragments of nondiagnostic lymph nodes.

C. Resection. Surgical resections of mediastinal contents are restricted in most cases to mass lesions in the anterior mediastinum with thymus-related neoplasms, the thymus gland in cases of myasthenia gravis, or a germ cell neoplasm, which may or may not be associated with the thymus. An enlarged substernal adenomatous thyroid or parathyroid adenoma may also present in the anterior superior mediastinum.

The other compartments with resectable specimens include the middle mediastinum with its bronchoenteric foregut cyst (most commonly the bronchogenic cyst), the posterior mediastinum with its enteric duplication cyst, and the entire morphologic spectrum of neurogenic neoplasms from neuroblastoma to schwannoma and paraganglioma.

A resected thymus may be represented by nondescript fibroadipose or adipose tissue, which on sectioning fails to demonstrate any mass lesion. In contrast, a mass lesion may be clearly evident by its size, shape, and weight; the latter three characteristics should be noted on the initial gross examination before any sectioning takes place. The external surface should be described as to whether it is smooth and/or glistening, or irregular by virtue of apparent fibrosis. The latter may reflect the presence of adhesions between the mass and contiguous structures such as the pericardium, lung, or pleura; some of these latter structures may be included as part of the resection specimen. Because surgical margins are important in pathologic staging, especially in the case of a thymoma, the surface of the tumor should be marked in such a manner that those margins can be identified microscopically. If the superior and inferior poles of the specimen can be identified, the specimen can be bisected along that plane and the salient features of the cut surface described, including the presence of a capsule or pseudocapsule, circumscription, diffuse or lobulated appearance, uniform or heterogeneous character, its solid, solid and/or cystic appearance, hemorrhage or necrosis, and any identifiable portion or remnant of uninvolved thymus. The selection of blocks for microscopic section should be directed to a thorough sampling of the margins. Sections of the apparent tumor should include any regional variations in the appearance of the mass.

If the mass is predominantly cystic, the differential diagnosis is teratoma, thymic cyst, or cystic thymoma. A solid mass may represent a thymoma, thymic carcinoma, seminoma or mixed germ cell neoplasm, HL, Castleman disease, mediastinal large B-cell lymphoma, Langerhans cell histiocytosis, granulocytic sarcoma (acute myeloid or monocytic leukemia), or localized sclerosing–fibrosing mediastinitis. Any one of the neoplastic entities may have both solid and cystic features.

III. INFLAMMATION OF THE MEDIASTINAL SOFT TISSUES (MEDIASTINITIS)

A. Acute and chronic inflammation. Acute mediastinitis with a purely neutrophilic reaction is a consequence of a contiguous infection, or a rupture or perforation of the esophagus, congenital duplication or foregut cyst, or bronchus. Other causes include a peritonsillar abscess, suppurative thyroiditis, periodontal abscess, and poststernotomy infection, notably by methicillin-resistant *Staphylococcus aureus*. In addition to the acute inflammatory reaction, the tissues may have a necrotizing appearance,

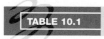

	CD15	CD30	ALK1	Smooth Muscle Actin	Factor XIIIa
TABLE 10.1 — Immunohistochemical Phenotypes of Fibroinflammatory Lesions of the Mediastinum					
Fibrosing mediastinitis	−	−	−	±	−
Hodgkin lymphoma	+	+	−	±	−
Inflammatory myofibroblastic tumor	−	−	+	+	−
Calcifying fibrous pseudotumor	−	−	−	±	+
Mediastinal large B-cell lymphoma	−	+	−	−	−
Fibromatosis (desmoid)	−	−	−	+	−

especially in those cases with the spread of an infection from the head and neck region into the mediastinum by so-called acute descending necrotizing mediastinitis. With the passage of time, acute inflammation is accompanied by a mixed inflammatory population with macrophages, a fibroblastic reaction, and microvascular proliferation.

B. **Chronic fibroinflammatory process (fibrosing–sclerosing mediastinitis).** This uncommon but well-documented clinicopathologic entity comes to attention with a persistent cough and fever in young to middle-age adults. A mass lesion is discovered in the right paratracheal or subcarinal region, often associated with punctuate calcifications. Less frequently, the presentation is as a more diffuse, infiltrative mass that is no longer confined to the middle mediastinum. An abnormal host response to the antigens of *Histoplasma capsulatum* is thought to account for most cases in endemic regions for this infection. A needle or wedge biopsy is the usual type of specimen for pathologic evaluation.

There are several microscopic stages through which this fibroinflammatory process evolves, from a reactive fibroblastic stage with an edematous background resembling nodular fasciitis, to dense hyalinized collagen with associated thickened blood vessels with similar hyalinized features (e-**Fig. 10.1**).* A dispersed population of lymphocytes and plasma cells is present throughout the biopsy. Granulomas are not a feature in most cases despite the association with *Histoplasma* infection. Dystrophic calcifications may or may not be present.

The differential diagnosis includes HL, inflammatory myofibroblastic tumor, calcifying fibrous pseudotumor, and fibromatosis (desmoid tumor). Appropriate immunohistochemical studies are helpful in the differential diagnosis if diagnostic or suspected cells are found in the biopsy (Table 10.1).

C. **Granulomatous mediastinitis.** A number of infectious etiologies are responsible for granulomatous inflammation in the mediastinum. It is generally the case that other sites in the thoracic cavity, including the lungs and regional lymph nodes, also harbor the particular infection, which is usually either tuberculous or fungal in nature. Unlike thoracic sarcoidosis, the active infectious granulomas show the presence of caseous necrosis. The granulomas are hyalinized, with or without dystrophic calcifications when the infection is inactive. In addition to *Mycobacterium tuberculosis*, fungal causes include *Histoplasma capsulatum*, *Blastomyces immitis*, and the rhizopus group. Sarcoidosis typically involves hilar lymph nodes without direct involvement of the mediastinal soft tissues.

IV. **MEDIASTINAL NEOPLASMS.** Intrathoracic, extrapulmonary, and nonmetastatic neoplasms arising in one of the mediastinal compartments are uncommon in the general experience of most institutions. No more than 5%–10% of intrathoracic neoplasms arise in the mediastinum. However, the number of different tumor types is a microcosm of neoplasms that are seen not only in intrathoracic sites but in extrathoracic organs and locations. The distribution and frequency of the different types of mediastinal tumors relate to the definition of particular lesions as neoplastic or non-neoplastic (especially in

*All figures are available online via the Solution Site Image Bank.

the case of some of the cysts), and whether the series includes benign as well as malignant tumors. Approximately 30%–35% of mediastinal tumors are thymic in origin, followed by lymphoma of HL and NHL types (25%–30%), germ cell neoplasms (10%–15%), neurogenic tumors (10%–15%), and a miscellaneous category (15%) consisting of soft tissue neoplasms of virtually all types. If consideration is restricted to those mediastinal tumors presenting in the first two decades of life, the general experience is that HL and NHL account for 40%–80% of cases, with neurogenic (20%–25%) and germ cell (15%–20%) neoplasms accounting for the remainder. Non-germ-cell thymic neoplasms are rare in children, but a variety of soft tissue neoplasms exclusive of schwannoma are seen in this young age group. The WHO classification of mediastinal tumors is shown in Table 10.2.

A. **Thymic neoplasms.** This category of neoplasms includes thymoma, thymic carcinoma, and neuroendocrine carcinoma including thymic carcinoid. These tumors arise from the thymic epithelium and are distinguished from lymphomas and germ cell neoplasms presenting within the thymus (although virtually every type of neoplasm in the thymus at one time or another has been regarded as a thymoma of one type or another). Thymomas with mixed thymomatous and neuroendocrine features support the argument that the thymic neuroendocrine carcinoma has its origin in thymic epithelium. Within the category of thymic neoplasms, approximately 80%–85% are thymomas, 10% are thymic carcinomas, and 5% are pure neuroendocrine carcinomas.

1. **Thymoma.** There are many potential approaches to the topic of thymomas and their classification; this topic is seemingly in some state of flux at all times. Thymomas are neoplasms of thymic epithelium with minimal to moderate atypia. If the tumor has features of a carcinoma in the traditional sense of cellular enlargement with hyperchromatic and mitotically active nuclei, the thymic neoplasm qualifies as a thymic carcinoma and may have the variety of patterns characteristic of carcinomas arising at other anatomic sites including the lung, salivary gland, nasopharynx, colon, and kidney.

Thymomas are neoplasms that tend to maintain to a greater or lesser degree the overall architectural and mixture of cell types present in the normal thymus (e-Figs. 10.2 and 10.3). Most thymomas have a multilobular growth pattern that is accentuated by the presence of fibrous bands that enclose the epithelial islands (e-Fig. 10.4). In the past, thymomas were differentiated on the basis of the prominence of the lymphocytic and/or epithelial elements. This descriptive classification was systematized in the World Health Organization (WHO) classification into a series of letter designations that reflect the morphology and correlate with prognosis in some studies (Table 10.3), although pathologic staging is the more significant determinant of outcome. There is also some correlation between the WHO type and the aggressiveness of the tumor into or through the capsule. Types A, AB, and B1 demonstrate invasive features in approximately 10%, 40%, and 45%, respectively, whereas types B2 and B3 are invasive in 70% and 85% of cases, respectively.

The salient microscopic features of the histologic subtypes of thymomas are summarized in Table 10.3. Thymic carcinoma or type C is regarded as separate and distinct from thymoma, and for this reason not all clinical series of thymic neoplasms include a type C. Types AB (e-Fig. 10.5) and B2 (e-Figs. 10.4 and 10.6) are the most common, and type A is the least common (e-Fig. 10.7). Regardless of the pathologic type, thymic neoplasms tend to have either macroscopic features of a solid circumscribed mass with a well-encapsulated appearance or evidence (either grossly or microscopically) that the tumor invades into or through the capsule into surrounding tissues of the mediastinum. If the thymoma has invaded the lung, pleura, pericardium, and/or great vessels, this finding is usually documented at the time of surgery with or without biopsy confirmation.

The clinical and/or pathologic staging of thymomas is complicated by the lack of standardization, but the National Cancer Institute Web site (www.cancer.gov) has included the Masaoka staging system, which was first proposed over 25 years ago, and is widely used in published clinical series despite

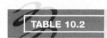

TABLE 10.2	WHO Histological Classification of Tumors of the Mediastinum

Epithelial tumors
Thymoma
  Type A (spindle cell; medullary)
  Type AB (mixed)
  Type B1 (lymphocyte-rich; lymphocytic;
    predominantly cortical; organoid)
  Type B2 (cortical)
  Type B3 (epithelial; atypical; squamoid;
    well-differentiated thymic carcinoma)
  Micronodular thymoma
  Metaplastic thymoma
  Microscopic thymoma
  Sclerosing thymoma
  Lipofibroadenoma

Thymic carcinoma (including neuroendocrine
    epithelial tumors of the thymus)
  Squamous cell carcinoma
  Basaloid carcinoma
  Mucoepidermoid carcinoma
  Lymphoepithelioma-like carcinoma
  Sarcomatoid carcinoma (carcinosarcoma)
  Clear cell carcinoma
  Adenocarcinoma
  Papillary adenocarcinoma
  Carcinoma with t(15;19) translocation
  Well-differentiated neuroendocrine
    carcinomas (carcinoid tumors)
    Typical carcinoid
    Atypical carcinoid
  Poorly differentiated neuroendocrine
    carcinoma
    Large cell neuroendocrine carcinoma
    Small cell carcinoma, neuroendocrine
    type
  Undifferentiated carcinoma
  Combined thymic epithelial tumors,
    including neuroendocrine carcinomas

**Germ cell tumors (GCT) of the
  mediastinum**
GCTs of one histological type (pure GCTs)
  Seminoma

Embryonal carcinoma
Yolk sac tumor
Choriocarcinoma
Teratoma, mature
Teratoma, immature
GCTs of more than one histological type
  (mixed GCT)
GCTs with somatic-type malignancy
GCTs with associated haematologic
  malignancy

**Mediastinal lymphomas and
  haematopoietic neoplasms**
B-cell lymphoma
T-cell lymphoma
Hodgkin lymphomas of the mediastinum
"Grey zone" between Hodgkin and
  Non-Hodgkin lymphoma
Histiocytic and dendritic cell tumors
Myeloid sarcoma and extramedullary acute
  myeloid leukaemia

**Mesenchymal tumors of the thymus and
  mediastinum**
Thymolipoma
Lipoma of the mediastinum
Liposarcoma of the mediastinum
Solitary fibrous tumor
Synovial sarcoma
Vascular neoplasms
Rhabdomyosarcoma
Leiomyomatous tumors
Tumors of the peripheral nerves

Rare tumors of the mediastinum
Ectopic tumors of the thymus
  Ectopic thyroid tumors
  Ectopic parathyroid tumors

**Metastasis to thymus and anterior
  mediastinum**

Modified from: Travis WD, Brambilla E, Müller-Hermelink HK, Harris CC, eds. *World Health Organization Classification of Tumours. Pathology and Genetics. Tumours of the Lung, Pleura, Thymus and Heart.* Lyon: IARC Press; 2004. Used with permission.

criticisms of its shortcomings (Table 10.4). Uncertainty may arise between stages II and III regarding the gross invasion of surrounding soft tissue, which may be difficult to document without a biopsy even though it was observed by the surgeon. It is also difficult to reconcile the equivalency of apparent extracapsular invasion and microscopic invasion by the thymoma into the capsule, but some have regarded the latter as stage IIa and the former stage IIb. Stage III disease is defined

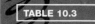

TABLE 10.3		World Health Organization Classification of Thymomas (A, B1, B2, B3, AB, and C System)	

Type	% Total	% Invasive	Microscopic features
A	8	10	Spindle to ovoid epithelial cells with diffuse or hemangiopericytomalike pattern, no lymphocytes
B1	16	45	Resembles normal thymus, with cortexlike features of immature thymocytes and scattered epithelial cells, with or without Hassall's corpuscles
B2	28	70	Lobules of large, polygonal epithelial cells separated by immature T lymphocytes
B3	11	85	Lobules of large, polygonal epithelial cells in sheets with a minimal lymphocytic component. Presence of mild epithelial atypia may question possibility of thymic carcinoma
AB	31	40	Lobules with mixed pattern of type A (lymphocyte poor) and type B (lymphocyte rich) with small spindled to ovoid shaped epithelial cells. Overall, lymphocytes more numerous than in type A. Type A and B equally represented or one pattern may dominate over the other
C	5	5	Any pattern of carcinoma with squamous, lymphoepithelial, clear cell, mucoepidermoid, basaloid, sarcomatoid, papillary, and mucinous features

as contiguous gross invasion of the pericardium, lung, and great vessels that is not necessarily confirmed by the pathologic examination of the resected thymoma. Stage IV disease represents noncontiguous, metastatic presence of tumor nodules or masses on the pleura, on the surface of the pericardium, or within the pericardial sac. The approximate 5-year survival without consideration of the specific histologic type is summarized in Table 10.4. Rather than metastatic spread, local control of tumor is a major impediment to long-term survival.

2. **Thymic carcinoma.** Only 5% or less of all primary thymic neoplasms are carcinomas. These neoplasms arise *de novo* in the thymus, but there are rare examples that may have evolved from a pre-existing thymoma. Unless a biopsy was taken of the tumor before resection, the carcinomatous nature may not be appreciated until microscopic examination. A solid, poorly differentiated carcinoma with or

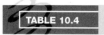

TABLE 10.4	Clinicopathologic Staging of Thymoma According to Masaoka with Added Comments	

Stage	Qualifying features	5-year survival (%)
I	Completely encapsulated without invasion of capsule	95–100
II	Gross invasion into surrounding soft tissues or mediastinal pleural and/or microscopic invasion into capsule	80–85
III	Gross invasion of pericardium, lung, and great vessels (established by biopsy or excision or intraoperative confirmation)	60–70
IVa	Dissemination to pericardium and/or pleura without contiguous spread as in stage III	40–50
IVb	Distant site metastasis (lung, skin, bone, liver)	25–30

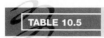

TABLE 10.5	Differential Diagnosis of Thymoma, Thymic Carcinoma, and Pulmonary Carcinoma						
Tumor Types	CK7	CD5	CD117	CD1a	TTF-1	CD205	FOXN1
Thymoma	+	−	−	+*	−	+	+**
Thymic carcinoma	+	+	+	−	−	+	±
Lung carcinoma	±	−	−	−	+	±	−

*CD1a positivity in immature thymic T lymphocytes.
**FOXN1 nuclear staining is diffuse in thymoma and focal in thymic carcinoma.

without squamous differentiation is the most common histologic appearance, but there is considerable diversity in the carcinomatous pattern (e-Figs. 10.8 and 10.9). In some cases, the distinction from an atypical appearing thymoma or carcinoma of the lung may be problematic; immunohistochemistry, as well as review of imaging studies, may provide assistance in this differential diagnosis (Table 10.5). Coexpression of CD5 and CD117 favors a thymic carcinoma, whereas thyroid transcription factor (TTF)-1 nuclear positivity is characteristic of most primary carcinomas of the lung (with exceptions).

Some points to remember about thymic epithelial neoplasms and their diagnosis and potential pitfalls follow:

a. Because the lymphocytes in a thymoma are immature T lymphocytes, they can be mistaken for lymphoblasts as in lymphoblastic lymphoma. These cells are immunopositive for CD1a and CD99.

b. Putative thymomas can measure only 1 to 2 mm in maximal dimension (microthymoma), so caution is warranted in thymic resections in cases of myasthenia gravis. The nodule must be distinguished from residual involuted thymus.

c. Sharply angulated, predominantly lymphoid lobules surrounded by fibrous stroma and widened perivascular spaces containing individual and small aggregates of lymphocytes are characteristic features of a thymoma.

d. Ectopic thymomas can present in the neck or on the pleura, and are primary tumors in both sites.

e. When a lymphocyte-rich thymoma metastasizes, the lymphocytes may be present in the metastatic focus.

f. Primary thymic hyperplasia can resemble type B1 thymoma; however, the presence of lymphoid follicles with germinal centers in the medulla is a useful differentiating feature in thymic hyperplasia, although it is not present in all cases.

g. Pathologic staging of a thymic carcinoma does not reliably predict the behavior of the tumor in the same sense as a thymoma because the carcinoma has a great potential to metastasize that is not necessarily correlated with the pathologic stage.

h. A thymoma may be a purely cystic mass. For those thymomas with liquefied, degenerated, and necrotic material within cystic spaces, demonstration of viable tumor is required to confirm the diagnosis.

i. A multicystic or multilobular thymic lesion may represent a multilocular thymic cyst, cystic thymoma, HL, mature cystic teratoma, or seminoma–germinoma.

3. Neuroendocrine carcinoma. This primary neoplasm of the thymus constitutes 5% or less of all thymic epithelial neoplasms. Cushing syndrome is one of the known clinical presentations, as is a manifestation of multiple endocrine neoplasia type I. These tumors are typically large and have usually invaded into the surrounding mediastinal tissues. The histologic features (e-Fig. 10.10) are those of neuroendocrine carcinomas elsewhere, including organoid profiles and/or rosettelike formations of uniform cells with finely distributed nuclear chromatin and central coagulative necrosis, to a small cell carcinoma resembling its pulmonary counterpart (the latter with involvement of the mediastinum is a consideration in the differential diagnosis, to which imaging studies are reliable in the localization of the mass to the hilum or thymus). It is worth noting that rosettelike profiles are seen in thymoma and mediastinal large B-cell lymphoma. The combination of thymoma and neuroendocrine carcinoma patterns in the same tumor supports the view that the latter neoplasm is fundamentally derived from thymic epithelium.

B. Germ cell tumors (GCT). The mediastinum, typically the anterior compartment, is one of the more common extranodal primary sites for this group of neoplasms, accounting for 10%–15% of all GCTs. As a primary neoplasm of the mediastinum, GCTs represent approximately 15%–20% of all mediastinal neoplasms. As a category of primary malignant neoplasms including seminoma, endodermal sinus tumor, embryonal carcinoma, choriocarcinoma, or a mixture of these patterns (with or without teratomatous elements), GCTs constitute 15%–20% of cases, equaling the proportion of invasive thymomas and thymic carcinomas. Individuals with Klinefelter syndrome are at an increased risk for mediastinal GCTs of various histologic types from teratomas to mixed GCTs, which may be heralded by the development of precocious puberty. Metastatic GCTs, from the testis more often than the ovary, can present as an apparent primary mediastinal neoplasm. Primary malignant GCTs of the mediastinum have a marked male predilection (80% or more of cases), whereas mature and immature teratomas do not have a similar male preference.

Teratomas, usually of the mature cystic type, and seminoma–germinoma are the two most common single pattern GCTs arising in the mediastinum and together represent 50%–60% of all mediastinal GCTs. Endodermal sinus tumor (yolk sac carcinoma) is next in frequency as a pure pattern GCT, and the remaining tumors have a mixture of teratomatous, seminomatous, and nonseminomatous features in a fashion similar to malignant mixed GCTs of the testis. Pure choriocarcinomas occur almost exclusively in males. The mediastinum is one site in which a GCT may engender a sarcomatous component including embryonal rhabdomyosarcoma, angiosarcoma, or other sarcomatous patterns. Granulocytic sarcoma and other hematologic malignancies (true malignant histiocytosis) are known to occur as well in this same pathologic setting.

Mature cystic teratoma presents over a broad age range from the neonatal period into early adulthood. The pathologic findings (e-Figs. 10.11 and 10.12) are the same as in the more common ovarian counterpart. As with teratomas elsewhere, especially in young children, the somatic components may have immature or fetal-like features, most commonly found in the neuroepithelium as embryolike neural tubes and neuroblastic foci. These findings should not be viewed with any more concern than they are in a sacrococcygeal teratoma in an infant; in the older child, adolescent, or young adult, a more cautious approach to the same findings is appropriate. Mature teratomas may also harbor foci of endodermal sinus tumor, as well as any one of the other malignant germ cell patterns. Therefore, it is important to widely sample any GCT of the mediastinum.

Seminoma, unlike teratoma, can present a diagnostic dilemma from other somewhat similar appearing neoplasms in the anterior mediastinum. Sheets of uniform polygonal tumor cells with a central round nucleus and clear cytoplasm, accompanied by lymphocytes and granulomas, is the classic microscopic appearance of a seminoma in the mediastinum or testis. However, the lymphocytic infiltrate or granulomas can obscure the tumor cells (e-Fig. 10.13). The differential diagnosis can include mediastinal large B-cell lymphoma, HL, sarcoidosis, and primary or metastatic clear cell carcinoma. Immunohistochemistry can be extremely helpful in most cases because mediastinal seminoma has a distinctive phenotype including CAM5.2 and vimentin (dot positive, 70%–80%), placentalike alkaline phosphatase (80%–90%), CD117 (>70%), CD30 (infrequent), and OCT4 (90%–100%) positivity. Cytokeratins AE1/AE3 and 7 are expressed in only approximately 5% of seminomas. If the seminoma is immunopositive for one or another cytokeratin, if the seminoma has arisen in the thymus, or if a thymoma, thymic carcinoma, or non-small-cell carcinoma of the lung is another diagnostic possibility, the diagnostic evaluation is more problematic (see Table 10.5).

C. Lymphoid neoplasms (lymphomas). Lymphomas in all categories account for approximately 15% of all mediastinal neoplasms overall, but 50%–60% of malignancies in the mediastinum. HL of the nodular sclerosis type is the most common, with a particular predilection for adolescent and young women (e-Figs. **10.14** and **10.15**). When there is extensive sclerosis–fibrosis, a definitive diagnosis can be difficult to establish as previously discussed in the section above on sclerosing–fibrosing mediastinitis. Lymphoblastic lymphoma with a mediastinal mass is the most common presentation of the latter neoplasm in children (50% of cases); with the exception of infrequent precursor B-cell lymphoblastic lymphomas, nearly all cases are examples of T-lymphoblastic lymphoma; if the bone marrow is involved, there is generally no need to biopsy the mediastinal mass. Mediastinal large B-cell lymphoma is specific to the mediastinum and is thought to be derived from the thymic medullary B cell. It is a neoplasm, which like HL, has a preference for young females; in fact, the differential diagnosis from HL may not be entirely clear as demonstrated by a small subset of cases referred to as "mediastinal grey zone lymphoma" that have hybrid features of nodular sclerosing HL and large B-cell lymphoma.

Castleman disease was originally characterized as a "pseudothymoma" or "localized mediastinal lymph node hyperplasia resembling thymoma." The unicentric form of the disease has two microscopic patterns: hyaline vascular and plasma cell types. Approximately 6%–10% of all unicentric cases present in the anterior mediastinum as a well-circumscribed mass consisting of one or more matted lymph nodes resembling nodular sclerosis HL (e-Fig. **10.16**). A penetrating small blood vessel extends into a germinal center composed of follicular dendritic cells surrounded by a mantle zone of concentrically arranged small lymphocytes in the hyaline vascular type of Castleman disease. In contrast, the follicles have hyperplastic germinal centers and mature plasma cells occupying the interfollicular zone in the plasma cell variant.

D. Neurogenic and neuroblastic neoplasms. These neoplasms in aggregate account for 20%–25% of all mediastinal neoplasms, and virtually all present in the posterior mediastinum. In children, these tumors are neuroblastic in nature, from neuroblastoma to ganglioneuroma (85%–90% of cases); in adults schwannoma, neurofibroma, and ganglioneuroma are the most commonly seen tumors. Other neoplasms in the posterior mediastinum include paraspinal Ewing sarcoma–primitive neuroectodermal tumor, paraganglioma (also found in middle mediastinum), and the rare cystic teratoma.

Neuroblastoma presenting in the posterior mediastinum represents 15%–20% of all neuroblastic tumors in children in all anatomic sites. These tumors tend to have favorable stages (stage 1, 2A, 2B), histology (e-Fig. **10.17**) (see Table 10.6), and biologic markers (nonamplified *MYCN* and no aberrations in chromosomes 1p and 11q).

Ganglioneuroma is often detected incidentally as a paraspinal, posterior mediastinal mass in later childhood and into adulthood. The presence of microscopic nests of neuroblasts in an otherwise ganglioneuromatous background is an example of the favorable histology maturing ganglioneuroma. Neuroblasts are not found in the mature ganglioneuroma.

V. CYSTIC LESIONS. Cysts of the mediastinum are a histogenetically diverse category, ranging from the earlier discussed cystic teratoma and thymoma, to developmental cysts including the bronchogenic and duplication cysts as manifestations of the so-called bronchopulmonary foregut or bronchoenteric malformation complex.

The bronchogenic cyst is typically a unilocular cyst arising in any one of the three mediastinal compartments, as well as in the heart, neck, and retroperitoneum. The cyst is lined by a ciliated respiratory-type epithelium with smooth muscle, accessory glands, and cartilage in the wall. However, the mucosal lining may have an enteric-like or an indeterminate simplified epithelial appearance, and a wall is not identified in all cases. An enteric duplication cyst of the esophagus is an intramural unilocular cyst that is lined by a squamous or enteric type mucosa; about 20% of all enteric duplications are found

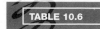

TABLE 10.6	Pathologic Types of Neuroblastic Tumors

Type	Histologic features
Undifferentiated NB (UF)	High-grade malignant round cell neoplasm, with high MKI and need for immunohistochemistry to differentiate from other malignant round cell tumors
Poorly differentiated NB (UF or FH on basis of age and MKI)	Malignant cells smaller than undifferentiated NB, with neurofibrillary processes, variable rosettes, low or high MKI, and absence of neuromatous or schwannian stroma
Diffuse or intermixed ganglioneuroblastoma (FH)	Individual nests or lobular foci of neuroblasts with prominent neurofibrillary processes, ganglion cell differentiation, and neuromatous stroma
Nodular ganglioneuroma (UH)	Distinct nodules of poorly differentiated neuroblasts with high or low MKI in a ganglioneuroma
Maturing ganglioneuroma (FH)	Microscopic foci of neuroblasts in an otherwise mature ganglioneuroma
Mature ganglioneuroma (FH)	Absence of neuroblasts

Abbreviations: NB, neuroblastoma; MKI, mitotic karyorrhectic index; UF, unfavorable histology; FH, favorable histology.

in the esophagus, and as a type of foregut malformation, the cyst may be associated with anomalies of the upper airway including a bronchogenic cyst, tracheoesophageal fistula, and communications of one type or another with the stomach.

VI. SOFT TISSUE NEOPLASMS unrelated to the heart or lungs, but presenting within the thoracic cavity in one of the mediastinal compartments, are exceedingly uncommon. That having been noted, virtually every soft tissue neoplasm of benign, indeterminate, or malignant type has been reported in the mediastinum as a single case or small series. Lipoma and schwannoma are the most common benign types arising, respectively, in the anterior and posterior mediastinum. Lipomatous involvement of the thymus results in so-called thymolipoma, the pathogenesis of which as a hamartoma or neoplasm remains uncertain; myoid cells have been observed in this tumefaction, which like the lipoma, can attain impressive dimensions. Lymphangioma and hemangioma of various subtypes are found in the mediastinum. Malignant peripheral nerve sheath tumor, angiosarcoma, leiomyosarcoma, liposarcoma, Ewing sarcoma–primitive neuroectodermal tumor, desmoplastic small round cell tumor, and embryonal rhabdomyosarcoma are just some of the soft tissue sarcomas that have been reported in the mediastinum. In a young child, the solid or solid and cystic pleuropulmonary blastoma with its complex multipatterned sarcoma may extend into one or more mediastinal compartments.

Suggested Readings

Shimosato Y, Mukai K. *Tumors of the Mediastinum*. Washington, DC: Armed Forces Institute of Pathology; 1997.

Travis WD, Brambilla E, Müller-Herkelink H, Harris CC. *Pathology and Genetics of Tumors of the Lung, Pleura, Thymus and Heart*. Lyon, France: IARC Press; 2004.

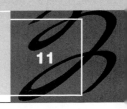

SEROSAL MEMBRANES
Jon H. Ritter and John D. Pfeifer

11

I. **INTRODUCTION.** The serosal membranes are derived from the mesoderm, and form the visceral and parietal surfaces of the pleural cavity, peritoneal cavity, pericardium, and tunica vaginalis testis. Histologically, the serosal membranes consist of a single layer of flat mesothelial cells that rest on a basement membrane, below which is a poorly delimited connective tissue layer. The parietal surfaces of the serosal membranes are perforated by numerous narrow stomas, the so-called lymphatic lacuna, which connects with the extensive lymphatic plexus, which drains the enclosed cavities. By electron microscopy, mesothelial cells show characteristic long slender surface microvilli; their demonstration can be used to support a mesothelial origin for a neoplasm that is indeterminate by other histopathologic methods.

II. **SPECIMEN PROCESSING**

  A. **Biopsy samples**, from procedures performed for diagnosis or in the context of staging procedures (most commonly for gynecologic malignancies), are usually small tissue fragments in the range of 1 to 5 mm in maximal dimension. Detailed gross descriptions are unnecessary, although documentation of the number and size is important to ensure that the tissue fragments are adequately represented on the slides. The tissue should be submitted in its entirety, and three hematoxylin and eosin (H&E) stain levels should be examined microscopically.

  B. **Excision specimens**, from procedures performed for benign or malignant diseases, include tissue from pleural decortication procedures (stripping procedures to remove thick visceral pleural peels that encase the lung and decrease ventilatory function), debulking procedures, and resections. The aggregate size of the tissue should be described, as well as its color and texture. The presence of gross lesions should also be documented. Gross abnormalities should be thoroughly sampled. When no gross lesions are identified, as a general rule, at least one section per centimeter of aggregate tissue should be submitted for microscopic examination.

III. **NON-NEOPLASTIC LESIONS OF THE SEROSAL MEMBRANES**

  A. **Acute serositis**

   1. **Acute pleuritis** is usually infectious in origin and is most commonly associated with pneumonia. Gram-positive bacteria are most commonly isolated, although a wide variety of pathogens can be responsible. Spontaneous bacterial pleuritis occurs occasionally in patients who have cirrhosis. Autoimmune pleuritis, although sterile, can produce clinical and pathologic findings that resemble infectious pleuritis.

   2. **Acute peritonitis** is usually associated with a perforated viscus. When due to gastric, biliary, or pancreatic rupture, it has a chemical etiology; when due to intestinal rupture, it has a bacterial etiology. Spontaneous bacterial peritonitis also occurs, usually in children, immunocompromised patients, or patients who have cirrhosis. Localized acute peritonitis is a feature of pelvic inflammatory disease.

   3. **Acute pericarditis** can have an infectious etiology or can be a manifestation of autoimmune disease.

  B. **Granulomatous serositis** can present in a number of different patterns; studding of the serosa by innumerable small nodules can be especially worrisome clinically for disseminated tumor.

1. **Infectious.** Although special stains can often demonstrate the offending pathogen, microbiologic cultures are a more sensitive and specific method for identification of the organism. Common causes include mycobacteria, fungi (including *Histoplasma, Cryptococcus,* and *Coccidioides*), and parasites (including *Schistosoma, Echinococcus,* and *Ascaris*).

2. **Noninfectious** etiologies include a reaction to foreign material from prior surgical procedure (such as starch granules and sutures) or from a perforated organ. In women, additional causes include retrograde introduction of foreign material through the fallopian tube (e.g., douche fluid, lubricants, radiographic contrast agents), and spillage of amniotic fluid from Cesarean section.

   Peritoneal granulomas can form as a response to implants of keratin produced by a neoplasm of the female reproductive tract, including mature cystic teratoma, endometrioid adenocarcinoma with squamous differentiation (of either endometrial or ovarian origin), squamous cell carcinoma of the cervix, or even atypical polypoid adenomyoma of the uterus. Microscopically, laminated deposits of keratin (sometimes including so-called ghost squamous cells) are present in the granulomas, but in the absence of viable tumor, these granulomas have no prognostic significance.

3. **Autoimmune** causes include Crohn disease and sarcoidosis.

4. **Meconium peritonitis** in a neonate can lead to a serosal granulomatous reaction.

C. **Mesothelial hyperplasia** is commonly seen in response to chronic serosal injury. Microscopically, hyperplasia has a number of different patterns, including solid, tubular, trabecular, papillary, or tubulopapillary, and often shows limited extension into the underlying connective tissue (e-**Fig. 11.1**).* The hyperplastic cells are often disbursed in linear, parallel, or thin layers in associated organizing fibrinous tissue. Cytologically, mild to moderate nuclear pleomorphism is present, and mitotic figures and even occasional multinucleated cells can be identified.

   Given these architectural and cytologic features, it is not surprising that mesothelial hyperplasia can be difficult to distinguish from well-differentiated diffuse malignant mesothelioma, especially epithelioid mesothelioma. The distinction is based on the degree of cellular proliferation and atypia; a diagnosis of mesothelioma should be suspected when deep infiltration of the underlying soft tissue is present, or when areas of necrosis are present. Knowledge of the clinical setting can be used to guide the diagnosis, although it is well established that slowly growing mesothelioma can initially present as a lesion that cannot be distinguished from mesothelial hyperplasia.

D. **Metaplasias** are predominantly features of the peritoneal serosal surfaces in women. Most originate from the so-called secondary Müllerian system, which by convention includes the pelvic and lower abdominal mesothelium and underlying mesenchyme. The close embryologic relationship of the mesothelium in these areas and the Müllerian ducts (which arise from invaginations of coelomic epithelium) provides an explanation for the fact that many of the metaplasias produce tissues that are a normal component of the female reproductive tract.

1. **Endometriosis** is thought to arise via a metaplastic process or through retrograde implantation of menstrual endometrium (the latter is the so-called metastatic theory). Rare cases of pleural endometriosis have been reported, as have cases of endometriosis in men who have been treated with long-term estrogen therapy (usually in the setting of adenocarcinoma of the prostrate).

   When endometriosis develops in association with viscera, such as the wall of the intestine, adjacent to the ureter, in the wall of the bladder, and so on, it can clinically present with signs and symptoms that resemble malignancy. Microscopically, the findings include endometrial glands and stroma, often associated with chronic inflammation, hemosiderin-laden macrophages, dense fibrosis, and adhesions (e-**Fig. 11.2**). Because a number of different malignancies, most commonly endometrioid adenocarcinoma and clear cell adenocarcinoma,

---

*All e-figures are available online via the Solution Site Image Bank.

can develop in endometriosis, areas of endometriosis in biopsy and excision specimens must be carefully examined.

2. **Endosalpingiosis** typically occurs in women during their reproductive years. Microscopically, multiple dilated cysts lined by a single layer of fallopian tube–type epithelium are present. The lack of endometrium-type stroma distinguishes endosalpingiosis from endometriosis.

3. **Endocervicosis,** consisting of benign glands with an endocervix-type epithelium, and squamous metaplasia, are both rare. Both primarily are metaplasias of the peritoneal mesothelium.

4. **Ectopic decidual reaction** is an incidental finding in women who are pregnant or on high-dose progestagen therapy. Most lesions are not evident grossly, but when they are, they consist of small gray–white nodules, which may be hemorrhagic, and often stud the peritoneal surfaces. Microscopically, the metaplasia involves the submesothelial stroma and consists of large epithelioid cells with prominent cell borders and abundant amphophilic cytoplasm (e-**Fig. 11.**3) morphologically identical to the cells composing the decidual reaction characteristic of the fallopian tube, cervix, and upper vagina in pregnant women. Diagnostic difficulty can arise on the rare occasions when the decidual cells assume a signet-ring appearance.

5. **Walthard nests,** usually found on the serosal surfaces of the fallopian tube or in the mesovarium as yellow–white nodules, are usually only several millimeters in greatest dimension. They may show cystic change, and are usually lined by mesothelial cells that have undergone transitional (urothelial) metaplasia.

6. **Disseminated peritoneal leiomyomatosis** (leiomyomatosis peritonealis disseminata) is an uncommon multifocal proliferation of smooth muscle–like cells that is thought to represent a hormone-induced metaplasia of the multipotential submesothelial mesenchymal cells of the peritoneum. Grossly, it appears as widely scattered nodules that often suggest metastatic malignancy. Microscopically, the lesion is characterized by bland, cytologically benign spindle cells centered in the submesothelial connective tissue (e-**Fig. 11.**4). A conservative approach to treatment is indicated because the condition tends to spontaneously regress.

E. **Fibrosis**
   1. **Pleura**
      a. **Reactive pleural fibrosis** is usually a consequence of prior inflammation or surgery. Often the fibrosis is associated with formation of dense adhesions. Because reactive mesothelial cells are entrapped within the fibrous tissue, careful microscopic examination with knowledge of the clinical history is required to avoid overinterpretation as mesothelioma.

      b. **Pleural plaques,** which primarily occur on the parietal pleura of the thoracic cavity, are raised, discrete, white to gray–white lesions that range from several millimeters to >6 centimeters in diameter. When pleural plaques are bilateral, they are almost always related to prior asbestos exposure, even very low fiber levels. Causes of unilateral plaques include asbestos, as well as any process that features pleural chronic effusions. Microscopically, they consist of paucicellular dense collagenous connective tissue, with a basket-weave pattern, sometimes associated with overlying organizing fibrinous deposits; asbestos bodies are essentially never seen within the plaques. Mesothelial cells are not a prominent component of the lesion; any significant cellularity in a putative pleural plaque should raise concern for desmoplastic mesothelioma. Finally, because mesothelioma and plaques may occur in individuals, it is not uncommon for blind biopsies to sample plaques; in this setting, additional biopsies are indicated if there is strong clinical suspicion for a pleural malignancy.

      c. **Diffuse visceral pleural fibrosis** has a number of etiologies. It is a feature of several occupational exposures (e.g., silicosis), and occurs as an advanced hypersensitivity reaction, as a component of connective tissue diseases, and as a sequela of bacterial pneumonia (especially as a result of empyema). Grossly, diffuse visceral pleural fibrosis may be difficult to distinguish from desmo-plastic mesothelioma. Microscopically, the fibrosis does not infiltrate the subjacent soft tissue. In addition, reactive pleural fibrosis also has a zonated appearance, with more cellular areas near the surface, whereas deeper tissue tends to be more paucicellular; mesothelioma has the reverse pattern. Nonetheless, careful microscopic examination, often accompanied by immunohistochemical studies, is often required to exclude mesothelioma.

2. **Peritoneum**
   a. **Reactive peritoneal fibrosis** is usually a consequence of recurrent bouts of peritonitis (often associated with long-term peritoneal dialysis), decompensated cirrhosis, or surgery, and is often associated with formation of dense adhesions. As is true with reactive pleural fibrosis, reactive mesothelial cells entrapped within the fibrous tissue must not be overinterpreted as mesothelioma.
   b. **Localized plaques,** composed of dense hyalinized fibrous tissue, are frequent incidental findings on the splenic capsule.
   c. **Sclerosing peritonitis** is due to hyperplasia of submesothelial mesenchymal cells, and manifests as diffuse sheets of white thickened visceral peritoneum that encase the small bowel and also involve the diaphragmatic, hepatic, and splenic peritoneum. Known etiologies include peritoneal dialysis, infections, autoimmune disorders, therapy with the beta adrenergic blocker practolol, and the carcinoid syndrome, although many cases are idiopathic.

F. **Cysts**
   1. **Emphysematous bullae** are the most frequent cystic lesions that involves the pleural cavity.
   2. **Peritoneal inclusion cysts** characteristically occur in the peritoneal cavity in women of reproductive age (although they also rarely occur in men, and also rarely occur in the pleural cavity). They are usually incidental findings at the time of surgery, and consist of single or multiple, thin-walled, translucent, unilocular cysts lined by a single layer of bland flattened mesothelial cells.
   3. So-called **pericardial cysts** are the most common cysts associated with the pericardium. They can achieve dimensions of 15 centimeters or more. Microscopically, they are lined by bland mesothelial cells.

G. **Splenosis** is an incidental finding, and usually represents implantation of splenic tissue as a result of traumatic splenic rupture. Grossly, innumerable red–blue nodules ranging from several millimeters to >5 centimeters in diameter are scattered widely throughout the abdomen.

H. **Eosinophilic peritonitis** arises in the context of a variety of medical diseases including childhood atopy, autoimmune disorders (especially collagen vascular diseases), and the hypereosinophilic syndrome. It also occurs in association with lymphoma, metastatic carcinoma, peritoneal dialysis, and ruptured hydatid cyst.

IV. **BENIGN SEROSAL NEOPLASMS**
   A. **Adenomatoid tumor** is of mesothelial origin, and usually arises in the peritoneum, also rarely from the pleura. It most commonly involves the serosal surfaces of the uterus or fallopian tubes, or paratesticular regions. Grossly, the tumor usually forms a tan 1- to 2-cm, well-circumscribed nodule. Microscopically, the tumor is composed of tubular and slitlike spaces lined by a single layer of flattened cuboidal cells with bland cytology (e-**Fig. 11.5**). The cells are immunopositive for cytokeratin, calretinin, and vimentin expression, but immunonegative for Factor VIII–related antigen and CD31 expression, a profile that can be used to distinguish the tumor from metastatic carcinoma and vascular tumors. Adenomatoid tumor is clinically asymptomatic, and complete excision is the appropriate management.
   B. **Multicystic peritoneal inclusion cysts** usually arise in the pelvis in women and are typically associated with lower abdominal pain. They form a palpable mass adherent to the pelvic organs that can grossly be indistinguishable from a cystic ovarian tumor, although a subset of cases arises in the upper adnominal cavity, in a hernia sac, or even in the retroperitoneum. Most cases are associated with a history of previous abdominal operation, endometriosis, or pelvic inflammatory disease.

Microscopically, the neoplasm consists of numerous thin-walled cysts lined by a single layer of bland, flat to cuboidal mesothelial cells. The septa and walls between the cysts are composed of loose fibrovascular connective tissue. The constitutive cells are immunophenotypically identical to those of other mesothelial cell lesions.

Some confusion exists regarding the proper classification of multicystic peritoneal inclusion cyst, as demonstrated by the fact that the lesion is also known as multicystic mesothelioma. Tumors in which the mesothelium has bland cytologic features with no significant atypia have an indolent course (*Cancer*. 1989;64:1336), although very rare cases may progress to conventional malignant mesothelioma (*Am J Surg Pathol*. 1988;12:737 and *J Surg Oncol*. 2002;79:243). However, cases in which the cysts are lined, even focally, by markedly atypical mesothelial cells and/or that harbor areas of conventional malignant mesothelioma are best considered low-grade mesotheliomas from the outset.

V. MALIGNANT PLEURAL NEOPLASMS. The World Health Organization (WHO) classification of tumors of the pleura is shown in Table 11.1.

A. Mesothelial

1. **Diffuse malignant mesothelioma (DMM).** The WHO recommends the terminology diffuse malignant mesothelioma when referring to malignant neoplasms arising from mesothelial cells. The association of the tumor with asbestos exposure is well established (*Ann Occup Hyg*. 2000;44:565). There is usually a long latency period between asbestos exposure and the onset of mesothelioma, of at least 15 to 20 years and as long as five or six decades. Although sequences from the highly oncogenic Simian vacuolating (SV40) virus have been reported in some cases (*Clin Lung Cancer*. 2003;5:177), an association with latent viral infection has yet to be established. Rare cases may be related to therapeutic radiation exposure or chronic pleural infections.

TABLE 11.1	WHO Histological Classification of Tumors of the Pleura

Mesothelial tumors
Diffuse malignant mesothelioma
Epithelioid mesothelioma
Sarcomatoid mesothelioma
Desmoplastic mesothelioma
Biphasic mesothelioma
Localized malignant mesothelioma
Other tumors of mesothelial origin
   Well-differentiated papillary mesothelioma
   Adenomatoid tumor

Lymphoproliferative disorders
Primary effusion lymphoma
Pyothorax-associated lymphoma

Mesenchymal tumors
Epithelioid hemangioendothelioma
   Angiosarcoma
Synovial sarcoma
   Monophasic
   Biphasic
Solitary fibrous tumor
Calcifying tumor of the pleura
Desmoplastic small round cell tumor

From: Travis WD, Brambilla E, Müller-Hermelink HK, Harris CC, eds. *World Health Organization Classification of Tumours. Pathology and Genetics. Tumours of the Lung, Pleura, Thymus and Heart.* Lyon: IARC Press; 2004. Used with permission.

Patients with mesothelioma usually present with dyspnea, chest wall pain, and a significant pleural effusion. Constitutional symptoms include weight loss, malaise, chills, sweats, weakness, and fatigue. Although the tumor may begin as multiple small nodules on the parietal and visceral pleura, it eventually encases the lung, invades the soft tissue of the chest wall, and often extends into the mediastinum with encasement of the pericardial sac and other midline structures. Diffuse malignant mesothelioma of the pleura remains a lethal disease, with essentially 100% mortality. Selected early-stage cases may benefit from extrapleural pneumonectomy and aggressive adjuvant therapy, although the role for therapy other than supportive care is controversial. The staging scheme for pleural diffuse malignant mesothelioma is shown in Table 11.2.

Several histopathologic types of mesothelioma have been described. While recognition of the various patterns is important for diagnosis, the patterns carry no clear prognostic significance. Immunohistochemically, diffuse malignant mesothelioma expresses calretinin, Wilms' tumor suppressor gene (WT1), and cytokeratin 5/6, but does not express carcinoembryonic antigen (CEA) (monoclonal), Ber72.3, and MOC-31; this panel of markers makes it possible to distinguish mesothelioma from adenocarcinoma of pulmonary or extrapulmonary origin in most cases (*Hum Pathol.* 2002;33:953 and *Am J Surg Pathol.* 2003;27:1031).

Nonetheless, no markers are available to reliably distinguish reactive from malignant mesothelial proliferations. It is this latter observation that suggests that a diagnosis of DMM based strictly on effusion cytology samples is difficult, because stromal invasion can not be definitively identified in such specimens. Given the gravity of the diagnosis of DMM, it is prudent to demand a tissue specimen in which invasion can be identified.

a. **Epithelioid mesothelioma,** as its name implies, has an epithelioid morphology, usually consisting of rather bland cells with abundant eosinophilic cytoplasm, although in some cases the cells have more anaplastic features. Architecturally, sheetlike, microglandular (adenomatoid), and tubulopapillary patterns are common (e-**Figs. 11.6** and **11.7**). Psammoma bodies are occasionally encountered.

b. **Sarcomatoid mesothelioma** is composed of spindle cells that have a haphazard distribution (e-**Fig. 11.8**). Some cases resemble fibrosarcoma, and others have a pattern that resembles undifferentiated pleomorphic sarcoma. Immunohistochemically, sarcomatoid mesothelioma is less likely to express cytokeratin 5 and/or 6; areas of chondrosarcomatous or osteosarcomatous differentiation may show positive staining for actin, desmin, vimentin, and/or S100. Many cases retain expression of calretinin. The potential overlap of histologic and immunohistologic features of sarcomatoid mesothelioma with sarcomatoid carcinoma and various soft tissue sarcomas highlights the necessity for correlation with clinical and radiographic findings; a solitary mass should raise concern for another nonmesothelial sarcomatoid process. Sarcomatoid mesothelioma is generally thought to have a more aggressive course than epithelioid varieties; patients with this subtype are generally excluded from consideration for surgical therapy.

c. **Desmoplastic mesothelioma.** By definition, this type of sarcomatoid mesothelioma consists of scattered atypical cells in a storiform or nonspecific pattern in more than 50% of the tumor, set in a dense collagenous background. This subtype is the most likely to be misdiagnosed as organizing pleuritis in small biopsy specimens.

d. **Biphasic mesothelioma.** This subtype contains a combination of the other patterns, in most cases a combination of the epithelioid and sarcomatous patterns (e-**Fig. 11.9**). By definition, each component should comprise at least 10% of the tumor.

2. **Well-differentiated papillary mesothelioma** is a rare type of mesothelioma that occurs in a wide range of patients, although most patients are elderly. An association with asbestos exposure has not been established. Patients usually

PRIMARY TUMOR (T)

TX	Primary tumor cannot be assessed
T0	No evidence of primary tumor
T1	Tumor involves ipsilateral parietal pleura, with or without focal involvement of visceral pleura
T1a	Tumor involves ipsilateral parietal (mediastinal, diaphragmatic) pleura. No involvement of visceral pleura.
T1b	Tumor involves ipsilateral parietal (mediastinal, diaphragmatic) pleura, with focal involvement of the visceral pleura.
T2	Tumor involves any ipsilateral pleural surfaces, with at least one of the following:
	Confluent visceral pleural tumor (including the fissure)
	Invasion of diaphragmatic muscle
	Invasion of lung parenchyma
T3[1]	Tumor involves any ipsilateral pleural surfaces, with at least one of the following:
	Invasion of endothoracic fascia
	Invasion into mediastinal fat
	Solitary focus of tumor invading soft tissues of the chest wall
	Nontransmural involvement of the pericardium
T4[2]	Tumor involves any ipsilateral pleural surfaces, with at least one of the following:
	Diffuse or multifocal invasion of soft tissues of chest wall
	Any involvement of rib
	Invasion through diaphragm to peritoneum
	Invasion of any mediastinal organ(s)
	Direct extension to contralateral pleura
	Invasion into the spine
	Extension to internal surface of pericardium
	Pericardial effusion with positive cytology
	Invasion of myocardium
	Invasion of brachial plexus

REGIONAL LYMPH NODES[3] (N)

NX	Regional lymph nodes cannot be assessed
N0	No regional lymph node metastasis
N1	Metastasis in ipsilateral bronchopulmonary and/or hilar lymph node(s)
N2	Metastasis in subcarinal lymph node(s) and/or ipsilateral internal mammary or mediastinal lymph node(s)
N3	Metastasis in contralateral mediastinal, internal mammary, or hilar node(s) and/or ipsilateral or contralateral supraclavicular or scalene lymph node(s)

DISTANT METASTASIS (M)

MX	Distant metastasis cannot be assessed
M0	No distant metastasis
M1	Distant metastasis

STAGE GROUPINGS

Stage	T	N	M
Stage IA	T1a	N0	M0
Stage IB	T1b	N0	M0
Stage II	T2	N0	M0
Stage III	T1, T2	N1	M0
	T1, T2	N2	M0
	T3	N0, N1, N2	M0
Stage IV	T4	Any N	M0
	Any T	N3	M0
	Any T	Any N	M1

1. T3 describes locally advanced, but potentially resectable tumor.
2. T4 describes locally advanced, technically unresectable tumor.
3. The regional lymph nodes are the intrathoracic, internal mammary, scalene, and supraclavicular nodes.

From: Greene FL, Page DL, Fleming ID, Fritz AG, Balch CM, Haller DG, Morrow M, eds. *AJCC Cancer Staging Manual.* 6th edition. New York: Springer; 2002. Used with permission. (A new AJCC TNM staging system is scheduled for release in 2009; after its publication, the new staging scheme will appear on the website for this book.)

present with dyspnea or a recurrent pleural effusion, but rarely with chest pain. At presentation, the tumor may be solitary and localized, multifocal, or widespread.

Microscopically, the tumor features fibrovascular cores (that often have a myxoid stroma) covered by a single layer of bland, cuboidal to flattened mesothelial cells. Focal areas of limited stromal invasion may be present; in cases with widespread invasion, diffuse malignant mesothelioma with papillary architecture must be excluded. The distinction is important, because when strictly defined, well-differentiated papillary mesothelioma has an indolent course with prolonged patient survival.

3. **Localized malignant mesothelioma** is a circumscribed nodular lesion attached to the parietal or visceral pleura that is usually <10 cm in greatest dimension. It is usually discovered incidentally on imaging studies. Microscopically, the tumor has architectural patterns that are identical to diffuse malignant mesothelioma. Some cases are cured by surgical excision (it is interesting to note that recurrent tumors often metastasize in a pattern more typical of sarcomas, without spread along the pleural surfaces).

B. Mesenchymal

1. **Epithelioid hemangioendothelioma** (so-called intravascular bronchioloalveolar tumor in the lung) is a low-grade malignant neoplasm of endothelial cells that can develop at virtually any anatomic site. Primary cases arising from the serosal surfaces occur, albeit rarely (*Int J Surg Pathol.* 2006;14:257).

Microscopically, the lesion is characterized by cords, short strands, and solid nests of bland, round to slightly spindled endothelial cells that have an epithelioid or histiocytoid morphology and a low mitotic rate (**e-Fig. 11.10**). Endothelial differentiation is evident by the formation of intracytoplasmic lumina (said to "blister" the cells), but distinct vascular channels are rarely formed. The neoplastic cells are classically embedded within a chondroidlike to hyalinized stroma. Immunohistochemically, epithelioid hemangioendothelioma typically expresses a variety of vascular antigens including CD31, CD34, and *Ulex Europaeus* antigen; expression of von Willebrand factor is more variable. Of note, 25%–30% of cases show focal cytokeratin expression, which can lead to an incorrect diagnosis of metastatic signet-ring cell carcinoma. In problematic cases, electron microscopy can be used to confirm the tumor's vascular origin by the demonstration of Weibel–Palade bodies.

2. **Solitary fibrous tumors** are classically considered pleural tumors, although they are now recognized to occur at virtually any anatomic location; most cases, in fact, occur in extrapleural sites. The tumor is most common in patients between 20 and 70 years old. It is classified as a tumor of intermediate (rarely metastasizing) biologic potential.

Grossly, pleural solitary fibrous tumors can be >20 cm in greatest dimension, although most tumors are <8 cm. The tumor is usually well circumscribed, although not encapsulated, and has a firm white cut surface that may show hemorrhage and areas of myxoid degeneration. Microscopically, the tumor is composed of bland, plump, spindled cells with a so-called patternless architecture that surround branching blood vessels of the type typically associated with hemangiopericytoma (**e-Fig. 11.11**). The cellularity often varies within individual tumors, and the background stroma can show areas of myxoid change or fibrosis. Immunohistochemically, the tumor cells express CD34 and CD99; in a subset of tumors, the cells also show immunoreactivity for smooth muscle actin, BCL2, and epithelial membrane antigen. Focal immunoreactivity for desmin, cytokeratin, and/or S100 may even be present. Significant cytokeratin expression should raise concern for sarcomatoid mesothelioma or carcinoma.

Malignant solitary fibrous tumors show an increased mitotic rate (≥4 mitoses per 10 high-power fields), areas of necrosis, increased cellularity, and focal marked cytologic atypia, usually with infiltrative margins (*Am J Surg Pathol.* 1998;22:1501), although the clinical behavior of an individual tumor is not absolutely correlated with its histologic features.

C. Lymphoid

1. **Primary effusion lymphoma** is a subtype of lymphoma that has a distinct clinical pathologic setting, presenting as an effusion without an associated tumor mass. It is defined by the presence of human herpesvirus-8 (*Adv Cancer Res.* 2001;80:115), and most cases arise in immunodeficient individuals in the setting of human immunodeficiency virus and acquired immunodeficiency syndrome. Immunohistochemically, primary effusion lymphoma is usually of null phenotype, although occasional cases express B-cell or T-cell markers (*Cancer.* 2007;111:224).

2. **Pyothorax-associated lymphoma** is a diffuse, large B-cell lymphoma that usually presents as a pleural mass in elderly individuals. As the name implies, it occurs in patients who have a longstanding history of pyothorax, usually in the setting of pulmonary tuberculosis or tuberculous pleuritis, and is strongly associated with Epstein–Barr virus infection. Immunohistochemically, representative B-cell markers other than CD20 are frequently negative, whereas aberrant expression of T-cell markers such as CD2 is present (*Adv Anat Pathol.* 2005;12:324).

D. Uncertain origin

1. **Desmoplastic small round cell tumors** were originally described as peritoneal tumors (see the section on malignant peritoneal tumors below). However, it is now recognized that the tumors arise at a wide variety of sites outside the peritoneum, including the pleura.

2. **Synovial sarcoma.** Both monophasic and biphasic primary pleural synovial sarcomas occur (despite the tumor's name, no biologic or pathologic relationship between synovial sarcoma and synovium has been demonstrated). Patients with biphasic tumors tend to be younger (third decade of life) than patients with monophasic tumors (fifth decade of life). The tumor is usually localized at presentation. Tumors that arise in the pleura have the same pathologic features as those that arise in the soft tissue (see Chapter 46).

E. Secondary neoplasms.
Although virtually any type of carcinoma can metastasize to the pleural serosal surfaces, secondary involvement is usually due to a peripheral adenocarcinoma of the lung. In western countries, the ovary, large intestine, pancreas, breast, thyroid, and stomach are as a group the second most common site of origin for metastatic tumors. Leukemias and lymphomas form the third most common group of tumors that secondarily involve the pleura. Because metastases to the thoracic cavity vastly outnumber mesotheliomas, metastatic malignancy must always enter into the differential diagnosis of a pleural tumor.

VI. MALIGNANT PERITONEAL NEOPLASMS.
The WHO classification of tumors of the peritoneum is shown in Table 11.3.

A. Mesothelial.
The low-grade tumors well-differentiated papillary mesothelioma and multicystic mesothelioma are far more common than diffuse malignant mesothelioma. Diffuse malignant mesothelioma and well-differentiated papillary mesothelioma appear to have an association with asbestos exposure.

1. **Well-differentiated papillary mesothelioma** is often discovered incidentally; about 80% of cases occur in women, usually of reproductive age. Grossly, the tumor is typically a solitary to multifocal, gray to white, nodular to papillary mass <2 cm in greatest dimension. Microscopically, papillary fronds with a fibrous core are covered by a single layer of bland cuboidal to flattened mesothelial cells.

    When the diagnosis is restricted to lesions with bland cytologic features and no invasion, well-differentiated papillary mesothelioma has an indolent course (*Cancer.* 1990;65:292). However, those cases that show evidence of invasion of organ walls or fat (emphasizing the need for thorough microscopic sampling) are associated with progressive disease and a worse prognosis, and so should be classified as diffuse malignant mesothelioma.

2. **Multicystic mesothelioma** is also known as multicystic peritoneal inclusion cyst. As suggested by the two very different names, there is confusion regarding the biologic potential of the neoplasm. Tumors in which the cysts are lined by mesothelium with bland cytologic features with at most only reactive atypia

TABLE 11.3   WHO Histological Classification of Tumors of the Peritoneum
Mesothelial tumors Diffuse malignant mesothelioma Well-differentiated papillary mesothelioma Multilocular peritoneal inclusion cyst Adenomatoid tumor **Smooth muscle tumor** Leiomyomatosis peritonealis disseminata **Tumor of uncertain origin** Desmoplastic small round cell tumor **Epithelial tumors** Primary peritoneal adenocarcinoma (specify type) Primary peritoneal borderline tumor (specify type) Others
From: Travis WD, Brambilla E, Müller-Hermelink HK, Harris CC, eds. *World Health Organization Classification of Tumours. Pathology and Genetics. Tumours of the Lung, Pleura, Thymus and Heart.* Lyon: IARC Press; 2004. Used with permission.

have an indolent course, consistent with a designation as multicystic peritoneal inclusion cysts (see section IV.B.). However, cases in which the cysts are lined, even focally, by markedly atypical mesothelial cells and/or that harbor areas of conventional malignant mesothelioma are best considered low-grade mesotheliomas (*Hum Pathol.* 1991;22:856).

3. **Diffuse malignant mesothelioma** arising in the peritoneum is rare; the ratio of pleural to peritoneal mesothelioma is approximately 10:1 in the United States.

   a. **The epithelioid subtype** is most common (e-**Fig. 11.12**). Rare cases, designated the deciduoid type, have a morphology that resembles an exuberant ectopic decidual reaction (*Am J Surg Pathol.* 2000;24:285). Immunohistochemically, peritoneal epithelioid mesothelioma expresses calretinin, thrombomodulin, and cytokeratin 5 and/or 6, but does not express MOC-31, Ber72.3, Ber-EP4, CA19-9, and CD15 (Leu-M1); this panel of markers is the most useful for distinguishing peritoneal epithelioid mesothelioma from peritoneal and ovarian serous carcinomas (*Am J Surg Pathol.* 1998;22:1203 and *Mod Pathol.* 2006;19:34).

   b. **The sarcomatoid and desmoplastic subtypes** are very uncommon in the peritoneum.

B. **Epithelial tumors of Müllerian type.** The architectural and cytologic features of these tumors are identical to those of their counterparts that arise within the ovary, fallopian tube, endometrium, and cervix. Their morphology is thought to represent another manifestation of the close embryologic relationship between the mesothelium and the secondary Müllerian system.

   The criteria for diagnosis of a tumor as of primary peritoneal origin include the following. First, the ovaries must be of normal size, or enlarged only as a result of a benign process. Second, the extraovarian involvement must be greater than the surface involvement of either ovary. Third, ovarian involvement must be absent, confined to the ovarian surface epithelium without stromal invasion, or involve the cortical stroma with a maximal tumor dimension of <5 × 5 mm (*Cancer Res.* 2000;60:1361). Primary peritoneal epithelial tumors are currently staged according to the scheme used for ovarian tumors (see Table 31.3).

   1. **Primary peritoneal carcinoma** occurs virtually only in women; the mean age of affected patients is the seventh decade. The most common type is serous adenocarcinoma (e-**Fig. 11.13**), but clear cell adenocarcinoma (e-**Fig. 11.14**), endometrioid adenocarcinoma, transitional cell carcinoma, and even squamous

cell carcinomas occur. Primary peritoneal carcinoma should possibly be included as a phenotype in familial breast and ovarian cancer syndromes, although the pattern of genetic abnormalities in primary peritoneal carcinomas seems to be distinct from the pattern that is characteristic of ovarian tumors.

2. **Primary peritoneal borderline tumors** (tumors of low malignant potential) are diagnosed by the same criteria as for their borderline counterparts arising in the ovary (see Chap. 31). Serous borderline tumors are by far the most common histologic type.

C. **Uncertain origin. Desmoplastic small round cell tumor** was originally described as a peritoneal tumor that arises in young men in their second or third decade, although the spectrum of disease is now known to include primary tumors arising at a wide variety of sites outside the peritoneum, including the pleura, extremities, viscera, bone, and brain, in patients of all ages.

Microscopically, the tumor is a primitive sarcoma with a growth pattern that includes variably sized sheets and nests of cells separated by a strikingly desmoplastic stroma (e-**Fig. 11.15**). Cytologically, the individual cells are small and round, and have minimal cytoplasm. Immunohistochemically, the cells show unique multilineage differentiation, including immunoreactivity for cytokeratins, epithelial membrane antigen, vimentin, desmin, and neuron-specific enolase.

The t(11;22) translocation that produces an *EWS-WT1* gene fusion is characteristic of the tumor. Demonstration of the translocation by molecular genetic techniques, or the encoded fusion protein by immunohistochemistry, can be used to aid diagnosis.

D. **Secondary neoplasms**
   1. **Carcinomas and adenocarcinomas** from virtually any primary site can metastasize to the peritoneal serosal surface. By far, the most common group of metastatic tumors in women is epithelial tumors of the reproductive tract, including the ovary, fallopian tube, endometrium, and cervix. Other tumors that commonly secondarily involve the peritoneum are carcinomas of the breast, pancreas and biliary tract, upper and lower gastrointestinal tract, and lung and sarcomas arising in the female reproductive tract.
   2. **Pseudomyxoma peritonei** is the clinical term used to designate masses of jellylike mucus in the pelvis and abdomen. In virtually all cases, the tumor producing the mucus originates from a low-grade mucinous neoplasm of the appendix or, much less commonly, the stomach, pancreas, or hepatobiliary tract (*Anat Pathol.* 1997;2:198). It has recently been suggested that classification of pseudomyxoma peritonei based on the cytologic features of the neoplastic epithelium (e-**Fig. 11.16**) provides important prognostic information (*Am J Surg Pathol.* 1995;19:1390). Cases in which the epithelium is benign or shows only mild atypia, classified as peritoneal adenomucinosis, have the best prognosis. Cases in which the epithelium is frankly malignant (classified as peritoneal mucinous carcinomatosis) are more often associated with metastatic spread to lymph nodes and liver, and have a much poorer prognosis.

   In all cases of presumed pseudomyxoma peritonei, the surgeon should be instructed to excise the appendix, regardless of its appearance; even if grossly normal, the appendix should be entirely submitted for microscopic examination. The surgeon should also be instructed to evaluate the pancreas, hepatobiliary tract, stomach, and intestines for any evidence of a primary neoplasm.

VII. **MALIGNANT PERICARDIAL NEOPLASMS.** The WHO classification of tumors of the pericardium is shown in Table 11.4.
   A. **Mesothelial.** By definition, the diagnosis of primary diffuse malignant mesothelioma of the pericardium is reserved for those cases in which there is no tumor outside the pericardium except for lymph node metastases. Histologically, diffuse malignant mesothelioma of the pericardium has the same histologic types as tumors arising from the pleura. The development of pericardial mesothelioma is also associated with asbestos exposure.
   B. **Germ cell tumors.** Intrapericardial germ cell tumors are rare, but occur over a wide age range, from neonates to elderly persons. Intrauterine tumors are increasingly being diagnosed in second and third trimester gestations due to the widespread use

TABLE 11.4	WHO Histological Classification of Tumors of the Pericardium

Solitary fibrous tumor
Malignant mesothelioma
Germ cell tumors
Metastatic pericardial tumors

From: Travis WD, Brambilla E, Müller-Hermelink HK, Harris CC, eds. *World Health Organization Classification of Tumours. Pathology and Genetics. Tumours of the Lung, Pleura, Thymus and Heart.* Lyon: IARC Press; 2004. Used with permission.

of prenatal ultrasound examination. Germ cell tumors of the pericardium, as with extragonadal germ cell tumors at other sites, are thought to arise from germ cells that lodge in midline structures early in embryogenesis along the normal route of migration from the yolk sack to the gonad.

Teratomas account for the vast majority of pericardial germ cell tumors. Over 75% of cases occur in children younger than 15 years. Teratomas can achieve remarkable sizes, up to 15 cm in greatest dimension. Grossly, they usually have a lobulated, smooth surface. Histologically, the vast majority are mature teratomas that resemble their counterparts arising in the gonads or mediastinum, in which case the differential diagnosis includes a bronchogenic cyst. Although teratomas are benign, tumors that contain other germ cell elements (e.g., embryonal carcinoma, choriocarcinoma, endodermal sinus tumor) are malignant; they are exceedingly rare, and most cases arise in adults.

   C. Secondary neoplasms. Metastases are the most common tumors of the pericardium. In a significant percentage of cases, a biopsy (often performed to establish the cause of pericarditis or life-threatening tamponade) provides the first evidence that the patient has a malignancy. The most common primary tumors that metastasize to the pericardium, in decreasing order of frequency, are carcinoma and adenocarcinoma of the lung, breast, and thyroid; lymphoma; and sarcoma. Although lymphatic or hematogenous spread is the most common route of involvement, direct extension (for example, by pleural mesothelioma or malignant thymoma) also occurs.

VIII. MALIGNANT TUNICA VAGINALIS TESTIS NEOPLASMS

   A. Diffuse malignant mesothelioma occasionally arises from the tunica, and rarely, even from hernia sacs. Grossly, the tumor forms nodules or papillary excrescences. Microscopically, the most common pattern consists of a prominent papillary architecture with associated tubular and solid areas.

   B. Epithelial tumors of Müllerian type have been reported.

   C. Secondary neoplasms. The tunica, as well as the lining of hernia sacs, can be involved by metastatic carcinoma. In some cases, the involvement of the tunica or hernia sac is the first manifestation of metastatic disease.

Suggested Readings

Battifora H, McCaughey WTE. *Tumors of the Serosal Membranes. Atlas of Tumor Pathology, 3rd Series, Fascicle 15.* Washington, DC: Armed Forces Institute of Pathology; 1995.

Clement PB. Diseases of the peritoneum. In *Blaustein's Pathology of the Female Genital Tract, 5th ed.* Kurman RJ, ed. New York: Springer; 2002.

Tavassoli FA, Devilee P, eds. *Pathology and Genetics of Tumors of the Breast and Female Genital Organs. World Health Organization Classification of Tumors.* Lyon, France: IARC Press; 2003.

Travis WD, Brambilla E, Müller-Hermelink HK, Harris CC, eds. *Pathology and Genetics of Tumors of the Lung, Pleura, Thymus and Heart. World Health Organization Classification of Tumors.* Lyon, France: IARC Press; 2004.

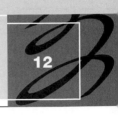

I. NORMAL ANATOMY. The esophagus begins at the level of cricoid cartilage and measures approximately 25 cm in length and 2 cm in diameter in an average adult. For endoscopists, however, the distance to the gastroesophageal (GE) junction is measured from the incisor teeth and is generally considered to be 40 cm (varying from 38 to 43 cm). Histologically, the esophagus is a muscular tube lined by nonkeratinizing stratified squamous epithelium. The basal layer of the squamous epithelium is normally one to three cells thick and occupies <15% of the full epithelial thickness, although it may be slightly thicker in the distal 2 to 3 cm. The lamina propria and submucosa are separated by a layer of longitudinally arranged smooth muscle cells that progressively becomes thicker distally. Mucin-producing glands, scattered lymphocytes and plasma cells, and occasionally lymphoid aggregates are normal findings in the lamina propria and submucosa. The muscularis propria is composed of inner circular and outer longitudinal layers. Striated muscle constitutes the upper third of the muscularis propria of the esophagus, gradually intermixes with smooth muscle in the middle third, and is entirely replaced by smooth muscle in the lower third. The esophagus does not have a serosa, except for the intra-abdominal portion. The connective tissue outside the muscularis propria, termed adventitia, merges with that in the mediastinum.

II. GROSS EXAMINATION AND TISSUE HANDLING

A. Endoscopic biopsies are usually received in 10% buffered formalin (Hollande's solution is preferred by some pathologists), with a copy of the endoscopy report. When processing the specimen, it is important to record not only pertinent clinical history, but also the endoscopic findings. The biopsies are typically small fragments of mucosal tissue in the range of 1 to 5 mm, which do not need to be inked or cut. Detailed gross descriptions, such as shape and color, are also unnecessary. However, the number of the biopsies should be recorded if they can be counted; if there are too many to count, an estimate should be made. The use of "multiple," "many," or "numerous" should be avoided. The dimension of the biopsies should also be documented. This can be done by giving either the size range of the biopsies, the greatest dimension of the largest tissue fragment, or the dimensions of the aggregate. Documentation of the number and size is important to ensure that the biopsies are adequately represented on the slides. Three hematoxylin and eosin (H&E)-stained slides are prepared for microscopic examination.

B. Endoscopic mucosal resection (EMR) has been increasingly used as a potentially curative therapy to replace esophagectomy for the treatment of Barrett's esophagus–associated high-grade dysplasia (HGD) and superficial carcinoma as determined by endoscopic ultrasound. EMR specimens are usually 1 to 2 cm in diameter and may or may not include a portion of the submucosa. Upon reception in the pathology laboratory, the specimen should be inked at the lateral and deep margins, stretched and pinned on a wax board with the mucosal side up, and fixed in 10% buffered formalin for at least 6 hours. The specimen is then sectioned at 2-mm intervals either along the longest axis or across the area where the lesion is grossly closest to the lateral margin so that the resection margins can be maximally evaluated microscopically (Fig. 12.1). The sections are sequentially submitted, and three H&E-stained slides are prepared from each tissue block for microscopic examination.

C. Esophagectomy specimens usually include the proximal stomach. After the staple line is removed, the specimen is opened longitudinally (avoiding cutting through any

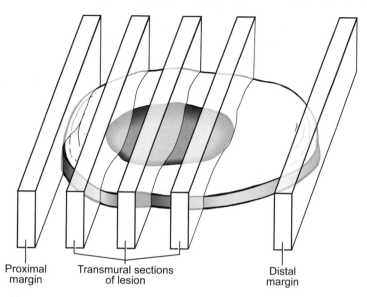

Proximal   Transmural sections   Distal
margin   of lesion   margin

Figure 12.1. Sectioning of endoscopic mucosal resection specimens.

palpable lesions), and the adventitia over the tumor is inked. After fresh tissue is taken from the tumor and nonneoplastic mucosa for the tumor bank, the specimen is pinned out on a wax board with the mucosal surface up, and fixed by submerging in 10% buffered formalin overnight. The esophagus and the attached portion of the stomach are then measured for length, circumference, and wall thickness. The size and appearance (polypoid, fungating, ulcerated, or diffuse thickening with narrowing of the lumen) of the lesion are recorded, as well as its relationship to the GE junction and distance from the proximal and distal margins. The length of Barrett's mucosa above the GE junction, if present, is also measured. Barrett's mucosa can be patchy and is recognized as salmon colored and finely granular, similar to gastric mucosa, in contrast to the gray-white, smooth, and glistening squamous cell lining of the normal esophagus (e-**Fig. 12.1**).* The grossly identified lesion is then longitudinally cross-sectioned to examine the depth of invasion (e-**Fig. 12.2**), and three to four longitudinal sections are submitted for microscopic examination. These sections should include the area of deepest penetration and demonstrate the relationship of the tumor to adjacent, grossly nonneoplastic esophageal and gastric mucosa (Fig. 12.2). Some patients may have received preoperative neoadjuvant radiation and/or chemotherapy, and the lesion may not be grossly evident, or there may be only slight roughening or shallow ulceration. In those cases, submission of the entire area of abnormal mucosa is necessary to demonstrate residual tumor. If the area of abnormal mucosa is too large, multiple sections should be taken with a map showing the location of the sections to guide additional sampling, if necessary. The previous biopsy site may be used to guide the selection of the area to sample. Any gross lesions in the esophagus and stomach should be sampled, including a representative section from the Barrett's mucosa. One random section is also submitted from grossly normal esophagus and stomach.

Additional sections of the proximal esophageal and distal gastric resection margins should also be submitted. One *en face* section from each margin is sufficient if the tumor is grossly distant from the margins. However, if tumor approximates the esophageal margin, the margin should be inked and perpendicular sections, which

*All e-figures are available online via the Solution Site Image Bank.

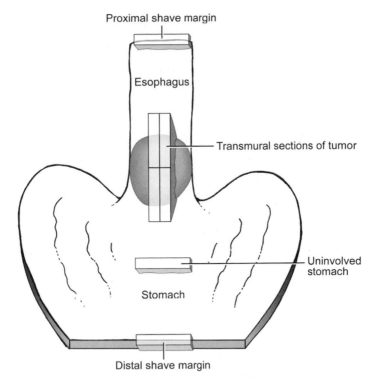

Proximal shave margin

Esophagus

Transmural sections of tumor

Uninvolved stomach

Stomach

Distal shave margin

Figure 12.2. Sectioning of esophagectomy specimens excised for malignancy.

may be multiple, should be submitted. If the inked adventitial margin is not included in the tumor sections described above, one separate section needs to be submitted.

After the above sections are taken, the adventitial and perigastric soft tissue is dissected for lymph nodes. The number and size range of identified nodes are recorded. Small lymph nodes can be submitted *in toto* without sectioning. Larger nodes are serially sectioned, and the cut surfaces are grossly examined. If metastatic carcinoma is grossly appreciated, as evidenced by a white and hard cut surface, the size of the metastatic deposit should be recorded; one representative section from each grossly positive node is submitted. If the cut surfaces of the nodes are tan, soft and homogeneous, and lack gross evidence of metastasis, the entire node should be submitted for microscopic evaluation. There is no need to separate the nodes around the esophagus from those around the stomach because they are all considered regional nodes.

III. DIAGNOSTIC FEATURES OF NONNEOPLASTIC CONDITIONS

A. **Reflux esophagitis** is the most common type of esophagitis. It occurs in patients with gastroesophageal reflux disease (GERD) secondary to dysfunction of the lower esophageal sphincter. It affects men and women equally and is seen in all age groups, including infants and children. The symptoms are diverse but typically include heartburn and regurgitation. The endoscopic appearance of the distal esophagus in patients with GERD is variable, and may be described as normal, erythematous, hemorrhagic, erosive, or ulcerative depending on the severity of the disease.

Histopathologic diagnosis of reflux esophagitis relies on a constellation of findings (**e-Fig. 12.3**), none of which is specific by itself. These include basal cell hyperplasia with a widened basal zone occupying >15% of the thickness of the squamous epithelium; elongation of the lamina propria papillae extending beyond two-thirds of the width of the mucosa; intra- and intercellular edema (spongiosis with ballooning squamous cells); intraepithelial infiltration by eosinophils, lymphocytes and neutrophils; and subepithelial vascular dilatation. The intraepithelial lymphocytes are also called "squiggle cells" because of their elongated and wavy nuclei (e-**Fig. 12.4**). In more severe cases, erosions and ulcerations are seen. Basal cell hyperplasia can be marked and may exhibit a pseudoepitheliomatous configuration (e-**Fig. 12.5**), which can be confused with invasive squamous cell carcinoma, particularly when the biopsy is tangentially sectioned and when mitotic figures are numerous.

B. **Candidal esophagitis** is the most common form of infectious esophagitis. It is characterized by the presence of yeast forms and pseudohyphae in a necroinflammatory background (e-**Fig. 12.6**). Recognition is facilitated by special stains, such as Gomori's Methenamine Silver (GMS) and periodic acid-Schiff (PAS), if needed.

C. **Herpetic esophagitis** is caused by herpes simplex virus, mainly type 1. The biopsy may show necrosis, ulceration, and neutrophilic infiltration. The infected squamous cells characteristically contain intranuclear viral inclusions with a "ground glass" appearance and margination of the chromatin. Multinucleation is common (e-**Fig. 12.7**). Immunohistochemical stains for herpes simplex virus types 1 and 2 may be performed in questionable cases.

D. **Eosinophilic esophagitis** is more frequently seen in children, but can also occur in adults. It can present as a distinct disease or as part of eosinophilic gastroenteritis, and is frequently associated with allergic disorders with or without peripheral eosinophilia. The patients may complain of progressive dysphagia, food impaction, vomiting, and chest pain. Refusal to feed and failure to thrive may be noted in children. Characteristic endoscopic findings include stricture, rings, corrugation, furrows, and granularity involving both the proximal and distal esophagus. Microscopically, eosinophilic esophagitis shares many of the histologic features with reflux esophagitis, including basal cell hyperplasia and mucosal edema. However, eosinophilic infiltration in the squamous mucosa is much more intense in eosinophilic esophagitis and usually >20 eosinophils per high-power field are present (e-**Fig. 12.8**). Eosinophilic microabscesses may be evident in some cases.

In addition to idiopathic eosinophilic esophagitis, intraepithelial eosinophils can be seen in other types of esophagitis, such as drug induced, infectious, and reflux. The main clinicopathologic features that may help distinguish eosinophilic esophagitis from reflux esophagitis are summarized in Table 12.1.

E. **Graft versus host disease (GVHD)** of the esophagus is similar to that of the skin. The squamous mucosa exhibits basal vacuolation and apoptosis, with or without lymphocytic infiltration. Desquamation may be evident.

F. **Ulcerative esophagitis** is a descriptive diagnosis when granulation tissue and necroinflammatory debris are the main histopathologic findings. The main reason

TABLE 12.1   Clinicopathologic Features of Eosinophilic and Reflux Esophagitis

	Eosinophilic esophagitis	Reflux esophagitis
Age	More common in children	More common in adults
Sex	More common in males	Equally in both sexes
Main symptom	Dysphagia	Heartburn
Endoscopic finding	Stricture, ring	Variable
Involvement	Entire esophagus	Distal esophagus
Microscopic finding	>20 eosinophils/HPF; eosinophilic microabscesses	<5 eosinophils/HPF
Therapy	Topical steroids	Anti-reflux
Complications	Stricture	Barrett's esophagus; stricture

HPF, High-power field.

to take a biopsy of an esophageal ulcer is to rule out malignancy, particularly in elderly patients. In the absence of malignancy, the differential diagnosis is broad, and includes reflux disease, infection (including human immunodeficiency virus), a drug reaction, chemotherapy- or irradiation-related change, Crohn's disease, and Behçet's disease. Clinical correlation is necessary to make a meaningful interpretation.

IV. DIAGNOSTIC FEATURES OF BARRETT'S ESOPHAGUS AND ASSOCIATED DYSPLASIA

A. Diagnosis of Barrett's esophagus.
Barrett's esophagus is currently defined as endoscopically visible salmon-colored mucosa of any length above the GE junction, which microscopically has specialized columnar epithelium characterized by the presence of goblet cells. Therefore, to make a diagnosis of Barrett's esophagus, pathologists not only need to recognize goblet cells, but also need to know the endoscopic findings.

Unequivocal goblet cells exhibit a distinctive morphology. Their nuclei are located at the base, and their cytoplasm is distended by acidic mucin, which gives a tincture of blue on H&E staining. PAS/Alcian blue at pH 2.5 also stains goblet cells blue, but this stain is usually unnecessary. In Barrett's esophagus, goblet cells are typically dispersed among gastric foveolar cells (incomplete intestinal metaplasia; e-Fig. 12.9). Goblet cells can also be flanked by epithelial cells with brush borders, identical to absorptive cells of the small intestine (complete intestinal metaplasia; e-Fig. 12.10). It has been suggested that Barrett's esophagus with incomplete intestinal metaplasia is more prone to develop dysplasia. Occasionally, gastric foveolar cells may show expanded cytoplasm with a goblet contour, but they contain neutral mucin and should not be confused with true goblet cells (e-Fig. 12.11). Some gastric epithelial cells that do not have a goblet shape may also contain blue mucin (e-Fig. 12.12). Recognition of these pseudogoblet cells is important because in the absence of goblet cells, replacement of the esophageal squamous lining by gastric mucosa alone should not be diagnosed as Barrett's esophagus by current definition.

If the endoscopist is uncertain about the endoscopic findings, pathologists should not make a definitive diagnosis of Barrett's esophagus. In this scenario, if goblet cells are identified in the biopsies from the GE junction, a descriptive diagnosis with a short comment is appropriate. For example, the diagnosis may read "cardiac-type gastric mucosa with goblet cells" or "cardiac-type gastric mucosa with intestinal metaplasia" with a comment that the findings of goblet cells in the biopsies may represent either intestinal metaplasia of the gastric cardia or a very short segment of Barrett's esophagus. The presence or absence of dysplasia should also be reported; when present, it should be graded using the same grading system as for Barrett's esophagus.

Intestinal metaplasia of the gastric cardia and GE junction may be associated with *Helicobacter pylori* infection, reflux disease, or aging. Although the biological significance is unknown, it has been suggested as a potential explanation for the increasing frequency of adenocarcinoma in this region. Immunohistochemical stains for cytokeratin (CK) 7 and CK20, or mucin core proteins (MUC), are not usually required to distinguish this type of intestinal metaplasia from Barrett's mucosa.

A relatively consistent microscopic finding in the GE junctional mucosa is mild to moderate lymphoplasmacytic infiltration of the lamina propria (carditis). Neutrophils may or may not be present. Although it is appropriate to mention this finding in the report, its significance is unclear.

B. Diagnosis and grading of dysplasia
are based on histopathologic evaluation of the architecture of the glands, cytologic features, surface maturation, inflammation, and ulceration.

1. **Negative for dysplasia.** The glandular architecture is within normal limits. Focal budding or branching and slight crowding of the glands are acceptable. Mild nuclear stratification, enlargement and pleomorphism, increased mitotic activity, mucin depletion, and small numbers of dystrophic goblet cells are also acceptable (e-Fig. 12.13). Architectural and cytologic atypia is characteristically seen in the deeper glands and may be enhanced in the setting of active inflammation, erosion, or ulceration. However, there is surface maturation, which can be appreciated at low magnification (e-Fig. 12.14). The nuclear polarity is also well maintained.

2. **Indefinite for dysplasia** is a category reserved for cases with worrisome cytologic and architectural alterations that are too abundant for the negative for dysplasia category, but still insufficient for the diagnosis of dysplasia. This may include cases with cytologic and architectural atypia in the deeper glands that would qualify for dysplasia if the atypia extended to the surface. This diagnosis is also applied to cases in which pathologists cannot determine whether the atypia is dysplastic or related to inflammation or regeneration (e-Fig. 12.15), and in which a comparative assessment between the surface and deeper glands cannot be made due to technical problems such as inappropriate embedding or tangential sectioning of the biopsies. The presence of abnormal mitotic figures in the absence of other dysplastic features may also belong to this category.

3. **Low-grade dysplasia (LGD).** Cytologic alterations are the main histologic feature that should at least focally extend to the surface so that the deeper glands and surface appear similar at low-power magnification (e-Fig. 12.16). In many cases, LGD is reminiscent of tubular adenomas of the colon. The nuclei are stratified, pencil-shaped, and hyperchromatic with irregular nuclear membranes, but still maintain their polarity, and lack prominent nucleoli. The normal glandular architecture is relatively well preserved or mildly distorted with crowding. Inflammation is typically minimal.

4. **High-grade dysplasia (HGD)** displays more advanced architectural complexity and more prominent cytologic atypia compared with LGD; either finding is sufficient for the diagnosis, although both are present in most cases. The glands are crowded with little intervening lamina propria and irregularly shaped with budding, branching, cribriforming, cystic dilation, and a villiform surface. Cytologically, dysplastic cells exhibit markedly enlarged, usually round or ovoid, and hyperchromatic nuclei (e-Fig. 12.17). Excessive nuclear stratification extending to the luminal surface and loss of nuclear polarity are evident. Abnormal mitotic figures may be numerous.

5. **Intramucosal carcinoma** is defined by invasion through the basement membrane into the lamina propria or muscularis mucosae, which can be difficult to distinguish from HGD or deeply invasive carcinoma in biopsies. Useful features include an extensive cribriform, back-to-back, or syncytial growth pattern, and individual or small clusters of dysplastic cells in the lamina propria (e-Fig. 12.18). Desmoplasia or necrosis is usually absent.

6. **General comment.** Diagnosis and grading of dysplasia in Barrett's esophagus is highly observer-dependent (*Hum Pathol* 2001;32:368 and *J Clin Pathol* 2006; 59:1029), and there are no reliable biomarkers to aid diagnosis. A conservative approach to diagnosis is recommended in the presence of active inflammation, but pathologists should be careful to not use "indefinite for dysplasia" for problematic cases merely as a default diagnosis. Confirmation by an experienced pathologist is also highly recommended. It is useful to clinicians to give a rough estimate of the extent of dysplasia in the report, e.g., in a total number of tissue fragments, how many are involved by LGD and how many by HGD.

V. **DIAGNOSTIC FEATURES OF COMMON NEOPLASMS.** The current World Health Organization (WHO) histologic classification of esophageal tumors is given in Table 12.2. The 2002 American Joint Committee on Cancer (AJCC) Tumor, Node, Metastasis (TNM) staging schema is given in Table 12.3.

A. **Adenocarcinoma** occurs predominantly in elderly white men in the setting of Barrett's esophagus, and is typically located in the distal third of the esophagus. Because it frequently involves the GE junction and the proximal stomach, it may be difficult to determine whether the tumor is esophageal or gastric in origin. By convention, a tumor is considered to be esophageal if the epicenter is in the esophagus and if Barrett's mucosa is present.

Like adenocarcinomas in other locations, esophageal adenocarcinoma consists of infiltrative tubular or papillary structures. Signet-ring cells and mucin production may be seen, but signet-ring-cell carcinoma (>50% of the tumor composed of signet-ring cells) is usually gastric in origin. As a general rule, adenocarcinoma of the gastrointestinal (GI) tract is graded into well differentiated (>95% of the tumor composed of glands), moderately differentiated (50% to 95%), and poorly differentiated

TABLE 12.2	**WHO Histologic Classification of Esophageal Tumors**

Epithelial tumors
Squamous cell papilloma
Intraepithelial neoplasia
   Squamous
   Glandular (adenoma)
Carcinoma
   Squamous cell carcinoma
   Verrucous (squamous) carcinoma
   Basaloid squamous cell carcinoma
   Spindle cell (squamous) carcinoma
   Adenocarcinoma
   Adenosquamous carcinoma
   Mucoepidermoid carcinoma
   Adenoid cystic carcinoma
   Small cell carcinoma
   Undifferentiated carcinoma
   Other
Carcinoid tumor

Nonepithelial tumors
Leiomyoma
Lipoma
Granular cell tumor
Gastrointestinal stromal tumor
   Benign
   Uncertain malignant potential
   Malignant
Leiomyosarcoma
Rhabdomyosarcoma
Kaposi's sarcoma
Malignant melanoma
Other

Secondary tumors

From: Hamilton SR, Aaltonen LA, eds. *World Health Organization Classification of Tumours. Pathology and Genetics. Tumours of the Digestive System.* Lyon: IARC Press; 2000. Used with permission.

(<50%). Well-differentiated adenocarcinoma may pose a diagnostic challenge in biopsy specimens (e-**Fig. 12.19**). More than 90% of esophageal adenocarcinomas express CK7, but 40% also express CK20.

- **B. Squamous cell carcinoma** is most common in the mid-esophagus and morphologically similar to squamous cell carcinoma elsewhere.
- **C. Leiomyoma** is the most common mesenchymal tumor of the esophagus.
- **D. GI stromal tumor (GIST)** of the esophagus is extremely rare, accounting for <1% of all GISTs. It typically occurs in the distal third of the esophagus and exhibits morphologic and immunophenotypic characteristics similar to that elsewhere in the GI tract (see Chapter 13).

CYTOLOGY OF THE ESOPHAGUS
Jing Zhai

- **I. INTRODUCTION.** Indications for cytologic examination of the esophagus include a suspected neoplasm, an infection, or surveillance for Barrett's esophagus. Cytology samples

TABLE 12.3	Tumor, Node, Metastasis (TNM) Staging Scheme for Esophageal Carcinoma

Primary tumor (T)

TX	Primary tumor cannot be assessed
T0	No evidence of primary tumor
Tis	Carcinoma in situ
T1	Tumor invades lamina propria or submucosa
T2	Tumor invades muscularis propria
T3	Tumor invades adventitia
T4	Tumor invades adjacent structures

Regional lymph nodes (N)

NX	Regional lymph nodes cannot be assessed
N0	No regional lymph node metastasis
N1	Regional lymph node metastasis

Distant metastasis (M)

MX	Distant metastasis cannot be assessed
M0	No distant metastasis
M1	Distant metastasis

For tumors of the lower thoracic esophagus:

M1a	Metastasis in celiac lymph nodes
M1b	Other distant metastasis

For tumors of the mid-thoracic esophagus:

M1a	Not applicable
M1b	Nonregional lymph node and/or other distant metastasis

For tumors of the upper thoracic esophagus:

M1a	Metastasis in cervical lymph nodes
M1b	Other distant metastasis

Stage grouping

Stage 0	Tis	N0	M0
Stage I	T1	N0	M0
Stage IIA	T2	N0	M0
	T3	N0	M0
Stage IIB	T1	N1	M0
	T2	N1	M0
Stage III	T3	N1	M0
	T4	Any N	M0
Stage IVA	Any T	Any N	M1a
Stage IVB	Any T	Any N	M1b

From: Greene FL, Page DL, Fleming ID, Fritz AG, Balch CM, Haller DG, Morrow M, eds. *AJCC Cancer Staging Manual.* 6th edition. New York: Springer; 2002. Used with permission. (A new AJCC TNM staging system is scheduled for release in 2009; after its publication, the new staging scheme will appear on the website for this book.)

can be obtained by endoscopic brushing of a mucosal surface abnormality or by endoscopic ultrasound–guided fine needle aspiration (EUS-FNA) of mucosal or intramural masses. Brushing cytology for malignancy has 79% sensitivity and 99% specificity, which are comparable to the sensitivity and specificity of endoscopic biopsy, but brushing cytology and endoscopic biopsy are best viewed as complementary for detection of malignancy (*Am J Clin Pathol* 1995;103:295 and *Acta Cytol* 1995;39:28). EUS-FNA for malignancy has 61% sensitivity, 79% specificity, and 67% accuracy (*Gastroentology* 1997;112:1087), which most likely reflect limitations of EUS-FNA due to inadequate sampling.

II. INFECTION. Reactive and reparative atypia are characterized by cohesive two-dimensional sheets of cells withoust marked nuclear crowding, but demonstrating slightly enlarged nuclei, smooth nuclear contours, conspicuous nucleoli, and a lack of single atypical cells. The background shows neutrophils.

   A. Candidal esophagitis displays pseudohyphae and yeast forms (e-**Fig. 12.20**). Oral contamination should be excluded, especially in the absence of inflammation.

   B. Herpetic esophagitis shows herpes viral cytopathic effect, including ground glass chromatin, thick nuclear membranes, multinucleation, and nuclear molding (e-**Fig. 12.21**). Cowdry type A viral inclusions are distinct eosinophilic nuclear inclusions surrounded by a clear halo and thick nuclear membrane (e-**Fig. 12.22**).

   C. Cytomegalovirus esophagitis demonstrates significantly enlarged mononuclear cells with a large intranuclear inclusion separated from a thickened nuclear membrane by a clear halo. Occasional cytoplasmic granular inclusions are also present.

III. BARRETT'S ESOPHAGUS. Cytological diagnosis relies on the identification of goblet cells in a honeycombing sheet of benign glandular cells. The goblet cells exhibit a single large cytoplasmic vacuole that displaces the nucleus, causing a crescent-shaped nucleus. The diameter of the vacuole is at least three times the width of a normal columnar cell (*Am J Clin Pathol* 1988;89:493 and *Hum Pathol* 1997;28:465).

   A. Dysplasia in Barrett's esophagus. Brushing cytology as a screening tool offers the advantage of sampling a wider area of abnormal mucosa as compared with biopsy. The presence of dysplasia and malignancy is evaluated based on architectural irregularities, cell cohesion, and cytological atypia. Because interobserver discrepancy can be high, any dysplasia identified in cytology specimens should be confirmed by biopsy (*Cancer* 1992;69:8; *Am J Clin Pathol* 1988;89:493; *Acta Cytol* 1991;35:199; and *Hum Pathol* 1997;28:465).

   B. LGD shows cohesive sheets of glandular cells with elongated nuclei, nuclear overlapping, and pseudostratification. The nuclear atypia, including an increased nucleus/cytoplasm (N/C) ratio and hyperchromasia, is mild.

   C. HGD displays crowded, three-dimensional clusters and occasional single atypical cells. Nuclear atypia and pleomorphism are easily identified, although marked atypia is not present. The cytologic findings include an increased N/C ratio, nuclear enlargement, hyperchromasia, and nuclear contour irregularity.

IV. NEOPLASMS

   A. Leiomyoma. The cellularity of the specimen is usually low. Findings include microfragments composed of spindle-shaped cells with oval to spindled nuclei, fine chromatin, and delicate cytoplasm. The distinction from GI stromal tumor requires immunostains (*Am J Clin Pathol* 2003;119:703).

   B. Adenocarcinoma. The specimen is highly cellular, consisting of haphazardly arranged three-dimensional clusters and abundant isolated atypical cells (e-**Fig. 12.23**). The nuclear atypia and pleomorphisms are marked. Necrosis may be present. The distinction from HGD is difficult by cytomorphology alone, and is quantitative rather than qualitative (*Cancer* 1992;69:8; *Am J Clin Pathol* 1988;89:493; *Acta Cytol* 1991;35:199; and *Hum Pathol* 1997;28:465).

   C. Squamous cell carcinoma. Well-differentiated squamous cell carcinoma displays abundant isolated cells with hyperchromatic and pyknotic nuclei, keratinized cytoplasm with sharp cytoplasmic borders, spindle- and/or tadpole-shaped malignant cells, and necrosis (e-**Fig. 12.24**). Poorly differentiated squamous cell carcinoma shows crowded groups and isolated cells with enlarged nuclei and coarsely clumpy chromatin; distinction from poorly differentiated adenocarcinoma may be difficult.

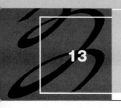

13 THE STOMACH
Hanlin L. Wang

I. **NORMAL ANATOMY.** The stomach is a distensible bag with a variable size, located a few centimeters below the diaphragm. By convention, it is divided into five regions. The cardia is an ill-defined area that connects with the gastroesophageal (GE) junction. The fundus is the superior portion of the stomach above the GE junction. The body or corpus is the main portion of the stomach below the fundus. The antrum is the distal portion separated from the body approximately at the incisura angularis. Finally, the pylorus is a 1- to 2-cm narrow channel that extends from the antrum and connects the stomach to the duodenum.

The gastric mucosa usually forms coarse folds (rugae), which are more prominent in the fundus and body and less prominent in the antrum. Histologically, the gastric mucosa varies in different regions but can be divided into fundic and antral types in general. Fundic-type mucosa is seen in the fundus and body and consists of tightly packed fundic (oxyntic) glands occupying approximately 80% of the mucosal thickness. The superficial 20% consists of foveolar cells that are tall and columnar and produce neutral mucin. The fundic glands contain acid-secreting cells (parietal cells) and zymogenic cells (chief cells) that stain pink and blue on hematoxylin and eosin (H&E), respectively. Antral-type mucosa is seen in the antrum, pylorus, and cardia, where the deeper glands are loosely packed and mucin-producing; in antral-type mucosa, the ratio of mucinous glands to overlying foveolae is roughly 1:1. The lamina propria of the stomach contains only a minimal number of lymphocytes, plasma cells, eosinophils, and mast cells. The submucosa, muscularis propria, and serosa of the stomach are histologically similar to those of the intestine.

II. **GROSS EXAMINATION AND TISSUE HANDLING**
   A. **Endoscopic biopsies.** When processing gastric biopsies, it is important to record not only pertinent clinical history, but also endoscopic findings. The biopsies are typically small fragments of mucosal tissue in the range of 1 to 5 mm, which do not need to be inked or cut. Detailed gross descriptions, such as shape and color, are also unnecessary. However, the number of biopsies should be recorded if they can be counted; if there are too many to count, an estimate should be given. The use of "multiple," "many," or "numerous" should be avoided. The dimension of the biopsies should also be documented by recording the size range of the biopsies, the greatest dimension of the largest tissue fragment, or the dimensions of the aggregate. Documentation of the number and size is important to ensure that the biopsies are adequately represented on the slides. Three H&E-stained slides are prepared for microscopic examination. Although some laboratories find it convenient to routinely order special stains for *Helicobacter pylori* at the time the specimen is processed, others perform stains for *H. pylori* only when necessary after examination of H&E-stained slides.
   B. **Gastrectomy** is performed for adenocarcinoma, gastrointestinal stromal tumor (GIST), and occasionally for benign ulcers. It can be total (including the cardia and pylorus), but usually partial (including a portion of either esophagus or duodenum). The spleen may sometimes be included. The serosal surface is examined for evidence of tumor penetration (e-**Fig. 13.1**),* and the area over the tumor is inked. The stomach

---

*All e-figures are available online via the Solution Site Image Bank.

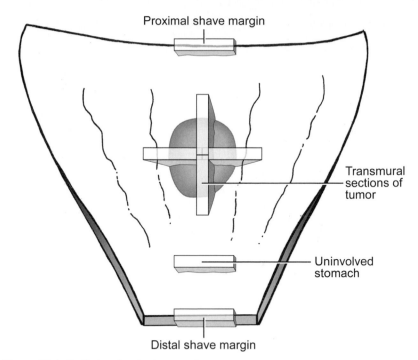

Proximal shave margin

Transmural sections of tumor

Uninvolved stomach

Distal shave margin

Figure 13.1. Sectioning of gastrectomy specimens.

is opened longitudinally along the greater curvature, unless a lesion is present at this location. The specimen is pinned out on a wax board with the mucosal side up and fixed by submerging in 10% buffered formalin overnight. The specimen is then measured, including the lengths of the greater and lesser curvatures, the circumferences of the proximal and distal resection margins, and the thickness of the gastric wall. The location, shape, and maximal dimension of the tumor or ulcer, and its distance to margins, are recorded. Any other gross abnormalities of the gastric mucosa should also be described. The grossly identified tumor is then cross-sectioned to examine the depth of invasion (e-**Fig. 13.2**). Three to four sections from the tumor are submitted for microscopic examination; these sections should include the area of deepest penetration and the relationship of the tumor to adjacent, grossly nonneoplastic gastric mucosa (**Fig. 13.1**).

If a diagnosis of adenocarcinoma has been established by a prior biopsy but the tumor or the biopsy site is not evident grossly, the mucosal surface needs to be carefully examined to search for subtle effacement of the mucosal folds or superficial erosions. This scenario often occurs in signet-ring-cell carcinoma, which may or may not exhibit diffuse thickening of the gastric wall (linitis plastica). Multiple sections may be needed; a map showing the location of the initial sections will help guide any additional sectioning that is necessary.

Additional sections include the proximal and distal resection margins. One *en face* section from each margin is sufficient if the tumor is grossly distant from the margins. However, if the tumor is close to a margin, the margin should be inked and multiple perpendicular sections should be submitted. If the inked serosal surface is not represented in the tumor sections described above, one separate section should be submitted. Any other gross lesions or areas of abnormal mucosa in the stomach also should be sampled. In addition, one random section from grossly normal antrum, one from grossly normal body/fundus, and one from the spleen (if present), are submitted.

After the above sections are taken, the perigastric and perisplenic soft tissue is dissected for lymph nodes. There is no need to separate the nodes into groups according to their different locations around the stomach because they are all considered to be regional nodes.

III. DIAGNOSTIC FEATURES OF NONNEOPLASTIC CONDITIONS OF THE STOMACH

A. **Gastritis.** There is no widely accepted classification for gastritis. The updated Sydney System has attempted to combine topographical, morphological, and etiological information into a schema that theoretically generates a reproducible and clinically useful diagnosis (*Am J Surg Pathol* 1996;20:1161). However, this schema is largely unused because of inadequate sampling and clinical information, poor endoscopic and histopathologic correlation, and ethnic, environmental, and geographical variations of disease.

1. **Chronic gastritis** is characterized by lymphoplasmacytic infiltration of the lamina propria, usually attributable to *H. pylori* infection. The inflammatory infiltrate is typically diffuse and superficial, and predominantly involves the antrum. However, it may become more extensive, involve the body and fundus, and infiltrate the full thickness of the lamina propria. Lymphoid follicles, intestinal metaplasia, and mucosal atrophy may be present. When neutrophils are present in the lamina propria, within the epithelium (pititis or cryptitis), or within gland lumens (crypt abscesses), the inflammation represents active (not "acute") chronic gastritis (e-**Fig. 13.3**) and is usually an indication of active *H. pylori* infection. In severe cases, erosion or ulceration may occur.

   Histology remains the gold standard for *H. pylori* detection. In many cases of active chronic gastritis, the microorganisms are visible on H&E-stained slides (e-**Fig. 13.4**); they are curved rods that colonize the mucus on the mucosal surface and in the pits. Detection sensitivity can be increased by using a number of special stains, such as Giemsa, Diff-Quik, Steiner, and Warthin–Starry, as well as by immunohistochemistry. By Steiner stain, the microorganisms are darkly coarse and easily recognized (e-**Fig. 13.5**). *H. pylori* are not tissue invasive, and do not colonize epithelium with intestinal metaplasia. In the absence of active inflammation, the chance of finding *H. pylori* microorganisms is minimal.

   After *H. pylori* eradication, neutrophils disappear quickly, usually within 6 to 8 weeks. Lymphoplasmacytic infiltrates disappear more slowly, usually after approximately 1 year in the body and 2 to 4 years in the antrum. Lymphoid follicles and intestinal metaplasia may be permanent changes or become reduced with time.

   Although we do not use the updated Sydney System for reporting, the following information should be included in the pathology report for gastric biopsies: the type of mucosa (antral or fundic), the grade of lymphoplasmacytic infiltration (minimal, mild, moderate, or marked), the presence or absence of active inflammation with the degree of activity (if present), the extent of intestinal metaplasia (if present), and the presence or absence of *H. pylori* microorganisms.

   Atrophic gastritis is a form of chronic gastritis that can be part of the morphologic spectrum of *H. pylori* gastritis as described above or mediated by other mechanisms such as an autoimmune process (e-**Fig. 13.6**). It is frequently associated with intestinal metaplasia and enterochromaffin cell–like (ECL) hyperplasia. Dysplasia, adenocarcinoma, or carcinoid tumor may develop in the background of atrophic gastritis. The clinicopathologic features separating autoimmune from nonautoimmune atrophic gastritis are summarized in Table 13.1. In general, histologic recognition of atrophy is more difficult in the antrum than in the body or fundus.

2. **Lymphocytic gastritis** is characterized by prominent lymphocytic infiltration of the surface and foveolar epithelium (>25 lymphocytes per 100 epithelial cells) as well as the lamina propria (e-**Fig. 13.7**).

3. **Collagenous gastritis** is extremely rare, featuring widening of the subepithelial collagen layer to a thickness exceeding 10 μm (e-**Fig. 13.8**).

4. **Eosinophilic gastritis** is usually part of the spectrum of eosinophilic gastroenteritis, and can involve any layer of the gastric wall. When the mucosa is involved,

TABLE 13.1 Clinicopathologic Features of Autoimmune and Nonautoimmune Atrophic Gastritis

	Autoimmune	Nonautoimmune
Patient population	Mainly older white women	Universal
Etiology and pathogenesis	Autoantibodies to parietal cells and intrinsic factor	*Helicobacter Pylori,* other environmental factors
Clinical manifestations	Hypochlorhydria, achlorhydria, pernicious anemia	Abdominal pain, dyspepsia, upper GI bleeding
Gastric involvement	Body and fundus only	Mainly antrum, or multifocal
Microscopic findings	Chronic gastritis, progressive destruction of fundic glands, intestinal metaplasia, pyloric metaplasia, ECL cell hyperplasia	Chronic gastritis, intestinal metaplasia, pyloric metaplasia if body is involved
Serum gastrin level	Elevated	Normal or low
Tumor development	Carcinoid, adenocarcinoma	MALT lymphoma

GI, gastrointestinal; ECL, enterochromaffin cell–like; MALT, mucosa-associated lymphoid tissue.

eosinophils are the dominant cell type and they intensely infiltrate the lamina propria. Eosinophilic cryptitis and crypt abscesses are evident. If the muscularis mucosa and submucosa are present in biopsies, infiltration by abundant eosinophils is a very helpful diagnostic feature (e-**Fig. 13.9**).

5. **Granulomatous gastritis** is not a specific entity. The majority of cases represent gastric involvement by Crohn's disease (e-**Fig. 13.10**). In the absence of granulomas, the diagnosis of Crohn's gastritis is difficult to make based on biopsy specimens; helpful features include the focal nature of inflammation (e-**Fig. 13.11**) and a suggestive clinical history. Other causes of granulomatous gastritis include sarcoidosis, infections, foreign body reaction, and vasculitis; some cases are idiopathic.

6. **Infectious gastritis** can be caused by a wide range of infectious agents. Examples include cytomegalovirus infection, Epstein-Barr virus infection, candidiasis, histoplasmosis, cryptococcosis, tuberculosis, syphilis, anisakiasis, and strongyloidiasis. Some of the infectious agents may be the causes of granulomatous or eosinophilic gastritis.

7. **Ischemic gastritis** is exceedingly rare, but may occur in the setting of hypoperfusion. Microscopic findings include necrosis, hemorrhage, erosion, or ulceration.

8. **Graft versus host disease** of the stomach exhibits apoptosis and glandular destruction. Granular eosinophilic debris in dilated glands with attenuated lining epithelium is quite characteristic (e-**Fig. 13.12**).

B. **Miscellaneous conditions**

1. **Foveolar hyperplasia** is not a specific diagnosis. Microscopically, the foveola of the mucosa is elongated with villiform transformation of the mucosal surface. Focal mild foveolar hyperplasia is a common finding in antral biopsies in the setting of chronic gastritis.

2. **Reactive or chemical gastropathy** is characterized by diffuse foveolar hyperplasia, most commonly seen in the antrum (e-**Fig. 13.13**). The glands may become tortuous, with a corkscrew appearance in more severe examples. The mucosa is typically noninflamed or only minimally infiltrated by inflammatory cells. Smooth muscle fibers may be prominent in the lamina propria. This condition is usually associated with bile reflux or medications, particularly nonsteroidal antiinflammatory drugs (NSAIDs). Of note, NSAIDs can also induce erosion and ulceration in the stomach.

3. **Ménétrier's disease** exhibits enlarged or giant gastric folds, mainly involving the body and fundus. Histologically, marked foveolar hyperplasia with tortuosity

and glandular atrophy are evident, reminiscent of the features seen in hyperplastic polyps of the stomach. The patients may present with protein-losing gastropathy and low acid production.

4. **Zollinger–Ellison syndrome** is the result of hypergastrinemia. The body and fundus exhibit enlarged mucosal folds due to hypertrophy and hyperplasia of parietal cells. However, foveolar hyperplasia is not present. The fundic glands may be cystically dilated, reminiscent of fundic gland polyps (e-**Fig. 13.14**).

5. **Gastric antral vascular ectasia (GAVE),** also known as watermelon stomach, is characterized by dilatation of mucosal capillaries, some of which may contain fibrin thrombi (e-**Fig. 13.15**). GAVE may or may not be associated with portal hypertension (portal hypertensive gastropathy features involvement of the body and fundus, without fibrin thrombi).

6. **Mucosal calcinosis** is usually an incidental finding in patients with renal failure or in organ transplant recipients (e-**Fig. 13.16**).

7. **Pseudomelanosis** of the stomach is caused by iron deposition in the mucosa (gastric siderosis) in patients taking ferrous sulfate (e-**Fig. 13.17**) or in patients with hemochromatosis. Mild inflammatory cell infiltration or erosions may be seen (iron pill gastritis). This condition can also be seen in other parts of the GI tract.

8. **Xanthelasma,** or xanthoma, is a clinically insignificant lesion consisting of aggregates of lipid-laden foamy histiocytes in the lamina propria (e-**Fig. 13.18**).

IV. **DIAGNOSTIC FEATURES OF COMMON GASTRIC POLYPS**
   A. **Hyperplastic polyp** is the most common polyp in the stomach and can be seen in any portion of the stomach. It consists of elongated, distorted, dilated, and branched foveola with an associated edematous and inflamed lamina propria (e-**Fig. 13.19**). Surface erosions, regenerative changes, and intestinal metaplasia may be evident. Dysplasia or even invasive carcinoma may be detected in approximately 2% of the cases, particularly in polyps >2 cm in size.
   B. **Fundic gland polyps** can be either syndromic (associated with familiar adenomatous polyposis [FAP] and Gardner's syndromes) or sporadic (occurring in the general population with or without proton pump inhibitor use). Morphologically, polyps that occur via a syndromic versus sporadic etiology are indistinguishable; both are characterized by cystically dilated fundic glands lined by hypertrophic or attenuated parietal cells (e-**Fig. 13.20**). They are typically small (average 5 mm) but can be multiple. Although a high frequency of epithelial dysplasia (approximately 25%) has been reported in syndromic polyps, the dysplasia is always classified as either low grade or indefinite; high-grade dysplasia and invasive carcinoma have only been described in rare case reports. Of note, fundic gland polyps (not adenomas) are the most common lesion in the stomach in patients with FAP.
   C. **Inflammatory fibroid polyp** occurs anywhere in the GI tract but is most common in the stomach, particularly the antrum. It is a submucosa-based lesion consisting of bland spindle cells, rich vasculature, and mixed inflammatory cells. Eosinophils are usually prominent (e-**Fig. 13.21**). The spindle cells are fibroblastic and myofibroblastic in nature and are immunoreactive for CD34 but not CD117 (c-kit).
   D. **Hamartomatous polyp** of the stomach is seen in Peutz–Jeghers' syndrome, juvenile polyposis, and Cowden's disease.

V. **DIAGNOSTIC FEATURES OF COMMON NEOPLASMS OF THE STOMACH.** The current World Health Organization (WHO) histologic classification of gastric tumors is given in Table 13.2. The 2002 American Joint Committee on Cancer (AJCC) Tumor, Node, Metastasis (TNM) staging schema is given in Table 13.3.
   A. **Adenoma and dysplasia** are separated by gross appearance; the former are localized polypoid or sessile lesions, the latter are flat diffuse lesions. The dysplasia seen in both lesions can be either low grade or high grade (carcinoma in situ), as determined by the degree of architectural complexity and cytologic atypia (e-**Fig. 13.22**). Adenomas can be divided into two types histologically. Intestinal type adenomas resemble adenomas of the colon and contain goblet cells and/or Paneth cells. Gastric type adenomas consist of foveolar epithelial cells containing neutral mucin. It has been reported that intestinal type adenomas have a higher chance of malignant transformation.

TABLE 13.2	WHO Histologic Classification of Gastric Tumors

Epithelial tumors
Intraepithelial neoplasia—Adenoma
Carcinoma
    Adenocarcinoma
        Intestinal type
        Diffuse type
    Papillary adenocarcinoma
    Tubular adenocarcinoma
    Mucinous adenocarcinoma
    Signet-ring-cell carcinoma
    Adenosquamous carcinoma
    Squamous cell carcinoma
    Small cell carcinoma
    Undifferentiated carcinoma
    Others
Carcinoid (well-differentiated endocrine neoplasm)

Nonepithelial tumors
Leiomyoma
Schwannoma
Granular cell tumor
Glomus tumor
Leiomyosarcoma
Gastrointestinal stromal tumor
    Benign
    Uncertain malignant potential
    Malignant
Kaposi's sarcoma
Other
Malignant lymphomas
    Marginal zone B-cell lymphoma of MALT type
    Mantle cell lymphoma
    Diffuse large B-cell lymphoma
    Other

Secondary tumors

From: Hamilton SR, Aaltonen LA, eds. *World Health Organization Classification of Tumours. Pathology and Genetics. Tumours of the Digestive System.* Lyon: IARC Press; 2000. Used with permission.

B. **Adenocarcinoma of the stomach** is traditionally divided into two major histologic types, intestinal and diffuse, according to the Lauren classification. The intestinal type is characterized by exophytic or ulcerative growth and a glandular pattern closely resembling colorectal adenocarcinoma. In contrast, the diffuse type exhibits widely infiltrative growth by poorly cohesive tumor cells without overt glandular formation as is typical of linitis plastica. In many diffuse cases, the tumor cells take on a signet-ring morphology with intracytoplasmic mucin pushing the nucleus aside.

Biopsy diagnosis of signet-ring-cell carcinoma can be difficult because the tumor cells that infiltrate the lamina propria can be inconspicuous and can resemble histiocytes (e-**Fig. 13.23**), and the associated gastric mucosa may be histologically unremarkable. Mucin stains and immunostains for pan-cytokeratin are helpful in these cases (e-**Fig. 13.24**). It should be noted that cytokeratin (CK) 7 and CK20 expression vary considerably in gastric adenocarcinomas; overall, 70% of cases express CK7, and 50% of the cases express CK20.

| TABLE 13.3 | **Tumor, Node, Metastasis (TNM) Staging Scheme for Gastric Carcinoma** |

PRIMARY TUMOR (T)

TX	Primary tumor cannot be assessed
T0	No evidence of primary tumor
Tis	Carcinoma in situ: Intraepithelial tumor without invasion of the lamina propria
T1	Tumor invades lamina propria or submucosa
T2	Tumor invades muscularis propria or subserosa*
T2a	Tumor invades muscularis propria
T2b	Tumor invades subserosa
T3	Tumor penetrates serosa (visceral peritoneum) without involvement of adjacent structures**,***
T4	Tumor invades adjacent structures**,***

REGIONAL LYMPH NODES (N)

NX	Regional lymph nodes cannot be assessed
N0	No regional lymph node metastasis
N1	Metastasis in 1 to 6 regional lymph nodes
N2	Metastasis in 7 to 15 regional lymph nodes
N3	Metastasis in >15 regional lymph nodes

DISTANT METASTASIS (M)

MX	Distant metastasis cannot be assessed
M0	No distant metastasis
M1	Distant metastasis

STAGE GROUPING

Stage 0	Tis	N0	M0
Stage IA	T1	N0	M0
Stage IB	T1	N1	M0
	T2a/b	N0	M0
Stage II	T1	N2	M0
	T2a/b	N1	M0
	T3	N0	M0
Stage IIIA	T2a/b	N2	M0
	T3	N1	M0
	T4	N0	M0
Stage IIIB	T3	N2	M0
Stage IV	T4	N1-3	M0
	T1-3	N3	M0
	Any T	Any N	M1

*A tumor may penetrate the muscularis propria with extension into the gastrocolic or gastrohepatic ligaments, or into the greater or lesser omentum, without perforation of the visceral peritoneum covering these structures. In this case, the tumor is classified T2. If there is perforation of the visceral peritoneum covering the gastric ligaments or the omentum, the tumor should be classified T3.
**The adjacent structures of the stomach include the spleen, transverse colon, liver, diaphragm, pancreas, abdominal wall, adrenal gland, kidney, small intestine, and retroperitoneum.
***Intramural extension to the duodenum or esophagus is classified by the depth of the greatest invasion in any of these sites, including the stomach.
From: Greene FL, Page DL, Fleming ID, Fritz AG, Balch CM, Haller DG, Morrow M, eds. *AJCC Cancer Staging Manual.* 6th edition. New York: Springer; 2002. Used with permission. (A new AJCC TNM staging system is scheduled for release in 2009; after its publication, the new staging scheme will appear on the website for this book.)

C. **Carcinoid tumors** occurring in the setting of chronic atrophic gastritis (type I) represent a continuum of nodular ECL cell hyperplasia due to hypergastrinemia. The distinction between carcinoid tumor and nodular ECL cell hyperplasia is arbitrary, and a cutoff of 0.5 mm in maximal dimension has been suggested, as has a cutoff of 5 mm. However, the distinction is not clinically important because there is no risk of metastasis from lesions of this size range; metastasis to the lymph nodes or liver generally occurs in tumors >1 cm in size. Even with metastasis, the prognosis is excellent.

Carcinoid tumor also occurs in association with Zollinger–Ellison syndrome secondary to gastrinoma (type II) and almost always in patients with multiple endocrine neoplasia (MEN) type I. Sporadic carcinoid tumor is designated as type III and is the most aggressive type in the stomach.

Carcinoid tumors of the stomach are histologically similar to those seen elsewhere in the body, characterized by microglandular, ribbonlike, trabecular, or insular growth patterns (e-Fig. 13.25). The diagnosis can be confirmed by immunostaining for neuroendocrine markers.

D. GISTs occur most commonly in the stomach; 60% of GISTs in the GI tract occur at this site. GIST occurs uniformly across all geographic and ethnic groups, and affects men and women equally. It is predominantly seen in patients >40 years old and is only rarely reported in children. Occasionally, GIST is part of a tumor syndrome, such as neurofibromatosis 1 and Carney's triad.

GIST is typically centered in the submucosa and muscularis propria. The tumor exhibits a broad spectrum of histologic features. Most are spindle cell tumors (e-Fig. 13.26), whereas others are epithelioid (e-Fig. 13.27). Tumors showing a pleomorphic morphology are indistinguishable from high-grade sarcomas.

A hallmark of GIST is the expression of c-kit protein, which can be detected in >95% of cases. Immunoreactivity to c-kit protein is typically global and strong, usually equivalent to that seen in mast cells present in the same tissue section. The staining pattern can be membranous (e-Fig. 13.28), cytoplasmic (e-Fig. 13.29), or cytoplasmic dotlike (e-Fig. 13.30). A fraction of GISTs are also immunoreactive for CD34 (80%), (smooth muscle actin [SMA]; 20%), desmin (<5%), and S100 protein (<5%). The positivity of these latter markers should not cause confusion between GIST and smooth muscle or nerve sheath tumors, the latter two of which are extremely rare now that the full clinicopathologic spectrum of GIST has been recognized. In 60% to 70% of GISTs, c-kit expression is associated with gain-of-function mutations of the *c-kit* gene. Mutations in a related gene, platelet-derived growth factor receptor α(*PDGFRA*), are detected in 35% to 67% of tumors lacking *c-kit* mutations. Immunostaining for *PDGFRA* is not currently available.

Approximately 5% of GISTs are immunohistochemically negative for c-kit. These tumors are diagnosed based on their typical clinical and histopathologic features (as well as mutational analysis of the *c-kit* or *PDGFRA* genes) and should not be confused with smooth muscle tumors even if they express SMA. A negative immunostain for desmin may be helpful in this regard. C-kit-negative GISTs tend to show an epithelioid morphology, to arise in extragastrointestinal locations, and to harbor *PDGFRA* mutations.

The biologic behavior of GIST is difficult to predict. Overall, approximately 20% to 30% of gastric GISTs show malignant behavior, although some authors believe that all GISTs should be considered to be of at least low-grade malignant potential. The consensus reached by the participants at a GIST workshop held at the National Institutes of Health in 2001 used tumor size and mitotic count as guides to predict malignant potential (*Hum Pathol* 2002;33:459). Table 13.4 presents proposed guidelines specifically for gastric GISTs based on a study of >1500 gastric GISTs with a long-term follow-up (*Am J Surg Pathol* 2005;29:52). Other histologic features that have been linked to aggressive behavior include mucosal invasion, tumor necrosis, cellularity, nuclear pleomorphism, and epithelioid histology.

E. Marginal zone B-cell lymphoma of mucosa-associated lymphoid tissue (MALT) type occurs in the entire GI tract, but the stomach is the most common location (*J Clin Pathol* 2007;60:361). The lymphoma cells are small to medium sized and typically have pale cytoplasm (monocytoid morphology); they expand the lamina propria and infiltrate around reactive lymphoid follicles, with colonization of the follicles by neoplastic cells. The malignant cells also invade the glandular epithelium to form highly distinctive lymphoepithelial lesions characterized by aggregates of three or more neoplastic cells that distort or displace the epithelial cells, often accompanied by eosinophilic degeneration of the epithelium and overt glandular

TABLE 13.4   **Proposed Guidelines for Assessing the Malignant Potential of Gastric GISTs**

Tumor	Predicted biologic behavior
≤2 cm, ≤5 mitoses/50 HPFs	Benign, metastasis rate or tumor-related mortality: 0
>2 ≤10 cm, ≤5 mitoses/50 HPFs	Very low malignant potential, metastasis rate or tumor-related mortality: <3%
>10 cm, ≤5 mitoses/50 HPFs, or ≤5 cm, >5 mitoses/50 HPFs	Low to moderate malignant potential, metastasis rate or tumor-related mortality: 12% to 15%
>5 cm, >5 mitoses/50 HPFs	High malignant potential, metastasis rate or tumor-related mortality: 49% to 86%

GISTs, gastrointestinal stromal tumors; HPFs, high-power fields.

destruction (e-**Fig. 13.31**). Plasmacytic differentiation is present in one third of the cases, usually seen in the superficial portion of the lamina propria.

The distinction between MALT lymphoma and chronic gastritis can sometimes be challenging (Table 13.5). Immunohistochemical stains for CD3, CD20, and CD43, and in situ hybridization for immunoglobulin light chain κ and λ expression, are helpful in difficult cases. In MALT lymphoma, the tumor cells express the B-cell marker CD20, and may aberrantly express the T-cell marker CD43; an immunostain for pan-cytokeratin can be used to highlight lymphoepithelial lesions, and special stains can be used to demonstrate associated *H. pylori* infection.

MALT lymphomas are indolent, low-grade neoplasms, many of which regress following *Helicobacter* eradication. Only a small subset of the tumors progresses to high grade, which may be indistinguishable from diffuse large B-cell lymphoma.

CYTOLOGY OF THE STOMACH
Jing Zhai

I. **INTRODUCTION.** The indications for cytological sampling include the presence of an inflammatory process or a neoplasm. Mucosal lesions can be sampled by endoscopic brushing cytology, and intramural lesions by endoscopic ultrasound–guided fine needle aspiration (EUS-FNA). Brushing cytology for malignancy has a sensitivity of 85% to 93% and a specificity of 99%, both comparable to the sensitivity and specificity of endoscopic biopsy. However, brushing cytology and biopsy are best considered complementary to each other for detection of malignancy (*Acta Cytol* 1988;32:461 and *Acta Cytol* 1990;34:217). EUS-FNA for malignancy has 61% sensitivity, 79% specificity, and 67% accuracy (*Gastroenterology* 1997;112:1087), which most likely reflects limitations of the technique due to inadequate sampling.

II. **INFLAMMATORY PROCESSES. H. *pylori* gastritis.** Antral mucosa brushing cytology with Papanicolaou stain is a sensitive, accurate, and simple procedure for investigating the presence of *H. pylori* infection. This bacterium presents as curved and S-shaped rods with basophilic staining properties (*World J Gastroenterol* 2005;11:2784).

III. **NEOPLASMS**

A. **Adenocarcinoma.** The smear of intestinal-type adenocarcinoma is hypercellular, consisting of haphazardly arranged, three-dimensional groups of cells and isolated cells. The malignant cells show nuclear enlargement, hyperchromasia, and irregular nuclear membrane contours (e-**Fig. 13.32**). A necrotic, dirty background is often present. The cytological diagnosis of diffuse type adenocarcinoma is difficult due to scarcity of the malignant cells; when present, the characteristic signet-ring cells show an intracytoplasmic vacuole abutting the nucleus and producing sharp angles (e-**Fig. 13.33**), with nuclear hyperchromasia. The differential diagnosis of the atypical

TABLE 13.5	Comparison of Histologic Features Between MALT Lymphoma and Chronic Gastritis	

Histologic feature	MALT lymphoma	Chronic gastritis
Lymphoid follicle	Frequent	May be present
Follicular colonization	May be present	Absent
Interfollicular lymphocytes	Small to intermediate in size, irregular nuclear contour, monocytoid	Small and round, mature
B lymphocytes (positive for CD20)	Predominant, present in lymphoid follicles and interfollicular spaces, may coexpress CD43	Sparse, usually limited to lymphoid follicles, do not coexpress CD43
T lymphocytes (positive for CD3)	Variable in number, scattered	Predominant, diffusely involve the lamina propria and interfollicular spaces
Plasma cells	Variable in number, usually seen beneath the surface lining epithelium, show light chain restriction	Usually prominent, diffusely present in the lamina propria, lack light chain restriction
Lymphoepithelial lesion	Usually prominent, the infiltrative lymphoid cells are B cells and form clusters, glandular destruction evident	Rare and inconspicuous, the infiltrative lymphoid cells are T cells and individually distributed, glandular destruction not evident
Helicobacter pylori microorganisms	May be present	May be present
Infiltration of muscularis mucosae by lymphoid cells	May be present	Absent

MALT, mucosa-associated lymphoid tissue.

cells in diffuse-type adenocarcinoma includes histiocytes and goblet cells (*Diagn Cytopathol* 2006;34:177).

B. GIST. The smear shows microfragments and sheets of spindle cells with moderate to high cellularity (**e-Fig. 13.34**), intact isolated spindle cells, and abundant stripped nuclei. The spindle cells have spindle-shaped to oval nuclei, fine chromatin, and abundant delicate cytoplasm with indistinct borders (**e-Fig. 13.35**). Nuclear atypia, mitosis, and necrosis can be identified occasionally. The epithelioid variant demonstrates large epithelioid cells with round nuclei and distinct cell borders. GIST cannot be graded based on cytologic specimens. Immunostains are required for a definitive diagnosis of GIST (*Cancer* 2001;93:269 and *Am J Clin Pathol* 2003;119:703).

C. Carcinoid tumors. The cytomorphology of carcinoid tumors (low-grade neuroendocrine carcinomas) is identical to that of the tumors when they occur at other locations. The smears are cellular and composed of loosely cohesive clusters and isolated cells with characteristic salt-and-pepper chromatin, small nucleoli and moderate granular cytoplasm. Focal and variable endocrine atypia, plasmacytoid cells, and spindle-shaped cells are easily identified.

D. Malignant lymphoma. The cytomorphology varies among the subtypes of gastric lymphoma. In general, the smears show isolated lymphoid cells exhibiting different degrees of atypia and monotony (the detailed cytomorphology of different lymphomas is discussed in the cytology section of Chapter 43). Precise diagnosis and classification require ancillary studies, which can be applied to EUS-FNA material (*Acta Cytol* 1994;38:169).

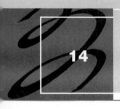

THE INTESTINES, APPENDIX, AND ANUS

Zong-Ming E. Chen and Hanlin L. Wang

I. NORMAL ANATOMY

  A. **The small intestine** starts distally from the gastric pylorus and ends proximally
     to the ileocecal valve, with an average length of 6 to 7 meters in adults. It is di-
     vided into the duodenum, jejunum, and ileum and is lined by villous mucosa. The
     villus is a slender, fingerlike projection, and its length-to-crypt ratio is 3:1 to 5:1
     (e-**Fig. 14.1**).* The epithelium consists mainly of tall, columnar absorptive cells
     that have basally situated nuclei, eosinophilic cytoplasm, and apical brush borders
     (microvilli). Other cell types include goblet cells, Paneth cells, and endocrine cells.
     Paneth cells are restricted to the base of the crypts and are recognized by their
     coarse supranuclear eosinophilic granules. Endocrine cells are also mainly seen in
     the lower portion of the crypts, but their cytoplasmic eosinophilic granules are
     smaller and infranuclear. The lamina propria always contains mixed inflammatory
     cells including abundant plasma cells, but neutrophils should only be seen within
     vascular channels. Intraepithelial lymphocytes (IELs) should be no more than one
     per five enterocytes. An increased IEL density may be seen in epithelium overlying
     lymphoid aggregates or Peyer's patches in the distal ileum, where shortened or even
     flattened villi may be evident. Shortened and broadened villi may also be seen in
     duodenal mucosa overlying Brunner's glands.
  B. **The large intestine, or colon,** is 1 to 1.5 meters long in adults. The right colon
     includes the cecum and the ascending and proximal transverse colon; the left colon
     consists of the distal transverse, descending, and sigmoid colon and the rectum.
     The mucosa contains evenly spaced, nonbranching, and perpendicularly arranged
     crypts extending from the surface to the muscularis mucosae, giving rise to a "rack
     of test tubes" appearance (e-**Fig. 14.2**). Occasional branching crypts or slight crypt
     architectural distortion may be seen in the rectum and sigmoid colon, and in areas
     adjacent to lymphoid aggregates. The epithelial and lamina propria components
     are similar to those of the small intestine, but goblet cells are more numerous,
     particularly in the left colon. Muciphages (mucin-containing macrophages) are also
     common in the lamina propria of the left colon. Paneth cells are only present in
     the right colon. As aforementioned, IELs can be prominent in epithelium overlying
     lymphoid aggregates. The lower portion of the rectum is not covered by visceral
     peritoneum (serosa).

     Bowel preparation for endoscopy may cause mucosal edema, hemorrhage, sur-
     face epithelial detachment, neutrophilic cryptitis, and increased apoptotic activity.
     These abnormalities are usually mild but may be confused with various colitides.
     Endoscopy may occasionally introduce air bubbles into the mucosa, mimicking
     adipose tissue (e-**Fig. 14.3**).
  C. **The appendix** is a tubular extension of the cecum with an average length of 7 to 10
     cm. Its structure is similar to that of the large intestine, except for more prominent
     lymphoid aggregates in the mucosa, often with well-formed germinal centers, and a
     poorly developed muscularis mucosae, which is frequently interrupted by lymphoid
     aggregates.
  D. **The anal canal** is the terminal 3 to 4 cm of the gastrointestinal (GI) tract, defined
     by the proximal and distal ends of the internal anal sphincter and centered by the

---

*All e-figures are available online via the Solution Site Image Bank.

dentate (pectinate) line. The mucosa lining the upper portion of the anal canal is a direct extension from the rectum (colorectal zone), often with shorter and more irregular crypts, and more conspicuous lamina propria smooth muscle fibers extended from the muscularis mucosae. These normal findings should not be viewed as evidence of chronic proctitis or mucosal prolapse. The middle portion, the anal transitional zone (ATZ), is a 0.5- to 1-cm segment above the dentate line. It is lined by variable types of epithelium, including rectal crypts and mature squamous epithelium. The typical ATZ epithelium, however, consists of 4 to 9 cell layers that have the features of both metaplastic squamous mucosa and urothelium. Submucosal and intramuscular anal glands open in the ATZ via anal ducts that are also lined by ATZ epithelium. The distal squamous zone extends from the dentate line downward to the anal verge and is lined by nonkeratinizing squamous mucosa with melanocytes. It is distinguished from the perianal skin by the lack of skin appendages.

II. GROSS EXAMINATION AND SPECIMEN HANDLING

A. Endoscopic biopsy. When processing the specimen, it is important to record not only pertinent clinical history, but also the endoscopic findings. Biopsies are typically small fragments of mucosal tissue in the range of 1 to 5 mm, which do not need to be inked or cut; gross descriptions of shape and color are usually unnecessary. The number of the biopsies should be recorded; if there are too many to count, an estimate should be given. The dimension of the biopsies should also be documented, which can be done by giving either the size range of the biopsies, the greatest dimension of the largest tissue fragment, or the dimensions of the aggregate. Documentation of the number and size is important to ensure that the biopsies are adequately represented on the slides. Routine microscopic examination of endoscopic biopsies usually entails examination of three hematoxylin and eosin (H&E)-stained levels.

B. Suction biopsy of the rectum is used for evaluation of Hirschsprung disease, which allows sampling of the submucosa. The biopsy is serially sectioned until the tissue is exhausted. Initially, every third level is H&E-stained; if no ganglion cells are identified in these slides, the remaining sections should be stained and examined. In some labs, frozen sections are performed for histochemical staining by the acetylcholinesterase reaction to identify proliferating nerve fibers in the lamina propria and muscularis mucosae.

C. Polypectomy specimens should be described (including their maximal dimension) and then inked at their cauterized base (although the stalk may retract and thus be difficult to identify). The specimen is bisected or serially sectioned depending on its size, and entirely submitted. The sectioning should follow the vertical plane of the stalk to maximize the evaluation of the polypectomy margin.

D. Bowel resections range from segmental resection, ileocolectomy, low anterior resection (LAR) and abdominoperineal resection (APR), to total colectomy. Once the portion of resected bowel is identified and oriented, the length and diameter (or circumference) are measured. The length and diameter of the appendix and the dimensions of mesentery are also measured, if present. The external surface (serosa in most cases) of the bowel is inspected for tumor involvement, perforation, adhesion, and fat wrapping. The bowel is opened longitudinally along the antimesenteric border, unless this would mean cutting through the tumor.

When resection is performed for a tumor, any nonperitonealized radial (circumferential) margin at the site of the tumor is inked. The maximal size of the tumor and the distance to the proximal and distal resection margins, or to the closest margin in unoriented specimens, are documented. After fresh tissue is taken for the tumor bank (as needed), the specimen is pinned out on a wax board with the mucosal side up and fixed by submerging in 10% formalin overnight. The tumor is then sectioned to assess the depth of invasion. Three to four sections from the tumor are submitted for microscopic examination; the sections should include the area of deepest penetration and the relationship to adjacent, grossly nonneoplastic mucosa. Additional sections include proximal and distal resection margins, either circumferential or longitudinal if tumor is grossly distant; however, if tumor approximates the margin, such as seen in APR or LAR specimens, the margin may be inked and perpendicular sections, which may be multiple, are submitted. If the inked radial margin is not included in the tumor sections, one separate radial margin section should be submitted. One random section from normal-appearing bowel and any additional gross lesions (such as separate polyps) should also be submitted. If an appendix is present, it is handled as an appendectomy specimen as described below.

After the above sections are taken, the mesentery and soft tissue are dissected for lymph nodes, and the number and size range of identified nodes are recorded. Small lymph nodes can be submitted in toto without sectioning. Larger nodes are serially sectioned, and the cut surfaces are grossly examined; if metastatic carcinoma is grossly appreciated, as evidenced by a white and hard cut surface, the size of the metastatic deposit(s) should be recorded, and one representative section from each grossly positive node should be submitted. If the cut surfaces of the nodes are tan, soft, and homogeneous, and lack gross evidence of metastasis, the entire node should be submitted for microscopic evaluation. Most of the nodes are located directly adjacent to the serosal surface and along large vessels. The mesenteric tissue may be stripped off and fixed in DisectAid solution (Decal Chemical Corp, Tallman, NY) for 1 to 4 hours to facilitate the node search. Although a minimum of 12 nodes is generally recommended, all nodes that can be found should be submitted. Fewer nodes are acceptable for short specimens, for cases that have received preoperative chemoradiation, and for APR or LAR specimens because the nodes are difficult to find below the peritoneal reflection.

For polyposis specimens, sampling should focus on large lesions and lesions with a distinct or worrisome gross appearance.

If resection is performed for inflammatory bowel disease (IBD), particularly for ulcerative colitis, sequential sections spaced every 10 cm should be submitted. The sections should include transition regions between normal-appearing and diseased segments, distal and proximal margins, and representative inflammatory polyps. Any focal lesions, such as areas with raised mucosa, fistula tract, or stricture, should be sampled. The appendix, if present, is handled as an appendectomy specimen as described below. Representative lymph nodes are submitted if they are easily located, but there is no need to spend too much time to search for them.

In the case of ischemia, the mesenteric vessels should be carefully examined and sampled to evaluate the possibility of thrombosis, embolization, or vasculitis. It is also important to microscopically examine the proximal and distal margins for tissue viability.

When proctectomy or rectosigmoid resection is performed with pull-through for Hirschsprung disease, the distal margin is usually indicated by suture by the surgeon. Sequential sections every 1 to 2 cm from distal to proximal should be submitted to achieve an accurate estimation of the aganglionic region.

E. **Appendectomy specimens** are described for length, diameter, surface appearance, and dimensions of the mesoappendix. For a nonneoplastic appendix, one half of the longitudinally bisected tip and two cross-sections are submitted in a single cassette. One of the cross-sections is taken from the middle portion of the specimen, or from areas with gross lesions such as perforation; the other is taken from the proximal margin in case a neoplastic process is detected by microscopy. For a neoplastic appendix, the entire appendix should be submitted; the proximal resection margin should be submitted in a separate cassette.

F. **Anal biopsy** is treated similarly to other GI biopsies. Resection for a neoplastic process may be handled as endoscopic mucosal resection as described in Chapter 12. If the procedure is performed for hemorrhoids, one representative section is sufficient.

III. **DIAGNOSTIC FEATURES OF NONNEOPLASTIC CONDITIONS OF THE SMALL IN-TESTINE**
   A. **Congenital anomalies**
      1. **Heterotopic gastric mucosa** typically presents as a small nodule or sessile polyp in the duodenal bulb, and consists of fundic-type mucosa. It should be distinguished from gastric surface metaplasia, where the surface absorptive and goblet cells of the duodenal mucosa are replaced by gastric foveolar mucin cells.

This latter condition is often associated with duodenitis secondary to *Helicobacter pylori* infection.

2. **Heterotopic pancreas** may present as a mass lesion, usually seen in the duodenum. It is composed of ducts and acini, with or without islets.

3. **Meckel's diverticulum** results from persistence of the proximal portion of the vitelline duct and is always located on the antimesenteric border of the ileum. Heterotopic pancreatic tissue or gastric mucosa is common. Congenital diverticulum can also occur in the duodenum and jejunum.

4. **Malrotation, stenosis, atresia, duplication, and defects of the musculature** are rare.

B. **Malabsorptive disorders**

1. **Celiac disease,** also known as gluten-sensitive enteropathy, celiac sprue, or nontropical sprue, is an immune-mediated disorder secondary to hypersensitivity to α-gliadin present in a gluten-containing diet. Classic histologic features in untreated celiac disease include villous atrophy, crypt hyperplasia, intraepithelial lymphocytosis, a dense lamina propria lymphoplasmacytic infiltrate, and enterocyte damage. Villous atrophy may range in severity from partial blunting or broadening, to complete flattening, but the overall thickness of the mucosa may not be reduced significantly due to crypt hyperplasia (e-**Fig. 14.4**). Eosinophils and neutrophils may be seen in celiac disease but are usually not prominent in number. Enterocyte damage is usually observed on the surface evidenced by flattening and/or cytoplasmic vacuolization.

An increased number of IELs is an important diagnostic feature of celiac disease. Although the increase is defined as >40 lymphocytes per 100 enterocytes, a formal count or immunostaining for T lymphocytes is unnecessary. Lymphocytosis is typically diffuse and evenly distributed along the entire length of the villi if the mucosa is not completely flattened (e-**Fig. 14.5**). In fact, an increased number of IELs may be the only histologic finding in patients with latent or partially treated celiac disease; serologic tests should be recommended in these cases. It should be emphasized, however, that, in addition to celiac disease, many other conditions can cause intraepithelial lymphocytosis (Table 14.1).

It is important to realize that a definitive diagnosis of celiac disease is not made by a pathologist; the typical histologic findings are best diagnosed as consistent with celiac disease because definitive diagnosis relies on clinical presentation, serologic tests, and clinical and histologic response to a gluten-free diet. More than 90% of patients have serum anti-gliadin, anti-endomysial, and/or anti-tissue transglutaminase antibodies (*Gastroenterology.* 2005;128:S38).

 TABLE 14.1 Conditions Causing Intraepithelial Lymphocytosis in the Small Intestine

Celiac disease
Tropical sprue
Autoimmune enteropathy
Common variable immunodeficiency
Viral enteritis
Cryptosporidiosis
Microsporidiosis
Giardiasis
Bacterial overgrowth
Food allergies
Crohn disease
Zollinger–Ellison syndrome
Systemic autoimmune diseases
Nonsteroidal anti-inflammatory drugs
Helicobacter pylori infection

2. **Refractory sprue** refers to unresponsiveness to a gluten-free diet or relapse of symptoms despite gluten restriction. It is histologically indistinguishable from classic celiac disease, although some gastroenterologists may regard it as a type of T-cell lymphoma. Neutrophils may be more numerous in some of the cases.
3. **Collagenous sprue** is characterized by villous flattening and subepithelial collagen deposition, which can be highlighted by trichrome stain.
4. **Autoimmune enteropathy** shares many clinical and histopathologic features with celiac disease, but often involves both the small and large intestines. A biopsy typically exhibits villous flattening and dense lamina propria lymphoplasmacytic infiltrates (e-Fig. 14.6). In contrast to celiac disease, intraepithelial lymphocytosis and crypt hyperplasia may not be evident, and neutrophils may be more numerous. Complete lack of goblet cells and/or Paneth cells may be seen in a fraction of the cases. Although some patients have anti-enterocyte and/or anti-goblet cell antibodies, these tests are not routinely available. The diagnosis may be confirmed by response to steroids and immunosuppressants.
5. **Eosinophilic gastroenteritis** involving the small intestine exhibits histologic features similar to those described for eosinophilic gastritis (Chap. 13). There may or may not be villous blunting, but IELs are usually not increased. Parasitic infestations, food allergy including cow's milk protein intolerance, drug reaction, connective tissue disorders, and neoplasms should be excluded.
6. **Common variable immunodeficiency** is characterized by the absence of lamina propria plasma cells (e-Fig. 14.7). Other features may include a variable degree of villous blunting, intraepithelial lymphocytosis, and lymphoid aggregates. Infectious agents, particularly Giardia, should be searched for in these biopsies.
7. **Microvillus inclusion disease** is a rare autosomal recessive disease causing intractable diarrhea in infancy. The hallmark of the disease is the loss of normal brush border on the luminal surface of the enterocytes. Instead, the brush border is incorporated into the cytoplasm as apical microvillus inclusions. The microscopic features can be best demonstrated by periodic acid–Schiff (PAS) stain, electron microscopy, and immunostains for carcinoembryogenic antigen (CEA), CD10, or villin. There is also diffuse villous atrophy, but an inflammatory response and intraepithelial lymphocytosis are not evident.
8. **Lymphangiectasia,** either primary (congenital) or secondary (due to obstruction), may present as a localized mass lesion or diffusely involve the bowel (e-Fig. 14.8). The diagnosis on small mucosal biopsies can be difficult because dilated lacteals can be easily overlooked or confused with artifactual spaces created by detachment of the lamina propria from the basement membrane.
9. **Abetalipoproteinemia** features lipid accumulation in enterocytes, giving rise to a clear or foamy appearance. The normal villous architecture is well preserved.

C. **Infectious diseases**
   1. **Tropical sprue and bacterial overgrowth** simulate celiac disease, but may involve the entire small intestine with more severe disease distally. Clinical and/or travel history is important in establishing the diagnosis.
   2. **Giardiasis** does not induce significant villous architectural change or an inflammatory response. The diagnosis is based on the identification of pear-shaped trophozoites at the luminal surface of normal-appearing mucosa (e-Fig. 14.9), which can be mistaken as cytoplasmic debris at a glance. The organisms are better recognized on trichrome and Giemsa stains.
   3. **Whipple disease** exhibits distended villi by lamina propria accumulation of foamy macrophages stuffed with the diastase-resistant PAS-positive, rod-shaped bacteria *Tropheryma whippelii*. The microorganisms can also be detected by polymerase chain reaction (PCR) analysis and electron microscopy. Gomori's methenamine silver (GMS), acid-fast bacilli (AFB), or Fite stains should be performed on these biopsies to rule out fungal (such as histoplasmosis) or mycobacterial (such as *Mycobacterium avium intracellulare*) infections because they are quite similar to Whipple disease on H&E stain.

4. **Cryptosporidiosis** is characterized by uniform, spherical, 2- to 4-μm bodies attached to the brush border that stain bluish on H&E (e-**Fig. 14.10**). The organisms should not be confused with mucin droplets.

5. **Strongyloidiasis** is diagnosed by identification of larvae, eggs, and adult worms embedded in the crypts (e-**Fig. 14.11**). Eosinophils, sometimes with Charcot–Leyden crystals, may be prominent. The nematodes most commonly infect the small intestine, and rarely the stomach and colon. It is interesting to note that gastric strongyloidiasis may sometimes be associated with infection by human T-lymphotropic virus type 1 that causes adult T-cell lymphoma/leukemia.

IV. **DIAGNOSTIC FEATURES OF POLYPS AND NEOPLASMS OF THE SMALL INTESTINE** (Table 14.2)

A. **Brunner's gland hyperplasia, hamartoma, and adenoma** (probably the same process) all consist of expanded lobules of benign Brunner's glands with delicate fibrous septa. They are typically located in the submucosa, but penetration into the mucosa is common. Cystic degeneration may occur, which has been termed Brunner's gland cyst.

B. **Peutz–Jeghers polyp** is most common in the small intestine but also occurs in the colon and stomach. It is a hamartomatous polyp characterized by an aborizing network of smooth muscle supporting benign-appearing mucosa that may be hyperplastic or form clusters (e-**Fig. 14.12**). Most polyps occur as part of an inherited cancer syndrome, but sporadic cases may be encountered. Because syndromic polyps carry an increased risk of cancer development, they should always be assessed for dysplasia.

C. **Adenomyoma of the ampulla of Vater,** also known as periampullary adenomyoma, adenomyomatous hyperplasia, or myoepithelial hamartoma, exhibits an orderly arranged lobular pattern of benign pancreaticobiliary ducts in a background of proliferating smooth muscle. It may coexist with heterotopic pancreas.

D. **Adenomas** are rare in the small intestine, usually occurring in the duodenum. Multiple adenomas are almost always associated with familial adenomatous polyposis (FAP). Histologically, they are essentially identical to their colorectal counterparts and are classified into tubular, tubulovillous, and villous types. The diagnostic pitfalls include gastric surface metaplasia and reparative change, which may mimic adenoma.

E. **Adenocarcinoma** of the small intestine is rare, accounting for only 2% of all primary GI tumors despite the fact that the small intestine constitutes ~75% of the length and ~90% of the mucosal surface of the GI tract. Adenocarcinoma of the small intestine is morphologically similar to or indistinguishable from its colorectal counterpart, but is immunophenotypically distinct. In contrast to colorectal adenocarcinomas, primary adenocarcinomas of the small intestine more frequently express cytokeratin (CK)7, and less frequently express CK20, α-methylacyl coenzyme A racemase (AMACR), nuclear β-catenin, caudal-related homeobox 2 (CDX2), villin, mucin-2 (MUC2), mucin-5AC (MUC5AC), and small intestinal mucin antigen (SIMA). The 2002 American Joint Committee on Cancer (AJCC) Tumor, Node, Metastasis (TNM) staging schema is given in Table 14.3.

F. **Ampullary carcinoma** is a heterogeneous group of tumors arising in the vicinity of the ampulla of Vater. Intestinal type adenocarcinoma is the most common histologic type, followed by pancreaticobiliary type. It appears that intestinal type has a more favorable outcome than pancreaticobiliary type, and that the overall survival of ampullary carcinoma is better than that of pancreatic ductal carcinoma probably due to its resectability. The 2002 AJCC TNM staging schema for ampullary carcinoma is given in Table 14.4.

G. **Carcinoid tumor,** or well-differentiated neuroendocrine neoplasm, accounts for one third of the small intestinal tumors. Duodenal carcinoids derive from endocrine cells of the foregut and tend to be <2 cm, whereas jejunoileal carcinoids derive from the midgut and tend to be >2 cm. Microscopically, these tumors are similar to those elsewhere in the body, and their potential for malignancy is generally independent of histologic features. The risk of metastasis, usually to the liver and regional lymph

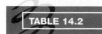

TABLE 14.2	WHO Histologic Classification of Tumors of the Small Intestine

Epithelial tumors
Adenoma
   Tubular
   Villous
   Tubulovillous
Intraepithelial neoplasia (dysplasia) associated with chronic inflammatory diseases
   Low-grade glandular intraepithelial neoplasia
   High-grade glandular intraepithelial neoplasia
Carcinoma
   Adenocarcinoma
   Mucinous carcinoma
   Signet-ring cell carcinoma
   Small cell carcinoma
   Squamous cell carcinoma
   Adenosquamous carcinoma
   Medullary carcinoma
   Undifferentiated carcinoma
Carcinoid (well-differentiated endocrine neoplasm)
   Gastrin cell tumor, functioning (gastrinoma) or nonfunctioning
   Somatostatin cell tumor
   EC cell, serotonin-producing neoplasm
   L-cell, glucagonlike peptide and PP/PYY-producing tumor
Mixed carcinoid–adenocarcinoma
Gangliocytic paraganglioma
Others

Nonepithelial tumors
Lipoma
Leiomyoma
Gastrointestinal stromal tumor
Leiomyosarcoma
Angiosarcoma
Kaposi sarcoma
Others

Malignant lymphomas
Immunoproliferative small intestinal disease (includes α-heavy chain disease)
Western type B-cell lymphoma of MALT
Mantle cell lymphoma
Diffuse large B-cell lymphoma
Burkitt lymphoma
Burkittlike/atypical Burkitt lymphoma
T-cell lymphoma
   Enteropathy associated
   Unspecified
Others

Secondary tumors

Polyps
Hyperplastic polyp (metaplastic)
Peutz–Jeghers
Juvenile

WHO, World Health Organization; EC, enterochromaffin cell; L,; PP, pancreatic polypeptide; PYY, polypeptide YY; MALT, mucosa-associated lymphoid tissue.
From: Hamilton SR, Aaltonen LA, eds. *World Health Organization Classification of Tumours. Pathology and Genetics. Tumours of the Digestive System.* Lyon: IARC Press; 2000. Used with permission.

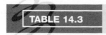

TABLE 14.3	**Tumor, Node, Metastasis (TNM) Staging Scheme for Small Intestinal Carcinomas**

Primary tumor (T)

TX	Primary tumor cannot be assessed
T0	No evidence of primary tumor
Tis	Carcinoma in situ
T1	Tumor invades lamina propria or submucosa
T2	Tumor invades muscularis propria
T3	Tumor invades through the muscularis propria into the subserosa, or into nonperitonealized perimuscular tissue (mesentery or retroperitoneum) with extension 2 cm or less*
T4	Tumor perforates the visceral peritoneum or directly invades other organs or structures (includes other loops of small intestine, mesentery, or retroperitoneum >2 cm, and abdominal wall by way of serosa; for duodenum only, invasion of pancreas)

Regional lymph nodes (N)

NX	Regional lymph nodes cannot be assessed
N0	No regional lymph node metastasis
N1	Regional lymph node(s) metastasis

Distant metastasis (M)

MX	Distant metastasis cannot be assessed
M0	No distant metastasis
M1	Distant metastasis

Stage grouping

Stage 0	Tis	N0	M0
Stage I	T1	N0	M0
	T2	N0	M0
Stage IIA	T3	N0	M0
Stage IIB	T4	N0	M0
Stage III	Any T	N1	M0
Stage IV	Any T	Any N	M1

AJCC, American Joint Committee on Cancer; TNM, Tumor, Node, Metastasis.
* The nonperitonealized perimuscular tissue is, for jejunum and ileum, part of the mesentery and, for duodenum in areas where serosa is lacking, part of the retroperitoneum.
From: Greene FL, Page DL, Fleming ID, Fritz AG, Balch CM, Haller DG, Morrow M, eds. *AJCC Cancer Staging Manual.* 6th edition. New York: Springer; 2002. Used with permission. (A new AJCC TNM staging system is scheduled for release in 2009; after its publication, the new staging scheme will appear on the website for this book.)

nodes, is determined by the size of the tumor and depth of invasion of the bowel wall. Poorly differentiated neuroendocrine tumors exhibit overt histologic features of malignancy.

Table 14.5 summarizes the classification and histologic grading of neuroendocrine tumors of the GI tract recommended by the World Health Organization (WHO; *World J Surg.* 1996;20:132).

H. Gangliocytic paraganglioma occurs almost exclusively in the periampullary region and is benign in the majority of cases. Similar to that in other locations, the tumor consists of a mixture of ganglionlike cells, Schwannian cells, and epithelioid endocrinelike cells. S-100 positivity is a useful marker to differentiate the neoplasm from a gastrointestinal stromal tumor (GIST).

I. GIST of the small intestine accounts for 30–40% of all GISTs of the GI tract, and tends to be more aggressive than its gastric counterpart as detailed in Table 14.6 (*Am J Surg Pathol.* 2006;30:477).

J. Immunoproliferative small intestinal disease (IPSID) is a distinct type of extranodal marginal zone B-cell lymphoma (mucosa-associated lymphoid tissue [MALT] lymphoma), typically seen in young adults in the Middle East and Mediterranean

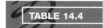

TABLE 14.4	Tumor, Node, Metastasis (TNM) Staging Scheme for Ampullary Carcinoma		

Primary tumor (T)

TX	Primary tumor cannot be assessed
T0	No evidence of primary tumor
Tis	Carcinoma in situ
T1	Tumor limited to ampulla of Vater or sphincter of Oddi
T2	Tumor invades duodenal wall
T3	Tumor invades pancreas
T4	Tumor invades peripancreatic soft tissues or other adjacent organs or structures

Regional lymph nodes (N)

NX	Regional lymph nodes cannot be assessed
N0	No regional lymph node metastasis
N1	Regional lymph node metastasis

Distant metastasis (M)

MX	Distant metastasis cannot be assessed
M0	No distant metastasis
M1	Distant metastasis

Stage grouping

Stage 0	Tis	N0	M0
Stage IA	T1	N0	M0
Stage IB	T2	N0	M0
Stage IIA	T3	N0	M0
Stage IIB	T1	N1	M0
	T2	N1	M0
	T3	N1	M0
Stage III	T4	any N	M0
Stage IV	Any T	Any N	M1

AJCC, American Joint Committee on Cancer; TNM, Tumor, Node, Metastasis.
From: Greene FL, Page DL, Fleming ID, Fritz AG, Balch CM, Haller DG, Morrow M, eds. *AJCC Cancer Staging Manual.* 6th edition. New York: Springer; 2002. Used with permission. (A new AJCC TNM staging system is scheduled for release in 2009; after its publication, the new staging scheme will appear on the website for this book.)

countries. About half of the patients exhibit characteristic α-heavy chain paraproteinemia without associated light chains (α-heavy chain disease).

  K. **Enteropathy-type T-cell lymphoma** typically develops in the setting of refractory sprue and ulcerative jejunitis or jejunoileitis. It most commonly affects the jejunum and is characterized by dense infiltration of atypical T lymphocytes in association with epithelial destruction. The prognosis is dismal.

V. DIAGNOSTIC FEATURES OF NONNEOPLASTIC CONDITIONS OF THE LARGE INTESTINE

  A. **Neuromuscular disorders**

   1. **Hirschsprung disease** affects approximately 1 in 5000 live births, mainly males. Germline mutations in *RET* and other genes play a central role in pathogenesis, which results in a failure of neural crest cells to appropriately migrate to the rectum or rectosigmoid colon or, rarely, the entire colon. The affected segment is narrowed because of the aganglionosis, whereas the upstream segment is dilated due to obstruction. The diagnosis is established by microscopic demonstration of a true absence of ganglion cells in the submucosa on a rectal suction biopsy, typically accompanied by hypertrophic nerve fibers (**e-Fig. 14.13**). Demonstration of acetylcholinesterase-positive nerve twigs in the muscularis mucosae and lamina propria in frozen sections also helps to confirm the diagnosis.

   The biopsy should be taken at least 2 cm above the pectinate line (because the distal 1.5- to 2-cm zone of the rectum is physiologically hypoganglionotic

TABLE 14.5	Classification and Grading of Neuroendocrine Neoplasms of the GI Tract		
Classification	**Grade**	**Biological behavior**	**Definition**
Well-differentiated neuroendocrine tumor	I	Benign	Nonfunctioning, cytologically bland, <1 cm, confined to the mucosa/submucosa, no angioinvasion
	II	Uncertain malignant potential	Nonfunctioning, cytologically bland, 1 to 2 cm, confined to the mucosa/submucosa, with or without angioinvasion
Well-differentiated neuroendocrine carcinoma	III	Low grade malignant	Nonfunctioning, cytologically bland, >2 cm, with or without angioinvasion, extension beyond the submucosa; or functional, well-differentiated tumor of any size
Poorly differentiated neuroendocrine carcinoma	IV	High grade malignant	Small cell carcinoma or large cell neuroendocrine carcinoma, functional or nonfunctional

GI, gastrointestinal.

and may even have prominent nerve fibers) and contain an adequate thickness of submucosa (equal in thickness to the mucosa). Thus, biopsies containing squamous or anal canal transitional mucosa, which indicates proximity to the pectinate line, should be considered inappropriate.

A potential diagnostic pitfall is that neonates may have immature ganglion cells with small nuclei, scanty cytoplasm, and inconspicuous nucleoli, which makes their recognition difficult. Immunohistochemical staining for neuron-specific enolase (NSE) or other neuronal markers may help in these cases.

2. **Pseudo-obstruction syndrome** encompasses a heterogeneous group of neuromuscular disorders characterized by colonic inertia with constipation. The diagnosis is essentially a clinical one and lacks specific histologic criteria. Melanosis coli (pigmented macrophages in the lamina propria) is a common finding in these patients due to excessive laxative use (e-**Fig. 14.14**). Brown bowel syndrome is

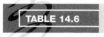

TABLE 14.6	Proposed Guidelines for Assessing the Malignant Potential of Small Intestinal GISTs
Tumor	**Predicted biologic behavior**
≤2 cm, ≤5 mitoses/50 HPFs	Benign, metastasis rate or tumor-related mortality: 0
>2 ≤5 cm, <5 mitoses/50 HPFs	Low malignant potential, metastasis rate or tumor-related mortality: 4%
>5 ≤10 cm, ≤5 mitoses/50 HPFs	Moderate malignant potential, metastasis rate or tumor-related mortality: 25%
>10 cm, or >5 mitoses/50 HPFs	High malignant potential, metastasis rate or tumor-related mortality: 50–90%

GIST, gastrointestinal stromal tumor; HPFs, high-power fields.
Modified from *Am J Surg Pathol*. 2006;30:477.

a unique condition believed to be caused by vitamin E deficiency, which leads to mitochondrial dysfunction and lipofuscin accumulation in smooth muscle cells.

B. **Ischemic bowel disease** occurs in a variety of clinical settings and does not always require a complete occlusion of the mesenteric vessels. However, acute ischemia is usually caused by mechanical alterations, which is particularly true for the small intestine (ischemic enteritis). The mucosa appears to be the most vulnerable layer of the bowel to acute ischemia, but transmural infarction can occur in more severe cases (e-**Fig. 14.15**) and is sometimes associated with hemorrhage or pseudomembranes. In acute ischemia, necrosis may be noted in the superficial mucosa while the deeper glands may exhibit regenerative changes with mucin depletion; the inflammatory infiltrate is usually insignificant. Chronic ischemia is more commonly seen in the colon (ischemic colitis) and is characterized by fibrosis and hyalinization of the lamina propria and atrophy (withering) of the crypts (e-**Fig. 14.16**).

Neonatal necrotizing enterocolitis (NEC) is a special form of ischemic bowel disease with a high mortality rate, typically occurring in the first week of life in premature infants. It classically affects the terminal ileum and the right colon with gangrenous necrosis. Pneumatosis intestinalis and segmental absence of the muscularis propria may be seen.

C. **IBD** is an idiopathic chronic inflammatory process with a genetic predisposition and familial clustering, and mainly refers to Crohn disease and ulcerative colitis. The disease is primarily characterized by its chronicity featuring crypt architectural distortion, basal plasmacytosis, basal lymphoid aggregates, mucosal atrophy, Paneth cell metaplasia, and pyloric metaplasia. Crypt architectural distortion often manifests as branching, shortening, irregular shape, irregular spacing, size variation, disarray, and parallel alignment (instead of perpendicular) to the muscularis mucosae (e-**Fig. 14.17**). Paneth cell metaplasia is defined by the presence of Paneth cells beyond the right colon. Pyloric metaplasia appears to be more commonly seen in the small bowel in Crohn disease, but also occurs in the colon in ulcerative colitis (e-**Fig. 14.18**).

The lamina propria in IBD is usually densely infiltrated by mixed inflammatory cells, mainly lymphocytes and plasma cells. Eosinophils can be abundant. Because of crypt shortening, a bandlike inflammatory infiltrate is often seen in the space above the muscularis mucosae, referring to basal plasmacytosis (e-**Fig. 14.18**). Lymphoid aggregates may be present in this space in some cases. The disease is active when neutrophils are present; in addition to infiltrating the lamina propria, neutrophils often infiltrate the crypt epithelium to cause cryptitis, and are present within the lumen of the crypt to cause crypt abscess (e-**Fig.14.19**). The inflammatory activity is graded as minimal, mild, moderate, or severe. Usually, minimally and mildly active disease feature the presence of cryptitis. When a significant number of crypt abscesses are seen, the disease is moderately active. Severely active disease is usually seen in cases with ulcerations. In the absence of neutrophilic infiltration, the disease is referred to as quiescent or inactive.

1. **Crohn disease** may involve any portion of the GI tract. Roughly, ~40% of patients have small bowel disease only, ~40% have small and large bowel involvement, and ~20% have colonic disease only. Grossly, the involved bowel segment typically has a rigid, strictured, or thickened wall with creeping fat. Upon opening, the segment usually maintains its cylindrical shape (e-**Fig. 14.20**). The mucosa may show crisscrossing linear and transverse ulcers with intervening edematous mucosa, generating a cobblestoning appearance. Deep fissuring ulcers and fistula tracts are common.

The microscopic hallmarks of Crohn disease are transmural inflammation, granulomas, and skip lesions. In resection specimens, lymphoid aggregates may be present in all layers of the bowel wall, but are characteristically seen in the subserosal fat where they typically follow the vasculature (e-**Fig. 14.21**). Granulomas are seen in up to 40% of the cases, and may be found in the mucosa, submucosa, and subserosa. In the mucosa, Crohn's granulomas are typically small, well-formed, and nonnecrotizing and lack multinucleated giant cells (e-**Fig. 14.22**). When they are located near or within the muscularis mucosae, they can be overlooked because of similarity to smooth muscle bundles. A diagnostic pitfall is the so-called "crypt granuloma," which represents a nonspecific pericryptal histiocytic response, sometimes with foreign body–type giant cells, to ruptured crypts (e-Fig. 14.23). In the subserosa, Crohn's granulomas can be larger, may contain giant cells, and are frequently associated with lymphoid aggregates (e-Fig. 14.21).

In the absence of granulomas, the diagnosis of Crohn disease in mucosal biopsies relies on microscopic skipping of the disease. If multiple tissue fragments are obtained from the same region, the disease may involve only a fraction of the specimens. Even in the same tissue fragment, the crypt architectural change and inflammatory activity may involve only a portion of the fragment while the rest is completely normal. Although focal or patchy colitis is characteristic of Crohn disease, it is also commonly seen in other conditions, such as infectious colitis, drug (particularly nonsteroidal anti-inflammatory drug [NSAID]) toxicity, and partially treated ulcerative colitis. Consequently, it is prudent to avoid labeling the patient with Crohn disease at the first biopsy, but rather to give a descriptive diagnosis (such as focal colitis) and to provide a differential diagnosis. Appropriate clinical follow-up and subsequent biopsies will usually resolve the diagnostic dilemma.

2. **Ulcerative colitis** classically involves the entire colon and has a tendency to be more severe distally. In some cases, the disease involves only the rectum (ulcerative proctitis), or presents as left-sided colitis with discontinuous patchy involvement of the cecum (cecal patch), ascending colon, and/or appendix. Grossly, the affected colon often has a thin and flaccid wall that becomes flattened upon opening. The mucosa looses its normal folds and becomes granular, friable, erythematous, and ulcerated (e-Fig. 14.24). Microscopically, the disease is characterized by its diffuseness in terms of crypt architectural distortion and inflammatory infiltration. In contrast to Crohn's colitis, crypt architectural distortion in ulcerative colitis is typically more dramatic, and inflammation is usually limited to the mucosa. Only in severely active disease with broad-based ulcers do inflammatory infiltrates extend into the submucosa and the muscularis propria in the ulcerated areas. It should be mentioned that patchy disease may be seen in pediatric patients with ulcerative colitis at initial presentation, and in biopsies from the advancing edge of the disease with gradual transition to normal mucosa. Treated ulcerative colitis may also show patchy disease, rectal sparing, or completely normal mucosa. These conditions should not be interpreted as evidence of Crohn disease.

Backwash ileitis is typically seen in severe pancolitis and is presumed to be caused by reflux of colonic contents. It features a mild degree of active inflammation in the distal few centimeters of the terminal ileum with relative preservation of the normal villous architecture. It differs from Crohn's ileitis, which usually involves a longer segment of the ileum with more severe inflammation and villous architectural distortion (e-Fig. 14.25). Table 14.7 summarizes the gross and histologic features that help distinguish ulcerative colitis from Crohn disease.

3. **Indeterminate colitis** is not a distinct entity, and the diagnosis should be applied only to those cases that are truly difficult to classify. Most cases will eventually evolve into ulcerative colitis or Crohn disease. The diagnosis is usually rendered because of insufficient clinical, radiologic, or endoscopic data, and because of prominent overlapping pathologic features. Fulminant colitis that lacks specific diagnostic features may also belong in this category. However, efforts should always be made to provide a more definitive diagnosis in atypical cases. For example, if severe ileal disease or well-formed granulomas are present, diffuse pancolitis without transmural inflammation should be diagnosed as Crohn disease rather than indeterminate colitis.

4. **Dysplasia** occurring in IBD is associated with the extent and duration of the disease and is a precursor of adenocarcinoma. Similar to that for Barrett's esophagus (Chap. 12), dysplasia in IBD is graded as indefinite, low grade, or high grade based on architectural complexity of the crypts and cytologic atypia. In general,

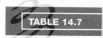

TABLE 14.7	Gross and Histologic Features Distinguishing Ulcerative Colitis from Crohn Disease	
Feature	**Ulcerative colitis**	**Crohn disease**
Distribution	Diffuse, continuous	Focal (skip), segmental
Depth of involvement	Mucosa, submucosa	Transmural
Mucosal appearance	Irregular ulcers, friable, atrophy	Cobblestoning
Bowel wall	Thin	Thickened or normal
Creeping fat	Absent	Common
Stricture	Usually absent	Maybe
Fistula	Usually absent	Maybe
Fissuring	Usually absent	Common
Ileal involvement	<10% (backwash)	Common
Upper GI involvement	Usually no	Maybe
Rectal involvement	100%	~15%
Anal involvement	5–10%	~75%
Well-formed granuloma	Absent	Common
Transmural lymphoid aggregates	Absent	Common

GI, gastrointestinal.

low-grade dysplasia simulates tubular adenoma, while high grade dysplasia is identical to adenocarcinoma in situ or intraepithelial carcinoma. However, it is always challenging to separate inflammatory or reactive atypia from dysplasia, and currently there are no reliable immunomarkers to assist in the distinction. Consulting with an experienced pathologist(s) in difficult cases is still the best solution.

IBD-associated dysplasia can be flat or polypoid. Distinguishing polypoid dysplasia, or a dysplasia-associated lesion or mass (DALM), from a sporadic adenoma is extremely difficult but appears unnecessary in practice because a DALM can also be adequately treated by simple polypectomy and continued surveillance, similar to a sporadic adenoma. Table 14.8 summarizes some of the potential differentiating features that may be used for cases in which a distinction is critically important in the decision-making of colectomy.

5. **Pouchitis** refers to inflammation of the ileal pouch created after total colectomy usually for ulcerative colitis. Active pouchitis features mixed neutrophilic and

TABLE 14.8	Features Distinguishing DALM from Sporadic Adenoma	
Feature	**Probable DALM**	**Probable adenoma**
Patient age	Younger	Older
Disease duration	Longer, usually >10 years	Shorter, usually <10 years
Background	Diseased area, usually with active inflammation	Usually nondiseased area
Association with flat dysplasia	Maybe	No
Involvement of stalk by dysplasia	Maybe	No
Involvement of surrounding mucosa by dysplasia	Maybe	No
Mixture of dysplastic and normal crypts on surface	Maybe	Usually no

DALM, dysplasia-associated lesion or mass.

TABLE 14.9	Comparison Between Lymphocytic Colitis and Collagenous Colitis	
	Lymphocytic	**Collagenous**
Female to male ratio	2:1	8:1
Symptom	Watery diarrhea	Watery diarrhea
Endoscopic finding	Normal	Normal
Involvement of the colon	Diffuse	Patchy or diffuse
Intraepithelial lymphocytosis	Diffuse and heavy	Patchy or diffuse, light
Subepithelial collagen	Absent	Patchy or diffuse
Epithelial injury	Mild, flattening	Prominent, sloughing
Crypt architecture	Normal	Normal
Lamina propria inflammatory cells	Increased	Increased

lymphoplasmacytic infiltrates in the ileal mucosa, and erosions or ulcerations in more severe cases. Chronic changes, such as villous architectural distortion, villous atrophy, and pyloric metaplasia, may be seen in long-term disease. An important differential diagnosis is recurrent Crohn disease in a case previously diagnosed as ulcerative colitis. Re-evaluation of a previous colectomy specimen may be necessary if granulomas, a fistula, a sinus tract, or a fissuring ulcer is detected in a pouch.

D. **Diversion colitis** refers to an inflammatory response in the blind segment, usually the rectum (Hartmann pouch) following ileostomy or colostomy. It is believed to be caused primarily by the deficiency of short-chain fatty acids because the rectum is excluded from the fecal stream. Although diversion colitis may exhibit variable histologic features, the classic finding is marked lymphoid hyperplasia in the mucosa, typically with well-formed germinal centers (e-**Fig. 14.26**).

E. **Microscopic colitis** includes mainly lymphocytic colitis and collagenous colitis, which share many clinicopathologic features (Table 14.9). The key feature of lymphocytic colitis is diffuse intraepithelial lymphocytosis defined by the presence of >20 lymphocytes within 100 epithelial cells (e-**Fig. 14.27**), although a formal count is unnecessary in typical cases. A focal increase in the number of IELs may be seen in IBD, infectious colitis, gluten-sensitive enteropathy, graft-versus-host disease (GVHD), and human immunodeficiency virus (HIV) infection and in areas with lymphoid aggregates.

The key feature of collagenous colitis is a thickened collagen layer at the subepithelial region, which can be patchy in distribution (e-**Fig. 14.28**). The thickness is highly variable but should be >10 μm. Small capillaries and scattered inflammatory cells are typically entrapped within the collagen layer. In fact, the entrapped lymphocytes can be used as an estimation of the thickness of the collagen band because small lymphocytes measure 7 to 10 μm in diameter. A pitfall is overinterpretation of the basement membrane as collagen deposition in tangentially sectioned biopsies. Evaluation should thus be performed at well-oriented regions. In difficult cases, a trichrome stain may be helpful. Another pitfall is mucosal fibrosis that involves the full thickness of the mucosa, which may be seen in ischemic colitis, a healed ulcer, and radiation colitis.

By definition, a large number of neutrophils should not be present in microscopic colitis. However, neutrophilic cryptitis or crypt abscesses may be seen in ~30% of patients. These patients may also have abnormal endoscopic findings including mucosal erythema or friability, or even ulceration. Occasionally, lymphocytosis or subepithelial collagen deposition extends into the terminal ileum, causing an abnormal appearance on endoscopy.

F. **Diverticular disease (diverticulosis)** refers to acquired outpouchings of the mucosa and submucosa through defects in weakened muscularis propria. Although it occurs throughout the colon, it is more commonly seen in the sigmoid colon. Approximately 10% of cases may become inflamed (diverticulitis), leading to abscess formation, perforation, and fistula formation. On biopsy, diverticulitis, particularly diverticular disease–associated segmental sigmoiditis, may be difficult to distinguish from IBD because of the presence of crypt architectural distortion in addition to active inflammation.

G. **Radiation colitis** is common in patients receiving radiation therapy for prostatic or cervical cancers. Biopsies are seldom taken of acute radiation injury, and may show increased apoptotic activity, nuclear atypia, mucin depletion, and decreased mitotic activity. Chronic radiation colitis is characterized by telangiectasia of the mucosal capillaries, lamina propria hyalinization, and atypical fibroblasts. Inflammatory cells are typically sparse (e-**Fig. 14.29**).

H. **Infectious colitis** is caused by a wide range of microorganisms including bacteria, viruses, parasites, and protozoa. Bacterial infection, such as that by *Campylobacter, Shigella,* and *Salmonella*, results in acute self-limited colitis characterized by neutrophilic infiltration in the lamina propria and epithelium with cryptitis and crypt abscesses. The inflammation tends to involve the upper portion of the mucosa more significantly, usually accompanied by damage of the surface lining epithelium with erosion and flattening. The normal crypt architecture is well-preserved in infectious colitis.

Pseudomembranous colitis is a potentially fatal mucosal reaction to toxins produced by *Clostridium difficile*. Most cases are associated with prior antibiotic exposure, which decreases normal bacterial flora. It is characterized by adherent yellow-white plaques consisting of necroinflammatory debris including neutrophils, fibrin, and mucin. The underlying crypts are ruptured, giving rise to the classic appearance of "volcano" lesions (e-**Fig. 14.30**). It should be stressed that pseudomembranous colitis is a morphologic diagnosis and can be seen in other conditions such as ischemic colitis. In contrast, ischemic colitis can also be attributed to an infectious etiology, such as *Escherichia coli* O157:H7.

Intestinal spirochetosis is not uncommon in HIV-infected patients, but can be an incidental finding in immunocompetent individuals. It may also be incidentally detected in appendectomy specimens. It is characterized by a fuzzy, purplish or bluish band of organisms carpeting the mucosal surface (e-**Fig. 14.31**). The organisms are more easily recognizable on silver stains, such as Warthin–Starry. There is no associated inflammatory response or epithelial damage.

I. **Drug-induced colitis** presents with a wide spectrum of histologic findings ranging from nonspecific colitis to ulceration (*Nat Clin Pract Gastroenterol Hepatol.* 2007;4:442). Interestingly, drug reactions have been well-documented to cause histologic changes similar to those of microscopic colitis, especially collagenous colitis. In fact, a large number of patients diagnosed as having microscopic colitis have a history of NSAID use, and neutrophilic infiltration tends to be more frequently seen in these cases.

J. **Irritable bowel syndrome (IBS)** is a common cause of abdominal pain and chronic diarrhea. Colonic biopsies from these patients are entirely normal on H&E stain. The current thinking is that IBS is a functional disorder related to food hypersensitivity, psychologic factors, or infection. In recent years, the pathogenesis has been linked to mast cell activation (*Scand J Gastroenterol.* 2005;40:129); supporting data for this association include increased number of mast cells in the colonic mucosa with increased mediator release and enhanced innervation. In the absence of systemic mastocytosis, increased mast cells in the lamina propria is defined by some authors as >20 mast cells per high-power field. Mast cells are difficult to recognize in H&E-stained sections, but can be easily identified by toluidine blue stain and tryptase or c-kit immunostain (e-**Fig. 14.32**).

K. **GVHD** commonly involves the intestine, and the histologic hallmarks are apoptosis and crypt damage (e-**Fig. 14.33**). The severity of acute colonic GVHD is graded as outlined in Table 14.10. Cytomegalovirus infection should always be evaluated by immunohistochemical staining in biopsies exhibiting histologic features of acute GVHD.

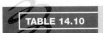

TABLE 14.10	Histologic Grading of Acute Colonic GVHD

Grade	Histologic features
1	Increased apoptotic activity
2	Increased apoptotic activity with crypt abscess
3	Necrosis of individual crypts
4	Total denudation of areas of mucosa

GVHD, graft-versus-host disease.

VI. DIAGNOSTIC FEATURES OF POLYPS AND NEOPLASMS OF THE LARGE INTESTINE (TABLE 14.11)

A. **Hyperplastic polyps** are typically small (usually <5 mm) and feature a serrated or sawtooth luminal configuration (e-**Fig. 14.34**). The serration is most prominent at the upper portion of the crypts, whereas the lower portion remains narrow and proliferative. Thus, there is a progressive maturation when the epithelial cells move up to the surface. There is no cytologic atypia, but occasional multinucleated cells may be noted. A thickened basement membrane may also be seen, which should not be confused with collagenous colitis.

Hyperplastic polyps are traditionally thought to be innocuous. However, recent studies have suggested that a subset of the polyps may possess a higher risk of malignant transformation, to which a number of new names have been assigned including sessile serrated polyp and sessile serrated adenoma. The distinction between a sessile serrated polyp and a hyperplastic polyp appears to rely primarily on the shape of the crypts, particularly at the base. In a sessile serrated polyp, the base is also serrated, dilated, flask-shaped, L-shaped, or branched (e-**Fig. 14.35**), but lacks the dysplastic features of a traditional adenoma. It is thus the architecture of the polyp that makes the distinction, although it should be pointed out that this is a highly controversial issue and the clinical significance of the distinction is really unknown.

Hyperplastic polyposis should be viewed as a precancerous syndrome, which is defined as at least 5 polyps proximal to the sigmoid colon, 2 of which are >1 cm; any number of polyps proximal to the sigmoid colon, with a first-degree relative having hyperplastic polyposis; or >30 polyps of any size throughout the colon. Thus, high-risk hyperplastic polyps are judged primarily by their large size, proximal location, multiplicity, and family history, which do not need detailed histologic analysis by pathologists.

B. **An adenomatous polyp** is traditionally categorized as tubular adenoma if the villous component accounts for <25% of the lesion, villous adenoma if >75%, and tubulovillous adenoma if between 25% and 75% (e-**Fig. 14.36**). By definition, adenomas display at least low-grade dysplasia, characterized by nuclear stratification, enlargement, elongation and hyperchromasia, and mucin depletion.

C. **Serrated adenoma** is a true adenomatous polyp, which is different from sessile serrated adenoma. Although serrated adenoma looks like a hyperplastic polyp with serration of the crypts, it also displays low-grade dysplasia with lack of surface maturation as is typical of traditional adenomas (e-**Fig. 14.37**). Cytoplasmic eosinophilia is characteristic of this lesion.

D. **Mixed hyperplastic and adenomatous polyp** contains discrete foci of hyperplastic and adenomatous components in a single polyp, often side by side.

E. **Familial adenomatous polyposis (FAP)** is an autosomal dominant disorder caused by germline mutations of the *APC* gene located at chromosome 5q21. A minimum of 100 colonic adenomas is required for the diagnosis, but an attenuated form with a reduced number is not uncommon. Adenomas of the upper GI tract, particularly in the ampullary region, and fundic gland polyps, are also common findings in FAP

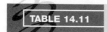

TABLE 14.11	WHO Histologic Classification of Tumors of the Colon and Rectum

---

Epithelial tumors
Adenoma
  Tubular
  Villous
  Tubulovillous
  Serrated
Intraepithelial neoplasia (dysplasia) associated with chronic inflammatory diseases
  Low-grade glandular intraepithelial neoplasia
  High-grade glandular intraepithelial neoplasia
Carcinoma
  Adenocarcinoma
  Mucinous carcinoma
  Signet-ring cell carcinoma
  Small cell carcinoma
  Squamous cell carcinoma
  Adenosquamous carcinoma
  Medullary carcinoma
  Undifferentiated carcinoma
Carcinoid (well-differentiated endocrine neoplasm)
  EC cell, serotonin-producing neoplasm
  L cell, glucagonlike peptide and PP/PYY-producing tumor
  Others
Mixed carcinoid–adenocarcinoma
  Others

Nonepithelial tumors
Lipoma
Leiomyoma
Gastrointestinal stromal tumor
Leiomyosarcoma
Angiosarcoma
Kaposi sarcoma
Malignant melanoma
  Others
Malignant lymphoma
  Marginal zone B-cell lymphoma of MALT type
  Mantle cell lymphoma
  Diffuse large B-cell lymphoma
  Burkitt lymphoma
  Burkittlike/atypical Burkitt lymphoma
  Others

Secondary tumors

Polyps
Hyperplastic polyp (metaplastic)
Peutz–Jeghers
Juvenile

WHO, World Health Organization; EC, enterochromaffin cell; L,; PP, pancreatic polypeptide; PYY, polypeptide YY; MALT, mucosa-associated lymphoid tissue.
From: Hamilton SR, Aaltonen LA, eds. *World Health Organization Classification of Tumours. Pathology and Genetics. Tumours of the Digestive System*. Lyon: IARC Press; 2000. Used with permission.

patients. Progression to colonic adenocarcinoma approaches 100% by midlife if prophylactic colectomy is not performed (e-**Fig. 14.38**).

Gardner and Turcot syndromes are considered variants of FAP. In addition to adenomas of the GI tract, extra-GI tumors are seen in these patients. These include osteoid osteoma, epidermal cyst, and intra-abdominal fibromatosis (desmoid tumor) for the former; and tumors of the central nervous system for the latter.

F. **Hereditary nonpolyposis colorectal cancer syndrome (HNPCC),** previously known as Lynch syndrome, is caused by mutations in at least one of the DNA mismatch repair enzymes, including hMLH1, hMSH2, hMSH6, and hPMS2, leading to microsatellite instability (MSI). This is also an autosomal dominant disorder with increased risk of colorectal cancer and extraintestinal malignancies such as endometrial carcinomas. MSI can be evaluated by immunohistochemical stains for DNA mismatch repair enzymes and DNA-based molecular analyses.

G. **Hamartomatous polyps** can occur sporadically or as part of syndromes such as juvenile polyposis, Peutz–Jeghers syndrome, Cowden syndrome, and Cronkhite–Canada syndrome. All these syndromes have an autosomal dominant inheritance except for Cronkhite–Canada, which is a nonhereditary disorder.

Juvenile polyps feature cystically dilated and tortuous crypts with edematous and inflamed lamina propria (e-**Fig. 14.39**). Dilated crypts often contain neutrophils and/or mucin, hence the name "retention polyp." The surface of the polyp may be eroded or ulcerated, with granulation tissue and epithelial regenerative changes. It should be pointed out that juvenile polyps can be seen in adults or even in elderly persons. The polyps in patients with Cowden and Cronkhite–Canada syndromes closely resemble juvenile polyps morphologically.

H. **High-grade dysplasia** is commonly seen in adenomatous polyps and occasionally in juvenile polyps. It is characterized by a cribriform or back-to-back growth pattern, rounded nuclei, coarse chromatin, prominent nucleoli, and loss of nuclear polarity (e-**Fig. 14.40**). High-grade dysplasia is usually focal and situated at the surface of the polyp, and thus requires no additional treatment beyond polypectomy if the polyp is completely removed. It should be noted that high-grade dysplasia in the colon is synonymous with carcinoma in situ or intraepithelial carcinoma. Intramucosal adenocarcinoma, defined by lamina propria invasion including invasion into (but not through) the muscularis mucosae, still belongs to the category of high-grade dysplasia because of its negligible potential of metastasis. Only those tumors that have frankly invaded into the submucosa are considered invasive carcinoma. If invasive carcinoma is detected in a polypectomy specimen, however, the distance of the invasive focus to polypectomy margin (e-**Fig. 14.41**), histologic grade, and the presence or absence of lymphovascular invasion should be reported. These data are important in determining whether segmental resection should be performed. A diagnostic pitfall is pseudoinvasion in which adenomatous elements are entrapped or herniated into the submucosa, usually secondary to traumatization (e-**Fig. 14.42**). Features that help to distinguish pseudoinvasion from true invasion include lack of overt malignant histology, presence of lamina propria inflammatory cells around entrapped elements, lack of a desmoplastic response, lack of direct contact with submucosal muscular vessels, and presence of hemosiderin or hemorrhage.

I. **Adenocarcinoma** is graded as well, moderately, or poorly differentiated based on glandular formation, and the majority of colorectal adenocarcinomas are moderately differentiated. The tumor size is primarily used for documentation and is not a prognostic factor by itself. As aforementioned, carcinoma of the large intestine is staged differently from those of the other parts of the GI tract because intramucosal carcinoma is still considered as high-grade dysplasia or carcinoma in situ (Table 14.12).

The radial resection margin may be the single most critical factor in predicting local recurrence, particularly for rectal carcinoma. It is the nonperitonealized surface including the perirectal soft tissue (adventitia) and the mesenteric pedicle. The radial margin should be inked before lymph node dissection is performed. A common mistake is to consider serosal surface as radial margin; a T3 tumor can have an involved radial margin (incomplete resection), and a T4 tumor (positive serosal surface) can have an uninvolved radial margin (complete resection).

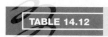

| TABLE 14.12 | Tumor, Node, Metastasis (TNM) Staging Scheme for Carcinoma of the Colon and Rectum |

Primary tumor (T)

TX	Primary tumor cannot be assessed
T0	No evidence of primary tumor
Tis	Carcinoma in situ: intraepithelial or invasion of lamina propria*
T1	Tumor invades submucosa
T2	Tumor invades muscularis propria
T3	Tumor invades through the muscularis propria into the subserosa or into nonperitonealized pericolic or perirectal tissues
T4	Tumor directly invades other organs or structures, and/or perforates visceral peritoneum**, ***

Regional lymph nodes (N)

NX	Regional lymph nodes cannot be assessed
N0	No regional lymph node metastasis
N1	Metastasis in 1 to 3 regional lymph nodes
N2	Metastasis in 4 or more regional lymph nodes

Distant metastasis (M)

MX	Distant metastasis cannot be assessed
M0	No distant metastasis
M1	Distant metastasis

Stage grouping

Stage 0	Tis	N0	M0
Stage I	T1	N0	M0
	T2	N0	M0
Stage IIA	T3	N0	M0
Stage IIB	T4	N0	M0
Stage IIIA	T1-T2	N1	M0
Stage IIIB	T3-T4	N1	M0
Stage IIIC	Any T	N2	M0
Stage IV	Any T	Any N	M1

AJCC, American Joint Committee on Cancer; TNM, Tumor, Node, Metastasis.
* Tis includes cancer cells confined within the glandular basement membrane (intraepithelial) or lamina propria (intramucosal) with no extension through the muscularis mucosae into the submucosa.
** Direct invasion in T4 includes invasion of other segments of the colorectum by way of the serosa; for example, invasion of the sigmoid colon by a carcinoma of the cecum.
*** Tumor that is adherent to other organs or structures, macroscopically, is classified T4. However, if no tumor is present in the adhesion, microscopically, the classification should be pT3.
From: Greene FL, Page DL, Fleming ID, Fritz AG, Balch CM, Haller DG, Morrow M, eds. *AJCC Cancer Staging Manual*. 6th edition. New York: Springer; 2002. Used with permission. (A new AJCC TNM staging system is scheduled for release in 2009; after its publication, the new staging scheme will appear on the website for this book.)

If a discrete tumor nodule is detected in the extramural adipose tissue that is discontinuous from the primary mass, it should be considered as a positive lymph node if the nodule has a smooth and round contour even without residual lymphoid tissue. If the nodule has an irregular contour, it is classified in the T category as T3 but should also be recoded as microscopic (V1) or macroscopic (V2) venous invasion. However, clear-cut microscopic lymphatic or vascular invasion discontinuous from the primary tumor should not be used as the farthest point of local invasion. In addition, the pure presence of acellular mucin in the bowel wall or regional lymph nodes should not be used to determine the extent of primary tumor or viewed as evidence of nodal metastasis. It has been recommended that if there is doubt concerning the correct staging, the less advanced category should be assigned (*CA Cancer J Clin* 54:295, 2004).

The majority of sporadic colorectal adenocarcinomas involve somatic mutations of the *APC* gene in tumorigenesis, and ~15% involve the MSI pathway. MSI tumors tend to be right-sided, mucinous, or poorly differentiated. Similar to those in the other parts of the GI tract, mucinous carcinoma and signet-ring cell carcinoma of the colon are defined by >50% of the tumor bulk consisting of a mucinous component or signet-ring cells. In poorly differentiated mucinous carcinoma, signet-ring cells can be numerous (e-**Fig. 14.43**).

Medullary carcinoma consists of sheets of poorly differentiated or undifferentiated tumor cells with a syncytial growth pattern and a pushing boarder. Characteristically, there is a marked inter- and intratumorous lymphocytic infiltrate. Crohnlike lymphoid aggregates may be present at the periphery in some cases. This variant of colorectal adenocarcinoma is frequently associated with DNA mismatch repair deficiency and is believed to bear a favorable prognosis despite its high-grade appearance.

Immunohistochemically, ~90% of colorectal adenocarcinomas exhibit a CK20-positive/CK7-negative staining pattern. Only ~10% of the tumors are CK20-negative/CK7-positive or CK20-negative/CK7-negative. Nearly 100% of the tumors express nuclear CDX2 and apical/luminal/cytoplasmic villin.

J. Carcinoid tumor and neuroendocrine carcinoma are rare in the colon, but focal neuroendocrine differentiation in conventional adenocarcinomas is not uncommon and may be associated with a poor prognosis. Neuroendocrine carcinoma of the colon is most commonly seen in the cecum and rectum, and is frequently associated with overlying adenomatous epithelium. Histologically, it is indistinguishable from small cell carcinoma or large cell neuroendocrine carcinoma elsewhere; immunomarkers such as CK20, CK7, and thyroid transcription factor-1 (TTF-1) do not help in the distinction from a metastasis.

K. GIST of the colon accounts for ~5% of all GISTs and is most commonly seen in the rectum. Its biological behavior is not well studied.

L. Leiomyoma is the most common mesenchymal tumor of the colon. It arises from the muscularis mucosae and presents as a well-demarcated nodular expansion in the submucosa. It is typically hypocellular, lacks cytologic atypia, and lacks c-kit expression.

M. Submucosal lipoma can be associated with hyperplastic change in the overlying colonic mucosa.

N. Inflammatory polyp is a heterogeneous group of polypoid lesions and includes the pseudopolyps seen in IBD. Inflammatory polyp features inflamed lamina propria and damaged or distorted crypts. Granulation tissue may be present. It may be indistinguishable from a juvenile polyp if cystic dilation of the crypts is prominent, and the distinction relies on clinical information. Occasionally, pseudosarcomatous stroma is noted, particularly in eroded or ulcerated areas, characterized by bizarre or multinucleated stroma cells simulating sarcoma (e-**Fig. 14.44**).

O. Mucosal prolapse occurs most commonly in the rectum but can be seen anywhere in the colon. The alternative name for this entity, solitary rectal ulcer, is apparently a misnomer. The characteristic histologic features include a fibromuscular lamina propria with vertical extension of the muscularis mucosae into the spaces between crypts, and elongated, hyperplastic, and distorted crypts (e-**Fig. 14.45**). It should be noted that lamina propria smooth muscle proliferation can be seen in any polypoid lesion, so the diagnosis of mucosal prolapse should not rely solely on this finding. It should also be pointed out that muscle fibers are normally present in the duodenal mucosa, which should not be viewed as evidence of mucosal prolapse in that location.

P. Colitis cystica profunda is a benign condition in which cystically dilated crypts are misplaced in the submucosa and/or deeper layers of the bowel wall (e-**Fig. 14.46**). The distinction from well-differentiated adenocarcinoma lies in the lobular arrangement of the displaced crypts, lack of dysplastic features, lack of desmoplasia, presence of surrounding lamina propria components, and presence of hemorrhage or hemosiderin. If the lesion is polypoid, colitis cystica polyposa appears to be a more appropriate diagnostic term.

Q. Mucosal ganglioneuroma resembles neurofibroma and features a bland Schwann cell proliferation with nerve fibers that expands the lamina propria, but individual or nests of ganglion cells are embedded in the spindle cell background (e-**Fig. 14.47**). Multiple (ganglioneuromatous polyposis) and diffuse (ganglioneuromatosis) lesions are usually seen in patients with multiple endocrine neoplasia (MEN) 2B or type 1 neurofibromatosis (NF1).

R. Fibroblastic polyps feature a bland spindle cell proliferation that expands the lamina propria. They are typically small mucosal lesions and only positive for vimentin immunohistochemically.

S. Mucosal folds and prominent lymphoid follicles can resemble polyps endoscopically. On biopsy, a mucosal fold consists of completely normal colonic mucosa.

VII. DIAGNOSTIC FEATURES OF COMMON NONNEOPLASTIC AND NEOPLASTIC CONDITIONS OF THE APPENDIX

A. Acute appendicitis usually occurs as the result of luminal occlusion (such as by a fecalith, lymphoid hyperplasia, or *Enterobius vermicularis*), followed by bacterial infection. Diverticulosis of the appendix is also a rare cause. Microscopically, acute appendicitis is characterized by diffuse neutrophilic infiltration of the appendiceal wall including the muscularis propria (e-**Fig. 14.48**). Abscess formation, gangrenous necrosis, and perforation may ensue. When inflammation extends into the mesoappendix and the serosa, periappendicitis is diagnosed. It should be cautioned, however, that in the absence of luminal inflammation, the pure presence of periappendicitis may signify another intra-abdominal or intrapelvic process, such as pelvic inflammatory disease.

B. Cystic fibrosis involving the appendix is characterized by thick, eosinophilic, and inspissated mucoid material in the lumen and in the crypts (e-**Fig. 14.49**).

C. Hyperplastic polyp of the appendix is histologically similar to that of the colorectum, but tends to be sessile. Hyperplasia can also diffusely involve the appendiceal mucosa (mucosal hyperplasia).

D. Adenoma of the appendix is also similar to that of the colorectum (Table 14.13). However, adenomas of the appendix may cause mucin retention with resultant cystic dilation of the appendix and flattening of the adenomatous mucosa. In that case, mucinous cystadenoma is a better diagnostic term and should be separated from mucocele that is lined by attenuated nonneoplastic appendiceal mucosa.

E. Adenocarcinoma of the appendix is classified, graded, and staged using the criteria for colorectal adenocarcinoma (Tables 14.12 and 14.13). It can be difficult to distinguish from mucinous cystadenoma when the adenocarcinoma is mucinous and/or well differentiated. A diagnosis of mucinous tumor of uncertain malignant potential has been suggested for cases in which histologic evidence of invasive growth is difficult to assess (*Adv Anat Pathol.* 2005;12:291).

F. Pseudomyxoma peritonei is primarily a clinical diagnosis, and its prognosis depends on the underlying lesion. Although appendiceal lesions are responsible for the majority of the cases, mucinous tumors of other sites can also be the cause.

  1. Disseminated peritoneal mucinosis (DPM) is defined by the presence of abundant acellular mucin on the peritoneal surfaces without a cellular component. This is likely caused by rupture of a mucocele or benign mucinous cystadenoma.

  2. Disseminated peritoneal adenomucinosis (DPAM) denotes the presence of adenomatous epithelium in the background of mucinous ascites. This is often caused by a mucinous cystadenoma, borderline mucinous tumor, or well-differentiated adenocarcinoma. A new term, mucinous carcinoma peritonei-low grade, has been proposed for this group of lesions (*Am J Surg Pathol.* 2006;30:551).

  3. Disseminated peritoneal carcinomatosis features the presence of frankly malignant epithelium similar to moderately and poorly differentiated adenocarcinomas. An alternative name for this category is mucinous carcinoma peritonei-high grade (*Am J Surg Pathol.* 2006;30:551).

G. Neuroendocrine tumors are the most common tumors of the appendix, and include a heterogeneous group of lesions with variable biologic behavior (Table 14.13).

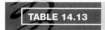

TABLE 14.13	WHO Histologic Classification of Tumors of the Appendix

Epithelial tumors
  Adenoma
  Tubular
  Villous
  Tubulovillous
  Serrated
Carcinoma
  Adenocarcinoma
  Mucinous adenocarcinoma
  Signet-ring cell carcinoma
  Small cell carcinoma
  Undifferentiated carcinoma
Carcinoid (well-differentiated endocrine neoplasm)
  EC cell, serotonin-producing neoplasm
  L cell, glucagonlike peptide and PP/PYY-producing tumor
  Others
Tubular carcinoid
Goblet cell carcinoid (mucinous carcinoid)
Mixed carcinoid–adenocarcinoma
Others

Nonepithelial tumors
Neuroma
Lipoma
Leiomyoma
Gastrointestinal stromal tumor
Leiomyosarcoma
Kaposi sarcoma
Others
Malignant lymphoma

Secondary tumors

Hyperplastic (metaplastic) polyp

WHO, World Health Organization; EC, enterochromaffin cell; L,; PP, pancreatic polypeptide; PYY, polypeptide YY; MALT, mucosa-associated lymphoid tissue.
From: Hamilton SR, Aaltonen LA, eds. *World Health Organization Classification of Tumours. Pathology and Genetics. Tumours of the Digestive System.* Lyon: IARC Press; 2000. Used with permission.

1. **Classic carcinoid tumors** are histologically identical to those seen in the other parts of the GI tract, and are typically found in the distal third of the appendix. However, they are distinguished from other GI carcinoids by their relatively benign behavior. Metastasis generally occurs in tumors >2 cm in size, and is almost never seen in those <1 cm.
2. **Goblet cell carcinoid** is a mixed endocrine–exocrine neoplasm, almost exclusively seen in the appendix. It is thought to represent a low-grade malignancy with a biologic behavior intermediate between classic carcinoid and adenocarcinoma. It has been synonymously called mucinous carcinoid, microglandular carcinoma, crypt cell carcinoma, and adenocarcinoid. It is currently recommended that the term adenocarcinoid be avoided because it historically also includes tubular carcinoid.
    Goblet cell carcinoid typically diffusely infiltrates the appendiceal wall, with relative sparing of the mucosa. The hallmark of the tumor is the presence of small, tight clusters or individual glands formed by tumor cells exhibiting a goblet or signet-ring morphology with a small compressed nucleus and conspicuous

intracytoplasmic mucin (e-**Fig. 14.50**). Small extracellular mucin pools may be seen. The presence of Paneth cells is also a useful diagnostic feature. Lack of significant cytologic atypia, lack of frank glandular formation, lack of necrosis and tissue destruction, and lack of a adenomatous or in situ carcinomatous component are features used to distinguish the neoplasm from mucinous or signet-ring cell carcinoma. The distinction should not depend on immunohistochemical stains for neuroendocrine markers because the immunoreactivity in goblet cell carcinoid varies widely from patchy to diffuse, and from weak to strong.

3. **Tubular carcinoid** is another mixed endocrine–exocrine neoplasm unique to the appendix. In contrast to goblet cell carcinoid, tubular carcinoid is a completely benign lesion with no potential to metastasize. It is typically a small lesion incidentally found at the tip of appendix, characterized by discrete tubules and/or short atubular nests within abundant stroma (e-**Fig. 14.51**). The orderly pattern, lack of cytologic atypia, and absence of mitotic activity should help in the distinction from metastatic adenocarcinoma.

4. **Mixed carcinoid–adenocarcinoma** consists of both carcinoid (usually goblet cell carcinoid) and conventional adenocarcinoma.

VIII. **DIAGNOSTIC FEATURES OF COMMON NONNEOPLASTIC AND NEOPLASTIC CONDITIONS OF THE ANUS**

A. **Hemorrhoids** are characterized by dilated thick-walled submucosal blood vessels, often with thrombi.

B. **Anal tag** is a fibroepithelial polyp, histologically identical to a skin tag (acrochordon).

C. **Inflammatory cloacogenic polyp** is a type of mucosal prolapse featuring fibromuscular proliferation of the lamina propria and villous hyperplasia of the mucosa that often contains mixed rectal and squamous epithelia (e-**Fig. 14.52**). The lesion may resemble a villous or tubulovillous adenoma at low-power view.

D. **Hidradenoma papilliferum** is a benign sweat gland tumor that can occur at the anal region. It histologically resembles intraductal papilloma of the breast.

E. **Condyloma acuminatum,** also known as genital warts, is caused by low-risk types of HPV. It features a papillomatous proliferation of the squamous epithelium with

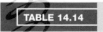

TABLE 14.14	WHO Histologic Classification of Tumors of the Anal Canal

Epithelial tumors
Intraepithelial neoplasia (dysplasia)
   Squamous or transitional epithelium
   Glandular
   Paget disease
Carcinoma
   Squamous cell carcinoma
   Adenocarcinoma
   Mucinous adenocarcinoma
   Small cell carcinoma
   Undifferentiated carcinoma
   Others
Carcinoid tumor

Malignant melanoma

Nonepithelial tumors

Secondary tumors

WHO, World Health Organization.
From: Hamilton SR, Aaltonen LA, eds. *World Health Organization Classification of Tumours. Pathology and Genetics. Tumours of the Digestive System.* Lyon: IARC Press; 2000. Used with permission.

parakeratosis and viral cytopathic (koilocytic) changes (e-**Fig. 14.53**). High-grade dysplasia may occasionally arise from this low-grade lesion.

F. Anal intraepithelial neoplasia (AIN) refers to a spectrum of squamous dysplasia strongly associated with high-risk types of HPV. Similar to cervical intraepithelial neoplasia (CIN), AIN is graded as mild (AIN I), moderate (AIN II), or severe (AIN III). AIN III is equivalent to squamous cell carcinoma in situ (e-**Fig. 14.54**).

G. Squamous cell carcinoma accounts for ~80% of anal carcinomas (Table 14.14). The majority of the tumors are nonkeratinizing and may exhibit basaloid features, but the term cloacogenic carcinoma appears to be obsolete.

H. Anal duct carcinoma is a unique type of adenocarcinoma arising from the anal duct. This is a slow-growing, well-differentiated tumor with glandular formation, bland cytology, and mucin production. The neoplastic glands are usually deeply

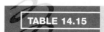

TABLE 14.15	Tumor, Node, Metastasis (TNM) Staging Scheme for Carcinoma of the Anal Canal

PRIMARY TUMOR (T)

TX	Primary tumor cannot be assessed
T0	No evidence of primary tumor
Tis	Carcinoma in situ
T1	Tumor ≤2 cm in greatest dimension
T2	Tumor >2 cm but not >5 cm in greatest dimension
T3	Tumor >5 cm in greatest dimension
T4	Tumor of any size invades adjacent organ(s), e.g. vagina, urethra, bladder*

REGIONAL LYMPH NODES (N)

NX	Regional lymph nodes cannot be assessed
N0	No regional lymph node metastasis
N1	Metastasis in perirectal lymph node(s)
N2	Metastasis in unilateral internal iliac and/or inguinal lymph node(s)
N3	Metastasis in perirectal and inguinal lymph nodes and/or bilateral iliac and/or inguinal lymph nodes

DISTANT METASTASIS (M)

MX	Distant metastasis cannot be assessed
M0	No distant metastasis
M1	Distant metastasis

STAGE GROUPING

Stage 0	Tis	N0	M0
Stage I	T1	N0	M0
Stage II	T2	N0	M0
	T3	N0	M0
Stage IIIA	T1	N1	M0
	T2	N1	M0
	T3	N1	M0
	T4	N0	M0
Stage IIIB	T4	N1	M0
	Any T	N2	M0
	Any T	N3	M0
Stage IV	Any T	Any N	M1

AJCC, American Joint Committee on Cancer; TNM, Tumor, Node, Metastasis.
* Direct invasion of the rectal wall, perirectal skin, subcutaneous tissue, or the sphincter muscle(s) is not classified as T4.
From: Greene FL, Page DL, Fleming ID, Fritz AG, Balch CM, Haller DG, Morrow M, eds. *AJCC Cancer Staging Manual*. 6th edition. New York: Springer; 2002. Used with permission. (A new AJCC TNM staging system is scheduled for release in 2009; after its publication, the new staging scheme will appear on the website for this book.)

situated without evidence of mucosal surface involvement (e-**Fig. 14.55**). It is important to separate true adenocarcinoma of the anal canal from adenocarcinoma of the lower rectum, because the former is T-staged based on the size of the tumor rather than the depth of invasion, and N-staged based on the location of involved lymph nodes rather than the number of involved nodes (Table 14.15).

I. **Paget disease** of the anus is histologically identical to that seen in the breast and vulva.

J. **Melanoma** of the anus is histologically identical to that seen in other parts of the body.

CYTOLOGY OF THE INTESTINES, APPENDIX, AND ANUS
Jing Zhai

I. **SMALL INTESTINE CYTOLOGY.** Usually, only the duodenum is sampled by endoscopic brushing or endoscopic ultrasound-guided fine needle aspiration for evaluation of inflammatory and neoplastic processes.

   A. **Infection.** *Giardia lamblia* trophozoites are pear-shaped with two mirror-shaped nuclei and flagella (*Am J Gastroenterol* 79:517, 1984). Atypical mycobacteria produce a negative image in the cytoplasm of foamy macrophages and in the background on Diff-Quik–stained smears (*Diagn Cytopathol.* 19:462, 1998). The cytomorphology of cryptosporidium (*Diagn Cytopathol* 6:193, 1990) and microsporidium (*N Engl J Med* 326:161, 1992) have also been described.

   B. **Adenoma.** The cells form two-dimensional small groups and papillary fragments. Individual cells exhibit elongated nuclei, nuclear stratification and palisading, and mild-to-moderate nuclear pleomorphism. There are no single cells or three-dimensional cell balls (*Cancer* 105:289, 2005).

   C. **Adenocarcinoma.** The sample is richly cellular, consisting of haphazardly arranged small clusters, three-dimensional cell balls, and isolated cells with enlarged nuclei, a high nuclear/cytoplasmic (N/C) ratio, and an irregular nuclear membrane (e-**Fig. 14.56**). Prominent nucleoli, unevenly distributed coarse chromatin, and necrosis are also seen (*Cancer* 105:289, 2005). The distinction between adenoma with high-grade dysplasia, intramucosal carcinoma, and invasive adenocarcinoma is difficult if not impossible cytologically.

II. **LARGE INTESTINE CYTOLOGY.** Endoscopic brushing of the colon is rarely used as an adjunct to endoscopic biopsy for IBD surveillance or diagnosis of neoplastic process (*Cancer* 66:1563, 1990). The distinction among reactive atypia, adenoma with high-grade dysplasia, intramucosal carcinoma, and invasive carcinoma is challenging by cytomorphology alone.

III. **ANAL CYTOLOGY.** Anal cytology has been used in those patients whose sexual history includes receptive anal intercourse to screen for HPV-related intraepithelial lesions. Bethesda System terminology for cervical/vaginal cytology, which is discussed in the cervical cytology section, has been adopted to report anal cytology (*The Bethesda System for Reporting Cervical Cytology.* New York: Springer-Verlag New York, Inc., pp 194, 2004).

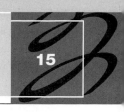

THE LIVER
Gustavo Alvarez and Hanlin L. Wang

15

I. NORMAL ANATOMY. The liver is the largest solid organ of the body and weighs from 1200 to 1600 grams in adults. It is topographically divided into right, left, caudate, and quadrate lobes, but functionally into right and left hemilivers of about equal size by an imaginary line running through the gallbladder fossa to the inferior vena cava. It is also divided into eight functional segments according to blood supply. The liver has a dual blood supply, with approximately two thirds from the portal vein (nonoxygenated) and one third from the hepatic artery (oxygenated). The venous return is via the left and right hepatic veins to the inferior vena cava.

Microscopically, the hepatic lobule is a hexagon composed of hepatocytes arranged in one-cell-thick plates with sinusoids on both sides, a centrally located terminal hepatic venule (central vein), and peripherally distributed portal tracts. A typical portal tract contains a branch of the hepatic artery, portal vein, and bile duct supported by a small amount of connective tissue (e-Fig. 15.1).* Larger portal tracts also contain lymphatics and autonomic nerve fibers. Inflammatory cells are typically lacking or minimal in number. The lobule is separated from the portal tract by a limiting plate, the first layer of hepatocytes directly adjoining the portal tract. The concept of a hepatic acinus is based on the oxygen gradient in the liver; according to this model, the portal tract lies at the center and the hepatic venules at the periphery, and the acinus is divided into three regions: zone 1 (periportal), zone 2 (mid-lobular), and zone 3 (centrilobular).

II. GROSS EXAMINATION AND SPECIMEN HANDLING

A. Needle core biopsy, performed either percutaneously or transjugularly, is undertaken to assess medical liver diseases that cause abnormal liver function tests, to establish the diagnosis of space-occupying lesions, and to evaluate the condition of allografts. The specimen should be promptly fixed in 10% buffered formalin. After the number and the length range of the cores are recorded, the specimen is wrapped in lens paper for submission; sponge pads are not recommended to protect needle cores from loss during processing because they tend to create histologic artifacts. Three hematoxylin and eosin (H&E)-, one trichrome-, and one reticulin-stained slides are routinely examined in many labs; some labs may also routinely perform a Prussian blue stain for iron, rhodanine stain for copper, periodic acid-Schiff (PAS) stain, and PAS stain with diastase digestion (PAS-D).

Frozen sections of needle biopsies are usually restricted to donor liver evaluation, clinical workup for acute fatty liver of pregnancy (where an oil red O stain may be needed), and intraoperative evaluation of liver lesions. When fresh tissue is submitted, it should never dry or be immersed in saline, but instead should be laid on a piece of saline-moisturized gauze in a closed container. If electron microscopic examination is expected for a potential metabolic disease, additional tissue should be fixed in 3% buffered glutaraldehyde. Most special analyses, such as iron or copper quantitation, can be performed on formalin-fixed tissue, and special handling of the biopsy is unnecessary.

B. Wedge biopsy or excision is commonly performed for small subcapsular lesions incidentally identified during an unrelated surgery, for which frozen section may be requested. Wedge biopsy is also performed for the diagnosis or treatment of small

---

*All e-figures are available online via the Solution Site Image Bank.

and superficial neoplasms (primary or metastatic). The specimen is measured and the surgical margin inked; any perforation or abutting of the liver capsule by an underlying lesion should be recorded. The wedge is then sectioned perpendicular to the capsule. If a lesion is grossly identified, its size, color, texture, relation to the capsule, and distance from the inked margin should be documented. If multiple lesions are present, their size range and their relation to the inked margin should also be described. If the specimen is small, it should be submitted in its entirety; otherwise, one section demonstrating the tumor in relation to the closest margin, one demonstrating the relationship to the capsule, and one additional section of the tumor will suffice.

Wedge biopsy is not recommended for the evaluation of diffuse liver parenchymal diseases because subcapsular regions may contain misleading fibrous septa extended from the capsule that may mimic cirrhosis or bridging fibrosis. The subcapsular regions also tend to show nonspecific necroinflammatory changes that may further confuse the histology.

C. Segmentectomy, lobectomy, or partial hepatectomy is commonly performed for large benign or malignant lesions that are not resectable by wedge excision. After the weight and size of the specimen and the appearance of the capsule are recorded, the resection margin is inked, and the specimen is sliced thinly at ~0.5-cm increments. The gross examination of the lesion(s) is similar to that for wedge specimens, and the nonlesional liver parenchyma should also be described, including color, texture, and nodularity. Three to four sections of the tumor, one section of nonneoplastic liver, and one section of inked resection margin (if not included in the previous sections) are submitted for histologic examination. If large vessels or bile ducts are present, their relation to the lesions and their margins should be sampled. Special stains, such as trichrome, reticulin, and iron stains, may be ordered on a nontumoral liver section either at the time of submission or after microscopic examination of the sections. If a tumor has been preoperatively embolized, the percentage of tumor necrosis should be assessed and reported.

D. Total hepatectomy (explant) is usually performed for end-stage liver disease, massive necrosis, or metabolic disorders followed by liver transplantation. The weight, size, and surface appearance of the liver should be recorded. The specimen is thoroughly sectioned at ~0.5-cm increments, and the appearance of the cut surface is described. Every slice should be carefully examined (especially in cirrhotic livers) to look for nodules that have a larger size or distinctive color or texture, and for those that bulge out upon sectioning. If detected, they should be described in terms of number, size, color, location in the liver, and relation with the capsule or hilum. Radiology reports may be consulted when processing the specimen to make sure that radiographically detected mass lesions are identified and sampled. In the absence of suspicious lesions, two random sections from the left lobe, two from the right lobe, one from the hilum, and one from the gallbladder (if present) are sufficient. If the underlying disease is primary sclerosing cholangitis (PSC), additional sections from the hilum (if not the entire hilar tissue) should be submitted to look for dysplasia in large ducts or early cholangiocarcinoma. Vascular and bile duct margins in the hilum should be sampled if suspicious nodules are present.

III. DIAGNOSTIC FEATURES OF COMMON NONNEOPLASTIC CONDITIONS. The liver has a limited repertoire of morphologic responses to various noxious stimuli. Although the patterns of injury can sometimes provide clues as to underlying etiology, there is frequent overlap between entities. The most common patterns of hepatic injury and response are listed in Table 15.1.

When liver specimens, particularly needle biopsies, are examined, it is important to understand the clinical question(s) to generate a meaningful report, so effective communication with clinicians is essential. Nonetheless, an initial blinded review of the slides is recommended to avoid bias or the overlooking of unexpected pathology; the histopathologic examination should undertake a systematic approach to include the evaluation of the overall hepatic architecture, portal structures, and lobules.

The adequacy of biopsy specimens depends on the disease. It is traditionally recommended that for accurate grading and staging of chronic hepatitis, an adequate needle

TABLE 15.1   Common Histologic Patterns of Hepatic Injury and Response

Apoptotic body (acidophil or Councilman body): Individual hepatocyte necrosis in which a dead hepatocyte is identifiable as a shrunken, intensely eosinophilic, round body with no or a pyknotic nucleus. It is usually not accompanied by inflammatory response. Rare apoptotic bodies may be observed in normal liver, and increased apoptotic activity is a nonspecific finding seen in a wide range of hepatic injury.

Ballooning (hydropic) degeneration: Reversible hepatocyte swelling and rounding with pale cytoplasm due to intracellular edema.

Cholestasis: Visible bile in the liver. The acute form is characterized by canalicular cholestasis with bile accumulation in dilated canaliculi between hepatocytes. Long-term canalicular cholestasis may cause pseudoglandular formation (cholestatic rosettes). In the chronic form, as seen in chronic biliary diseases, bile accumulates in periportal hepatocytes to cause pseudoxanthomatous change (cholate stasis); increased deposition of copper and copper-binding protein in the hepatocytes may occur. Cytoplasmic cholestasis may also cause feathery degeneration in individual hepatocytes within the lobules, characterized by pale, swollen, and feathery cytoplasm, secondary to the toxic effect of bile salts.

Ductular reaction (proliferation): An increase in the number of ductules or cholangioles, which are small tubular structures without an apparent lumen typically found at the periphery of portal tracts or fibrous septa. It is virtually always associated with inflammatory cell infiltrates, particularly neutrophils, and should not be interpreted as acute cholangitis.

Fibrosis: Deposition of collagen fibers. When fibrous bands link portal tracts and/or central veins, it is referred to as **bridging fibrosis. Cirrhosis** is the end stage of chronic liver diseases, characterized by diffusely nodular replacement and remodeling of the normal hepatic architecture due to septal formation and hepatocyte regeneration. Traditionally, cirrhosis is classified as micronodular if nearly all the nodules are <0.3 cm in diameter, and macronodular if >0.3 cm.

Interface hepatitis (piecemeal necrosis): Breakdown of the limiting plate by inflammatory cells accompanied by individual hepatocyte necrosis. It is a common finding in chronic hepatitis.

Lobular activity (lobulitis): Small clusters of inflammatory cells within the lobules, accompanied by hepatocyte damage.

Mallory hyaline (bodies): Irregular, dense eosinophilic cytoplasmic aggregates of cytokeratins, usually seen in ballooning hepatocytes. They stain positive for ubiquitin.

Necrosis: Death of hepatocytes in various patterns. Widespread necrosis of single or small groups of hepatocytes is referred to as **spotty** or **focal necrosis.** When dead hepatocytes degenerate, the gap in the cell plates may be replaced by inflammatory cells (hepatocyte drop-out). **Confluent necrosis** refers to death of adjacent hepatocytes in substantial areas, which usually leads to collapse of the reticulin framework. When confluent necrosis spans the distance between vascular structures (central veins and portal tracts), it is referred to as **bridging necrosis.** Confluent necrosis may be zonal in distribution. When occurring around the terminal hepatic venule (centrilobular or zone 3 necrosis), it is often due to ischemia. Massive or submassive necrosis refers to panlobular or multilobular necrosis involving the entire liver or a substantial portion of the liver. This is commonly associated with fulminant hepatitis that leads to liver failure. Grossly, massive necrosis may be suggested by decreased organ weight, flaccidness, and wrinkling of the capsule.

Steatosis (fatty change): Excessive accumulation of lipid in hepatocytes. Microvesicular steatosis is characterized by numerous densely packed fine fat droplets that fill the cytoplasm but do not displace the nucleus. Macrovesicular steatosis is characterized by a single large fat droplet or several small droplets that occupy a large portion of the cytoplasm and push the nucleus to the periphery. Focal or multifocal fat accumulation in the liver may simulate nodular or mass lesions radiographically.

biopsy should be at least 1.5 cm in length or contain at least five portal tracts. More recent data suggest that at least 11 complete portal tracts are needed (*Semin Liver Dis* 2004; 24:89). Clinicians need to be informed if a biopsy is inadequate or suboptimal for histopathologic evaluation.

A. Infectious liver diseases

   1. Viral hepatitis is caused by one of the hepatotropic viruses in most cases. These include hepatitis A, B, C, and E viruses, as well as hepatitis D viral coinfection in hepatitis B patients. Other nonhepatotropic viruses may also cause liver injury as part of a systemic disease.

     a. Acute viral hepatitis results from an immunologic response directed to viral antigens expressed on the membrane of infected hepatocytes. The liver is expected to be heavy, diffusely red, and edematous, with a tense capsule. The diagnosis of acute viral hepatitis usually does not require a biopsy given the ready availability and reliability of serologic tests. If liver tissue is available for histopathologic examination, it is characterized by ballooning degeneration, spotty necrosis, inflammatory cell infiltration in the lobules and portal tracts, Kupffer cell hyperplasia, and regenerative activity. The inflammatory infiltrates consist predominantly of mononuclear cells, mainly lymphocytes and macrophages. Occasionally, plasma cells, eosinophils, and neutrophils may be seen. The necroinflammatory process typically diffusely involves the lobules and disrupts the orderly arrangement of the plates and sinusoids, resulting in lobular disarray (e-**Fig. 15.2**). In severe cases, bridging, submassive or massive necrosis may occur (e-**Fig. 15.3**). Trichrome and reticulin stains can be helpful in distinguishing from bridging fibrosis or cirrhosis in these cases, particularly in the presence of ductular reaction as part of the regenerative process (e-**Fig. 15.4**). Acute canalicular cholestasis is not a typical finding in acute viral hepatitis; if prominent, it may be diagnosed as acute cholestatic hepatitis (e-**Fig. 15.5**).

      Complete resolution is the common outcome of patients with hepatitis A and E. If the connective tissue scaffolding remains intact, regeneration can lead to restoration of normal lobular architecture. In contrast, the inflammation in patients with hepatitis B and C may evolve to chronic hepatitis or a carrier state.

      Acute viral hepatitis needs to be differentiated from autoimmune hepatitis, Wilson's disease, and drug- or toxin-induced hepatitis. Clinical history and laboratory investigation are important in this regard. In most cases, histologic recognition of acute hepatitis is sufficient, and a specific etiologic diagnosis is usually not expected.

     b. Chronic viral hepatitis is defined as persistent clinical symptoms or abnormal liver tests for >6 months caused by hepatitis B or C virus, or B and D coinfection. It features portal mononuclear cell infiltrates rich in T lymphocytes. Plasma cells, macrophages, eosinophils, and neutrophils may be present but are typically few in number. The portal inflammation may be accompanied by varying degrees of piecemeal necrosis (e-**Fig. 15.6**), lobular activity with acidophil bodies (e-**Fig. 15.7**), and fibrosis (e-**Fig. 15.8**).

      A few histologic features are characteristic of specific types of chronic viral hepatitis. In particular, hepatitis B can be recognized by the presence of so-called ground glass hepatocytes characterized by finely granular or homogeneous eosinophilic cytoplasm due to expanded smooth endoplasmic reticulum stuffed with viral surface antigen (e-**Fig. 15.9**). Intranuclear inclusions containing hepatitis B core antigen (known as sanded nuclei) can also be seen in some cases (e-**Fig. 15.10**); these cells can be easily identified by immunohistochemical stains for hepatitis B surface and core antigens. In B- and D-coinfected cases, the necroinflammation tends to be more severe, and delta antigen can also be demonstrated in the nuclei by immunostaining.

      Although not pathognomonic, the presence of portal lymphoid aggregates, often with well-formed germinal centers, strongly suggests chronic hepatitis C (e-**Fig. 15.11**). Steatosis and mild bile duct injury are also common findings in chronic hepatitis C; the steatosis is usually large and small droplet macrovesicular and focal, and is thought to be the direct cytopathic effect

TABLE 15.2   **Grading and Staging Chronic Hepatitis**

Grade

Grade 0	No significant portal or lobular inflammation, or hepatocyte damage
Grade 1	Mononuclear cell infiltrates are limited to the portal tracts. Piecemeal necrosis and lobular activity are minimal, if any
Grade 2	Piecemeal necrosis and lobular inflammation are mild, with piecemeal necrosis involving >50% of the circumference of the portal tracts
Grade 3	Piecemeal necrosis and lobular inflammation are moderate, with piecemeal necrosis involving ≥50% of the circumference of the portal tracts
Grade 4	Piecemeal necrosis and lobular inflammation are severe; bridging necrosis may be evident

Stage

Stage 0	No fibrosis
Stage 1	Fibrosis confined to the portal tracts, with portal expansion
Stage 2	Portal and periportal fibrosis; occasional portal-to-portal septal formation is allowable
Stage 3	Bridging fibrosis
Stage 4	Cirrhosis

of the virus, particularly genotype 3. However, a small subset of the patients may concurrently have steatohepatitis of alcoholic or nonalcoholic etiology; in those cases, steatosis tends to involve more hepatocytes. Nonnecrotizing granulomas may be detected in ~10% of the biopsies from hepatitis C patients.

Needle biopsies are frequently performed to grade and stage chronic hepatitis. A number of grading and staging systems have been developed, all of which share the assessment of portal and lobular necroinflammation for grade and fibrosis for stage (*Hepatology* 2000;31:241); most systems use a scale of 0 to 4 for both grade and stage as defined in Table 15.2 and illustrated in Figs. 15.1 and 15.2 (*Am J Surg Pathol* 1995;19:1409). Necroinflammation in chronic hepatitis C is typically mild, usually grade 1 or 2, but tends to be more severe in chronic hepatitis B.

  c. **Epstein-Barr virus hepatitis** is characterized by a diffuse lymphocytic infiltrate in the sinusoids in a "beads on a string" pattern (e-**Fig. 15.12**). The diagnosis can be confirmed by in situ hybridization for viral RNA and serologic tests.

  d. **Cytomegalovirus hepatitis** features neutrophilic microabscesses surrounding infected cells that may have characteristic intranuclear and intracytoplasmic viral inclusions (e-**Fig. 15.13**). The presence of microabscess should prompt immunostaining for cytomegalovirus if viral inclusions are not evident.

  e. **Adenovirus hepatitis** causes random foci of coagulative necrosis with minimal inflammatory response. The infected hepatocytes show smudgy nuclei with chromatin margination (e-**Fig. 15.14**). The diagnosis can be confirmed by immunohistochemical staining for viral proteins.

  f. **Herpesvirus hepatitis** is morphologically similar to adenovirus hepatitis, but multinucleation is more common. Immunohistochemical stains can be used to distinguish herpesvirus hepatitis from adenovirus hepatitis.

  2. **Bacterial infections** can cause liver abscess (pyogenic bacteria) and granulomatous inflammation (mycobacterium). Sepsis may lead to microabscess formation, centrilobular canalicular cholestasis, and an unusual form of cholestasis known as cholangitis lenta that is characterized by ductular cholestasis with inspissated bile in dilated ductules at the periphery of the portal tracts (e-**Fig. 15.15**).

  3. **Fungal infections** are usually part of systemic diseases, such as candidiasis, aspergillosis, and histoplasmosis.

  4. **Parasitic infections** include hydatid cyst, amebic abscess, and schistosomiasis.

B. **Metabolic and toxic liver diseases**

  1. **Alcoholic liver disease** encompasses the clinicopathological spectrum of fatty liver, alcoholic hepatitis, and alcoholic cirrhosis. Steatosis may be predominantly

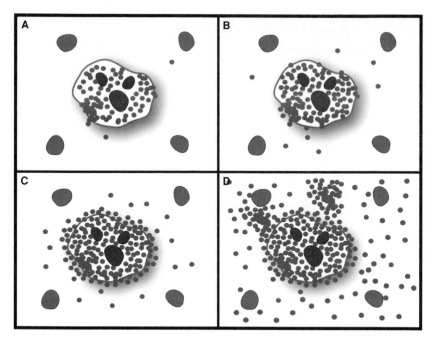

Figure 15.1. Grading schema of chronic hepatitis. **(A)** grade 1; **(B)** grade 2; **(C)** grade 3; **(D)** grade 4.

macrovesicular and initially involves zone 3 hepatocytes. The entire hepatic lobule may be involved in severe cases, but the steatosis is reversible with cessation of alcohol consumption. The histologic hallmarks of alcoholic hepatitis are hepatocyte ballooning, spotty necrosis, and neutrophilic infiltration of the lobules commonly around hepatocytes containing Mallory bodies (**e-Fig. 15.16**). The pattern of fibrosis in alcoholic hepatitis is characteristic; it is usually patchy and perisinusoidal/pericellular, giving rise to a distinct "chicken-wire" pattern. A trichrome stain is particularly useful in recognizing this unique type of fibrosis (**e-Fig. 15.17**). Perivenular fibrosis is also common, which may obliterate the terminal hepatic venule leading to central hyaline necrosis (**e-Fig. 15.18**). Alcoholic cirrhosis is typically micronodular.

2. **Nonalcoholic fatty liver disease (NAFLD)** resembles alcoholic liver disease, but occurs in patients who are not heavy drinkers but who may suffer from obesity, hypertension, diabetes, or hyperlipidemia. It is also associated with the use of a variety of medications. Unlike alcoholic hepatitis, however, nonalcoholic steatohepatitis (NASH) usually exhibits a milder degree of parenchymal necroinflammation and less prominent Mallory hyaline, and typically does not obliterate the central vein. Steatosis may become insignificant when the liver becomes cirrhotic. In fact, "burnt-out" NASH may be the most likely cause of cryptogenic cirrhosis. In NASH, the hepatocytes may show prominent glycogenated nuclei, particularly when associated with diabetes (**e-Fig. 15.19**). Portal inflammation, when present, is usually mild and less intense than lobular inflammation, although pediatric cases may show more prominent portal mononuclear cell infiltration.

3. **Diabetic glycogenosis,** or glycogenic hepatopathy, is a rare condition of marked glycogen overload in hepatocytes in association with poor control of diabetes mellitus. The hepatocytes exhibit expanded cytoplasm, show pale staining in H&E sections, and are similar to those seen in glycogen storage diseases. There is usually no or little fat, nor evidence of hepatitis. Megamitochondria and glycogenated nuclei may be prominent (**e-Fig. 15.20**).

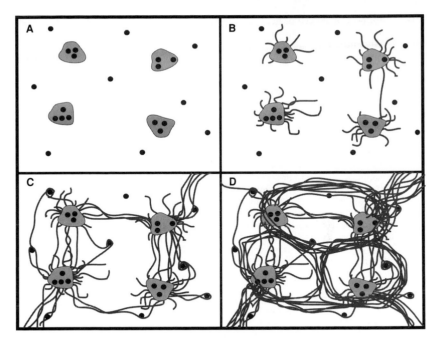

Figure 15.2. Staging schema of chronic hepatitis. **(A)** stage 1; **(B)** stage 2; **(C)** stage 3; **(D)** stage 4.

4. **Iron overload** can be primary (hereditary hemochromatosis) or secondary. In hereditary form, iron deposition initially occurs in zone 1 hepatocytes and is best demonstrated by an iron stain, which usually shows 3+ or 4+ staining intensity using a 4-point semiquantitative scale (e-**Fig. 15.21**). The diagnosis is established by biochemical quantitation of hepatic iron concentration (hepatic iron index >2) and mutational analysis of the *HFE* gene. Secondary iron overload occurs in a variety of conditions and primarily involves Kupffer cells.

5. **Wilson's disease** is caused by copper accumulation in the liver and other organs. The histologic findings in the liver lack specificity and range from steatosis, chronic hepatitis, cirrhosis, and acute hepatitis to fulminant hepatitis with massive or submassive necrosis. Glycogenated nuclei and Mallory hyaline may be seen. Excessive copper and copper-binding protein deposition, mainly in zone 1 hepatocytes, may be demonstrated by special techniques such as rhodanine and orcein stains (e-**Fig. 15.22**); however, these stains are not diagnostic because copper accumulation may also result from other chronic cholestatic liver diseases such as primary biliary cirrhosis (PBC). It is important to recognize that the absence of stainable copper does not exclude the diagnosis of Wilson's disease, nor does a normal serum ceruloplasmin value. Copper quantitation in hepatic tissue is the current diagnostic test (>250 μg/g dry hepatic tissue). Genetic testing for *ATP7B* gene mutations has not yet become available for diagnosis.

6. **α1-Antitrypsin deficiency** is characterized by the presence of cytoplasmic eosinophilic hyaline globules in zone 1 hepatocytes, best demonstrated by PAS-D stain (e-**Fig. 15.23**). The diagnosis can be confirmed by immunostaining for α1-antitrypsin and serum protein electrophoresis. In infants and young children, hyaline globules may not be evident; instead, the disease may manifest in this population as giant cell or neonatal hepatitis with hepatocyte rosetting and giant cell transformation (e-**Fig. 15.24**). Cytoplasmic and canalicular cholestasis, ductular reaction, and bile duct loss may occur, reminiscent of biliary atresia.

Of note, giant cell or neonatal hepatitis is a descriptive diagnosis and may result from a variety of etiologies.

7. **Glycogen storage diseases,** or **glycogenoses,** are characterized by abnormal accumulation of glycogen in hepatocytes, giving rise to a pale, distended, and mosaic appearance. PAS stains and electron microscopy may help confirm the diagnosis.

8. **Lysosomal storage diseases** feature accumulation of partially digested and insoluble metabolites in lysosomes. The most common is Gaucher's disease, in which distended Kupffer cells, known as Gaucher cells, fill the sinusoids and compress hepatocytes. The cytoplasm of Gaucher cells is characteristically pale and finely striated like wrinkled tissue paper.

9. **Reye's syndrome** is characterized by panlobular microvesicular steatosis, which may require an oil red O stain on a frozen section to recognize. Electron microscopic findings of abnormal mitochondria are essentially diagnostic.

10. **Total parenteral nutrition (TPN)** may cause canalicular cholestasis, steatosis, steatohepatitis with perisinusoidal fibrosis, bridging fibrosis, and ultimately cirrhosis.

11. **Amyloidosis** primarily involves the portal arteries and sinusoids. In severe cases, the sinusoids may be completely blocked by pink amorphous material with compression and atrophy of the hepatocytes (e-**Fig. 15.25**). A Congo red stain (which demonstrates apple-green birefringence in the amyloid deposits) may or may not be needed for the diagnosis.

12. **Cystic fibrosis** involves the liver in ∼20% of patients. The histologic hallmark is the presence of dense inspissated mucous material in dilated bile ducts, in association with ductular proliferation and fibrosis.

13. **Drug- and toxin-induced liver injury** can be direct (predictable, intrinsic) or indirect (unpredictable, idiosyncratic). Direct toxicity occurs with drugs or toxins known to produce liver damage in a dose-dependent manner in a high percentage of patients. Indirect toxicity is usually immune-mediated and dose-independent. Acute injury is exemplified by cholestasis, bile duct damage, acute hepatitis, and focal or massive necrosis. Chronic injury may assume the form of chronic hepatitis, granulomatous hepatitis, steatosis, steatohepatitis, vascular injury, fibrosis, cirrhosis, or neoplasia. Drug toxicity should always be included in the differential diagnosis when investigating an unexplained liver abnormality.

C. **Autoimmune and bile duct disorders of the liver**

1. **Autoimmune hepatitis** typically affects women who often have other types of immunologic disorders. Autoimmune hepatitis is characteristically associated with hypergammaglobulinemia and/or high titers of antinuclear, anti-smooth muscle, anti-liver-kidney microsomal type 1, or antisoluble liver antigen autoantibodies. In classic cases, there is a dense portal and lobular mononuclear cell infiltrate enriched in plasma cells (e-**Fig. 15.26**). Marked interface hepatitis, centrilobular or bridging necrosis, and hepatitic resetting are common findings. Fibrosis may develop rapidly in untreated patients. Although autoimmune hepatitis is usually regarded as a chronic disease, acute or fulminant hepatitis sometimes occurs; in these cases, plasma cells may not predominate.

2. **PBC** is a progressive cholestatic disease that leads to the destruction of intrahepatic bile ducts. It occurs mainly in middle-aged women. The early stage of the disease (stage 1) is defined by mixed portal inflammatory cell infiltrates and the pathognomonic florid duct lesion characterized by granulomatous or lymphocytic infiltration of the duct epithelium (e-**Fig. 15.27**). In the setting of positive antimitochondrial antibody (AMA) serology, the florid duct lesion is essentially diagnostic. The granulomas in PBC are epithelioid and lack necrosis, and are typically poorly formed; if the granulomas are large and well formed, and do not damage the bile duct, stains for fungal and acid-fast organisms should be performed even in the setting of positive AMA serology. As PBC progresses, ductular reaction, interface hepatitis, and chronic cholestasis develop (stage 2), with eventual progression to bridging fibrosis (stage 3) and biliary cirrhosis (stage 4). Florid duct lesions and portal granulomas are usually undetectable when

ductopenia becomes evident. The areas of native bile ducts may be replaced by foamy macrophages.

Autoimmune cholangiopathy, autoimmune cholangitis, and AMA-negative PBC are synonymous terms used to describe a small subset of patients who present with typical clinical and histopathologic findings of PBC but are seronegative for AMA. These patients may have autoantibodies more typical of patients with autoimmune hepatitis.

3. **PSC** is a fibroinflammatory disorder that affects the extra- and intrahepatic biliary tree leading to biliary strictures and cirrhosis. It is strongly associated with inflammatory bowel disease (particularly ulcerative colitis) and autoimmune pancreatitis. The definitive diagnosis of PSC rests on characteristic cholangiographic findings; liver biopsy may or may not reveal diagnostic features because of the segmental nature of the disease. The relatively specific findings include concentric periductal fibrosis with an "onion-skin" appearance and degenerative changes of the duct epithelium (e-**Fig. 15.28**). Portal inflammation is usually mild, although the bile ducts are eventually replaced by an obliterative scar. The explanted liver should be carefully evaluated for occult cholangiocarcinoma.

4. **Overlap syndrome** refers to cases of autoimmune hepatitis with the simultaneous presence of diagnostic features of PBC or PSC.

5. **Secondary biliary cirrhosis** results from mechanical obstruction of the extrahepatic biliary tree. The common causes in adults are lithiasis, tumors, and surgical stenosis; in children, the common causes are biliary atresia and choledochal cysts. Histologically, large duct obstruction may cause portal edema, canalicular cholestasis, bile plugs in dilated ducts, bile lakes, feathery degeneration of the hepatocytes, and ductular reaction. Long-standing obstruction leads to portal and periductal fibrosis similar to that seen in PSC. Biliary cirrhosis may ensue. Biliary atresia in infants may simulate neonatal or giant cell hepatitis when lobular damage is extensive.

6. **Ascending cholangitis** is diagnosed when neutrophils are present within the lumen of the bile ducts. The duct epithelium may show degenerative change or necrosis. Abscess formation may occur.

7. **Ductal plate malformation** results from developmental arrest with persistence of the embryologic ductal plate, which assumes an anastomosing ringlike structure lining the periphery of the portal tracts (e-**Fig. 15.29**). It is often associated with von Meyenburg complexes, congenital hepatic fibrosis, Caroli's disease, and polycystic liver disease.

In congenital hepatic fibrosis, the portal tracts are expanded by connective tissue with an increased number of aberrant duct profiles. Inspissated bile may be noted in ectatic ducts, and there may be bridging fibrosis. The portal vein branches may be hypoplastic or absent, but the branches of hepatic artery may be hypertrophic and abnormally numerous.

Caroli's disease is characterized by segmental cystic dilatation of the larger intrahepatic ducts, usually accompanied by recurrent bacterial cholangitis and biliary lithiasis. When associated with congenital hepatic fibrosis, it is termed Caroli's syndrome.

8. **Paucity of intrahepatic bile ducts,** or **intrahepatic biliary atresia,** is defined by a ratio of <0.5 between the number of interlobular ducts and portal tracts (the normal range is 0.9 to 1.8). When a biopsy is evaluated, at least five intact portal tracts should be present to be considered adequate. Multiple sections and immunostains for cytokeratin 7 or 19 may help identify hypoplastic ducts in difficult cases. Unlike extrahepatic biliary atresia or obstruction, ductular reaction is absent in this condition. In pediatric patients, paucity of intrahepatic bile ducts may be syndromic (Alagille syndrome) or nonsyndromic; the nonsyndromic variant may be associated with viral infections or α1-antitrypsin deficiency in some patients. In adults, ductopenia may be seen in PBC, PSC, chronic allograft rejection, chronic graft versus host disease (GVHD), viral infections, or drug reactions or may be idiopathic (idiopathic adulthood ductopenia or vanishing bile duct syndrome).

TABLE 15.3	Vascular Disorders of the Liver

Hepatic artery
Atherosclerosis
Thrombosis
Embolization
Stricture
Vasculitis
Amyloidosis
Systemic hypotension (ischemic or shock liver)

Portal vein
Thrombosis
Pyelophlebitis
Allograft rejection
Osler–Weber–Rendu syndrome (hereditary hemorrhagic telangiectasia)
Nodular regenerative hyperplasia
Hepatoportal sclerosis

Hepatic vein
Congestive heart failure
Budd–Chiari syndrome
Veno-occlusive disease

Sinusoids
Peliosis hepatis
Sinusoidal dilatation
Amyloidosis

D. Vascular disorders of the liver (Table 15.3)
   1. **Venous outflow obstruction** ranges etiologically from congestive heart failure, to narrowing or occlusion of large hepatic veins (Budd–Chiari syndrome), to obliteration of the terminal or larger intrahepatic veins (veno-occlusive disease). Liver injury caused by congestive heart failure is characterized by zone 3 sinusoidal dilatation and congestion; in long-standing cases, the hepatocytes become atrophic and perivenular fibrosis develops. Cardiac cirrhosis with reverse lobulation may result. Budd–Chiari syndrome produces similar histopathologic features, but acute onset may give rise to a hemorrhagic appearance at zone 3 with more significant hepatocyte necrosis and red cell extravasation. Veno-occlusive disease (also termed sinusoidal obstruction syndrome), which rarely results in cirrhosis, is characterized by collagen deposition in the subendothelial space and sinusoids, leading to thickening, narrowing, and eventual obliteration of the intrahepatic veins (e-**Fig. 15.30**).
   2. **Nodular regenerative hyperplasia (NRH)** is a common condition underlying noncirrhotic portal hypertension. The liver is diffusely nodular, with nodules ranging from 0.1 to 1 cm in diameter. The nodularity is better appreciated at low magnification and with a reticulin stain (e-**Fig. 15.31**), which highlights the regenerative hepatocytes within the nodules and the atrophic hepatocytes between the nodules. NRH differs from cirrhosis in that there is no or only minimal fibrosis, and the portal structures are usually unaltered.
   3. **Hepatoportal sclerosis,** also known as idiopathic portal hypertension or noncirrhotic portal fibrosis, is characterized by an abnormal hepatic architecture. The portal tracts are either abnormally approximated to each other or are widely separated. The central veins may be eccentrically located adjacent to portal tracts, or multiple ectatic tributaries may be seen in a single lobule. Portal fibrosis is usually conspicuous, and the portal veins may show marked wall thickening with

luminal narrowing or obliteration (e-Fig. 15.32). Because abnormal portal vasculature can sometimes be seen in the absence of portal hypertension (*Am J Surg Pathol* 2005;29:1382), interpretation requires clinical correlation.

E. Miscellaneous

1. **Granulomas** are a common finding in the liver. Underlying etiologies include PBC, sarcoidosis, a drug reaction, hepatitis C, fungal or mycobacterial infection, foreign bodies, autoimmune hepatitis, and neoplasia; many cases are idiopathic (granulomatous hepatitis). Gomori's Methenamine Silver (GMS) and acid-fast stains may be performed to rule out unexpected fungal or mycobacterial infection.

2. **Pregnancy** is occasionally associated with liver injury. Acute fatty liver of pregnancy typically occurs in the late third trimester and is potentially fatal to the mother and fetus. The histologic hallmark is zone 3 or diffuse microvesicular steatosis that may require an oil red O stain on a frozen section to confirm. Preeclampsia/eclampsia and HELLP syndrome (hemolysis, elevated liver enzymes, and low platelets) may cause hemorrhage, necrosis, and fibrin deposition.

F. Transplantation pathology

1. **Donor liver evaluation** is often performed on frozen sections to evaluate the extent of steatosis. The percentages of the liver parenchyma involved by total steatosis, and by large droplet macrovesicular steatosis, are estimated on H&E stains and separately reported. In many centers, 30% large droplet fat is used as a cutoff (a 50% cutoff is used in other centers). An important pitfall is frozen artifact, in which sinusoidal spaces may be misinterpreted as large fat vacuoles. An oil red O stain is not recommended because it may result in an overrepresentation of small droplet fat that is not associated with graft dysfunction or nonfunction. The degree of portal inflammation, fibrosis, and preservation injury should also be recorded as the baseline for comparison with subsequent posttransplant biopsies.

2. **Preservation/reperfusion injury** is caused by ischemic damage sustained during the process of graft harvesting, transportation, or reperfusion. It features hepatocyte ballooning, spotty necrosis, and cholestasis; centrilobular necrosis may occur in more severe cases. The injury usually resolves spontaneously within a few weeks after transplantation but may persist for a few months.

3. **Humoral (hyperacute) rejection** is rare, and is mediated by preformed or subsequently formed antibodies to an ABO blood group–incompatible liver. It may occur immediately after reperfusion or within the first few days after transplantation. The liver shows extensive coagulative and hemorrhagic necrosis with fibrin thrombi.

    Late-onset humorally mediated rejection, evidenced by immunohistochemical demonstration of vascular C4d deposition, is a well-established complication of heart and kidney transplantation. Its role in liver allograft rejection has not been well studied.

4. **Acute (cellular) rejection** is directed at duct epithelium and endothelium. It is usually first recognized between 5 and 30 days after transplantation, but late onset also occurs if immunosuppression is reduced or discontinued. The histologic triad includes mixed portal inflammation, bile duct damage, and endotheliitis (or endothelialitis). The portal infiltrates consist mostly of lymphocytes admixed with eosinophils, histiocytes, plasma cells, and neutrophils. Although eosinophils are virtually always present, the diagnosis of acute rejection should not rely on their presence. Bile duct damage is characterized by lymphocytic infiltration of the duct epithelium, accompanied by cytoplasmic vacuolation, nuclear overlapping, enlargement or pyknosis, and breakdown of the basement membrane (e-Fig. 15.33). Endotheliitis takes the forms of subendothelial lymphocytic infiltration; lifting, detachment, and sloughing of endothelial cells; or attachment of lymphocytes to the luminal aspect of the endothelium (e-Fig. 15.34). Endotheliitis most frequently involves portal veins, but central veins can also be similarly affected, with resultant centrilobular necrosis.

    Acute rejection is usually graded using the Banff schema recommended by an international panel (Table 15.4). If portal inflammation is the only finding,

TABLE 15.4	Banff Scheme for Grading Acute Liver Allograft Rejection

Global assessment	Criteria
Indeterminate	Portal inflammatory infiltrate that fails to meet the criteria for the diagnosis of acute rejection
Mild	Rejection infiltrate in a minority of the triads that is generally mild and confined within the portal spaces
Moderate	Rejection infiltrate expanding most or all of the triads
Severe	As above for moderate, with spillover into periportal areas and moderate to severe perivenular inflammation that extends into the hepatic parenchyma and is associated with perivenular hepatocyte necrosis

it may be interpreted as indeterminate for rejection if recurrent diseases have been ruled out. Mild rejection is diagnosed if <50% of the portal tracts are involved by inflammation accompanied by bile duct damage and/or endotheliitis. Moderate rejection is diagnosed if ≥50% of the portal tracts are affected. If centrilobular necrosis and/or significant piecemeal necrosis are also present, severe rejection is diagnosed. Alternatively, the Rejection Activity Index (RAI) may be used (*Hepatology* 1997;25:658).

5. **Chronic rejection** may become evident as early as 2 months after transplantation. It is defined by ductopenia and obliterative vasculopathy. Vascular rejection, characterized by subintimal accumulation of foamy histiocytes in large caliber arteries, is usually not seen in needle biopsies; its presence can only be inferred when perivenular necrosis and fibrosis are present. Therefore, the diagnosis of chronic rejection is primarily based on the evaluation of bile ducts. As shown in Table 15.5, chronic rejection is divided into early and late stages (*Hepatology* 2000;31:792). The early stage is defined by bile duct dystrophy/degeneration in >50% of portal tracts, and/or duct loss in >20% but <50% of portal tracts (**e-Fig. 15.35**). The late stage features duct loss in ≥50% of portal tracts (**e-Fig. 15.36**). Portal inflammation and ductular reaction are typically insignificant in the late stage.

6. **Technical complications** usually occur during the first few months after transplantation. Hepatic artery or portal vein thrombosis or stricture may cause hepatocyte necrosis and infarction. Ischemic damage of the biliary tree may also occur as a complication of hepatic artery complications, with resultant necrosis, stricture, or loss of the bile ducts. Hepatic vein thrombosis or stricture leads to outflow obstruction. Stenosis or obstruction of the bile duct anastomosis causes morphologic changes similar to those of secondary biliary cirrhosis.

7. **Recurrent diseases** can be difficult to diagnose as they share some histopathologic features with allograft rejection and technical complications. Many diseases can recur, but the frequency and timeframe vary. Recurrent diseases include viral hepatitis (B, C, and D), alcoholic hepatitis, NASH, autoimmune hepatitis, PBC, PSC, vascular disorders, and malignant tumors.

Recurrent viral hepatitis is virtually universal. It can recur as early as the first 1 to 2 weeks after transplantation, but usually only becomes evident after 4 weeks. Features favoring recurrent hepatitis C include prominent lobular activity, numerous acidophil bodies, steatosis, lymphoid aggregates, ductular proliferation, bridging fibrosis, and cirrhosis. Although bile duct damage and endotheliitis can be seen in hepatitis C, they are neither severe nor widespread. In typical cases, lymphocytic infiltrates in the portal tracts avoid the bile ducts and vasculature (**e-Fig. 15.37**). In difficult cases, measurement of blood viral load may help differentiate recurrent hepatitis C from acute rejection. In the acute phase of recurrent hepatitis B, ground glass hepatocytes may be absent and immunostains for surface and core antigens may be negative.

Structure	Early CR	Late CR
Small bile ducts	Degenerative changes involving a majority of ducts: Eosinophilic transformation of the cytoplasm; increased nuclear to cytoplasmic (N/C) ratio; nuclear hyperchromasia; uneven nuclear spacing; ducts only partially lined by biliary epithelial cells Bile duct loss in <50% of portal tracts	Degenerative changes in remaining bile ducts Loss in ≥50% of portal tracts
Terminal hepatic venules and zone 3 hepatocytes	Intimal/luminal inflammation Lytic zone 3 necrosis and inflammation Mild perivenular fibrosis	Focal obliteration Variable inflammation Severe (bridging) fibrosis
Portal tract hepatic arterioles	Occasional loss involving <25% of portal tracts	Loss involving >25% of portal tracts
Other	So-called "transition" hepatitis with spotty necrosis of hepatocytes	Sinusoidal foam cell accumulation; marked cholestasis
Larger perihilar hepatic artery branches	Intimal inflammation, focal foam cell deposition without luminal compromise	Luminal narrowing by subintimal foam cells Fibrointimal proliferation
Large perihilar bile ducts	Inflammation damage and focal foam cell deposition	Mural fibrosis

TABLE 15.5 Banff Criteria for Chronic Liver Allograft Rejection (CR)

Fibrosing cholestatic hepatitis is a rare but rapidly progressive disease seen in recurrent hepatitis B and C, often resulting in graft loss. It typically occurs within the first few months after transplantation, and features marked portal and periportal fibrosis with perisinusoidal extension, canalicular and intracellular cholestasis, hepatocyte ballooning, and ductular reaction. Inflammatory changes are generally mild. In recurrent hepatitis B, the viral surface and core antigens are highly expressed in reinfected hepatocytes.

PBC and PSC may recur several years after transplantation. In the absence of granulomatous duct lesions, recurrent PBC can be difficult to distinguish from acute rejection. Recurrent PSC needs to be distinguished from technical complications such as hepatic artery or biliary stricture, or obstruction.

8. **De novo autoimmune hepatitis** infrequently develops in recipients whose original liver disease is not autoimmune hepatitis. The disease mimics autoimmune hepatitis both histologically and serologically. In addition to the classic features described above, centrilobular necrosis may be a cardinal finding in some cases.

9. **GVHD** occurs following bone marrow or stem cell transplantation, and is only rarely associated with orthotopic liver transplantation. Histologically, acute GVHD resembles acute rejection (with less frequent endotheliitis) and chronic hepatitis. Chronic GVHD typically occurs after 100 days and histologically simulates ductopenic chronic rejection.

IV. DIAGNOSTIC FEATURES OF COMMON NEOPLASTIC AND TUMORLIKE CONDITIONS. The current World Health Organization (WHO) histologic classification of tumors of the liver and intrahepatic bile ducts is given in Table 15.6. The 2002 American

TABLE 15.6	WHO Histologic Classification of Tumors of the Liver and Intrahepatic Bile Ducts

Epithelial tumors
Benign
  Hepatocellular adenoma (liver cell adenoma)
  Focal nodular hyperplasia
  Intrahepatic bile duct adenoma
  Intrahepatic bile duct cystadenoma
  Biliary papillomatosis
Malignant
  Hepatocellular carcinoma (liver cell carcinoma)
  Intrahepatic cholangiocarcinoma (peripheral bile duct carcinoma)
  Bile duct cystadenocarcinoma
  Combined hepatocellular and cholangiocarcinoma
  Hepatoblastoma
  Undifferentiated carcinoma

Nonepithelial tumors
Benign
  Angiomyolipoma
  Lymphangioma and lymphangiomatosis
  Hemangioma
  Infantile hemangioendothelioma
Malignant
  Epithelioid hemangioendothelioma
  Angiosarcoma
  Embryonal sarcoma (undifferentiated sarcoma)
  Rhabdomyosarcoma
  Other

Miscellaneous tumors
Solitary fibrous tumor
Teratoma
Yolk sac tumor (endodermal tumor)
Carcinosarcoma
Kaposi sarcoma
Rhabdoid tumor
Other

Hematopoietic and lymphoid tumors
Secondary tumors
Epithelial abnormalities
Liver cell dysplasia (liver cell change)
  Large cell type (large cell change)
  Small cell type (small cell change)
Dysplastic nodules (adenomatous hyperplasia)
  Low grade
  High grade (atypical adenomatous hyperplasia)
Bile duct abnormalities
  Hyperplasia (bile duct epithelium and peribiliary glands)
  Dysplasia (bile duct epithelium and peribiliary glands)
  Intraepithelial carcinoma (carcinoma in situ)

Miscellaneous lesions
Mesenchymal hamartoma
Nodular transformation (nodular regenerative hyperplasia)
Inflammatory pseudotumor

From: Hamilton SR, Aaltonen LA, eds. *World Health Organization Classification of Tumours. Pathology and Genetics. Tumours of the Digestive System.* Lyon: IARC Press; 2000. Used with permission.

TABLE 15.7	Tumor, Node, Metastasis (TNM) Staging Scheme for Carcinoma of the Liver and Intrahepatic Bile Duct

PRIMARY TUMOR (T)

TX	Primary tumor cannot be assessed
T0	No evidence of primary tumor
T1	Solitary tumor without vascular invasion
T2	Solitary tumor with vascular invasion or multiple tumors none >5 cm
T3	Multiple tumors >5 cm or tumor involving a major branch of the portal or hepatic vein(s)
T4	Tumor(s) with direct invasion of adjacent organs other than the gallbladder or with perforation of visceral peritoneum

REGIONAL LYMPH NODES (N)

NX	Regional lymph nodes cannot be assessed
N0	No regional lymph node metastasis
N1	Regional lymph node metastasis

DISTANT METASTASIS (M)

MX	Distant metastasis cannot be assessed
M0	No distant metastasis
M1	Distant metastasis

STAGE GROUPING

Stage I	T1	N0	M0
Stage II	T2	N0	M0
Stage IIIA	T3	N0	M0
Stage IIIB	T4	N0	M0
Stage IIIC	Any T	N1	M0
Stage IV	Any T	Any N	M1

From: Greene FL, Page DL, Fleming ID, Fritz AG, Balch CM, Haller DG, Morrow M, eds. *AJCC Cancer Staging Manual.* 6th edition. New York: Springer, 2002. Used with permission. (A new AJCC TNM staging system is scheduled for release in 2009; after its publication, the new staging scheme will appear on the website for this book.)

Joint Committee on Cancer (AJCC) Tumor, Node, Metastasis (TNM) staging schema is given in Table 15.7.

A. Hepatocellular

1. **Focal nodular hyperplasia (FNH)** is a well-demarcated tumorlike lesion characterized by a central stellate scar (e-**Fig. 15.38**) that contains large, thick-walled blood vessels and a variable number of proliferating bile ductules. True bile ducts are absent. The lesion is nodular in appearance, resembling cirrhosis (e-**Fig. 15.39**). The telangiectatic variant exhibits marked sinusoidal dilatation and may simulate hepatocellular adenoma.

2. **Hepatocellular adenoma,** or **liver cell adenoma,** is almost exclusively seen in women of childbearing age with a history of prolonged use of oral contraceptives. It is also associated with anabolic/androgenic steroids and metabolic disorders including glycogenosis, tyrosinemia, and galactosemia. Adenomas arising in the setting of metabolic disorders may have an increased risk of transformation into hepatocellular carcinoma (HCC).

   Hepatocellular adenoma is usually solitary but can be multiple (adenomatosis). Adenomas consist solely of bland appearing hepatocytes, arranged in plates of 1 to 3 cells thick. Small arterioles and thin-walled vessels are common within the tumor, but bile ducts or ductules are absent (e-**Fig. 15.40**). Hemorrhage, necrosis, and fat accumulation are common findings. Mitosis is virtually never seen. Occasional pseudoacinar formation may be present, but should not be viewed as evidence of well-differentiated HCC. The lesion may or may not be encapsulated, but variable sized blood vessels, some of which may show fibromyxoid intimal thickening, are often present at the boundary.

3. **HCC** arises in a cirrhotic background in the majority of the cases and is usually distinctive from the adjacent cirrhotic nodules. HCC commonly assumes a trabecular growth pattern with thickened cell plates (>3 cells thick). The trabeculae are lined by endothelial cells that are immunoreactive to anti-CD34 antibody. The tumor cells may also form pseudoacinar structures or solid sheets, or exhibit clear cell change. A reticulin stain is extremely useful for highlighting distorted architecture and widened cell plates, and for showing a reduction or loss of reticulin fibers (e-Fig. 15.41). Bile production by tumor cells is also a useful feature that can be used to distinguish HCC from cholangiocarcinoma or metastatic tumors (e-Fig. 15.42). The presence of vascular invasion should always be carefully evaluated because it is an important parameter for tumor staging.

Although not prognostically important, HCC is conventionally graded by differentiation. Most tumors are moderately or poorly differentiated, featuring a high N/C ratio, increased nuclear pleomorphism, prominent nucleoli, and frequent mitoses. Well-differentiated HCC may be difficult to distinguish from hepatocellular adenoma and dysplastic nodule; thickened trabecular cords, frequent pseudoacinar formation, invasive growth at the periphery, vascular invasion, and metastasis are important differentiating features in this regard. The immunomarker glypican-3 (GPC3) may also be useful because it shows cytoplasmic, membranous, and/or canalicular staining in 70% to 80% of HCCs but is negative in hepatocellular adenoma and other benign hepatocellular lesions; only a small fraction of dysplastic and cirrhotic nodules are immunopositive for the marker.

Additional immunomarkers may be used to support the diagnosis of HCC. Hepatocyte antigen (Hep Par 1) stains benign hepatocytes and ~90% of HCCs. Polyclonal CEA and CD10 show a characteristic canalicular staining pattern in HCC. α-Fetoprotein (AFP) is relatively specific for HCC but has low sensitivity because it stains only ~40% of tumors. HCC is typically negative for cytokeratin (CK)7, CK19, and CK20.

4. **Fibrolamellar HCC** may occasionally resemble FNH grossly when a central scar is present. Histologically, the tumor consists of large polygonal oncocytic cells that are separated into groups by hyalinized, paucicellular collagen bands in a parallel (lamellar) fashion (e-Fig. 15.43). Some of the tumor cells may contain cytoplasmic pale bodies due to the presence of fibrinogen. This variant of HCC is generally believed to have a better prognosis, probably because of the younger age of the patient population and lack of accompanying cirrhosis, with a consequent higher rate of resectability. Serum AFP is seldom elevated.

5. **Dysplastic nodule** is a poorly defined premalignant lesion arising in the background of cirrhosis (*Hepatology* 1995;22:983 and *Semin Liver Dis* 2005;25:133). It is diagnosed based on a constellation of gross and microscopic features, but primarily on the basis of the presence of a clonelike expansion of cells with an increased N/C ratio and increased nuclear atypia. Resistance to iron accumulation, clear cell change, and the presence of isolated arterioles unaccompanied by bile ducts are also useful diagnostic features. Unlike HCC, dysplastic nodules do not have cords thicker than three cell layers or invasive growth. Although it has been classified into low and high grades, low-grade dysplastic nodules are seldom diagnosed given that it is difficult to distinguish them from large regenerative nodules.

Dysplastic nodules are rarely >2 cm in size. When the lesion is <0.1 cm, it is termed a dysplastic focus, lesions which are further divided into those with large cell change and those with small cell change (Table 15.6). Large cell change may or may not be considered a precursor lesion; it is characterized by cellular and nuclear enlargement with nuclear atypia, but a normal N/C ratio is maintained. Small cell change is strongly associated with HCC, and is characterized by nuclear enlargement and hyperchromasia with an increased N/C ratio.

6. **Hepatoblastoma** is most common in children <3 years of age. An elevated serum AFP is present in 90% of cases.

The epithelial type consists of fetal and/or embryonal liver cells. Fetal cells, resembling adult hepatocytes but smaller in size, contain variable amounts of cytoplastic fat and glycogen, giving rise to an alternating light-and-dark pattern (e-**Fig. 15.44**). Embryonal cells have a higher N/C ratio and may form nests, rosettes, or small tubules. Both fetal and embryonal cells may also exhibit a macrotrabecular growth pattern reminiscent of HCC.

The mixed epithelial-mesenchymal type contains mesenchymal components, such as cartilage and osteoid, in addition to the epithelial element. It may also show teratoid features.

The anaplastic type consists of small, undifferentiated primitive cells and has the worst prognosis.

B. Biliary

  1. Solitary unilocular biliary cysts are lined by a single layer of benign flattened, cuboidal, or columnar biliary-type epithelium, surrounded by a variable amount of fibrous tissue.

  2. Bile duct hamartoma, also known as **von Meyenburg complex** or **biliary micro-hamartoma,** is composed of a cluster of irregularly dilated bile ducts in a fibrotic background (e-**Fig. 15.45**). It is a small lesion (typically 1 to 2 mm) and usually an intraoperative incidental finding for which a frozen section may be requested. The importance of this lesion lies in the fact that it may be confused with metastatic carcinoma.

  3. Bile duct adenoma is composed of closely packed, well-formed, and relatively uniform small ducts that form a 1- to 20-mm diameter, sharply demarcated nodule (e-**Fig. 15.46**). When the lesion is >10 mm in diameter, careful microscopic examination is necessary to exclude the atypia, mitosis, and evidence of invasive growth that are indicative of cholangiocarcinoma. Large lesions may also be difficult to distinguish from metastatic carcinoma on frozen sections.

  4. Biliary cystadenoma consists of cystic structures lined by a layer of mucin-producing columnar cells. In women, ovarian-type stroma may be evident.

  5. Intrahepatic cholangiocarcinoma is a mucin-secreting adenocarcinoma usually arising in noncirrhotic livers. Cirrhosis should not be used as evidence to exclude the diagnosis, however. The tumor is characterized by a glandular, duct-like, papillary, or solid growth pattern in a prominent desmoplastic background; the latter feature is responsible for the firm, white or gray gross appearance. The tumor cells are cuboidal or columnar, and may not have prominent nucleoli. Immunophenotypically, >90% of the cases express CK7 and CK19, and ~40% also express CK20. Most cases are also positive for expression of monoclonal CEA and CA19-9. Intrahepatic cholangiocarcinoma is essentially indistinguishable from metastatic ductal adenocarcinoma of the pancreas on histologic and immunohistochemical grounds.

C. Mesenchymal

  1. Cavernous hemangioma is the most common benign tumor of the liver and only becomes clinically relevant when large. It is histologically similar to hemangiomas seen elsewhere, but tends to show thrombosis, calcification, and hyalinization.

  2. Infantile hemangioendothelioma occurs in the first 6 months of life in 90% of cases, and can be solitary or multifocal. This tumor has been traditionally divided into 2 types. Type I is characterized by intercommunicating vascular channels lined by a single layer of pump endothelial cells (e-**Fig. 15.47**). Type II is an aggressive variant now considered to represent angiosarcoma; the neoplastic endothelial cells exhibit multilayering, budding, papillary or solid growth, nuclear pleomorphism and hyperchromasia, and brisk mitotic activity.

  3. Epithelioid hemangioendothelioma is a low- or intermediate-grade malignancy. The tumor cells appear epithelioid (with abundant eosinophilic cytoplasm) or dendritic (stellate and spindle shaped), and are arranged as single cells or small clusters in a dense or myxoid fibrous stroma. Some tumor cells contain an intracytoplasmic vascular lumen simulating signet-ring-cell carcinoma (e-**Fig. 15.48**). Sinusoidal growth of the tumor cells at the periphery of the lesion is also characteristic, often accompanied by hepatocyte atrophy. The tumor may also grow into and occlude veins, a finding which should not be confused with veno-occlusive disease. The tumor cells should express at least one endothelial marker such as CD34, CD31, or factor VIII.

4. **Angiosarcoma** is the most common mesenchymal malignancy of the liver. A unique histologic feature of the tumor is a sinusoidal growth pattern by pleomorphic malignant endothelial cells with little stromal response (e-**Fig. 15.49**). Tumors with solid growth may pose diagnostic difficulty, but immunostains can help demonstrate their vascular nature. Kaposi sarcoma consists of a pure spindle-cell proliferation with slitlike spaces containing extravasated red cells, and is almost always seen in human immunodeficiency virus (HIV)-infected patients.

5. **Mesenchymal hamartoma** is an uncommon childhood tumor characterized by a mixture of hepatocytes, bile ducts, stellate mesenchymal cells, blood vessels, and cystic spaces in a loose, edematous, or myxoid stroma (e-**Fig. 15.50**). Rarely, embryonal (undifferentiated) sarcoma arises in this lesion, evidenced by markedly increased cellularity and cytologic features of malignancy.

CYTOLOGY OF THE LIVER
Jing Zhai

I. **INTRODUCTION.** Virtually the only indication for cytological sampling of the liver is the presence of a mass lesion. Mass lesions can be targeted by percutaneous ultrasound or computed tomography (CT)-guided fine needle aspiration (FNA); lesions in the left lobe can be aspirated by endoscopic ultrasound-guided FNA (EUS-FNA) (*Gastrointest Endosc* 2002;55:859). Liver FNA is a very safe procedure; fatal complications are rare, occurring at a rate of 0.006% to 0.031% (*Radiology* 1991;178:253), and most are associated with hemorrhage. The sensitivity for malignancy ranges from 76% to 95%, and specificity is close to 100% (*Diagn Cytopathol* 2002;26:283 and *Diagn Cytopathol* 2000;23:326).

II. **HEPATIC ABSCESS.** The aspirate of a pyogenic abscess shows abundant neutrophils and necrotic debris (e-**Fig. 15.51**). Amebic abscesses contain more necrotic debris and fewer inflammatory cells. Culture and special stains are usually necessary to identify microorganisms (e-**Fig. 15.52**). For cases of suspected abscess, it is always necessary to rule out the presence of a necrotic, infected neoplasm by extensive sampling and careful cytological evaluation.

III. **HYDATID CYST.** The aspirated cyst fluid can be clear or turbid. Laminated cyst walls, scolices, and hooklets are observed. Neutrophils can be present. Although aspiration of a hydatid cyst poses a risk of anaphylactic reaction, successful procedures are the norm (*Diagn Cytopathol* 1995;12:173).

IV. **HEMANGIOMA.** The aspirate usually shows abundant blood. Scattered stromal fragments with bland elongated spindle cells are characteristic (*Diagn Cytopathol* 1998; 19:250). Cell block preparations are helpful to identify the vascular channels.

V. **FNH.** The aspirate shows both abundant benign hepatocytes and benign biliary epithelial cells (*Acta Cytol* 1989;33:857). Clinical and radiological correlation is necessary.

VI. **HEPATOCELLULAR ADENOMA.** The aspirate contains abundant benign hepatocytes without biliary epithelial cells (*Acta Cytol* 1989;33:857). Clinical and radiological correlation is necessary.

VII. **HCC.** The most characteristic and specific features are thickened hepatocyte trabeculae rimmed by spindle-shaped endothelial cells (e-**Fig. 15.53**), hepatocyte tissue fragments with well-defined traversing capillaries (e-**Fig. 15.54**), increased cellular nucleus/cytoplasm (N/C) ratio (e-**Fig. 15.55**), and frequent atypical naked nuclei (e-**Fig. 15.56**) (*Diagn Cytopathol* 1999;21:370 and *Cancer* 1999;87:270). Poorly differentiated HCC demonstrates loose nests, three-dimensional fragments, and occasional glandlike structures of malignant hepatocytes with marked pleomorphism, macronucleoli, necrosis, and numerous mitoses (*Cancer* 2004;102:247). Features that favor hepatocyte origin include polygon-shaped cells with centrally placed nuclei, abundant granular cytoplasm, and bile pigment (e-**Fig. 15.56**); however, distinction from cholangiocarcinoma and metastatic adenocarcinoma is challenging and may require immunostains.

The fibrolamellar variant of HCC has a distinct cytomorphology that includes poorly cohesive clusters of cells and singly dispersed large monotonous cells with abundant granular cytoplasm, a low N/C ratio, prominent nucleoli, and intracytoplasmic hyaline globules. Fragments of lamellar collagen bands with benign, spindle-shaped cells are present. The thickened trabeculae are not identified (*Diagn Cytopathol* 1999;21:180).

VIII. CHOLANGIOCARCINOMA. The aspirate is composed of crowded sheets of cells, three-dimensional clusters of cells, acinar structures, and singly dispersed cells. The malignant cells show a high N/C ratio, irregular nuclear membranes, prominent nucleoli, and occasional intracytoplasmic mucin (*Cancer* 2005;105:220) (e-**Figs. 15.57** and **15.58**). Poorly differentiated carcinoma displays marked nuclear pleomorphism and necrosis.

IX. EPITHELIOID HEMANGIOENDOTHELIOMA. The aspirate is paucicellular, containing single cells and small tissue fragments. Cytomorphology displays a spectrum of small, bland appearing epithelioid and spindle cells, to malignant large tumor cells. The epithelioid cells have abundant cytoplasm and may contain characteristic intracytoplasmic lumens or sharply defined intranuclear cytoplasmic inclusions.

X. ANGIOSARCOMA. The aspirate shows abundant blood in which there are loose clusters of cells and isolated cells. The malignant cells are spindle shaped to epithelioid, and have hyperchromatic nuclei and abundant but ill-defined cytoplasm. Necrosis is present. Scattered malignant cells may show hemosiderin-laden cytoplasm or erythrophagocytosis (*Diagn Cytopathol* 1998;18:208).

XI. METASTATIC MALIGNANCY. The most common malignancy that involves the liver is a metastatic tumor from another site. The most common primary tumors that metastasize to the liver are colorectal adenocarcinoma (e-**Fig. 15.59**) and pancreatic adenocarcinoma. Comparison with the primary malignancy in cases of metastases is essential for diagnosis.

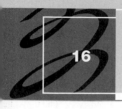

THE GALLBLADDER AND EXTRAHEPATIC BILIARY TREE

16

Hanlin L. Wang

I. NORMAL ANATOMY. The gallbladder is a pear-shaped sac measuring up to 10 cm in length, 3 to 4 cm in width, and 1 to 2 mm in wall thickness. It is divided into the fundus, body, and neck. The free surface of the gallbladder is covered by serosa; at the hepatic bed, the subserosal connective tissue merges with liver parenchyma. The mucosa is usually folded and lined by a single layer of columnar epithelium. The lamina propria consists of loose connective tissue, which usually contains a small number of lymphocytes and plasma cells. Ganglion cells may also be present, which should not be confused with ganglioneuromatosis. There is no muscularis mucosae or submucosa; the muscularis propria layer consists of haphazardly arranged bundles of smooth muscle. Accessory mucous glands are seen only in the neck, typically arranged in a lobular pattern.

The cystic duct connects the gallbladder with other components of the extrahepatic biliary system, including the right, left, and common hepatic ducts and the common bile duct. These ducts are lined by a single layer of columnar cells resting directly on dense connective tissue. The distribution patterns of the smooth muscle fibers vary in different portions of the duct, but they are usually arranged longitudinally and are intermingled with collagen bundles. Small groups of periductal mucous glands are embedded in the connective tissue; the lobular arrangement and lack of cytologic atypia in these mucous glands are useful features to distinguish them from invasive adenocarcinoma, particularly on frozen sections (e-**Fig. 16.1**).*

II. GROSS EXAMINATION AND TISSUE HANDLING

A. Cholecystectomy is most commonly performed for gallstone-related diseases. The gallbladder should be opened longitudinally and promptly fixed in 10% formalin to avoid bile-related autolysis. On gross examination, the length, maximal diameter (or circumference), and wall thickness of the gallbladder, the size of the cystic duct, and the size of cystic duct lymph node (if present) are measured. The appearance of the outer surface and mucosa is described. If stones are present, the approximate number, size range, color, shape, and firmness should be documented. Three full-thickness sections, one each from the fundus, body, and neck, are submitted in one cassette. Additional sections from cystic duct lymph node or any gross lesions are also submitted, if present. If a tumor is grossly identified, the location in the gallbladder, size, and appearance should be recorded, and the serosal surface or hepatic bed over the tumor should be inked and submitted for microscopic examination. If a tumor is identified, the cystic duct margin should also be taken.

B. Biopsy of the bile duct is usually performed for biliary stricture or overt neoplastic lesions during endoscopic retrograde cholangiopancreatography (ERCP). When processing biopsies in the gross room, it is important to record not only pertinent clinical history, but also the endoscopic findings. The biopsies are typically small fragments of mucosal tissue in the range of 1 to 5 mm, and do not need to be inked or cut. Detailed gross descriptions, such as shape and color, are also unnecessary. However, the number of the biopsies should be recorded and the use of "multiple," "many," or "numerous" should be avoided. The dimension of the biopsies should also be documented. This can be done by giving either the size range of the biopsies, the

---

*All e-figures are available online via the Solution Site Image Bank.

greatest dimension of the largest tissue fragment, or the dimensions of the aggregate. Documentation of the number and size is important to ensure that the biopsies are adequately represented on the slides. Three hematoxylin and eosin (H&E)-stained slides are prepared for microscopic examination.

Intraoperative frozen section examination of the bile duct margin on Whipple specimens is also commonly performed.

III. DIAGNOSTIC FEATURES OF NONNEOPLASTIC CONDITIONS

A. Cholecystitis is associated with gallstones (cholelithiasis) in >90% of cases. In acute cholecystitis, the gallbladder is often edematous and congested, with diffuse wall thickening and a serosal exudate. Neutrophilic infiltration may be prominent. Erosion, ulceration, hemorrhage, transmural necrosis (gangrenous cholecystitis), and/or perforation may be seen (e-**Fig. 16.2**).

Chronic cholecystitis is characterized by a variable degree of mononuclear cell infiltration and fibrosis. Intestinal, pyloric, or gastric surface metaplasia, or rarely, squamous metaplasia, may be present. Rokitansky-Aschoff sinuses, which represent herniations or diverticula of the gallbladder mucosa into the muscle layer, may be evident in chronic cholecystitis (e-**Fig. 16.3**). When exaggerated and accompanied by muscular hypertrophy, the herniations develop into an adenomyoma (when localized usually at the fundus); when the process is more diffuse, the herniations develop into adenomyomatosis. Rupture of Rokitansky–Aschoff sinuses, or mucosal ulceration with bile extravasation, may result in accumulation of foamy macrophages to give rise to xanthogranulomatous cholecystis (e-**Fig. 16.4**).

Acalculous cholecystitis may be acute or chronic. The acute form typically occurs in patients with debilitating conditions or systemic infections. The chronic form may exhibit distinct morphologic features, such as eosinophilic cholecystitis (e-**Fig. 16.5**) or follicular cholecystitis (e-**Fig. 16.6**).

B. Cholesterolosis of the gallbladder (strawberry gallbladder) is characterized by linear yellow streaks on gross examination and lipid-laden macrophages in the lamina propria microscopically. Occasionally, the process protrudes focally to form a cholesterol polyp (e-**Fig. 16.7**), which is usually an incidental finding that has no clinical significance and is not associated with hypercholesterolosis.

C. Choledochal cyst is a fusiform or spherical dilatation of the common bile duct. Thorough sampling is recommended (ideally, the entire lesion should be submitted for microscopic examination) because the cyst may harbor dysplasia or invasive adenocarcinoma.

D. Biliary atresia is a congenital anomaly in which the extrahepatic ducts and gallbladder may be completely absent or replaced by fibrous cords with no or only a very small lumen.

E. Primary sclerosing cholangitis involving the extrahepatic biliary system is diagnosed based primarily on cholangiographic findings. Biopsy is seldom diagnostic of sclerosing cholangitis because of the difficulty in assessing the fibrotic region of the duct wall. However, biopsy is still useful to determine if the stricture is associated with a neoplastic process.

F. Secondary sclerosing cholangitis has a variety of etiologies, including obstructive processes, exposure to toxins, ischemia, and infections. Histologic features of sclerosing cholangitis with biliary stricture are also commonly seen in human immunodeficiency virus (HIV)-infected patients (acquired immunodeficiency syndrome [AIDS] cholangiopathy).

IV. DIAGNOSTIC FEATURES OF SELECTED NEOPLASMS.
The current World Health Organization (WHO) histologic classification of tumors of the gallbladder and extrahepatic bile ducts is given in Table 16.1. The 2002 American Joint Committee on Cancer (AJCC) Tumor, Node, Metastasis (TNM) staging schemas are given in Table 16.2 (for gallbladder carcinoma) and Table 16.3 (for carcinoma of the extrahepatic bile ducts).

A. Adenoma is typically a small polypoid lesion that can be divided into tubular, papillary (villous), and tubulopapillary (tubulovillous) patterns architecturally, and pyloric, intestinal, and biliary types cytologically. Adenomas are more common in the gallbladder than in the extrahepatic bile ducts. Adenomas of the gallbladder are

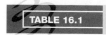 TABLE 16.1	WHO Histologic Classification of Tumors of the Gallbladder and Extrahepatic Bile Ducts

Epithelial tumors
Adenoma
  Tubular
  Papillary
  Tubulopapillary
  Biliary cystadenoma
  Papillomatosis (adenomatosis)
Intraepithelial neoplasia (dysplasia and carcinoma in situ)
Carcinoma
  Adenocarcinoma
  Papillary adenocarcinoma
  Adenocarcinoma, intestinal type
  Adenocarcinoma, gastric foveolar type
  Mucinous adenocarcinoma
  Clear cell adenocarcinoma
  Signet-ring-cell carcinoma
  Adenosquamous carcinoma
  Squamous cell carcinoma
  Small cell carcinoma
  Large cell neuroendocrine carcinoma
  Undifferentiated carcinoma
  Biliary cystadenocarcinoma
Carcinoid tumor
Goblet cell carcinoid
Tubular carcinoid
Mixed carcinoid-adenocarcinoma
Other

Nonepithelial tumors
Granular cell tumor
Leiomyoma
Leiomyosarcoma
Rhabdomyosarcoma
Kaposi sarcoma
Other
Malignant lymphoma

Secondary tumors

From: Hamilton SR, Aaltonen LA, eds. *World Health Organization Classification of Tumours. Pathology and Genetics. Tumours of the Digestive System.* Lyon: IARC Press; 2000. Used with permission.

usually incidental findings, and commonly of pyloric type composed of tightly packed tubular glands similar to pyloric glands. This type of adenoma tends to show insignificant cytologic atypia, seldom harbors high-grade dysplasia or carcinoma, and is sometimes confused with pyloric metaplasia. Adenomas of the extrahepatic bile ducts may cause biliary obstruction and are commonly of intestinal type, closely resembling their colonic counterparts; high-grade dysplasia is frequently present. Papillomatosis or adenomatosis is diagnosed when adenomas are multiple and extensively involve the extrahepatic bile ducts.

B. **Flat dysplasia** (intraepithelial neoplasia) is usually not grossly recognizable. It is characterized by nuclear enlargement and hyperchromasia, with nuclear stratification and loss of nuclear polarity (e-Fig. 16.8). When dysplasia is incidentally detected in a cholecystectomy specimen, multiple sections of the mucosa should be examined; in the case of high-grade dysplasia (carcinoma in situ), the entire gallbladder should

TABLE 16.2	Tumor, Node, Metastasis (TNM) Staging Scheme for Gallbladder Carcinoma

PRIMARY TUMOR (T)

TX	Primary tumor cannot be assessed
T0	No evidence of primary tumor
Tis	Carcinoma in situ
T1	Tumor invades lamina propria or muscle layer
	T1a Tumor invades lamina propria
	T1b Tumor invades muscle layer
T2	Tumor invades perimuscular connective tissue; no extension beyond serosa or into liver
T3	Tumor perforates the serosa (visceral peritoneum) and/or directly invades the liver and/or one other adjacent organ or structure, such as the stomach, duodenum, colon, or pancreas, omentum or extrahepatic bile ducts
T4	Tumor invades main portal vein or hepatic artery or invades multiple extrahepatic organs or structures

REGIONAL LYMPH NODES (N)

NX	Regional lymph nodes cannot be assessed
N0	No regional lymph node metastasis
N1	Regional lymph node metastasis

DISTANT METASTASIS (M)

MX	Distant metastasis cannot be assessed
M0	No distant metastasis
M1	Distant metastasis

STAGE GROUPING

Stage 0	Tis	N0	M0
Stage IA	T1	N0	M0
Stage IB	T2	N0	M0
Stage IIA	T3	N0	M0
Stage IIB	T1	N1	M0
	T2	N1	M0
	T3	N1	M0
Stage III	T4	Any N	M0
Stage IV	Any T	Any N	M1

From: Greene FL, Page DL, Fleming ID, Fritz AG, Balch CM, Haller DG, Morrow M, eds. *AJCC Cancer Staging Manual.* 6th edition. New York: Springer, 2002. Used with permission. (A new AJCC TNM staging system is scheduled for release in 2009; after its publication, the new staging scheme will appear on the website for this book.)

be submitted to rule out invasive carcinoma. The main challenge in the diagnosis of dysplasia is differentiation from the reactive atypia frequently associated with inflammation and ulceration.

C. **Adenocarcinoma of the gallbladder** may infiltrate the wall (mimicking chronic cholecystitis grossly) or grow as an intraluminal polypoid lesion. Microscopically, conventional adenocarcinoma is usually well to moderately differentiated, and characterized by well-formed glands lined by one or more layers of highly atypical cuboidal or columnar cells embedded in a desmoplastic stroma (e-**Fig. 16.9**). Mucin production and perineural invasion are common. Immunohistochemically, these tumors consistently express cytokeratin (CK) 7 and variably express CK20; they are usually immunoreactive for CA19-9 and carcinoembryonic antigen (CEA).

Papillary adenocarcinoma of the gallbladder is characterized by a predominantly papillary architecture. The tumor may fill the gallbladder lumen. It is important to recognize this variant because it tends to be noninvasive or only superficially invasive (e-**Fig. 16.10**), and thus may have a better prognosis. Tumor extension to Rokitansky–Aschoff sinuses should not be interpreted as deep infiltration.

D. **Adenocarcinoma of the extrahepatic bile ducts** (cholangiocarcinoma) develops at any level of the biliary tree, but is most common around the hilum of the liver (Klatskin tumor). The histologic features of the tumor are essentially the same as those

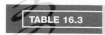

TABLE 16.3	Tumor, Node, Metastasis (TNM) Staging Scheme for Carcinoma of the Extrahepatic Bile Ducts

PRIMARY TUMOR (T)

TX	Primary tumor cannot be assessed
T0	No evidence of primary tumor
Tis	Carcinoma in situ
T1	Tumor confined to the bile duct histologically
T2	Tumor invades beyond the wall of the bile duct
T3	Tumor invades the liver, gallbladder, pancreas, and/or unilateral branches of the portal vein (right or left) or hepatic artery (right or left)
T4	Tumor invades any of the following: main portal vein or its branches bilaterally, common hepatic artery, or other adjacent structures, such as the colon, stomach, duodenum, or abdominal wall

REGIONAL LYMPH NODES (N)

NX	Regional lymph nodes cannot be assessed
N0	No regional lymph node metastasis
N1	Regional lymph node metastasis

DISTANT METASTASIS (M)

MX	Distant metastasis cannot be assessed
M0	No distant metastasis
M1	Distant metastasis

STAGE GROUPING

Stage 0	Tis	N0	M0
Stage IA	T1	N0	M0
Stage IB	T2	N0	M0
Stage IIA	T3	N0	M0
Stage IIB	T1	N1	M0
	T2	N1	M0
	T3	N1	M0
Stage III	T4	Any N	M0
Stage IV	Any T	Any N	M1

From: Greene FL, Page DL, Fleming ID, Fritz AG, Balch CM, Haller DG, Morrow M, eds. *AJCC Cancer Staging Manual*. 6th edition. New York: Springer, 2002. Used with permission. (A new AJCC TNM staging system is scheduled for release in 2009; after its publication, the new staging scheme will appear on the website for this book.)

of adenocarcinoma of the gallbladder. Loss of lobular architecture and high-grade nuclear atypia are useful features to distinguish cholangiocarcinoma from reactive atypia; perineural invasion is an indication of malignancy and is a particularly useful feature when the tumor is well differentiated. For resection specimens, the proximal, distal, and radial (circumferential) margins should be thoroughly evaluated.

CYTOLOGY OF THE GALLBLADDER AND EXTRAHEPATIC BILIARY TREE
Jing Zhai

I. **GALLBLADDER CYTOLOGY.** Cytological sampling of gallbladder mass lesions is not routinely performed, but can be achieved by ultrasound-guided transabdominal fine needle aspiration (FNA) and endoscopic ultrasound–guided FNA (*Diagn Cytopathol* 1998;18:258; *Gastrointest Endosc* 2003;57:251; *Acta Cytol* 1997;41:1654; and *Endoscopy* 2005;37:751). The diagnostic accuracy is 95% (*Acta Cytol* 1997;41:1654).
   A. **Inflammatory lesions. Acute cholecystitis** yields abundant neutrophils and necrotic debris. Bacterial colonies can be seen occasionally. The aspirate of **xanthogranulomatous cholecystitis** exhibits abundant foamy histiocytes and multinucleated giant cells (*Diagn Cytopathol* 1998;18:258).

B. Neoplasms

1. **Adenocarcinoma.** The malignant cells form crowded sheets, microacini, and papillae and exhibit enlarged nuclei, prominent nucleoli, and an irregular nuclear membrane contour. Nuclear pleomorphism and cell dissociation are more abundant in more poorly differentiated tumors. Mucin secretion can be prominent (*Diagn Cytopathol* 1998;18:258).

2. **Squamous cell carcinoma.** The aspirate contains malignant cells with cytoplasmic keratinization and hyperchromatic and pyknotic nuclei. Spindle-shaped fiber cells and tadpole cells are common.

II. **EXTRAHEPATIC BILIARY TREE CYTOLOGY.** The indication for cytological sampling of extrahepatic biliary tract lesions is the presence of a biliary stricture. Biliary brush cytology, obtained by ERCP, has a high specificity (up to 98%) but rather low sensitivity (average of 44%) (*Clin Gastroenterol* 2004;2:209). Endoscopic ultrasound–guided FNA achieves an increased sensitivity (86%) and high specificity (100%) (*Clin Gastroenterol* 2004;2:209).

A. **Reactive atypia.** The cytologic features of reactive ductal epithelial atypia in the presence of a stent include monolayer sheets with minimal nuclear crowding, slightly enlarged nuclei, smooth nuclear membranes, fine chromatin, and small nucleoli. It is important not to overdiagnose reactive atypia as evidence of dysplasia or malignancy.

B. **Dysplasia.** Low-grade dysplasia shows monolayer sheets of cells with slight nuclear crowding, or palisading strips of cells with nuclear pseudostratification. The dysplastic cells have mild to moderate nuclear enlargement, small nucleoli, and smooth nuclear membranes. High-grade dysplasia shows sheets of cells with more prominent nuclear crowding, an increased nuclear/cytoplasmic (N/C) ratio, clumpy chromatin, and prominent nucleoli. Single atypical cells and necrosis are uncommon (*Arch Pathol Lab Med* 2000;124:387). Although criteria for diagnosis of dysplasia have been proposed, they show poor interobserver reproducibility (*Acta Cytol* 1995;39:11).

C. **Adenocarcinoma.** The aspirate is hypercellular. Well-differentiated adenocarcinoma shows crowded sheets with loss of honeycombing. The malignant cells display nuclear enlargement, an increased N/C ratio, nuclear membrane irregularity, clumpy chromatin, and prominent nucleoli (e-**Figs. 16.11** and **16.12**). Poorly differentiated adenocarcinoma exhibits marked nuclear pleomorphism, more individual cells, and necrosis (*Arch Pathol Lab Med* 2000;124:387; *Mod Pathol* 1995;8:498; and *Am J Clin Pathol* 1998;110:635).

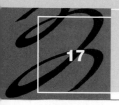

THE PANCREAS
17
Namsoo Suh and Hanlin L. Wang

I. NORMAL ANATOMY. The pancreas is a deep seated retroperitoneal organ ranging 15 to 20 cm in length and 85 to 120 grams in weight in adults. The pancreas shows distinct and uniform lobulation and is divided into four rather indistinct regions: the head (including the uncinate process), neck, body, and tail.

The exocrine component comprises the majority of the pancreatic parenchyma and consists of lobular units of acini. The acinar cells are large and polarized, with basally situated nuclei; the apical cytoplasm is eosinophilic due to the presence of abundant zymogen granules, whereas the basal portion is basophilic and contains abundant rough endoplasmic reticulum. The acini empty into small ducts that merge into the main pancreatic duct of Wirsung and the accessory duct of Santorini. The ductal lining epithelium has a low columnar shape with no detectable cytoplasmic mucin by hematoxylin and eosin (H&E) staining.

The endocrine component, constituting 1% to 2% of the pancreas in adults, is represented mainly by islets of Langerhans that are distributed throughout the pancreas. They contain four major cell types: insulin-secreting β cells (60% to 70%), glucagon-secreting α cells (15% to 20%), somatostatin-secreting δ cells, and pancreatic polypeptide-secreting PP cells.

II. GROSS EXAMINATION AND TISSUE HANDLING

A. Biopsy, fine needle aspiration, and **brushing cytology** specimens may be obtained percutaneously, intraoperatively, or via endoscopic retrograde cholangiopancreatography (ERCP). Needle core biopsies should be immediately fixed in 10% formalin. When processed in the gross room, the number and the length or length range of the biopsies should be recorded. Documentation of the number and length is important to ensure that the biopsies are adequately represented on the slides. Three H&E-stained slides are prepared for microscopic examination.

Aspiration smears are processed with alcohol fixation for Papanicolaou staining or air dried for Diff-Quik staining. Brushings are handled by routine liquid-based cytology methods.

B. Distal pancreatectomy specimens consist of the pancreatic tail (usually with attached spleen) and a portion of the pancreatic body. The specimen is oriented to identify the proximal resection margin and main pancreatic duct. After the dimensions and the surface appearance of the pancreas and the spleen are recorded, the soft tissue margins around the pancreas are inked (use of different colors of ink for different margins is helpful for maintaining specimen orientation microscopically). The pancreas is then serially sectioned into sagittal planes, and the size, location, nature, and relation to margins of the tumor or cyst are described. After fresh tissues are sampled for tumor bank, the specimen is fixed in 10% formalin overnight. Sections from the lesion should include samples that demonstrate the relation of the lesion to margins and uninvolved pancreas. If the pancreatic lesion is cystic and small, it should be submitted in its entirety. For large lesions (e.g., >5 cm), at least one section per centimeter is recommended, which should focus on thickened, solid, or irregular areas. An *en face* section of the proximal pancreatic margin, which may also contain the pancreatic duct margin, is submitted if it has not already been performed as part of an intraoperative frozen section evaluation. A perpendicular section from inked posterior (retroperitoneal) soft tissue margin should also be submitted. One representative section from the spleen is sufficient unless gross abnormalities are detected.

After the above sections are submitted, the peripancreatic and splenic hilar soft tissue is searched for lymph nodes; all identified lymph nodes should be submitted in their entirety for microscopic examination.

C. **The Whipple procedure,** performed for tumors of the pancreatic head, common bile duct, ampullary or periampullary region, involves excision of a composite specimen usually consisting of the pancreatic head, a portion of the common bile duct, the duodenum, the distal stomach, and the gallbladder. The various surgical margins of the pancreas (pancreatic neck, posterior, portal vein groove, and uncinate) are inked with different colors in the operating room with the surgeon's aid; frozen section evaluation of the pancreatic neck and bile duct margins are almost always requested intraoperatively.

After the specimen is properly oriented, the stomach is opened along the greater curvature and the duodenum is opened along the border opposite the pancreas. The dimensions and surface appearance of various organs are recorded. The pancreas may be sectioned along the plane defined by the pancreatic duct and bile duct using probes as a guide, or cut perpendicularly. The size, location, and nature of the tumor are recorded, as is the relation of the tumor to the surgical margins. The specimen is then pinned out and fixed in 10% formalin overnight. In general, one section per centimeter of the tumor is then submitted; if tumor diffusely involves the pancreatic duct and is noninvasive in the initial sections, it is necessary to return to the gross specimen and submit the entire duct to ensure that invasive tumor is not missed. Additional sections should demonstrate the relation of the tumor to the various margins, uninvolved pancreas, ducts, ampulla, duodenum, and soft tissue; one section from the gastric resection margin, one from duodenal resection margin, and one from the gallbladder margin should also be submitted. One section from uninvolved pancreas and one from uninvolved ampulla are also submitted if not already sampled in the tumor sections. All identified lymph nodes in the soft tissue should be submitted for microscopic examination; there is no need to separate the nodes into groups because they are all considered regional. Microscopic examination of a minimum of 10 nodes has been recommended for Whipple specimens.

III. DIAGNOSTIC FEATURES OF NONNEOPLASTIC CONDITIONS

A. **Acute pancreatitis** is most commonly associated with biliary tract disease (such as gallstones) and alcohol abuse. The pancreas is swollen and edematous, and hemorrhagic in more severe cases. Chalky white fat necrosis may be evident. Histologically, mild pancreatitis is characterized by interstitial edema and leukocytic infiltration. The pancreatic parenchyma may be well preserved, with only limited necrosis. In severe cases, extensive necrosis and hemorrhage are seen (e-Fig. 17.1).* Calcification and secondary infection may occur.

B. **Chronic pancreatitis** is also frequently associated with alcoholism and ductal obstruction. A small fraction of the cases may be idiopathic, associated with genetic factors (hereditary pancreatitis), hyperlipidemia, hyperparathyroidism, or autoimmune disorders (autoimmune pancreatitis). Chronic pancreatitis is characterized by acinar atrophy, mixed inflammatory cell infiltrates, and fibrosis with relative sparing of the islets of Langerhans (e-Fig. 17.2). Dilatation of the pancreatic ducts with proteinaceous, often calcified, secretions is characteristic. Preservation of the normal lobular architecture is an important histologic feature to distinguish chronic pancreatitis from infiltrating ductal adenocarcinoma.

Autoimmune pancreatitis is a distinct type of chronic pancreatitis frequently associated with systemic autoimmune diseases, including inflammatory bowel disease and primary sclerosing cholangitis. Autoimmune pancreatitis may mimic pancreatic cancer radiographically and endoscopically when it presents as a mass lesion in the pancreatic head and/or strictures of the pancreatic and common bile ducts. Histologically, autoimmune pancreatitis shares many features of conventional chronic pancreatitis, but is distinguished by the presence of a dense lymphoplasmacytic infiltrate, particularly in the periductal regions (e-Fig. 17.3), and the presence of obliterative phlebitis (e-Fig. 17.4). In addition to various autoantibodies, selective elevation of

---

*All e-figures are available online via the Solution Site Image Bank.

serum immunoglobulin G (IgG) 4 level helps establish the diagnosis (*Arch Pathol Lab Med* 2005;129:1148 and *J Gastroenterol* 2006;41:613). Patients often respond well to steroid therapy.

C. Pseudocyst is the most common cystic lesion of the pancreas and usually develops as a result of pancreatitis or trauma. The cyst is lined by granulation or fibrous tissue but lacks an epithelial lining.

D. Lymphoepithelial cysts are lined by squamous epithelium with abundant underlying lymphocytes that occasionally form germinal centers (**e-Fig. 17.5**).

IV. DIAGNOSTIC FEATURES OF TUMORS OF THE EXOCRINE PANCREAS. The current World Health Organization (WHO) histologic classification of tumors of the exocrine pancreas is given in Table 17.1. The 2002 American Joint Committee on Cancer (AJCC) Tumor, Node, Metastasis (TNM) staging schema is given in Table 17.2.

A. Serous cystadenoma is a benign cystic neoplasm usually found in the body or tail of the pancreas in elderly patients. It is usually multilocular (microcystic cystadenoma), but occasionally unilocular or oligocystic (macrocystic). Grossly, the tumor has a spongy appearance (**e-Fig. 17.6**) with cysts that are filled with clear serous fluid. Frequently there is a stellate scar within the tumor. Microscopically, the individual cysts are lined by a single layer of flat to cuboidal epithelial cells with pale to clear glycogen-rich cytoplasm (**e-Fig. 17.7**).

Serous cystadenocarcinoma is exceedingly rare in the pancreas and is morphologically indistinguishable from serous cystadenoma in reported cases. The diagnosis is established by invasive growth and distal metastasis.

B. Mucinous cystic neoplasms tend to occur in the tail or body of the pancreas in women about 50 years of age. The neoplasm is a solitary, multilocular (rarely unilocular) cystic mass filled with gelatinous mucin (**e-Fig. 17.8**). The cysts typically do not communicate with the ductal system.

Mucinous cystic neoplasms exhibit a spectrum of cytologic and architectural atypia (dysplasia) similar to that seen in their ovarian counterparts. Tumors with no or only mild epithelial atypia are benign, and are termed mucinous cystadenomas. The cyst wall, which may be partially denuded, is lined by tall columnar mucin-producing cells with characteristic underlying ovarian-type stroma (**e-Fig. 17.9**). The

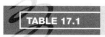

TABLE 17.1	WHO Histologic Classification of Tumors of the Exocrine Pancreas

Epithelial tumors	Undifferentiated carcinoma with
Benign	osteoclastlike giant cells
Serous cystadenoma	Mixed ductal-endocrine carcinoma
Mucinous cystadenoma	Serous cystadenocarcinoma
Intraductal papillary mucinous adenoma	Mucinous cystadenocarcinoma
Mature teratoma	Noninvasive
	Invasive
Borderline (uncertain malignant potential)	Intraductal papillary mucinous carcinoma
Mucinous cystic neoplasm with moderate dysplasia	Noninvasive
	Invasive (papillary mucinous carcinoma)
Intraductal papillary mucinous neoplasm with moderate dysplasia	Acinar cell carcinoma
Solid pseudopapillary neoplasm	Acinar cell cystadenocarcinoma
	Mixed acinar-endocrine carcinoma
Malignant	Pancreatoblastoma
Ductal adenocarcinoma	Solid pseudopapillary carcinoma
Mucinous noncystic carcinoma	Other
Signet-ring-cell carcinoma	
Adenosquamous carcinoma	**Nonepithelial tumors**
Undifferentiated (anaplastic) carcinoma	**Secondary tumors**

From: Hamilton SR, Aaltonen LA, eds. *World Health Organization Classification of Tumours. Pathology and Genetics. Tumours of the Digestive System.* Lyon: IARC Press; 2000. Used with permission.

TABLE 17.2	Tumor, Node, Metastasis (TNM) Staging Scheme for Exocrine Pancreas*

Primary tumor (T)
TX   Primary tumor cannot be assessed
T0   No evidence of primary tumor
Tis   Carcinoma in situ
T1   Tumor limited to the pancreas, ≤2 cm or less in greatest dimension
T2   Tumor limited to the pancreas, >2 cm in greatest dimension
T3   Tumor extends beyond the pancreas but without involvement of the celiac axis or the superior mesenteric artery
T4   Tumor involves the celiac axis or the superior mesenteric artery (unresectable primary tumor)

Regional lymph nodes (N)
NX   Regional lymph nodes cannot be assessed
N0   No regional lymph node metastasis
N1   Regional lymph node metastasis

Distant metastasis (M)
MX   Distant metastasis cannot be assessed
M0   No distant metastasis
M1   Distant metastasis

Stage grouping

Stage 0	Tis	N0	M0
Stage IA	T1	N0	M0
Stage IB	T2	N0	M0
Stage IIA	T3	N0	M0
Stage IIB	T1	N1	M0
	T2	N1	M0
	T3	N1	M0
Stage III	T4	Any N	M0
Stage IV	Any T	Any N	M1

*Endocrine tumors arising from the islets of Langerhans and carcinoid tumors are not included.
From: Greene FL, Page DL, Fleming ID, Fritz AG, Balch CM, Haller DG, Morrow M, eds. *AJCC Cancer Staging Manual.* 6th edition. New York: Springer, 2002. Used with permission. (A new AJCC TNM staging system is scheduled for release in 2009; after its publication, the new staging scheme will appear on the website for this book.)

stromal cells are frequently positive for estrogen and progesterone receptors and inhibin, and can be luteinized. Interestingly, ovarian-type stroma is also seen in tumors occurring in male patients. Tumors with moderate dysplasia are borderline mucinous cystic neoplasms, and those with severe dysplasia or carcinoma in situ are noninvasive mucinous cystadenocarcinomas. Severe dysplasia is characterized by papillary, cribriform, branching, and budding growth patterns, marked nuclear stratification and atypia, mucin depletion, and frequent mitosis (e-**Fig. 17.10**); the prognosis is excellent for noninvasive tumors regardless of the degree of cytologic atypia if the tumor is completely resected. Invasive mucinous cystadenocarcinoma is characterized by invasion of malignant glands into the stroma, and the tumor may resemble conventional ductal adenocarcinoma histologically. Mucinous tumors of large size, with papillary excrescences, or areas of solid growth have an increased likelihood of malignancy, and extensive or complete sampling of these tumors is critical in the identification of small foci of invasive carcinoma.

C. **Intraductal papillary mucinous neoplasms (IPMNs)** arise in the main pancreatic duct or its major branches, typically in the head of the pancreas. The involved ducts are often cystically dilated and contain copious amounts of mucin, which may be detected at the ampulla of Vater by endoscopy. An IPMN is classified as an adenoma, borderline tumor, or as carcinoma in situ based on the degree of cytoarchitectural atypia by criteria that are similar to those for mucinous cystic neoplasms. Typically, the papillary fronds are lined by mucin-producing columnar cells (e-**Fig. 17.11**) with

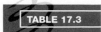

TABLE 17.3	Distinction Between Intraductal Papillary Mucinous Neoplasm (IPMN) and Mucinous Cystic Neoplasm (MCN)	
Features	**IPMN**	**MCN**
Patient population	Older women and men	Predominantly middle-aged women
Location in pancreas	Head	Tail or body
Communication with ductal system	Yes	No
Ovarian-type stroma	No	Yes

occasional Paneth and goblet cells. Tumor extension into smaller branches and mucin extravasation into surrounding parenchyma may simulate invasive carcinoma, and examination of deeper levels may be necessary to clarify classification. Similar to mucinous cystic neoplasms, IPMNs should be extensively (or, ideally, completely) submitted for histologic examination to rule out focal invasion (papillary mucinous carcinoma) because the presence or absence of invasive carcinoma is the most important prognostic factor. Invasive carcinoma is present in about one third of the cases, and may be mucinous or of conventional ductal morphology. IPMN should be distinguished from mucinous cystic neoplasm (Table 17.3).

Intraductal oncocytic papillary neoplasm (IOPN) is a recently described variant of IPMN. It is characterized by oncocytic cells, more architectural complexity and cytologic atypia, and intraepithelial lumina (e-**Fig. 17.12**).

D. Solid-pseudopapillary neoplasm is most commonly seen in young women of child-bearing age. This tumor can be quite large at the time of diagnosis but is typically well demarcated and encapsulated; grossly, it exhibits variable solid and cystic areas with hemorrhage and necrosis. Microscopically, solid-pseudopapillary neoplasm is a cellular neoplasm consisting of sheets of small, relatively uniform tumor cells, sometimes surrounding delicate, often hyalinized, fibrovascular stroma to form pseudopapillae (e-**Fig. 17.13**). The tumor cells have eosinophilic or clear vacuolated cytoplasm, indented or grooved nuclei, and inconspicuous nucleoli (e-**Fig. 17.14**). Intra- and extracellular eosinophilic, diastase-resistant periodic acid–Schiff (PAS)-positive hyaline globules may be evident. Foamy cells, cells with cholesterol crystals, and foreign body giant cells may be present within the tumor. In necrotic areas, the tumor cells lose their cohesiveness and may undergo cystic degeneration. Mitotic figures are rare.

Patients with solid-pseudopapillary neoplasm usually have an excellent prognosis if the tumor is completely excised. However, rare malignant cases have been reported; these cases are characterized by unequivocal perineural invasion, venous invasion, invasion into surrounding soft tissue, a high nuclear grade, a high mitotic count, and metastasis. In general, solid-pseudopapillary neoplasm is regarded as a low-grade malignancy.

The most frequently positive immunomarkers in solid-pseudopapillary neoplasm are vimentin, neuron-specific enolase (NSE), α_1-antitrypsin, α_1-antichymotrypsin, progesterone receptor, CD10, and nuclear β-catenin. The expression of epithelial and neuroendocrine markers is highly variable (*Am J Surg Pathol* 2000; 24:1361). Positive CD10 and nuclear β-catenin stains are useful in the distinction from pancreatic endocrine neoplasms (PENs).

E. Acinar cell carcinoma accounts for 1% to 2% of exocrine pancreatic neoplasms. The tumor usually occurs in late adulthood, but can be seen in children. Approximately 15% of the patients develop a lipase hypersecretion syndrome characterized by extrapancreatic fat necrosis, polyarthralgia, and peripheral eosinophilia.

Acinar cell carcinoma frequently presents as a well-circumscribed mass with or without necrosis and cystic degeneration. Microscopically, tumor cells are arranged in acinar or solid patterns and typically lack desmoplastic stroma (e-**Fig. 17.15**). The individual tumor cells typically have basally located nuclei, single prominent nucleoli, and moderate amounts of amphophilic or eosinophilic granular cytoplasm (e-**Fig. 17.16**). Mitotic activity and nuclear pleomorphism are variable. Most acinar cell carcinomas are composed of cells that contain zymogen granules in their cytoplasm, which can be demonstrated by PAS stain with diastase or by electron microscopy. The tumor cells also exhibit abundant rough endoplasmic reticulum by electron microscopy.

Immunohistochemically, the tumor cells are reactive to antibodies against trypsin, chymotrypsin, and lipase. Approximately one third of the tumors also express neuroendocrine markers, such as chromogranin or synaptophysin, usually in only a small portion of the cells. If >25% of the tumor cells show neuroendocrine differentiation by immunostains, the tumor should be designated as a mixed acinar–endocrine carcinoma.

F. **Ductal adenocarcinoma** accounts for 85% to 90% of pancreatic neoplasms and is most frequently found in the head of the pancreas in patients 60 to 80 years of age. Numerous genetic alterations have been detected in this tumor, including activation of the *K-ras* oncogene by point mutations in >90% of cases, Her2/neu overexpression in 70% of cases, and inactivation of the tumor suppressor genes *TP53* and *DPC4* in more than one half of cases. The prognosis is extremely poor in most cases, with an overall 5-year survival rate of <5%. Grossly, ductal adenocarcinoma is usually poorly demarcated, firm, and yellowish grey or white due to its infiltrative growth and strong desmoplasia.

Most tumors are well to moderately differentiated, and are characterized by glandular structures haphazardly distributed in desmoplastic stroma (e-Fig. 17.17). In well-differentiated tumors, the neoplastic glands are well formed and usually large or medium sized; however, the neoplastic glands may show rupture or are incomplete, features that are not observed in normal ducts. Mucin production may be evident. The most important histologic features that can be used to distinguish well-differentiated adenocarcinoma from chronic pancreatitis are a haphazard growth pattern (Table 17.4), perineural invasion (e-Fig. 17.18), vascular invasion, and close approximation to muscular vasculature (e-Fig. 17.19).

The neoplastic glands in moderately differentiated adenocarcinoma are often incompletely formed, of medium size, or tubular. Cribriform and papillary growth patterns are not uncommon (e-Fig. 17.20). Mitotic activity is more brisk and nuclear pleomorphism is more prominent, with nuclear sizes varying by > 3:1 in the same glands. Mucin production is usually decreased.

In poorly differentiated adenocarcinoma, the tumor cells form solid sheets or nests, or infiltrate as single individual cells. Neoplastic glands, if present, are typically small and irregular. Tumor cells exhibit marked nuclear pleomorphism and a high mitotic count. There is usually little mucin production.

The majority of pancreatic ductal adenocarcinomas are immunohistochemically positive for pancytokeratin (CK) (AE1/AE3), CK7, CK19, carcinoembryonic antigen (CEA), CA19-9, MUC1, MUC4, MUC5AC, claudin-4, cyclooxygenase (COX)-2, mesothelin, and KOC (K homology domain containing protein overexpressed in cancer). These markers may be useful in distinguishing ductal from nonductal pancreatic neoplasms, but are less useful in separating from adenocarcinomas of nonpancreatic origins.

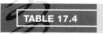

TABLE 17.4	Distinction Between Ductal Adenocarcinoma and Chronic Pancreatitis	
Features	**Ductal adenocarcinoma**	**Chronic pancreatitis**
Histologic pattern	Haphazard	Lobular
Ruptured or incomplete glands	Yes	No
Companion muscular vessel	Yes	No
Nuclear pleomorphism	>3:1 in the same glands	Insignificant
Perineural invasion	Yes	No
Angioinvasion	Yes	No
Mitosis	Frequent	Infrequent

G. Variants of ductal adenocarcinoma

1. **Ductal adenocarcinoma** frequently displays focal squamous differentiation. If the squamous component exceeds 30% of the tumor volume, a diagnosis of **adenosquamous carcinoma** is made, although this diagnosis does not alter the clinical outcome of the patient.

2. **Mucinous noncystic carcinoma** (colloid carcinoma) is often associated with IPMN or mucinous cystic neoplasm, and is believed to have a better prognosis than conventional ductal adenocarcinoma. Histologically, this tumor is similar to mucinous carcinoma in other locations and is defined by >50% of the tumor consisting of mucin.

3. **Signet-ring-cell carcinoma** is a rare variant with an extremely poor prognosis; a metastasis from the stomach should always be investigated.

4. **Undifferentiated carcinoma** exhibits little epithelial differentiation histologically, but some or most of the tumor cells express cytokeratins by immunohistochemistry; the tumor cells usually also express vimentin. This tumor is essentially indistinguishable from a sarcoma and has been variably termed anaplastic, sarcomatoid, spindle cell, pleomorphic large cell, and giant cell carcinoma (**e-Fig. 17.21**).

5. **Undifferentiated carcinoma with osteoclastlike giant cells,** which should be separated from undifferentiated carcinoma, may have a more favorable prognosis. This tumor is characterized by the presence of nonneoplastic osteoclastlike giant cells, which are histiocytic in origin, within the tumor (**e-Fig. 17.22**).

H. Pancreatic intraepithelial neoplasia. Proliferative epithelial changes are frequently encountered in small-caliber ducts adjacent to carcinoma. These proliferative changes are believed to be neoplastic based on molecular studies, and so are regarded as precursor lesions. A new nomenclature of pancreatic intraepithelial neoplasia (PanIN) has been introduced to describe the entire spectrum of epithelial changes in the small ducts (*Am J Surg Pathol* 2001;25:579) based on the degree of architectural and cytologic atypia (Table 17.5). A further description of PanIN, as well as numerous examples of PanIN, can be found at http://162.129.103.56/N/n.web?EP=N&URL=/MCGI/SEND`WEBUTLTY(12774)/526590275.

PanIN-1A includes flat epithelial lesions without atypia, such as mucinous hyperplasia and pyloric metaplasia. It is composed of tall columnar cells with small and round to oval, basally located nuclei with abundant supranuclear mucin (**e-Fig. 17.23**). The neoplastic nature of many cases of PanIN-1A has not been established.

PanIN-1B is an intraductal epithelial lesion that has a papillary, micropapillary, or basally pseudostratified architecture, but is otherwise identical to PanIN-1A (**e-Fig. 17.24**).

PanIN-2 may be flat but is usually papillary. By definition, these lesions must have some degree of architectural and cytologic atypia, such as nuclear crowding, enlargement, pseudostratification and hyperchromatism, and loss of nuclear polarity.

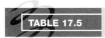

TABLE 17.5	Pancreatic Intraepithelial Neoplasias (PanIN) and Corresponding Older Synonyms

Squamous metaplasia: Epidermoid metaplasia, multilayered metaplasia

PanIN-1A: Pyloric gland metaplasia, goblet cell metaplasia, mucinous hypertrophy, mucinous ductal hyperplasia, mucinous cell hyperplasia, mucoid transformation, simple hyperplasia, flat duct lesion without atypia, flat ductal hyperplasia, ductal hyperplasia grade 1, nonpapillary epithelial hypertrophy, nonpapillary ductal hyperplasia

PanIN-1B: Papillary hyperplasia, papillary ductal hyperplasia, papillary ductal lesion without atypia, ductal hyperplasia grade 2, adenomatous ductal hyperplasia, adenomatoid hyperplasia

PanIN-2: Atypical hyperplasia, papillary duct lesion with atypia, low-grade dysplasia, any PanIN lesions with moderate dysplasia

PanIN-3: Carcinoma in situ, intraductal carcinoma, severe ductal dysplasia, high-grade dysplasia, ductal hyperplasia grade 3, atypical hyperplasia

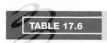

TABLE 17.6	Distinction Between Pancreatic Intraepithelial Neoplasias (PanIN) and Intraductal Papillary Mucinous Neoplasm (IPMN)		
Features	**PanIN**		**IPMN**
Radiographically detectable	No		Yes
Grossly visible	No		Yes
Grossly visible mucin	No		Yes
Size of involved duct	Usually <5 mm		Usually >10 mm
Well-formed papillae	No		Yes
Association with colloid carcinoma	No		Yes

Mitotic figures are rare and not atypical. This category represents low-grade dysplasia, and the degree of atypia is insufficient for the diagnosis of PanIN-3.

PanIN-3 is usually papillary or micropapillary, and is only rarely flat. It is a high-grade intraductal lesion and synonymous with carcinoma in situ. True cribriforming, budding or tufting of small clusters of epithelial cells into the lumen, and luminal necroses should all suggest the diagnosis of PanIN-3. Cytologically, these lesions are characterized by the loss of nuclear polarity, dystrophic goblet cells, abnormal mitoses, nuclear irregularities, and prominent nucleoli (e-**Fig. 17.25**).

PanIN should not be confused with IPMN, particularly when IPMN extends into small branches (Table 17.6). PanIN is a microscopic lesion typically occurring in ducts <5 mm in diameter; in contrast, IPMN is a grossly visible lesion usually involving ducts >10 mm in diameter (*Am J Surg Pathol* 2004;28:977).

On frozen section of pancreatic margins, PanIN-3 lesions should be reported, but the significance of lower grade PanIN in this context has not been established. However, if the preoperative diagnosis or intraoperative findings suggest IPMN, the presence of PanIN-1 and PanIN-2 lesions should be reported because of the difficulty in differentiating low-grade PanIN from small duct extension by IPMN on frozen sections.

I. Pancreatoblastoma is the most common pancreatic neoplasm of childhood, usually occurring in the first decade of life (mean age: 4 years), although the neoplasm also rarely occurs in adults. Interestingly, the prognosis is very good for pediatric patients in the absence of metastasis, but poor for adults. Pancreatoblastoma is a highly cellular tumor composed of sheets or islands of small monotonous cells divided by cellular stromal bands. The tumor cells may exhibit acinar differentiation and form small acinar lumina, although a lesser degree of endocrine and ductal differentiation may also be seen. A histologic hallmark of pancreatoblastoma is the presence of squamoid corpuscles, which are present in virtually every case (e-**Fig. 17.26**); they serve as a useful feature to distinguish the tumor from other pancreatic neoplasms, particularly acinar cell carcinoma. Squamoid corpuscles consist of an aggregate of plump epithelioid cells, a whorled nest of spindle cells, or a cluster of frankly keratinized squamous cells, and are usually located in the center of the tumor lobules. The cells forming the squamoid corpuscle are usually larger than surrounding tumor cells. The stroma in pancreatoblastoma can also be neoplastic in appearance and may contain heterologous elements such as bone and cartilage.

V. DIAGNOSTIC FEATURES OF PANCREATIC ENDOCRINE NEOPLASMS (PENs).
Most PENs are well or moderately differentiated (differentiated PENs), and are traditionally divided into functional (syndromic) and nonfunctional (nonsyndromic) categories. Functional tumors produce clinical symptoms corresponding to the hormones they produce, which allows their clinical diagnosis even when they are small in size. Among this group, insulinoma is the most common type, and is benign in 90% to 95% of the cases; in contrast, gastrinoma, glucagonoma, somatostatinoma, and VIPoma tend to be malignant. Nonfunctioning PENs are usually larger in size when first diagnosed, probably because they do not produce clinical syndromes. A PEN <0.5 cm in maximal dimension is called a microadenoma by convention, and is almost always an incidental finding and clinically benign. In some cases, differentiated PENs are part of the multiple endocrine neoplasia type I (MEN I) syndrome.

Differentiated PENs are well circumscribed, soft, homogeneous, yellow to pink lesions. Cystic spaces may be present in some cases. The tumor cells are uniformly round with "salt and pepper" chromatin and a moderate amount of cytoplasm. The cells are arranged in trabecular, gyriform, acinar, rosettelike, or solid patterns with a rich vasculature. Hyalinized fibrovascular stroma, sometimes with amyloid deposition, is characteristic (e-Fig. 17.27). Psammoma bodies may be seen, particularly in somatostatinomas. Immunohistochemically, PENs typically show diffuse and strong staining for neuroendocrine markers such as synaptophysin, chromogranin, NSE, and CD56. Immunostaining for various pancreatic peptides is mainly of academic interest because functional tumors are defined by clinical syndromes rather than by immunohistochemical findings. Nonfunctional tumors may stain positive for one or more peptides, but detection of peptides does not have prognostic value.

An important issue in the diagnosis of PENs is determination of their malignant potential. In addition to the types of syndromes the tumors produce, malignancy is also defined by vascular invasion, extrapancreatic invasion, and distal metastasis (usually to lymph nodes and liver). Tumor size >2 cm, a mitotic rate of >2 mitoses per 10 high-power fields, and a Ki-67 labeling index >2% are also features suggestive of malignancy.

Poorly differentiated (undifferentiated or high-grade) pancreatic neuroendocrine tumors include small cell carcinoma and large cell neuroendocrine carcinoma. These extremely rare tumors are morphologically similar to their counterparts in the lungs, so metastasis should be excluded before a pancreatic primary is diagnosed. Another related rare tumor, primitive neuroectodermal tumor (PNET), can also occur in the pancreas and typically expresses CD99.

CYTOLOGY OF THE PANCREAS
Jing Zhai

I. **INTRODUCTION.** The indications for cytological sampling of the pancreas include the presence of a solid mass, common bile duct stricture, or cystic lesion. Percutaneous ultrasound, computed tomography (CT)-guided fine needle aspiration (FNA), or endoscopic ultrasound (EUS)-guided FNA are most often used to target the lesion, although common bile duct brushing via ERCP is occasionally performed to evaluate common bile duct strictures (*Endoscopy* 1993;25:143). Brushing cytology for malignancy has high specificity (98%) but only modest sensitivity (44% to 72%) (*Acta Cytol* 1995;39:11 and *Gastrointest Endosc* 1996;44:300). Percutaneous image- and EUS-guided FNA demonstrate high sensitivity and specificity for solid masses (EUS-FNA: 92% sensitivity and 100% specificity; percutaneous FNA: 98% sensitivity and 100% specificity) (*Gastrointest Endosc* 1997;45:387 and *Diagn Cytopathol* 1998;19:423); however, the performance of EUS-FNA for cystic lesions is poor due to sampling errors (56% sensitivity and 45% specificity) (*Gastroentrol* 2004;126:1330). The most common diagnostic pitfall for EUS-FNA is contamination by normal gastrointestinal surface epithelial cells and luminal mucin.

II. **REACTIVE LESIONS.** Aspiration of **acute pancreatitis**, which is rarely performed, shows abundant necrotic debris, neutrophils, macrophages, fat necrosis, and a variable number of ductal epithelial cells with degenerative changes and reactive atypia. **Chronic pancreatitis** is more frequently aspirated due to its clinical similarity to adenocarcinoma; the aspirate contains lymphocytes, neutrophils, a variable number of ductal and acinar cells, and debris; the reactive ductal epithelial cells may show nuclear enlargement, mild hyperchromasia, prominent nucleoli, and mitosis. The distinction between reactive ductal epithelial cells and well-differentiated adenocarcinoma can be difficult; in general, reactive ductal epithelial cells retain smooth nuclear membrane contours, cell cohesion, and form two-dimensional cohesive sheets with rare single atypical cells (*Diagn Cytopathol* 2005;32:65).

III. **NEOPLASMS**
   A. **Ductal adenocarcinoma**
      1. **The minimal diagnostic criteria** for well-differentiated adenocarcinoma include sheets of ductal epithelial cells with nuclear crowding, overlapping, and loss of a honeycombing pattern; three-dimensional clusters of atypical cells; and anisonucleosis, nuclear membrane irregularity, and nuclear enlargement (e-Fig. 17.28).

Poorly differentiated adenocarcinoma usually shows more nuclear pleomorphism, single malignant cells, clumpy chromatin, and necrosis (e-**Fig. 17.29**) (*Cancer* 2003;99:44; *Acta Cytol* 1995;39:1; and *Cancer* 2002;96:362).

2. **Adenosquamous carcinoma** shows both squamous differentiation (cytoplasmic keratinization) (e-**Fig. 17.30**) and glandular differentiation (acinar structures and mucin production) (*Cancer* 2003;99:372).

3. **Mucinous noncystic adenocarcinoma** shows malignant ductal epithelial cells and abundant extracellular mucin. Distinction from mucinous cystadenocarcinoma and intraductal papillary mucinous carcinoma is impossible on cytology material alone (*Cancer* 2004;102:92).

4. **Undifferentiated (anaplastic) carcinoma** demonstrates poorly cohesive clusters of cells and singly dispersed bizarre malignant cells with marked atypia. Multinucleated tumor giant cells and malignant spindle cells are common (e-**Fig. 17.31**) (*Am J Clin Pathol* 1988;89:714).

B. **Pancreatic endocrine tumor.** The aspirate is hypercellular and composed mainly of isolated and poorly cohesive clusters of uniform cells with small round nuclei, small nucleoli, finely granular and evenly distributed salt-and-pepper chromatin, and moderate amounts of granular cytoplasm (e-**Figs. 17.32** and **17.33**). Plasmacytoid cells with eccentrically located nuclei (e-**Fig. 17.32**), spindle-shaped cells, binucleated cells, and focal atypia are frequently seen (*Diagn Cytopathol* 1996;15:37 and *Diagn Cytopathol* 1997;16:112).

C. **Acinar cell carcinoma.** The aspirate shows loosely cohesive clusters of cells and an increased number of single cells. The neoplastic cells have uniform nuclei, an increased nuclear/cytoplasmic (N/C) ratio, prominent nucleoli, and finely granular cytoplasm (*Diagn Cytopathol* 1997;16:112).

D. **Solid-pseudopapillary neoplasm.** The aspirate is richly cellular, composed of branching papillary structures with central fibrovascular cores, poorly cohesive clusters of cells, and isolated single cells. The neoplastic cells show uniform round nuclei, nuclear grooves, finely granular chromatin, small nucleoli, and poorly defined pale cytoplasm (e-**Fig. 17.34**). Hyaline globules surrounded by neoplastic cells are frequently identified (e-**Fig. 17.35**). Degenerative changes, such as foamy histiocytes, multinucleated giant cells, and debris, are frequently present (e-**Fig. 17.36**) (*Diagn Cytopathol* 2002;27:325).

IV. **CYSTIC LESIONS.** The cytological findings are more suggestive than definitive; false-negative diagnoses are not uncommon due to sampling errors. If EUS-FNA is performed, the distinction among serous cystadenoma, mucinous cystic neoplasm, IPMN, and contaminating gastrointestinal epithelium and mucin is very difficult if not impossible (*Am J Clin Pathol* 2003;120:398).

A. **Pseudocyst.** The aspirate yields turbid watery fluid. It is sparsely cellular, and contains debris, foamy histiocytes, and scattered lymphocytes without ductal epithelial cells (e-**Fig. 17.37**).

B. **Serous cystadenoma.** The aspirated fluid is thin, watery, and proteinaceous. The specimen shows scant cellularity, with rare two-dimensional sheets and small groups of uniform cells with minimal atypia and a moderate amount of cytoplasm with occasional clearing or vacuolization (e-**Fig. 17.38**). Microfragments of acellular fibrovascular stroma are occasionally seen (*Cancer* 2004;102:288).

C. **Mucinous cystic neoplasm.** The aspirate shows singly dispersed, small clusters and flat sheets of columnar mucinous cells in a background of foamy histiocytes and abundant extracellular mucin (e-**Fig. 17.39**). The neoplastic cells exhibit a spectrum of cytological atypia; Benign, dysplastic, and frankly malignant epithelial cells are identified in cystadenoma, borderline neoplasm, and cystadenocarcinoma, respectively (*Cancer* 2004;102:92 and *Arch Pathol Lab Med* 1991;115:571).

D. **IPMN.** The aspirate displays papillary arrangements and flat sheets of tall columnar cells with goblet cell morphology that is characterized by intracellular mucin and basally located nuclei. The neoplastic cells exhibit a spectrum of cytological atypia; benign, dysplastic, and frankly malignant epithelial cells are identified in adenoma, borderline neoplasm, and carcinoma, respectively (*Cancer* 2004;102:92 and *Arch Pathol Lab Med* 1991;115:571). There are foamy histiocytes and abundant extracellular mucin in the background (e-**Fig. 17.40**).

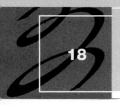

THE BREAST
Omar Hameed

18

I. NORMAL MICROSCOPIC ANATOMY. The breast represents a modified skin adnexal structure composed of major lactiferous ducts that originate from the nipple and progressively branch. In postpubertal women, these ducts end in terminal duct lobular units (TDLUs), from which most pathological processes are thought to arise. The TDLUs are composed of lobules, which are groups of alveolar glands embedded in loose intralobular connective tissue that connect to a single terminal lobular duct (e-**Fig. 18.1**)* (Mills SE, ed. *Histology for Pathologists*, 2nd ed. Philadelphia: Lippincott Williams & Wilkins; 2007). The lining throughout the duct/lobular system of the breast is composed of two distinct layers: an inner (luminal) epithelial layer, and an outer (basal) myoepithelial layer (e-**Fig. 18.2**). Identification of these two layers is very important in the assessment of breast lesions as they are almost always preserved in benign lesions, as well as in noninvasive malignant lesions. Immunohistochemistry can also be used toward this end as myoepithelial cells are usually positive for S-100 protein, actin, calponin, p63, CD10, and high-molecular-weight cytokeratins such as CK5/6, CK14, and CK17, whereas luminal cells express low-molecular-weight cytokeratins including CK7, CK8, and CK18 (e-**Fig. 18.3**). In addition, a proportion of luminal epithelial cells almost always expresses estrogen and/or progesterone receptors. The intralobular stroma is sharply demarcated from a denser, collagenized paucicellular interlobular stroma and stromal adipose tissue. The proportion of dense stroma to adipose tissue is variable, with younger women having denser connective tissue (which explains why mammography is less sensitive in younger individuals). During pregnancy, there is a progressive increase in both the number and size of TDLUs, and by late pregnancy, lobular myoepithelial cells become inconspicuous while the cytoplasm of the luminal epithelium becomes vacuolated as secretions accumulate in the expanded lobules. These florid changes, including the frequent presence of luminal cells with atypical nuclei protruding into the lumen (hobnail cells), can be alarming to the inexperienced observer (e-**Fig. 18.4**). In contrast, due to lack of hormonal stimulation, TDLUs do not develop to a significant extent in men, and lobular acini cannot usually be seen.

II. SPECIMEN PROCESSING
A. Importance of clinical presentation. Most patients with breast pathology present with a clinically or radiologically detected mass and/or a mammographically detected abnormality, most often in the form of microcalcification. Pain, skin and nipple abnormalities, and nipple discharge are less common presentations, but can help narrow the differential diagnosis. The manner of presentation often dictates the approach to specimen processing.
B. Gross examination and tissue sampling. Because most breast specimens lack natural anatomical landmarks, careful specimen processing, especially margin assessment, is crucial for accurate pathological interpretation. In addition, because of the importance of pathological–radiological correlation, evaluation of specimen radiographs represents an integral part of examination of breast specimens. Review of specimen radiographs can provide valuable information as to the nature (ill-defined vs. well-defined mass; microcalcification; both) (e-**Fig. 18.5**) and location of the lesion(s) present, including provisional information about margin status (obviously limited to only four margins in two-dimensional radiographs). This information is

---

*All e-figures are available online via the Solution Site Image Bank.

useful at the time of gross examination and is essential for planning sectioning of the specimen, as well as for estimating the number of sections needed to adequately sample the lesion or a specific margin. It should be noted that even examination of radiographs of needle core biopsy specimens can be useful to determine the amount and size of microcalcifications present in these specimens, as such an examination may influence the decision to subsequently radiograph the paraffin block and/or examine further sections when no such microcalcifications are seen in the initial set of slides. Accordingly, specimen radiographs, when available, should always be submitted with the specimen(s) to be reviewed by the pathologist. Most breast specimens received for pathological evaluation are in one of the following forms:

1. **Needle core biopsies.** These have almost totally replaced fine needle aspiration biopsy specimens for the initial pathological evaluation of localized breast lesions. The size of these specimens ranges from the 14-gauge (or sometimes 18-gauge) needle core samples obtained directly or with ultrasound guidance from mass and mass-like lesions, to larger 11-gauge (and more recently 9-gauge) needle core specimens obtained through vacuum–assisted stereotactic biopsy devices (such as the Mammotome) for mammographically detected abnormalities.

   After describing the shape, size, and color of the tissue cores, they should be aligned in parallel and placed in the cassette between two sponges (preferable) or wrapped in tissue paper. Similar to biopsies from other organs, overstuffing of cassettes should be avoided. Although some laboratories mark these needle cores (especially the smaller ones) with permanent ink, nonpermanent stains (such as hematoxylin) still facilitate identification of the core in the paraffin block but do not compromise histological interpretation that can occur when excessive permanent ink paints significant portions of the biopsy material. At least three histological levels should be obtained from each paraffin block with needle core biopsy material to ensure adequate representation of the lesion(s). As for all other breast specimens, the histological findings should always be correlated with the clinical and radiological findings, and, if discrepant (such as when microcalcifications are not seen in original sections of a biopsy performed for microcalcifications), then radiographic images of the paraffin block and/or additional sections need to be examined to resolve the discrepancy. Saving interval unstained sections, especially for smaller samples, is often beneficial for subsequent immunohistochemistry.

2. **Excisional biopsies.** These are either oriented or nonoriented specimens. Nonoriented specimens are those in which evaluation of the status of specific margins is not required by the surgeon (such as excisions of benign lesions or malignant lesions with separate margin specimens); nonetheless, these specimens should be inked. Oriented specimens need to be inked differentially to facilitate specific margin orientation; any approach using from two to six ink colors can be used to accurately "map" the margins. After the specimen has been inked, it should be serially sectioned (at 3- to 5-mm intervals) as soon as possible to allow for good penetration of fixative. Such sectioning may be performed in any direction (usually perpendicular to the long axis of the specimen); however, sectioning may be influenced by the proximity of the lesion(s) to particular margins. In addition, it is preferable to section subareolar excision specimens parallel of the skin surface (perpendicular to the anterior–posterior axis), as intraductal lesions such as papillomas are best detected by sections that facilitate examination of numerous duct cross-sections.

   a. **Mass lesions.** The size of the mass (accurate to nearest millimeter), consistency (gelatinous, rubbery, firm, or hard), growth pattern (well-circumscribed, infiltrative, rounded), and distance from margins should all be described. The presence and size of a biopsy cavity should also be noted. For well-circumscribed lesions thought to be benign (such as fibroadenomas), one section per centimeter of lesion is usually sufficient. Ill-defined and suspicious lesions need to be entirely submitted if <1 to 1.5 cm in greatest dimension; otherwise, four sections of the tumor usually suffice. When such tumors approximate one or more margins, these margins should be sampled in a radial fashion along with the tumor; representative shave sections of distant

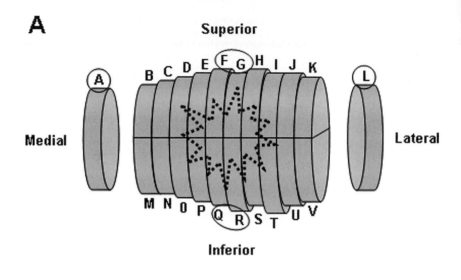

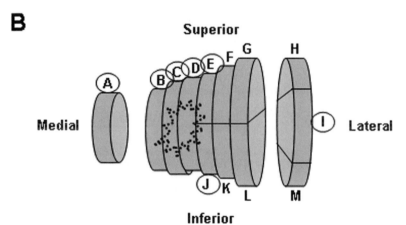

Figure 18.1. Schematic representation of "bread-loafing" and sampling of mass lesions. **A:** Specimen was serially sectioned perpendicular to its long axis, and an irregular mass was identified in the center of the specimen. Given the size of the specimen and the mass, submission of sections F, G, Q, and R would appear to adequately represent the mass, as well as the immediately adjacent superior, inferior, anterior, and posterior (deep) margins. Sections A and L would be submitted as the shaved medial and lateral margins, respectively. Given the smaller size of the specimen and mass in **(B)**, submission of sections B, C, D, E, and J would insure that the entire mass and the same immediately adjacent margins could be examined histologically. Section A would be submitted as the shaved medial margin, and section I as representative of the shaved lateral margin.

margins are all that is required (Fig. 18.1). In general, it is preferable to entirely submit for histological examination smaller specimens that fit into fewer than 10 cassettes.

b. Specimens excised for microcalcifications. Most of these specimens show no significant gross pathology. Specimen radiographs, especially for larger specimens, can be used to preferentially sample areas of microcalcification, immediately adjacent areas, as well as the margins. For smaller specimens, however, it is preferable to entirely submit the specimen as this facilitates

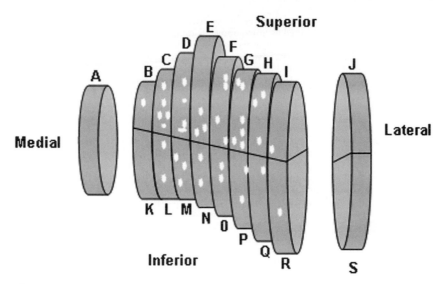

Figure 18.2. Schematic representation of "bread-loafing" and sampling of a specimen excised for microcalcifications. Especially given the scattered widespread distribution of the microcalcifications and their proximity to several margins (both determined by examination of the specimen radiograph), the specimen should be entirely submitted for histological examination. An example of a section code (block summary) that would permit three-dimentional reconstruction of the lesion might read as follows: *A*, shaved medial margin; *B–J*, superior half of specimen, sequential serial sections from medial to lateral; *K–S*, inferior half of specimen, corresponding sequential serial sections from medial to lateral. An advantage of such an approach would be that three (or even two) colors of ink would be sufficient to map and evaluate the margins histologically.

accurate estimation of the extent of disease present. In general, fibrous areas should be entirely submitted for examination. If possible, the specimen should be sectioned in a way that facilitates some inference of the three-dimensional aspects of the lesion when histological sections are evaluated (Fig. 18.2).

3. **Margin and biopsy re-excisions.** These cases range from unorientated flat portions of tissue that should be laid flat in a cassette (the presence of any malignancy seen histologically would thus be indicative of a positive margin), to larger, variably oriented specimens that should be inked preferentially, bread-loafed perpendicular to the new margin, and submitted in a manner to examine the new margin. For re-excisions following invasive carcinoma, the status of gross residual disease should be evaluated as well as its relationship to different excision margins; in the absence of such gross disease, the specimen need only to be representatively sampled. For re-excisions following a diagnosis of in situ carcinoma, the specimen may need to be more widely sampled to detect residual disease and/or associated invasive carcinoma.

4. **Mastectomies.** These range from simple skin-sparing mastectomy (which only removes the nipple–areola complex), to modified radical mastectomy (including axillary lymph nodes; see below), to radical mastectomy (including pectoral muscles). Subcutaneous mastectomies (without skin) are only performed in men. Mastectomies may be prophylactic or therapeutic; in the former case, as well as in therapeutic mastectomies following core needle biopsy with or without neoadjuvant chemotherapy, it may be difficult to find a localized lesion and/or site of the prior biopsy. Accordingly, review of the medical and pathology records as well as radiography of the specimen after sectioning may be necessary to locate any lesions. After describing its external appearance, including the nipple–areola complex and the presence of orienting sutures and/or clips, the specimen should be inked, serially sectioned from the posterior aspect at 5-mm intervals, and

examined for gross findings before or after overnight fixation. All lesions should be carefully described as noted above. Sampling should include the nipple (preferentially via cross-section as well as radial sections), representative sections from grossly detected lesions, as well as representative sections (one to two) from breast quadrants not involved by the primary pathological process. A search for lymph nodes should always be performed even in simple mastectomies and, if found, sampled accordingly (see below).

5. **Mammary implants.** These should be inspected grossly for any evidence of leakage. One or two sections are usually sufficient to evaluate the surrounding fibrous "capsule" that is usually submitted with the implant(s).

6. **Sentinel lymph nodes.** Specimens designated as sentinel lymph nodes should be dissected carefully because not infrequently more than one lymph node is present. Although there are different methods to process sentinel lymph nodes removed for breast carcinoma, intraoperative evaluation (frozen sections and/or touch preparations) is usually limited to lymph nodes grossly suspicious for malignancy. Otherwise, each node is serially sectioned at 1-mm intervals and, in the absence of gross evidence of metastatic carcinoma, entirely submitted for histological examination. Although there are many different protocols for microscopic evaluation, one common approach involves examination of three hematoxylin and eosin (H&E)-stained sections from each paraffin block, and, if negative for malignancy, examination of two additional cytokeratin-stained sections.

7. **Nonsentinel (axillary) lymph nodes.** After carefully dissecting grossly benign appearing nodes from the fat, nodes smaller than 0.4 cm can be submitted intact, whereas larger nodes need to be bisected or trisected and submitted in a manner that permits accurate enumeration (either by submitting them in individual cassettes or by differential inking). If possible, the size of the largest grossly positive node or metastatic deposit should be measured, in which case only one section needs to be submitted per each grossly positive lymph node.

III. DIAGNOSTIC FEATURES OF COMMON DISEASES OF THE BREAST

A. Inflammatory lesions

1. **Acute bacterial infections.** These most frequently develop in pregnant or lactating women but may also complicate duct ectasia (see below). Incision and drainage is performed if an abscess develops, and submitted tissue usually shows granulation tissue with mixed acute and chronic inflammation; suppuration may also be evident, and fibrosis is seen in later stages.

2. **Granulomatous inflammation.** There are several disease processes that cause granulomatous inflammation in the breast, most of which present as a mass.

   a. **Idiopathic granulomatous mastitis.** This is characterized by a perilobular granulomatous inflammation that includes epithelioid macrophages, Langerhans giant cells, lymphocytes, and plasma cells. Eosinophils may also be identified. The disease usually presents in parous premenopausal women as a variably sized mass that may be suspicious for carcinoma both clinically and mammographically. By definition, evidence of vasculitis or an infectious process (as detected by special stains and/or cultures) is lacking.

   b. **Sarcoidosis.** This disease can rarely involve the breast and, if so, produces clinical, radiographical, and microscopic findings very similar to idiopathic granulomatous mastitis. A history of sarcoidosis elsewhere is usually present.

   c. **Infectious granulomas.** The breast may occasionally be the site of mycobacterial, fungal, or parasitic infections resulting in necrotizing or non-necrotizing granulomas. In contrast to idiopathic granulomatous mastitis, a lobulocentric pattern of growth is usually lacking, and there is often evidence for an infectious etiology elsewhere. The diagnosis often rests on identifying the causative organism by special stains and/or cultures.

   d. **Fat necrosis.** Although fat necrosis can result from trauma, most cases are idiopathic (secondary to prior surgery or radiotherapy). Histologically, foamy macrophages and foreign body giant cells are seen as infiltrating fat (e-**Fig. 18.6**). In later stages, fibrosis and dystrophic calcification may be seen. It should be noted that lobular carcinoma can invade adipose tissue in a manner mimicking fat necrosis and, accordingly, is an important differential diagnosis.

e. **Silicone granuloma.** Leakage of silicone from breast implants leads to a foreign body giant cell reaction. Most of the silicon dissolves during tissue processing, leaving variably sized clear spaces and vacuolated macrophages, although residual refractile material may occasionally be seen. It should be noted that silicone granulomas may also be seen in axillary lymph nodes.

3. **Duct ectasia.** This usually presents in middle-aged women as nipple discharge, with or without an associated mass lesion. It is characterized by dilation of the major duct system, often with luminal amorphous material and foamy macrophages (with or without calcification) (e-Fig. **18.7**). There is usually associated fibrosis and periductal inflammation, often including numerous plasma cells (plasma cell mastitis). Periductal granulomas (as opposed to the perilobular granulomas seen in idiopathic granulomatous mastitis) may also be identified.

4. **Lymphocytic mastitis (sclerosing lymphocytic lobulitis).** Given its frequent association with longstanding insulin-dependant diabetes mellitus (among other autoimmune diseases), this lesion has also been termed diabetic mastopathy. Patients usually present with a painless mass that on excision is rubbery to firm and composed of fibrous stroma in which scattered, well-circumscribed breast lobules are seen. These lobules have a dense lymphocytic infiltrate that is polyclonal. Recognition of this lesion on needle biopsy may prevent unnecessary surgical excision.

5. **Amyloidosis.** This is usually secondary in nature and may present as a mass lesion in middle-aged to elderly patients. Similar to its appearance elsewhere, amorphous eosinophilic deposits of amyloid are seen in the fat, stroma, and blood vessel walls. Deposits may also be indentified around atrophic ducts and lobules. The diagnosis can be confirmed by a Congo red stain or other special techniques.

6. **Vasculitis.** The breast is rarely the site of different forms of vasculitis, including giant cell arteritis, polyarteritis nodosa, and Wegener's granulomatosis. Granulomas may also be evident (e-Fig. **18.8**). As for vasculitis elsewhere, clinical, pathological, and serological findings must be integrated for a specific diagnosis.

7. **Other inflammatory reactions.** It is important to note that an inflammatory reaction can be associated with both in situ and invasive carcinomas (see below) and be of an intensity that may mask the presence of carcinoma.

B. **Intraepithelial lesions.** As the name indicates, these lesions are confined within the basement membrane of the ducts and/or lobules involved. Nonproliferative lesions are usually incidental findings, but may be a component of a mass lesion. Most proliferative lesions present as mammographic abnormalities, usually as microcalcification with or without an associated mass.

1. **Nonproliferative lesions**

   a. **Apocrine metaplasia.** This is a very common benign finding that is almost always seen in premenopausal women and is often part of so-called fibrocystic changes, a constellation of benign breast changes which usually includes fibrosis, cysts, and ductal hyperplasia (DH). Apocrine metaplasia can be seen in ducts or lobules and is characterized histologically by eosinophilic cells with finely granular cytoplasm and rounded nuclei, often with prominent nucleoli (e-Fig. **18.9**). A papillary architecture is sometimes evident.

   b. **Squamous metaplasia.** This is most frequently seen in association with intraductal papillomas, especially if infarcted. The lack of cytological atypia or infiltration of surrounding tissues helps to distinguish it from low-grade adenosquamous carcinoma, which can be seen in association with intraductal papillomas. Squamous metaplasia can also be seen within biopsy cavities in rare instances.

   c. **Secretory/lactational changes.** Although usually a normal physiological change seen in reproductive-aged women, such changes are occasionally identified in postmenopausal women possibly as a reaction to certain medications (such as digitalis) and can also rarely produce a mass lesion. Given the atypical cytological features sometimes present (e-Fig. **18.10**), it is important not to mistake these changes for a more significant intraepithelial neoplastic process.

   d. **Cystic lesions.** Cystic dilation of the breast TDLUs (as opposed to the major duct system in duct ectasia) is quite common and can produce marked expansion and, especially when associated with microcalcification or fibrosis, can result in mammographically detectable and/or palpable lesions. Histologically, these cysts are usually lined by flat nonatypical epithelium (e-Fig. 18.11). Occasionally these cysts are filled by mucin (so-called mucocele-like lesions), which can rupture and resemble the extracellular mucin seen with invasive mucinous carcinoma (e-Fig. 18.12), a differential diagnosis that should always be considered when mucocele-like lesions are seen on needle core biopsy.

The galactocele is another cystic lesion that usually presents in pregnant women as a well-circumscribed mass with a characteristic radiological appearance. Histologically, a cuboidal or flat epithelial lining, often with vacuolated cells, is seen surrounding amorphous secretions. Inflammation may also be present.

e. Columnar cell change. This is characterized by dilation of the TDLUs, which become lined by columnar cells that usually display cytoplasmic projections at the apex of the cells, termed apical snouts; intraluminal secretions are also present (e-Fig. 18.13). This alteration represents one end of the spectrum of columnar cell lesions of the breast (see below) that are increasingly being recognized due to their frequent association with microcalcifications.

f. Collagenous spherulosis. This is an incidental histological finding characterized by TDLUs displaying rounded or fibrillary material surrounded by myoepithelial or epithelial cells (e-Fig. 18.14). The finding of collagenous spherulosis is nonspecific; it can be associated with a number of proliferative lesions, including DH, ductal carcinoma in situ (DCIS), adenoid cystic carcinoma, and lobular carcinoma in situ (LCIS). The cytoarchitectural features of the cells surrounding the spherules usually suggest the correct diagnosis.

2. Proliferative lesions. Most breast epithelial proliferations have their origin in the TDLUs. However, based on their morphological, epidemiological, and molecular features, they have traditionally been divided into ductal and lobular lesions, a distinction that is easily made in most situations. Of note, ductal lesions tend to present mammographically as mass lesions, whereas most lobular lesions are incidental (Table 18.1).

a. Ductal lesions

i. Ductal hyperplasia. This is characterized by increased numbers of cells within the duct epithelium; the increase ranges from ducts lined by three layers of cells, to ducts almost filled by proliferating plump epithelial cells (termed florid DH). Haphazard placement of cells of variable size and shape (both epithelial and myoepithelial), often with prominent streaming and/or swirling, indistinct cell borders, and irregular and usually peripheral secondary spaces are all features of DH (e-Fig. 18.15) that distinguish it from low-grade DCIS. Immunohistochemically, DH is usually positive for high-molecular-weight-keratin (e-Fig. 18.16), unlike most examples of DCIS. A unique form of hyperplasia, gynecomastoid hyperplasia, is seen with gynecomastia (in both women and men) and is characterized by a micropapillary intraductal proliferation that tends to taper toward the lumen and is often associated with increased cellularity of the intralobular connective tissue.

ii. Columnar cell hyperplasia. The clinicopathological features of this lesion are similar to columnar cell change except that, instead of a single layer of the characteristic columnar cells, the TDLUs are lined by two or more layers of such cells (e-Fig. 18.17). This lesion is also seen in association with DH.

iii. Low-grade DCIS (LG-DCIS). This is characterized by a uniform population of small epithelial cells that replaces the normal ductal epithelial cells. These cells can fill the duct spaces (solid DCIS) or even extend into the lobular units (so-called lobular cancerization). Constituent cells are characterized by rounded to oval nuclei, regularly distributed chromatin, and inconspicuous nucleoli. In contrast to DH, there is an orderly placement of these monomorphic cells with minimal overlap and streaming, with well-formed solid, papillary, micropapillary, or cribriform (sieve-like) architectural patterns (e-Fig. 18.18) in which the cells are polarized around secondary spaces. Because these lesions, as well as higher grade DCIS, are

TABLE 18.1 Salient Clinical and Pathological Features of Different Intraepithelial Lesions of the Breast

Presentation	DH	CCC/H	ADH	FEA	LG-DCIS	I/HG-DCIS	LCIS
Microcalcification	+/-	+	-	+	+; granular	Branching	-
Mass lesion	+/-	Rare	Rare	Rare	+/-	+/-	-
Morphological features							
Cell type	Mixed	Monotonous	Monotonous	Monotonous	Monotonous	Monotonous	Monotonous
Swirling of cells	+	-	Rare	-	-	+/-	Discohesive
Polarization of cells	-	+/-	+/-	-	+	Variable	Indistinct
Cell borders	Indistinct	Indistinct	Distinct	Indistinct	Distinct	Variable	Indistinct
Nuclear shape	Variable	Oval	Round/oval	Oval	Round/oval	Irregular	Round
Hyperchromasia	-	-	+/-	+	+	+	+/-
Nucleoli	Indistinct	Indistinct	Indistinct	Small	Indistinct	Often large	Indistinct
Necrosis	Rare	-	-	Rare	Rare	+/-	Rare
HMWK expression	+	-	-	-	-	+/-	+/-

DH, ductal hyperplasia; CCC/H, columnar cell change/hyperplasia; ADH, atypical ductal hyperplasia; FEA, flat epithelial atypia; LG-DCIS, low-grade ductal carcinoma in situ; I/HG-DCIS, intermediate-/high-grade ductal carcinoma in situ; LCIS, lobular carcinoma in situ (classic type); HMWK, high-molecular-weight cytokeratin.

TABLE 18.2	Pathological Findings that Should be Evaluated and Reported for Cases of Ductal Carcinoma in Situ (DCIS)
Feature	**Key points**
Nuclear grade	Report as low, intermediate, or high (use Nottingham scheme for nuclear grading; see Table 18.5)
Necrosis	Report as present/absent
Architectural type(s)	Report as solid/cribriform/micropapillary/papillary/comedo
Extent	Report size (in greatest dimension) or ratio of slides involved/noninvolved
Microcalcification	Report as absent/present (associated with DCIS/benign epithelium/stroma)
Margin status	Report as positive/negative/distance from closest (designated/undesignated) margin(s)
ER and PR status (if requested)	Report as positive/negative for each ± perform semiquantitative score

ER, estrogen receptor; PR, progesterone receptor.

often associated with microcalcifications, they are increasingly detected in mammographically directed needle biopsies, so a statement regarding associated microcalcification should always be part of the pathological report of DCIS (Table 18.2). In the absence of an invasive component, DCIS is associated with an excellent prognosis following conservative excision (with or without radiotherapy).

iv. **Intermediate and high-grade DCIS.** These lesions often have architectural patterns similar to their low-grade counterparts; however, as the name indicates, they are composed of cells with moderate to marked cytological atypia (e-**Fig. 18.19** and e-**Fig. 18.20**). Compared to LG-DCIS, these lesions are less often estrogen and progesterone receptor positive, more frequently positive for amplification of the *HER2-neu* oncogene (see below), and more likely to be associated with central "comedo-type" necrosis (e-**Fig. 18.21**) and higher recurrence rates (especially when necrosis is present).

v. **Atypical Ductal Hyperplasia (ADH).** This lesion has some, but not all, of the features of LG-DCIS (Table 18.1). Morphologically, ADH is characterized by a cellular proliferation very similar to that seen in LG-DCIS (e-**Fig. 18.22**) except that it does not entirely involve two duct spaces and/or is <2 mm in greatest dimensions (*Hum Pathol.* 1992;23:1095). Given that this distinction is mostly quantitative (rather than qualitative), it is not surprising that the immunohistochemical and molecular features of ADH are very similar to those of LG-DCIS. A diagnosis of ADH on needle biopsy is usually followed by excision due to the relatively high incidence of finding DCIS on excision.

vi. **Flat epithelial atypia (FEA).** This can be thought of as representing the neoplastic counterpart of columnar cell change and columnar cell hyperplasia; one alternative term (among many others) is columnar cell change (or hyperplasia) with atypia, nomenclature that reflects the atypical cytological features of the component epithelial cells (e-**Fig. 18.23**). FEA is frequently associated with ADH, LG-DCIS, LCIS, and invasive carcinoma (usually tubular carcinoma) (*Am J Surg Pathol.* 2007;31:417) and shares many of the immunophenotypic and molecular features of LG-DCIS. Given its frequent association with more significant proliferative lesions, the finding of FEA on needle biopsy is also an indication for follow-up excision. At this point, the literature does not suggest that the finding of FEA at the margin of an excisional biopsy is an indication for further excision.

b. **Papillary lesions.** Although papillary lesions are technically ductal proliferative lesions, their unique nature merits separate consideration.

TABLE 18.3 Salient Pathological Features of Papilloma and Noninvasive Papillary Carcinoma

Histological feature	Papilloma	Papillary carcinoma
Myoepithelial cells	Present	Absent/markedly reduced
Nuclei	Oval/normochromatic	Round to elongated/ hyperchromatic
Apocrine metaplasia	Present	Absent
Gland pattern	Complex; haphazard	Cribriform/trabecular; regular/ polarized
Stroma	Prominent; fibrosis and entrapment	Delicate or absent
Adjacent ducts	Hyperplasia	Ductal carcinoma in situ
Sclerosing adenosis	Sometimes present	Usually absent

i. **Intraductal papillomas (and related lesions).** These usually show an arborizing growth pattern and fibrovascular cores covered by myoepithelial cells and overlying nonatypical epithelial cells (e-**Fig. 18.24**). Secondary hemorrhagic infarction, squamous metaplasia, and extensive sclerosis (sclerosing papilloma) can sometimes be seen (e-**Fig. 18.25**) (Table 18.3). Intraductal papillomas can progressively increase in size resulting in tumorous lesions and/or bloody nipple discharge. So-called nipple adenoma and ductal adenoma can also be considered variants of intraductal papilloma and sclerosing papilloma, respectively, whereas multiple papillomas (papillomatosis) can be considered a variant of DH with a prominent papillary architecture. Intraductal papillomas and related lesions can secondarily be involved by other different intraepithelial proliferations including DH, ADH, DCIS, and LCIS, and atypical papilloma has been used to designate some of these lesions (see below). In the absence of any secondary neoplastic proliferation, primary excision is adequate treatment for papillomas.

ii. **Noninvasive (intraductal, intracystic, encapsulated) papillary carcinoma.** The architectural structure of papillary carcinoma is similar to that of a benign papilloma; however, the papillary fronds tend to be delicate with minimal sclerosis. Although additional histological differences exist between papilloma and papillary carcinoma (Table 18.3), the single most important differentiating feature is the absence, or only minimal presence, of myoepithelial cells in the latter (e-**Fig. 18.26**). Considering that papillary carcinoma is in reality a variant of DCIS, it is not surprising that predominantly cribriform, micropapillary, and solid patterns of papillary carcinoma exist; the latter (e-**Fig. 18.27**) is usually associated with neuroendocrine differentiation (sometimes with spindle-cell morphology) and mucin production and can also be seen in association with invasive mucinous carcinoma and invasive solid neuroendocrine carcinoma. Although displaced cells along a tract of prior biopsy and entrapped epithelial elements can be seen in the fibrous tissue around both papillomas and papillary carcinomas (e-**Fig. 18.28**), distinguishing such elements from invasive carcinoma is critical. In the absence of evidence of prior biopsy changes such as hemorrhage and foamy macrophages, the presence of a desmoplastic reaction (e-**Fig. 18.29**) as well as extension into adipose tissue supports a diagnosis of invasion. In the absence of associated invasive carcinoma, papillary carcinoma is associated with an excellent long-term outcome.

iii. **Atypical papilloma.** This term has been mostly used to designate intraductal papillomas that display, at least focally, areas of ADH or DCIS (e-**Fig. 18.30**). Considering that there is no consensus regarding the quantity of ADH or DCIS required for the atypical designation, it is important to quantify such components in the pathology report. In the absence of adjacent ADH or DCIS, the behavior of atypical papilloma is identical to that of benign papillomas.

c. Lobular lesions

i. Lobular carcinoma in-situ. This is characterized by a neoplastic proliferation that fills (and often distends) most of the lobules in the involved TDLUs. Atypical lobular hyperplasia is the term that has been used for lesser degrees of involvement; however, most authorities now consider such lobular proliferations under the rubric of "lobular neoplasia" or "lobular intraepithelial neoplasia". In contrast to solid LG-DCIS, the cells of LCIS are usually small and discohesive, and often display intracytoplasmic lumina (e-**Fig. 18.31**) (as opposed to extracellular secondary spaces in DCIS). It is sometimes difficult to distinguish between LCIS and LG-DCIS; in such situations, the fact that loss of membranous expression of E-cadherin by immunohistochemistry is quite characteristic for LCIS (cytoplasmic expression may still be evident) can be helpful for diagnosis (e-**Fig. 18.32**). Most cases of classic LCIS are treated by steroid hormone receptor antagonists, and most data do not support re-excision for positive surgical margins. Although pagetoid extension of neoplastic cells into the major ductal system is usually seen with LCIS, it can also be seen in association with DCIS; such extension undermines the normal ductal epithelium and produces a clover leaf–like appearance (e-**Fig. 18.33**).

ii. Pleomorphic LCIS. This lesion shares with classic LCIS distension of the TDLUs by discohesive malignant cells; however, as the name indicates, it is composed of cells with far more cytological atypia, occasionally with apocrine features (e-**Fig. 18.34**). The main differential diagnosis for pleomorphic LCIS is intermediate- or high-grade DCIS, a differential confounded by the not infrequent presence of central comedo-like necrosis in all these lesions. Lack of membranous E-cadherin expression by immunohistochemistry (e-**Fig. 18.35**) can be very useful in confirming the diagnosis. Similar to classic LCIS, pleomorphic LCIS can also spread along the duct system in a pagetoid fashion. Given the clinical, radiological, and pathological similarities of pleomorphic LCIS to DCIS, including the frequent extension into larger ducts, it is managed in a manner similar to DCIS; nevertheless, it is still important to correctly identify pleomorphic LCIS due to the occasional co-existence of invasive lobular carcinoma (ILC) that can be focal and quite subtle (e-**Fig. 18.36**), especially on needle biopsy.

C. Pseudoinfiltrative lesions. These proliferative lesions are characterized by an apparent infiltrative growth pattern that can simulate invasive carcinoma. However, they usually maintain some degree of lobular architecture, are usually composed of both epithelial and myoepithelial cells, and rarely invade adipose tissue, features that are all useful in avoiding an overdiagnosis of malignancy.

1. Sclerosing adenosis. This relatively common lesion is often incidental and admixed with proliferative lesions, but can also present mammographically with calcification and/or distortion, or clinically as a mass termed "adenosis tumor" or "nodular sclerosing adenosis". Sclerosing adenosis is characterized by an increased number of tubular glands (adenosis) surrounded by a fibrotic (sclerosing) stroma (e-**Fig. 18.37**). The fact that these glands/tubules are markedly compressed and often obliterated renders identification of a dual cell layer sometimes difficult. Accordingly, the main differential diagnosis is invasive (usually tubular) carcinoma, which may be difficult to exclude on small biopsies, especially in the rare examples of sclerosing adenosis associated with perineural invasion and/or areas in which sclerosing adenosis is secondarily involved by a neoplastic intraepithelial proliferation such as ADH, DCIS (e-**Fig. 18.38**), or LCIS. Elongated and compressed (as opposed to angulated) tubules, lack of a cellular desmoplastic stroma, a lobulocentric pattern of growth (e-**Fig. 18.39**), and immunohistochemical demonstration of myoepithelial cells (e-**Fig. 18.40**) are all features that can support the diagnosis of sclerosing adenosis. Occasionally, the epithelium in sclerosing adenosis undergoes apocrine metaplasia, termed apocrine adenosis, which may also be difficult to distinguish from a neoplastic proliferation.

2. Radial scar/complex sclerosing lesions. These are characterized by a central fibrous/fibroelastotic scar from which a stellate arrangement of ducts/lobules radiates (e-**Fig. 18.41**). Associated hyperplastic or neoplastic epithelial proliferations are often identified (e-**Fig. 18.42**). In addition to their microscopic pseudoinfiltrative nature, these lesions may also be clinically, radiologically, or grossly confused with invasive carcinoma due to their fibrotic nature and their characteristic stellate/spiculated appearance. Nevertheless, excisional biopsy is still recommended after a diagnosis of radial scar of needle biopsy because of the occasional presence of associated unsampled DCIS or invasive carcinoma at the periphery of the lesions.

3. **Microglandular adenosis (MGA).** This uncommon lesion is characterized by a proliferation of small rounded glands surrounded by a collagenous stroma (e-**Fig. 18.43**). Characteristically, these glands contain eosinophilic periodic acid–Schiff (PAS)-positive material in their lumens, but in contrast to other pseudoinfiltrative lesions, the glands are composed of only a single S-100–positive epithelial layer without a myoepithelial layer. The lesion is not always lobulocentric and can extend into adipose tissue; consequently, identification of the characteristic luminal eosinophilic material and lack of a desmoplastic stroma is very important to distinguish MGA from invasive carcinoma, especially when it presents as a palpable mass. It should be noted, however, that carcinomas (both in situ and invasive) can rarely arise from MGA (e-**Fig. 18.44**).

D. **Invasive carcinoma.** Most carcinomas present as a palpable mass and/or as a mammographic abnormality. However, in some cases the primary tumor is occult, and the patient presents with lymph node or distant metastasis. Determination of pathological stage (Table 18.4) is vital to determine prognosis and to guide therapy; the status of axillary lymph nodes is the single most important prognostic factor in invasive carcinoma. Tumor size is usually determined grossly or microscopically (the latter is more accurate, especially when there is a significant in situ component that should not be included for staging purposes). Radiological estimation of size can be used when pathological size cannot be determined (such as when the entire tumor is removed during needle core biopsy). Although the aggregate size of multifocal tumors has been reported to better correlate with the risk of lymph node metastasis than the size of the largest focus (*Cancer.* 2004;100:20), the sizes of the different foci should be individually reported and only the largest focus should be used for staging purposes. In addition to pathological stage, the prognosis of breast carcinoma is greatly dependant on additional prognostic and predictive factors (Table 18.5) that should be evaluated and reported for all breast carcinomas. Such factors are most significant in lymph node–negative breast carcinoma and include:

1. **Histological grade.** Invasive carcinomas have variable degrees of glandular differentiation (degree of gland/tubule formation), nuclear pleomorphism, and mitotic activity (e-**Fig. 18.45**). Variation in these three elements is the basis for the universally accepted Nottingham grading scheme for breast carcinoma (Table 18.5). Given the strength of histological grade as a prognostic marker (second only to axillary lymph node status), it should be reported for all carcinomas, even those of special histological type (see below).

2. **Vascular invasion.** The presence of angiolymphatic invasion (e-**Fig. 18.46**) is an independent prognostic factor in invasive carcinomas and should be evaluated in the breast tissue immediately adjacent to the tumor.

3. **Hormone receptor status.** Estrogen receptor (ER) and progesterone receptor (PR) expression are weak prognostic factors (but excellent predictive factors; see below) and are seen in approximately 70–80% of breast carcinomas (e-**Fig. 18.47**). Because of better fixation and the potential for guiding subsequent therapy, immunohistochemical assessment of hormone receptor status (and other predictive markers) is best performed on needle biopsy material if available; concordance with subsequent excisional material, as well as with recurrent and metastatic foci, is excellent. Several scoring schemes incorporating both strength and percentage of staining have been devised to evaluate expression; however, it has been shown that weak expression in only 1–10% of tumor cells can still predict response to hormonal therapy (*J Clin Oncol.* 1999;17:1474). It is important to report the expression of both ER and PR separately as the response rates to hormonal treatment are also dependant on the pattern of expression, being

TABLE 18.4 Tumor, Node, Metastasis (TNM) Staging Scheme for Breast Carcinoma

PRIMARY TUMOR (T)

TX	Primary tumor cannot be assessed
T0	No evidence of primary tumor
Tis	Carcinoma in situ (ductal, lobular, and/or Paget disease of the nipple without invasive carcinoma)
T1	Tumor <2 cm in greatest dimension
T1mic	Microinvasion $\leq$0.1 cm in greatest dimension
T1a	Tumor >0.1 cm but $\leq$0.5 cm in greatest dimension
T1b	Tumor >0.5 cm but $\leq$1 cm in greatest dimension
T1c	Tumor >1 cm but $\leq$2 cm in greatest dimension
T2	Tumor >2 cm but $\leq$5 cm in greatest dimension
T3	Tumor >5 cm in greatest dimension
T4	Tumor of any size with direct extension to chest wall or skin, only as described below
T4a	Extension to chest wall, not including pectoralis muscle
T4b	Edema (including *peau d'orange*) or ulceration of the skin of the breast, or satellite skin nodules confined to the same breast
T4c	Both T4a and T4b
T4d	Inflammatory carcinoma

REGIONAL LYMPH NODES (pN)*

pNX	Regional lymph nodes cannot be assessed
pN0	No regional lymph node metastasis or lymph node metastasis <0.2 mm. pN0 can be further classified as
	pN0(i+): Isolated tumor cells (<0.2 mm) detected by hematoxylin and eosin or immunohistochemistry
	pN0(mol+): Tumor cells detected by positive molecular findings (reverse transcription–polymerase chain reaction)
pN1	Metastasis in 1 to 3 axillary lymph nodes, and/or in internal mammary nodes with microscopic disease detected by sentinel lymph node dissection but not clinically apparent (not detected clinically or by noninvasive imaging techniques)
pN1mi	Micrometastasis (>0.2 mm, none <2.0 mm)
pN1a	Metastasis in 1 to 3 axillary lymph nodes
pN1b	Metastasis in internal mammary nodes
pN1c	Metastasis in 1 to 3 axillary lymph nodes and in internal mammary lymph nodes. If associated with >3 positive axillary lymph nodes, the internal mammary nodes are classified as pN3b to reflect increased tumor burden
pN2	Metastasis in 4 to 9 axillary lymph nodes or in clinically apparent internal mammary lymph nodes in the absence of axillary lymph node metastasis
pN2a	Metastasis in 4 to 9 axillary lymph nodes (at least one deposit >2 mm)
pN2b	Metastasis in clinically apparent internal mammary lymph nodes in the absence of axillary lymph node metastasis
pN3	Metastasis in $\geq$10 axillary lymph nodes, or in infraclavicular lymph nodes, or in clinically apparent ipsilateral internal mammary lymph nodes in the presence of $\geq$1 positive axillary lymph nodes; or in >3 axillary lymph nodes with clinically negative microscopic metastasis in internal mammary lymph nodes; or in ipsilateral supraclavicular lymph nodes
pN3a	Metastasis in $\geq$10 axillary lymph nodes (at least one deposit >2 mm), or metastasis to the infraclavicular lymph nodes
pN3b	Metastasis in clinically apparent ipsilateral internal mammary lymph nodes in the presence of $\geq$1 positive axillary lymph nodes; or in >3 axillary lymph nodes and in internal mammary lymph nodes with microscopic disease detected by sentinel lymph node dissection but not clinically apparent
pN3c	Metastasis in ipsilateral supraclavicular lymph nodes

(*continued*)

TABLE 18.4	Tumor, Node, Metastasis (TNM) Staging Scheme for Breast Carcinoma (*Continued*)		

DISTANT METASTASIS (M)

MX	Distant metastasis cannot be assessed		
M0	No distant metastasis		
M1	Distant metastasis		

AJCC STAGE GROUPINGS

Stage 0	Tis	N0	M0
Stage I	T1	N0	M0
Stage IIA	T0	N1	M0
	T1	N1	M0
	T2	N0	M0
Stage IIB	T2	N1	M0
	T3	N0	M0
Stage IIIA	T0	N2	M0
	T1	N2	M0
	T2	N2	M0
	T3	N1	M0
	T3	N2	M0
Stage IIIB	T4	N0	M0
	T4	N1	M0
	T4	N2	M0
Stage IIIC	Any T	N3	M0
Stage IV	Any T	Any N	M1

*Sentinel nodes are indicated by adding (sn) to the designation.
From: Tavassoli FA, Devilee P, eds. *World Health Organization Classification of Tumours. Pathology and Genetics. Tumours of the Breast and Female and Genital Organs.* Lyon: IARC Press; 2001. Used with permission.

highest in ER+/PR+ tumors, followed by ER−/PR+ tumors, and then ER+/PR− tumors, and lowest in ER−/PR− tumors.

4. **Human epidermal growth factor receptor-2 (HER2) status.** The *HER2/neu* oncogene is involved in the regulation of cell proliferation, survival, motility, and invasion. Gene amplification and/or protein overexpression of HER2 is present in approximately 20% of all breast carcinomas and is associated with a worse clinical outcome. More importantly, such amplification or overexpression can predict response (or lack thereof) to certain chemotherapeutic agents, hormonal therapy, and to trastuzumab (Herceptin), a humanized monoclonal antibody directed against cells that express HER2. Accordingly, HER2 status should be evaluated in all cases of invasive breast carcinoma. An algorithmic approach is recommended whereby cases are initially tested by immunohistochemistry. Cases positive for overexpression (3+) are characterized by a strong membranous reaction visible on 10× magnification in at least 30% of tumor cells (e-**Fig. 18.48**) and negative cases characterized by absent (0) or only weak (1+) membranous expression (e-**Fig. 18.49**). Well-calibrated immunohistochemistry can identify the majority of cases as positive or negative; equivocal cases (2+), characterized by moderate membranous staining (e-**Fig. 18.50**), are then evaluated for gene amplification, most frequently using fluorescence in situ hybridization (e-**Fig. 18.51**). Given the prognostic and predictive impact of HER2 status, guidelines for standardized testing and reporting have been developed (*Arch Pathol Lab Med.* 2007;131:18).

5. **Other immunohistochemical prognostic markers.** Proliferation markers, such as Ki67/MIB1 and p53, have been variably been used as prognostic markers in the evaluation of invasive breast cancer. However, the list of potential prognostic markers for breast carcinoma continues to expand, and thus far routine use of these other markers is rarely indicated.

| TABLE 18.5 | Pathological Features of Invasive Carcinoma that Should be Reported |

Feature	Key points
Histological type	Need >90% of characteristic morphology for special types Need 50–90% of characteristic morphology to be considered mixed
Size	Do not include in situ component in measurement Report individual sizes of multifocal tumors; use largest for Tumor, Node, Metastasis (TNM) category
Grade	Evaluate entire tumor for percentage of tubule formation (structures with clearly defined central lumina surrounded by polarized epithelial cells) • >75%: score of 1 • 10–75%: score of 2 • <10%: score of 3 Access nuclear pleomorphism based on worst area: • Minimal (no significant size ↑; uniform chromatin): score of 1 • Moderate (variable size and shape; open chromatin; nucleoli): score of 2 • Marked (marked variation in size and shape ± bizarre nuclei; prominent nucleoli): score of 3 Assign mitotic score (1–3) by assessing most active/peripheral area of tumor for unequivocal mitotic figures per high-power field; at least 10 fields should be counted; score cutoffs depend on microscope field diameter (FD):*

FD (mm)	Score 1	Score 2	Score 3
0.40	≤4	5–8	≥9
0.44	≤5	6–10	≥11
0.50	≤6	7–13	≥14
0.55	≤8	9–16	≥17
0.60	≤9	10–19	≥20
0.65	≤11	12–23	≥24
0.70	≤13	14–27	≥28

	Add up scores to arrive at final grade: • 3–5 points: Grade I • 6–7 points: Grade II • 8–9 points: Grade III
Margin status	Report as positive (designated/undesignated) or provide distance from closest (designated/undesignated) margin(s)
Vascular invasion	Report when present (routine immunohistochemistry for endothelial/lymphatic markers not necessary)
ER and PR status	Report as positive/negative for each ± perform semiquantitative score
HER2 status	Report as positive/negative/equivocal for overexpression/amplification
In situ component	Report features of ductal carcinoma in situ separately (see Table 18.2)

* Among other methods, the FD can be measured using an objective scale or calculated. ER, estrogen receptor; PR, progesterone receptor.

6. **Histological type.** Although recent gene expression studies (*Nature.* 2000;406:747) have been able to stratify breast carcinomas into different types or classes with different prognostic implications, histological typing remains the gold standard for classification of breast carcinoma and provides useful prognostic information. The World Health Organization has recently published its histological classification (Table 18.6) that includes tumors as well as intraepithelial proliferations (Tavassoli FA, Devilee P. *Pathology and Genetics of Tumors of the Breast and Female Genital Organs.* Lyon, France: IARC Press; 2003). The

TABLE 18.6 | WHO Histological Classification of Breast Tumors

Epithelial tumors	**Myoepithelial lesions**
Invasive ductal carcinoma, not otherwise specified	Myoepitheliosis
Invasive lobular carcinoma	Adenomyoepithelial adenosis
Tubular carcinoma	Adenomyoepithelioma
Invasive cribriform carcinoma	Malignant myoepithelioma
Medullary carcinoma	
Mucinous carcinoma and related tumors	**Mesenchymal tumors**
Neuroendocrine tumors	Hemangioma
Invasive papillary carcinoma	Angiomatosis
Invasive micropapillary carcinoma	Hemangiopericytoma
Apocrine carcinoma	Pseudoangiomatous stromal hyperplasia
Metaplastic carcinomas	Myofibroblastoma
Lipid-rich carcinoma	Fibromatosis (aggressive)
Secretory carcinoma	Inflammatory myofibroblastic tumor
Oncocytic carcinoma	Lipoma and angiolipoma
Adenoid cystic carcinoma	Granular cell tumor
Acinic cell carcinoma	Neurofibroma
Glycogen-rich clear cell carcinoma	Schwannoma
Sebaceous carcinoma	Angiosarcoma
Inflammatory carcinoma	Liposarcoma
Lobular neoplasia	Rhabdomyosarcoma
Lobular carcinoma in situ	Osteosarcoma
Intraductal proliferative lesions	Leiomyoma
Usual ductal hyperplasia	Leiomyosarcoma
Flat epithelial atypia	
Atypical ductal hyperplasia	**Fibroepithelial tumors**
Ductal carcinoma in situ	Fibroadenoma
Microinvasive carcinoma	Phyllodes tumor
Intraductal papillary neoplasms	Periductal stromal sarcoma, low grade
Papilloma	Mammary hamartoma
Atypical papilloma	
Intraductal/intracystic papillary carcinoma	**Tumors of the nipple**
Adenomas	Nipple adenoma
Tubular adenoma	Syringomatous adenoma
Lactating adenoma	Paget disease of the nipple
Apocrine adenoma	
Pleomorphic adenoma	**Malignant lymphoma**
Ductal adenoma	
	Metastatic tumors

From: Tavassoli FA, Devilee P, eds. *World Health Organization Classification of Tumours. Pathology and Genetics. Tumours of the Breast and Female Genital Organs.* Lyon: IARC Press; 2001. Used with permission.

majority (>70%) of invasive mammary carcinomas are invasive ductal carcinomas (IDC) of no special type (NST) or not otherwise specified (NOS) (e-**Fig. 18.52**). Nevertheless, there are multiple special histological types of invasive mammary carcinoma, some of which have outcomes significantly different from IDC NOS and/or have fairly distinct clinicopathological features (see below). For a carcinoma to be considered of special type, at least 90% of the tumor should have the characteristic morphology of that particular type, whereas those containing 50–90% of the characteristic morphology are considered mixed NOS/special type carcinomas, and those containing <50% of the characteristic morphology are classified as NOS carcinomas. Mixed carcinomas tend to have outcomes intermediate between NOS carcinoma and the "pure" special type component. The special histological types or variants of invasive mammary carcinoma (Table 18.7) include the following:

a. **Special types of carcinomas with clear-cut glandular differentiation**

   i. **Tubular carcinoma.** This tumor type constitutes 1–3% of invasive carcinomas (up to 8% of cancers detected by screening programs), and is composed of angulated tubules lined by a single layer of cells that often display eosinophilic to amphophilic cytoplasm with apical snouts and oval nuclei with only mild to moderate nuclear pleomorphism (e-**Fig. 18.53**). A cellular desmoplastic stroma is characteristic. As discussed earlier, tubular carcinoma needs to be differentiated from pseudoinfiltrative sclerosing lesions. Tubular carcinoma is associated with an excellent prognosis.

   ii. **Invasive cribriform carcinoma.** This is an uncommon histological type of carcinoma that is closely related to and often mixed with tubular carcinoma. It is composed of somewhat similar tumor cells, although they form cribriform structures (e-**Fig. 18.54**) rather than angulated tubules; these structures are often also surrounded by a desmoplastic stromal response. The differential diagnosis of invasive cribriform carcinoma includes cribriform DCIS as well as adenoid cystic carcinoma. Invasive cribriform carcinoma has a good prognosis.

   iii. **Adenoid cystic carcinoma.** This rare tumor is histologically identical to that of salivary gland origin. It has solid nests or cribriform structures composed of a biphasic population of cells: small basaloid cells surrounding eosinophilic basal lamina-like material, and larger epithelial cells lining true acinar spaces (e-**Fig. 18.55**). Among the features that distinguish it from invasive cribriform carcinoma, adenoid cystic carcinoma is ER and PR negative. This tumor type is associated with an excellent prognosis.

   iv. **Secretory carcinoma.** This rare histological type is characterized by a multicystic/honeycombed pattern of growth with abundant intracellular and extracellular eosinophilic secretions (e-**Fig. 18.56**). Although characteristically seen in younger patients including children, secretory carcinoma has also been seen in postmenopausal women as well as in men. The prognosis is very good.

   v. **Apocrine carcinoma.** As the name suggests, this tumor displays cytological and immunohistochemical evidence of apocrine differentiation. The cytological features of apocrine differential include abundant granular eosinophilic cytoplasm and central large vesicular nuclei with prominent nucleoli (e-**Fig. 18.57**). The immunohistochemical evidence of apocrine differentiation includes a lack of ER and PR expression, but expression of androgen receptor and gross cystic disease fluid protein 15 (GCDFP-15).

b. **Special types of carcinomas with characteristic growth patterns**

   i. **Invasive lobular carcinoma.** This comprises 5–15% of all invasive carcinomas, with a reportedly increased incidence in patients receiving postmenopausal combined hormone replacement therapy. Histologically, ILC is composed of scattered noncohesive individual cells often arranged in a single file or concentrically around benign epithelial elements, termed Indian file and targetoid patterns of growth, respectively (e-**Fig. 18.58**). Although intracytoplasmic lumina can be frequently seen, there is no glandular or tubular differentiation; occasionally, these intracytoplasmic lumina contain abundant mucin-producing signet-ring cells, which, when abundant, support the diagnosis of signet-ring carcinoma. Because tumor cells usually have intermediate score nuclei, most ILCs tend to be histological grade 2; however, the pleomorphic variant of ILC, characterized by more pleomorphic nuclei and increased mitoses (e-**Fig. 18.59**), is usually grade 3. Most cases of ILC show reduced or absent expression of E-cadherin by immunohistochemistry. As suggested by their higher grade, pleomorphic ILCs (as well as the solid variant) do not share the somewhat better outcome (compared to IDC-NOS)

TABLE 18.7 Frequency and Key Features of Most Prevalent Special Histological Types of Invasive Mammary Carcinoma

| Histological types | Frequency | Key microscopic features and usual receptor status | | |
		Microscopic features	ER/PR	HER2
Special types of carcinomas with clear-cut glandular differentiation:				
Tubular carcinoma	1–8%	Angulated tubules; cellular desmoplastic stroma	Positive	Negative
Invasive cribriform carcinoma	1–3%	Punched out spaces ± cellular desmoplastic stroma	Positive	Negative
Adenoid cystic carcinoma	Rare	Dual population; basal lamina material	Negative	Negative
Secretory carcinoma	Very rare	Prominent secretion	Positive	Negative
Apocrine carcinoma	0.5–4%	Granular eosinophilic cytoplasm; prominent nucleoli	Negative	Negative
Special types of carcinomas with characteristic growth patterns:				
Invasive lobular carcinoma	5–15%	Individual cells; Indian files; targetoid pattern	Positive	Negative
Tubulolobular carcinoma	Uncommon	Mixture of tubular and lobular patterns	Positive	Negative
Invasive papillary carcinoma	2%	Intraductal papillary carcinoma with invasion	Positive	Negative
Invasive micropapillary carcinoma	2%	Tumor within clear spaces	Variable	Variable
Mucinous carcinoma	1–5%	Extracellular mucin	Positive	Negative
Medullary carcinoma	1–7%	Syncytial growth; high grade; lymphoplasmacytic infiltrate	Negative	Negative
Solid neuroendocrine carcinoma	~2–5%	Alveolar/nested/trabecular growth pattern with "salt and pepper" nuclei; associated solid papillary carcinoma	Positive	Negative
Metaplastic carcinomas:				
Squamous, adenosquamous, spindle cell, and matrix-producing	Rare	Characteristic cell type or extracellular matrix	variable	Usually negative

ER, estrogen receptor; PR, progesterone receptor.

that characterizes classic ILC. Other differences from IDC-NOS include the higher incidence of parenchymal and isolated tumor cell metastatic patterns in minimally involved axillary lymph nodes (as opposed to the usual finding of tumor cell clusters in the subcapsular sinus) as well as characteristic metastatic spread to certain organs such as the ovary and stomach (where the metastases can resemble primary signet-ring adenocarcinoma).

ii. **Tubulolobular carcinoma.** As the name suggests, this uncommon histological subtype is a mixture of the two histological patterns (e-**Fig. 18.**60) and has a prognosis intermediate between classical tubular and lobular carcinoma. It should be noted that mixed tumors with both ductal (NOS) and lobular features are much more common than tubulolobular carcinomas.

iii. **Invasive papillary carcinoma.** This is essentially intraductal/intracystic papillary carcinoma in situ with associated invasive carcinoma (e-**Fig. 18.29**). The invasive component can be of any histological type. Given that a significant proportion of the published literature evaluating outcomes in "papillary carcinoma" do not make a distinction between in situ and invasive components or do not quantify the latter when present (usually a minor component), it is not surprising that "papillary carcinoma" is associated with a very good prognosis.

iv. **Invasive micropapillary carcinoma.** In a pure form, invasive micropapillary carcinoma accounts for approximately 2% of invasive carcinoma; however, it is much more frequently a component of a mixed carcinoma. Histologically, this variant is composed of small solid clusters of malignant cells lying within clear stromal spaces (e-**Fig. 18.61**). The importance of recognizing this variant of invasive carcinoma (as well as mixed tumors with a micropapillary component) is the associated high incidence of axillary lymph node metastasis. It should be noted, however, that when matched for stage, this variant does not necessarily have a worse prognosis than IDC-NOS.

v. **Mucinous carcinoma.** Depending on the series and stringency of diagnostic criteria, this variant comprises 1–6% of all invasive carcinomas. Characteristically, these are rounded/well-circumscribed gelatinous tumors composed of tumor cell nests and trabeculae floating within lakes of mucin (e-**Fig. 18.62**). This tumor is frequently associated with solid noninvasive papillary carcinoma, and often shows neuroendocrine differentiation. This tumor type is associated with a very good prognosis. It should be noted that signet-ring carcinoma (discussed above), and a few other very rare tumors, can also be classified as primary invasive carcinomas with mucinous differentiation.

vi. **Medullary carcinoma.** This comprises 1–7% of all invasive carcinomas and is characteristically a rounded/well-circumscribed neoplasm composed of highly pleomorphic (nuclear score 3) tumor cells arranged in a syncytial pattern of growth (>75% of tumor) with a moderate to intense associated lymphoplasmacytic infiltrate (e-**Fig. 18.63**). Medullary carcinomas, and related tumors also having a prominent syncytial pattern of growth but lacking other features of medullary carcinoma, are associated with familial mutations in the *BRCA1* tumor suppressor gene. Classic medullary carcinoma is associated with an excellent prognosis.

vii. **Solid neuroendocrine carcinoma.** Together with small cell carcinoma and large cell neuroendocrine carcinoma (both very rare), these carcinomas comprise 2–5% of primary breast carcinomas. Solid neuroendocrine carcinoma, usually seen in older individuals and often associated with solid intraductal papillary carcinoma, has a characteristic alveolar, nested, or trabecular carcinoid-like growth pattern, with granular or spindle cells displaying finely granular chromatin (e-**Fig. 18.64**) and immunohistochemical evidence of neuroendocrine differentiation in at least 50% of the tumor cells. It is always important to include metastatic neuroendocrine carcinoma in the differential diagnosis. The behavior of solid neuroendocrine carcinoma is mostly dependant on histological grade.

c. **Metaplastic carcinomas.** These include a heterogeneous group of carcinomas that contain, or are totally composed of, definable non-adenocarcinomatous (epithelial and/or mesenchymal) elements.
   i. **Adenosquamous carcinoma.** Although all adenosquamous carcinomas contain a squamous component, there is a spectrum of differentiation. Low-grade adenosquamous carcinoma, frequently associated with papillary and sclerosing lesions, is characterized by angulated glands embedded in a cellular stroma composed of cells with low-grade cytological atypia and focal squamous differentiation (e-**Fig. 18.65**). In contrast to higher grade tumors that resemble adenosquamous carcinoma elsewhere, low-grade adenosquamous carcinomas rarely metastasize. It should be noted that, compared to adenosquamous carcinoma, pure squamous cell carcinoma of the breast (of non-skin origin) is very rare.
   ii. **Metaplastic spindle cell carcinoma.** This includes carcinomas with abundant spindle cell transformation and/or frank sarcomatoid elements (e-**Fig. 18.66**). The diagnosis is relatively straightforward when glandular elements are easily evident, but when absent, may only be made by demonstrating cytokeratin immunoreactivity in the spindle cells. It should be noted that spindle cell carcinoma can be histologically bland and show minimal cytological atypia (such as in so-called fibromatosis-like spindle cell carcinoma). Accordingly, immunohistochemistry for cytokeratin or p63 (another marker frequently positive in metaplastic spindle cell carcinoma) should be performed in the evaluation of spindle cell breast lesions.
   iii. **Matrix-producing carcinoma.** Another form of metaplastic carcinoma, these tumors are characterized by production of extracellular chondroid (most common) or osteoid matrix. Some of these tumors show prominent spindle cells and thus overlap with spindle cell carcinomas.
d. **Other rare types of carcinoma.** Such carcinomas include, among others, myoepithelial carcinoma, sebaceous carcinoma, lipid-rich carcinoma, clear cell/glycogen-rich carcinoma, acinic cell carcinoma, and oncocytic carcinoma.
e. **Inflammatory carcinoma.** This is not a specific histological type of invasive carcinoma, but rather any carcinoma that has a characteristic clinical presentation consisting of diffuse erythema, induration, and tenderness of breast skin associated with nonpitting edema (*peu d'orange*). A breast mass may or may not be evident. Histologically, there is extensive dermal lymphatic invasion by carcinoma, which is believed to be the underlying mechanism for the clinical features. Inflammatory carcinoma is a form of locally advanced breast cancer (stage T4d) and is associated with an unfavorable outcome.

E. **Other epithelial tumors**
   1. **Tubular adenoma.** This uncommon lesion shares the clinical and radiological features of fibroadenomas (see below) and is composed of closely packed benign epithelial tubules separated by little intervening tubules.
   2. **Lactating adenoma.** This benign lesion is usually identified during pregnancy or lactation. It has a basic architecture that resembles tubular adenoma but the glandular component displays prominent secretory/lactational changes.
   3. **Pleomorphic adenoma.** This rare tumor is histologically identical to its salivary gland counterpart. The well-circumscribed nature of the lesion and the lack of a sarcomatous or malignant epithelial component are useful in distinguishing pleomorphic adenoma from matrix-producing metaplastic carcinoma with chondroid differentiation.
   4. **Metastatic tumors.** The breast may rarely be the site of metastatic involvement. Most metastases are either melanomas, or carcinomas originating from the lung or gastrointestinal tract. Such lesions, especially if isolated, may occasionally be sampled to exclude a primary breast neoplasm.
      In the absence of an in situ component, it is always possible that a malignant epithelial proliferation that appears to represent one of the many histological variants of invasive breast carcinoma is in reality a metastasis from elsewhere. A few metastatic tumors are in fact histologically identical to primary breast

carcinoma, such as gastric signet-ring adenocarcinomas and intestinal carcinoid tumors, which resemble primary breast signet-ring carcinoma and solid neuroendocrine carcinoma, respectively. In such situations, the correct diagnosis cannot be made without the full clinical history.

F. Myoepithelial lesions. In addition to adenoid cystic carcinoma, myoepithelial carcinoma, and pleomorphic adenoma (discussed above), there are a few other rare lesions in which myoepithelial cells represent a significant component.

    1. Myoepitheliosis. This nonneoplastic, often incidental microscopic lesion is characterized by proliferation of the myoepithelial cells surrounding benign breast lobules. Such a proliferation may also accompany sclerosing adenosis.

    2. Adenomyoepithelioma. This rare tumor is usually well circumscribed and is characterized by a solid proliferation of myoepithelial cells that usually surround epithelium-lined spaces. The component myoepithelial cells may be spindle, clear, or plasmacytoid in appearance. Occasional adenomyoepitheliomas are associated with malignant foci.

G. Fibroepithelial lesions. These are biphasic lesions composed of both epithelial and stromal elements.

    1. Fibroadenoma. This is a very common lesion that presents as a mass or radiographic abnormality, more commonly in younger women. Grossly, fibroadenomas are grayish-white, firm, well-circumscribed masses. Histologically, they are composed of a variably cellular spindle-cell stroma, in which benign cleft-like or tubular glandular elements are present (e-Fig. 18.67). These glandular elements are usually composed of a single basal cell and a single luminal cell layer. Some fibroadenomas, especially those arising in the second decade, can grow rapidly and appear quite cellular (an appearance that overlaps with benign phyllodes tumor); such lesions have been termed cellular fibroadenomas. Myxoid fibroadenomas display prominent myxoid changes in the stroma and may be a component of Carney's complex (which also includes myxomas, spotty pigmentation, and endocrine overactivity).

    Fibroadenomas may undergo secondary changes such as infarction or prominent hyalinization of the stroma, with or without calcification (the former is usually seen with pregnancy, whereas the latter is more often seen in elderly patients with longstanding lesions). In addition, almost all of the epithelial changes that arise in the breast can secondarily develop in fibroadenomas including various metaplasias, epithelial hyperplasia, sclerosing adenosis, DCIS, LCIS, and invasive carcinoma. Fibroadenomas with significant epithelial proliferation have been termed complex fibroadenomas. The main differential diagnosis of fibroadenoma is a benign phyllodes tumor. Among other differential features (Table 18.8), fibroadenomas lack the leaf-like architecture characteristic of phyllodes tumors, but it may still be difficult to distinguish between the two in needle core biopsy specimens. In such cases, a diagnosis of "fibroepithelial lesion" with an explanatory comment is a prudent approach.

    2. Phyllodes tumor. This tumor is much less common than fibroadenoma, accounting for <3% of fibroepithelial lesions. As mentioned above, the main feature distinguishing phyllodes tumor from fibroadenoma is the presence of the characteristic leaf-like architectural pattern produced by extensive branching of the epithelial component. Stromal hypercellularity is the rule, often with accentuation near the epithelial clefts. Phyllodes tumor can be divided into benign (e-Fig. 18.68), borderline (e-Fig. 18.69), and malignant (e-Fig. 18.70) categories; the first two are only distinguished by the degree of cellular atypia and mitotic activity, whereas the latter usually displays an infiltrative border, unequivocal sarcomatous areas, and stromal overgrowth (areas of stroma devoid of epithelium) (Table 18.8). Heterologous sarcomatous elements may also be occasionally present in malignant tumors (e-Fig. 18.70). Similar to fibroadenomas, phyllodes tumors can also harbor areas of epithelial hyperplasia, carcinoma in situ, or invasive carcinoma; the presence of the latter component (or the presence of a cytokeratin-positive spindle cell component) might suggest metaplastic carcinoma as an alternative diagnosis, albeit not necessarily prognostically different. Overall, about 20% of phyllodes tumors recur (ranging from 17% for benign tumors to 27% in

TABLE 18.8 Salient Pathological Features of Fibroadenoma and Phyllodes Tumor (PT) of Different Grades

Feature	Fibroadenoma	Benign PT	Borderline PT	Malignant PT
Architecture	Lobulated	Leaf-like	Leaf-like	Leaf-like
Margins	Round	Pushing	Pushing	Infiltrative
Cellularity	Usually hypocellular ± hyalinization	Cellular; can be heterogeneous	Cellular; can be heterogeneous	Cellular; can be heterogeneous
Zonal hypercellularity*	Not present	May be present	May be present	May be present
Epithelial spaces	Tubular or short slit-like	Elongated/ branching cleft-like or cystic	Elongated/ branching cleft-like or cystic	Elongated/ branching cleft-like or cystic
Stromal overgrowth	Not present	Not present	Not present	Often present; may obscure architecture
Cellular atypia	Rare atypical stromal cells may be found	Mild; atypical stromal cells can be found	Mild-moderate; resembles fibrosarcoma	Moderate to marked
Mitotic activity	Rare but variable	<5 per 10 HPFs	5–10 per 10 HPFs	>10 per 10 HPFs
Heterologous elements	Benign rarely present	Benign, may be present	Benign, may be present	Malignant, may be present

* Tumors with zonal hypercellularity show a zone of stromal hypercellularity immediately adjacent to epithelial spaces.
HPF, high power field.

malignant tumors) and 10% metastasize (0%, 4%, and 22% of benign, border-line, and malignant tumors, respectively). Recurrences can be associated with grade progression.

3. **Periductal stromal sarcoma.** This very rare tumor histologically resembles a low-grade phyllodes tumor, except that it tends to grow around rounded epithelial structures and lacks the leaf-like pattern seen with phyllodes tumors.

4. **Mammary hamartoma.** This uncommon lesion usually appears as a rubbery, well-circumscribed mass composed of a poorly organized variable admixture of ductal and lobular elements, mammary stroma, and adipose tissue. Smooth muscle may also be present, and if prominent, the term myoid hamartoma may be used. Mammary hamartomas are benign.

H. Stromal/mesenchymal lesions

1. **Fibroblastic/myofibroblastic lesions**

   a. **Pseudoangiomatous stromal hyperplasia (PASH).** This myofibroblastic proliferation is often an incidental histological finding, but may present as a mass lesion. Most patients are premenopausal; PASH has also been reported in postmenopausal women on hormone replacement therapy. Mass lesions are rubbery and well demarcated. Histologically, PASH appears on slit-like spaces lined by variably plump spindle cells surrounded by dense collagenized stroma (e-**Fig. 18.71**). The component myofibroblasts are usually vimentin, CD34, and actin positive by immunohistochemistry. The somewhat connecting slit-like spaces with their plump "endothelium-like" lining can occasionally resemble the anastomosing vascular channels of low-grade angiosarcoma, an important differential diagnosis (which can be further confounded by the occasional presence of large atypical cells in PASH). The lack of true vascular channels or destruction of breast lobules can be helpful in excluding angiosarcoma. The lack of cytokeratin expression in PASH can also be used to exclude ILC, another potential differential diagnosis. PASH is completely benign but may occasionally recur.

   b. **Myofibroblastoma.** This rare benign tumor is almost as common in men as in women. It appears as a well-circumscribed rubbery to firm mass that is composed of bland spindle cells arranged in small clustered fascicles separated by thick collagen bands (e-**Fig. 18.72**). An epithelioid variant has also been described. The spindle cells are usually immunoreactive for vimentin, CD34, desmin, and actin, but negative for cytokeratin. Among other features, the well-circumscribed nature of the lesion helps to distinguish it from fibromatosis and spindle-cell metaplastic carcinoma.

   c. **Fibromatosis.** This infiltrative fibroblastic/myofibroblastic lesion is similar to its nonmammary counterpart, and presents as an irregular firm to hard mass that resembles carcinoma clinically and/or radiologically. Histologically, fibromatosis is composed of sheets or fascicles of plump spindle cells with poorly defined cell borders (e-**Fig. 18.73**); a storiform or herringbone pattern and occasional mitoses are sometimes present. There are several differential diagnoses (in addition to myofibroblastoma) that need to be considered: A prior history of surgery would suggest a hyperplastic scar reaction; better circumscription, an inflammatory infiltrate, extracellular mucin, and extravasated red blood cells would suggest nodular fasciitis; hypercellularity, nuclear pleomorphism, and prominent mitotic activity are more in keeping with a diagnosis of fibrosarcoma, or in the presence of a prominent storiform pattern, malignant fibrous histiocytoma; and finally, a histological similarity to fibromatosis would suggest low-grade spindle cell metaplastic carcinoma.

   d. **Solitary fibrous tumor, spindle cell lipoma, and hemangiopericytoma.** These related tumors have all been reported in the breast. Lack of muscle marker expression helps distinguish these CD34-positive lesions from myofibroblastoma, the most important differential diagnosis.

   e. **Other tumors.** These include, among others, inflammatory myofibroblastic tumor, fibrosarcoma, and malignant fibrous histiocytoma. The latter two tumors are more often seen as part of a malignant phyllodes tumor.

2. **Vascular lesions**
   a. **Hemangiomas.** These breast lesions of the breast occur in both men and women with a wide age distribution. They can be microscopic and incidental, termed perilobular hemangioma, or present as a mass and/or radiographic abnormality. Nonincidental hemangiomas appear grossly as well-circumscribed spongy lesions, and microscopically may be capillary, cavernous, or venous in nature.
   b. **Angiomatosis.** This rare vascular lesion displays an extensive proliferation of irregular vascular channels that do not dissect breast lobules, or shows anastamosing channels or endothelial atypia.
   c. **Atypical vascular lesions.** These present as solitary or multiple skin or breast nodules 2 to 5 years after radiotherapy. Histologically, the findings include dilated anastamosing vascular spaces lined by plump endothelium with occasional projections or epithelial tufting. Unlike angiosarcoma, the major differential diagnosis, these lesions are well circumscribed, and lack the nuclear atypia, mitotic activity, blood lakes, and degree of endothelial proliferation seen in angiosarcoma.
   d. **Angiosarcoma.** Angiosarcomas rarely involve the breast and may be primary or develop secondary to radiotherapy. Primary angiosarcomas can present anytime between the second and eighth decades, usually as a breast mass with or without skin discoloration. Postradiation angiosarcomas that arise after mastectomy usually involve the chest wall, whereas those developing after conservation surgery usually involve the skin with or without the underlying breast. Almost all patients with postradiation angiosarcomas are older than 60 years, with the interval between radiotherapy and tumor development ranging from 3 to 13 years.

   Angiosarcomas appear grossly as spongy hemorrhagic lesions, but are usually less well-demarcated than other vascular lesions. Microscopically, the histological hallmark of angiosarcoma is the presence of freely anastamosing vascular channels that dissect the involved tissue, whether skin collagen, interlobular breast stroma, intralobular breast stroma (e-**Fig. 18.74**), or soft tissues of the chest wall. Low-grade angiosarcomas display atypical endothelial cells with prominent hyperchromatic nuclei and minimal endothelial tufting or mitotic activity; there should be no papillary formations, solid areas, necrosis, or blood lakes. Intermediate-grade tumors display more prominent endothelial tufting and mitotic activity; papillary and cellular foci should not constitute >25% of the tumor. High-grade tumors display extensive solid areas (usually >50% of tumor), often with prominent nuclear atypia and mitotic activity; necrosis and blood lakes are often present. Because the 5-year survival rates for low-, intermediate-, and high-grade angiosarcomas are 91%, 68%, and 14%, respectively, extensive sampling of low-grade tumors should always be performed to exclude higher grade foci.
3. **Adipocytic tumors**
   a. **Lipoma.** Intramammary lipoma is a rare lesion and presents as a slowly growing doughy mass, which appears well circumscribed grossly and microscopically. Angiolipoma can also be rarely encountered in the breast.
   b. **Liposarcoma.** Similar to other mammary sarcomas, liposarcoma most frequently arises as component of a malignant phyllodes tumor. The appearance is similar to liposarcomas at other sites.
4. **Rhabdomyosarcoma.** Alveolar rhabdomyosarcoma is a rare primary tumor that arises in children and young adults; metastatic involvement from elsewhere is more common. Rhabdomyosarcomatous differentiation is more frequently seen as a heterologous component in a malignant phyllodes tumor.
5. **Hematolymphoid lesions.** Primary breast lymphoma is rare; secondary involvement by systemic lymphoma or leukemia is more common. Most cases present with a mass, but constitutional symptoms may also be present. Diffuse large B-cell lymphoma and Burkitt's lymphoma are the most frequent types of primary B-cell lymphomas; T-cell lymphomas are much less frequent, and Hodgkin lymphoma is very rare. It is important to note that a diffuse lymphomatous infiltrate

(e-Fig. 18.75) that extends into fat, especially in low-grade tumors, may mimic ILC. Accordingly, lack of ER and PR expression in what superficially appears to be an ILC should always prompt careful examination and/or additional immunostains (such as cytokeratin and/or leukocyte common antigen) to confirm the diagnosis. Other differential diagnostic considerations include a benign intramammary lymph node and lymphocytic mastitis. Plasmacytomas and Rosai–Dorfman disease are among other hematolymphoid lesions that can sometimes involve the breast.

6. **Granular cell tumor and nerve sheath tumors.** Granular cell tumor is most often seen in women between 30 and 50 years of age. It usually presents as a firm or hard mass, often close to the nipple. Histologically, it appears as an infiltrative tumor composed of solid nests of cells with granular eosinophilic cytoplasm (e-Fig. 18.76). Diffuse strong immunoreactivity for S-100 protein and a lack of reaction with epithelial markers can confirm the diagnosis and exclude invasive carcinoma. Most granular cell tumors of the breast behave in a benign fashion. Other tumors of nerve sheath origin that can arise in the breast include schwannomas and neurofibromas.

I. **Diseases of the nipple**
   1. **Developmental anomalies.** The most common abnormality is polythelia, which is characterized by the presence of one or more accessory nipples anywhere along the primitive milk line that runs from the mid-axillary line to the vulva.
   2. **Inflammatory conditions.** Eczema and other inflammatory dermatoses can involve the nipple and the adjacent skin. The pathological findings are similar to those elsewhere (see Chap. 38).
   3. **Paget disease of the nipple.** This is characterized by the presence of malignant glandular epithelial cells scattered between the squamous epithelial cells of the nipple (e-Fig. 18.77). Such cells can often also be identified tracking between the normal epithelial cells of an underlying lactiferous duct, and in most cases, Paget disease is a pattern of intraductal spread from an underlying in situ and/or invasive carcinoma. Paget disease may be discovered incidentally in the course of a mastectomy, or may present as an erythematous to eczematous lesion with or without an underlying mass. The presence of intracytoplasmic PAS-positive, diastase-resistant mucin globules is a characteristic, but not a universal, finding. Immunohistochemical stains can also help confirm the diagnosis, as Paget cells are positive for epithelial membrane antigen, low-molecular-weight cytokeratin, and carcinoembryonic antigen. Paget cells are immunonegative for melanoma markers (HMB45, Melan-A, and S-100), which is important from a differential diagnostic standpoint.
   4. **Nipple adenoma.** As discussed earlier, this can be considered a form of intraductal papilloma arising within lactiferous ducts and localized to the nipple. Most patients are older than 40 years and present with an irregular firm mass with or without erosion or ulceration of the overlying nipple. Histologically, there is an expansile, cellular, adenomatous and papillary proliferation in which both epithelial and myoepithelial cells are seen. Especially when ulceration is present, the cellularity of the lesion and the occasional presence of epithelial atypia may lead to confusion with a malignant process.
   5. **Syringomatous adenoma.** This is a locally aggressive tumor of the nipple/areola complex that is histologically identical to syringoma of the skin. It presents as an irregular firm mass and is composed of irregular glands, cords, and nests of cells displaying both basal and luminal layers.

J. **Diseases of the male breast.** A significant number of breast lesions can arise in the male breast. These include papillary lesions, fibroepithelial tumors, myofibroblastoma, duct ectasia, benign proliferative disease, gynecomastia, and invasive carcinoma. The appearances of invasive carcinomas are very much similar to those seen in the female breast.

K. **Pathology of axillary (and intramammary) lymph nodes**
   1. **Metastatic carcinoma.** Involvement of axillary lymph nodes by metastatic breast carcinoma is most frequently manifested within the subcapsular sinuses with or without parenchymal involvement (e-Fig. 18.78). Especially with ILC, metastases

may sometimes appear as scattered individual tumor cells within the parenchyma. In all of these situations, the size of the largest deposit should be measured and reported. In addition, because extracapsular extension of carcinoma often dictates additional radiotherapy directed to the axilla, its presence or absence should also be documented.

2. **Silicone lymphadenitis.** As mentioned earlier, silicone granulomas can sometimes be seen in axillary lymph nodes.

3. **Heterotopic epithelial elements.** Heterotopic breast tissue can occasionally be seen in the axilla adjacent to lymph nodes. Less frequently, various epithelial inclusions can be seen within axillary lymph nodes, including cystic lesions lined by squamous or apocrine epithelium and heterotopic breast tissue. The obvious differential diagnosis for heterotopic breast tissue is metastatic carcinoma; heterotopic breast tissue tends to preferentially involve the capsule and/or parenchyma and spare the sinuses, and myoepithelial cells and even specialized intralobular stroma are present (e-Fig. 18.79). In the absence of a myoepithelial cell component, any glandular lesion within axillary lymph nodes should be regarded as evidence of metastatic carcinoma regardless of how well differentiated.

4. **Nevus cell aggregates.** Capsular aggregates of nevus cells are not infrequently identified in axillary lymph nodes (e-Fig. 18.80). Several features, not all of which are always present, help to distinguish these aggregates from metastatic carcinoma, including pigmentation, a nested growth pattern, extension into perinodal fat, a cellular component characterized by a somewhat spindled shape, ill-defined cell borders, and intranuclear inclusions. The diagnosis of nevus aggregates can easily be substantiated by S-100 and/or HMB45 immunoreactivity and a negative reaction with cytokeratin antibodies.

5. **Displaced epithelial cells.** As discussed earlier, displacement of epithelial cells into the stroma can occur with papillary lesions and can simulate invasion. More problematic is the evaluation of epithelial elements of papillary lesions in axillary lymph nodes as displaced cells versus metastatic carcinoma, as displacement has been reported to occur following needle biopsy and other surgical procedures involving papillomas and papillary carcinomas (*J Clin Oncol.* 2006;24:2013) (e-Fig. 18.81).

L. **Pathology of treated breast cancer.** Neoadjuvant chemotherapy and radiotherapy are increasingly being used in the management of breast cancer. Response to treatment is often categorized clinically as complete, partial, or no response. Treatment may affect the primary tumor and lymph nodes involved by metastatic disease producing various histological changes in the tumor morphology, including necrosis, decreased cellularity, cytoplasmic eosinophilia, and nuclear aberrations. Fibrosis, a foamy histiocytic infiltrate, and hemosiderin deposition are other common manifestations (e-Fig. 18.82). In up to 10% of cases, no residual tumor cells are detected by routine H&E-stained sections (immunohistochemistry is rarely indicated), indicating a complete histological response. The effect of such neoadjuvant treatment is not limited to invasive carcinomas, and normal breast epithelium may show atrophy, hyalinization, and nuclear aberrations in response to therapy.

CYTOLOGY OF THE BREAST
Lourdes R. Ylagan

I. METHODS OF SPECIMEN PROCUREMENT

A. **Fine needle aspiration** (FNA) of palpable and non-palpable breast lesions through mammographic guidance is currently accepted as a cost-effective, reliable, and accurate tool in the evaluation of breast lesions. The combination of mammographic features, clinical findings, and cytologic evaluation of breast FNA specimens (the so-called triple test) has considerably decreased the false diagnosis rate of breast cancer (*Cancer* 1987;60:1866).

B. **Ductal lavage** has recently been employed as a screening method in women with a personal history of breast cancer, but the sensitivity and accuracy of the approach for detecting premalignant lesions of the breast ductal epithelium is still under investigation (*Am J Surg* 2006;191:57 and *Clin Lab Med* 2005;25:787).

II. **SPECIMEN ADEQUACY.** There is no uniform criterion on which specimen adequacy can be determined, even in the presence of well-preserved and well-visualized breast epithelium (e-**Fig. 18.83**), without taking into consideration the experience of the aspirator and/or interpreter, clinical presentation, and mammographic findings of the individual mass.

III. **DIAGNOSTIC CATEGORIES**
   A. **Negative for malignancy.** This diagnosis is generally rendered for benign breast lesions, including inflammatory or infectious lesions, that are without clinical or mammographic findings suspicious for malignancy.
   B. **Atypical cytology.** This diagnosis is rendered on cellular lesions showing some degree of nuclear atypia; the cells generally maintain a well-organized pattern (e-**Fig. 18.84**).
   C. **Suspicious for malignancy.** This diagnosis is rendered when the aspirate shows cells with worrisome cytologic features that fall short of those required for a diagnosis of malignancy.
   D. **Positive for malignancy.** This diagnosis is rendered when both the quality of the cytologic changes and the quantity of the malignant cells are sufficient for an unequivocal diagnosis of malignancy.

IV. **CYTOLOGIC FEATURES OF COMMON BREAST LESIONS**
   A. **Fibroadenoma** is a clinically well-circumscribed nodule with a homogeneous mammographic appearance. Cytologically, it is composed of benign ductal cells arranged in a staghorn pattern with abundant myoepithelial cells (e-**Fig. 18.85**). Abundant stromal fragments may be seen.
   B. **Gynecomastia** is clinically a well-circumscribed and often painful subareolar lesion in a man. The lesion has mammographic and cytologic findings that are similar to those of a fibroadenoma (e-**Fig. 18.85**).
   C. **Fibrocystic changes** typically present as a palpable, ill-defined lesion which may have mammographically detectable microcalcifications. Cytologically, the lesion is composed of apocrine, ductal cells, mucus, and muciphages in varying amounts (e-**Fig. 18.86**).
   D. **Subareolar abscess** is a clinically painful, palpable subareolar mass typically associated with lactation. Cytologically, it consists of neutrophils and benign anucleate squamous epithelium (e-**Fig. 18.87**).
   E. **Ductal adenocarcinoma** usually presents as a clinically palpable, mammographically suspicious mass which cytologically shows a cellular smear containing large ductal cells which maybe poorly cohesive, without a myoepithelial component. The cells have pleomorphic nuclei, vesicular chromatin, and prominent nucleoli. Individual cells may have intracytoplasmic vacuoles containing inspissated material (e-**Fig. 18.88**).
   F. **Lobular adenocarcinoma** may not be clinically palpable, but presents mammographically as an ill-defined mass lesion. Cytologic preparations show siingly dispersed small plasmacytoid cells with vacuolated cytoplasm often containing inspissated material. The nuclei are uniformly small, round-to-oval, and not much bigger than a neutrophil (e-**Fig. 18.89**).

V. **SPECIAL STUDIES.** Immunocytologic evaluation of estrogen and progesterone receptor studies can be performed on cytospin slide preparations; immunocytologic evaluation of HER2 on cytospin slide preparations is limited due to the requirement of an intact cell membrane for proper assessment. Immunohistochemical evaluation of three of these markers can also be performed on paraffin-embedded cell block samples prepared from fine needle aspirates. FISH for *HER2* gene amplification can be performed on cytospin slide preparations or paraffin-embedded cell blocks.

Suggested Readings

Mckee GT. *Cytopathology of the Breast with Imaging and Histologic Correlation.* Oxford University Press. 2002.

Zakhou H, Wells C, and Perry NM. *Diagnostic Cytopathology of the Breast.* Churchill Livingstone. 1999.

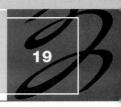
I. RENAL BIOPSY HANDLING AND PROCESSING. Renal biopsy is performed for various reasons, among which is monitoring the status of renal allografts, diagnosis of renal masses, and diagnosis of medical renal diseases. Renal allograft and medical renal biopsies are usually received in transport media, allowing distribution of tissue for light microscopy (LM), immunofluorescence (IF), and electron microscopy (EM).

    A. Light microscopy. The LM evaluation requires a minimum of three hematoxylin & eosin (H&E), one trichrome, two periodic acid–Schiff (PAS), and one Jones silver–stained sections. A minimum of seven glomeruli and one artery is required.

    B. Immunofluorescence. A minimum of two glomeruli is required. A direct IF method is routinely used employing a panel of antibodies, including anti-immunoglobulin (Ig)G, IgA, IgM, C3, C1q, fibrinogen, albumin, and κ and λ light chains. It is important to document the staining pattern (linear vs granular) and distribution (mesangial, loop, or combined).

    C. Electron microscopy. Ultrastructural evaluation of two glomeruli is recommended. EM allows for evaluation of cellular and extracellular abnormalities in the glomeruli, tubules, interstitium, and vessels. EM is very useful in confirming the presence and distribution of electron-dense deposits. Deposits can be located in the mesangium or glomerular capillary basement membrane. In the basement membrane they can be subepithelial, subendothelial, or intramembranous (surrounded by basement membrane).

II. GLOMERULAR DISEASES. Glomerular diseases may be primary or secondary (associated with systemic diseases). Patients can be grouped into those that present with the nephrotic syndrome (>3 g urine protein/day), nephritic syndrome (proteinuria + hematuria), or isolated hematuria. It is important to the pathologist to have access to the patient's clinical and laboratory data. For example, minimal change disease, focal segmental glomerulosclerosis, and membranous glomerulonephritis (GN) usually present with nephrotic syndrome. In contrast, postinfectious GN usually presents with nephritic syndrome.

    A. Minimal change disease and focal segmental glomerulosclerosis. Minimal change disease (MCD) and focal segmental glomerulosclerosis (FSGS) are the most common causes of nephrotic syndrome in children and are also common in adults, affecting ~10% to 20% of patients with kidney disease. Primary FSGS may be idiopathic, secondary, or familial (*Am J Nephrol* 23:353, 2003). Less than nephrotic range proteinuria may be present in advanced cases. Some patients have concurrent hematuria and hypertension (HTN). The classic findings in MCD are (Table 19.1):

        LM: Normal appearing glomeruli
        IF: Negative
        EM: Extensive foot process effacement (e-**Fig. 19.1**).*
    The diagnostic features of FSGS are:
        LM: Segmental sclerosis in some but not all glomeruli. Accurate diagnosis of FSGS depends on the extent of the disease and the number of glomeruli present in the biopsy. The diagnosis may be missed because of sampling error, particularly with the smaller size needles currently used. It has been estimated that in a biopsy containing 10 glomeruli, there is a 35% chance of missing FSGS. Notably, even one glomerulus

---

*All e-figures are available online via the Solution Site Image Bank.

TABLE 19.1 Major Glomerular Patterns and Differential Diagnosis on Light Microscopy

Minimal changes	FSGS	Mesangial hypercellularity	Thick loops	Tram-track	Proliferative	Crescents	Nodular pattern
MCD	Primary NOS	IgA-HSP, MCD/FSGS	Membranous	MPGN	Postinfectious GN	>50% is crescentic	Diabetes
Thin membrane disease	Secondary NOS	Lupus	Diabetes	HSP	Lupus	<50% is other GN	MPGN
Early lupus	Cellular type	IgM nephropathy	Alport	Lupus	HSP		Amyloidosis
Early/mild IgA	Perihilar	C1q nephropathy	Amyloidosis				MIDD
Early diabetes	Tip lesion	C3/IgG glomerulopathy					
	Collapsing						

FSGS, focal segmental glomerulosclerosis; NOS, not otherwise specified; Ig, immunoglobulin; HSP, Henoch–Schonlein purpura; MCD, minimal change disease; MPGN, membranoproliferative glomerulonephritis; MIDD, monoclonal immunoglobulin deposition disease.

with FSGS is sufficient for diagnosis. The corticomedullary glomeruli are the first to be sclerosed; therefore, needle biopsies should opt to sample this region.

IF: Is either entirely negative or has focal and weak mesangial C3 or IgM deposits.

EM: Shows focal foot process effacement (e-**Fig. 19.2**), the degree of which may depend on the degree of proteinuria. Other EM findings in MCD/FSGS include microvillus transformation of foot processes, endothelial cell edema, podocyte detachment, and glomerular basement membranes (GBM) wrinkling (e-**Fig. 19.2f**).

Beyond this classic presentation, light and electron microscopic findings may be similar in MCD and FSGS. For example, glomeruli may appear normal in FSGS, and focal foot process effacement may be present in MCD.

Glomerular hypercellularity and enlargement (glomerulomegaly) is thought to represent an early lesion of FSGS. A recent FSGS classification scheme describes various histologic patterns with significantly different prognosis (*Kidney Int* 38:115, 1990). The cellular variant is rare (seen in only ~3% of FSGS), but the following variants are more frequent: perihilar FSGS (26%), tip lesion (17%), usual type not otherwise specified (NOS) (42%), and collapsing FSGS (11%) (e-**Fig. 19.2, a–e**) (*Am J Kidney Dis* 43:368, 2004). The tip and cellular lesions have the best prognosis and collapsing FSGS the worst (*Kidney Int* 69:920, 2006). Tubulointerstitial damage and vascular thickening indicate chronic disease. Pathologic similarities between MCD and FSGS suggested that they are one disease with a spectrum of findings, but recent clinical and molecular studies demonstrate that FSGS has a worse prognosis and different pathogenesis than MCD.

B. Collapsing FSGS is a distinct FSGS variant considered by some to be an entirely different disease. Clinically, the disease is characterized by black racial predominance, a high incidence of nephrotic syndrome, and rapidly progressive renal failure. First identified in human immunodeficiency virus (HIV) patients, the disease was later recognized in association with viruses such as parvovirus 19, hepatitis B, hepatitis C, and pamidronate chemotherapy (*Semin Diagn Pathol* 19:106, 2002). The disease may also involve allograft kidneys. It is an aggressive disease that is difficult to treat (*Semin Nephrol* 23:209, 2003). Pathogenesis involves podocyte cell-cycle dysregulation resulting in proliferation.

LM: Characterized by segmental glomerular capillary collapse and podocyte hypertrophy, often accompanied by microcystic tubular dilatation and interstitial inflammation (e-**Fig. 19.2e**). The main difference from usual FSGS is the collapse of the capillary loops versus sclerosis, and podocyte proliferation versus podocyte loss.

IF: Nonspecific

EM: Shows proliferating podocytes and wrinkled/collapsed capillary loops.

C. Membranous GN is the most common cause of nephrotic syndrome in adults (30% to 50% of cases). It may occur at any age, but accounts for <5% of childhood nephrotic syndrome. Most cases are idiopathic, but approximately 10% are associated with identifiable causes such as malignancy, autoimmune diseases (systemic lupus erythematosis [SLE]), drugs, and infections (hepatitis B, syphilis). Glomerular lesions resemble those seen in Heymanns' nephritis, an animal model in which antibodies react with the Heymann antigen, a complex of **megalin** and the **receptor-associated protein,** expressed in the tubular brush border and the basal surface of the visceral epithelial cells.

LM: Membranous GN is a diffuse process in which the glomeruli are not hypercellular but usually exhibit thickening of the capillary basement membrane while maintaining luminal patency. In Jones silver–stained sections, the basement membrane can show "spikes" projecting from the epithelial side of the basement membrane. Spikes result from the presence of subepithelial electron-dense deposits (silver stain negative) and deposition of basement membranelike material on the sides of the deposits (e-**Fig. 19.3**). Glomeruli appear essentially normal in early cases.

IF: Diffuse, granular staining for IgG and C3 is present along the glomerular capillary loops by IF. Other immunoglobulins can be present but have lower intensity.

EM: At early stages, the electron-dense deposits are subepithelial. As the disease progresses, deposition of basement membranelike material at the sides of the electron-dense deposits occurs so that with time the electron-dense deposits are surrounded by basement membrane and so become intramembranous. The deposits eventually become electron lucent, suggesting their degeneration or reabsorption (e-Fig. 19.3).

D. **Mesangial proliferative GN (IgA, IgM, IgG, and C3).** Mesangial hypercellularity is defined as > 3 mesangial cells per glomerular segment. Many glomerular diseases may have increased mesangial cells (Table 19.1) including variants of MCD and FSGS. Mesangial hypercellularity indicates the presence of associated mesangial immune deposits and/or reactive proliferation. The most common disease is the IgA form, clinically characterized by micro- or macrohematuria and varying proteinuria (rarely nephrotic syndrome or crescentic GN) (*Nephrol Dial Transplant* 16 Suppl 6:77, 2001).

LM: Mesangial hypercellularity varies from focal to diffuse.

IF: Diagnosis is made by the presence of predominant or codominant IgA mesangial deposits (e-Fig. 19.4). Mild IgG and IgM deposits may also be present, particularly in Henoch-Schonlein purpura (HSP), which is thought of as the systemic form of IgA disease.

EM: Shows mesangial/paramesangial deposits, and occasionally capillary loop subendothelial deposits, that may extend to the GBM and cause splitting (more common in HSP) or "humps."

Histologic parameters which negatively affect prognosis in IgA disease include glomerular sclerosis, capillary wall IgA deposits, and vascular and tubulointerstitial fibrosis. Glomerular sclerosis is the best independent predictor of adverse outcome and renal failure. HSP mimics IgA disease pathologically, but clinically is a systemic disease that presents with skin rash, arthritis, and abdominal pain in addition to nephritis. IgA is the most common glomerular disease worldwide with variable prognosis (~30% develop end-stage renal disease [ESRD]); HSP tends to be self-limiting with only about 18% of patients progressing to ESRD. Both may recur in transplant kidneys, but clinical symptoms are mild despite IgA deposition.

Mesangial hypercellularity not infrequently accompanies the various types of GN. For example, MCD and/or FSGS with mesangial hypercellularity are generally thought to have a worse prognosis. Focal IgM deposits are seen in some such cases. Rarely, diffuse IgM deposits are detected (which have raised considerable debate as to whether they represent a separate entity named IgM nephropathy).

An entity known as **C1q nephropathy** is characterized by predominant C1q deposits and is considered a variant of MCD/FSGS (*Am J Clin Pathol* 83:415, 1985). C1q nephropathy is primarily a disease of children and young adults. Other glomerulopathies characterized by isolated C3 or IgG mesangial deposits in patients without lupus stigmata have been described recently and named accordingly. IgG glomerulopathy is a pediatric disease that may be an aberrant manifestation of lupus nephritis (LN) (*JASN* 13:379, 2002).

E. **Postinfectious GN.** Postinfectious GN (PIGN) is a classic complication of streptococcal pharyngitis and presents acutely with nephritic syndrome. However, classic PIGN is currently infrequent; most cases now follow staphylococcal skin infections and other bacterial, viral, fungal, or parasitic infections, and are more frequently chronic or atypical (*Hum Pathol* 34:3, 2003). Erythrogenic toxin type B is thought to be the target antigen for immune complexes that are implanted in the GBM.

LM: The pathology is unique, characterized by white cells in the glomeruli (predominantly neutrophils in the acute phase), and lymphocytes or macrophages in chronic cases.

IF: There are large granular IgG and C3 deposits along capillary loops (e-Fig. 19.5). Occasionally, deposits are located predominantly in the mesangium (instead of in the loops) and are C3 or IgA/ IgM instead of IgG (*Semin Diagn Pathol* 19:146, 2002).

EM: Shows characteristic bell-shaped deposits (humps).

F. Membranoproliferative GN. Patients with membranoproliferative GN (MPGN) can present with features of nephrotic and/or nephritic syndrome, and most patients have a low serum C3 level. Although MPGN can affect patients of all ages, it is more common in children. Three types of MPGN have been described; because all types can have similar histologic findings, EM is used to differentiate them. Type I is the most common type, followed by types II and III. It is important to note that MPGN type I can be associated with other diseases such as viral hepatitis, so patients should have a work-up for secondary causes of MPGN when the pathologic diagnosis is established.

LM: MPGN is a diffuse glomerulopathy with endocapillary proliferation that results in lobular accentuation (e-**Fig. 19.6**). The GBMs are thick, and the capillary lumens are not evident. The Jones silver stain reveals double GBM contours, also known as "tram-tracking." These findings are more commonly seen in MPGN type I. MPGN type II tends to have a less consistent histologic pattern.

IF: A strong and diffuse granular staining for C3 is observed along the glomerular capillary walls and the mesangium. Approximately 60% of type I MPGN also exhibit positive IgG and/or C1q immunostains. Negative immunostains for immunoglobulins and C1q are usually observed in MPGN type II.

EM: This is the most useful tool for differentiating MPGN types. MPGN type I shows mesangial interposition (extension of mesangial cell cytoplasm into the capillary wall) and subendothelial electron-dense deposits. When the mesangial cell cytoplasm extends into the glomerular capillary wall, basement membranelike material is laid down by the mesangial and endothelial cells, creating a second "new" basement membrane. This process results in the "tram-tracking" observed by LM. MPGN type II is also known as dense deposit disease because it has ribbonlike, electron-dense deposits along the capillary walls, often replacing the lamina densa. These deposits are not necessarily present in all capillary loops and may only be present in some segments and the mesangium. The composition of these electron-dense deposits remains uncertain (e-**Fig. 19.6**). The ultrastructural findings of MPGN type III are similar to those of MPGN type I, but with subendothelial and subepithelial electron-dense deposits.

G. Crescentic GN. The term crescentic GN refers to the presence of cellular crescents in >50% of glomeruli available in a renal biopsy. Its usual clinical presentation is that of rapidly progressive GN. Patients can have renal limited or systemic disease (Table 19.2).

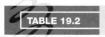

TABLE 19.2	Findings That Help in Subclassification of Crescentic Glomerulonephritis		
Light microscopy	**Renal biopsy where 50% or more glomeruli have cellular crescents**		
Immunofluorescence	Smooth linear staining along glomerular capillary loops for IgG	Negative glomerular immunostain for immunoglobulins	Granular glomerular immunostain for immunoglobulins
Electron microscopy	No electron-dense deposits	No electron-dense deposits	Electron-dense deposits present
Diagnostic category	Antiglomerular basement membrane disease; Goodpasture's disease	Pauci-immune glomerulonephritis	Immune-complex glomerulonephritis (primary or secondary)

IgG, immunoglobulin G.

LM: Cellular crescents are identified in >50% of glomeruli (**e-Fig. 19.7**). Necrotizing glomerular lesions are commonly seen. Additional morphologic findings are dependent on the type of renal limited or systemic disease.

IF: Is used to further classify crescentic GN. In anti-GBM disease or Goodpasture's disease, glomeruli exhibit smooth linear IgG staining along the capillary basement membrane (**e-Fig. 19.7**). Immune-complex GN has a granular staining pattern for one or more immunoglobulins. Pauci-immune GN has negative immunostains for all immunoglobulins.

EM: The glomerular changes noted by EM correspond to the necrosis, disruption of the GBM, and crescents that are seen in all crescentic GN. The smooth linear IgG staining of anti-GMB or Goodpasture's disease does not have a morphologic correlate that can be detected by EM. Cases of immune-complex GN will show electron-dense deposits. Similar findings are also identified in pauci-immune GN.

H. Lupus nephritis. SLE is a multisystemic autoimmune disorder with a peak incidence in the second and third decade of life and a female predominance (male/female ratio of 1:9). It is more common in African Americans. The clinical diagnosis of lupus is based on clinical and laboratory criteria established by the American Rheumatism Association. Renal involvement by the disease is relatively common; approximately half of lupus patients develop LN during the first year of the disease. Although this chapter emphasizes the glomerular findings of LN, it is important to note that interstitial, tubular, and vascular lesions can also accompany the glomerular changes. Use of the International Society of Nephrology/Renal Pathology Society (ISN/RPS) classification of LN (Table 19.2), which is a modification of the World Health Organization (WHO) classification (*Kidney Int* 65:521, 2004.), is recommended.

LM: LN can present with various light microscopic patterns (Tables 19.3 and 19.4). With time and/or treatment, the renal lesion can evolve into a different class. Membranous LN can occur in combination with Class III or IV. The glomerular active lesions include endocapillary hypercellularity with or without leukocyte infiltration and with substantial luminal reduction, karyorrhexis, fibrinoid necrosis, rupture of GBM, cellular or fibrocellular crescents, wire loops, and hyaline thrombi (**e-Fig. 19.8**). The glomerular chronic lesions include segmental or global glomerulosclerosis, fibrous adhesions, and fibrous crescents.

TABLE 19.3   **ISN/RPS Classification of Lupus Nephritis (LN)**

Class I	Minimal mesangial LN	
Class II	Mesangial proliferative LN	
Class III	Focal LN (involvement of <50% glomeruli)	
	III (A)	Focal proliferative LN (purely active lesions)
	III (A/C)	Focal proliferative and sclerosing LN (active and chronic lesions)
	III (C)	Focal sclerosing LN (chronic inactive with glomerular scars)
Class IV	Diffuse LN (Active or inactive diffuse, segmental and/or global endocapillary and/or extracapillary GN involving ≥50% glomeruli)	
	IV-S (A) or IV-G (A)	Diffuse segmental or global proliferative LN
	IV-S(A/C) or IV-G (A/C)	Diffuse segmental or global proliferative and sclerosing LN
	IV-S(C) or IV-G(C)	Diffuse segmental or global sclerosing LN
Class V	Membranous LN	
Class VI	Advanced sclerosing LN (≥90% glomeruli globally sclerosed)	

ISN/RPS, International Society of Nephrology/Renal Pathology Society; S, segmental; G, global; A, active lesions; C, chronic lesions.

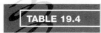

| **TABLE 19.4** | Summary of Pathologic Findings of Lupus Nephritis |

Class	Light microscopy	Immunofluorescence	Electron microscopy
I	Minimal mesangial hypercellularity	Mesangial +	Mesangial deposits
II	Mesangial hypercellularity and increased matrix	Mesangial +	Mesangial deposits
III	Endocapillary and/or extracapillary proliferation in <50% of glomeruli	Mesangial and loop +	Mesangial and subendothelial deposits
IV	Endocapillary and/or extracapillary proliferation in ≥50% of glomeruli	Mesangial and loop +	Mesangial and subendothelial deposits
V	Thick loops and mesangial hypercellularity	Mesangial and loop +	Numerous subepithelial and scattered mesangial deposits

IF: A glomerular IgG-positive immunostain is almost universal in LN; the term "full house" is used when IgG, IgA, and IgM immunostains are positive. C3 and C1q are usually present.

I. Diabetes mellitus. In the kidney, diabetes mellitus increases the propensity to pyelonephritis, papillary necrosis, arteriosclerosis, and glomerular disease. Hyperglycemia induces biochemical changes in the GBM, nonenzymatic glycosylation of proteins, and hemodynamic changes with glomerular hypertrophy. Diabetic glomerulosclerosis in the absence of vascular changes in the eye fundus is unlikely to develop.

LM: GBM thickening develops in early stages. Increased mesangial matrix eventually results in diffuse glomerulosclerosis and nodular diabetic glomerulosclerosis, also known as Kimmelstiel-Wilson disease (e-**Fig. 19.9**).

IF: Immunofluorescence studies of the renal biopsy are essentially negative. However, glomeruli exhibit a nonspecific IgG linear staining that has the same or less intensity than that observed in the albumin immunostain.

EM: Shows thickening of the GBM and various degrees of mesangial expansion. Electron-dense deposits are not identified by EM.

J. Amyloidosis. Renal amyloidosis can be primary or secondary. Patients often present with nephrotic syndrome (~50%), peripheral neuropathy (carpal-tunnel syndrome), heart failure, and/or liver disease due to amyloid deposits. There are many different proteins that form amyloid, including AA, AL amyloid, transthyretin (ATTR), and familial types, which confer a different prognosis (for example, worse for AL amyloid compared with ATTR). Amyloid is composed of proteins forming β-pleated sheets.

LM: Varies from GBM thickening to nodular or segmental sclerosis. Amorphous material is often apparent in the mesangium or the capillary loops. A Congo red stain is diagnostic, revealing apple green fluorescence under polarized light (e-**Fig. 19.10**).

IF: May show κ or λ light chains. Deposits of immunoglobulin fragments, such as heavy chains of IgG, IgM, IgA, or κ or λ light chains, may not form amyloid; in these latter cases a Congo red stain is negative, and the term "Congo red–negative amyloidosis" or monoclonal immunoglobulin deposition disease (MIDD) is used.

EM: Is characteristic and consists of randomly arranged 4- to 12-nm fibrils (e-**Fig. 19.10c**). EM shows either finely granular or filamentous deposits in the mesangium or the GBM (*Semin Diagn Pathol* 19:116, 2002).

The pathologic differential diagnosis of MIDD includes other nodular GN such as diabetes and fibrillary and immunotactoid glomerulopathy; the latter may have overlapping IF, but the EM findings are distinct from amyloid (*Kidney Int* 62:1764, 2002). The characteristic findings in MIDD are as follows.

LM: Glomeruli may appear nodular or have nonspecific changes. Diagnosis is usually (but not always) made by IF.

IF: Identifies the specific type of immunoglobulin fragment as either heavy or light chain (e-**Fig. 19.11**) (*J Am Soc Nephrol* 12:1482, 2001).

EM: Is often not specific, but in a typical use fine granular deposits (powder-like) are seen within the glomerular basement membrane.

K. **Alport's syndrome/thin membrane disease.** Classic X-linked (A-L) Alport's syndrome presents with microscopic or gross hematuria and deafness. Deafness and/or proteinuria are indications of severe disease. Mutations in *COLIVA3* cause X-L Alport's syndrome; *COLIVA4* mutations cause autosomal dominant (AD) and *COLIVA3* mutations cause autosomal recessive (AR) Alport's syndrome. Fifteen percent of X-L Alport's patients have no family history and are thought to represent a new mutation. There are very few patients with AD Alport's. Patients with AR Alport's are clinically similar to X-L Alport's. The organs that are affected in Alport's syndrome reflect the sites where these collagen IV chains are normally expressed ($\alpha 3$, $\alpha 4$, and $\alpha 5$ are exclusively found in the kidney, eye, and ear). Renal biopsy is performed for diagnosis as well as assessment of disease progression.

LM: Is not specific; it varies from unremarkable glomeruli, to FSGS, to chronic scarring. Foamy interstitial cells were once thought to be characteristic of Alport's, but they are in fact seen in many types of proteinuria.

IF: Routine stains are negative. Diagnosis of Alport's is facilitated by collagen IV chain immunostaining. The $\alpha 5$ chain of collagen IV is distinctly absent in X-L Alport's, and it is accompanied by absent $\alpha 3$ and $\alpha 4$ chains in glomeruli (collagen IV monomers are incorporated into basement membrane as triple helices to form the structural meshwork (*Kidney Int* 65:1109, 2004); when one chain is mutated, all three chains may degenerate because they become susceptible to enzymatic proteolysis). Typically, women with X-L Alport's have mosaic IV$\alpha 5$ linear staining in the glomeruli or skin (e-**Fig. 19.10**) (*Hum Pathol* 33:836, 2002). However, some women may have positive staining, making it difficult to distinguish from thin membrane disease (TMD, see below). The diagnostic pattern in men is absent collagen IV$\alpha 5$ and mosaic staining (linear interrupted positivity) in X-L women carriers (e-**Fig. 19.12**, **b–d**). A screening test for families with potential X-L Alport's is skin biopsy (IV$\alpha 5$ is the only chain found in skin).

EM: The cardinal pathologic findings of X-L Alport's are seen on EM and consist of abnormal splitting, widening, or thinning of the GBM with degeneration of collagen IV in the lamina densa in a pattern known as "bread crumbs" (e-**Fig. 19.12**). The lesions may involve tubular basement membranes as well. However, the specificity of the EM findings is only moderate (*Kidney Int* 56:760, 1999); for example, young children and women with Alport's nephritis may only manifest uniformly thin GBM that is indistinguishable from TMD (*Semin Nephrol* 25:149, 2005). About 30% of Alport's heterozygotes have uniformly thin GBM, but have *COLIVA3, COLIVA4,* or *COLIVA5* mutations by genetic testing; others have GBM lamellation in thin segments. Routine genetic testing is not required for diagnosis; testing is not only technically difficult (a number of different genes must be evaluated and mutational hot-spots do not exist), but also does not strictly correlate with pathology or prognosis. In contrast, a good family history of close relatives is very helpful.

TMD is defined as GBM thinning <250 nm in adults and <200 nm in children. These values are approximate as there is no true consensus as to how thin the GBM should be for the diagnosis of TMD. It is also debated as to whether GBM thinning must be diffuse or focal; most cases diagnosed as TMD have focal GBM thinning involving <50% of loops.

LM: In TMD is usually unremarkable.

IF: Routine stains are negative. Collagen IV$\alpha 3$, IV$\alpha 4$, and IV$\alpha 5$ immunostains are positive.

EM: Shows GBM diffuse or segmental thinning without lamellation (e-**Fig. 19.12f**).

III. TUBULOINTERSTITIAL DISEASES

A. Infectious processes. Infectious agents can result in tubulointerstitial nephritis by colonizing the renal parenchyma, or by triggering a systemic immunologic response that will target the renal tubules and interstitium. Bacterial agents are responsible for most cases of **acute pyelonephritis.** Most cases of acute pyelonephritis are ascending infections caused by gram-negative bacteria, particularly *Escherichia coli.* When bacteria reach the kidney using a hematogenous route, *Staphylococcus aureus* is usually the responsible agent. Acute pyelonephritis is characterized by an abundance of neutrophils in the lumen of tubules and the interstitium. Neutrophils are usually accompanied by other inflammatory cells.

Viral agents are also associated with tubulointerstitial nephritis. **Polyoma virus** and **cytomegalovirus (CMV)** are particularly important in renal allografts. The polyoma virus, also known as the BK virus, is a DNA virus with high prevalence during childhood, causing respiratory infections. Respiratory infection leads to hematogenous spread, with the virus reaching organs including the kidney, where it remains dormant; when the patient later becomes immunosuppressed, the virus reactivates. Kidneys with either of these viral infections show chronic interstitial inflammation sometimes associated with tubulitis, a pattern that is difficult to distinguish from acute cellular rejection. Both viruses elicit cytopathic changes that are seen in endothelial and tubular epithelial cells; polyoma virus forms an intranuclear basophilic inclusion, and CMV forms cytoplasmic and intranuclear basophilic inclusions with a perinuclear halo. It is useful to confirm the morphologic findings of viral infection using antibodies against the specific microorganism.

A granulomatous inflammatory response is usually seen with mycobacterial and some fungal infections. Histochemical stains like acid-fast bacillus (AFB), PAS, and silver stains are needed to visualize the microorganisms.

B. Acute tubular necrosis. Acute tubular necrosis (ATN) is the most common cause of acute renal failure and is usually due to toxins or ischemia. Regardless of the cause, the proximal tubule is the main target in ATN. The histologic changes are mainly confined to the tubules, with necrosis of the lining epithelium; epithelial necrosis is more extensive and confluent in the toxic type of ATN and tends to be patchy in the ischemic type. Because necrotic tubular epithelium will exfoliate into the tubular lumen, focal denudation of the tubular basement membrane is common (e-Fig. 19.13). Epithelial cells can also exhibit regenerative changes with nuclear enlargement, prominent nucleoli, and mitotic activity. Interstitial edema is usually present.

C. Allergic interstitial nephritis. Most cases of allergic interstitial nephritis are drug related; renal manifestations develop approximately 2 weeks after drug exposure. The typical presentation includes fever, skin rash, and eosinophilia, but this triad is only present in approximately 1/3 of patients. Interstitial eosinophils are the most important histologic clue for diagnosis. Eosinophils are accompanied by other inflammatory cells, mainly lymphocytes, and may be seen only focally (e-Fig. 19.14). Tubulitis and tubular injury usually accompany interstitial changes. Nonsteroidal anti-inflammatory drugs (NSAIDs) can also cause allergic interstitial nephritis, but interstitial eosinophils are usually rare. Patients taking NSAIDs can also develop nephrotic syndromes, and their glomeruli exhibit changes indistinguishable from minimal change disease.

D. Cast nephropathy. Amyloidosis, cast nephropathy, and light chain deposition disease are renal complications of patients with multiple myeloma. Casts are usually located in the collecting ducts, but due to retrograde filling casts can even be seen in the proximal tubules. Casts are composed of light chains and Tamm–Horsfall protein, and tend to have a fractured appearance. A granulomatous response with multinucleated macrophages and reactive epithelial cells is typically found at the periphery of myeloma casts (e-Fig. 19.15); other inflammatory cells, such as neutrophils and lymphocytes, can also be part of the inflammatory process. Nonspecific changes, such as tubular atrophy and interstitial fibrosis, are commonly present. Immunofluorescence studies often exhibit a monoclonal light chain in the casts.

IV. VASCULAR DISEASES

A. Vasculitides. The kidney has a dense arterial, venous, and lymphatic network. Vasculitides affect all these vessels, but most commonly the arteries. They are usually classified as large, medium, and small vessel vasculitides based on the predominant vessel size affected, but this classification is controversial because there is variability in the size of affected vessels. Vasculitides are also classified by the underlying pathogenetic mechanism as either immune-complex–mediated or pauci-immune (absence of immune deposits). The following are the most common vasculitides affecting the kidney, grouped by size:

1. **Takayasu's aortitis** affects large branches of the abdominal aorta and the renal arteries. Mural inflammation with giant cells is the distinct feature.

2. **Polyarteritis nodosa, scleroderma lupus, rheumatoid arthritis,** and **Wegener's granulomatosis** affect medium to small size vessels. These are systemic diseases and, with the exception of lupus, are pauci-immune systemic vasculites. The renal pathology is variable and includes interstitial granulomas, arterial acute inflammation, fibrinoid necrosis, and thrombotic occlusion. The inflammation can lead to aneurysm formation or fibrous wall thickening. Involvement of glomerular capillaries leads to crescentic GN. The diagnosis largely depends on the clinical syndrome, not the pathological findings. For example, Wegener's granulomatosis is associated with serum autoantibodies against components of neutrophils known as circulating antineutrophil cytoplasmic antibodies (ANCA); these antibodies correlate with disease activity and underscore the pathogenesis of vascular injury.

3. Of the small vessel systemic vasculitides, some are referred to as **thrombotic microangiopathies (TMAs).** A typical presentation is with hemolytic anemia and thrombocytopenia, known as hemolytic uremic syndrome (HUS). Entities under TMA include diarrhea associated (classic) HUS, thrombotic thrombocytopenic purpura, eclampsia, pre-eclampsia, thrombosis due to drugs (contraceptives, chemotherapy drugs such as bleomycin), cryoglobulinemia, idiopathic hypereosinophilia, antiphospholipid syndrome, hereditary deficiency of blood clotting factors, and malignant HTN (*J Am Soc Nephrol* 14:1072, 2003). Renal biopsy shows arterial intimal thickening (called mucoid degeneration) and luminal fibrin thrombi (e-**Fig. 19.16a**); all these entities may also show characteristic arteriolar thickening (also known as onion skinning, e-**Fig. 19.16b**), endothelial swelling, and/or luminal thrombosis.

B. Systemic HTN. Vascular diseases of the kidney are often associated with systemic HTN. The most common cause of HTN is idiopathic, which, despite modern pharmacologic therapies, remains a primary cause of renal failure. High blood pressure damages parenchymal arteries causing wall thickening; the arterioles show characteristic acellular eosinophilic material due to increased intravascular pressure and endothelial injury that allows leaking and deposition of plasma proteins. Glomeruli beyond damaged arterioles undergo sclerosis (e-**Fig. 19.16c**).

1. **Malignant HTN,** defined as diastolic pressure >120 mm Hg, complicates ~10% of patients with benign HTN, and presents acutely with papilledema, nausea, vomiting, convulsions, and coma. Renal function declines rapidly, and patients develop gross hematuria, albuminuria, and hemolytic anemia. Onion skinning is characteristic (e-**Fig. 19.16b**).

2. A small fraction (5% to 10%) of benign HTN is secondary to specific causes, some of which may be amenable to surgical therapy, that together are known as renovascular HTN. Most common is renal artery stenosis due to atherosclerotic aneurysms in older mostly diabetic men. Patients with abdominal or renal artery atherosclerosis may present with acute renal failure or proteinuria due to cholesterol embolism in parenchymal arteries (e-**Fig. 19.16d**). Fibromuscular dysplasia, an idiopathic mural thickening of the renal artery, is seen in young women (*Am J Kidney Dis* 29:167, 1997).

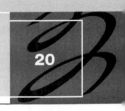

PEDIATRIC RENAL NEOPLASMS
Jason A. Jarzembowski and Frances V. White

I. **INTRODUCTION.** There are approximately 500 pediatric renal neoplasms diagnosed each year in the United States, the majority of which are unique to childhood or occur only rarely in adults (Table 20.1). Protocols for specimen processing, the staging system, and differential diagnosis differ from that of adult tumors. At present, the majority of pediatric renal tumors in the United States are centrally reviewed by the Children's Oncology Group (COG), and procurement of snap-frozen tumor for molecular studies has become important for placement of patients in specific treatment protocols (*Pediatr Dev Pathol* 8:320, 2005).

II. **GROSS EXAMINATION AND TISSUE SAMPLING.** A radical nephrectomy is the usual specimen. In cases of bilateral nephroblastoma, partial resections (kidney-sparing procedures) are performed. Pretreatment biopsies may be obtained for unresectable tumors; however, intraoperative biopsies are discouraged due to risk of tumor spillage, unless diagnosis will alter operative course.

Pediatric renal tumors are often large, friable tumors that bulge beyond the normal renal contour. The capsule should be carefully examined for sites of rupture and inked before incisions are made. The initial plane of section is taken to demonstrate the relationship of tumor to capsule and renal sinus. At this point, fresh tissue from each tumor nodule, nephrogenic rests, and normal kidney is snap frozen for protocol studies. Tissue may also be taken for cytogenetics, flow cytometry, and electron microscopy, depending on clinical history. Following initial cuts to facilitate fixation, overnight fixation is recommended before histologic sampling to decrease tumor friability and capsule retraction. Tissue for histology should be mainly taken from the tumor's periphery, as histology of the interface of tumor and renal parenchyma is often important in identifying type of tumor. Each separate tumor nodule should be sampled, with at least one section per centimeter of tumor diameter. Sections should also demonstrate the relationship of tumor to capsule and renal sinus. The hilum is a common route of tumor spread, necessitating adequate sampling of this area. Ureteral and vascular margins, lymph nodes, nephrogenic rests, and normal kidney are also sampled. Tumor sections are mapped, using either a diagram or photograph of the specimen; mapping is necessary for nephroblastoma, as the presence of diffuse versus focal anaplasia alters type of treatment (*Arch Pathol Lab Med* 127:1280, 2003).

III. **DIAGNOSTIC FEATURES OF PEDIATRIC RENAL TUMORS.** Pediatric renal neoplasms are notorious for their variant histologic patterns, many of which overlap with those of other pediatric renal neoplasms. Most tumors, however, have at least focal areas with classic histology. Correct diagnosis depends on knowledge of both classic and variant histology, along with adequate sampling. There should be careful examination of the tumor-kidney interface for pattern of infiltration, which is characteristic for each tumor type. Immunohistochemical studies may be useful for certain tumors (e.g., INI1 in rhabdoid tumor) or for excluding a diagnosis in specific cases; however, immunohistochemical stains are usually not needed. Molecular studies may confirm specific diagnoses

279

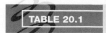

TABLE 20.1	Pediatric Renal Neoplasms: Percentages and Age Distribution (Compiled from References in Suggested Readings)		
Tumor	**Mean age**	**% Pediatric renal neoplasms**	**Age distribution (y)**
Classic mesoblastic nephroma	7 d	1%	0 to 2
Cellular mesoblastic nephroma	4 mo	3%	0 to 2
Malignant rhabdoid tumor	18 mo	2%	0 to 3
CCSK	2 y	4%	0 to 9; rare after 9 y of age
Nephroblastoma	36.5 mo (boys) 42.5 mo (girls)	85%	0 to 10; rare in first 3 mo and after 10 y of age
Metanephric stromal tumor	2 y	Rare	0 to 15
Ewing sarcoma / PNET	28 y	Rare	0 to 18 +
Papillary RCC	10 y	<5%	1 to 18 +
Translocation carcinomas	Wide range	<5%	1 to 18 +
Metanephric adenoma	41 y	Rare	5 to 18 +
Renal medullary carcinoma	22 y	Rare	11 to 18 +
Angiomyolipoma	50 y	Rare	17 to 18 +
Synovial sarcom	37 y	Rare	18

PNET, primitive neuroectodermal tumor; RCC, renal cell carcinoma; CCSK, clear cell sarcoma of kidney.

(Table 20.2). Knowledge of the differential diagnosis of pediatric tumors is essential, along with correlation with patient age and other clinical information.

A. Nephroblastoma (Wilms tumor) and nephrogenic rests. Nephroblastoma (Wilms tumor) accounts for 85% of pediatric renal tumors. Most patients present before 10 years of age, with a peak between 2 and 5 years. Rare examples have been reported in adults. The tumor is more common in children of African descent than of other races, and is slightly more common in girls than boys.

Although genetic abnormalities have been identified in only a minority of nephroblastomas, multiple genetic abnormalities and syndromes are associated with the tumor. Abnormalities of *WT1* on chromosome 11p13, a gene involved in renal and gonadal development, occurs in aniridia and genital anomalies syndrome (WAGR), Denys-Drash, and Frasier syndromes, all associated with a high risk for nephroblastoma. Molecular alterations of imprinted genes at the *WT2* locus on chromosome 11p15 are associated with Beckwith-Wiedemann syndrome, which has an increased risk for nephroblastoma. Both *WT1* and *WT2* locus gene alterations are found in a minority of sporadic tumors. In addition, 1% of patients with nephroblastoma have a family history of nephroblastoma. Two familial genes, *FWT1* and *FWT2*, have been identified; transmission in this setting is autosomal dominant with variable penetrance (*Curr Opin Pediatr* 14:5, 2002). Other molecular alterations that are associated with tumor progression or aggressiveness have been identified. *TP53* is implicated in progression to anaplastic nephroblastoma. Loss of heterozygosity of 1p and 16q is associated with poor prognosis in favorable histology nephroblastoma (*J Clin Oncol* 23:7312, 2005, *J Clin Oncol* 24:2352, 2006).

Nephroblastomas are usually solitary masses; however 10% are multicentric and 5% are bilateral at presentation (e-**Fig. 20.1**).* The cut surface is typically pale

---

*All e-figures are available online via the Solution Site Image Bank.

Tumor	Cytogenetic abnormality	Implicated genes	Protein role	Related assay(s)
Nephroblastoma	Deletions or mutations involving 11p13, 11p15 or Xq11.1	*WT1, WT2, WT3, WTX*	Zinc-finger DNA-binding protein; tumor suppressor genes	IPOX for WT1
Cellular mesoblastic nephroma	t(12;15)(p13;q25)	*ETV6-NTRK3*	Receptor tyrosine kinase	RT–PCR, FISH
Ewing sarcoma / PNET	Translocations of 22q11, usually t(11;22)(q24;q12)	*EWS-FLI1*	Transcriptional activator	RT–PCR, FISH; IPOX for CD99 or FLI-1
Synovial sarcoma	t(X;18)(p11;q11)	*SYT* and *SSX1, 2, or 4*	Chromatin remodeling, transcriptional regulation, β-catenin signaling pathways	RT–PCR, FISH
CCSK	t(10;17), del 14q	Undetermined	Undetermined	Karyotyping
Malignant rhabdoid tumor	Deletions or mutations involving 22q11.2	*hSNF5/INI1*	Chromatin remodeling and transcriptional regulation	IPOX for INI1 and cytokeratin
Translocation carcinomas	t(X;1)(p11.2;q25) t(6;11)(p21;q12)	*ASPL-TFE Alpha-TFEB*	Transcriptional activators	Karyotyping, IPOX for TFE
Renal medullary carcinoma	Constitutional 11p15.5 mutation; possible 22q11.2 involvement	*HBB hSNF5/INI1*	Hemoglobin S Chromatin remodeling and transcriptional regulation	IPOX for INI1
Angiomyolipoma	9q34, 16p13.3, 5q mutations	*TSC1, TSC2*	Tumor suppressor genes	Constitutional karyotype

IPOX, immunoperoxidase; RT–PCR, reverse transcription–polymerase chain reaction; FISH, fluorescence in situ hybridization; PNET, primitive neuroectodermal tumor; CCSK, clear cell sarcoma of kidney.

gray and friable, and may be hemorrhagic or cystic. Stromal predominant tumors often have a myomatous appearance. The tumor is derived from nephrogenic blastema and is composed of varying proportions of blastemal, epithelial, and stromal elements (e-Fig. 20.2). Nephroblastomas have a pushing border surrounded by a fibrous pseudocapsule; one exception, however, is the diffuse blastemal type, which infiltrates adjacent renal parenchyma. Other blastemal types include serpentine, nodular, and basaloid patterns. Epithelial differentiation includes tubular, papillary, and glomeruloid patterns; squamous cell, mucinous, and neural differentiation can also occur. The stroma may be primitive mesenchyme or show differentiation into skeletal muscle or, less frequently, smooth muscle, adipose tissue, and cartilage. Tumors with prominent heterologous elements are sometimes referred to as **teratoid Wilms tumor**.

Nephroblastomas are designated favorable or unfavorable based on the presence and distribution of anaplasia, rather than type of differentiation. **Anaplasia** is defined by the presence of large multipolar mitotic figures and large hyperchromatic nuclei (three times the size of other tumor nuclei) (e-Fig. 20.2). **Focal anaplasia** is defined by one or more focal areas of anaplasia surrounded by nonanaplastic tumor and limited to the kidney. Anaplasia that does not meet the definition of focal is considered **diffuse anaplasia**; anaplasia in a biopsy is also considered diffuse. Approximately 5% of tumors have diffuse anaplasia (unfavorable histology). The incidence of anaplasia is higher in posttreatment nephrectomies (*J Clin Oncol* 24:2352, 2006).

Nephrogenic rests are the precursor lesions of nephroblastoma (e-Figs. 20.1B, 20.3). **Perilobar nephrogenic rests** are located at the periphery of the renal lobule, are well demarcated from adjacent renal parenchyma, and have predominantly blastemal and epithelial elements. The cells in hyperplastic perilobar rests are cytologically identical to malignant tumor cells; however, the rests tend to be ovoid in shape rather than spherical, and they lack a tumor pseudocapsule. **Intralobar nephrogenic rests** occur anywhere in the kidney and have a prominent stromal component that intermixes with normal renal parenchyma. The presence of multiple nephrogenic rests or nephroblastomas is consistent with nephroblastomatosis and increases the risk for tumor in the contralateral kidney, especially in infants. In **diffuse hyperplastic perilobar nephroblastomatosis**, the renal parenchyma is extensively replaced by nephrogenic tissue (e-Fig 20.1). The diagnosis is made by imaging studies and is treated without biopsy. Tumors that grow despite chemotherapy are removed with kidney-sparing surgical procedures (*Med Pediatr Oncol* 21:158, 1993, *Pediatr Blood Cancer* 46:203, 2006).

Nephroblastomas with prominent cysts are designated **cystic nephroblastomas**. Multiloculated renal cysts with microscopic areas of nephroblastoma in the cyst walls, without any expansile septal mass, are designated **partially differentiated cystic nephroblastomas** (e-Fig. 20.1). Multilocular cysts with only mature elements and no expansile nodules are designated **cystic nephroma** and, in children, are thought to represent end-stage differentiation of nephroblastoma (*Semin Diagn Pathol* 15:2, 1998, *Cancer* 64:466, 1989).

Following chemotherapy, biopsied or partially resected (usually bilateral) nephroblastomas are categorized according to histologically observed treatment effect (*Pediatr Dev Pathol* 8:320, 2005) (summarized in Table 20.3). Most tumors will fall into the "intermediate" grade with subtotal necrosis and classic triphasic elements observed in the remaining viable tumor. Under current protocols, these patients will receive an additional 6 weeks of chemotherapy. Less frequently, tumors may show complete necrosis, in which case surgical resection can be performed. Biopsy specimens demonstrating worrisome histologic features such as predominance of blastemal elements or anaplasia after initial treatment are switched to more aggressive chemotherapeutic regimens.

B. **Metanephric tumors** are well-differentiated nephroblastic tumors containing varying proportions of epithelial and stromal cells. Metanephric tumors are benign; however, both nephroblastoma and papillary renal cell carcinoma (RCC) have been reported in tumors with epithelial elements.

TABLE 20.3	Pathologic Staging of Nephroblastoma and Other Pediatric Renal Neoplasms

Stage	Pathologic criteria
I	Tumor limited to the kidney and completely resected Intact renal capsule No rupture nor previous biopsy Renal sinus vessels not involved No evidence of tumor at or beyond margins of resection

II	Tumor completely resected
	Tumor extends beyond the kidney, due to one of the following:
	    Penetration of the renal capsule
	    Extensive invasion of the soft tissue of the renal sinus
	    Tumor within blood vessels outside the renal parenchyma, including those of the renal sinus
	No evidence of tumor at or beyond the margins of resection

III	Residual nonhematogenous tumor confined to the abdomen, as evidenced by:
	    Involvement of lymph nodes within the abdomen or pelvis
	    Penetration through the peritoneal surface
	    Tumor implants on the peritoneal surface
	    Tumor present at the margin of surgical resection
	    Tumor not respectable because of local infiltration into vital structures
	    Tumor spillage of any degree or localization occurring before or during surgery
	    Tumor removed in more than one piece
	Biopsy by any method prior to removal

IV	Hematogenous metastases (lung, liver, bone, brain, etc.) Lymph node metastases outside the abdomen or pelvis
V	Bilateral renal involvement at diagnosis Stage each side separately using above criteria

Modified from *Pediatr Dev Pathol.* 2005;8:320.

1. **Metanephric stromal tumors (MSTs)** occur throughout childhood, but most commonly in infancy (**e-Fig. 20.4**). Historically, these tumors were considered to be mesoblastic nephromas (MNs), but are now considered a distinct entity. The tumor is usually solitary and extends out from the renal medulla as an unencapsulated mass that may be solid or cystic. The cut surface is firm and myomatous. Microscopically, the tumor is composed of spindled to stellate cells with indistinct cytoplasm. Under low-power microscopy, the tumor has a distinct nodular appearance due to alternating areas of hypocellularity and hypercellularity. The tumor is unencapsulated, and bands of tumor cells extend outward to entrap adjacent glomeruli and tubules, resulting in cysts and epithelial embryonal and juxtaglomerular hyperplasia. Distinguishing features include concentric cuffs of spindled cells around blood vessels and renal tubules ("collarettes") and angiodysplasia of arterioles with epithelioid transformation of smooth muscle. Heterologous elements such as cartilage and glial tissue are infrequently present (*Am J Surg Pathol* 24:917, 2000).

2. **Metanephric adenofibromas (MAFs)** occur in both children and adults. In children, the tumor has been reported as early as 5 months of age. MAFs are centrally located and contain varying proportions of stroma resembling MST and epithelial nodules of metanephric adenoma. The peripheral stromal component merges with normal renal parenchyma in a manner similar to intralobar nephrogenic rests (see section on adult tumors below) (*Am J Surg Pathol* 25:433, 2001).

3. **Metanephric adenoma** occurs most frequently in adults; however, the tumor has been reported in children as young as 5 years of age (see section on adult tumors below). In children, the main differential diagnosis is epithelial nephroblastoma. Unlike nephroblastoma, however, mitoses are rare, and there is no pseudocapsule, blastemal component, or vascular invasion. Immunohistochemical stains are helpful in distinguishing metanephric adenoma from papillary RCC, but not for distinguishing metanephric adenoma from epithelial nephroblastoma.

C. **Mesoblastic nephroma (MN)** is a distinct neoplasm of infancy which may present antenatally as fetal hydrops (e-**Fig. 20.5**). Tumors diagnosed in a child older than 2 years most likely represent MST, clear cell sarcoma of the kidney (CCSK), or other tumor. The tumors are unencapsulated and solitary, and they infiltrate the renal sinus. Microscopically, they are characterized as cellular, classic, or mixed. **Classic MNs** contain intersecting fascicles of spindled cells resembling infantile fibromatosis. Long fascicles of tumor cells extend into the adjacent renal parenchyma, entrapping tubules and glomeruli and resulting in cysts and epithelial embryonal metaplasia. Dysplastic change with cartilage may be present in adjacent parenchyma. Consistent molecular abnormalities have not been identified with classic histology tumors. **Cellular MN** is composed of plump cells with vesicular nuclei, variable amounts of cytoplasm, and increased mitoses. The tumor has a well-demarcated interface with adjacent renal parenchyma, although it lacks a pseudocapsule. Cellular MN is histologically similar to infantile fibrosarcoma, both of which have the t(12;15)(p13;q25) chromosomal translocation that produces the fusion gene *ETV6-NTRK3*. **Mixed MNs** contain both cellular and classic areas. MNs are treated by complete surgical resection, with adjuvant chemotherapy for positive margins. The recurrence rate is 5% to 10%, and the tumor rarely metastasizes, usually to lung (*Adv Anat Pathol* 10:243, 2003).

D. **Clear cell sarcoma of kidney (CCSK)** represents 4% of pediatric renal tumors. It is a primitive mesenchymal neoplasm not associated with any consistent chromosomal or genetic abnormality. CCSK occurs usually from 1 to 4 years of life, but is also seen in infants (including stillborns) and rarely in adults. It is a high-risk neoplasm, with a tendency for metastases (lung, bone, brain, and soft tissue) and late recurrences. Boys are affected more often than girls. The tumor is unilateral, solitary, well circumscribed, and located in the renal medulla. Its cut surface is typically tan-grey and mucoid, although the surface may have a firm, whorled appearance (e-**Fig. 20.6**). Cysts are often present. Microscopically, areas with classic histology contain nests and cords of uniform polygonal to spindled cells with ovoid nuclei with finely granular to vesicular chromatin, inconspicuous nucleoli, and indistinct cytoplasm, in a background of clear extracellular matrix. A delicate, arborizing fibrovascular network separates groups of tumor cells. The tumor interface is well circumscribed under low-power microscopy, however, a pseudocapsule is not present and tumor extends a short distance into adjacent parenchyma, entrapping tubules that may be cystic or have epithelial metaplasia. Almost all tumors have at least focal classic histology, however, numerous variant histologies may also be present and may predominate (e-**Fig. 20.6**). These include myxoid, sclerosing, cellular, epithelioid, palisading, spindle cell, pericytomatous, storiform, and anaplastic patterns. CCSK tumor cells are positive for vimentin and negative for epithelial markers. Although immunohistochemical stains may be useful in ruling out other tumors on an individual basis, there are no specific markers for CCSK (*Am J Surg Pathol* 24:4, 2000, *Virchows Arch* 446:566, 2005).

E. **Rhabdoid tumor of the kidney (RTK)** is a highly aggressive malignant neoplasm of infancy, accounting for 2% of pediatric renal tumors (e-**Fig. 20.7**). Most patients present at younger than 1 year with metastatic disease, and almost all patients present by 3 years of age. Approximately 10% to 15% of RTKs are associated with rhabdoid tumors of the central nervous system. Both renal and extrarenal infantile rhabdoid tumors contain molecular alterations of the *hSNF5/INI1* gene at chromosome 22q11. Grossly, the renal tumor is pale tan and unencapsulated, and arises from the renal medulla. Multicentric or bilateral tumors are considered metastatic lesions. In areas of classic histology, there are sheets of discohesive tumor cells with large vesicular nuclei, prominent nucleoli, and abundant eccentric cytoplasm containing large eosinophilic inclusions. Ultrastructurally, these inclusions consist of whorls of intermediate filaments that are characteristic but not specific for the tumor. Cells with smaller nuclei and less cytoplasm may sometimes predominate. Variant histology includes sclerosing, epithelioid, spindled, and lymphomatoid patterns. Tumor cells have a polyphenotypic immunostaining pattern, with diffuse vimentin positivity and patchy positivity for other markers, including epithelial markers. An immunostain for INI1 (negative nuclear staining in RTK) is now available (*Adv Anat Pathol* 10:243, 2003, *Am J Surg Pathol* 13:439, 1989, *Am J Surg Pathol* 28:1485, 2004).

F. **Pediatric renal cell carcinoma (RCCs).** Although **pediatric RCCs** bear a strong morphologic resemblance to their adult counterparts, they often possess unique clinical, pathologic, and genetic features that distinguish them from the adult versions (*Adv Anat Pathol* 10:243, 2003). The mean age at presentation is between 9 and 10 years, and the sentinel symptoms include a palpable mass, flank and/or abdominal pain, hematuria, polycythemia, and hypertension. Children tend to have a slightly better prognosis than adults, primarily due to their presentation at earlier stages; metastatic disease has a poor prognosis (<10% 5 year survival) in both groups.

1. In adults, **clear cell RCC** is the most common malignant epithelial renal neoplasm, but in children this tumor is less common and probably only occurs in patients with von Hippel–Lindau syndrome or another predisposing genetic background. (Many previously reported/diagnosed cases of pediatric clear cell RCC are now thought to be associated with Xp11.2 translocations and therefore likely represent different entities.) The histopathologic features are identical to those in adult clear cell RCC.

2. In children, **papillary RCC** is the most common malignant epithelial neoplasm of the kidney (*Am J Surg Pathol* 23:795, 1999). The histologic, molecular, and genetic findings are identical to those of the adult tumors. The tumor is microscopically composed of a single layer of columnar cells lining a papillary stalk, often with clusters of foamy macrophages, hemosiderin, and necrosis in the surrounding background. This neoplasm is often surrounded by a pseudocapsule with an associated lymphoid infiltrate. The tumor cells are strongly positive for cytokeratin 7 and EMA, which can help differentiate papillary RCC from Wilms tumor and metanephric adenoma.

3. Recently, the category of **renal tumors with Xp11.2 translocations** has been developed to describe a group of neoplasms that, despite diversity in their histologic features, share common molecular and genetic abnormalities (*Pediatr Dev Pathol* 8:168, 2005, *Proc Natl Acad Sci* USA 93:15294, 1996, *Am J Clin Pathol* 126:349, 2006, *Med Pediatr Oncol* 31:153, 1998). Although a variety of chromosomal alterations underlie these tumors, the common end result is a chimeric fusion gene involving *TFE3*, a basic helix–loop–helix transcription factor located at Xp11.2. Histologically, these translocation carcinomas exhibit voluminous cells with clear to eosinophilic cytoplasm arranged in papilla or nests with thin intervening fibrous septa (e-**Fig. 20.8**). Psammoma bodies and hyaline nodules are frequently seen. The tumor cells show variable positivity for cytokeratins and EMA, as well as CD10 and RCC marker antigen. The most common mimicker, epithelioid angiomyolipoma, shows positivity for HMB-45 and Melan-A, which is not seen in the translocation carcinomas.

   The most consistent and specific finding is nuclear positivity for the TFE3 protein using an antibody directed towards the C-terminal end of the protein, which is retained in various gene fusion products. The morphologic similarity to alveolar soft part sarcoma (ASPS) is not surprising as the latter entity also has a characteristic translocation involving *TFE3*; in fact, the *ASPL-TFE3* rearranged renal carcinomas [which harbor the t(X;1)(p11.2;p34) translocation] bear the greatest resemblance to ASPS (*Am J Pathol* 21:621, 1997). Other fusion partners include *PRCC* [in which t(X;1)(p11.2;q21) is the most common] and *PSF* [in which t(X;1)(p11.2;q25) is present]. Also, a group of tumors exists with similar morphology including large, polygonal clear and eosinophilic cells in nests and acini with intervening hyaline material; these are **renal tumors with t(6;11)**

translocations that involve the *TFEB* gene, a member of the *TFE3* family (*Am J Surg Pathol* 29:230, 2005).

Overall, the translocation carcinomas have a propensity for lymph node metastasis, but while children and adults with RCC fare similarly stage for stage, children with lymph node involvement have a significantly better prognosis than adults (*Cancer* 101:1575, 2004, *Med Pediatr Oncol* 19:33, 1991, *Med Pediatr Oncol* 23:36, 1994). The best predictors of outcome and the true prognosis for pediatric RCC patients have yet to be determined.

4. **Renal medullary carcinoma** is an extremely rare, highly malignant neoplasm which occurs only in patients with sickle cell hemoglobin trait (**e-Fig 20.9**) (*Am J Surg Pathol* 19:1, 1995, *Urology* 60:1083, 2002, *J Urol Pathol* 4:191, 1996). The etiologic relationship between medullary carcinoma and sickle cell trait is unknown. Patients typically present as teenagers or young adults, usually at late stages with widely disseminated disease; survival is measured in weeks or months.

   Renal medullary carcinoma grows in an aggressive, infiltrative, and often sarcomatoid pattern, often entrapping nascent structures. Intrarenal spread occurs hematogenously and gives the appearance of multifocal lesions. The tumor can be morphologically heterogeneous with yolk sac-like, cribriform, microcystic, and solid patterns; it often has rhabdoid cytology. Common mimics include **collecting duct carcinoma** (CDC), **endodermal sinus tumor** (EST), and RTK; however, CDC typically occurs in older patients, and EST has a distinguishing immunoprofile. Like RTK, renal medullary carcinoma shows loss of nuclear hSNF5/INI1 staining. Immunohistochemical staining of renal medullary carcinoma is otherwise nonspecific, but the tumor cells usually express cytokeratin and are variably reactive for carcinoembryonic antigen (CEA) and EMA.

5. **Postneuroblastoma RCC** is exceedingly rare, occurring in children and teenagers 3 to 12 years old after being diagnosed with neuroblastoma (*Pathol* 35:499, 2003, *Am J Surg Pathol* 23:772, 1999). These tumors exhibit morphologic diversity including solid and papillary growth patterns, a characteristic oncocytic cytology, and areas resembling clear cell RCC with occasional psammoma bodies and/or collections of foamy histiocytes. Immunohistochemically, they are positive for vimentin, EMA, and cytokeratin CAM 5.2. No specific genetic aberrations have been identified. Invasive and metastatic behavior is common. Interestingly, postneuroblastoma RCC does not appear to be secondary to treatment; no common chemotherapeutic or radiotherapeutic regimen has been implicated, and at least two cases have been reported in patients with previously untreated, spontaneously-resolving stage IVS neuroblastoma. The pathogenesis of this neoplasm therefore remains unclear.

6. The other renal epithelial neoplasms of adulthood—**oncocytoma, chromophobe RCC,** and others—have all been rarely reported in children. Although the histopathologic features are identical to those in adults, these entities occur too infrequently in the pediatric population to ascertain whether the clinical course is also similar.

G. **Other small round cell tumors.** Small round cell tumors that are usually extrarenal but can occur as a primary renal tumor include neuroblastoma, primitive neuroectodermal tumor (PNET), synovial sarcoma, and lymphoma. All can be mistaken for one of the relatively more common pediatric renal tumors.

1. **Undifferentiated neuroblastoma** and **PNETs** can mimic blastemal predominant nephroblastoma, and neural pseudorosettes may resemble primitive tubule formation in nephroblastoma (**e-Fig. 20.10**). Features favoring neuroblastoma over nephroblastoma include diffuse infiltration, hemorrhage, calcification, and nonoverlapping nuclei with "salt and pepper" chromatin (*Lab Invest* 83:4P, 2003). PNETs are distinguished from nephroblastoma by diffuse infiltration, immunoreactivity for CD99 and FLI1, nonreactivity for WT1, and by chromosomal translocations involving the *EWS* gene detected by fluorescence in situ hybridization (FISH) and reverse transcription–polymerase chain reaction (RT-PCR) (*Am J Surg Pathol* 25:133, 2001, *Am J Surg Pathol* 26:320, 2002).

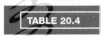

TABLE 20.4	Classification of Postchemotherapy Nephroblastoma

Category	%	Pathologic features
Completely necrotic tumors	10%	Less than 1% viable tumor tissue (the presence of scattered mature tubules is allowed) Multiple blocks available taken from different areas of a well-sampled tumor (at least 1 block per cm of greatest tumor dimension)
Intermediate tumors	70%	Tumors may contain a variety of histologic features, including epithelial, stromal, and blastemal differentiation. A spectrum of proliferative changes may be present, and a spectrum of necrosis and regressive changes may likewise be present but fall short of complete necrosis. Less than 66% of the viable tumor should be blastemal if the tumor is >1/3 viable grossly
Blastema-predominant tumors	10%	Viable tumor must comprise >1/3 of the tumor mass. At least 2/3 of the viable tumor consists of blastema. Other components of nephroblastoma may be present in varying proportions.
Anaplastic tumors	10%	Tumors demonstrating the usual criteria of focal or diffuse anaplasia

Modified from *Pediatr Dev Pathol.* 8:320, 2005.

2. **Synovial sarcomas** present in older adolescents. In the kidney, they are usually monophasic and may resemble blastemal nephroblastoma or PNET. Synovial sarcomas have the t(X;18) translocation resulting in the SYT-SSX fusion transcript (*Am J Surg Pathol* 24:1087, 2000).

3. **Non-Hodgkin lymphoma** rarely presents in the kidney as bilateral or multicentric masses. Both B- and T-cell lymphomas have been reported in children. Immunohistochemical markers for lymphoma are used for diagnosis (*Pediatr Pathol Lab Med* 17:449, 1997).

H. **Miscellaneous tumors. Ossifying renal tumor of infancy** is an extremely rare tumor that typically presents as a calcified abdominal mass in male infants with hematuria. The tumor is attached to the renal papilla and protrudes into the calyceal lumen and pelvis. Microscopically, it consists of spindled cells surrounding a partially mineralized osteoid matrix. The tumor is benign, and recurrences have not been reported (*Pediatr Pathol Lab Med* 15:745, 1995).

IV. **PATHOLOGIC STAGING.** Most pediatric renal tumors are pathologically staged using the National Wilms Tumor Study Group (NWTS) staging system. This system has been recently modified by the COG (Table 20.4). In the current system, any pretreatment biopsy or intraoperative tumor spillage automatically upstages the tumor to stage III. Lymph node sampling and triaging of tumor for molecular studies is required for specific treatment protocols. Pediatric RCCs are staged using the Tumor, Node, Metastasis (TNM) system (*Pediatr Dev Pathol* 8:320, 2005).

V. **REPORTING PEDIATRIC RENAL NEOPLASMS.** The histologic type should be reported for resections, along with pathologic stage and margin status. For pediatric RCC, Fuhrman nuclear grade should be reported. For Wilms tumor, presence of multicentric tumors, presence and extent of anaplasia, presence and type of adjacent nephrogenic rests, and grade of treatment effect postchemotherapy, should be reported.

Suggested Readings

Argani P, Beckwith JB. Renal neoplasms of childhood. In: Mills SE, ed. *Sternberg's Diagnostic Surgical Pathology*. 4th ed. New York: Lippincott, Williams & Wilkins; 2004;2001–2033.

Argani P, Ladanyi M. Recent advances in pediatric renal neoplasia. *Adv Anat Pathol.* 2003;10:243–260.

Murphy WM, Grignon DJ, Perlman EJ. AFIP Atlas of Tumor Pathology, Fourth Series, *Fascicle 1: Tumors of the Kidney, Bladder, and Related Urinary Structures*. Washington, D.C.: American Registry of Pathology; 2004.

Perlman EJ. Pediatric renal tumors: practical updates for the pathologist. *Pediatr Dev Pathol.* 2005;8:320–338.

Ramphal R, Pappo A, Zielenska M, Grant R, Ngan BY. Pediatric renal cell carcinoma: clinical, pathologic, and molecular abnormalities associated with the members of the mit transcription factor family. *Am J Clin Pathol.* 2006;126:349–364.

ADULT RENAL NEOPLASMS
Maria F. Serrano and Peter A. Humphrey

I. **NORMAL ANATOMY.** The normal weight of a kidney is 115 to 155 g for women and 125 to 170 g for men. Anatomically, the kidneys are composed of an outer cortex and an inner medulla that has 8 to 18 pyramids. The base of each pyramid is at the corticomedullary junction, and the apex extends toward the renal pelvis, forming a papilla where the collecting ducts open. The minor calyces receive the papillae, which in turn join to form the major calyces that end in the dilated upper portion of the ureter in the renal pelvis. Histologically, the components of the kidney include glomeruli, tubules, blood vessels, and interstitium (SE Mills, ed. *Histology for Pathologists*, 2e. Philadelphia: Lippincott Williams and Wilkins, 2007).

II. **GROSS EXAMINATION AND TISSUE SAMPLING. Renal tissue sampling** for tumor includes partial and radical nephrectomies and, less commonly, needle biopsies and fine needle aspirates.

A. **Needle cores. Needle core biopsy** is being performed in some centers, particularly prior to use of percutaneous ablative therapies such as radiofrequency heat ablation or cryosurgery. It can also be done if there is a clinical concern for lymphoma or metastatic disease. The cores can usually be submitted in 10% formalin, with generation of H&E-stained slides. If lymphoma is in the differential diagnosis, additional core(s) should be submitted fresh for lymphoma work-up. Histopathologic diagnosis of needle core biopsy tissue from renal masses is highly accurate in establishing a malignant diagnosis (*Am J Roentgenol* 188:563, 2007) and in renal tumor typing. In the future, FISH (*BJU Int* 99:290, 2007) and/or immunohistochemistry may aid in typing.

B. **Partial nephrectomy.** The surgical resection margin is inked, and the specimen is serially sectioned; the distance to the resection margin should be recorded. Sections demonstrating the relationship of the mass to the surgical resection margin and perirenal fat are taken. Intraoperative consultation for gross or frozen section examination of the margin may be requested (*Arch Pathol Lab Med* 129:1505, 2005).

C. **Radical nephrectomy.** A radical nephrectomy includes the kidney, a portion of the ureter, renal vein and artery, perinephric fat, and Gerota's fascia. The adrenal gland may also be present. Intraoperative consultation is most commonly requested to grossly confirm presence of a renal or pelvic mass in the nephrectomy specimen (*Arch Pathol Lab Med* 129:1586, 2005).

After weighing the entire specimen, the renal hilum is examined to identify the ureter, renal vein, and artery, and cross-sections of these margins are taken (Fig. 20.1). The renal vein and ureter are opened longitudinally. Areas suspicious for tumor involvement of the perirenal soft tissue are inked selectively. Rarely, lymph nodes are found in the hilar region.

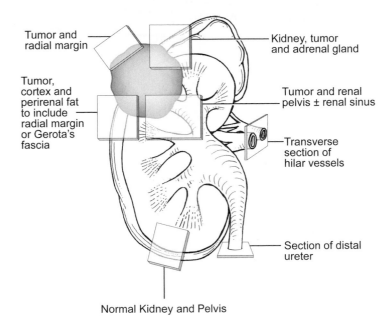

Normal Kidney and Pelvis

Figure 20.1. Sampling of radical nephrectomy specimen for adult renal tumors. Sections through renal masses should demonstrate relationship of mass to capsule, peripheral fat, renal parenchyma, and renal pelvis. Modified from WA Schmidt. *Principles and Techniques of Surgical Pathology.* Menlo Park, CA: Addison-Wesley; 1983.

The kidney is then sectioned sagittally. Tumor size, location (upper or lower pole, cortex or medulla), involvement of calyceal or pelvic mucosa, invasion of the capsule or perirenal soft tissue, and involvement of the adrenal gland are recorded. The uninvolved parenchyma is then examined: Color, cortical thickness, additional focal lesions, and renal pelvis appearance are described. One section per centimeter of tumor, demonstrating its relationship to adjacent capsule, renal parenchyma, and pelvis, are submitted, as well as sections of any additional lesions, uninvolved renal parenchyma, and adrenal gland (Fig. 20.2). Nephroureterectomy for urothelial carcinomas are described in Chapter 21.

III. DIAGNOSTIC FEATURES OF COMMON TUMORS OF THE ADULT KIDNEY

A. Carcinoma. RCC arises from the epithelium of the renal tubules, and represents approximately 90% of all renal malignancies in adults.

1. **Risk factors.** The most important risk factor is tobacco smoking. Additional risk factors include obesity, hypertension, unopposed estrogens, and exposure to arsenic, asbestos, cadmium, organic solvents, pesticides, and fungal toxins. Patients with tuberous sclerosis, chronic renal failure, and acquired cystic disease of the kidney have an increased incidence of RCC (about 5% of patients with acquired cystic disease of the kidney develop renal cell tumors; the most common tumor in this setting is characterized by microcystic growth of high-grade eosinophilic cells, often with intratumoral oxalate crystals) (*Am J Surg Pathol* 30:141, 2006). Most RCCs are sporadic; however, there are several inherited cancer syndromes that affect the kidney (*N Eng J Med* 353:2477, 2005).

   a. **Von Hippel-Lindau (VHL) disease** is inherited in an autosomal dominant manner and is characterized by hemangioblastomas of the cerebellum and retina, clear cell RCC, pheochromocytoma, pancreatic cysts, and inner ear tumors. Typically, renal tumors are multiple and bilateral. Numerous renal cysts, lined by neoplastic clear cells, are also characteristic. This disease is caused by

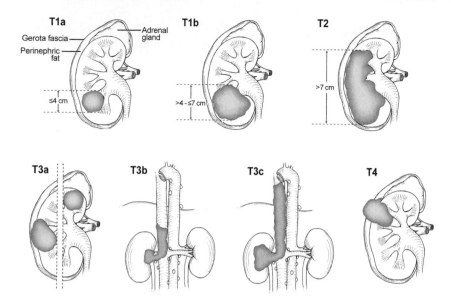

Figure 20.2. Renal cell carcinoma pathologic primary tumor (pT) stages. Modified from FL Greene, CC Compton, AG Fritz, JP Shah, DP Winchester, eds. *AJCC Cancer Staging Atlas.* New York: Springer; 2006.

germline mutations of the *VHL* tumor suppressor gene on chromosome 3p25-26.

- **b. Hereditary papillary RCC** is also inherited in an autosomal dominant manner and is characterized by multiple, bilateral papillary RCCs with a type I-like papillary or tubulopapillary architecture. The disease is caused by activating mutations of the *MET* oncogene on chromosome 7q31.

- **c. Hereditary leiomyomatosis and renal cell cancer** is an autosomal dominant disease caused by mutations in the fumarate hydratase gene. It is characterized by benign leiomyomas of the skin and uterus. Patients are predisposed to RCC and uterine leiomyosarcoma. Tumors have papillary type 2 large eosinophilic cells with large nuclei and nucleoli.

- **d. Birt–Hogg–Dubé syndrome** is characterized by cutaneous fibrofolliculomas, trichodiscomas, and acrochordons. Multiple and bilateral diverse types of renal tumors are present. The chromophobe type is most common; oncocytoma, papillary, clear cell, and "hybrid" chromophobe-oncocytic tumors can also be seen (*Arch Pathol Lab Med* 130:1867, 2006). This syndrome is autosomal dominant with incomplete penetrance. The responsible gene, folliculin, is located on chromosome 17p 11.2.

- **e. Constitutional chromosome 3 translocations** are related to an increased risk of RCC. Tumors are typically of the clear cell type.

2. **Clinical diagnosis.** Hematuria, pain, and flank mass are the classical triad of presenting symptoms, but in North America most renal tumors are now detected as incidental findings by radiological studies. Other presentations include weight loss, anorexia, fever, hypercalcemia, erythrocytosis, hypertension, gynecomastia, anemia, and hepatosplenomegaly. Radiological studies, especially ultrasound and computed tomography (CT), are excellent for detection and characterization of renal masses, but up to 15% of renal masses thought to be malignant by radiology are histologically benign, typically oncocytomas or angiomyolipomas.

3. **Histological typing and diagnosis of renal epithelial malignancies.** The 2004 World Health Organization (WHO) classification of neoplasms of the kidney is given in Table 20.5.

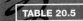

| **TABLE 20.5** | WHO Histological Classification of Tumors of the Kidney |

Renal cell tumors
Clear cell renal cell carcinoma
Multilocular clear cell renal cell carcinoma
Papillary renal cell carcinoma
Chromophobe renal cell carcinoma
Carcinoma of the collecting ducts of Bellini
Renal medullary carcinoma
Xp11 translocation carcinomas
Carcinoma associated with neuroblastoma
Mucinous tubular and spindle cell carcinoma
Renal cell carcinoma, unclassified
Papillary adenoma
Oncocytoma

Metanephric tumors
Metanephric adenoma
Metanephric adenofibroma
Metanephric stromal tumor

Nephroblastic tumors
Nephrogenic rests
Nephroblastoma
  Cystic partially differentiated
  nephroblastoma

Mesenchymal tumors
Occurring mainly in children
  Clear cell sarcoma
  Rhabdoid tumor
  Congenital mesoblastic nephroma
  Ossifying renal tumor of infants
Occurring mainly in adults
  Leiomyosarcoma (including renal vein)
  Angiosarcoma

Rhabdomyosarcoma
Malignant fibrous histiocytoma
Hemangiopericytoma
Osteosarcoma
Angiomyolipoma
Epithelioid angiomyolipoma
Leiomyoma
Hemangioma
Lymphangioma
Juxtaglomerular cell tumor
Renomedullary interstitial cell tumor
Schwannoma
Solitary fibrous tumor

Mixed mesenchymal and epithelial tumors
Cystic nephroma
Mixed epithelial and stromal tumor
Synovial sarcoma

Neuroendocrine tumors
Carcinoid
Neuroendocrine carcinoma
Primitive neuroectodermal tumors
Pheochromocytoma

Hematopoietic and lymphoid tumors
Lymphoma
Leukemia
Plasmacytoma

Germ cell tumors
Teratoma
Choriocarcinoma

Metastatic tumors

From: Ebele JN, Sauter G, Epstein JI, Sesterhenn IA, eds. *World Health Organization Classification of Tumours. Pathology and Genetics. Tumours of the Urinary System and Male Genital Organs.* Lyon: IARC Press; 2004. Used with permission.

a. **Clear cell RCC** is the most common histologic type. Grossly, these tumors often have a variegated appearance (e-**Fig 20.11**). Bright yellow areas are due to the high lipid content of the cells, whereas red and white-yellow regions are due to hemorrhage, fibrosis, and necrosis. Calcification and cystic change are also fairly common. Histologic sections show round or polygonal cells with clear or eosinophilic cytoplasm and centrally located nuclei. The cells are arranged in nests within a fine vascular network (e-**Fig. 20.12**). Tumor cells react with antibodies to low-molecular-weight keratins, RCC marker (RCC Ma), epithelial membrane antigen, and CD10. Clear cell RCCs are associated with 3p deletions, and *VHL* gene mutations are found in up to 60% of sporadic cases.

Fuhrman nuclear grading is the most important prognostic factor after staging. (Table 20.6). Grade 1 cells have small, round, uniform nuclei without visible nucleoli. Grade 2 cells have larger nuclei with irregular outlines and nucleoli seen only at 400 ×. Grade 3 cells have recognizable nucleoli at 100×, and grade 4 cells exhibit nuclear pleomorphism, hyperchromasia, with bizarre, often multilobed nuclei. Tumors should be graded according to the highest

TABLE 20.6	Fuhrman Nuclear Grading of Renal Cell Carcinoma
Grade 1	Small, round and uniform nuclei. No evident nucleoli
Grade 2	Nuclei with irregular outlines. Inconspicuous nucleoli
Grade 3	Irregular nuclei with identifiable nucleoli at 100× magnification
Grade 4	Large, hyperchromatic, pleomorphic nuclei. Single or multiple nucleoli

grade present even if focal (defined as occupying at least one 400× high-power field). (e-**Figs. 20.13** to **20.16**).

Clear cell RCC spreads locally into the renal sinus or perinephric fat by direct extension, and by venous invasion into the renal vein and vena cava. Lymphatic spread to lymph nodes can occur. Hematogenous spread to lungs, liver, and bone are most frequent, although spread to unusual sites is a well-known characteristic. Metastasis can be found many years after primary diagnosis. A prognostic nomogram predicting clear cell RCC recurrence after nephrectomy incorporates tumor size, pT stage, Fuhrman grade, necrosis, vascular invasion, and mode of clinical presentation (*J Urol* 173:48, 2005).

b. Multilocular cystic RCC is composed of multiple cysts separated by thin septa with a neoplastic clear cell epithelial lining, with clear tumor cells in the septa (e-**Fig. 20.17**). Grossly, this tumor is well circumscribed and contains cysts of variable size filled with clear or hemorrhagic fluid. Calcification is frequent. Tumor cells are reactive with antibodies to cytokeratins and epithelial membrane antigen; such immunostains can be useful in the distinction of tumor cells from macrophages in the septa. No recurrences or metastasis have been reported for this tumor type.

c. Papillary RCC comprises about 10% of RCCs. Grossly, the tumor can be cystic, hemorrhagic, and necrotic, with a fibrous pseudocapsule. Multifocality and bilaterality are more common than for other RCCs. Microscopically, there is papillary or tubulopapillary architecture with papillae formed by thin fibrovascular cores, which may harbor aggregates of foamy macrophages. Cholesterol crystals may be present. There are two types of papillary RCC. Type 1 tumors have papillae lined by a single layer of cuboidal cells with scant cytoplasm (e-**Fig. 20.18**) that has a basophilic quality. Type 2 tumors have taller cells with more abundant, eosinophilic cytoplasm, higher nuclear grade, and pseudostratified nuclei (e-**Fig. 20.19**). Fuhrman grading may be applied. (*Am J Clin Pathol* 118:877, 2002), but nucleolar grading may also be useful (*Am J Surg Pathol* 30:1091, 2006). Genetically, there is characteristic trisomy of chromosomes 7 and 17, and loss of chromosome 4, but chromosomal analysis is not used diagnostically. Papillary RCC, especially type 1, has a better outcome than clear cell RCC.

d. Chromophobe RCC accounts for approximately 5% of RCCs. Grossly, chromophobe RCCs are well-circumscribed with slightly lobulated surfaces. Tumors are composed of pale, eosinophilic polygonal cells with prominent cell borders, often wrinkled nuclear membranes, and perinuclear halos (e-**Fig. 20.20**). Fuhrman grading can be applied, but its usefulness is controversial (*Am J Surg Pathol* 31:957, 2007). Diffuse cytoplasmic positivity with Hale's colloidal iron is characteristic, and these tumors show extensive aneusomy with loss of chromosomes 1, 2, 6, 10, 13, 17, and 21, which can be detected by FISH (*Mod Pathol* 18:320, 2005). Hale's colloidal iron and FISH can be used to address the differential diagnosis of the eosinophilic variant of chromophobe RCC versus oncocytoma. Chromophobe RCC has a much better prognosis than clear cell RCC.

e. Collecting duct carcinoma is thought to arise from the collecting ducts of Bellini. It accounts for <1% of renal cell tumors. These tumors are centered in the medulla, have tubular or tubulopapillary architecture, and have a surrounding desmoplastic reaction (e-Fig. 20.21). Tumor cells are typically of high nuclear grade and can have hobnail cytology. Use of immunostains in diagnosis has limitations. When needed, alpha-methylacyl coenzyme A racemase (AMACR), CD10, and RCC Ma negativity would favor CDC over papillary RCC, which figures prominently in the differential diagnosis, and which would usually be positive for these three markers (*Semin Diag Pathol* 22:51, 2005). Most tumors present at an advanced stage with metastatic disease. The prognosis is poor.

  f. Renal medullary carcinoma is very rare. Tumors in adults are identical to those in the pediatric age group as discussed above.

  g. Renal carcinomas associated with Xp11.2 translocations/*TFE3* gene fusions are defined by various translocations affecting chromosome Xp11.2, resulting in gene fusions involving the *TFE3* gene. Although rare in adults, they are histologically identical to those in the pediatric age group as discussed above.

  h. RCC associated with neuroblastoma is exceedingly rare and occurs in long-term survivors of childhood neuroblastoma.

  i. Mucinous tubular and spindle cell carcinoma is an uncommon low-grade renal epithelial neoplasm composed of elongated tubules separated by a mucinous stroma (e-Fig 20.22). The tumor cells are cuboidal or spindle shaped with low-grade nuclear features. Uncommonly, necrosis, clear cells, papillations, foamy macrophages, and inflammation can be present (*Am J Surg Pathol* 30:1554, 2006). In the past, some cases have been mistaken for sarcomatoid RCC. Loss of chromosomes 1, 4, 6, 8, 13, and 14 and gains of chromosomes 7, 11, 16, and 17 are characteristic of these tumors, but molecular analysis is not currently used diagnostically. This tumor type has a good prognosis.

  j. Unclassified RCC is a diagnosis that should be reserved for those tumors that do not fit into other categories. It is a diagnosis rendered in about 5% of RCC cases. Features that place tumors in this group include the following: a combination of different histologic types, mucin production, sarcomatoid appearance, presence of epithelial and stromal elements, and nonidentifiable patterns. This designation is linked to a worse prognosis than clear cell RCC (*BJU Int* 100:802, 2007).

  Sarcomatoid change can be associated with a specific type of carcinoma or can overgrow the pre-existing carcinoma type and exist in pure form. The percentage of the tumor that is sarcomatoid should be specified as being less than or greater than 50%. Heterologous malignant bone, cartilage, fat, and skeletal muscle, or homologous undifferentiated malignant spindle cells can be seen. Rhabdoid cells can be found in about 5% of RCC cases, usually clear cell carcinoma (*Am J Surg Pathol* 24:1329–1338, 2000). Both sarcomatoid and rhabdoid features all associated with a poor prognosis.

B. Benign epithelial tumors

  1. Papillary adenoma of the kidney is the most common benign epithelial neoplasm of renal cells. Grossly, the tumor consists of single or multiple well-defined white nodules in the renal cortex. The tumors have papillary architecture, low nuclear grade, and measure ≤5 mm in diameter. The cytoplasm is scant, and nuclear grooves can be present. Psammoma bodies and foamy macrophages are common.

  2. Oncocytoma is a benign epithelial neoplasm that comprises approximately 5% of all neoplasms of the renal tubular epithelium. Tumors are more frequent in men, and the peak incidence is during the seventh decade of life. Grossly, the tumors are well circumscribed and the cut-surface is typically mahogany-brown. A central scar is seen in up to 33% of cases, generally with larger tumors; such scarring, although characteristic, is not specific for oncocytoma. Hemorrhage is frequent, but necrosis is almost always absent.

  Microscopically, these tumors are composed of nests and tubules of round or polygonal cells with granular eosinophilic cytoplasm, round nuclei, and single central nucleoli (e-Fig. 20.23). Scattered larger cells with a higher nuclear/cytoplasmic ratio and hyperchromatic nuclei can be seen; scant, atypical mitotic figures are allowed. A hyalinized or edematous stromal background is frequent. Microscopic (but not gross) extension into perirenal fat and vessels has been described. Rare cases of numerous oncocytic tumors (oncocytosis) exist. Chromosomal abnormalities in oncocytoma include t(5;11) and loss of chromosomes 1 and 14, but assessment for these abnormalities is not usually necessary. No cases of death due to metastatic disease have been reported.

C. Metanephric tumors (see also the pediatric renal neoplasm section above)

1. **Metanephric adenoma** occurs in children and adults during the fifth and sixth decades. It is more frequent in women. About 50% of cases are incidental. Tumors are usually well circumscribed, gray to tan to yellow, and firm or soft. Hemorrhage, necrosis, calcification, and cyst formation are common. Microscopically, metanephric adenomas are composed of small, uniform round acini with small lumens (e-Fig 20.24). The cells are uniform with small nuclei and inconspicuous nucleoli. Branching and tubular configurations are common, as well as papillary architecture with numerous psammoma bodies. In the differential diagnosis with papillary RCC, immunostains that are positive for WT1, negative for EMA, with focal positivity for cytokeratin (CK)7 favor metanephric adenoma.

2. **Metanephric adenofibroma** is more common in men. Grossly, it is solitary and partially cystic. Histologically, its cells are similar to those of a metanephric adenoma but are embedded in a stroma of fibroblastlike spindle cells. Psammoma bodies are also common.

D. Mesenchymal tumors

1. **Leiomyosarcoma** is the most common renal sarcoma; it occurs mainly in adults and affects women and men equally. Leiomyosarcomas can arise from the renal capsule, parenchyma, pelvis muscularis, or the renal vein. They are solid, gray-white, and focally necrotic. Histologically, these tumors are composed of spindle cells with a fascicular growth pattern (e-Fig. 20.25). Necrosis, nuclear pleomorphism, and numerous mitotic figures indicate malignancy. Leiomyosarcoma is an aggressive tumor with a 5-year survival rate of 29% to 36%, and most patients die within 1 year of diagnosis. Sites of metastasis include lung, liver, and bone. Sarcomatoid RCC is in the differential diagnosis and is more common, and so must be excluded; diffuse desmin and smooth muscle actin immunoreactivity would favor leiomyosarcoma.

2. **Rare primary sarcomas** include rhabdomyosarcoma, angiosarcoma, malignant fibrous histiocytoma, chondrosarcoma, low-grade fibromyxoid sarcoma, malignant mesenchymoma, and osteosarcoma.

3. **Angiomyolipoma** is a benign clonal mesenchymal neoplasm tumor composed of thick-walled blood vessels, smooth muscle cells, and adipose tissue. This tumor belongs to the perivascular epithelioid cell tumor (PEComa) family. The mean age at presentation is 45 to 55 years for patients without tuberous sclerosis and 25 to 35 year for patients with this disease. Patients with tuberous sclerosis tend to have multiple, bilateral renal tumors, and can have associated pulmonary lymphangioleiomyomatosis. Tumors are nonencapsulated, yellow to pink masses depending on the content of the tissue components. Rarely, angiomyolipomas can extend into the renal vein or the vena cava. Vascular invasion and lymph node involvement can be present; however, these features are considered to be evidence of direct extension and multifocality, respectively, rather than metastatic disease.

Microscopically, the limits between the tumor and the kidney are well defined. The smooth muscle cells are generally spindled but can appear round or epithelioid in some cases (e-Fig. 20.26). Nuclear atypia can be present. Characteristically, these tumors coexpress melanocytic markers such as HMB45 and smooth muscle markers such as smooth muscle actin and muscle-specific actin. Epithelial markers including cytokeratin are always negative. Classic angiomyolipomas are benign.

4. **Epithelioid angiomyolipoma** is a potentially malignant mesenchymal neoplasm that presents more commonly in patients with tuberous sclerosis. It is much less

common than usual angiomyolipoma. Grossly, these tumors are usually large with tan-gray or hemorrhagic cut surfaces and necrosis. The cells are epithelioid with abundant granular cytoplasm. Multinucleated cells, nuclear pleomorphism, mitotic activity, vascular invasion, necrosis, and involvement of perinephric fat can be present. These tumors express melanocytic markers with variable expression of smooth muscle markers. These tumors can metastasize to lymph nodes, liver, lungs, and spine.

5. **Leiomyoma** is a benign smooth muscle neoplasm that can arise from the renal capsule, the muscularis of the renal pelvis, or from cortical vascular smooth muscle. Most are found incidentally. Grossly, they are firm, well-defined masses, although calcification and cysts can be present. Necrosis should be absent. Leiomyomas are composed of spindled cells arranged in fascicles, with minimal nuclear pleomorphism and no mitotic activity. They demonstrate a smooth muscle immunophenotype, with actin and desmin immunopositivity.

6. **Hemangioma** is a benign vascular tumor that presents in young and middle-aged adults. The tumor is usually unilateral and single, with a red spongy gross appearance. Microscopically, the lesion is characterized by irregular blood-filled spaces lined by a single layer of endothelial cells. No mitoses or nuclear pleomorphism should be present.

7. **Lymphangiomas** are more common in adults, and can represent a lymphatic malformation or can develop secondary to urinary tract infections. Grossly, these are cystic, encapsulated lesions that can overgrow the entire renal parenchyma. The cysts are filled with clear fluid and lined by a single layer of flat endothelium.

8. **Juxtaglomerular cell tumors** are benign renin-secreting tumors that occur in younger individuals and are more common in women. Clinically, the tumor manifests with severe hypertension and hypokalemia. Tumors are solid, well circumscribed, and composed of sheets of polygonal or spindled cells with central regular nuclei, well-defined borders, and granular eosinophilic cytoplasm. Mast cells, hyalinized vessels, and tubular elements are common. Tumor cells are immunoreactive for renin, actin, vimentin, and CD34.

9. **Renomedullary interstitial cell tumors** are commonly found during autopsy. They are present in about 50% of men and women, and frequently they are multifocal. They are 1 to 5 mm in diameter, white or gray, and located within the renal pyramids. Histologically, they contain small polygonal cells in a basophilic background. Renal tubules can be entrapped within the tumor nodules (e-Fig. 20.27).

E. **Mixed mesenchymal and epithelial tumors**

1. **Cystic nephroma** is a benign neoplasm that presents after age 30, more commonly in women. It is associated with pleuropulmonary blastoma in the patient or other family members. Grossly, the tumor is well defined, encapsulated, and entirely composed by cysts. Solid areas and necrosis are not present. These cysts are lined by cuboidal epithelium that often assumes a hobnail appearance. The fibrous septa may contain tubules but not blastema or clear neoplastic cells.

2. **Mixed epithelial and stromal tumor** predominates in adult perimenopausal women. A history of estrogen therapy is common. Grossly, the tumor is composed of solid and cystic areas. Microscopically, the tumor shows tubules and cysts lined by flattened to cuboidal to columnar epithelium. The stromal component is variably cellular and may exhibit myxoid, smooth muscle, ovarian stromal-like, and collagenous features. Fat can be present. The behavior is benign.

F. **Neuroendocrine tumors**

1. **Renal carcinoid tumors** are very rare and present between the fourth and seventh decades. There is a tendency for occurrence in horseshoe kidneys, and there is an association with renal teratomas. They are solid, lobulated, and well circumscribed, and are histologically similar to carcinoids in other organs. (*Am J Surg Pathol* 31:1539, 2007).

2. **Neuroendocrine carcinoma,** including small cell carcinoma, can rarely arise within the adult kidney. A primary tumor elsewhere should be clinically and radiologically excluded. Grossly, the tumor is usually a white, friable, and

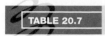

TABLE 20.7	Tumor, Node, Metastasis (TNM) Staging Scheme for Renal Cell Carcinoma

PRIMARY TUMOR (T)

TX	Primary tumor cannot be assessed
T0	No evidence of primary tumor
T1	Tumor ≤7 cm in greatest dimension, limited to the kidney
T1a	Tumor ≤4 cm in greatest dimension, limited to the kidney
T1b	Tumor >4 cm but not >7 cm in greatest dimension, limited to the kidney
T2	Tumor >7 cm in greatest dimension, limited to the kidney
T3	Tumor extends into major veins or invades adrenal gland or perinephric tissues but not beyond Gerota's fascia
T3a	Tumor directly invades adrenal gland or perirenal and/or renal sinus fat but not beyond Gerota's fascia
T3b	Tumor grossly extends into the renal vein or its segmental (muscle-containing) branches, or vena cava below the diaphragm
T3c	Tumor grossly extends into vena cava above the diaphragm or invades the wall of the vena cava
T4	Tumor invades beyond Gerota's fascia

REGIONAL LYMPH NODES (N)*

NX	Regional lymph nodes cannot be assessed
N0	No regional lymph nodes metastases
N1	Metastases in a single regional lymph node
N2	Metastasis in more than one regional lymph node

*Laterality does not affect the N classification

DISTANT METASTASIS (M)

MX	Distant metastasis cannot be assessed
M0	No distant metastasis
M1	Distant metastasis

STAGE GROUPING

Stage I	T1	N0	M0
Stage II	T2	N0	M0
Stage III	T1	N1	M0
	T2	N1	M0
	T3	N0	M0
	T3	N1	M0
	T3a	N0	M0
	T3a	N1	M0
	T3b	N0	M0
	T3b	N1	M0
	T3c	N0	M0
	T3c	N1	M0
Stage IV	T4	N0	M0
	T4	N1	M0
	Any T	N2	M0
	Any T	Any N	M1

From: Greene FL, Page DL, Fleming ID, Fritz AG, Balch CM, Haller DG, Morrow M, eds. *AJCC Cancer Staging Manual.* 6th edition. New York: Springer, 2002. Used with permission. (A new AJCC TNM staging system is scheduled for release in 2009; after its publication, the new staging scheme will appear on the website for this book.)

necrotic mass. Microscopically, the tumor is composed of small round cells with hyperchromatic nuclei and inconspicuous nucleoli, arranged in sheets and trabeculae. Centrally located tumors can be admixed with urothelial carcinoma. Tumor cells show dotlike cytoplasmic immunostaining with cytokeratin antibodies, and are variably positive for synaptophysin and chromogranin. The prognosis is poor.

3. **PNETs** are rare primary renal tumors, and are discussed above in the pediatric renal neoplasm section.
4. **Neuroblastoma and paragangliomas/pheochromocytomas** are very rare.

G. **Hematopoietic and lymphoid tumors.** Primary renal lymphomas usually arise in transplanted kidneys and are Epstein–Barr virus (EBV)-associated B-cell lymphoproliferations. Secondary involvement of the kidney by lymphoma is more common. Plasmacytoma can occur as a manifestation of disseminated multiple myeloma. Diffuse infiltration of the kidney secondary to acute leukemias has also been reported.

H. **Germ cell tumors** include choriocarcinomas and teratomas, and are very rare.

I. **Metastatic tumors** to the kidney include tumors of lung, breast, gastrointestinal tract, pancreas, ovary, and testis and malignant melanoma. Involvement is usually in the setting of known, widely metastatic disease. Only infrequently does metastatic tumor mimic a primary renal tumor. Most metastatic masses are multiple and bilateral.

IV. **HISTOLOGIC GRADING OF RCC** should be reported for all RCCs of clear cell, papillary, and chromophobe types, as described above and in Table 20.6.

V. **PATHOLOGIC STAGING** applies only to RCCs. The 2002 TNM American Joint Committee on Cancer (AJCC)/International Union Against Cancer (UICC) staging classification is given in Table 20.7.

VI. **REPORTING OF ADULT KIDNEY CARCINOMA** should follow suggested guidelines (College of American Pathologists kidney, cancer protocol and checklists 2005 at http://www.cap.org).

A. For a **fine needle aspiration biopsy,** report the presence or absence of a neoplasm, and the type of neoplasm (by WHO classification), if present.

B. For a **core needle biopsy,** report the histologic type, histologic grade (Fuhrman nuclear grade, scale of 1 to 4), and any additional pathologic findings (such as inflammation and glomerular disease).

C. For a **nephrectomy,** partial or radical, report the tumor site (upper pole, middle pole, lower pole), focality (unifocal or multifocal), tumor size (largest, if multiple) in greatest dimension (cm), macroscopic extent of tumor (tumor limited to kidney, tumor extension into perinephric tissues, tumor extension beyond Gerota's fascia, tumor extension into adrenal gland, tumor extension in major veins (intraluminal, with or without vein wall invasion), histologic type, histologic grade (Fuhrman nuclear grade), pathologic TNM stage, and margin status (cannot be assessed, margins uninvolved by invasive carcinoma, margins involved by invasive carcinoma). The adrenal gland, if present, should be reported as uninvolved by tumor, involved by direct invasion, or involved by metastasis. Venous (large vessel) invasion (excluding renal vein and inferior vena cava) should be specified as absent, present, or indeterminate. Lymphatic (small vessel) invasion should also be designated as absent, present, or indeterminate. Additional pathologic findings worth noting, if present, include inflammation (type), glomerular disease (type), interstitial disease (type), acquired cystic disease, and adenoma.

CYTOLOGY OF THE KIDNEY
Rosa M. Dávila

I. **CYTOLOGY OF THE NEOPLASTIC KIDNEY.** Neoplasms involving the renal parenchyma are amenable to sampling by fine needle aspiration biopsy. When the renal pelvis is involved, sampling can also be performed endoscopically. Because the endoscopic biopsies are usually small, cell block processing has been advocated, particularly in low-grade lesions where the architectural features are of diagnostic importance. Cytologic evaluation of ureteral catheterization samples is also useful in detecting high-grade urothelial lesion of the upper urinary tract (*J Urol* 164:1901, 2000).

II. **BENIGN NEOPLASMS**

A. **Angiomyolipoma.** Mature adipose tissue, smooth muscle, and blood vessels are the main components of this tumor (e-**Fig** 20.28). Identification of adipose tissue in the fine needle aspiration biopsy is an important clue in making this diagnosis.

The smooth muscle component may have an epithelioid appearance with nuclear atypia, so it is important not to misinterpret the findings as a malignant process. Immunostains for HMB45 and smooth muscle actin are used to differentiate angiomyolipoma from RCC (*Acta Cytol* 50:466, 2006).

B. Oncocytoma can be solitary or multifocal and usually has a characteristic radiologic appearance that includes good demarcation, a central scar, and a density similar to that of the uninvolved renal parenchyma. Cytologic samples show numerous large cells with abundant granular cytoplasm, round nuclei, and distinct cell borders. The nucleolus can be prominent, but no necrosis or mitoses are present.

III. MALIGNANT NEOPLASMS

A. RCC is the most common renal malignancy. The cytologic findings of these tumors vary according to the histologic type. In the conventional clear cell variant, the fine needle aspiration samples are usually richly cellular and bloody. The neoplastic cells have abundant vacuolated cytoplasm that may be more noticeable in air-dried, Romanowski-stained slides (**e-Fig 20.29**). It is not unusual to see naked nuclei from disrupted tumor cells in the background. When tumor microfragments are available, a rich capillary network is seen. The degree of nuclear abnormalities and the presence of prominent nucleoli are dependent on the nuclear grade of the tumor.

Papillary structures, macrophages, and psammoma bodies are identified in the **papillary RCC** (**e-Fig 20.30**). Additionally, nuclear pseudoinclusions, nuclear grooves, and cytoplasmic hemosiderin can be identified (*Diagn Cytopathol* 334:797, 2006).

Chromophobe RCC consists of cells with abundant cytoplasm, well-defined cell borders, and a perinuclear halo. The nuclei usually have irregular contour borders and hyperchromasia, resulting in a raisinoid appearance, nuclear features that allow for differentiation from oncocytoma. Nuclear grooves and/or pseudoinclusions and necrotic debris can also be present.

B. Urothelial carcinoma is the most common tumor arising in the renal pelvis. It is morphologically similar to urothelial carcinomas arising in other sites. The cytologic findings of these tumors vary according to their grade. Cells from low-grade tumors lack nuclear atypia and may have a spindle shape (**e-Fig 20.31**).

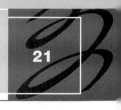

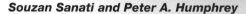

I. **NORMAL ANATOMY.** The upper tract of the urinary collecting system is composed of the renal calyces, pelves, and ureters. Renal papillae protrude into the minor calyces, which expand into two or three major calyces, which in turn are outpouchings of the renal pelvis, a saclike expansion of the upper ureter.

The mucosa is normally arranged in folds. The urothelium of the renal pelvis is three to five cell layers thick and five to seven layers thick in the ureter. The lamina propria is composed of highly vascularized connective tissue, without a muscularis mucosa; it is absent beneath the urothelium lining the renal papillae and is thin along the minor calyces. The thickness and amount of muscularis propria in the collecting system within renal sinus fat can be variable; ureteral muscularis propria is composed of interlacing bundles of smooth muscle, without inner or outer layers (SE Mills ed., *Histology for Pathologists* 2nd ed., Philadelphia: Lippincott Williams and Wilkins, p. 839–907, 2007).

II. **GROSS EXAMINATION AND TISSUE SAMPLING.** Tissue samples include ureteroscopic biopsies, needle biopsies, segmental ureterectomy specimens, and radical nephroureterectomy with urinary bladder cuff resection specimens.

A. **Ureteroscopic biopsies** are entirely submitted. Because these are often minute in size, one approach to processing is to submit the biopsy sample for cytology cell block preparation (*Urology* 50:117, 1997).

B. **Needle core biopsies** of renal masses, including urothelial carcinoma involving the kidney, should be completely-submitted, with generation of three levels on each of three hematoxylin and eosin (H&E)-stained slides.

C. **Segmental ureterectomy** is performed for tumors of the proximal or mid-ureter. The length and diameter of the intact ureter is recorded, with a search for a mass by palpation and visual inspection. Proximal and distal cross-sectional margins are taken, and the outer aspect of the ureter is inked. The ureter is then opened longitudinally and assessed for mucosal abnormalities. After overnight fixation in 10% formalin, sections are taken to demonstrate the deepest invasion of any lesion(s). At least one section of uninvolved ureter should be submitted.

D. **Radical nephroureterectomy with bladder cuff.** Gross examination and sampling should document the relationship of tumor to adjacent renal parenchyma, peripelvic fat, nearest soft tissue margin, and ureter. Sections of grossly unremarkable kidney, pelvis, and ureter should be obtained. The important urothelial margin is the urinary bladder cuff, which can be sampled as shave sections.

III. **DIAGNOSTIC FEATURES OF COMMON DISEASES**

A. **Benign conditions** that involve the urothelium in the upper tract have an appearance similar to those in the urinary bladder. Examples are ureteritis, pyelitis cystica and glandularis, malakoplakia, nephrogenic adenoma, and squamous metaplasia.

B. **Benign epithelial neoplasms** are rare and include urothelial papilloma, inverted papilloma, villous adenoma, and squamous papilloma.

C. **Benign nonepithelial neoplasms** include the distinctive fibroepithelial polyp, which is most frequently seen in the proximal ureter of young males. Microscopically, these are exophytic intraluminal projections of a variably inflamed fibrovascular stroma lined by a normal urothelium. Benign mesenchymal neoplasms such as leiomyoma, hemangioma, neurofibroma, and fibrous histiocytoma are rare.

D. **Urothelial dysplasia** in isolated form is rare and displays the same features as in the urinary bladder, where it is defined as low-grade intraurothelial neoplasia.

E. Renal pelvic and ureteral cancers are in the vast majority of cases, as in the urinary bladder, of urothelial type (*Am J Surg Pathol* 28:1545, 2004, *Mod Pathol* 19:494, 2006).

Upper tract tumors differ from those in the urinary bladder in the following ways: Upper tract tumors are found at a lower frequency; have a stronger association with long-term analgesic (such as phenacetin) abuse and urinary tract obstruction; are associated with an increased frequency (in up to 65% of patients) of synchronous or metachronous urothelial neoplasms elsewhere in the urinary tract (WM Murphy, DJ Grignon, EJ Perlman. *Tumors of the Kidney, Bladder, and Related Urinary Structures.* Washington, DC: American Registry of Pathology, 2004); and tend to present with higher histologic grade and at higher stage.

1. **Risk factors.** The main risk factor, as for urinary bladder malignancies, is smoking. Other risk factors are analgesics (as just noted); occupation in chemical, petrochemical, or plastics industries; exposure to tar, coal, or asphalt; papillary necrosis; Balkan nephropathy; thorium contrast exposure; hereditary nonpolyposis colorectal cancer (HNPCC) syndrome (Lynch syndrome II); and urinary tract infections or stones (JN Eble, G Sauter, JI Epstein, IA Sesterhenn, eds. Tumours of the urinary system and male genital organs. Lyon: IARC Press, 2004).

2. **Clinical features.** Most patients are around 70 years of age, and the chief presenting symptoms are hematuria and flank pain. In the majority of patients, there is a prior history of a bladder cancer, which means that many upper tract tumors are detected during the course of clinical surveillance after diagnosis of a bladder tumor.

3. **Histologic typing and diagnosis of upper tract tumors** are accomplished by examination of H&E-stained sections. Typing of upper tract urothelial neoplasia is the same as that for the urinary bladder as defined in the 2004 World Health Organization (WHO) classification of neoplasms (Table 22.1).

4. **Urothelial carcinoma** is by far the most common type of upper tract tumor.
    a. **Gross diagnosis** is possible in resection specimens. Patterns of growth include papillary, polypoid, nodular, ulcerative, and infiltrative. Exophytic tumors can fill and distend the pelvis (e-**Fig. 21.1**),* with or without hydronephrosis and stones. High-grade invasive tumors can grossly involve soft tissue and/or renal parenchyma (e-**Fig. 21.2**). Extensive renal parenchymal involvement can mimic a primary renal parenchymal neoplasm; in these cases there is often a request for an intraoperative consultation to determine whether the mass is a urothelial carcinoma or a renal cell carcinoma (RCC), because the distinction alters the extent of surgery. The correct diagnosis can usually be determined by straightforward gross examination alone, but in some cases a frozen section may be required. The average size of renal pelvic tumors is just under 4 cm, with a range of 0.3 to 9 cm (*Am J Surg Pathol* 28:1545, 2004). Multifocality in the pelvis and ureter is seen in about one quarter of cases. In the ureter, the tumor may be associated with a stricture and hydroureter.
    b. **Microscopically,** the full range of urothelial carcinoma may be seen from flat intraepithelial neoplasia, including carcinoma in situ, to noninvasive papillary neoplasia, including papillary urothelial neoplasm of low malignant potential, low-grade papillary urothelial carcinoma (e-**Fig. 21.3, A and B**), and high-grade papillary urothelial carcinoma (e-**Fig. 21.4, A and B**). The full spectrum of invasive urothelial carcinoma and its variants as found in the urinary bladder may also be found in the upper tract. Of note, unusual histomorphological variants seem to be more common in the upper tract (*Mod Pathol* 19:494, 2006), including carcinomas with micropapillary, lymphoepithelioma-like, sarcomatoid, squamous, clear cell, glandular, rhabdoid, signet-ring, and plasmacytoid features or areas.

    Primary resections done for renal pelvic urothelial carcinoma show high-grade carcinoma in >70% of cases, with deep invasion (pT2 or greater) in 45% of cases and with lymph node metastases in one quarter of patients.

---

*All e-figures are available online via the Solution Site Image Bank.

Cancerization of the distal renal collecting ducts is common in high-grade urothelial carcinoma (**e-Fig. 21.5**). Levels of invasion include lamina propria invasion (**e-Fig. 21.6**); extension into muscularis propria (**e-Fig. 21.7**), renal sinus and hilar fat, and periureteral fat (**e-Fig. 21.8**); and renal parenchymal infiltration. Metastatic sites include lymph nodes, peritoneum, and liver. When the differential diagnosis of a centrally located high-grade carcinoma centers on urothelial carcinoma versus RCC, extensive mucosal sampling is important because identification of urothelial carcinoma in situ (CIS) is in keeping with a urothelial primary.

   c. Immunohistochemical studies are not usually needed, but can be useful in the differential diagnosis of urothelial carcinoma versus RCC, when the diagnosis is not clear by standard gross and microscopic examination. A useful marker panel includes cytokeratin (CK)7, CK20, p63, thrombomodulin, uroplakin III, and RCC marker (RCC Ma). Positivity for the first five favors urothelial carcinoma, whereas RCC Ma immunoreactivity is seen in RCC rather than urothelial carcinoma (*Semin Diagn Pathol.* 22:51, 2005).

   d. Molecular studies. The most promising test is fluorescence in situ hybridization done on cells in urine from the upper tract. In this test (UroVysion/Vysis/Abbott), a mixture of fluorescent probes to chromosomes 3, 7, 17, and

TABLE 21.1	Tumor, Node, Metastasis (TNM) Staging Scheme for Carcinoma of Renal Pelvis and Ureter

Primary tumor (T)

TX	Primary tumor cannot be assessed
T0	No evidence of primary tumor
Ta	Noninvasive papillary carcinoma
Tis	Carcinoma in situ
T1	Tumor invades subepithelial connective tissue
T2	Tumor invades muscularis
T3	Renal pelvis tumors: Tumor invades beyond muscularis into peripelvic fat or renal parenchyma
	Ureteral tumors: Tumor invades beyond muscularis into periureteric fat
T4	Tumor invades adjacent organs or through the kidney into perinephric fat

Regional lymph nodes (N)

NX	Regional lymph nodes cannot be assessed
N0	No regional lymph node metastasis
N1	Metastasis to a single lymph node ≤2 cm in greatest dimension
N2	Metastasis in a single lymph node 2 to 5 cm in greatest dimension
N3	Metastasis in a lymph node >5 cm in greatest dimension

Distant metastasis (M)

MX	Distant metastasis cannot be assessed
M0	No distant metastasis
M1	Distant metastasis

Stage grouping

Stage 0a	Ta	N0	M0
Stage 0is	Tis	N0	M0
Stage I	T1	N0	M0
Stage II	T2	N0	M0
Stage III	T3	N0	M0
Stage IV	T4	N0	M0
	Any T	N1–3	M0
	Any T	Any N	M1

From: Greene FL, Page DL, Fleming ID, Fritz AG, Balch CM, Haller DG, Morrow M, eds. *AJCC Cancer Staging Manual.* 6th edition. New York: Springer; 2002. Used with permission. (A new AJCC TNM staging system is scheduled for release in 2009; after its publication, the new staging scheme will appear on the website for this book.)

9p21 locus is used to detect numerical chromosomal abnormalities associated with urothelial carcinoma (*Expert Rev Mol Diagn.* 7:11, 2007). The precise clinical indications for its use for upper tract tumors are not yet established.

5. **Squamous cell carcinoma** is rare, is more common in the pelvis, is frequently associated with nephrolithiasis and/or infection, and often presents with high-stage and high-grade disease (e-**Fig. 21.9, A and B**). Pure squamous cell carcinomas should be distinguished from urothelial carcinoma with squamous differentiation.

6. **Adenocarcinoma** is rare and may display enteric, mucinous, and/or signet-ring features. Pure adenocarcinomas should be separated from urothelial carcinoma with glandular differentiation. Intestinal metaplasia, nephrolithiasis, and infection are predisposing factors.

7. **Small cell carcinomas** in very rare cases arise from the renal pelvis. There may be admixed urothelial carcinoma.

8. **Malignant mesenchymal neoplasms** are rare. The most common is leiomyosarcoma. Exceedingly rare types include osteosarcoma, rhabdomyosarcoma, fibrosarcoma, angiosarcoma, and Ewing sarcoma.

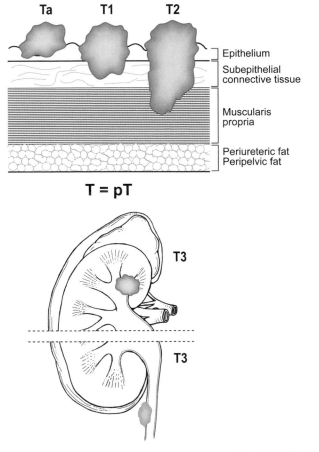

Figure 21.1. Depiction of pT stages pTa, pT1, pT2, and pT3. Modified from Greene FL, Compton CC, Fritz AG, Shah JP, Winchester DP, eds. *AJCC Cancer staging Atlas.* New York: Springer; 2006.

9. **Hematolymphoid neoplasms** in the ureter and renal pelvis typically are due to secondary involvement.

10. **Miscellaneous neoplasms** rarely encountered include paraganglioma, carcinoid tumor, Wilms tumor, malignant melanoma, and choriocarcinoma.

11. **Secondary malignancies** include carcinomas of the cervix, prostate, colon, breast, and urinary bladder.

IV. **HISTOLOGIC GRADING** should be performed for all carcinomas, with urothelial carcinoma grade being assigned as low grade or high grade, as for the urinary bladder. Pure squamous cell carcinoma and adenocarcinoma may be graded as well-differentiated, moderately differentiated, or poorly differentiated.

V. **PATHOLOGIC STAGING** applies only to carcinomas of the ureter and renal pelvis. Stage is the most important prognostic factor for upper tract carcinoma. The 2002 Tumor, Node, Metastasis (TNM) American Joint Committee on Cancer/International Union Against Cancer (AJCC/UICC) staging classification is given in Table 21.1; pT stages pTa through pT3 are shown in Fig. 21.1. Clinical staging should be distinguished from pathologic staging. One important note is that renal pelvic carcinoma extending into the renal collecting ducts does not represent renal parenchymal invasion, which is pT3 disease.

VI. **REPORTING CARCINOMA OF THE URETER AND RENAL PELVIS.** In addition to typing, grading, staging, and assessing size and margins, pertinent pathologic features that should be reported include the following: For ureteroscopic biopsies, the amount of sampled stroma available to allow for evaluation of invasion should be specified (*Arch Path Lab Med.* 127:1263, 2003). For nephroureterectomy or ureterectomy specimens, gross characteristics such as tumor location, focality (unifocal vs. multifocal), gross appearance (papillary, solid/nodule, flat, ulcerated), gross depth of invasion, and distance to margins should be given. Additional gross abnormalities such as other mucosal lesions, renal parenchymal lesions, stones, hydronephrosis, and hydroureter should be documented, when present. Microscopically, additional relevant pathologic findings, if present, include lymphovascular space invasion by carcinoma, flat urothelial carcinoma in situ (focal vs. multifocal), inflammation, renal epithelial neoplasia or medical renal disease (glomerulopathy), and metaplasias of the urothelium, including keratinizing squamous metaplasia and intestinal metaplasia.

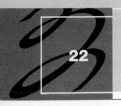

THE URINARY BLADDER

22

Omar Hameed and Peter A. Humphrey

I. **NORMAL MICROSCOPIC ANATOMY.** The wall of the urinary bladder is formed by four layers (e-**Fig. 22.1**)* (SE Mills ed., *Histology for Pathologists*, 2nd ed. Philadelphia: Lippincott Williams & Wilkins; 2007). The thickness of the innermost layer, the urothelium, depends on the degree of bladder distension, and the shape of its constituent urothelial cells ranges from smaller cuboidal cells at the base to larger polyhedral cells toward the surface. Umbrella cells, the most superficial cells, have abundant eosinophilic cytoplasm and are often binucleated. Separated from the urothelium by a thin basement membrane, the underlying lamina propria is composed of loose connective tissue with blood vessels, nerves, adipose tissue, and a variable amount of smooth muscle fibers forming a discontinuous muscularis mucosae. Aggregates of urothelium termed von Brunn nests (e-**Fig. 22.2**), are often seen as invaginations or separate clusters in the lamina propria. The term cystitis cystica is used when these nests become prominent and undergo cystic change (e-**Fig. 22.3**). Cystitis glandularis is similar to cystitis cystica except that the cells lining the cysts are mucin-secreting cuboidal or columnar cells, or true goblet cells, in which case the term cystitis glandularis with intestinal metaplasia is used. These proliferative lesions, although sometimes seen associated with local inflammation, represent variants of normal histology. Their main importance lies in the fact that they can occasionally cause visible lesions simulating a bladder neoplasm. The third layer, the muscularis propria or detrusor muscle, is composed of large bundles of muscle fibers and is covered by the outermost adventitial layer, including perivesical adipose tissue. It is important to note that adipose tissue can also be found in the submucosa and wall, such that identification of fat does not equate to a specific layer of the bladder wall.

II. **GROSS EXAMINATIONS AND TISSUE SAMPLING OF THE BLADDER.** The most common samples submitted for surgical pathology examination include small biopsies, larger transurethral resection specimens, as well as partial and radical (complete) cystectomies.

A. **Biopsy specimens.** These are usually obtained without cautery ("cold-cup") and should be immediately immersed in formalin. If multiple biopsies are submitted separately, as in mapping procedures, they should be processed separately. After gross examination, bladder biopsies should be marked with ink or hematoxylin, then placed in a cassette after being put in a fine mesh envelope, wrapped in lens paper, or sandwiched between sponge pads. After processing, three hematoxylin and eosin (H&E)-stained slides should be prepared, each with a strip of 3 to 4 levels.

B. **Transurethral resection of bladder specimens.** These specimens are usually obtained with the aid of thermal cautery, often for the transurethral resection of bladder tumors (TURBT). Because of the significant prognostic and therapeutic implications for the presence of muscularis propria invasion by the bladder neoplasms, it is often necessary to process all of the submitted tissue to ensure that such foci of invasion are not overlooked.

C. **Partial cystectomy specimens.** Partial or segmental cystectomy is indicated in only a minority of bladder cancer patients, typically those who suffer a first time tumor recurrence with a solitary tumor, and tumor location that allows for a 1- to 2-cm margin of resection, such as at the dome. Urachal carcinomas at the dome and above, with extension toward the umbilicus, may also be treated by partial cystectomy, as

---

*All e-figures are available online via the Solution Site Image Bank.

can carcinoma in a bladder diverticulum. Carcinoma in situ elsewhere in the bladder (or multifocal tumors) is an absolute contraindication. The specimens usually consist of a sheetlike portion of tissue that should be pinned down and fixed overnight. In addition to describing and sampling any gross tumor(s) as described for cystectomy specimens, the status of the margins is most important; these could be shaved off or sampled by perpendicular sections, depending on their relationship and proximity to the tumor(s) present. Frozen section of the mucosal margin may be requested.

D. Total cystectomy and cystoprostatectomy specimens. Radical cystoprostatectomy in men and anterior exenteration in women, along with pelvic lymphadenectomy, are standard surgical approaches for muscle wall–invasive bladder carcinoma in the absence of metastatic disease. Cystectomy may be performed in some cases for nonmuscle wall-invasive bladder carcinoma if the bladder is nonfunctional, or for high-grade pT1 carcinoma that is not responsive to intravesical therapy. If not sampled separately, a request to perform frozen sections on the ureteric and urethral margins may be received (*Arch Pathol Lab Med* 129:1585–1601, 2005), and these should be shaved off for that purpose. After orientation and inking, one of two methods can be used to fix the specimen. The first entails filling the bladder with formalin (through the urethra, or by using a large bore needle through the dome) and fixing overnight, and the second entails opening the bladder (usually through the urethra extending upward on the anterior surface) and pinning it down, then fixing it overnight. After opening the bladder (in the fresh or fixed state), the mucosa is examined for tumors(s) and, if present, the size, location, pattern of growth (exophytic, endophytic, and/or ulcerated), and depth of invasion are recorded. The mucosa of the adjacent bladder should also be examined for areas of hemorrhage and discoloration that may represent areas of carcinoma in situ. In addition to sampling of any tumor(s) (3 to 4 sections of each), representative sections need to be submitted from the different areas of the bladder including the trigone; posterior, lateral, and anterior walls; and dome (Fig. 22.1). If ureteric and urethral shave margins were not submitted for frozen section examination, they should be sampled for permanent sections, as should any possible lymph nodes identified in the perivesical fat. In cystoprostatectomy specimens, additional blocks from the prostate and seminal vesicles should be submitted, the extent of which depends on whether a preoperative diagnosis or suspicion of prostatic carcinoma exists (see Chapter 29). When the bladder (with or without the prostate) is removed as part of larger pelvic exenteration specimens (that may include portions of the rectum and/or the gynecological tract in females), then it becomes imperative to document the presence or absence of involvement of these additional organs by preferentially sampling suspicious areas, as well as by sampling the resection margins of these organs.

III. DIAGNOSTIC FEATURES OF COMMON DISEASES OF THE BLADDER

A. Congenital malformations

1. Urachal abnormalities. The urachus is a vestigial structure that connects the dome of the bladder to the umbilicus; it normally closes by the fourth month of fetal life. Persistence or malformations of the urachus can present in childhood and occasionally in adulthood. They include patent urachus, urachal cysts, and urachal sinuses, all of which can result in secondary infection, as well as the development of secondary tumors, most frequently adenocarcinoma. (Foster CS, Ross JS, eds. *Pathology of the Urinary Bladder.* Philadelphia: Saunders; pp. 49–66, 2004).

2. Exstrophy. This is a rare congenital anomaly characterized by failure of development of the anterior wall of the bladder and abdominal wall, usually resulting in severe secondary infection if left untreated.

B. Inflammatory conditions.

Cystitis is most frequently infectious in nature. There are, however, specific variants of cystitis that produce somewhat characteristic cystoscopic and/or microscopic appearances. The latter include hemorrhagic, granulomatous, eosinophilic, and interstitial variants, as well as malakoplakia.

1. Infectious cystitis. Acute and chronic cystitis is most frequently secondary to bacterial infection (usually by enteric organisms). The incidence is higher in females as well as when intermittent urinary obstruction or stasis is present. Biopsy

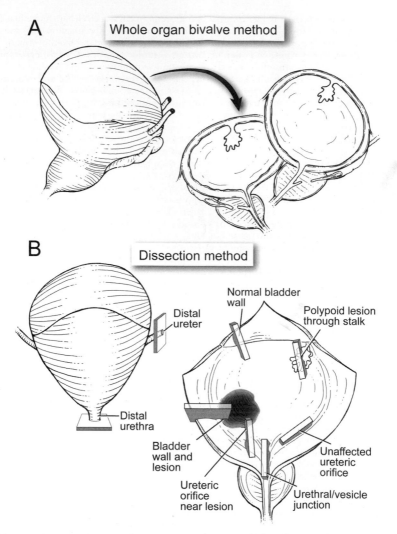

Figure 22.1. Gross dissection of radical cystectomy specimens by whole organ bivalve method **(A)** and by opening along urethra and anterior wall, with demonstration of sections to be taken **(B)**. Three to four sections, or complete embedding, of masses should be performed (Modified from Schmidt WA. *Principles and Techniques of Surgical Pathology.* Menlo Park, California: Addison-Wesley Publishing Co.; p.525, 1983).

during active infection is contraindicated, but biopsy may be performed in cases of chronic cystitis to rule out neoplasia, especially carcinoma in situ. The histopathological features include a nonspecific acute and/or chronic inflammatory infiltrate occasionally with lymphoid aggregates/follicles (follicular cystitis) (**e-Fig. 22.4**), and a variable degree of lamina propria edema. Of note, similar findings may be seen in the absence of infection such as following radiation or cytotoxic chemotherapy. Other infections can produce specific histological findings such as viral inclusions (polyoma and herpesviruses) or granulomas (tuberculosis, fungal infections, and schistosomiasis).

2. **Granulomatous cystitis.** As noted above, bacterial, fungal, or parasitic infections can lead to granuloma formation. The most frequent cause, however, is iatrogenic, either secondary to intravesical Bacille Calmette-Guerin (BCG) immunotherapy for urothelial carcinoma in situ and superficially invasive carcinoma (e-**Fig. 22.5**), or following TURBT (e-**Fig. 22.6**).

3. **Hemorrhagic cystitis.** This is an uncommon side effect of cyclophosphamide therapy that results in extensive ulceration and hemorrhage that, if severe, may require cystectomy. Adenovirus infection (in immunocompromised individuals) may also produce such a picture.

4. **Papillary and polypoid (bullous) cystitis.** These related forms of cystitis are characterized by fingerlike (papillary) or broad (polypoid) projections of edematous, variably inflamed lamina propria covered by reactive nonneoplastic urothelium (e-**Fig. 22.7**). These forms of cystitis are most frequently seen with prolonged indwelling catheter use. The presence of such an inflammatory component in papillary cystitis can help in making the occasionally difficult distinction from a low-grade papillary urothelial neoplasm.

5. **Eosinophilic cystitis.** This is characterized by dense infiltration of eosinophils in the bladder wall. Such infiltrates are most frequently seen adjacent to invasive urothelial carcinoma, but they also occur in patients with allergic conditions and rarely in patients with parasitic infections, both often in association with peripheral eosinophilia.

6. **Interstitial cystitis.** This is an uncommon inflammatory disorder that predominantly affects middle-aged and elderly women and results in severe intractable symptoms of culture-negative cystitis. Petechial submucosal hemorrhages or ulcers (termed Hunner's ulcers) are usually evident cystoscopically. The microscopic features are nonspecific and include a mixed inflammatory infiltrate in the lamina propria, often with an increased number of mast cells that can also involve the muscularis propria and nerves. Clinical correlation is required in these cases because the histological findings are, at most, consistent with the clinical impression of interstitial cystitis.

7. **Malakoplakia.** This is an uncommon form of cystitis characterized by the presence of soft yellowish mucosal plaques composed of inflammatory cells including abundant epithelioid histiocytes (known as von Hansemann histiocytes) having granular eosinophilic cytoplasm, and characteristic 3- to 10-micron, rounded, basophilic intracytoplasmic inclusions (Michaelis–Gutmann bodies) that contain iron and calcium, best demonstrated by Prussian blue and von Kossa special stains, respectively. The condition is thought to result from a defect in the ability of histiocytes to degrade phagocytosized bacteria. Control of urinary tract infection can help control the disease.

C. **Reactive and metaplastic urothelial lesions**

1. **Squamous metaplasia.** This can be of two types, nonkeratinizing and keratinizing. The former is considered a normal finding in the trigone and bladder neck of females, but can rarely be seen in males receiving estrogen treatment for prostate cancer. In contrast, keratinizing squamous metaplasia is more common in males in association with chronic irritation, and is considered a significant risk factor for the subsequent development of carcinoma (*Eur Urol* 42:469, 2002, *Am J Surg Pathol* 20:883, 2006).

2. **Intestinal metaplasia.** In addition to the intestinal metaplasia occasionally seen in cystitis glandularis, intestinal metaplasia in the presence of a chronically irritated bladder can involve the bladder mucosa and lamina propria in a focal or diffuse manner, resulting in an appearance almost indistinguishable from colonic mucosa.

3. **Nephrogenic metaplasia (adenoma).** This is a benign epithelial proliferation composed of cells resembling renal tubular epithelium (hence the name), which usually arises in the setting of chronic irritation or injury such as infection or calculi (*Adv Anat Pathol* 13:247, 2006). The lesion was believed to be metaplastic; however, more recent evidence has demonstrated that, at least in renal transplant recipients, nephrogenic metaplasia is derived from shed renal tubular

epithelial cells that may attach to areas of prior injury. Although most frequently seen in the bladder, it is also quite common in the urethra, and less so in the ureters and renal pelvis. Nephrogenic metaplasia is usually an incidental finding, but it may also present as a mass lesion simulating cancer. Histologically, papillae (e-**Fig. 22.8**), small tubules, or cystically dilated tubules lined by cuboidal, low columnar, or flattened hobnail cells are seen. The importance of nephrogenic metaplasia lies in the fact that in the bladder it can be confused with adenocarcinoma (especially clear cell adenocarcinoma) and glandular variants of urothelial carcinoma, and in the urethra it can be confused with prostatic adenocarcinoma. The immunohistochemical reactivity of nephrogenic metaplasia with cytokeratin 7, alpha-methylacyl coenzyme A racemase (AMACR), and PAX2 (a transcription factor present in renal tubular epithelial cells) antibodies and the lack of reactivity with high-molecular-weight cytokeratin (e.g., 34βE12) and prostate-specific antigen (PSA) help in distinguishing it from its mimickers.

4. **Urothelial hyperplasia.** An increase in the thickness of the urothelium (>7 layers) is usually reactive in nature and most frequently seen secondary to chronic inflammatory conditions. Flat urothelial hyperplasia (e-**Fig. 22.9**) is more common than papillary urothelial hyperplasia, which some authors have also found to be associated with papillary urothelial neoplasms.

5. **Reactive urothelial atypia.** Usually seen in a setting of acute and/or chronic inflammation, reactive atypia may be associated with hyperplastic or thin urothelium. Nuclear enlargement, often with vesicular chromatin and a single prominent nucleolus, are the most prominent findings (e-**Fig. 22.10**). Mitotic figures may be increased and cell crowding may be observed; however, polarity, cell uniformity, and maturation are usually well preserved. Acute or chronic inflammation is often identified.

D. **Miscellaneous nonneoplastic conditions**

1. **Endometriosis.** Most frequently seen on the serosal aspect of the bladder in women with a previous history of pelvic surgery, foci of endometriosis can also involve the lamina propria or muscularis propria and may be visible cystoscopically. As elsewhere, at least two of the three histological features of endometriosis–endometrial glands, endometrial stroma, and hemosiderin-laden macrophages–are required for the diagnosis.

2. **Endocervicosis and endosalpingiosis.** These are characterized by the presence of glands within the bladder wall lined by columnar endocervical-type mucinous cells or ciliated tubal epithelial cells, respectively. When both are present with endometriosis, the term "Müllerianosis" has been used. Lack of significant nuclear atypia, mitoses, and a stromal tissue reaction help distinguish these benign lesions from invasive adenocarcinoma.

3. **Diverticula.** These outpouchings of mucosa through the muscularis propria are mostly due to increased pressure. Diverticula are frequently complicated by secondary inflammation, squamous metaplasia, and lithiasis, and in less than 10% of cases by secondary neoplastic development.

4. **Amyloidosis.** The bladder may rarely be involved by amyloidosis (usually as part of systemic amyloidosis) and as a primary localized form limited to the bladder, where it may present as a localized lesion.

5. **Ectopic prostatic tissue.** These are usually small polypoid projections most frequently seen in the trigone area. They are composed of benign prostatic epithelium (very similar to so-called "prostatic urethral polyps" in the urethra).

E. **Neoplastic urothelial lesions.** Urothelial neoplasms are the most common neoplasms that can involve the bladder. Histologic typing and diagnosis of urothelial abnormalities are accomplished by examination of H&E-stained sections. The 2004 World Health Organization (WHO) classification is given in Table 22.1.

1. **Flat urothelial lesions with atypia.** In addition to reactive atypia discussed above, such lesions include urothelial dysplasia and urothelial carcinoma in situ.

a. **Urothelial dysplasia.** Dysplasia is an intraepithelial neoplastic urothelial proliferation characterized by variable degrees of loss of polarity, nuclear enlargement, and chromatin clumping (e-**Fig. 22.11**), all of which fall short of the degree seen in carcinoma in situ. Dysplasia is often identified in patients with

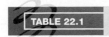

TABLE 22.1	WHO Histologic Classification of Tumors of the Urinary Tract (Including Bladder)

Urothelial tumors
Infiltrating urothelial carcinoma
  With squamous differentiation
  With glandular differentiation
  With trophoblastic differentiation
  Nested
  Microcystic
  Micropapillary
  Lymphoepithelioma-like
  Lymphoma-like
  Plasmacytoid
  Sarcomatoid
  Giant cell
  Undifferentiated
Noninvasive urothelial neoplasias
  Urothelial carcinoma in situ
  Noninvasive papillary urothelial
    carcinoma, high grade
  Noninvasive papillary urothelial
    carcinoma, low grade
  Noninvasive papillary urothelial
    neoplasm of low malignant potential
  Urothelial papilloma
  Inverted urothelial papilloma

Squamous neoplasms
Squamous cell carcinoma
Verrucous carcinoma
Squamous cell papilloma

Glandular neoplasms
Adenocarcinoma
  Enteric
  Mucinous
  Signet-ring cell
  Clear cell
Villous adenoma

Neuroendocrine tumors
Small cell carcinoma
Paraganglioma
Carcinoid

Melanocytic tumors
Malignant melanoma
Nevus

Mesenchymal tumors
Rhabdomyosarcoma
Leiomyosarcoma
Angiosarcoma
Osteosarcoma
Malignant fibrous histiocytoma
Leiomyoma
Hemangioma
Other

Hematopoietic and lymphoid tumors
Lymphoma
Plasmacytoma

Miscellaneous tumors
Carcinoma of Skene, Cowper, and Littre glands
Metastatic tumors and tumors extending from
  other organs

From: Ebele JN, Sauter G, Epstein JL, Sesterhenn IA, eds. *World Health Organization Classification of Tumors. Pathology and Genetics. Tumours of the Urinary System and Male Genital Organs.* Lyon, IARC Press; 2004. Used with permission.

urothelial neoplasms. Occasionally it may be difficult to distinguish urothelial dysplasia from reactive atypia; in such situations a diagnosis of atypia of unknown significance may be warranted. Isolated urothelial dysplasia progresses to bladder carcinoma in about 15% of cases (*Cancer* 88:625, 2000).

b. Urothelial carcinoma in situ. This is a high-grade, often multifocal intraurothelial neoplastic proliferation characterized by the presence of unequivocal malignant urothelial cells within the bladder epithelial lining (Fig. 22.2, e-Fig. 22.12). The urothelial proliferation need not involve the entire thickness of the urothelium, and pagetoid and undermining patterns of growth are not uncommon. Another common feature is the discohesive nature of the neoplastic cells that often leads to denudation and a "clinging" pattern of growth in which only scarce malignant cells remain attached to the bladder wall. In difficult cases where the differential diagnosis includes reactive urothelial atypia, immunostains for cytokeratin 20, p53, CD44, and Ki-67 can be useful (*Semin Diagn Pathol* 22:69, 2005). Urothelial carcinoma in situ is often associated with invasive urothelial carcinoma, and carries a significant risk of death from bladder carcinoma (*Cancer* 85:2469, 1999).

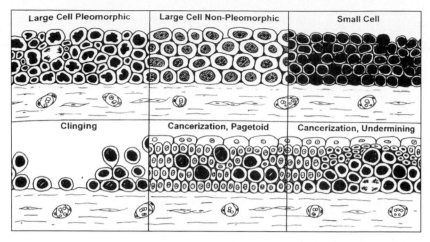

Figure 22.2. Patterns of urinary bladder carcinoma in situ (From McKenney JK, et al. *Am J Surg Pathol* 25:356, 2001, with permission).

2. **Papillary urothelial neoplasms**
   a. **Urothelial papilloma.** This uncommon benign neoplasm is composed of delicate papillary urothelial fronds with no or minimal branching or fusion. The constituent cells are identical to normal urothelial cells, and no mitoses are present (e-**Fig. 22.13**). The classic cystoscopic finding is a solitary lesion in a younger patient with hematuria. Papillomas may recur or progress to higher grade disease (in 0% to 8%, and 2% of cases, respectively).
   b. **Inverted papilloma.** Another uncommon neoplasm, an inverted papilloma has a polypoid or sessile appearance cystoscopically. It is composed of anastamosing islands and cords of bland urothelial cells that invaginate and grow downward in the lamina propria with peripheral palisading, no to rare mitoses, and no to minimal cytological atypia (e-**Fig. 22.14**) (*Am J Surg Pathol* 28:1615, 2004, *Cancer* 107:2622, 2006). These latter two features help distinguish this lesion from other papillary neoplasms that may also occasionally have an inverted growth pattern. Inverted papillomas rarely recur.
   c. **Papillary urothelial neoplasm of low malignant potential (PUNLMP).** This neoplasm shares the clinical and endoscopic features of papilloma; however, it is characterized histologically by occasionally fused papillae and ordered, yet larger nuclei than are seen in papillomas (e-**Fig. 22.15, A and B**). Mitotic figures are rare and basal in location. Compared to papillomas, PUNLMP has higher recurrence and progression rates (25% to 35%, and 0% to 4%, respectively), and thus close follow-up is warranted.
   d. **Noninvasive papillary urothelial carcinoma, low grade.** In contrast to PUNLMP, this urothelial neoplasm shows frequent branching and fusion of papillae and variations in nuclear size, shape, and contour (e-**Fig. 22.16**). Mitoses are occasional and may be found at any level. These tumors tend to be larger than papillomas and PUNLMPs and are more likely to be multiple. They are also more likely to recur and progress (64% to 71%, and 2% to 10%, respectively).
   e. **Noninvasive papillary urothelial carcinoma, high grade.** These are uncommon noninvasive papillary neoplasms; more frequently there is associated invasion. They are characterized by frequent branching and fusion with moderate to marked cytoarchitectural disorder and nuclear pleomorphism (e-**Fig. 22.17**). Mitoses are frequent. Similar to low-grade tumors, these tumors frequently recur (56%), and 18% progress to invasive carcinoma.

3. **Invasive urothelial neoplasms.** Invasive urothelial carcinomas can have papillary, polypoid, nodular, or ulcerative configurations. Most of them are cytologically high-grade tumors. Determination of anatomic depth of invasion by carcinoma is vital, because pathological stage is the single most important prognostic feature in urothelial carcinoma.

Recognition of diagnostic patterns of lamina propria invasion can facilitate pT1 stage assignment (Table 22.2). There are several different patterns of lamina

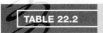

TABLE 22.2	Tumor, Node, Metastasis (TNM) Staging Scheme for Bladder Carcinoma

Primary tumor (T)

TX	Primary tumor cannot be assessed
T0	No evidence of primary tumor
Ta	Noninvasive papillary carcinoma
Tis	Carcinoma in situ (i.e., flat tumor)
T1	Tumor invades subepithelial connective tissue
T2	Tumor invades muscle
pT2a	Tumor invades superficial muscle (inner half)
pT2b	Tumor invades deep muscle (outer half)
T3	Tumor invades perivesical tissue
pT3a	Microscopically
pT3b	Macroscopically (extravesical mass)
T4	Tumor invades any of the following: prostate, uterus, vagina, pelvic wall, or abdominal wall
T4a	Tumor invades the prostate, uterus, vagina
T4b	Tumor invades the pelvic wall, abdominal wall

Note: The suffix "m" should be added to the appropriate T category to indicate multiple lesions. The suffix "is" may be added to any T to indicate the presence of associated carcinoma in situ.

Regional lymph nodes (N)

NX	Regional lymph nodes cannot be assessed
N0	No regional lymph node metastasis
N1	Metastasis in a single lymph node, ≤2 cm in greatest dimension
N2	Metastasis in a single lymph node, >2 cm but ≤5 cm in greatest dimension; or multiple lymph nodes, ≤5 cm in greatest dimension
N3	Metastasis in a lymph node, >5 cm in greatest dimension

Distant metastasis (M)

MX	Distant metastasis cannot be assessed
M0	No distant metastasis
M1	Distant metastasis

AJCC stage groupings

Stage 0a	Ta	N0	M0
Stage 0is	Tis	N0	M0
Stage I	T1	N0	M0
Stage II	T2a	N0	M0
	T2b	N0	M0
Stage III	T3a	N0	M0
	T3b	N0	M0
	T4a	N0	M0
Stage IV	T4b	N0	M0
	Any T	N1	M0
	Any T	N2	M0
	Any T	N3	M0
	Any T	Any N	M1

From: Greene FL, Page DL, Fleming ID, Fritz AG, Balch CM, Haller DG, Morrow M, eds. *AJCC Cancer Staging Manual.* 6th edition. New York: Springer, 2002. Used with permission. (A new AJCC TNM staging system is scheduled for release in 2009; after its publication, the new staging scheme will appear on the website for this book.)

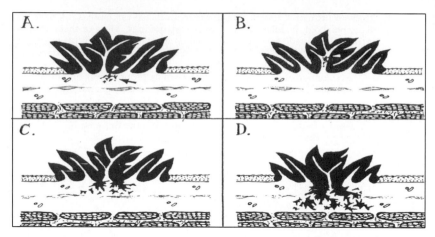

Figure 22.3. Patterns of invasion from papillary carcinoma. **A:** Microinvasive carcinoma at base. **B:** Stalk invasion. **C:** Lamina propria invasion up to muscularis mucosae. **D:** Lamina propria invasion beyond muscularis mucosae. (From Amin MB, et al. *Am J Surg Pathol* 21:1057, 1997, with permission.)

propria invasion, including those seen with papillary urothelial carcinoma (Fig. 22.3, e-Figs. 22.18, 22.19) and carcinoma in situ (CIS) (e-Fig. 22.20), nested carcinoma, and inverted pattern carcinoma (Fig. 22.4) (*Am J Surg Pathol* 21:1057, 1997). Recently emphasized pitfalls in the diagnosis of lamina propria invasive urothelial carcinoma include tangential sectioning, thermal artifact, obscuring inflammation, carcinoma in situ involving von Brunn nests, deceptively bland urothelial carcinoma, invasion into indeterminate type of muscle, and invasion into adipose tissue within lamina propria (Epstein JI, Amin MB, Reuter VE. *Bladder Biopsy Interpretation.* Philadelphia: Lippincott Williams & Wilkins; 2004).

The level of invasion of carcinoma in pT1 disease is related to patient outcome, with a worse prognosis for patients with tumors that invade the muscularis mucosae (pT1b) or deeply into the subepithelial connective tissue, as quantitated using an ocular micrometer. The WHO 2004 group recommended that some

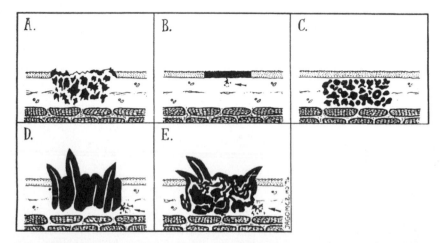

Figure 22.4. Patterns of lamina propria invasion. **A** and **B:** From carcinoma in situ. **C:** Nested variant. **D:** Endophytic growth and invasion. **E:** Inverted growth and invasion. (From Amin MB, et al. *Am J Surg Pathol* 21:1057, 1997, with permission.)

estimate of extent of lamina propria invasion (e.g., pT1a [invasion above muscularis mucosae] vs. pT1b tumors) be provided, but this is currently not a formal part of the 2002 Tumor, Node, Metastasis (TNM) system and it is not universally reported because there is no established method that is consistently applicable and reproducible.

Invasion by bladder carcinoma into muscularis propria (muscle wall, detrusor) (e-Fig. 22.21) is an ominous finding that makes the patient a candidate for aggressive surgical therapy (radical cystectomy) or radiation therapy, with or without adjuvant chemotherapy.

Determination of the type of muscle (muscularis mucosae vs. muscularis propria) invaded by carcinoma can occasionally be difficult because of small tissue-sample size, tissue distortion, cautery artifact, poor orientation, fibrosis, inflammation elicited by destructive growth of invasive tumor, or even hypertrophy of the normally thin, wispy, and discontinuous muscularis mucosae. The designation of "muscle type indeterminate" is a viable description in a few cases. Substaging of pT2 (pT2a, invasion of "superficial" muscle = inner half vs. pT2b, invasion of "deep" muscle = outer half) and distinction of pT2 versus pT3 can only be performed on radical cystectomy specimens and not samples from transurethral resections of bladder tumor. Even in cystectomy specimens it can be a challenge at times to determine extravesical (pT3) spread because the boundary between muscularis propria and its fat is not well demarcated from perivesical fat. Moreover, this boundary can be distorted, obscured, or obliterated by fibrosis and inflammation associated with infiltrating tumor.

Histologic variants of urothelial carcinoma with divergent differentiation (*Hum Pathol* 37:1371, 2006).

a. **Invasive urothelial carcinoma with squamous differentiation.** Focal squamous differentiation, to be distinguished from pure squamous cell carcinoma, can be seen in approximately 20% of invasive urothelial carcinomas. It appears that squamous differentiation predicts a poor response to radiotherapy and systemic chemotherapy.

b. **Invasive urothelial carcinoma with glandular differentiation.** True glandular spaces with or without mucin production and/or signet cells is seen in approximately 6% of invasive urothelial carcinomas (e-Fig. 22.22). Although this variant needs to be distinguished from adenocarcinoma, it is not clear whether it behaves any different from classic invasive urothelial carcinoma.

c. **Urothelial carcinoma with trophoblastic differentiation.** Trophoblastic differentiation can be manifested by the presence of any of the following: syncytiotrophoblastic giant cells, immunoreactivity for human chorionic gonadotropin (hCG), or choriocarcinoma. hCG immunoreactivity can be found in about one third of high-grade urothelial carcinomas and can be associated with serum elevations of hCG, but because such immunoreactivity is not of prognostic significance hCG immunostains should not be performed. Very few (about 30) cases of urothelial carcinoma with hCG-positive syncytiotrophoblasts (e-Fig. 22.23) have been reported; these giant cells should be distinguished from the tumoral giant cells of giant cell carcinoma and osteoclastlike giant cells, and recognized as examples of divergent differentiation and not a primary germ cell tumor of the urinary bladder. Nonetheless, this variant should be reported because the prognosis is extremely poor, with most patients dead of disease within 1 year. Very rare cases of pure choriocarcinoma of the urinary bladder have been described, but most likely represent urothelial carcinoma with trophoblasts.

d. **Sarcomatoid variant.** This is a biphasic neoplasm displaying morphologic and/or immunophenotypic evidence of both epithelial and mesenchymal differentiation (*Am J Surg Pathol* 18:241, 1994). Because there is a monoclonal origin for both components, this tumor is another example of a neoplasm with divergent differentiation. This variant accounts for <1% of bladder malignancies. Previous radiation and cyclophosphamide treatment are predisposing factors. Carcinosarcoma was previously used as a diagnostic term. Grossly, the tumor is often exophytic, polypoid, and deeply invasive into muscularis propria. Microscopically, the growth is typified by a biphasic neoplastic population of cells with the epithelial and mesenchymal-like components often in continuity (e-**Fig. 22.24, A and B**). The carcinomatous component is usually urothelial (85%), but can (in a small percentage of cases) be adenocarcinoma, squamous cell carcinoma, or small cell carcinoma. The amount of the malignant epithelial element varies and in some cases is only represented by carcinoma in situ; consequently, apparently pure malignant spindle cell tumors of the bladder should be sampled extensively in an attempt to find epithelioid areas. The sarcomatous component is usually an undifferentiated high-grade spindle cell proliferation, arranged in fascicles, a storiform pattern, or a patternless pattern. The most common heterologous element is osteosarcoma, followed by chondrosarcoma (e-**Fig. 22.25**), rhabdomyosarcoma, leiomyosarcoma, liposarcoma, angiosarcoma, or mixtures thereof. These sarcomatous regions are almost always high-grade. Immunohistochemical staining of the sarcomatoid variant shows strong, diffuse immunopositivity for pan-cytokeratin (e-**Fig. 22.24B**), although epithelial membrane antigen immunostaining (EMA) is characteristically weak. Note, however, that epithelial markers can be negative and focal immunoreactivity for desmin and smooth muscle actin may be present. The opposite pattern of staining would favor a leiomyosarcoma, in the correct histopathological context. Anaplastic lymphoma kinase (ALK)-1 immunostaining, which typifies inflammatory myofibroblastic tumor, is negative in sarcomatoid carcinoma. For cases of sarcomatoid carcinoma, the pathology report should include whether the sarcomatoid carcinoma is homologous or heterologous, although to date this does not appear to be of prognostic importance. Surgery and radiation result in 25% survival at 2 years.

Histologic variants of urothelial carcinoma with unusual growth patterns

e. Nested variant. This variant is characterized by the presence of infiltrating small nests and tubules of urothelial carcinoma (e-**Fig. 22.26**). Despite its relatively bland cytological features (low grade), this variant is often aggressive. Because of its cytoarchitectural features, florid von Brunn nests, cystitis cystica and glandularis, inverted papilloma, nephrogenic adenoma, and paraganglioma are all in the differential diagnosis. Clues that are of aid in establishing the diagnosis are the high-density, nearly confluent nests that can anastomose and invade muscularis propria. Nuclear atypia may be only focally present, and is often found in the deeper aspects of the proliferation. Although the nested variant of urothelial carcinoma has a higher proliferation index than florid von Brunn nests by MIB-1 immunostaining (8.8% vs. 2.8%), and a higher p53 immunopositivity (4.2% vs. 1.5%), the degree of overlap precludes use of these markers as diagnostic tools (*Am J Surg Pathol* 27:1243, 2003).

f. Microcystic variant. This variant is also deceptively bland and somewhat similar to the nested variant, except for characteristic prominent cystic change (e-**Fig. 22.27**). It is uncommon, accounting for only about 1% of bladder carcinomas. Microscopically, there are variable-sized cysts ranging up to 1 to 2 mm in diameter. The cysts are round to oval and may contain necrotic material or pink secretions. The layer of lining cells may be flattened or denuded. The differential diagnosis includes cystitis cystica, cystitis glandularis, and nephrogenic adenoma. The correct diagnosis is achieved by the detection of an association with usual urothelial carcinoma, haphazard and infiltrative growth, and cyst size and shape variability. In the largest series, 25% of cases had invasion of muscularis propria and 11 of 12 were high grade (*J Urol* 74:722, 1997).

g. Micropapillary variant. This rare pattern of urothelial carcinoma resembles papillary serous carcinoma of the ovary, an important differential diagnosis in women. It is characterized by the presence of small nests of cells and filiform papillae that have retracted from the surrounding stroma leaving an empty space reminiscent of angiolymphatic invasion (e-**Fig. 22.28**). This variant is characteristically aggressive; the percentage of urothelial carcinoma that is micropapillary influences outcome. While muscle wall invasion is commonly detected, some cases, especially those with a low percentage (<10%) of micropapillary component, and surface micropapillary growth, can be low stage (pTa or pT1). It has been argued that early cystectomy should be offered to patients with such low-stage, nonmuscle-invasive micropapillary urothelial carcinoma (*J Urol* 195:881, 2006).

h. **Lymphoepithelioma-like variant.** This is characterized by sheets and nests of poorly differentiated malignant cells that grow in a syncytial pattern with an admixed dense lymphoplasmacytic infiltrate (e-**Fig. 22.29**). It may be pure or mixed with usual urothelial carcinoma. There is a tendency for patients to present with muscularis propria–invasive disease. The differential diagnosis centers on large cell lymphoma and severe chronic cystitis, including follicular cystitis; immunostains for pan-cytokeratin and CD45 are confirmatory. Epstein–Barr virus has not been detected. These are aggressive carcinomas with a 26% mortality at 3 years. These tumors should be treated as other bladder carcinomas—that is, based on stage—although they do also appear to be chemoresponsive.

Histologic variants of urothelial carcinoma with unusual cytologic features

i. **Lymphoma-like and plasmacytoid variants.** These variants are exceedingly rare and are usually admixed with conventional urothelial carcinoma. However, the diagnosis of urothelial carcinoma in small biopsies composed solely of such variants (e-**Fig. 22.30**) may only be achieved with the help of immunohistochemistry (positive reactivity to cytokeratin with negative reactivity to CD45 and other lymphoid markers).

j. **Giant cell variant.** This high-grade variant is characterized by numerous pleomorphic and bizarre tumor giant cells (e-**Fig. 22.31**), and needs to be distinguished from urothelial carcinoma with osteoclastlike giant cells, which represents an unusual stromal response to invasive carcinoma. Outcome is poor, with median survival of 11 months (*Br J Urol* 75:167, 1995).

k. **Glycogen-rich (clear-cell) and lipid-rich variants.** The main importance of these rare variants is the fact that they may be confused with clear-cell adenocarcinoma of the bladder or kidney, and liposarcoma or signet-ring carcinoma, respectively. The lipid-rich (also known as lipoid-cell) variant carries a poor prognosis (*Br J Urol* 75:167, 1995).

F. **Squamous neoplasms**

1. **Squamous papilloma.** This is a very rare papillary lesion that typically presents in elderly women and, unlike condyloma accuminatum (which can also involve the bladder), has not been associated with human papilloma virus infection or with subsequent development of carcinoma (*Am J Surg Pathol* 20:883, 2006, *Cancer* 88:1679, 2000). Recurrence is rare.

2. **Squamous cell carcinoma.** In areas of the world where schistosomiasis is endemic (parts of Africa and the Middle East), this type of carcinoma is the most common primary neoplasm of the bladder. Elsewhere, squamous cell carcinoma is relatively rare, representing <5% of bladder carcinomas. Other predisposing conditions include ones of chronic irritation, such as cystitis, vesical lithiasis, and long-term indwelling catheters. Smoking is also a significant risk factor (as for conventional urothelial carcinoma). Squamous cell carcinomas are represented at a higher percentage in patients with nonfunctioning bladders (50% of carcinomas) or diverticula (20%), and in renal transplant patients (15%). Keratinizing squamous metaplasia is a potential precursor and is a risk factor for subsequent detection of carcinoma; 20% to 42% of patients with keratinizing squamous metaplasia were later diagnosed with carcinoma.

Squamous cell carcinoma typically presents as invasive carcinoma, although in a few cases, pure squamous cell carcinoma in situ may be detected (*Am J Surg Pathol* 20:883, 2006). Squamous cell carcinoma in situ is a strong risk factor for subsequent detection of invasive carcinoma, with 5 of 11 (45%) patients diagnosed with invasive squamous cell or urothelial carcinoma at follow-up intervals of 2 to 12 months (*Am J Surg Pathol* 20:883, 2006). Grossly, squamous cell carcinomas are often large, solid necrotic masses that can fill the entire bladder lumen (e-Fig. **22.32**). Some, however, may be flat and infiltrative, with ulceration. Microscopically, the carcinoma should be purely squamous, with keratin production and/or intercellular bridges (e-Fig. **22.33**). Adjacent keratinizing squamous metaplasia strongly supports a diagnosis of squamous cell carcinoma; such metaplasia is seen in 20% to 60% of cases of invasive squamous cell carcinoma. Histological variants of squamous cell carcinoma of the bladder include the exceptionally rare basaloid variant and the uncommon verrucous variant.

Grading is three tiered (well, moderately, or poorly differentiated), and histologic grade may correlate with stage and outcome. However, stage is the most important determinant of outcome. Many patients with squamous cell carcinoma of the bladder present with muscularis propria-invasive disease, and this accounts for the poor outcome for most patients. No molecular genetic abnormalities are currently used for diagnosis or prognosis. Treatment is radical cystectomy, with or without radiation therapy and chemotherapy.

3. **Verrucous squamous cell carcinoma.** This variant of squamous cell carcinoma is seen almost exclusively in patients with schistosomiasis and appears as an exophytic "warty" mass composed of thickened papillary squamous epithelium with minimal cytoarchitectural atypia and a rounded pushing border. This tumor is considered to be clinically indolent.

G. Glandular neoplasms

1. **Villous adenoma.** An uncommon exophytic papillary neoplasm histologically resembling its colonic counterpart, villous adenoma is usually located in the trigone and, unless associated with an invasive component, does not recur following excision.

2. **Adenocarcinoma.** Primary adenocarcinomas are rare, representing 2% of malignant bladder neoplasms, and may be of urachal or nonurachal origin. The latter are more common and usually arise in patients with a nonfunctional bladder or with exstrophy. Urachal adenocarcinomas usually arise from the dome or anterior wall of the bladder but may also involve urachal remnants in the anterior abdominal wall. Characteristics of these tumors that are helpful in differentiating them from nonurachal adenocarcinomas are as follows: (a) their bulk is in the wall rather than the lumen of the bladder, (b) they lack an associated in situ component or cystitis glandularis, and (c) they are sharply demarcated from surface urothelium. Identification of these tumors is important because, unlike nonurachal tumors, surgical management of urachal adenocarcinomas usually includes excision of the median umbilical ligament and umbilicus. Bladder adenocarcinomas (of urachal or nonurachal type) may have different morphological appearances including enteric (e-Fig. **22.34A,B**), mucinous, signet-ring cell, clear cell (similar to its gynecological counterpart), and mixed. The main differential diagnosis for most of these patterns is the more common secondary extension (or metastasis) from another primary tumor site, most notably the prostate and the colon. Immunohistochemistry may be helpful in this situation, especially when the clinical findings are not helpful or available. Immunoreactivity with PSA and prostatic acid phosphatase, β-catenin (nuclear), or thrombomodulin supports a diagnosis of prostate, colon, or bladder adenocarcinoma, respectively; cytokeratin 7 and 20 immunostains are not very useful in this context because of significant overlap (*Semin Diagn Pathol* 22:69, 2005). Adenocarcinoma of the bladder has a generally poor prognosis with 5-year survival rates ranging from 18% to 47%.

H. Neuroendocrine neoplasms

1. **Paraganglioma.** Derived from bladder paraganglia, paragangliomas are typically found in the muscularis propria and are not infrequently associated with hypertension and/or headaches, palpitations, and sweating that may be precipitated by micturition. The tumor is composed of cells with abundant amphophilic, clear, or eosinophilic cytoplasm arranged in a diffuse or nested (Zellballen) pattern of growth with an associated thin capillary network (e-Fig. **22.35**). Nuclear atypia can occasionally be prominent. The tumor is frequently immunopositive for neuroendocrine markers and negative for cytokeratin (useful in distinguishing

the tumor from nested urothelial carcinoma), whereas the spindle cells surrounding tumor nests (sustentacular cells) are positive for S100 protein. The majority (85% to 90%) of bladder paragangliomas are benign and do not recur following surgical excision.

2. **Small cell carcinoma.** This is a rare neoplasm, which is diagnosed even when mixed with other bladder carcinomas (urothelial, squamous, or adenocarcinomas) because the presence of any small cell carcinoma component has a significant negative impact on prognosis. As with other bladder carcinomas, hematuria is the most common presentation; however, almost half of patients present with metastatic disease, with or without a paraneoplastic syndrome. Histologically, the tumor cells are characteristically small with scant cytoplasm, stippled chromatin, and inconspicuous nucleoli with nuclear molding. The diagnosis can often be confirmed by immunoreactivity with one or more neuroendocrine markers such as neuron-specific enolase, chromogranin, synaptophysin, and CD56, with or without cytokeratin expression (which is usually seen in a dot-like paranuclear pattern).

3. **Rare neuroendocrine tumors.** Large cell neuroendocrine carcinomas and carcinoid tumors are rare as primary tumors in the urinary bladder.

I. **Mesenchymal lesions and neoplasms**

1. **Myofibroblastic proliferations.** These spindle cell proliferations can develop a few weeks to several months following bladder instrumentation (for which the term "postoperative spindle cell nodule" has been used), or may be unrelated to trauma. They can grow up to 9 cm in diameter. These neoplasms are composed of myofibroblasts, and have been variously termed inflammatory myofibroblastic tumor (*Am J Surg Pathol* 20:592–603, 2007) and pseudosarcomatous myofibroblastic proliferation (*Am J Surg Pathol* 30:787, 2006). It is unsettled as to whether these are all the same entity or a heterogeneous group of proliferations. Histologically, these lesions are composed of elongated spindle or stellate cells resembling tissue-culture fibroblasts, embedded in a myxoid matrix that contains a variable chronic inflammatory infiltrate and extravasated red blood cells. Although enlarged nuclei with prominent nucleoli (as well as prominent mitotic activity) can be observed, the presence of significant nuclear atypia and/or abnormal mitotic figures should suggest an alternative diagnosis such as sarcomatoid carcinoma or leiomyosarcoma. Immunohistochemistry can sometimes be a useful diagnostic tool as the spindle cells are often positive for cytokeratin, actin, and vimentin. In addition, more than two thirds of cases display expression of ALK, often associated with a translocation involving its locus on the short arm of chromosome 2 (2p23). Although recurrences can be seen and the proliferations can be locally aggressive, there have been no reports of metastatic spread.

2. **Smooth muscle neoplasms.** Leiomyomas and leiomyosarcomas represent the most common benign and malignant mesenchymal neoplasms of the bladder, respectively. Leiomyomas usually present as well-circumscribed lamina propria (two thirds of cases), intramural, or subserosal masses and are composed of intersecting fascicles of spindle cells with abundant eosinophilic cytoplasm and oval/elongated nuclei with blunt ends. By definition, there should be no significant nuclear atypia (hyperchromasia, nuclear membrane irregularities, pleomorphism) or evidence of an infiltrative growth pattern. In contrast, leiomyosarcomas (e-**Fig. 22.36**) are infiltrative tumors with or without significant nuclear atypia, coagulative tumor cell necrosis, and brisk mitotic activity (usually >5 mitoses per 10 high-power fields), the latter being a typical feature of high-grade tumors. In addition to being immunoreactive with one or more smooth muscle markers (actins, desmin, caldesmon), leiomyosarcomas can also be positive for cytokeratin and EMA, although the staining is usually focal. Most patients with leiomyosarcoma develop recurrences and/or metastasis resulting in mortality in almost one half of cases.

3. **Rhabdomyosarcoma.** Almost a quarter of all childhood rhabdomyosarcomas arise in the genitourinary tract, and a significant proportion are of bladder origin. Almost all of these cases are of the embryonal type. Grossly, most embryonal rhabdomyosarcomas of the bladder present as polypoid intraluminal masses

(e-**Fig.** 22.37) resembling a cluster of grapes (hence the alternative name "botryoid" type), with the remainder being deeply invasive tumors. Histologically, these tumors are mostly composed of small round tumor cells with a variable admixture of spindle cells embedded in a myxoid stroma, often with cell condensation under the surface urothelium forming the so-called "cambium layer" (e-**Fig.** 22.38). The latter feature, as well as the identification of rhabdomyoblasts and cross-striations, is particularly useful for diagnosis. Immunohistochemistry can confirm the diagnosis as these tumors are usually positive for myogenin and myoD1, among other muscle markers. The prognosis of embryonal rhabdomyosarcoma has greatly improved with multimodality treatment, although the alveolar type, as well as rare rhabdomyosarcomas presenting in adulthood, is associated with a worse outcome.

4. **Other spindle cell neoplasms.** There are other spindle cell neoplasms that can occasionally involve the bladder including hemangioma, neurofibroma, solitary fibrous tumor, angiosarcoma, osteosarcoma, and malignant fibrous histiocytoma. These tumors are histologically identical to their nonbladder counterparts.

J. **Other miscellaneous neoplasms.** As discussed earlier, the bladder can be involved by metastatic carcinomas and those extending from adjacent organs, where clinical data and immunohistochemical findings can help resolve the diagnosis. Hematolymphoid neoplasms can also involve the bladder, either primarily or secondarily (more common), and may present as mass lesions. Finally, there are a few reported primary bladder melanomas in the literature.

IV. **HISTOLOGIC GRADING OF UROTHELIAL CARCINOMA** is done as low grade or high grade, as discussed above. Histologic grade of primary adenocarcinoma or squamous cell carcinoma of the urinary bladder can be reported as well-, moderately-, or poorly differentiated.

V. **PATHOLOGIC STAGING OF URINARY BLADDER CANCER** applies to carcinomas only. Pathologic primary tumor (pT) 2002 TNM AJCC stage categories are given in Table 22.2 and illustrated in Fig. 22.5. pN and pM groupings are also listed in Table 22.2.

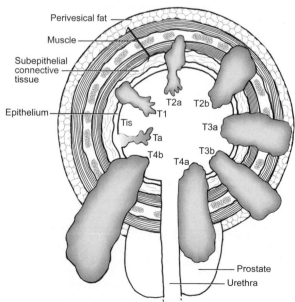

Figure 22.5. Pathologic T staging of carcinoma of the urinary bladder. Modified from Greene FL, et al., eds. *AJCC Cancer Staging Atlas.* New York: Springer; 2006.

VI. REPORTING URINARY BLADDER CARCINOMA. (*Arch Pathol Lab Med* 127:1263, 2003). For urinary bladder biopsy and transurethral resections, report histologic type, grade, and depth of invasion, if present. The presence or absence of muscularis propria should also be noted for each biopsy sample. Carcinoma in situ, when present in flat urothelium adjacent to papillary tumor, should also be reported. If lymphovascular space invasion by carcinoma is seen, it should be reported.

For cystectomy (partial or total), radical cystoprostatectomy, and pelvic exenteration specimens, report tumor location, size in three dimensions, gross growth pattern (papillary, nodular/solid, flat, ulcerated), gross depth of invasion, gross involvement of adjacent structures (prostate, vagina, uterus, colon), and relation to surgical margins. Microscopic features that should be reported include histologic type, grade, site(s) of involvement, growth pattern, extent of invasion, involvement of other structures, lymphovascular invasion, and margin status. Important margins include the ureters, distal urethra, perivesical soft tissue (for cystectomy specimens), and pelvic soft tissue (for exenteration specimens). For regional lymph nodes, document the total number examined, number positive for carcinoma, presence of extranodal extension, and size of largest metastatic deposit.

CYTOLOGY OF THE URINARY BLADDER
Rosa M. Dávila

I. TYPES OF SPECIMENS
   A. Voided urine normally has a mixture of benign urothelial cells and squamous cells. Although the squamous cells may be a vaginal or skin contaminant, they can also be derived from areas of squamous metaplasia that often develop in the bladder trigone. When urothelial cells are present in papillary-like clusters, the possibility of a low-grade urothelial neoplasm should be raised. Similar clusters may also be due to recent instrumentation or lithiasis.
   B. Catheterized urine normally has papillary-like clusters of urothelial cells resulting from the mechanical disruption of the urothelial mucosa. They should not be confused with low-grade urothelial carcinoma.
   C. Bladder washings are obtained by irrigating the bladder with saline instilled via a catheter, or during cystoscopic evaluation. The cytologic findings in this specimen type are similar to those seen in catheterized urine.
   D. Neobladder or ileal conduit samples have abundant degenerated cells, some of which are arranged in clusters and have vacuolated cytoplasm. Well-preserved intestinal-type epithelium is rarely present. A variable number of inflammatory cells, macrophages, and bacteria are seen (e-Fig. 22.39).

II. INFLAMMATORY/INFECTIOUS PROCESSES
   A. Eosinophils. Detection of eosinophils may be difficult in Papanicolaou-stained slides because the cytoplasmic granules do not stain prominently. Therefore, identification of eosinophils is based on their bilobed nucleus. Patients with allergic interstitial nephritis or eosinophilic cystitis or those who have had recent bladder biopsies can display urinary eosinophils.
   B. Human polyoma virus (BK virus) is an important cause of morbidity in renal transplant patients. This DNA virus initially infects children and becomes dormant until the patient becomes immunosuppressed. Because it infects the renal tubular epithelial cells and urothelial cells, the cellular changes can be detected by urine cytology. Infected cells are usually arranged singly and have a blackish–blue inclusion that occupies most of the nucleus. The cellular changes can resemble those of high-grade urothelial carcinoma; therefore, infected cells are also known as "decoy cells." In contrast to high-grade urothelial carcinoma, "decoy cells" have a round nucleus with smooth contours and a dark, homogenous nucleus (*Am J Transplant* 1:373, 2001).
   C. Acute inflammation is common in patients with lower urinary tract infections that do not require cytologic evaluation. However, urine samples with acute inflammation may be submitted to cytology when an underlying pathology is clinically suspected.

In addition to the acute inflammation, urothelial cells may display reactive changes characterized by cellular and nuclear enlargement, a normal nucleus/cytoplasm ratio, and prominent nucleoli.

D. Trichomonas is commonly identified in cervical–vaginal samples, and occasionally it is identified in urine samples from female and male patients. Because men are often asymptomatic carriers, the infection is often initially detected by urine cytology. This protozoa is small (1.5 to 50 μm) and pear shaped, and has a small nucleus, eosinophilic cytoplasmic granules, and flagella. Flagella are often difficult to visualize in cytologic samples (e-**Fig. 22.40**).

III. NEOPLASMS

A. Urothelial carcinomas can be divided into the following groups: low-grade neoplasms composed of normal-appearing urothelial cells, and high-grade neoplasms composed of overtly abnormal urothelial cells. Urine cytology has a poor sensitivity (approximately 30%) in diagnosing low-grade urothelial neoplasms (*Acta Cytol* 40:676, 1996). Papillary urothelial clusters in a voided sample, even in the absence of nuclear atypia, can be a manifestation of low-grade papillary neoplasm (e-**Fig. 22.41**). In high-grade urothelial neoplasms, the sensitivity of urinary cytology is approximately 80%, and the specificity >90% (*Urol Clin North Am* 27:25, 2000). High-grade urothelial carcinoma cells exhibit nuclear enlargement, a high nucleus/cytoplasm ratio, and nuclear hyperchromasia with a coarse chromatin pattern (e-**Fig. 22.42**); in addition, the cells have a tendency to be arranged singly or in small, poorly cohesive clusters.

One particularly promising method as an adjunct to urinary cytology is fluorescence in situ hybridization (FISH) to detect chromosomal aneusomy, where chromosomal centromeric probes (and one locus-specific probe) are used to analyze chromosomes 3, 4, 17, and 9p21 in voided urine specimens fixed on glass slides. Compared to cytology, FISH seems to be more sensitive and slightly less specific. In conjunction with cytology, it is likely that FISH can lengthen the interval between surveillance cystoscopy in evaluation of patients with urothelial carcinoma.

B. Squamous cell carcinoma can occur as a primary bladder tumor or can arise in adjacent organs, such as the uterine cervix, and extend into the bladder. A more common scenario is to have a urothelial carcinoma with a squamous component. Cytologic features that will indicate the presence of squamous differentiation include neoplastic cells with variable amount of dense and eosinophilic cytoplasm, pyknotic nuclei, and bizarre cell shapes (e-**Fig. 22.43**). Parakeratotic and/or anucleated cells are often seen in the background. Poorly differentiated squamous cell carcinoma that is nonkeratinizing may be confused with high-grade urothelial carcinoma.

C. Adenocarcinoma of the bladder can be primary or metastatic. Although most (87%) of adenocarcinomas of the bladder can be identified as malignant by urine cytology, only 67% will be additionally classified as adenocarcinoma (*Cancer Cytopathol* 84:335, 1998). Columnar or cuboidal cell shapes and cytoplasmic vacuoles of the neoplastic cells are some cytologic features that support the diagnosis of adenocarcinoma.

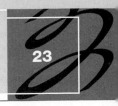
I. NORMAL ANATOMY. The male urethra is divided into three anatomic regions: prostatic (bladder neck to apex of the prostate), bulbomembranous (apex of the prostate to inferior surface of urogenital diaphragm), and penile (inferior surface of urogenital diaphragm to the urethral meatus). The prostatic portion is lined by urothelium, the bulbomembranous portion is lined by pseudostratified or stratified columnar epithelium, and the penile portion shows a transition from the stratified columnar epithelium at its origin to squamous epithelium at the meatus. The female urethra is lined by urothelium in the proximal one third and squamous epithelium in the distal two thirds.

The urethra contains periurethral glands. Skene glands are present in females, and are concentrated distally. Present in males are the bulbourethral (Cowper glands) and glands of Littre, located in the bulbomembranous portion and along the penile urethra, respectively.

II. GROSS EXAMINATION AND TISSUE SAMPLING

   A. Urethroscopic biopsy tissue samples should be entirely submitted for histologic examination, and three levels should be examined.

   B. Surgical excision of urethral carcinoma: For men, the type of surgery is dependent on tumor location and extent, and includes transurethral resection (TUR), local segmental excision, partial or radical penectomy, and cystoprostatectomy. TUR chips should be submitted in their entirety. Segmental excision specimens should be sampled to include sections of the proximal and distal margins and area of deepest growth. (Handling of penectomy and cystoprostatectomy specimens is covered in Chaps. 30 and 29, respectively.) Urethrectomy (primary or secondary) involves stripping of all or part of the urethra with preservation of the penis, and is performed for patients with primary urethral carcinoma or secondary involvement by bladder carcinoma.

   For women, local excision of distal urethra and adjacent vaginal wall is often sufficient surgical therapy for carcinoma of the urethra; sections of the mass, and urothelial, radial soft tissue, and vaginal mucosal margins should be submitted. For proximal urethral cancer in women, cystourethrectomy (anterior exenteration, with excision of part or all of the vagina) is often necessary; sections of the mass demonstrating relationships with adjacent structures and depth of invasion, grossly uninvolved urethra and urinary bladder, and ureteral and radial soft tissue margins should be submitted.

III. DIAGNOSTIC FEATURES OF BENIGN DISEASES

   A. Congenital anomalies

   1. Urethral valves are mucosal folds lined by normal urothelium that project into the urethral lumen causing obstruction, hematuria, or inflammation. Posterior urethral valves are usually seen in men and are associated with bladder neck hypertrophy.

   2. Diverticula are invaginations of urethral mucosa usually seen in women as a result of infection, trauma, or obstruction. They are lined by urothelium that may undergo squamous or glandular metaplasia (e-Fig. 23.1).*

---

*All e-figures are available online via the Solution Site Image Bank.

3. Fibroepithelial polyp is a congenital anomaly usually in the posterior urethra of male infants and young boys. It consists of a fibrous connective tissue stalk lined by urothelium.

B. Inflammation and infection

1. Urethritis is an inflammatory response in the urethra usually occurring secondary to sexually transmitted agents. Diagnosis is made by examination of a urethral smear that shows neutrophils. Polypoid urethritis is usually seen in the prostatic urethra near the verumontanum, and is the result of inflammation that induces multiple polypoid lesions with edematous stroma, distended blood vessels, and chronic inflammation (e-**Fig. 23.2**).

2. Caruncle is a pedunculated or sessile polypoid inflammatory mass in the distal urethra in postmenopausal women showing a mixed inflammatory infiltrate with rich vascularity (e-**Fig. 23.3, A and B**).

3. Malakoplakia is a rare urethral granulomatous inflammatory process more commonly seen in women, showing histiocytes containing characteristic Michaelis–Gutmann bodies.

4. Condyloma acuminatum of the urethra is caused by human papilloma virus (HPV), usually serotypes 6, 11, 16, and 18. Condyloma acuminatum can primarily involve the urethra, but more commonly arises by direct extension from similar lesions in adjacent sites including the external genitalia, perineum, or anus. Histologically, there is a flat or polypoid proliferation of squamous epithelium (e-**Fig. 23.4**) with koilocytic atypia. Multiplicity and recurrence are common.

C. Metaplasia

1. Squamous metaplasia can occur as a response to chronic inflammatory insults secondary to infection, diverticula, calculi, or instrumentation.

2. Urethritis cystica and glandularis are small cysts lined by urothelial and glandular cells, respectively.

3. Nephrogenic adenoma (metaplasia) is rare in the urethra. It occurs at the site of previous damage, often related to a previous surgical procedure. Microscopically, there is a proliferation of tubular and papillary structures, sometimes with cystic change, lined by flattened to cuboidal to hobnail cells with bland nuclear features. Some cases may be due to implantation and growth of tubular epithelial cells shed from the kidney.

D. Hyperplasia

1. Urothelial hyperplasia is a reactive thickening of cytologically bland urothelium, and can be flat or papillary. In the papillary form the mucosa can be undulating but still lacks a well-developed fibrovascular core.

2. Prostatic urethral polyp is seen in the verumontanum in young men and consists of benign prostatic tissue arranged in a polypoid or papillary configuration, with projection into the urethral lumen.

IV. DIAGNOSTIC FEATURES OF NEOPLASTIC DISEASES

A. Benign neoplasms are exceedingly rare and have the same appearance as in the urinary bladder.

1. Benign epithelial neoplasms include villous adenoma, squamous papilloma, and urothelial (including inverted) papilloma.

2. Benign mesenchymal neoplasms include leiomyoma and hemangioma.

B. Malignant neoplasms originating in the urethra are very rare and are carcinomas in the vast majority of cases (*Semin Diagn Pathol* 14, 1997, *Urology* 68:1164, 2006). Compared with urinary bladder carcinomas, urethral carcinomas are more often found in women; a much higher percentage are squamous cell carcinomas; there is a greater percentage of high-grade and -stage tumors; and there is a poorer prognosis. Primary urethral carcinoma histologic type corresponds to the anatomic site of origin in the urethra. In general, proximal neoplasms (prostatic urethra in men; proximal one third in females) tend to be urothelial carcinomas, whereas distal tumors (membranous, bulbous, or penile in men; distal two thirds in women) are frequently squamous cell carcinomas. Often it is difficult to ascertain the precise site of origin of a urethral carcinoma due to infiltrative growth and destruction of normal cells by tumor.

1. Squamous cell carcinoma is the most common urethral carcinoma in both sexes. HPV infection has a significant role in its etiology; 30% of squamous cell carcinomas in men and 60% in women test positive for high-risk HPV, although molecular HPV typing is not necessary for diagnosis. Grossly, squamous cell carcinoma can be verruciform or grayish-white and scirrhous, with necrosis (e-Fig. 23.5, A and B). Microscopically, most are moderately differentiated and deeply invasive. Squamous cell carcinomas of the distal penile urethra frequently invade the corpus cavernosum; more proximal tumors in men may penetrate directly into the urogenital diaphragm, prostate, rectum, and bladder neck. In women, tumors arising in the distal third of the urethra are commonly low-grade squamous cell carcinoma (e-Fig. 23.6) or verrucous carcinomas.

2. Urothelial carcinoma rarely primarily involves the urethra, but more commonly results from secondary involvement by bladder carcinoma. This so-called secondary involvement could represent direct extension, multifocal disease, and/or lymphovascular invasion. For primary and secondary urothelial neoplasia, the 2004 World Health Organization (WHO) urinary bladder classification is used for typing purposes (Table 22.1). Grossly, carcinoma in situ (CIS) can be erythematous and/or ulcerative. Carcinomas can be papillary, nodular, ulcerative, and/or infiltrative. Histopathologically, primary or secondary urothelial tumors can present as pure CIS, noninvasive papillary neoplasia (e-Fig. 23.7, A and B), or invasive carcinoma, with or without a papillary component. In men there is a propensity for high-grade carcinoma (CIS or invasive) to involve the prostate, which can represent in situ duct/acinar spread and/or stromal-invasive disease. In women, CIS can cancerize suburethral glands, which can mimic invasion.

3. Adenocarcinoma is usually seen in the proximal urethra and can originate in a diverticulum. Grossly, the tumor is often infiltrative, with or without an exophytic component, with mucinous, gelatinous, and/or cystic cut surfaces (e-Fig. 23.8, A and B).

   Microscopically, glandular metaplasia, and urethritis cystica and glandularis, are frequently seen in adjacent epithelium. In women, the most common subtype is clear cell adenocarcinoma (40% of cases). In men, enteric, colloid, or signet-ring histomorphological features are common but clear cell type is rare.

   a. Clear cell adenocarcinoma is a rare tumor that is almost always found in women. Histologically, it is similar to clear cell adenocarcinoma of the vagina or uterus. A distinct feature of this tumor is pattern heterogeneity within the same neoplasm with solid, tubular, tubulocystic, micropapillary, or papillary structures lined by hobnailed cells (e-Fig. 23.9, A and B). Necrosis and mitoses are frequent. The neoplastic cells are uniform and ovoid with well-defined borders and amphophilic, acidophilic, or clear cytoplasm containing glycogen. Nuclei are large and hyperchromatic with prominent nucleoli. Clear cell adenocarcinoma should be differentiated from nephrogenic adenoma (metaplasia), which lacks an infiltrative pattern, sheet-like growth, mitotic figures, necrosis, and significant nuclear atypia.

   b. Nonclear cell adenocarcinoma includes enteric, mucinous (e-Fig. 23.10, A and B), signet-ring-cell, and not otherwise specified subtypes. Extension of adenocarcinoma from adjacent organs should be excluded.

4. Paraurethral gland carcinomas usually develop in paraurethral (Skene glands in females; glands of Littre in males) and bulbourethral (Cowper's) glands. Establishing the origin of adenocarcinoma can be difficult because of mucosal ulceration and obliteration of landmarks by the time of diagnosis.

5. Other rare carcinomas include small cell carcinoma, adenosquamous carcinoma, sarcomatoid carcinoma, and lymphoepithelioma-like carcinoma.

6. Melanoma. The urethra is the most common site of primary melanoma of the genitourinary tract (*Am J Surg Pathol* 24:785, 2000), but secondary involvement as a result of spread from the glans penis or vulvar lesions is more common. Amelanotic melanoma is commonly seen in this location. Evaluation of margin

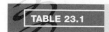

TABLE 23.1	Tumor, Node, Metastasis (TNM) Staging Scheme for Urethral Carcinoma

PRIMARY TUMOR (T)

TX	Primary tumor cannot be assessed
T0	No evidence of primary tumor

Urethra (male and female)

Ta	Noninvasive papillary, polypoid, or verrucous carcinoma
Tis	Carcinoma in situ
T1	Tumor invades subepithelial connective tissue
T2	Tumor invades any of the following: corpus spongiosum, prostate, periurethral muscle
T3	Tumor invades any of the following: corpus cavernosum, beyond prostatic capsule, anterior vagina, bladder neck
T4	Tumor invades other adjacent organs

Urothelial (transitional cell) carcinoma of prostate

Tis pu	Carcinoma in situ, involvement of prostatic urethra
Tis pd	Carcinoma in situ, involvement of prostatic ducts
T1	Tumor invades subepithelial connective tissue
T2	Tumor invades any of the following: prostatic stroma, corpus spongiosum, periurethral muscle
T3	Tumor invades any of the following: corpus cavernosum, beyond prostatic capsule, bladder neck (extra-prostatic extension)
T4	Tumor invades other adjacent organs (invasion of bladder)

REGIONAL LYMPH NODES (N)

NX	Regional lymph nodes cannot be assessed
N0	No regional lymph node metastasis
N1	Metastasis in a single lymph node ≤2 cm in greatest dimension
N2	Metastasis in a single lymph node >2 cm in greatest dimension, or multiple lymph nodes

DISTANT METASTASIS (M)

MX	Distant metastasis cannot be assessed
M0	No distant metastasis
M1	Distant metastasis

STAGE GROUPING

Stage 0a	Ta	N0	M0
Stage 0is	Tis	N0	M0
	Tis pu	N0	M0
	Tis pd	N0	M0
Stage I	T1	N0	M0
Stage II	T2	N0	M0
Stage III	T1, T2	N1	M0
	T3	N0, N1	M0
Stage IV	T4	N0, N1	M0
	Any T	N2	M0
	Any T	any N	M1

From: Greene FL, Page DL, Fleming ID, Fritz AG, Balch CM, Haller DG, Morrow M, eds. *AJCC Cancer Staging Manual.* 6th edition. New York: Springer 2002. Used with permission. (A new AJCC TNM staging system is scheduled for release in 2009; after its publication, the new staging scheme will appear on the website for this book.)

status and the absence of skip lesions are important in determining the prognosis (e-**Fig. 23.11**).

7. Hematopoietic neoplasms. Case reports exist of non-Hodgkin's lymphoma, mucosal associated lymphoid tissue (MALT) lymphoma, and plasmacytoma in the urethra.

V. HISTOLOGIC GRADING OF URETHRAL CARCINOMA. For squamous cell carcinoma and adenocarcinoma, well-, moderately, or poorly differentiated grades may be applied. Urothelial carcinomas are graded as low or high grade.

VI. PATHOLOGIC STAGING OF URETHRAL CARCINOMA is presented in Table 23.1. Pathologic stage and tumor location are the most significant pathologic prognostic indicators for urethral carcinoma. Proximal tumors have a worse outcome.

VII. REPORTING URETHRAL CARCINOMA. The pathology report of a urethral malignancy should include the histologic type, histologic grade, anatomic location (proximal versus distal), extent of invasion (depth and involvement of adjacent anatomic structures, if resected), presence or absence of lymphovascular space invasion and perineural invasion, and pathologic Tumor, Node, Metastasis (TNM) staging for resection specimens. The status of the margins should also be indicated, if applicable, including identification of the number and location of positive sites. Any additional findings such as inflammation, metaplasia, presence of a diverticulum, or presence of a stricture, should also be reported.

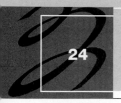

24 THYROID
James S. Lewis Jr.

I. **NORMAL ANATOMY.** The thyroid gland is a bilobed and encapsulated organ in the lower neck surrounding, and in intimate contact with, the trachea. It consists of right and left lobes connected by a small isthmus in the midline (Fig. 24.1). Two functioning cell types, the follicular cells and C (calcitonin) cells, comprise the thyroid follicle. The follicular component develops from invaginating tissue from the tongue (foramen cecum) and pharynx at 5 to 6 weeks' gestation. Through differential embryonic growth and migration, the bilobed gland assumes its definitive location in the neck. A hollow tube, known as the thyroglossal duct, connects the foramen cecum to thyroid remnants along its inferior course. The C-cells develop from the branchial clefts/pouches of the ultimobranchial body, and they are distributed in a density gradient, being most prominent in the upper lobes and least in the lower portion of the lobes.

The normal gland has a relatively firm consistency, is light brown, and lacks any obvious nodules. Microscopically, it consists of follicles lined by epithelial cells that are low cuboidal and relatively inconspicuous; this follicular epithelium surrounds a central core of eosinophilic colloid. In normal glands, the follicles are relatively consistent and regular in size (e-**Fig. 24.1**).* The C-cells lie within the follicular epithelium and are invested by the basement membrane. They are inconspicuous in normal thyroid.

II. **GROSS EXAMINATION, TISSUE SAMPLING, AND HISTOLOGIC SLIDE PREPARATION**

    A. **Biopsy.** Tissue needle biopsies of the thyroid gland are only very rarely performed because fine needle aspiration is technically easy to perform, has low morbidity, and is effective for triaging lesions for further management (see separate section at the end of this chapter).

    B. **Resection.** Hemithyroidectomy and total thyroidectomy are common procedures for management of thyroid disease. The specimens from both types of procedure are handled in a similar manner. The gland is oriented, if possible, based just on the anatomy alone or with markings by the surgeon. It is then measured and weighed. The surface (capsule) is inspected for any disruptions or attached soft tissue. Small nodules of tissue situated in the adjacent tissues may represent lymph nodes, parathyroid glands, or sequestered thyroid in cases of multinodular goitrous thyroid. The gland should be inked, sectioned in the axial plane ("breadloafed") for each lobe at intervals of 3 to 5 mm, and described clearly including masses and their size(s), color, and consistency. For diffuse or inflammatory lesions, three sections from each lobe should be taken, along with one of the isthmus. For a solitary, encapsulated mass, the entire circumference of the capsule should be sampled, including the surrounding thyroid tissue because the distinction of adenoma from carcinoma relies on features seen in the capsule; at least one section per centimeter should be submitted. Some sections should demonstrate the closest inked margin (Fig. 24.1). For multinodular glands (nodular hyperplasia), each major nodule should be sectioned, including the edge and/or adjacent soft tissue margin. Any attached perithyroidal soft tissue should be removed and sampled. Any lymph nodes or parathyroid glands should be removed and sampled as well. Oftentimes, the parathyroid gland(s) are first detected by microscopic examination. Their number should be recorded in one of the final diagnostic lines to highlight their presence.

---

*All e-figures are available online via the Solution Site Image Bank.

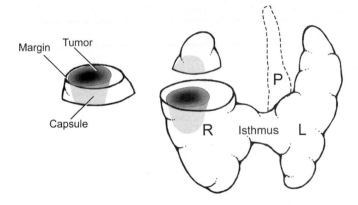

Figure 24.1. Thyroid anatomy/grossing (R = right lobe; L = left lobe; P = pyramidal lobe).

III. DIAGNOSTIC FEATURES OF COMMON DISEASES

A. Developmental. Residual thyroid tissue can be present anywhere along the path of thyroid migration during development. Carcinomas can rarely develop outside of the thyroid gland in these residual tissue sites.

1. The most common development remnant is a pyramidal lobe, a linear projection of thyroid tissue from the isthmus pointing cranially (Fig. 24.1).

2. Failure of closure of the thyroglossal duct commonly results in a midline cyst known as a thyroglossal duct cyst (TDC). Excision specimens generally consist of several often nondescript fragments of tissue, and a visible cyst is not always appreciated. Because remnants of the midline tract pass through the hyoid bone, the latter should be identified; failure to resect the bone often results in persistence of the TDC. If a cyst is identified grossly, it should be sampled in a few cassettes to document the type of epithelial lining, which is often obscured by acute inflammation. Because TDCs develop from a hollow tube, not all of them have thyroid tissue in their walls (only approximately 5% do on routine sections; 40% on serial sectioning). Otherwise, microscopically, these lesions have a squamous or respiratory-type lining epithelium without a muscular wall (e-**Fig. 24.2**). TDCs can get infected and inflamed with associated granulation tissue.

3. Thyroid tissue can be present at the base of the tongue at the site of developmental invagination, referred to as lingual thyroid. Microscopically, the thyroid tissue is normal.

B. Inflammation (thyroiditis)

1. Acute thyroiditis is caused predominantly by bacteria, but rarely can be fungal. It is usually seen in the setting of neck trauma or as spread from infection of adjacent structures. Microscopically, the gland is infiltrated by neutrophils with microabscesses and necrotic foci. Organisms can often be seen with or without special stains. Patients usually recover with antibiotics.

2. Subacute thyroiditis: de Quervain's thyroiditis. Technically referred to as granulomatous thyroiditis or subacute thyroiditis, deQuervain's thyroiditis is a disease primarily of women and is thought to be due to systemic viral infection. There is linkage to human leukocyte antigen (HLA) Bw35. Patients present with fever, malaise, and neck pain. The disease consists of three phases: hyperthyroidism, hypothyroidism, and recovery.

Grossly, the gland is usually asymmetrically enlarged and slightly firm. Microscopically, in the hyperthyroid phase, there is disruption of the follicles, with depletion of colloid and associated acute inflammation with microabscesses. Aggregates of neutrophils in the follicles are a characteristic feature; multinucleated giant cells are rare. In the hypothyroid phase, the follicular epithelium may be very scarce, and there is a florid mixed inflammatory response with lymphocytes, plasma cells, and multinucleated giant cells. Finally, in recovery, there is regeneration of follicles with fibrosis. Virtually all patients recover thyroid function after a few months without specific treatment.

3. Chronic thyroiditis

   a. Focal lymphocytic thyroiditis. Also termed nonspecific thyroiditis or focal autoimmune thyroiditis, this is a common disorder usually discovered incidentally in surgically excised thyroids or at autopsy. It is found in 25% to 60% of patients in autopsy studies, and is most common in older women. Patients are asymptomatic but often have a low level of antithyroid antibodies.

     There are no significant gross findings. Microscopically, focal lymphocytic thyroiditis consists of aggregates of lymphocytes, occasionally with germinal centers, between the follicles (e-**Fig. 24.3**). The lymphocytes can infiltrate follicles, but there is no significant destruction or damage. The disease is not progressive.

   b. Hashimoto's thyroiditis. Hashimoto's thyroiditis, or chronic autoimmune thyroiditis, is an autoimmune disease with thyroid enlargement and antithyroglobulin antibodies. It occurs most often in middle-aged women and is caused by antibodies to thyroglobin and thyroid peroxidase that lead to inflammation and destruction of the follicles. There is a familial association, and Hashimoto's thyroiditis is often associated with other autoimmune diseases. There is also an association with HLA subtypes, specifically HLA DR3 and DR5. Patients can present with a goiter, hypothyroidism, or both, and are typically in their sixth decade. The gland is symmetrically enlarged; ultrasound shows an enlarged gland with a hypoechogenic pattern, and antithyroglobulin and antithyroid microsomal antibodies are present in approximately 60% and 95% of cases, respectively.

     Grossly, the thyroid is diffusely enlarged and firm with a mildly nodular surface. On sectioning, lobulation is accentuated due to fibrosis, and the gland is tan-yellow or off-white rather than the usual brown due to the abundant lymphoid tissue. Microscopically, there are sheets of lymphocytes and plasma cells with abundant germinal centers. Florid inflammation often renders the residual follicles and follicular epithelium inconspicuous. The follicles are atrophic with minimal colloid. Characteristic Hürthle cell change is present, consisting of large cells with abundant, granular, eosinophilic cytoplasm and large, round nuclei with vesicular chromatin and prominent nucleoli (e-**Fig. 24.4**). The inflammatory infiltrate may extend into the perithyroidal soft tissue causing adherence of the gland at the time of surgery. Finally, there may be fibrons septa between the lobules, and the follicular epithelium may develop squamous metaplasia.

     A number of variants of Hashimoto's thyroiditis occur, including fibrous (sclerosing), fibrous atrophy, juvenile, and cystic forms. Both of the fibrous variants show the same histologic findings, namely retention of a lobulated pattern with extensive and severe fibrosis. Atrophic follicular cells are more scattered but show Hurthle cell change, and there is abundant chronic inflammation with germinal centers. In the fibrous variant, the gland is markedly enlarged throughout; in the fibrous atrophy variant, the gland is small and shrunken. Both of the latter variant forms have marked hypothyroidism and high titers of antithyroid antibodies.

     The differential diagnosis for Hashimoto's thyroiditis includes Riedel's thyroiditis and lymphoma. The fibrous variant of Hashimoto's may simulate Riedel's thyroiditis with an enlarged fibrotic gland; however, the fibrosis in Hashimoto's is typically limited to the gland itself, whereas in Riedel's there is severe adherence of the fibrotic gland to the neck soft tissues. The dense inflammation in Hashimoto's thyroiditis can simulate lymphoma, and most thyroid lymphomas do arise in the setting of Hashimoto's; the distinction lies in the absence of sheets of atypical lymphocytes, the lack of a strikingly prominent lymphoepithelial pattern, and the lack of clonality of the lymphocytes by flow cytometry or molecular studies.

The issue of whether there is an increased risk of papillary carcinoma in Hashimoto's thyroiditis is a controversial topic. Whether or not this is the case, nuclear features that can simulate those of papillary carcinoma, such as clear chromatin, crowding, and occasional grooves, develop frequently in the inflamed follicular epithelium.

c. **Graves' disease.** Graves' disease is also known as diffuse hyperplasia and is an autoimmune condition resulting in excess thyroid hormone production. It causes the majority of cases of spontaneous hyperthyroidism, occurs most often in the third and fourth decades, and is 5 to 10 times more common in women. Thyroid-specific autoantibodies, specifically thyroid-stimulating immunoglobulin (TSI), are present in Graves' disease patients. TSI binds to and stimulates thyrocytes through the thyroid-stimulating hormone (TSH) receptor, resulting in thyrotoxicosis. Patients also develop a characteristic infiltrative ophthalmopathy with proptosis.

Grossly, the thyroid gland is diffusely and symmetrically enlarged. Post-treatment or after long-standing disease, the gland may be somewhat nodular or fibrotic. Microscopically, the gland typically shows a low-power lobular accentuation due to increased septal fibrous tissue. Inflammation varies from none, to patchy lymphocytic, to lymphocytic with formation of germinal centers. The follicular epithelium is convoluted and irregular, and often assumes an almost papillary appearance. Colloid is decreased or absent and typically has a 'scalloped' appearance from clearing at the interface with the follicular epithelium (e-Fig. 24.5). Treated cases have a variable morphology and often have cellular nodules mimicking adenomas. After radioactive iodine treatment, there can be marked nuclear atypia. The differential diagnosis includes papillary carcinoma when the stellate outlines of follicles resemble papillae; keys to correct diagnosis of Graves' disease lie in the lack of cytologic changes of papillary carcinoma and the diffuse gland involvement.

d. **Riedel's thyroiditis.** A peculiar form of fibrosing disease, Riedel's thyroiditis is a chronic thyroiditis of unknown etiology which is more common in women, occurs most commonly in the fifth decade, and is commonly associated with fibrosing disease at other sites such as the mediastinum, retroperitoneum, and lung. Patients present with firm thyroid enlargement and local symptoms such as dysphagia, stridor, or dyspnea. Recurrent laryngeal nerve or sympathetic trunk involvement can lead to hoarseness or Horner's syndrome; compression of the large vessels can lead to superior vena cava syndrome. Most patients are euthyroid at presentation, but many subsequently develop hypothyroidism.

Grossly, the thyroid gland is usually received in irregular pieces because the fibrosis makes it difficult to remove surgically. It is tan to white, firm, and may have attached muscle. Microscopically, the characteristic finding is dense and hypocellular eosinophilic fibrous tissue with scattered and patchy aggregates of lymphocytes, plasma cells, neutrophils, and eosinophils, without germinal centers or granulomas. Rare entrapped and atrophic thyroid follicles are seen without Hürthle cell change. A characteristic finding is small veins with infiltrating lymphocytes and myxoid intimal thickening. Marked fibrosis extends into and involves the surrounding soft tissue as well.

The differential diagnosis includes hypocellular anaplastic thyroid carcinoma and fibrous or sclerosing Hashimoto's thyroiditis. The lack of necrosis or markedly atypical cells rules out anaplastic carcinoma. The lack of Hürthle cell change and germinal centers, and the profound degree of perithyroidal fibrosis, rule out fibrous Hashimoto's disease.

C. **Nodular hyperplasia.** Nodular hyperplasia (or multinodular goiter) is an extremely common disorder of the thyroid gland. It consists of enlargement of the gland with varying degrees of nodularity. The pathogenesis is complex but has been classically related to iodine deficiency with impaired thyroid hormone synthesis and subsequent

TSH stimulation. With supplementation of iodine in the diet, nodular hyperplasia has also been related to either excess iodine intake with impaired organification or to genetic factors. It is much more common in women than men and typically presents in middle age as asymptomatic enlargement. Large goiters, however, can cause dysphagia, hoarseness, or stridor, and can extend into the upper mediastinum. A small percentage of patients present with hyperthyroidism (toxic multinodular goiter).

Grossly, the thyroid gland is diffusely but irregularly enlarged. Some glands can attain a weight of several hundred grams. Parasitic nodules that have only a tenuous connection to the gland can develop. On sectioning, the nodules may be fleshy, red-brown, tan, and solid or, more commonly, show varying degrees of degeneration with cystic change, hemorrhage, fibrosis, and calcification. Heterogeneity of the nodules is typical.

Microscopically, nodular hyperplasia is also heterogeneous. The common appearance is nodules composed of variably sized follicles (e-**Fig. 24.6**). The nodules may be quite cellular with tightly packed follicular epithelium and little colloid, resembling follicular adenomas or carcinomas. Around cystic areas there is often fibrosis with variably-sized foci of dystrophic calcification and hemorrhage, with abundant hemosiderin-laden macrophages. Hürthle cell change is common. Pseudopapillary and truly papillary structures (Sanderson's polsters) can project into the cystic areas. The surrounding grossly normal thyroid tissue usually demonstrates microscopic nodularity as well.

The differential diagnosis for cellular nodules includes follicular adenoma or carcinoma. Hyperplastic nodules have a fibrous capsule that is not as well developed or continuous as those of adenomas and carcinomas. Follicular adenomas are discrete lesions, are microscopically different from the surrounding thyroid tissue, do not show cystic change or degeneration, and have a monotonous cell population—all features that are not characteristic of hyperplastic nodules. Papillary areas in nodular hyperplasia show basally oriented nuclei without the crowding or other features of papillary carcinoma.

D. Neoplasms. The World Health Organization (WHO) classification of tumors of the thyroid gland is listed in Table 24.1.

1. Adenoma. Follicular adenomas are benign, encapsulated tumors that are clonal. They are seen mostly in young to middle-aged adults and are more common in women than men. There is a relationship with previous irradiation or radiation exposure, just as with follicular carcinoma. Most follicular adenomas are asymptomatic and are detected by careful physical examination or incidentally by imaging performed for other reasons.

Grossly, follicular adenomas are very well-defined, round to oval lesions with a thin capsule. They are typically very soft and homogeneous with a color ranging from gray-white to tan or dark brown depending on the amount of colloid. Cystic change and hemorrhage are uncommon. Microscopically, they are encapsulated without, by definition, capsular or vascular invasion. They show a monotonous follicular or trabecular arrangement. The microfollicular pattern features trabeculae with only scattered small follicles with colloid. The macrofollicular pattern has prominent, large follicles with abundant colloid. The cells typically have a small amount of eosinophilic cytoplasm and are quite regular with uniform, round nuclei with condensed chromatin and inconspicuous nucleoli. There is a well developed and moderately thick capsule (e-**Fig. 24.7**). As with all endocrine organ tumors, there can be a marked degree of nuclear pleomorphism which is not necessarily an indication of malignancy or aggressive behavior. Mitotic figures are rare.

A number of adenoma variants are recognized, most notably the oncocytic or Hürthle cell adenoma, which has cells with abundant granular eosinophilic cytoplasm and vesicular nuclei with nucleoli and pleomorphism (e-**Fig. 24.8**). Lipoadenoma (with intratumoral fat), signet-ring-cell adenoma, and follicular adenoma with papillary hyperplasia are others.

Follicular adenomas are benign, so surgical removal is curative. The differential diagnosis includes hyperplastic nodules of nodular hyperplasia, follicular

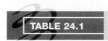

TABLE 24.1	WHO Histological Classification of Thyroid Tumors

Thyroid carcinomas
Papillary carcinoma
Follicular carcinoma
Poorly differentiated carcinoma
Undifferentiated (anaplastic) carcinoma
Squamous cell carcinoma
Mucoepidermoid carcinoma
Sclerosing mucoepidermoid carcinoma with eosinophilia
Mucinous carcinoma
Medullary carcinoma
Mixed medullary and follicular carcinoma
Spindle cell tumor with thymus-like differentiation
Carcinoma showing thymus-like differentiation

Thyroid adenoma and related tumors
Follicular adenoma
Hyalinizing trabecular tumor

Other thyroid tumors
Teratoma
Primary lymphoma and plasmacytoma
Ectopic thymoma
Angiosarcoma
Smooth muscle tumors
Peripheral nerve sheath tumors
Paraganglioma
Solitary fibrous tumor
Follicular dendritic cell tumor
Langerhans cell histiocytosis
Secondary tumors

From: DeLellis RA, Lloyd RV, Heitz P, Eng C, eds. *World Heath Organization Classification of Tumours. Pathology and Genetics. Tumours of Endocrine Organs.* Lyon: IARC Press; 2004. Used with permission.

variant of papillary thyroid carcinoma (PTC), and minimally invasive follicular carcinoma. Consequently, it is critical to sample tumors well, including sectioning of the entire capsule to look for microscopic capsular penetration or vascular invasion (see Table 24.2). The follicular variant of papillary carcinoma can present as an encapsulated mass but will manifest at least some of the cellular, nuclear, and colloid features of papillary carcinoma.

2. **Follicular carcinoma.** Follicular carcinomas account for approximately 10 to 15% of thyroid malignancies, and are best thought of as occurring in two types that have vastly different clinical behavior: minimally invasive and widely invasive. Follicular carcinomas are more common in women than men, occur in middle-aged adults, and usually present as asymptomatic masses. There is some association with iodine deficiency and prior irradiation.

Grossly, follicular carcinomas are usually round to oval, well encapsulated, solid tumors. They are bulging, and tan to brown. Minimally invasive follicular carcinomas are grossly indistinguishable from follicular adenomas, but widely invasive follicular carcinomas show extensive invasion of the surrounding gland and/or soft tissue beyond the capsule. They are almost always unifocal.

Microscopically, they range from tumors with well-formed follicles throughout, to solid, to trabecular. The nuclei of follicular carcinomas tend to be round to oval with granular chromatin. The oncocytic form has prominent nucleoli. Mitotic activity is present, but rarely brisk, and necrosis is lacking. The oncocytic

TABLE 24.2	Histologic Features Differentiating the Solitary Benign from the Malignant Follicular Lesion

Benign	Malignant
Complete but delicate capsule	Dense, circumferential fibrosis
Entrapped or sequestered thyroid in/near capsule	Transcapsular "mushrooming" invasion
Juxtaposed or prolapsed thyroid tissue near vessels, but with intact endothelium	Adherence of thyroid tissue to endothelium with associated thrombus

variant (Hürthle cell) is somewhat controversial, but consists of cells with voluminous eosinophilic and granular cytoplasm and nuclei that are characteristically vesicular with prominent, single nucleoli.

By immunohistochemistry, follicular carcinomas are positive for thyroglobulin, thyroid transcription factor-1 (TTF-1), and low-molecular-weight cytokeratins, but these are rarely necessary or useful for diagnosis except occasionally to assess distant metastases. In addition, molecular rearrangements in the *PPARγ* gene, most commonly with fusion to the *PAX8* gene, have been detected in 25% to 50% of cases, but this finding is not currently useful in diagnosis or management.

The differential diagnosis includes follicular adenoma, medullary carcinoma (MTC), and poorly differentiated (insular) carcinoma. The distinction of follicular carcinoma from adenoma lies in capsular and/or vascular penetration alone (Table 24.2). Capsular invasion is defined by the WHO as tumor penetration through the capsule not caused by previous fine needle aspiration. This invasion needs to be definitive and classically takes the form of "mushrooming" of the tumor outward (e-**Fig. 24.9**). Vascular invasion is defined by the WHO as the presence of intravascular tumor cells either covered by endothelium or associated with thrombus. Strict adherence to these criteria is necessary to assure that the diagnosis of carcinoma is correct. Tumors that show only focal capsular penetration and/or vascular invasion are defined as minimally invasive.

The distinction of follicular carcinoma from MTC is based on morphology (MTCs are rarely follicular in their growth patterns and their nuclei tend to be more spindle shaped, even if only focally) and immunohistochemical findings (neuroendocrine markers, carcinoembryogenic antigen [CEA], and calcitonin are positive in MTC and not in follicular carcinomas, whereas immunohistochemistry for thyroglobulin is positive in follicular carcinoma and negative in MTC). Finally, poorly differentiated (insular) carcinomas can be similar to widely invasive follicular carcinomas, but the former have cells with less cytoplasm, marked mitotic activity, and necrosis.

Unlike PTC, follicular carcinomas only uncommonly involve regional lymph nodes. Instead, metastasis is hematogenous to lung and bone. In general, minimally invasive follicular carcinomas have an excellent prognosis with an approximately 5% long-term mortality. Widely invasive follicular carcinomas, however, have a long-term mortality approaching 50%.

3. **Poorly differentiated (insular) carcinoma.** This type of thyroid carcinoma shows evidence of follicular differentiation but fits morphologically and biologically in between well-differentiated and undifferentiated thyroid carcinomas (UTCs). Some prefer to group this variant under the follicular carcinoma heading, but the WHO recognizes it as a separate entity.

Because the classification of insular carcinoma is somewhat controversial, epidemiologic data are difficult to obtain. In general, however, it represents much less than 5% of thyroid carcinomas in the United States, but between 4% to 7% in Italy and some Latin American countries. It is more common in women, particularly after age 50. Most insular carcinomas present as sizable asymptomatic masses, with or without pathologically enlarged regional lymph nodes. There is occasionally a history of a long-standing mass with recent, rapid growth.

Grossly, most tumors are large with solid gray to white nodules. Necrosis is common. Extrathyroidal extension is present in some cases, but is much less common than in undifferentiated carcinomas. Microscopically, the tumor consists of sheets, trabeculae, or nests (insula) of cells with central rounded nuclei. Most cells have only a small amount of cytoplasm giving the tumor a decidedly neuroendocrine look, although the tumor nuclei typically do not have a 'salt and pepper' cytology and often have prominent nucleoli (e-**Fig. 24.10**). There is prominent mitotic activity. Occasional follicles with colloid can be seen. It is not uncommon for well-formed capsules to be present around some of the nodules. Vascular invasion is often a prominent feature. Although rarely useful for diagnosis, by immunohistochemistry the tumors are positive for thyroglobulin and TTF-1, although the thyroglobulin reactivity may be focal.

The differential diagnosis includes MTC, the solid variant of papillary carcinoma, and metastasis (particularly from a carcinoid tumor). The mean 5-year survival is approximately 50%.

4. **Papillary carcinoma.** PTC is defined by the WHO as a carcinoma showing evidence of follicular differentiation and characterized by distinct nuclear features. The terminology has become somewhat confusing because papillary architecture, although very commonly present, is not necessary for diagnosis. PTC is the most common malignant thyroid tumor (representing 85% to 90% of differentiated thyroid carcinomas) and has been increasing in incidence, but its prognosis is excellent (the mean 5-year survival is >90%). The commonality of the tumor relative to its indolent behavior makes the appropriate management of PTC controversial. PTC occurs across all ages, and women are affected four times more commonly than men. There is a close link with previous radiation exposure, particularly in younger patients.

Grossly, most tumors are tan or white with infiltrative borders and a firm, often gritty cut surface. Cystic change is relatively common, particularly in lymph node metastases, and the bulk of nodal metastatic disease may far outstrip the volume of tumor in the thyroid gland. Microscopically, PTC is diagnosed based on a constellation of architectural and cytologic features (Table 24.3). Architectural patterns include papillary, trabecular, micro- and macrofollicular, solid, and cystic. The stroma around the tumor is often fibrotic or sclerotic. In tumors with follicles, the colloid is typically described as 'bright' or dark red relative to the normal thyroid. Another very typical feature is the psammoma body, a small, round, laminated form of calcification (e-**Fig. 24.11**); psammoma bodies are not pathognomonic of PTC but are an extremely typical feature. Distinct nuclear features include marked crowding with overlapping of adjacent nuclei, pale or clear chromatin, irregular nuclear contours, grooves (e-**Fig. 24.12**), and intranuclear cytoplasmic inclusions, which are a fixation artifact where round nodules of cytoplasm

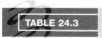

TABLE 24.3   **Diagnostic Histologic Features of Papillary Thyroid Carcinoma**

True papillae
Psammoma bodies
Dark red colloid
Crowded nuclei
Optically clear ("Orphan Annie") chromatin
Irregular nuclear contours
Nuclear grooves
Intranuclear cytoplasmic inclusions

indent the nucleus. Grading is not important because PTC is, by definition, well differentiated. PTC is very frequently multifocal (in up to 40% to 50% of cases), which often can be appreciated grossly.

Although rarely needed for diagnosis, immunohistochemistry in PTC is positive for pancytokeratin, cytokeratin 7, thyroglobulin, and TTF-1. Other markers that have been reported to be useful for differentiating the follicular variant of PTC from follicular adenoma include HBME-1, CK19, and galectin 3; however, these markers have not gained widespread acceptance, and the diagnosis ultimately rests on hematoxylin and eosin (H&E) morphology. More recently, molecular analysis has demonstrated translocations, inversions, or other chromosomal rearrangements involving the receptor tyrosine kinase gene *RET* in approximately 20% to 30% of cases; in addition, approximately 70% of PTC will have point mutations in *BRAF*, and 10% of cases harbor chromosomal rearrangements of the *TRK* gene. However, none of these molecular changes are useful currently for diagnosis or management.

A number of morphologic variants of PTC have been described, with the diagnosis of those without a papillary architecture based on the typical nuclear features. The follicular variant (e-**Fig. 24.13**) is often encapsulated and consists of follicles throughout without papillae. The oncocytic variant has lining cells with abundant eosinophilic and granular cytoplasm akin to Hürthle cells. So-called papillary microcarcinoma is a focus (or foci) of PTC <1 cm in maximal diameter; papillary microcarcinoma is an extremely common incidental finding and, although capable of metastasizing, the vast majority of these tumors pursue a benign course. The clear cell variant has a partially or completely clear cytoplasm, often admixed with oncocytic features. Both a tall cell (tumor cells at least 3 times as tall as they are wide) and columnar cell variant exist, both of which have been reported to be more aggressive than classic PTC. Finally, the diffuse sclerosing variant tends to occur in younger patients, shows diffuse involvement of one or both lobes without a dominant mass, and has numerous psammoma bodies, dense lymphocytic infiltration, and stromal fibrosis. Because there is an element of subjectivity in the assessment of the morphologic variants of PTC, disagreement often arises in the diagnosis among different observers.

The prognosis for PTC is excellent, with a 10-year survival approaching 100% for younger patients, and >90% overall. Patients older than 45 years typically have more aggressive tumors. The American Joint Committee on Cancer (AJCC) staging system strongly reflects this age-related difference (see Table 24.4).

5. **Undifferentiated (anaplastic) carcinoma.** UTCs are extremely aggressive malignant tumors composed, at least in part, of pleomorphic cells that show evidence of epithelial differentiation either by light microscopy, immunohistochemistry, or ultrastructural analysis. UTC is a tumor of the elderly, with 75% of cases occurring in patients older than 60 years. There is a slight female preponderance. Patients classically present with a rapidly growing neck mass with local signs and symptoms such as hoarseness, dysphagia, pain, vocal cord paralysis, or dyspnea.

At surgery, the tumor is usually large, ill defined, and difficult to excise due to extensive surrounding soft tissue invasion. Grossly, UTC is usually fleshy and tan-white with areas of hemorrhage and necrosis. Microscopically, it is typically composed of a variable admixture of spindle cells, epithelioid cells, and giant cells. The cells have a moderate amount of eosinophilic cytoplasm and almost always show brisk mitotic activity with abundant apoptosis (e-**Fig. 24.14**). There is often geographic necrosis, and typically the remaining thyroid gland is obliterated by tumor. On thorough examination, a residual, more well-differentiated carcinoma, either papillary or follicular, is sometimes identified. Predominantly spindled tumors mimic true sarcomas.

Immunohistochemistry for cytokeratin is positive in approximately 80% of cases, and for epithelial membrane antigen in 30% to 50%. Immunohistochemistry is useful for diagnosis of tumors in which no clear carcinomatous differentiation is present on H&E in order to confirm that the neoplasm is a carcinoma rather than a high-grade sarcoma. TTF-1 and thyroglobulin are typically negative in UTC. The prognosis for UTC is very poor with a median survival of <6 months despite aggressive surgery, radiation and chemotherapy.

6. **Medullary thyroid carcinoma.** MTC is a carcinoma with C-cell differentiation and represents a neuroendocrine neoplasm of the thyroid. C-cells secrete calcitonin, a peptide that causes increased renal excretion of calcium and inhibits osteoclasts to prevent calcium liberation from bone.

MTC represents approximately 5% to 10% of thyroid tumors. Although 80% are sporadic, there is a strong association with multiple endocrine neoplasia (MEN) type 2, which must always be considered in the work-up of patients with MTC. The clinical presentation of MTC strongly depends on the familial or nonfamilial nature of the tumor. Sporadic MTC presents in middle age with a unilateral thyroid mass; a high percentage of patients have associated cervical lymphadenopathy. Familial MTCs associated with MEN type 2A are frequently identified in the work-up of other MEN-related diseases (such as hyperparathyroidism or pheochromocytomas) or are identified in the work-up of relatives of MEN patients. As such, they are detected at a younger age (mean, third decade) and are multicentric and bilateral. When associated with MEN type 2B, MTC is usually identified in even younger patients due to other manifestations such as mucosal neuromas. Virtually all patients with MTC have an elevated serum calcitonin level. MTC is strongly associated with activating point mutations of the *RET* proto-oncogene; all cases of hereditary MTC, as currently detectable, have such mutations. A precursor lesion, C-cell hyperplasia, is often present in familial forms (see section below) and sometimes can be observed in sporadic cases.

Grossly, MTC is circumscribed but unencapsulated, and is tan-yellow to white. Sporadic tumors are solitary, whereas familial tumors are characteristically multifocal and bilateral. Microscopically, MTC shows great variability. The typical features are sheets, nests, or trabeculae of polygonal, round to oval cells with moderate to generous amounts of eosinophilic to amphophilic cytoplasm. The nuclei are round to oval with a coarse and somewhat granular neuroendocrine chromatin. Nucleoli are usually not prominent. A great number of variants have been described, including papillary or pseudopapillary, plasmacytoid, glandular, giant cell, spindle cell, small cell or neuroblastoma-like, paraganglioma-like, and oncocytic. Another characteristic feature of MTC is the presence of amyloid, which is formed from the deposition of calcitonin in the peritumoral stroma (e-**Fig. 24.15**); the amyloid is positive by Congo red staining.

Neoplastic C-cell hyperplasia, a precursor lesion to MTC, is identified in the middle third to upper third of the thyroid lobes where C-cells are preferentially located; it is characterized by groups of intrafollicular atypical C-cells that may begin to obliterate the normal follicular epithelium. Reactive, or nonneoplastic C-cell hyperplasia, occurs in a number of other thyroid diseases, most notably hyperparathyroidism and lymphocytic thyroiditis. Although the histology of C-cell hyperplasia is somewhat controversial, a few generalities apply. First, reactive C-cell hyperplasia is usually not identifiable by H&E examination alone. Second, if there are aggregates of C cells >50 in number, in nodules, bilaterally, or diffusely, neoplastic C-cell hyperplasia is diagnosed.

Immunohistochemistry is useful for diagnosis of MTC. C-cells and MTC tumor cells are usually strongly positive for calcitonin, synaptophysin, chromogranin-A, and CEA, but negative for thyroglobulin. The differential diagnosis includes thyroid paraganglioma, intrathyroidal parathyroid adenoma, follicular adenoma, follicular carcinoma, poorly differentiated (insular) carcinoma, and oncocytic tumors. All of these tumors can be differentiated by histology and immunohistochemistry.

The behavior of MTC is highly stage dependent. Patients who do not have metastatic disease are usually cured by total thyroidectomy—their 10-year survival approaches 100%. Lymph node metastases are very common, and favored distant metastatic sites include the lungs, liver, and bone. The overall 10-year survival for patients with cervical lymph node metastases is approximately 70% to 80%, and for patients with distant metastases 40% to 50%. Because C-cell

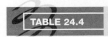

TABLE 24.4	Tumor, Node, Metastasis (TNM) Staging Scheme for Tumors of the Thyroid

PRIMARY TUMOR (T)

TX	Primary tumor cannot be assessed
T0	No evidence of primary tumor
T1	Tumor ≤2 cm greatest dimension limited to the thyroid
T2	Tumor >2 cm but not >4 cm limited to the thyroid
T3	Tumor >4 cm in greatest dimension limited to the thyroid or any tumor with minimal extrathyroid extension (e.g., extension to sternothyroid muscle or perithyroid soft tissues)
T4a	Tumor of any size extending beyond the thyroid capsule to invade subcutaneous soft tissues, larynx, trachea, esophagus, or recurrent laryngeal nerve
T4b	Tumor invades prevertebral fascia or encases carotid artery or mediastinal vessels *All anaplastic carcinomas are considered T4 tumors* Intrathyroidal anaplastic carcinoma–surgically resectable Extrathyroidal anaplastic carcinoma–surgically unresectable

REGIONAL LYMPH NODES (N)

NX	Regional lymph nodes cannot be assessed
N0	No regional lymph node metastasis
N1a	Metastasis to Level VI (pretracheal, paratracheal, and prelaryngeal/Delphian lymph nodes
N1b	Metastasis to unilateral, bilateral, or contralateral cervical or superior mediastinal lymph nodes

DISTANT METASTASIS (M)

MX	Distant metastasis cannot be assessed
M0	No distant metastasis
M1	Distant metastasis

STAGE GROUPING

Separate stage groupings are recommended for papillary or follicular, medullary, and anaplastic carcinoma.

Papillary or Follicular (<45 years)

Stage I	Any T	Any N	M0
Stage II	Any T	Any N	M1

Papillary or Follicular (45 years and older)

Stage I	T1	N0	M0
Stage II	T2	N0	M0
Stage III	T3	N0	M0
Stage III	T1	N1a	M0
Stage III	T2	N1a	M0
Stage III	T3	N1a	M0
Stage IVA	T4a	N0	M0
Stage IVA	T4a	N1a	M0
Stage IVA	T1	N1b	M0
Stage IVA	T2	N1b	M0
Stage IVA	T3	N1b	M0
Stage IVA	T4a	N1b	M0
Stage IVB	T4b	Any N	M0
Stage IVC	Any T	Any N	M1

(Continued)

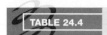

TABLE 24.4	Tumor, Node, Metastasis (TNM) Staging Scheme for Tumors of the Thyroid (*Continued*)		
Medullary Carcinoma			
Stage I	T1	N0	M0
Stage II	T2	N0	M0
Stage III	T3	N0	M0
Stage III	T2	N1a	M0
Stage III	T2	N1a	M0
Stage III	T3	N1a	M0
Stage IVA	T4a	N0	M0
Stage IVA	T4a	N1a	M0
Stage IVA	T1	N1b	M0
Stage IVA	T2	N1b	M0
Stage IVA	T3	N1b	M0
Stage IVA	T4a	N1b	M0
Stage IVB	T4b	Any N	M0
Stage IVC	Any T	Any N	M1
Anaplastic Carcinoma			
All anaplastic carcinomas are considered Stage IV			
Stage IVA	T4a	Any N	M0
Stage IVB	T4b	Any N	M0
Stage IVC	Any T	Any N	M1

From: Greene FL, Page DL, Fleming ID, Fritz AG, Balch CM, Haller DG, Morrow M, eds. *AJCC Cancer Staging Manual.* 6th edition. New York: Springer; 2002. Used with permission. (A new AJCC TNM staging system is scheduled for release in 2009; after its publication, the new staging scheme will appear on the website for this book.)

hyperplasia and MTC occur early in life in hereditary cases, prophylactic thyroidectomy and central node dissection should be performed as early as possible in MEN type 2B, although it may be delayed somewhat in MEN type 2A. Among the different clinical settings in which it arises, the prognosis is best for MTC in patients with non-MEN familial inheritance, slightly worse for those with MEN type 2A or sporadic tumors, and worst for those patients with MEN type 2B.

IV. **PATHOLOGIC REPORTING OF THYROID CARCINOMA.** American Joint Committee on Cancer (AJCC) staging of thyroid carcinomas is quite different than for other organ sites because the histologic type and age of the patient are critical for prognosis (Table 24.4). Patients with papillary carcinoma that has not metastasized distantly have an excellent prognosis, particularly those younger than 45 years, in whom survival approaches baseline. Any nonepithelial tumor type is excluded from staging.

CYTOLOGY OF THE THYROID
Jing Zhai

I. **INTRODUCTION.** Ultrasound or palpation guided thyroid fine needle aspiration (FNA) is considered to be the most sensitive and most specific non-surgical screening and diagnostic test in the management of patients with thyroid nodules with 95% accuracy, 43–98% sensitivity, and 72–100% specificity (*J Endocrinol Invest* 20:482, 1997).

II. **BENIGN DISEASES**
  A. **Acute thyroiditis.** Acute thyroiditis is rarely sampled given its typical clinical presentation. The aspirate shows predominantly neutrophils and necrotic debris with scattered histiocytes and scant reactive follicular cells. Special stains and culture are required for microorganism identification.
  B. **Chronic lymphocytic (Hashimoto's) thyroiditis.** The aspirate is usually cellular and it consists of two major components: an abundant mixed population of

lymphoid cells (including predominant small mature lymphocytes, plasma cells, lymphohistiocytic aggregates, and tingible body macrophages) and scattered, two-dimensional clusters of Hurthle cells with variable nuclear atypia (e-Fig. 24.16). Occasional multinucleated giant cells can be identified. Normal follicular cells and colloid are scant (*Diagn Cytopathol*, 11:141, 1994).

   C. Subacute granulomatous (de Quervain's) thyroiditis. The aspirate can be hypocellular due to fibrosis. The diagnostic feature is the granuloma consisting of cohesive aggregates of epithelioid histiocytes with elongated and kidney-shaped nuclei, granular chromatin, small nucleoli, and abundant pale cytoplasm with ill-defined borders (e-Fig. 24.17). Multinucleated giant cells and lymphocytes are usually present (*Diagn Cytopathol*, 16:214, 1997).

   D. Riedel's thyroiditis. The aspirate is marked hypocellular, containing microfragments of stroma with bland spindle shaped cells. Other cellular components are absent.

III. FOLLICULAR LESION. The diagnosis of "follicular lesion" is the most common diagnosis of thyroid FNA specimens. The cytological differential diagnosis includes nodular hyperplasia, follicular adenoma, follicular carcinoma, and follicular variant of papillary carcinoma. Thyroid FNA is considered a screening test to identify patients with a high risk of having follicular carcinoma. The architectural arrangement of the follicular cells in the lesion is the key to the correct classification (*Cancer* 71:2598,1993).

   A. Nodular hyperplasia is characterized by its heterogeneity. The aspirate is usually low to moderately cellular. The follicular cells form two dimensional honey-comb sheets and macrofollicles. Intermixed are small clusters of Hurthle cells with variable atypia, foamy histiocytes, and hemosiderin-laden macrophages (e-Fig. 24.18). Colloid is usually abundant; watery colloid forms a thin layer of filmy lavender material with occasional characteristic linear cracks (e-Fig. 24.18), and dense colloid forms deep purple blobs with sharp edges (e-Fig. 24.19).

   B. Follicular neoplasm yields richly cellular smears. The follicular cells predominantly form microfollicles and trabeculae (e-Fig. 24.20) and are slightly enlarged and crowded, with loss of a honey-comb architecture, without significant nuclear atypia. Colloid is absent or scant. The diagnosis of follicular carcinoma is based on the assessment of capsular and vascular invasion in surgical specimens, which cannot be evaluated in cytology specimens.

IV. HÜRTHLE CELL LESIONS. Hürthle cells are present in both neoplastic and non neoplastic processes (*Am J Clin Pathol* 100:231,1993). Thyroid FNA can be a useful screening test to identify patients with a high risk of having a Hürthle cell neoplasm.

   A. Benign Hürthle cell nodules are quite common in nodular hyperplasia and Hashimoto's thyroiditis. These non-neoplastic Hürthle cells form cohesive groups with only rare single cells. Features characteristics of nodular hyperplasia and Hashimoto's thyroiditis are also evident, including normal follicular cells, colloid, lymphocytes and plasma cells.

   B. Hürthle cell neoplasms yield hypercellular specimens composed of an almost pure population of Hürthle cells. The Hürthle cells are dyshesive single cells with prominent nucleoli (e-Fig. 24.21), and the background contain an insignificant number of normal follicular cells, lymphocytes, and colloid. The diagnosis of Hürthle cell carcinoma is based on assessment of capsular and vascular invasion in surgical specimen, which cannot be evaluated in cytology specimens.

V. MALIGNANT NEOPLASMS

   A. Papillary carcinoma. The specimen is richly cellular, consisting of large sheets with occasional papillary structures (e-Fig. 24.22). The follicular cells are slightly enlarged and have crowded nuclei. The characteristic nuclear features are fine open chromatin with nuclear membrane prominence, small and peripherally located nucleoli, intranuclear cytoplasmic inclusions, and longitudinal nuclear grooves (e-Fig. 24.23). Other associated features include dense cytoplasm, "bubble gum" like dense colloid, psammoma bodies (e-Fig. 24.24), and multinucleated giant cells (*Diagn Cytopathol* 7:462,1991).

   B. Hyalinizing trabecular adenoma. This lesion is regarded as a variant of papillary carcinoma by some investigators based on identification of *RET-PTC* gene rearrangements, although its classification remains controversial. The cytomorphology exhibits a great similarity to papillary carcinoma, including pale chromatin, longitudinal nuclear grooves, and intranuclear cytoplasmic inclusions. Hyalinizing stroma is suggestive of the diagnosis. The distinction from papillary carcinoma is based on histological examination (*Am J Clin Pathol* 91:115, 1989).

C. **Poorly differentiated (insular) carcinoma.** The aspirate is richly cellular and composed of monomorphic follicular cells with scant colloid. The follicular cells are present predominantly as single cells, with only occasional crowded clusters and microfollicles (**e-Fig. 24.25**). The necrosis and mitosis seen in tissue biopsy specimens are rare in smears. There are no distinct cytological features to render definitive diagnosis (*Diagn Cytopathol*, 25:325, 2001).

D. **Anaplastic carcinoma.** The aspirate is highly cellular and contains single cells exhibiting marked nuclear atypia. Necrosis is common. The malignant cells show diverse morphology, including epithelioid (**e-Fig. 24.26**), spindle shaped, and giant pleomorphic cells (*Acta Cytol* 40:953, 1996).

E. **Medullary carcinoma.** Medullary carcinoma typically generates highly cellular specimens, predominantly consisting of single cells and loose clusters of cells. The cell morphology is variable, ranging from monotonous with little atypia to highly atypical. The characteristic features are mixtures of plasmacytoid and spindle shaped cells with characteristic salt-and-pepper chromatin (**e-Fig. 24.27**). Amyloid is usually present, but its distinction from colloid is impossible without a Congo red stain (*Pathologica* 90:5, 1998).

F. **Lymphoma.** Most primary thyroid lymphomas develop in the background of Hashimoto's thyroiditis. Diffuse large B-cell lymphoma (DLBCL) is the major type, followed by extranodal marginal zone B-cell lymphoma of mucosa-associated lymphoid tissue (*Am J Surg Pathol* 24:623, 2000). DLBCL exhibits monotonous large atypical lymphoid cells with irregular nuclear contours, vesicular chromatin, single prominent nucleoli (immunoblast-like cells) or multiple nucleoli (centroblast-like cells) (**e-Fig. 24.28**). Marginal zone B-cell lymphoma shows a heterogeneous population of lymphoid cells with a predominance of small lymphoid cells, and intermixed plasmacytoid cells and immunoblasts; monocytoid cells with abundant pale cytoplasm are frequently seen. Demonstration of light chain restriction by flow cytometry is critical for diagnosis.

VI. **METASTATIC MALIGNANCY.** Metastasis to the thyroid is uncommon. The kidney is the most common primary site of metastatic tumors, followed by lung and breast. In a patient with a history of malignancy, the differentiated diagnosis for a new thyroid nodule should include metastasis. Comparison of the aspirate with the slides of the primary malignancy, together with immunostains, is critical for diagnosis.

Suggested Readings

Adair C. Non-neoplastic lesions of the thyroid gland. In: Thompson LDR, ed. *Endocrine Pathology*. New York: Churchill Livingstone; 2006.

DeLellis RA, Guiter G, Henley JD. Thyroid and parathyroid glands. In: Gnepp DR, ed. *Diagnostic Surgical Pathology of the Head and Neck*. Philadelphia: W.B. Saunders Publishers; 2001.

Lloyd RV, Douglas BR, Young WF. Thyroid gland. In: King DW, ed. Fascicle #1 - Endocrine Diseases, First Series. Armed Forces Institute of Pathology Atlas of Non-Tumor Pathology. Washington, DC: American Registry of Pathology; 2002.

Thompson LDR. Benign neoplasms of the thyroid gland. In: Thompson LDR, ed. *Endocrine Pathology*. New York: Churchill Livingstone; 2006.

Thompson LDR. Malignant neoplasms of the thyroid gland. In: Thompson LDR, ed. *Endocrine Pathology*. New York: Churchill Livingstone; 2006.

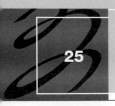

25 PARATHYROID GLANDS
James S. Lewis Jr.

I. **NORMAL ANATOMY.** The endodermally derived parathyroid glands develop from the third (inferior parathyroids) and fourth (superior parathyroids) pharyngeal pouches. They produce parathyroid hormone (PTH) which acts to increase the circulating calcium level. They are normally found along the posterior surface of the thyroid gland, but given their complex embryologic development, normal variations in location range from within the substance of the thyroid gland, superiorly to the hyoid bone, inferiorly into the mediastinum, within the thymus gland, or within the pericardium. Furthermore, 2% to 7% of the population has more than the usual four glands.

Most normal parathyroid glands are from 0.3 to 0.6 cm in largest dimension, and the normal aggregate weight of all glands is 120 to 140 mg. They are brown to light yellowish-brown and oval, and have a thin capsule. Histologically, they consist of chief (or principal) cells and oxyphil cells. The former have round nuclei with granular chromatin and slightly eosinophilic to clear cytoplasm; the latter have round nuclei and more abundant brightly eosinophilic and granular cytoplasm (e-**Fig. 25.1**).* Both types of cells are arranged in sheets, nests, and cords. Occasional pseudoglandular or pseudoacinar foci with central eosinophilic proteinaceous material can also be seen in the normal parathyroid. Oxyphil cells may also form small nodules in adults. Intraparenchymal adipose tissue is a normal feature of the parathyroid glands; it is usually scant in children but progressively increases with age to constitute about 50% of the gland by the fifth decade and plateaus beyond that time.

Parathyroid cells, both chief and oxyphil, are positive by immunohistochemistry for PTH, chromogranin-A, and cytokeratins; this immunoprofile is maintained in virtually all pathologic processes of the parathyroid glands. Parathyroid cells are negative for thyroglobulin and thyroid transcription factor-1 (TTF-1).

II. **GROSS EXAMINATION, TISSUE SAMPLING, AND HISTOLOGIC SLIDE PREPARATION**
- A. **Fine needle aspiration.** Fine needle aspiration of parathyroid lesions is rarely ever performed. The two exceptions are, first, when an adenoma arises within the substance of the parathyroid gland and thus a biopsy is taken as part of the evaluation of a presumed thyroid lesion, and second, when parathyroid carcinoma presents as a large neck mass.
- B. **Biopsy.** Intraoperative biopsies (frozen sections) are frequently performed to confirm that the excised tissue is a parathyroid gland, because lymph nodes, thymus, thyroid, and fat may all be mistaken clinically for parathyroid tissue. The tissue should be weighed, but no other special handling is required.
- C. **Excision.** The gross examination of parathyroid glands begins with recording their weight and measurement in three dimensions. The glands should be closely examined and, if firm, ragged, or irregular, inked around their periphery. They should then be sectioned and their color and consistency described. One section should be taken for histologic examination or, if the gland is 2 cm or larger, two to three sections should be taken.

---

*All e-figures are available online via the Solution Site Image Bank.

III. DIAGNOSTIC FEATURES OF COMMON DISEASES

A. Nonneoplastic

1. **Abnormal.** Abnormal development of the parathyroid glands sometimes occurs. The classic example is DiGeorge's syndrome, in which there is failure in the development of several of the branchial pouches with resulting absence of at least the thymus and parathyroid glands; neonates develop hypocalcemia due to lack of parathyroid hormone. Albright's hereditary osteodystrophy is due to pseudohypoparathyroidism as a result of target organ unresponsiveness to PTH; neonates present with hypocalcemia, hyperphosphatemia, and blunted responses to PTH.

2. **Inflammatory.** Parathyroiditis is a rare and poorly understood condition thought to be autoimmune in nature. It is characterized by extensive infiltration of the glands by lymphocytes. It is usually idiopathic and isolated, but may be associated with a rare autoimmune polyglandular syndrome in which two or more endocrine glands are affected. Between one quarter and three quarters of patients will have circulating antiparathyroid tissue antibodies; most patients have hypoparathyroidism, but parathyroiditis is sometimes associated with parathyroid hyperplasia. Histologically, the glands are infiltrated by clusters of lymphocytes, often with germinal center formation. Plasma cells and fibrosis with clear parenchymal destruction are sometimes seen.

3. **Cysts.** Cysts of the parathyroid glands are relatively uncommon. They occur in the neck and less commonly in the mediastinum. Most patients do not have clinical hyperparathyroidism. Grossly, they are often loosely attached to the thyroid gland, range from microscopic up to as large as 10 cm, have thin walls, and contain watery fluid. Microscopically, they are lined by a cuboidal layer of epithelial cells with round, hyperchromatic nuclei (e-Fig. 25.2). The cyst wall consists of fibrous tissue with entrapped islands of parathyroid chief cells.

4. **Hyperplasia.** Hyperplasia is an increase in the overall mass of parathyroid cells, and accounts for approximately 15% of all cases of primary hyperparathyroidism. Hyperplasia is divided into primary (where there is no known clinical stimulus), secondary (usually due to renal failure or another known metabolic cause), and tertiary (where there is an autonomously increased parathyroid mass in patients who have had secondary hyperparathyroidism and now are on dialysis or have had a renal transplant) (Table 25.1). A significant minority of cases of primary hyperparathyroidism (up to 40%) have been shown to be monoclonal, indicating that some cases represent true neoplasia; however, the clinical and pathophysiologic importance of this finding is unclear.

    Approximately 75% of patients are women, and 20% present with familial disease (most commonly due to multiple endocrine neoplasia [MEN] type 1 or 2A). Many patients are asymptomatic and are identified only indirectly through clinical evaluation for other reasons. The symptoms and signs of hyperparathyroidism can be vague such as fatigue, lethargy, nausea, constipation, arthralgias, or anorexia. The classic "bones, stones, and abdominal moans" (osteitis fibrosa cystica, kidney stones, and peptic ulcer disease) presentation is rare, and patients rarely present with a neck mass. Psychological disorders such as depression, psychosis, emotional instability, and confusion are sometimes the presenting symptoms.

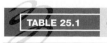

TABLE 25.1	Classification of Parathyroid Hyperplasia
Primary hyperparathyroidism	No known stimulus
Secondary hyperparathyroidism	Known stimulus such as chronic renal failure, malabsorption, or vitamin D metabolism abnormality
Tertiary hyperparathyroidism	After long-standing renal failure with development of autonomous parathyroid hyperfunction

In hyperplasia, all of the glands are involved but to varying degrees, leading to asymmetric findings. Grossly, the glands are usually enlarged and are soft and brown; they may also be nodular or cystic. The total weight is above normal, but is still usually <1 g. Microscopically all of the glands show similar findings, but to different degrees, including increased parenchymal cells and a commensurate decrease in fat (e-**Fig. 25.3**). Both chief and oxyphil cells are usually increased, although usually chief cells predominate, in a nodular, multimodular, or diffuse pattern; only rarely is a follicular pattern present. Cytologic atypia can be seen but is rarely widespread. There is minimal mitotic activity. A rare type of hyperplasia termed 'water-clear cell hyperplasia' is sometimes encountered, in which all the cells have abundant, perfectly clear cytoplasm and no adipose tissue is present.

The differential diagnosis of hyperplasia includes parathyroid adenoma; because the histologic features of an adenoma are not consistently different than those of hyperplasia, examination of more than one gland is necessary, as is correlation with the clinical findings, to distinguish between the two entities. Water-clear cell hyperplasia must be distinguished from metastatic renal cell carcinoma (RCC). RCC will show diffuse nuclear atypia and will be negative for PTH and neuroendocrine marker expression by immunohistochemistry.

- **a. Autotransplantation.** A common surgical approach to hyperplasia is to remove three glands, entirely and then a remnant of the fourth. Alternatively, all four glands are excised, and a portion of one gland is implanted (often the skeletal muscle of the forearm or neck) to facilitate surgery in case of recurrent hyperparathyroidism. Because the cells of a hyperplastic autotransplanted gland can be mitotically active and infiltrate the skeletal muscle, and thus imitate a malignant process, clinical history is required for correct diagnosis.

- **b. Parathyromatosis.** This is a rare condition that presents as a primary or, more commonly, secondary disease in which numerous nests of parathyroid tissue are present throughout the neck and/or mediastinum. When it is a primary condition, it is commonly associated with an MEN syndrome. Secondary parathyromatosis is thought to occur after parathyroid surgery as a result of spillage of cells into the soft tissues which then become hyperplastic. The morphology of the nodules in parathyromatosis is similar to that of the glands hyperplasia.

B. Neoplasms. The World Health Organization (WHO) classification of tumors of the parathyroid gland is listed in Table 25.2.

- **1. Adenoma.** Parathyroid adenomas are benign neoplasms composed of chief cells, oxyphil cells, or a mixture of both. They occur in approximately 0.1% of the population and account for approximately 80% of cases of hyperparathyroidism. They are more common in women and have a peak incidence in the 6th and 7th decades of life. Adenomas are sometimes (albeit rarely) familial; in these cases they are associated with MEN type 1 or 2, or the uncommon hyperparathyroidism-jaw tumor syndrome. Adenomas involve a single gland (it is controversial as to whether patients with more than one adenoma actually suffer from hyperplasia). Patients present with signs and symptoms related to hypercalcemia (as detailed above in the section on parathyroid hyperplasia). Technetium is concentrated in parathyroid tissue, so technetium sestamibi scans are often used to detect and localize the abnormal gland.

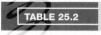

TABLE 25.2   **WHO Histological Classification of Parathyroid Tumors**

Parathyroid carcinoma
Parathyroid adenoma
Secondary tumors

From: DeLellis RA, Lloyd RV, Heitz P, Eng C, eds. *World Health Organization Classification of Tumours. Pathology and Genetics. Tumours of Endocrine Organs.* Lyon: IARC Press; 2004. Used with permission.

Grossly, adenomas are rounded, encapsulated, and tan to reddish-brown, with an average weight of 1 g. On sectioning, they are soft and homogeneous, although degeneration and cystic change may occur. Microscopically, adenomas are a well-circumscribed, thinly-encapsulated mass with little stroma and no, or very minimal, fat, often with a rim of normal appearing parathyroid gland. The cell population is uniform and usually of one cell type, chief or oxyphil (e-**Fig. 25**.4), usually arranged in solid sheets although pseudoglandular (pseudoacinar or follicular) areas may be seen (e-**Fig. 25**.5), sometimes containing central eosinophilic material mimicking thyroid follicles. The nuclei in chief cell adenomas are small, round, regular, and hyperchromatic. The nuclei in oxyphilic adenomas are round and may have prominent eosinophilic nucleoli. Nuclear pleomorphism can be seen although it is usually very localized. Mitotic figures are scarce (1 or fewer per 10 high-power fields).

The differential diagnosis of an adenoma includes parathyroid hyperplasia; adenomas simply cannot be distinguished from hyperplasia without sampling more than a single gland because the morphologic features of adenomas overlap those of large hyperplastic glands. If only one gland is available for evaluation, it is best to diagnose "hypercellular parathyroid consistent with adenoma." Adenomas can be distinguished from cellular nodules of thyroid tissue (particularly from patients with nodular hyperplasia of the thyroid) by finding convincing colloid in thyroid lesions, finding a rim of definite parathyroid tissue in adenomas, or immunostaining for thyroglobulin, PTH, and/or TTF-1.

2. **Carcinoma.** Parathyroid carcinoma is rare, estimated to be the cause of <1% of hyperparathyroidism, and is by far the least common lesion of the parathyroid glands. The average age of patients is between 45 and 55 years, and the sex distribution is roughly equal. The etiology is unknown, and there is no significant association with any of the familial syndromes that cause parathyroid disease. Most patients present with profound hyperparathyroidism and hypercalcemia (with calcium levels often >16 mg/dL with secondary nephrolithiasis, renal insufficiency, and bone involvement with osteopenia and/or "brown tumors"), and have typical nonspecific symptoms such as weakness, fatigue, nausea, and depression.

Grossly, parathyroid carcinomas are usually large, poorly circumscribed, and adherent to surrounding tissues, particularly the thyroid gland. They range from 1.5 to 6.0 cm or larger, and average 6.7 grams. Their cut surface is usually gray-white and firm. Microscopically, they usually have a thick, hypocellular, and collagenous capsule and intratumoral fibrous bands. Capsular invasion by the tumors is common, and invasion through the capsule as tongue-like or mushroom-like extensions is typical (e-**Fig. 25**.6). Tumors often extensively invade soft tissue and nearby structures, but vascular and perineural invasion are relatively uncommon. The growth pattern is usually solid, occasionally with areas of necrosis. The individual cells may have clear cytoplasm or be exclusively oxyphilic, but most often they have an intermediate eosinophilic color. Most carcinomas have nuclei that show mild to moderate variability, but occasional tumors will show marked nuclear pleomorphism (e-**Fig. 25**.7). Mitotic activity can be quite low, but most tumors have >5 mitoses per 50 high-power fields.

The differential diagnosis is primarily with parathyroid adenoma. Although there is no single diagnostic feature other than metastasis that is considered completely diagnostic of carcinoma, the overall constellation of findings is usually definitive. Vascular invasion, capsular penetration, invasion of the thyroid gland, and/or perineural invasion are indicative of carcinoma (Table 25.3). Thyroid neoplasms, as well as metastases from RCC or thyroid medullary carcinoma, can be excluded by immunohistochemical results.

Surgery is the mainstay of treatment, and complete surgical excision at presentation offers the best chance for cure. The 5-year survival is approximately 85%, and 10-year survival is 50%. Patients frequently develop local recurrence, as well as metastases to neck lymph nodes, lung, liver, and bone. The associated hypercalcemia is a cause of significant comorbidity and death.

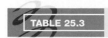

TABLE 25.3	Pathologic Features of Parathyroid Carcinoma

Thick capsule	*Vascular invasion
Fibrous bands	*Perineural invasion
*Capsular penetration	Marked cytologic atypia
*Soft tissue extension	Mitotic activity
Necrosis	Tumor cell spindling

*Most useful and specific features.

3. **Metastatic tumors.** The parathyroid glands are an uncommon site for metastases, although they are sometimes involved by direct extension from thyroid or laryngeal tumors. The rare metastases from distant sites most commonly arise from breast, kidney, and lung carcinomas or melanoma.

IV. **HISTOLOGIC GRADING, STAGING, AND REPORTING OF PARATHYROID CARCINOMA.** Grading of parathyroid carcinoma based on cytologic features or degree of differentiation has not been found to predict behavior. Similarly, there is no durable staging system for parathyroid carcinoma, so no American Joint Committee on Cancer (AJCC) guidelines are available in this regard; neither tumor size nor lymph node status at presentation is predictive of outcome.

For excision specimens, the surgical pathology report should include tumor size in three dimensions, growth pattern, involvement of adjacent structures, and relation to surgical margins. Although lymph node status is not predictive of outcome, the number of regional lymph nodes examined, and the number positive for carcinoma, should also be reported.

CYTOLOGY OF THE PARATHYROID GLANDS
Jing Zhai

I. **INTRODUCTION.** The parathyroid glands can be sampled by ultrasound- or palpation-guided fine needle aspiration, although cytological sampling of a parathyroid mass to confirm that the lesion is of parathyroid origin is usually not indicated.

II. **MICROSCOPIC FINDINGS.** Parathyroid cells in aspirates tend to form cohesive tissue fragments, papillary structures, and microacinar structures, although scattered single cells are also present. The cells are uniform with small, round nuclei and granular chromatin (e-**Fig. 25.8**), with great similarity to thyroid follicular cells. Consequently, measurement of PTH level in the aspirated material and/or immunostains for PTH are necessary to confirm the cell origin (*Hum Pathol* 26:338–343, 2005; *Diagn Cytopathol* 16:476–484, 1997). Cytologic findings alone cannot be used to differentiate hyperplasia, adenoma, and carcinoma.

Suggested Readings
DeLellis RA, Guiter G, Henley JD. Thyroid and parathyroid glands. In: Gnepp DR, ed. *Diagnostic Surgical Pathology of the Head and Neck*. Philadelphia: W.B. Saunders Publishers; 2001.

Lloyd RV, Douglas BR, Young WF. Parathyroid gland. In: King DW, ed. *Fascicle #1 - Endocrine Diseases, First Series*. Armed Forces Institute of Pathology Atlas of Non-Tumor Pathology. Washington: American Registry of Pathology; 2002.

Thompson LDR. Benign neoplasms of the parathyroid gland. In: Thompson LDR, ed. *Endocrine Pathology*. China: Churchill Livingstone, 2006.

Thompson LDR. Malignant neoplasms of the parathyvoid gland. In: Thompson LDR, ed. *Endocrine Pathology*. China: Churchill Livingstone; 2006.

Thompson LDR. Non-reoplastic lesions of the parathyroid gland. In: Thompson LDR, ed. *Endocrine Pathology*. China: Churchill Livingstone; 2006.

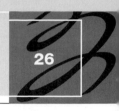

I. **NORMAL ANATOMY AND HISTOLOGY.** The adrenal glands are located anterior to the upper poles of the kidneys. The glands are pyramidal on the right and crescentic on the left. In adults, the normal combined weight should not exceed 6 grams. Each adrenal gland is divided into head (most medial), body (middle), and tail (most lateral).

The adrenal gland is composed an outer cortex and an inner medulla. Microscopically, the cortex consists of three zones: the outer zona glomerulosa (secreting aldosterone), middle zona fasciculata (secreting mainly cortisol and minor amounts of sex steroids), and inner zona reticularis (secreting mainly sex steroids) (e-**Fig. 26.1**).*
The zona glomerulosa is composed of a thin, usually discontinuous layer of cells with a ball-like arrangement and less cytoplasm than cells in other cortical zones. The zona fasciculata consists of radial cords or columns of cells with abundant lipid-rich cytoplasm. The zona reticularis cells have compact, finely eosinophilic cytoplasm with or without lipofuscin pigment. Normally the medulla accounts for 10% of the adrenal volume. The medulla is limited to the head and body, and grossly has a gray-white color. The predominant cells in the medulla are chromaffin cells (pheochromocytes) organized in nests and cords (e-**Fig. 26.2**). The cytoplasm of the chromaffin cells is usually basophilic but may be amphophilic or even eosinophilic. These cells have indistinct cell borders and usually a single nucleus that may show variation in size and hyperchromasia. The chromaffin cells are peripherally surrounded by the sustentacular cells. The medulla may also contain rare ganglion cells (e-**Fig. 26.3**). The major function of adrenal medulla is to secrete catecholamines (epinephrine and norepinephrine).

II. **GROSS EXAMINATION OF ADRENAL GLAND SPECIMEN.** The adrenal glands are removed either as part of a radical nephrectomy or for excision of an adrenal tumor. Less often biopsy is performed, especially for the diagnosis of metastatic tumors.

A. **Needle biopsy.** The entire tissue should be submitted for histologic examination.

B. **Adrenal gland removed as part of radical nephrectomy.** After gross examination of the kidney, the gland should be measured and weighed. Then the gland should be serially sectioned at 2- to 3-mm intervals perpendicular to its long axis; the thickness of the cortex and medulla should be noted. Infrequently, the adrenal may be invaded directly by renal cell carcinoma or be the site of discontinuous metastases.

C. **Adrenectomy for a pathologic process of the adrenal gland.** The first step is to orient the specimen and examine the contour of the adrenal gland. If it is apparent that the gland has been largely replaced by a mass, the periphery should be inked because the margins may be important (assuming that the mass has not already invaded surrounding structures such as the liver). If the cortex and medulla maintain their normal relationship to each other, the thickness of each should be recorded. Serial sectioning should be done at intervals appropriate for the pathology. If the disease process is apparently diffuse hyperplasia, the periadrenal soft tissue should be removed and the gland should be measured and weighed. If the adrenal contains a solitary mass or multiple nodules, three-dimensional measurements should be obtained. The cut surface of the lesion and its relationship to any identifiable normal tissue should be described, including color, consistency, any hemorrhage or

---

*All e-figures are available online via the Solution Site Image Bank.

necrosis, degree of circumscription, and degree of encapsulation. If any portions of adjacent organs such as liver, kidney, spleen, or abdominal wall (usually for adrenal tumors) are attached, their appearance and relationship to adrenal gland and tumor should be noted. A large, en bloc resection will require numerous sections from the peripheral margins. For diffuse and/or nodular hyperplasia, representative sections are sufficient.

For a neoplasm, the following sections should be taken: tumor, including sections demonstrating the relationship of the tumor to the associated soft tissues and adjacent organs, and relationship of the tumor to uninvolved adrenal gland; tumor capsule, if present; margins; periadrenal fatty tissue overlying a bulging mass; representative section from uninvolved adrenal gland, if any; and regional lymph nodes. The gross description should clearly document the site of the sections. For large specimens, a gross illustration is extremely helpful in that it depicts the specimen at time when landmarks are still maintained with some anatomic orientation.

D. Neuroblastoma specimens. Neuroblastic tumors (NBs) present some special issues regarding acquisition of neoplastic tissue for a variety of special studies required to biologically profile the tumor for those children enrolled in a Children Oncology Group (COG) protocol. If the specimen is an adrenal gland–based neuroblastoma, then generally the amount of available tumor is sufficient for pathologic diagnosis as well as for all other ancillary studies. However, when the specimen is only a portion of the total mass or consists of largely necrotic and hemorrhagic tumor, sampling is more complicated.

A resected primary neuroblastoma of the adrenal, or extra-adrenal retroperitoneal mass, should be examined fresh if at all possible. The aspects of the gross examination do not differ from those discussed in the previous section. The COG reference laboratory requests at least 1 gram of snap-frozen tumor tissue, but will accept any frozen sample of tumor; the snap freezing should occur as soon as the specimen becomes available following resection. Tumor samples should be labeled "primary" or "metastatic"; involved bone marrow is required as well. Storage at $-70°C$ is preferable to $-20°C$.

Fresh tissue should also be collected for local institutional studies including conventional cytogenetic studies. Snap-frozen fresh tissue should be saved for possible molecular studies. Multiple air-dry touch preparations should be prepared for in situ hybridization.

III. ADRENAL CORTICAL LESIONS

A. Congenital abnormalities. The most common congenital anomaly of the adrenal gland is often an incidental finding of heterotopia consisting of microscopic foci of cortical tissue or nodule(s) along the so-called inguinoscrotal path. The spermatic cord, inguinal hernia sac, or adjacent to the epididymis are the three common sites of heterotopic nodules (*Int Surg.* 2006;91:125). Heterotopias are identified in 1.5–2.7% of groin procedures in males, but not in females (*BJU Int .* 2005;95:407). Only cortical tissue is identified as a rule (e-**Fig. 26.4**), but cortex and medulla have been seen in the celiac axis. Other congenital abnormalities include adrenal union/fusion, adrenal cytomegaly, intra-adrenal heterotopic tissue, and congenital adrenal hyperplasia. Adrenal cytomegaly is characterized by the presence of foci of bizarre cells with eosinophilic granular cytoplasm and large hyperchromatic nuclei with pseudoinclusions; this finding is detected in Beckwith–Wiedemann syndrome. Heterotopic tissues within the adrenal gland include liver, thyroid, and ovarian stroma.

B. Incidental adrenal cortical nodules. Nonfunctional cortical nodules are found in 1–10% of autopsies, are usually multiple and bilateral, and can protrude into adjacent fat. These variably sized nodules have a yellow appearance on cut surface. Circumscribed, but nonencapsulated nodules consist of fasciculata-type cells with various patterns. Myelolipomatous metaplasia, osseous metaplasia, and secondary changes (hyalinization, calcification, or hemorrhage) may be present. Pigmented nodules are composed of zona reticularis–type cells with lipofuscin or neuromelanin.

C. Lesions leading to adrenal cortical hypofunction (insufficiency). Adrenal cortical insufficiency is divided into primary and secondary type.

1. **Primary adrenal cortical insufficiency** (Addison disease) is due to destruction of the adrenal cortex. In developed countries, >80% of cases are due to autoimmune adrenalitis as an isolated manifestation of autoimmune polyendocrinopathy (*Lancet.* 2003;361:1881). This T-cell–mediated immunologic destructive process of the cortex results in small glands that have a mixed inflammatory infiltrate of lymphocytes, plasma cells, and histiocytes. Lymphoid follicles with germinal centers may be present in a pattern similar to that in Hashimoto's thyroiditis. Cortical cells may be difficult to identify, but the medulla remains intact. Various inborn errors of metabolism, hemorrhage, and neoplastic infiltrates or replacement are other etiologies.

   Adrenal cortical insufficiency may occur on the basis of infectious etiologies including tuberculosis, other bacterial infections (including *Meningococcus, Pseudomonas, Streptococcus pneumoniae,* and *Haemophilus influenzae*), fungal infections, cytomegalovirus, herpes simplex virus, and toxoplasmosis (in human immunodeficiency virus [HIV]-infected individuals). These infections lead to destruction of the entire gland.

   Other causes of primary insufficiency include amyloidosis and drugs. Treatment with mitotane may cause adrenal atrophy with fibrosis.

2. **Secondary and tertiary adrenal cortical insufficiencies** are due to the failure of the pituitary gland to secrete adrenocorticotropic hormone (ACTH; secondary) or of the hypothalamus to secrete corticotropin-releasing hormone (CRH; tertiary). The gland size is decreased. Histologically, the zona fasciculata is atrophic, whereas the zona glomerulosa and medulla are usually relatively normal.

D. **Adrenal cortical hyperplasia can be divided into congenital and acquired types.**

1. **Congenital adrenal hyperplasia** is an autosomal recessive disorder caused by one of five enzymatic defects that cause a failure in cortisol synthesis; 21-hydroxylase deficiency accounts for 90–95% of cases (*Lancet.* 2005;365:2125). Marked diffuse hyperplasia of the zona fasciculata results from ACTH stimulation, whereas cells of the zona fasciculata are lipid depleted due to their conversion into zona reticularis–type cells with compact eosinophilic cytoplasm. Persistent ACTH stimulation may also give rise to adrenal cortical neoplasms. Nodules resembling hyperplastic adrenal cortical tissue in testis can develop into the so-called testicular tumors of the adrenogenital syndrome (*Am J Surg Pathol.* 1988;12:503).

2. **Acquired adrenal cortical hyperplasia** is a nonneoplastic bilateral process characterized by a gland weighing in excess of 6 grams. The gland has a diffuse, nodular, or combined appearance.

   a. **Diffuse hyperplasia** is usually ACTH dependent and caused by a hyperfunctional pituitary (most often pituitary adenoma, less often CRH from the hypothalamus) or an ectopic ACTH/CRH-producing tumor. The latter neoplasms include small cell carcinoma (usually from the lung), carcinoid (usually from the lung or thymus), medullary thyroid carcinoma, pancreatic endocrine neoplasm, and pheochromocytoma (PHEO). Both glands are symmetrically enlarged. The zonae fasciculata and reticularis are expanded with their relative proportions varying from case to case. The zona fasciculata is lipid depleted and converted into zona reticularis–type cells with compact eosinophilic cytoplasm.

   b. **Nodular cortical hyperplasia** is ACTH independent in most cases. The glands are markedly enlarged, in excess of 15 to 20 grams in some cases. The cortical nodules may constitute a transformation from diffuse hyperplasia in its late stage; these nodules are yellowish and vary from 0.2 cm to >4.0 cm. Fasciculata-type clear cells, reticularis-type cells, or a mixture of these two cell types characterize the nodules.

   c. **Primary pigmented nodular adrenocortical disease (PPNAD),** an uncommon but specific form of ACTH-independent nodular hyperplasia, is usually recognized in the second decade of life with or without the other stigmata of Carney complex (*Horm Res.* 2005;64:132 and *Orphanet J Rare Dis.*

TABLE 26.1	**WHO Histological Classification of Tumors of Adrenal Gland and with Additional Entities**

Adrenal cortical tumors	**Extra-adrenal paraganglioma**
Adrenal cortical adenoma	Jugulotympanic
Adrenal cortical carcinoma	Vagal
Adrenal medullary tumors	Laryngeal
Benign pheochromocytoma	Orbital nasopharyngeal
Malignant pheochromocytoma	Carotid body
Composite pheochromocytoma	Aorticopulmonary
Other adrenal tumors	Gangliocytic
Adenomatoid tumor	Cauda equine
Sex cord–stroma tumor	Cervical paravertebral
Soft tissue and germ cell tumors	Intrathoracic
Myelolipoma	Intra-abdominal
Teratoma	Superior para-aortic
Schwannoma	Inferior para-aortic
Ganglioneuroma	Urinary bladder
Angiosarcoma	
Leiomyoma	
Wilms tumor (extrarenal)	
Secondary or metastatic tumors	

From: DeLellis RA, Lloyd RV, Heitz P, Eng C, eds. *World Health Organization Classification of Tumours. Pathology and Genetics. Tumours of Endocrine Organs.* Lyon: IARC Press; 2004. Used with permission.

2006;1:21). A germline-heterozygous inactivating mutation of *PRKR1A* is found in the Carney complex and may also have a role in primary PPNAD (*Pituitary.* 2006;9:211). The glands are of normal size, and their cut surface has scattered pigmented micronodules or, less often, macronodules measuring 1 to 4 mm in size. Uniform compact cells with eosinophilic cytoplasm and some balloon cells are features of the nodules. Pigmentation is due to intracytoplasmic lipofuscin. The same cells are strongly positive for synaptophysin. The nodules may abut the cortical medullary junction, extend into the periadrenal fat, or involve the entire thickness of the cortex.

    d. Adrenal cortical hyperplasia with hyperaldosteronism (Conn syndrome) is due to an adenoma in 70% of cases; the remainder have bilateral cortical hyperplasia. The size, weight, and appearance of the glands are variable, and the size may be within normal range. The zona glomerulosa has tongue-like projections toward the underlying zona fasciculata. Micronodules may be present with fasciculata-type cells.

  E. Adrenal cortical neoplasms are traditionally divided into adenomas and carcinomas (Table 26.1).

    1. Adrenal cortical adenomas are typically unilateral, solitary, rarely larger than 50 grams or 5 cm in size, and heterogeneous with or without clinical manifestations due to hyperfunction. The hormone-associated syndromes are hyperaldosteronism, Cushing syndrome, and adrenogenital syndrome in descending order of frequency.

      a. Hyperaldosteronism (Conn syndrome) is associated with an adenoma, <2 cm in size in most cases. A yellowish, circumscribed, but encapsulated nodule is composed of zona fasciculata–type cells, zona reticularis–type cells, zona glomerulosa–type cells, or cells showing hybrid features (e-**Fig. 26.5**). Occasionally the adjacent cortex may show hyperplasia of the zona glomerulosa (paradoxical hyperplasia). If there has been treatment with spirolactone (an aldosterone antagonist), characteristic spirolactone bodies are usually present, consisting of small, intracytoplasmic, 2- to 6-um round to oval inclusions with a slightly eosinophilic appearance and two to six concentric rings within the tumor cells and the adjacent zona glomerulosa (*Am J Clin Pathol.* 1970;54:22). A halo separates the spirolactone bodies from the surrounding cytoplasm.

b. **Cushing syndrome** is characterized by an adenoma that is sharply demarcated or even capsulated, and has a homogeneous yellow to golden-yellow appearance or irregular foci of dark discoloration on cut surface. Solid nests or alveola-like profiles are present, composed of cells that are usually larger than the normal cortical cells. The cells of the adenoma have features of zona fasciculata–type cells with the occasional presence of foci of smaller zona reticularis–type cells (e-**Fig. 26.6**); both types of tumor cells usually have single, round to oval nuclei with a small nucleolus. In some cases, there are scattered cells with larger, hyperchromatic nuclei with pseudoinclusions; they have no prognostic importance. Mitotic figures are rare. Fibrosis, organizing thrombi within sinusoids, and lipomatous and myelolipomatous metaplasia are other features. The compressed residual cortex is invariably atrophic.

c. **Adrenogenital syndrome** with sex hormone production is infrequently caused by an adenoma, but is more often associated with cortical carcinomas that produce estrogen. Androgen-producing adenomas are generally larger than those in Cushing syndrome and are also sharply demarcated from the adjacent cortex. The tumor cells have the features of zona reticularis cells with compact, eosinophilic cytoplasm.

d. **Morphologic variants** of adrenal cortical adenoma include pigmented or black adenoma, oncocytic adenoma, and myxoid variant of adrenal cortical adenoma.

   i. **Black (pigmented) adenoma** is associated with Cushing syndrome, and rarely with Conn syndrome. In most cases the tumor is composed predominantly or entirely of cells resembling zona reticularis cells with a variable amount of intracytoplasmic brown or golden brown pigment (lipofuscin).

   ii. **Oncocytic adrenal cortical adenoma** or oncocytoma is a rare entity with only about 20 cases reported in the literature. Most of them are nonfunctioning, but occasionally they can be associated with Cushing syndrome (*Ann Diagn Pathol.* 2005;9:295). Similar to oncocytomas at other sites, they may have a mahogany color on cut surface. The tumor is composed exclusively of polygonal oncocytes with abundant granular eosinophilic cytoplasm. The tumor cells contain sparse or no lipid.

   iii. **Myxoid adrenal cortical adenoma** is a recently described entity (*Am J Surg Pathol.* 2000;24:396). These tumors have a prominent, often grossly evident, myxoid stroma. The tumor cells in the myxoid area often form thin anastomosing cords, clusters, nests, and pseudogland-like structures (e-**Fig. 26.7**). The tumor cells in myxoid areas are often smaller than those in conventional areas, with predominantly eosinophilic cytoplasm and occasional clear cells. The myxoid variant is also seen in cortical carcinomas.

2. **Adrenal cortical carcinoma (ACC)** is a rare neoplasm with an incidence of about 1 per million population in the United States. This tumor can occur at any age, but it appears to have a bimodal age distribution with one peak in children younger than 5 years and another peak in adults in the fourth or fifth decade of life. ACCs are seen in association with several syndromes including Li–Fraumeni syndrome and Beckwith–Wiedemann syndrome. Most patients present with distant metastases at the time of diagnosis. ACCs are more likely to be nonfunctional than adenomas. The symptoms associated with functional tumors include virilization, Cushing syndrome, and rarely feminization and hyperaldosteronism.

   ACC is not a subtle neoplasm in terms of its pathologic features. The tumor is usually a mass in excess of 10 cm and weighing >100 grams (often >500 grams) with an irregular external appearance. Cut sections show a complex collage of reds and yellows, obvious necrosis with or without cystic degeneration, and hemorrhage (e-**Fig. 26.8**). Direct extension into the liver may be grossly obvious. Like renal cell carcinoma, ACC invades major vessels.

Microscopically, large, often pleomorphic epithelioid cells with abundant eosinophilic cytoplasm are arranged in trabecular, alveolar, or nested profiles (e-Fig. 26.9). Rarely a sarcomatoid or spindle cell pattern may be seen. Some tumors contain abundant lipid-rich cells. The tumor cells may contain intracytoplasmic hyaline globules (also seen in cortical adenomas). Rarely, the entire tumor is composed of oncocytes (oncocytic ACC) (*Mod Pathol.* 2002;15:973). Occasionally, hyperlobated or multinucleated tumor cells may be seen, some with nuclear pseudoinclusions. Mitotic figures are found without difficulty, and atypical forms may be present (e-Fig. 26.9). Necrosis is either multifocal (either grossly or microscopically) or extensive and confluent. Within the stroma there may be prominent fibrous bands intersecting the tumor and foci of dystrophic calcification. The stroma can be myxoid.

The distinction between adenoma and carcinoma is established without much difficulty in most cases, but in some cases can be challenging; several histopathologic systems have been proposed to distinguish the two lesions. The three main systems are those of Hough (*Am J Clin Pathol.* 1979;72:390), of van Slooten (*Cancer.* 1985;55:76), and of Weiss (*Am J Surg Pathol.* 1989;13:202). The Weiss system is probably the simplest and the most widely used; according to this system, the presence of 3 or more of the following features in an adrenal cortical neoplasm is highly correlated with subsequent malignant behavior: (i) high nuclear grade (Fuhrman grade system), (ii) more than five mitotic figures per 50 high-power fields, (iii) atypical mitotic figures, (iv) eosinophilic cytoplasm in >75% of tumor cells, (v) diffuse architecture in more than one third of the tumor, (vi) necrosis, (vii) venous (smooth muscle in the wall) invasion, (viii) sinusoidal (no smooth muscle in the wall) invasion, and (ix) capsular invasion. Immunohistochemically, ACC shows a greater level of vimentin expression and a lesser level of expression of low-molecular-weight cytokeratin than adenomas. Ki-67 labeling index and p53 expression are less helpful than pathologic assessment in the differential diagnosis of adenomas and ACC (*Mod Pathol.* 2003;16:742).

It is important to note that children, especially those younger than 5 years, can have adrenal cortical neoplasms that weigh <100 grams (often <50 grams) with marked nuclear enlargement, hyperchromatism, and minimal mitotic activity that are best regarded as "atypical adenomas" rather than well-differentiated ACC (*Am J Surg Pathol.* 2003;27:1005 and *Am J Surg Pathol.* 2003;27:867).

IV. ADRENAL MEDULLARY LESIONS. Major categories of adrenal medullary lesions include medullary hyperplasia, PHEO, and neuroblastic tumors (NBs).

A. Adrenal medullary hyperplasia (AMH) is defined as an increase in the mass of medullary cells with expansion of these cells into areas of the gland that normally do not contain medullary cells, such as the tail. Multiple endocrine neoplasia (MEN) (type IIA, IIB) is the most common setting of AMH, but it is also seen in association with Beckwith–Wiedemann syndrome, neurofibromatosis, somatostatin-rich duodenal carcinoid, cystic fibrosis, and sudden infant death syndrome. Sporadic examples are rare. Diffuse or nodular hyperplasia with multiple nodules is present in both glands in MEN IIA and IIB; medullary tissue is present in both alae (normally it is present in only one ala) or in the tail (normally not present), with increased medullary volume. The microscopic distinction between AMH and normal medulla can be difficult, requiring morphometric evaluation (>10% of adrenal volume is indicative of medullary hyperplasia). Differentiation of medullary hyperplasia from PHEO is more important; some investigators have recommended a size distinction with 1 cm as the demarcation, with nodules >1 cm considered PHEOs (as arbitrary as that may be).

B. PHEO, arising from the chromaffin cells of the adrenal medulla, occurs in all age groups with a peak in the fifth decade of life. By convention, PHEO refers to adrenal, extra-adrenal, and thoracic neoplasms that are hormonally active, whereas paraganglioma refers to neoplasms of the head and neck that are largely inactive (see below). PHEO has been referred to as the "10% tumor": 10% bilateral, 10% extra-adrenal, 10% malignant, 10% in children, and 10% hereditary, although the latter figure may be too low. Hereditary PHEO is characterized by bilaterality and multiplicity; MEN type II, von-Hippel–Lindau disease, neurofibromatosis 1, tuberous sclerosis, and Sturge–Weber syndrome are PHEO-associated syndromes (*Endocr Relat Cancer.* 2007;14:935). Germline mutations in succinate dehydrogenase genes are found in familial PHEO (*Lancet.* 2001;357:1181 and *JAMA.* 2004; 292:943).

Grossly, a sharply circumscribed gray-tan or hemorrhagic mass, measuring 4 cm and weighing 90 grams on average, is present, confined to the gland with remnants of the cortex at the periphery. A nested/nesting pattern with the formation of so-called zellballen is the classic morphology of PHEO (e-**Fig. 26.10**), but other patterns include trabecular, mixed alveolar and trabecular, solid and diffuse, and (rarely) spindle cell formations (usually focal). The chromaffin cells often have slightly eosinophilic and finely granular cytoplasm, but they may be amphophilic to basophilic or even oncocytic (e-**Fig. 26.11**). A finely vacuolated cytoplasm is present in some cases due to lipid accumulation (e-**Fig. 26.12**). Intracytoplasmic periodic acid–Schiff–positive and diastase-resistant hyaline globules are yet another finding (e-**Fig. 26.13**). Melanin-containing PHEOs are rare but well documented (*Hum Pathol.* 1993;24:420). The polygonal cells can vary in size and nuclear detail, with marked enlargement and hyperchromasia, although less impressive cytologic atypia is often present (e-**Fig. 26.14**). Prominent nucleoli and nuclear pseudoinclusions are additional but inconsistent findings (e-**Fig. 26.14**). Mitotic figures, if seen, are not an indication of malignancy. The stroma may exhibit extensive hyalinization, fibrosis, or rarely amyloid deposition, and the vasculature may be prominent. The chromaffin cells are positive for chromogranin A, synaptophysin, and cytokeratin in 25% of cases (*Arch Pathol Lab Med.* 1990;114:506); these cells do not express epithelial membrane antigen (EMA), melan A, or inhibin. S-100 labels sustentacular cells that are usually located at the periphery of the nests.

Only the presence of metastatic disease to the skeletal system (ribs and spine), liver, lung, or regional lymph nodes establishes the malignancy of a PHEO (e-**Fig. 26.15**). Even capsular and/or vascular invasion is not a completely reliable indication of a malignant PHEO. However, the presence of confluent necrosis and a size in excess of 100 grams should cause concern regarding the malignant potential of that particular PHEO.

Composite PHEO (e-**Fig. 26.16**), a rare variant, is defined in most cases as a PHEO with a ganglioneuromatous (80%), ganglioneuroblastomatous (20%), neuroblastomatous (<1%), malignant peripheral nerve sheath tumor, or neuroendocrine carcinoma (extremely rare) component. These tumors are reported in the clinical settings of neurofibromatosis I and MEN IIA (*Am J Surg Pathol.* 1993;17:837 and *Am J Surg Pathol.* 1997;21:102).

C. **Neuroblastic tumors,** embryonal tumors arising from the sympathoadrenal neuroendocrine system, are the most common extracranial solid malignancies of childhood (*Nat Rev Cancer.* 2003;3:203). About 600 new cases are diagnosed each year in the United States. Approximately 98% of NBs are diagnosed by 10 years of age, and 85–90% are detected before 5 years of age. The abdomen and retroperitoneum is the site of clinical presentation in 65% of cases, and 50% of these arise in the adrenal medulla.

1. **Neuroblastoma (NB)** is best characterized as having a variegated appearance because the tumor's gross features are dependent on its morphologic composition and on secondary changes such as hemorrhage, yellowish foci of necrosis and calcification, cystic degeneration, and fibrosis; some or all of these findings may be found in any one tumor. It is often difficult to judge whether some of the gross changes are spontaneous because the resection may be preceded by chemotherapy and/or radiation therapy. A well-circumscribed soft gray-tan tumor, measuring 2 to 10 cm in dimension, with or without hemorrhage and calcifications, is the common appearance of a poorly differentiated NB, differentiating NB, or a ganglioneuroblastoma (GNB) with intermixed features. A neuroblastic tumor with one or more discrete nodules with variable dimensions in a background of grayish-tan, firm tissue is the gross appearance of nodular GNB. Some NBs are entirely hemorrhagic, and have undergone near total cystic degeneration (with or without calcifications).

Histologically, the tumor cells are small with hyperchromatic nuclei and scanty cytoplasm, and are arranged in sheets (e-**Fig. 26.17**). The cell borders are indistinct. A lobular appearance at low power is associated with thin fibrovascular septa between nests of tumor cells. Homer Wright rosettes or pseudorosettes (e-**Fig. 26.18**) have a central collection of neuropil surrounded by a mantle of neuroblasts. Based on the presence of neuropil and the proportion of tumor cells differentiating toward ganglion cells, NBs are further divided into undifferentiated, poorly differentiated, and differentiating subtypes; neuropil is not present in undifferentiated NBs but is present in poorly differentiated and differentiating NBs (e-**Fig. 26.19**). Poorly differentiated and differentiating NBs are distinguished by the percentage of tumor cells showing ganglionic differentiation, which by definition is <5% in the former and at least 5% in the latter. Ganglionic differentiation is recognized by the presence of enlarged cells with eccentric nuclei with vesicular chromatin and a single prominent nucleolus, with increased eosinophilic or amphophilic cytoplasm; the diameter of the differentiating neuroblasts must be at least twice that of the nucleus. In all subtypes of NBs, the Schwannian stroma must account for <50% of the tumor (Schwannian stroma-poor); Schwannian stroma is not neuropil, but has a spindle cell, almost fibrous appearance with features resembling those of a schwannoma.

An undifferentiated NB is composed of a relatively monotonous population of malignant round cells without a fibrillary network. These tumors must be differentiated from other similar appearing round cell neoplasms, especially malignant rhabdoid tumor. Undifferentiated NB expresses vimentin and chromogranin, and clinically can be nonfunctioning.

The prognosis of neuroblastoma is based on multiple factors: age, primary site, pathologic subtype, mitosis–karyorrhexis index (MKI), biologic markers, and stage of disease (localization and metastasis) (Table 26.2). Despite all of the pathologic and molecular refinements in the characterization of NBs, age (<1 year old) and pathologic stage are the most significant determinants of outcome (*Lancet*. 2007;369:2106). Patients with extra-adrenal tumors do better than those with adrenal-based NBs, and undifferentiated NBs generally have a worse outcome than the other subtypes, although such differences are influenced by age.

NBs are categorized into favorable and unfavorable pathologic groups based on features that incorporate age at diagnosis and the MKI (Table 26.3). The latter is calculated on the number of mitotic or karyorrhectic tumor cells based on 5,000 cells in random fields; in all practicality, "high" or "low" MKI NB is easily recognized after a high magnification examination of several

TABLE 26.2   International Neuroblastoma Staging System

Stage	Definition
1	Localized tumor with gross complete excision, with or without microscopic residual disease, negative lymph nodes
2A	Unilateral tumor with incomplete gross excision, negative lymph nodes
2B	Unilateral tumor with complete or incomplete gross excision, positive ipsilateral lymph nodes, but negative contralateral lymph nodes
3	Unresectable unilateral tumor infiltrating cross the midline (positive or negative lymph nodes) or localized unilateral tumor with positive contralateral lymph nodes
4	Tumor disseminated to distant lymph node groups, bone, bone marrow, liver, skin, and/or other organs (except as defined in 4s)
4s	Stage 1 to 2 tumor but with dissemination that is limited to skin, bone marrow, and/or liver

TABLE 26.3	International Neuroblastoma Pathology Committee Age-Linked Prognostic Classification

Age group	Favorable histology	Unfavorable histology
Any age	Ganglioneuroma Ganglioneuroblastoma, intermixed subtype	Neuroblastoma, undifferentiated subtype (any mitosis–karyorrhexis index [MKI])
<1.5 years	Neuroblastoma, poorly differentiated with low or intermediate MKI (≤4% or 200/5,000 cells) Ganglioneuroblastoma, nodular, with poorly differentiated nodule(s) or differentiating nodule(s) with low to intermediate MKI	Neuroblastoma, poorly differentiated with high MKI Neuroblastoma, differentiating with high MKI (>4% or 200/5,000 cells) Ganglioneuroblastoma, nodular, with undifferentiated nodules or nodules with high MKI
1.5 to 5 years	Neuroblastoma, differentiating with low MKI Ganglioneuroblastoma, nodular, with differentiating nodule(s) with low MKI	Neuroblastoma, poorly differentiated (any MKI) Neuroblastoma, differentiating with intermediate or high MKI (>2% or >100/5,000 cells) Ganglioneuroblastoma, nodular, with undifferentiated or differentiating nodule(s) or nodule(s) with intermediate to high MKI
>5 years		Neuroblastoma, any subtype ganglioneuroblastoma, nodular type

References: *Cancer.* 2003;298:2274; *Arch Pathol Lab Med.* 2005;129:874.

microscopic fields. Tumors with favorable histopathology on the basis of histologic subtype and low MKI have better outcomes. The molecular genetic markers associated with a poor prognosis are *N-myc* amplification and several chromosomal abnormalities (1p deletion, 14q deletion, 11q deletion, 17q gain) (*Lancet Oncol.* 2003;4:472 and *Gene.* 2004;325:1).

2. **GNB,** seen in young children, tends to present in the retroperitoneum or mediastinum more often than in the adrenal gland. Intermixed GNB has a uniform grayish-white to tan mucoid appearance, whereas nodular GNB has grossly visible nodules or discrete microscopic foci of poorly differentiated neuroblasts. The Schwannian stroma accounts for at least 50% of the tumor in both types, and well-defined microscopic foci of neuroblastic cells show various stages of neuroblastic maturation to ganglionic differentiation in a fibrillary and neuromatous or Schwannian background (e-**Fig. 26.20**). The macroscopic nodules are composed of neuroblasts in varying phases of differentiation; these are sharply demarcated from the surrounding stroma. Tumors in which the nodules have a high MKI have a worse prognosis than those with nodules that have a low MKI; the other parameters used to group NBs into favorable and unfavorable categories also apply to GNB in general (*Cancer.* 2003;98:2274). The overall favorable prognosis of GNB is related to the fact that most tumors are localized and have intermixed rather than nodular features.

3. **Ganglioneuroma (GN)** is the most common neoplasm of the sympathetic nervous system in adults, and occurs in posterior mediastinum, retroperitoneum, and rarely in the adrenal gland. The tumor is grossly a solid, circumscribed, encapsulated homogenous gray-white mass, measuring 5 to 10 cm. Mature GN is characterized by mature scattered single cells or groups of cells in a neuromatous stroma (e-**Fig. 26.21**), whereas the maturing GN has a similar pattern of

cellular distribution of differentiating neuroblasts and ganglion cells. The differential diagnosis of maturing GN is intermixed GNB, but the stroma should constitute >50% of the tumor in the former.

V. OTHER ADRENAL PARENCHYMAL LESIONS

A. Myelolipoma accounts for <5% of primary adrenal tumors and is usually detected incidentally on imaging studies of the abdomen. Hemorrhage with pain is a rare presentation. Grossly, the tumor is a unilateral mass with a soft yellow to red surface, depending on the fat content and amount of hemorrhage. The usual microscopic appearance includes varying proportions of mature adipose tissue admixed with hematopoietic elements showing normal trilineage hematopoiesis (e-Fig. 26.22). Clonality has been demonstrated (*Am J Surg Pathol.* 2006;30:838). Lipoma, angiomyolipoma, and liposarcoma are in the differential diagnosis. Extra-adrenal presentations include the lung, mediastinum, renal hilum, and retro-peritoneum.

B. Adenomatoid tumor, like myelolipoma, is detected as an "incidentaloma." Grossly, the tumor is a well-circumscribed solid (or solid and cystic) mass that measures from 0.5 to 9 cm. Microscopically, the tumor is composed of tubules, cysts, papillary structures, and occasional solid sheets of flattened or cuboidal cells (e-Fig. 26.23). The tumor cells may have cytoplasmic vacuoles with signet-ring features (e-Fig. 26.24), but are mucicarmine negative for mucin. The tumor cells have the same immunophenotype as mesothelial cells: positive for expression of cytokeratin, calretinin, and WT-1. Adenomatoid tumor is believed to arise from mesothelial inclusions within the adrenal gland. The main differential diagnoses include lymphangioma, metastatic carcinoma, and vascular tumors.

C. Adrenal mesenchymal tumors include lipoma, Schwannoma, hemangioma, leiomyoma, and solitary fibrous tumor, among others. Hemangioblastoma of the adrenal gland has features of its cerebellum counterpart (*Am J Surg Pathol.* 2007;31:1545). Primary malignant mesenchymal tumors include leiomyosarcoma, angiosarcoma, malignant peripheral nerve sheath tumor, and Wilms tumor.

VI. ADRENAL CYSTS

are relatively uncommon and are divided into four categories: parasitic cysts (7%), epithelial cysts (9%), pseudocysts (39%), and endothelial cysts (45%) (*Arch Surg.* 1966;92:131).

A. Pseudocysts are discovered more frequently due to increased use of imaging examination. They are well-defined cysts with water-like density and a median size of 6 to 10 cm in diameter. Some pseudocysts are associated with cortical or medullary neoplasms including neuroblastoma and PHEO (*Cancer.* 2004;101:1537). Grossly, pseudocysts are unilocular and filled with yellow-brown or bloody amorphous material. The cyst wall has a thickness of 1 to 5 mm, and is composed of dense hyalinized connective tissue that may contain focal calcifications or even metaplastic bone formation. Entrapped cortical tissue may also be present in the cyst wall. The smooth muscle in the wall is continuous with the smooth muscle of the adrenal vein. By definition, the cyst does not contain a lining.

B. Endothelial or vascular cysts including lymphangiomas and hemangiomas are extremely rare. Endothelial cysts are usually well circumscribed and are surrounded by a capsule. Lymphangiomatous cysts are composed of numerous small cysts of varying size lined by a single layer of flat endothelial cells. Most hemangiomas are discovered at autopsy and are small. Clinically detected hemangiomas are unilateral and have cavernous features.

C. Epithelial cysts are divided into true glandular cysts and embryonal cysts. Some investigators consider cystic adrenal tumors in the category of epithelial cysts.

D. Parasitic cysts are a manifestation of echinococcal infection.

VII. HEMATOLYMPHOID TUMORS

are represented by secondary leukemic or lymphomatous involvement. Rare examples of primary B or T lymphomas have been reported.

VIII. METASTATIC NEOPLASMS

to the adrenal gland are common. The primary sites of the metastatic tumors in decreasing order are from the breast and lung (e-Fig. 26.25), kidney, stomach, and colon (e-Fig. 26.26). Other primary neoplasms that metastasize to the adrenal gland include melanoma (e-Fig. 26.27), hepatocellular carcinoma, and urothelial carcinoma. About 40% of metastasis to the adrenal are bilateral, and they cause adrenal cortical insufficiency in 20–30% of cases. The gland may or may not be enlarged, but the cortex may be inapparent because the cortex is preferentially involved.

Metastatic hepatocellular and renal cell carcinomas can be mistaken for or included in the differential diagnosis of ACC. Immunohistochemistry can be used to distinguish these neoplasms. ACCs express vimentin, melan A (MART-1), and inhibin, but do not express cytokeratin or EMA. Hepatocellular carcinoma is positive for hepar-1 and has a canalicular pattern if labeled with polyclonal carcinoembryogenic antigen (CEA) and CD10. Renal cell carcinoma, especially the clear cell type, is usually positive for RCC and CD10. Malignant melanoma is HMB45 and S-100–positive, but negative for inhibin (although primary adrenal melanoma has been reported, it is extremely rare).

IX. EXTRA-ADRENAL PARAGANGLIOMAS

A. Normal anatomy and histology. The extra-adrenal paraganglia are divided into two broad categories: those related to the parasympathetic system and those of the sympathetic nervous system. The former are concentrated in the head, neck, and mediastinum and can be further divided into jugulotympanic, vagal, carotid body, laryngeal, and aorticopulmonary paraganglia; among these, the carotid body and at least some of the aorticopulmonary paraganglia have chemoreceptor function. The aorticopulmonary paraganglia are distributed in parallel to the sympathetic nervous system along the paravertebral and para-aortic axis and are divided into cervical, intrathoracic, and intra-abdominal groups. Paraganglia are also distributed in the bladder, prostate, and gallbladder. All paraganglia have a similar composition of chief cells arranged in well-defined nests or Zellballen surrounded by peripheral sustentacular cells.

B. Extra-adrenal paragangliomas, named according to their anatomic location, include tumors arising in the head and neck but exclude PHEOs, although there remains some discussion about the proper designation of intrathoracic and extra-adrenal neoplasms as PHEO or paraganglioma (*JAMA.* 2004;292:943 and *Endocr Pathol.* 2006;17:321). Extra-adrenal paragangliomas (e-**Fig. 26.28**) have the same architecture as PHEOs. Cytokeratin may be expressed in 20–25% of PHEOs, but is not expressed in extra-adrenal paragangliomas with the exception of gangliocytic paraganglioma and paraganglioma of the cauda equina.

1. Paragangliomas of the extra-adrenal sympathetic nervous system include those of the cervical, intrathoracic, and intra-abdominal groups.

  a. Cervical sympathetic paragangliomas are extremely rare (fewer than 10 cases reported). They must be distinguished from a carotid body tumor.

  b. Intrathoracic sympathetic paragangliomas, typically arising in the posterior mediastinum along the sympathetic chain, are different from aorticopulmonary paragangliomas, which present in the anterior mediastinum. Distant metastases occur in 7–12% of cases.

  c. Intra-abdominal paragangliomas account for 85% of extra-adrenal sympathetic paragangliomas and are classified in three major groups: superior para-aortic (45% of cases; in the vicinity of the adrenal gland and renal hilum or pedicle), inferior para-aortic (30% of cases; below the inferior pole of the kidney and along the iliac vessels and from the organ of Zuckerkandl), or urinary bladder (10% of cases).

  d. Other rare sites include gallbladder, kidney, urethra, prostate, spermatic cord, ovary, and vagina.

2. Paragangliomas in the head, neck, and mediastinum include several groups based on their anatomic location: jugulotympanic, vagal, and laryngeal. Only 1% of these tumors are functional, and 10–50% are familial. The rate of malignancy varies from site to site; it is lowest (1–3%) in jugulotympanic and laryngeal paragangliomas, and highest (20%) in aorticopulmonary paragangliomas.

  a. Jugulotympanic paragangliomas include the jugular type (present at the jugular foramen with compression of the cranial nerves IX–XII) and the tympanic type (present with hearing disturbance). Small tympanic paragangliomas can present as an aural polyp or extend into the external ear canal.

b. Vagal paragangliomas present as a lateral neck mass with extension to the skull base. Approximately 30% have vagal manifestations of vocal cord paralysis, hoarseness, and dysphagia.

c. Laryngeal paragangliomas arise more often from the superior than the inferior laryngeal paraganglia. The most common symptom of laryngeal paragangliomas is hoarseness.

d. Carotid body paragangliomas present as a slowly growing painless mass in the middle or upper neck.

e. Aorticopulmonary paragangliomas can cause chest pain, dysphagia, or hoarseness due to compression. The pericardium or heart may be involved.

3. **Gangliocytic paraganglioma,** arising in the periampullary portion of the duodenum, is also rarely seen in the nasopharynx, lung, esophagus, mediastinum, pancreas, and appendix. It occurs in patients over a wide age range as a solitary, polypoid mass that projects into the lumen of the intestine and measures up to 7 cm in diameter. It is an infiltrative neoplasm composed of three cell types in variable proportions, namely spindle cells, ganglion cells, and epithelioid cells (**e-Fig. 26.29**). The spindle cells are elongated and have wavy nuclei resembling Schwannian cells, with S-100 and neurofilament immunopositivity; these cells can envelope the ganglion and epithelioid cells, analogous to sustentacular cells. The larger epithelioid cells (**e-Fig. 26.30**) are arranged in solid nests, ribbons, or pseudoglandular or papillary structures and have neuroendocrine features including granular eosinophilic to amphophilic cytoplasm with uniform oval nuclei and finely stippled chromatin; these cells express cytokeratin, chromogranin, and synaptophysin. Ganglion cells have typical features, but there may be an apparent morphologic continuum with the epithelioid cell population. Recurrences are rare, but metastatic behavior is restricted to regional lymph nodes (*J Gastrointest Surg.* 2007;11:1351). The only reported case with distant metastasis (to bone) is a pancreatic gangliocytic paraganglioma (*Ann Chir.* 2003;128:336).

CYTOLOGY OF THE ADRENAL GLAND
Jing Zhai

I. **INTRODUCTION.** Fine needle aspiration (FNA) is frequently used to evaluate adrenal gland mass lesions, and is performed under percutaneous computed tomography (CT) and ultrasound guidance, or endoscopic ultrasound guidance for left adrenal lesions (*Diagn Cytopathol.* 2005;33:26). FNA diagnosis of adrenal lesions has an accuracy of 98% and specificity of 100% (*Diagn Cytopathol.* 1999;21:92). FNA biopsy of PHEO is regarded as a relative contradiction due to possible induction of hypertensive crisis (*Radiology.* 1986;159:733).

II. **SPECIFIC NEOPLASMS**

A. **Myelolipoma.** The aspirate shows a mixture of mature adipose tissue and hematopoietic elements, including nucleated red blood cells, granulocytes and precursors, and megakaryocytes (*Acta Cytol.* 1991;35:353).

B. **Adrenal cortical neoplasms.** The cytological distinction between adrenal cortical hyperplasia, adrenal cortical adenoma, ACC, and normal adrenal cortical cells is not always possible. Radiological correlation is essential.

1. **Adrenal cortical adenoma** yields moderately cellular smears that contain poorly cohesive sheets of epithelial cells with ill defined and vacuolated cytoplasm and abundant stripped small round uniform nuclei. Bubbly and vacuolated lipid background is prominent (**e-Fig. 26.31**). Scattered cells show nuclear atypia. Some cells may have cytoplasmic lipofuscin (*Diagn Cytopathol.* 1999;21:92; *Acta Cytol.* 1995;39:843; *Acta Cytol.* 1998;42:1352).

2. **ACC** yields richly cellular aspirates. It consists of more frequent single cells that have marked nuclear atypia, intact granular cytoplasm, eccentric nuclei, and

necrosis (e-**Fig. 26.32**). The cytological diagnosis of a well-differentiated ACC is difficult (*Acta Cytol.* 1997;41:385).

C. PHEO. The cytomorphology shows similarity to that of other neuroendocrine tumors. The aspirate contains abundant isolated and loose clusters of malignant cells with intervening vasculature (e-**Fig. 26.33**). The isolated polygonal or spindle shaped cells exhibit poorly defined fragile cytoplasm and fine granular salt-and-pepper chromatin (e-**Fig. 26.34**). Red cytoplasmic granules can be seen on Romanowsky-type stains (*Acta Cytol.* 1999;43:207).

D. Metastatic malignancy. The most common malignancies metastatic to the adrenal gland are adenocarcinoma of the breast or lung (e-**Fig. 26.35**). The confirmation of metastasis is straightforward given a known malignant history. It is important to integrate clinical, laboratory, radiological, cytological, and immunocytochemical findings to differentiate primary neoplasms from metastasis (*Acta Cytol.* 1995;39:843).

Suggested Readings

DeLellis RA, Mangray S. The adrenal glands. In: Mills SE, ed. *Steinberg's Diagnostic Surgical Pathology*, 4th ed. Philadelphia: Lippincott Williams &Wilkins; 2004:621–668.

DeLellis RA, Lloyd RV, Heitz PU, Eng C, eds. The Adrenal Gland. In: *Pathology and Genetics of Tumors of Endocrine Organs* (WHO Classification of Tumors). Lyon, France: IACR Press; 2004:135–173.

Lack EE. Tumors of the adrenal gland and extra-adrenal paraganglia. In: *Atlas of Tumor Pathology, Third Series*. Washington, DC: American Registry of Pathology; 1997.

Rosai J. Adrenal gland and other paraganglia. In: Rosai J, ed. *Rosai and Ackerman's Surgical Pathology*, 9th ed. St. Louis, MO: Mosby; 2004:1115–1147.

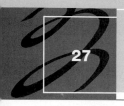

27 PITUITARY GLAND
Sushama Patil and Arie Perry

I. **NORMAL ANATOMY AND HISTOLOGY.** The pituitary gland, composed of adenohypophysis (anterior pituitary) and neurohypophysis (posterior pituitary or pars nervosa), is located at the base of the brain, beneath the hypothalamus within the sella turcica of the sphenoid bone. Most of the pituitary gland (about 75%) is made up of adenohypophysis, which in turn is divided into pars tuberalis (infundibular), pars intermedia, and pars distalis. Located between the two lobes is the vestigial intermediate lobe, which contains remnants of Rathke's cleft (glandlike cystic spaces).

Microscopically, normal adenohypophysis (**e-Fig. 27. 1**)* is composed of three different cell types, namely, acidophilic, basophilic, and chromophobic cells, all of which are arranged in an acinar pattern. These acini are separated by a delicate fibrovascular stroma best visualized on reticulin stains. Occasionally with aging, basophilic and chromophobic cells extend into the neurohypophysis; this phenomenon is termed basophilic invasion, and it should not be misinterpreted as infiltration into the neurohypophysis. The posterior pituitary is largely composed of axons and axon terminals and sometimes axonal swellings (spheroids) called Herring bodies, which contain vasopressin and oxytocin. Specialized glial cells are also part of the posterior pituitary and they accompany the axons. Ectopic pituitary tissue can be found in the nasal cavity, sphenoid sinus, or rarely within ovarian teratomas.

II. **INTRAOPERATIVE EVALUATION AND TISSUE HANDLING.** Intraoperative evaluations are frequently requested for pituitary neoplasms, most often to confirm the clinical diagnosis of pituitary adenoma. Although frozen sections provide adequate information to make an intraoperative diagnosis, imprint smears or touch preps are particularly useful in this instance. Smears provide similar information, but in a more timely fashion, and without nuclear freezing artifacts (**e-Fig. 27.2**). More importantly, the minimal tissue needed for preparing smears makes it possible to submit the remaining tissue for paraffin embedding free from freeze artifacts. During the intraoperative evaluation, part of the tissue (1 mm) should also be submitted in 3% glutaraldehyde for possible electron microscopic studies, particularly for adenomas with unusual clinical or immunohistochemical features.

III. **NONNEOPLASTIC LESIONS**
- A. **Pituitary hyperplasia.** Diffuse expansion of pituitary acini is the histologic hallmark of pituitary hyperplasia, although histologic documentation is often difficult. Reticulin stains show expanded acini. Nodular expansion of acini with one single hormonal cell type is noted in a variety of clinical scenarios, including pregnancy and estrogen therapy.
- B. **Pituitary apoplexy.** Spontaneous hemorrhage and infarction of nonneoplastic or neoplastic pituitary results in hypopituitarism and represents a medical emergency. Reticulin and immunohistochemical stains are sometime helpful in partially preserved regions of markedly necrotic specimens.
- C. **Lymphocytic hypophysitis** is a rare autoimmune disorder of the adenohypophysis that results in its destruction with resulting panhypopituitarism. Lymphocytic hypophysitis occurs exclusively in postpartum women. Subsets of patients also have other associated autoimmune disorders. Microscopically, the anterior pituitary

---

*All e-figures are available online via the Solution Site Image Bank.

demonstrates lymphoplasmacytic infiltrates without granuloma formation. The disease is often fatal if untreated.

D. Rathke's cleft cyst is a developmental abnormality located between the anterior and posterior lobes, often detected incidentally. Lesions larger than 1 cm are usually symptomatic (i.e., cause hyperprolactinemia, visual disturbances). The cyst is lined by cuboidal to columnar epithelium that may or may not be ciliated. Often goblet cells are noted, and the cyst contents are mucoid. Surgical resection is curative.

E. Other. The pituitary is also occasionally involved by systemic histiocytic disorders, such as Langerhans cell histiocytosis, Rosai–Dorfman disease, Erdheim–Chester disease, and xanthoma disseminatum.

IV. BENIGN NEOPLASMS

A. Pituitary adenomas are by far the most common sellar neoplasms. Tumors <1 cm are typically identified as microadenomas, and those >1 cm are categorized as macroadenomas. Microadenomas are most often functional (hormone producing) and therefore draw clinical attention early, particularly with Cushing disease. Nonfunctional tumors account for one third of all adenomas, are typically silent, and grow to a large size. Often, large tumors produce so-called stalk effect, in which mild to moderate elevations of prolactin (PRL) hormone result from stalk compression caused by the growing tumor mass. This mass blocks the transport of dopamine and thus releases the anterior pituitary from the inhibitory control by the hypothalamus. Macroadenomas compress normal pituitary tissue and cause panhypopituitarism. Nonfunctioning adenomas are often referred to as null cell adenomas based on their morphologic features, immunoprofile (hormonal), and ultrastructural analysis. However, most clinically nonfunctional adenomas are now known to be silent gonadotroph adenomas, based on evidence of limited production of gonadotrophic hormones using sensitive immunohistochemical or in situ hybridization methods of detection.

Microscopically (e-**Fig. 27.3**), adenomas are composed of patternless sheets of monomorphic tumor cells (typically larger than normal pituicytes) with round and regular nuclei, a delicate stippled chromatin pattern (salt and pepper), and inconspicuous nucleoli. In comparison with normal pituitary, they are relatively reticulin-poor, the latter stain highlighting large nodules rather than small acini. Occasionally, adenomas exhibit moderate to marked cytologic atypia, but this does not translate into aggressive behavior unless accompanied by elevated mitotic and proliferation indices. Mitotic figures are typically rare. Immunohistochemically, the majority of pituitary adenomas show reactivity for synaptophysin. Hormone immunoprofiles and ultrastructural analyses are used to subtype adenomas. The vast majority of pituitary adenomas follow a benign clinical course.

Rough histologic clues toward adenoma biology (hormonal secretion patterns) include the presence of calcium and amyloid bodies (rare) in prolactinoma. High nuclear to cytoplasmic (N/C) ratios and fibrosis are common in medically treated prolactinoma. Perivascular pseudorosettes usually indicate a gonadotrophic or null cell adenoma (e-**Fig. 27.4**). Crooke's hyaline (ringlike cytoplasmic cytokeratin inclusions) is most commonly accumulated in nonneoplastic corticotrophic cells in patients with hypercortisolism of any cause (see section on corticotroph adenoma). Strong periodic acid–Schiff (PAS) staining suggests a corticotroph adenoma, whereas weak PAS positivity is a sign of glycoprotein adenoma such as follicle-stimulating hormone (FSH), luteinizing hormone (LH), and thyroid-stimulating hormone (TSH) secreting tumors. Cytokeratin positive, paranuclear fibrous bodies most often indicate a growth hormone (GH)-producing adenoma.

B. Atypical pituitary adenomas are similar to benign pituitary adenomas histologically and in their clinical presentations except for elevated mitotic and proliferative indices (nuclear Ki-67/MIB-1 labeling >3%). These tumors also show elevated nuclear p53 labeling, and clinically recur more often than benign adenomas. The tumor cells are often positive for PRL, GH, or adrenocorticotrophic hormone (ACTH).

C. Prolactinoma. Also called lactotrophic adenoma, prolactinoma occurs commonly in women and presents clinically with amenorrhea and galactorrhea. In contrast, men with prolactinoma are either asymptomatic or present with decreased libido.

Patients with prolactinomas are often treated medically with a dopamine agonist (e.g., bromocriptine) that is cytostatic rather than cytotoxic. Tumors resected post-therapy usually show interstitial fibrosis and reduced cell size with shrunken cytoplasm resulting from cellular growth arrest or atrophy. Microscopically, tumor cells have a high N/C ratio and may at first glance resemble a small cell carcinoma. However, they are usually at least focally positive for PRL and display a low mitotic/proliferative index.

D. Corticotroph (ACTH-producing) adenoma. Corticotroph adenomas most often present as microadenomas and account for 20% of all pituitary adenomas. The tumors may be so small and soft that they are often inadvertently aspirated by the surgeon before any tissue can be collected for pathologic evaluation. In such cases in which there are no abnormal histopathologic findings, a postoperative drop in the patient's ACTH levels nonetheless implies that the tumor was removed. ACTH adenomas arise in the central region of the gland, where most corticotrophic cells are located. Microscopically, they are composed of monomorphic cells that are usually basophilic and deeply PAS positive. Crooke's hyaline results from hypercortisolism relentlessly stimulating nonneoplastic corticotrophic cells via a negative feedback loop (e-**Fig. 27.5**). A subset of adenomas are immunopositive for ACTH but biochemically and clinically negative for Cushing's syndrome; such adenomas are termed silent corticotroph adenoma and are often invasive and large (macroadenomas).

E. Somatotroph (GH cell) adenoma. This subgroup of pituitary adenomas includes tumors with exclusive GH production (PAS negative), tumors producing GH and PRL (mammosomatotroph adenomas), and plurihormonal adenomas (most positive for GH, PRL, and TSH). Somatotroph adenomas (e-**Fig. 27.6**) have two different cell types: tumor cells (with sparse granulation, weak GH immunoreactivity, and paranuclear whorls known as fibrous bodies) and densely granulated cells (with strong GH immunoreactivity).

F. Gonadotroph adenomas. These adenomas are often nonfunctional, grow to a very large size, and produce mass effects. These tumors exhibit marked variability for hormonal markers. Some tumors exhibit immunoreactivity for the β subunits of FSH and LH, with or without immunoreactivity for the α subunits. The nonfunctionality of these tumors is thought to result from failure to incorporate α and β subunits of the two hormones.

V. PITUITARY CARCINOMA. Pituitary carcinoma is a very rare neoplasm diagnosed by the presence of brain invasion or extracranial metastasis. The Ki-67/MIB-1 and p53 labeling indices are typically high, and the tumors are usually PRL, GH, or ACTH immunopositive.

TESTIS AND PARATESTIS
Kiran R. Vij and Peter A. Humphrey

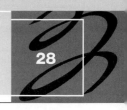

I. NORMAL ANATOMY. The normal adult testis is an ovoid paired organ, each measuring 4.5 × 2.5 × 3 cm, and weighing approximately 20 grams. They are suspended within scrotal sacs by spermatic cords. The testis is covered by a capsule composed of an outer tunica vaginalis lined by mesothelium, the collagenous tunica albuginea, and the inner tunica vasculora. The tunica vaginalis forms a sac filled with serous fluid. The posterior portion of the testis not covered by a capsule is called the mediastinum and contains blood vessels, nerves, lymphatics, and the extratesticular rete testis.

The testicular parenchyma is subdivided into lobules containing seminiferous tubules separated by fibrous septae. The terminal portions of the seminiferous tubules drain into the tubuli recti that connect to the tubules of the rete testis at the mediastinum. The tubules of the rete testis anastomose with the ductuli efferentes, which form the head of the epididymis and empty into the vas deferens, which traverses the inguinal canal as a component of the spermatic cord. The testicular artery arises from the aorta and is the major source of vascular supply to the testes. The venous drainage occurs through numerous small veins that form a convoluted mass known as the pampiniform plexus that surrounds the testicular artery. These small veins anastomose to form the right testicular vein, which drains into the inferior vena cava, and two left testicular veins, which drain into the left renal vein.

Histologically, prepubertal and postpubertal seminiferous tubules are quite different. Prepubertal tubules are small, with few or no lumina, and contain mostly Sertoli cells with a few primordial germ cells (e-Fig. 28.1).* Postpubertal seminiferous tubules are larger and harbor Sertoli cells and germ cells at varying stages of maturation (e-Fig. 28.2). The Sertoli cells abut the basement membrane and are aligned perpendicular to the membrane; their nuclei are round to oval with prominent nucleoli, and the cytoplasm has Charcot–Bottcher crystals, which can occasionally be seen by light microscopy. Within the seminiferous tubules, the least mature germ cells—spermatogonia—are present along the basement membrane, with the most mature cells—elongate spermatids—found at the luminal border. Primary and secondary spermatocytes are found in an adluminal position.

The interstitial tissue between the seminiferous tubules contains Leydig cells, vessels, and connective tissue. Leydig cells are arranged singly and in clusters (e-Fig. 28.3), and can be associated with nerves. They are large and irregularly spherical to polyhedral, with small spherical nuclei and abundant acidophilic cytoplasm. The cytoplasm can exhibit lipofuscin and rod-shaped Reinke crystals.

II. GROSS EXAMINATION, TISSUE SAMPLING, AND HISTOLOGIC SLIDE PREPARATION. Tissue samples of the testes received for surgical pathologic examination include testicular biopsies, and unilateral and bilateral orchiectomy specimens. Retroperitoneal lymph node dissection can be performed as part of a staging maneuver for testicular cancer.

    A. Fine needle aspiration biopsy of the testis in infertile patients (with sperm aspiration and cytopathologic examination) is occasionally performed. Cytological touch imprints or wet preparations may be made at the time of open testicular biopsy in infertile patients to rapidly identify the presence of sperm. The role of cytology in the evaluation of testicular tumors is limited to diagnosis of lymph node metastases by

---

*All e-figures are available online via the Solution Site Image Bank.

fine needle aspiration. Although seminomas can usually be differentiated from non-seminomatous tumors, subtyping of nonseminomatous tumors can not be reliably performed by cytology.

B. **Testicular biopsies,** which can be open or percutaneous, are typically performed for evaluation of infertility. They are usually contraindicated in the evaluation of solid testicular masses, with the possible exception of epidermoid cysts, which can be removed by excisional biopsy. Testicular biopsy specimens are usually received in Bouin's fixative. An accurate documentation of the number and size of the biopsy fragments and exact site(s) of the biopsy for each container should be made during gross dictation. The biopsy fragments should be inked with hematoxylin to facilitate identification during embedding, wrapped in lens paper, placed between sponges, and processed entirely. Three hematoxylin and eosin (H&E)-stained slides, each with three to four serial sections, are prepared from each block.

C. **Unilateral simple orchiectomy** is performed in cases of testicular torsion. Gross examination of the testis similar to that for tumor cases should be performed. One section of the testicular parenchyma in relation to the capsule, and a section each of the epididymis and spermatic cord, should be submitted with description and sampling of focal lesions.

D. **Radical orchiectomy** is performed for testicular tumors. The specimen consists of the testis and paratesticular organs (surrounding tunica vaginalis, epididymis, soft tissue, and a segment of spermatic cord). In cases of tumor resection, the specimen should ideally be sent fresh and intact to the surgical pathology laboratory for immediate gross examination. Alternatively, when delay is anticipated, the specimen is placed in 10% buffered formalin and sent intact. In such cases, tumor morphology is often suboptimal due to poor fixation. The surgeon may occasionally bisect the specimen to aid fixation. This approach is not recommended as it prevents evaluation of involvement of the tunica by the tumor as well as procurement of fresh tissue for ancillary studies.

The specimen is weighed, and measurements are recorded in three dimensions. The length and diameter of the resected segment of spermatic cord are noted separately. The external surfaces of the testis and spermatic cord are examined for involvement by tumor. The proximal shave resection margin of the spermatic cord is submitted in a separate cassette. The cord is then serially sectioned and inspected for tumor involvement; representative sections are then submitted proximal to distal. The tunica vaginalis is opened anteriorly to show the tunica albuginea; presence of fluid, if any, within the sac is noted. The testis is then bisected anteroposteriorly through the epididymis. Serial sections are made parallel to this plane. Each slice is examined, and the tumor is described in relation to the epididymis and the tunica albuginea. The size, color, and consistency of the tumor should be noted. Foci of hemorrhage, necrosis, and variegation, as well as multifocality, if present, should be described. Photographs or digital images should be taken and tissue procured for tumor bank and ancillary studies such as flow cytometry and karyotyping, if necessary. The specimen should then be fixed overnight in an adequate amount of 10% buffered formalin before submission of one section per centimeter of tumor. Representative sections should include heterogenous areas and sections of tumor in relation to uninvolved parenchyma, epididymis, and tunica albuginea. One section of grossly normal-appearing parenchyma should be included. If correlation of identified histologic tumor type with serum markers (alpha-fetoprotein [AFP] and human chorionic gonadotropin [hCG]) is not achieved, additional sections should be submitted (note that such correlation will not always be perfect because metastatic deposits may harbor different elements than the primary tumor).

E. **Retroperitoneal lymph node dissection** is performed as a separate procedure. The specimen is received in 10% buffered formalin. During gross examination the tissue fragments should be measured in aggregate and carefully dissected to harvest as many lymph nodes as possible, and the size of the largest and the smallest putative nodes should be noted. Possible foci of tumor encountered during dissection should be measured and sampled. An effort should be made to sample any area(s) suspicious for viable tumor.

F. **Bilateral orchiectomy specimens** may be submitted as part of treatment of carcinoma of the prostate. Gross examination and sectioning are similar to that for unilateral simple orchiectomy. Prostate cancer is rarely encountered within these specimens.

III. **DIAGNOSTIC FEATURES OF BENIGN DISEASES OF THE TESTIS**
   A. **Congenital abnormalities**
      1. **Cryptorchidism** is maldescent of the testis, where the testis is found, after 1 year of age, to be located high in the scrotum, within the inguinal canal, or in an intra-abdominal location. Grossly, the prepubertal undescended testis differs little from normal, but after puberty the undescended testis is smaller. Histologically, there is a progressive loss of germ cells with age, along with decreased size of seminiferous tubules and increased thickness of tubular tunica propria. Often seen in cryptorchid testes are Sertoli cell nodules (e-**Fig. 28.4**), which are foci of tubules containing immature Sertoli cells and laminated calcific deposits. These are likely hyperplastic foci, although they have also been termed tubular adenoma of Pick. The major complications of cryptorchidism are infertility and germ cell neoplasia, ranging from intratubular germ cell neoplasia (IGCN) to invasive germ cell tumors, particularly seminoma, embryonal carcinoma, and embryonal carcinoma/teratoma. For patients >1 year of age, PLAP and CD117 immunostains can be useful in highlighting intratubular germ cell neoplastic cells.
      2. **Anorchism and polyorchism** are absence of testis and more than two testes, respectively.
      3. In **testicular-splenic fusion,** encapsulated splenic tissue is found adjacent to the left testis, which can show germ cell aplasia in the seminiferous tubules.
      4. **Adrenal cortical rests** are usually incidental, millimeter-sized nodules of adrenal cortical tissue that are detected along the pathway of descent of the testis, including along the spermatic cord and testis.
   B. **Infertility.** The causes of infertility may be pretesticular, which include endocrine disorders involving the pituitary and adrenal glands; testicular, including genetic disorders; or posttesticular, which are mainly obstructive and include varicocele and cystic fibrosis. The evaluation of the patient includes a detailed clinical history, physical examination, semen analysis, tests of endocrine function, analysis of sperm function, and serology for antisperm antibody. Testicular biopsy (preferably open biopsy) is indicated in cases where an endocrine dysfunction has been ruled out. Biopsies from patients with azoospermia may show germ cell aplasia (Sertoli cell only) (e-**Fig. 28.5**), maturation arrest (e-**Fig. 28.6**), and/or a normal spermatogenesis that points to an obstructive etiology (Levin HS. In Zhou M, Magi-Galluzzi C, eds. *Genitourinary Pathology.* Philadelphia: Churchill Livingstone Elsevier; 2007: pp. 491–503). Patients with oligospermia show a combination of one or more of the following: tubular hyalinization, fibrosis, hypospermatogenesis, normal or arrested spermatogenesis, and sloughing or disorganization. Although testicular biopsies are rarely performed in cases of endocrine dysfunction, the findings include: small tubules with fibrosis and basement membrane thickening, and Leydig cell aplasia or hyperplasia. Synoptic-style reporting of testicular biopsies for infertility is described in Table 28.1.
   C. **Inflammation and infection.** Most cases of orchitis are due to infection that spreads from the vas deferens and epididymis. Epididymitis is typically more common and severe than orchitis, and is commonly related to urinary tract infection (from the urinary bladder, urethra, or prostate) by *Chlamydia, Neisseria, Escherichia coli,* and *Pseudomonas.* Tissue sampling is not needed for the diagnosis of orchitis and/or epididymitis.
      Infectious agents that can cause orchitis include bacteria, mycobacteria, fungi, viruses, or spirochetes.
      1. **Tuberculous orchitis** always emanates from another site and spreads into the testis from the epididymis or bloodstream. Both testes are usually involved. The testicular inflammatory infiltrate varies from nonspecific to caseating granulomas.
      2. **Mumps orchitis** is caused by a paramyxovirus. Microscopically, there is an initial interstitial lymphocytic inflammatory infiltrate, followed by a mixed infiltrate that can result in tubular atrophy and peritubular fibrosis.

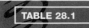

TABLE 28.1	Reporting Infertility Biopsies

1. Method of obtaining sample
   a. Percutaneous testis sperm aspiration
   b. Incisional testis sperm extraction
   c. Orchiectomy/other
2. Presence/absence of testicular tissue
3. Seminiferous tubules
   a. Number
   b. Tunica propria: Normal/thickened
   c. Mean number of spermatozoa/tubule (count 20 tubules)
   d. Most advanced stage of spermatogenesis
   e. Sertoli cells: Present/absent
4. Interstitium
   a. Leydig cells: Present/absent/hyperplastic
   b. Amount of interstitial inflammation
   c. Presence of macrophages and mast cells
5. Extratesticular/Other comments
   a. Epididymis: Present/absent
   b. Vas deferens: Present/absent
   c. Immunohistochemical/special stains
6. Histological diagnoses
   a. The most advanced histological pattern is:
   b. The predominant histological pattern is:

   3. **Syphilitic orchitis** occurs prior to infection of the epididymis. Histologically, peritubular lymphocytes and plasma cells can be seen along with obliterative endarteritis and perivascular plasma cells. Gummas can form an intratesticular mass with central necrosis.
      Other types of orchitis include nonspecific granulomatous orchitis and malakoplakia. Before diagnosing nonspecific granulomatous orchitis, a specific infectious orchitis, sarcoidosis, lymphoma, and exuberant granulomatous inflammation associated with a germ cell neoplasm should be excluded.
   D. **Vascular disorders**
      1. **Systemic vasculitis** can affect the testis, but isolated vasculitis involving only the testis is rare.
      2. **Varicocele** is an abnormal dilatation and tortuosity of veins of the pampiniform plexus of the spermatic cord.
      3. **Torsion and infarction** generally occur in young men and in the setting of abnormal testicular descent. Initially, there is congestion, edema, and hemorrhage, followed by hemorrhagic infarction (e-**Fig. 28.7**).
   E. **Atrophy** can be caused by many factors, but the morphological findings are similar. Grossly, the testis is small. Microscopically, the tubules are decreased in size and the tunica propria is thickened and hyalinized. End-stage atrophic tubules are completely hyalinized, without intraluminal cells (e-**Fig. 28.8**).
IV. **TUMORS OF THE TESTIS.** These are of germ cell origin in the vast majority of cases, with sex cord/gonadal stromal tumors occurring in 4% to 6% of cases. The highest incidence is found in Europe and parts of New Zealand. Populations in Africa and Asia show a much lower incidence. The 2004 World Health Organization classification of the neoplasms of the testis is given in Table 28.2.
   A. **Germ cell tumors.** Clinical diagnosis is usually made when the patient presents with a painless mass in the testis. Associated symptoms such as a dull ache in the scrotum or lower abdomen may be present. Less commonly, patients may present with gynecomastia and thyrotoxicosis. In 10% of cases metastatic disease may produce presenting signs and symptoms. Patients with cryptorchidism are at an increased risk

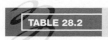

TABLE 28.2	WHO Histological Classification of Tumors of the Testis and Paratestis

Germ cell tumors
Intratubular germ cell neoplasia, unclassified
Other types

Tumors of one histologic type (pure forms)
Seminoma
   Seminoma with syncytiotrophoblastic cells
Spermatocytic seminoma
   Spermatocytic seminoma with sarcoma
Embryonal carcinoma
Yolk sac tumor
Trophoblastic tumors
   Choriocarcinoma
   Trophoblastic neoplasms other than choriocarcinoma
   Monophasic choriocarcinoma
   Placental site trophoblastic tumor
Teratoma
   Dermoid cyst
   Monodermal teratoma
   Teratoma with somatic type malignancies

Tumors of more than one histologic type (mixed forms)
Mixed embryonal carcinoma and teratoma
Mixed teratoma and seminoma
Choriocarcinoma and teratoma / embryonal carcinoma
Others

Sex cord / gonadal stromal tumors
Pure forms
Leydig cell tumor
Malignant Leydig cell tumor
Sertoli cell tumor
   Sertoli cell tumor, lipid-rich variant
   Sclerosing Sertoli cell tumor
   Large cell–calcifying Sertoli cell tumor
Malignant Sertoli cell tumor
Granulosa cell tumor
   Adult type granulosa cell tumor
   Juvenile type granulosa cell tumor
Tumors of the thecoma/fibroma group
   Thecoma
   Fibroma
Sex cord/gonadal stromal tumor
Incompletely differentiated
Sex cord/gonadal stromal tumors, mixed forms
Malignant sex cord/gonadal stromal tumors
Tumors containing both germ cell and sex cord/gonadal stromal elements
   Gonadoblastoma
   Germ cell sex-cord/gonadal stromal tumor, unclassified

(Continued)

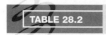

| TABLE 28.2 | WHO Histological Classification of Tumors of the Testis and Paratestis (*Continued*) |

Miscellaneous tumors of the testis
Carcinoid tumor
Tumors of ovarian epithelial types
  Serous tumor of borderline malignancy
  Serous carcinoma
  Well-differentiated endometrioid carcinoma
  Mucinous cystadenoma
  Mucinous cystadenocarcinoma
  Brenner tumor
Nephroblastoma
Paraganglioma

Hematopoietic tumors

Tumors of collecting ducts and rete
Adenoma
Carcinoma

Tumors of paratesticular structures
Adenomatoid tumor
Malignant mesothelioma
Benign mesothelioma
  Well-differentiated papillary mesothelioma
  Cystic mesothelioma
Adenocarcinoma of the epididymis
Papillary cystadenoma of the epididymis
Melanotic neuroectodermal tumor
Desmoplastic small round cell tumor

Mesenchymal tumors of the spinal cord and testicular adnexae

Secondary tumors of the testes

From: Ebele JN, Sauter G, Epstein JI, Sesterhenn IA, eds. *World Health Organization Classification of Tumours. Pathology and Genetics. Tumours of the Urinary System and Male Genital Organs.* Lyon: IARC Press; 2004. Used with permission.

(~3- to 5-fold) of developing germ cell neoplasia both in the cryptorchid as well as the normal contralateral testis. Patients with testicular atrophy, infertility, a family history of germ cell neoplasia, 46,XY or 45,X/46,XY gonadal dysgenesis, and a previous history of germ cell neoplasia are also at an increased risk. The age of the patient as well as characteristic elevations in the levels of serum tumor markers in different subtypes of germ cell tumors can be very helpful in predicting tumor type. Yolk sac tumor and/or teratoma are seen in infants and children; seminomas and nonseminomatous germ cell neoplasms (including embryonal carcinoma, teratoma, yolk sac tumor, and choriocarcinoma) are found in adolescents and young adults; and spermatocytic seminoma is detected in patients older than 50 years. Serum AFP levels can be elevated in nonseminomatous germ cell tumors, especially with a yolk sac tumor component, whereas serum beta-hCG levels are increased in choriocarcinoma and tumors with syncytiotrophoblasts, which include about 10% of seminomas. The levels of these tumor markers are monitored posttreatment and are indicators of residual disease.

    Imaging studies such as ultrasound are extremely sensitive and inexpensive in evaluating testicular masses. Localization of the mass, including evaluation of extratesticular versus intratesticular sites of involvement, and presence of heterogeneity within the tumor, can be determined with accuracy. Epididymal lesions cannot be characterized with a similar degree of sensitivity. Computed tomography and magnetic resonance imaging are not used as primary diagnostic tools but can be helpful in tumor staging.

1. **Histologic typing and diagnosis of germ cell tumors** is made by examination of H&E-stained sections (*J Clin Pathol* 60:866, 2007). Gross examination can provide useful diagnostic clues as to tumor type. For instance, a tan-yellow, solid, homogenous, well-circumscribed appearance is characteristic of classic seminoma. Choriocarcinomas show extensive areas of hemorrhage and necrosis, whereas teratomas are multicystic and nodular, and may have grossly visible cartilage or bone. Embryonal carcinomas are smaller, soft, tan-white with hemorrhage and necrosis, and yolk sac tumors may show gelatinous, mucoid, and often cystic areas. Lymphomas are fleshy and ill-defined, and more often exhibit extratesticular extension. Scarring may represent a regressed germ cell tumor. Because many germ cell tumors are of mixed type, the importance of adequate sampling of heterogenous areas cannot be overemphasized.

2. **Histopathologic diagnosis** is based on the presence of one (pure) or more (mixed) histologic types.

    a. **IGCN, unclassified type (IGCNU),** a precursor of invasive germ cell neoplasia, may be found in isolated form or adjacent to invasive germ cell tumors. Patients with infertility, cryptorchidism, intersex syndrome, gonadal dysgenesis, a history of invasive germ cell tumor in the contralateral testis, or a retroperitoneal germ cell tumor have an increased likelihood of development of IGCNU. The high sensitivity of testicular biopsy in detecting IGCNU makes it a useful screening tool in these subgroups of patients. IGCNU is not recognizable grossly. Histologically, the seminiferous tubules show enlarged neoplastic cells with clear cytoplasm and prominent nucleoli, and often a thickened tunica propria (e-**Fig. 28.9**). Mitoses may be seen. Normal spermatogenesis is lacking. The surrounding stroma may show a prominent lymphocytic response. The presence of scattered neoplastic germ cells in the surrounding stroma qualifies as microinvasion (e-**Fig. 28.10**). Occasionally, the neoplastic cells spread along the tubules or the rete testis in a pagetoid fashion. Periodic acid–Schiff histochemical stains highlight glycogen in the cytoplasm of IGCNU cells; immunohistochemically, PLAP, CD117 (c-kit), and OCT4 positivity are observed (*Semin Diagn Pathol* 22:33, 2005). In infants up to 1 year of age, prepubertal germ cells can resemble IGCNU morphologically and by PLAP staining, so caution is advised in diagnosing IGCNU in this age group. Molecular genetic studies are not currently used in the diagnosis of IGCNU. About 90% of pure IGCNU cases progress to invasive disease in 7 years.

    b. **Seminoma** comprises almost 40% to 50% of all testicular germ cell tumors. Grossly, it has a homogeneous white to gray cut surface (e-**Fig. 28.11**). Necrosis may be seen, but hemorrhage and cystic change are uncommon. Histologically, it is composed of a diffuse sheet of uniform cells. These may be separated into nests, clusters, or columns by delicate fibrous septae infiltrated by mature lymphocytes (e-**Fig. 28.12**). A parenchymal or intratubular granulomatous reaction may be present. The granulomatous inflammation can be so extensive, both in the testis and draining lymph nodes, that the tumor cells are nearly obscured, resulting in a misdiagnosis of granulomatous orchitis. The tumor may entirely replace the normal testicular parenchyma, and may show an intratubular and less commonly an interstitial growth pattern. Other morphologic patterns include pseudoglandular, tubular, cribriform, and occasionally microcystic appearances (*Am J Surg Pathol* 29:500, 2005). In these latter cases, membranous PLAP and c-kit positivity, together with a negative staining pattern for AFP, inhibin, pan-cytokeratin, and CD30, can be useful for differentiation from nonseminomatous germ cell tumors (Table 28.3). An OCT4 immunostain will mark seminoma and embryonal carcinoma, but not other germ cell tumor types (*Am J Surg Pathol* 28:935, 2004). Foci of scarring

| TABLE 28.3 | Immunophenotype of Testis Neoplasms |

Tumor Type	PLAP	c-kit (CD117)	OCT4	CD30	AFP	AE1/ AE3	CK7	EMA	Inhibin	CD45 (LCA)
Seminoma	+	+	+	−	−	v	v	−	−	−
Spermatocytic seminoma	−	v	−	−	−	−	nd	−	nd	−
Embryonal carcinoma	+	−	+	+	v	+	+	−	−	−
Yolk sac tumor	+	−	−	v	+	+	−	−	−	−
Sertoli/Leydig cell tumor	−/v	−	−	nd	nd	−/v	nd	v	v/+	−
Lymphoma	−	−	−	v	nd	−	nd	−	−	+

Modified from: *Semin Diagn Pathol.* 2005;22:333.
+ ≥ 80% of cases positive; v = variable staining (20% to 80% of cases); ≤ 20% of cases positive; nd = no data.

may indicate a regressed germ cell tumor, and areas of calcification should prompt a search for possible foci of gonadoblastoma. Although brisk mitotic activity (>6 mitoses per high-power field) is observed in some tumors, there is little evidence to support that this denotes a worse prognosis, although it has been hypothesized that this finding may indicate progression to embryonal carcinoma. Marked cytologic atypia and mitoses have been used in the past to define "anaplastic seminoma," but this is not a currently recognized subtype of seminoma. Scattered multinucleated, syncytiotrophoblasts are seen in up to 10% of seminomas (e-**Fig. 28.13**); this finding has no prognostic significance, but is important to diagnose such cases as seminoma with syncytiotrophoblastic cells because this may correlate with a mildly elevated serum hCG level. However, seminoma with syncytiotrophoblastic cells does need to be differentiated from choriocarcinoma; the lack of a cytotrophoblastic component is helpful in this regard. Other important entities in the differential diagnosis of seminoma include inflammatory conditions (especially in the presence of a prominent lymphocytic response), spermatocytic seminoma, and sex cord stromal tumors.

c. **Spermatocytic seminoma** is rare and lacks the associations (i.e., cryptorchidism and IGCNU) commonly seen with classic seminoma. This neoplasm is seen in older patients, and is more often than not unilateral. Extratesticular extension is rare. The tumor cells are noncohesive and arranged in sheets, and are of three types: small lymphocyte-like with dark nuclei and scant cytoplasm, intermediate with round nuclei and moderate eosinophilic cytoplasm, and large with single or multiple nuclei (e-**Fig. 28.14**). The presence of stromal edema may cause the tumor cells to appear to be nested or pseudoglandular. Mitoses are frequent, but a lymphocytic and granulomatous response is usually not present. The main differential diagnosis is with classic seminoma and lymphoma. Clinicomorphologic features and, if necessary, PLAP and OCT4 immunostains are useful in the distinction from classic seminomas (Table 28.3). Lymphomas are more often bilateral and extratesticular, and have a more monomorphic cell population. Only one case of metastatic pure spermatocytic seminoma has been reported, and so radical orchiectomy alone is curative for almost all patients with spermatocytic seminoma. Spermatocytic seminoma with sarcoma is an aggressive variant of spermatocytic seminoma associated with a high-grade sarcomatous component such as rhabdomyosarcoma or chondrosarcoma, and has been described in about a dozen cases; no known etiology or familial predisposition has been reported, and most patients present with metastatic disease.

d. **Embryonal carcinoma** occurs in young adults, most commonly as a component of a mixed germ cell tumor. Grossly, hemorrhage and necrosis are common (e-**Fig. 28.15**). The tumor cells are large and undifferentiated with an 'epithelial' appearance, and are arranged in a solid, papillary, and/or glandular pattern (e-**Fig. 28.16**). Nuclei are polygonal and vesicular with coarse chromatin. Mitotic activity and necrosis are extensive. Intratubular germ cell neoplasia can be present at the periphery and frequently displays intratubular necrosis. Vascular invasion can be seen and should be differentiated from retraction artifact and artificial implantation during sampling. Pan-cytokeratin, OCT4, and CD30 positivity is seen in tumor cells; PLAP and AFP are only focally positive in pure tumors. Epithelial membrane antigen (EMA) is negative, which is important in the differential diagnosis with somatic carcinomas (Table 28.3). Evaluation of H&E-stained slides is usually sufficient to establish the diagnosis; in occasional cases, immunohistochemistry is needed to help differentiate embryonal carcinoma from yolk sac tumor, large cell anaplastic lymphoma, and/or choriocarcinoma.

e. **Yolk sac tumor (endodermal sinus tumor)** shows differentiation reminiscent of embryonic yolk sac, allantois, and extraembryonic mesenchyme. In infants and young children it tends to occur in pure form, whereas in adults it is found as a component of mixed malignant germ cell tumors. The morphologic appearance is varied and includes reticular (most common), microcystic, endodermal sinus-like (with Schiller–Duval bodies), papillary, solid, glandular, alveolar, enteric, polyvesicular vitelline, and hepatoid patterns (e-**Fig. 28.17**). Rarely, a neoplastic spindle cell component has been observed in association with the myxomatous and reticular variants. The immunoprofile reveals AFP, PLAP, and low-molecular-weight cytokeratin positivity. IGCNU is commonly seen in adult yolk sac tumors but not as frequently in childhood yolk sac tumors. Embryonal carcinoma may, in certain foci, be difficult to tell apart from yolk sac tumor, and indeed the two tumor types can appear to merge; however, embryonal carcinoma nuclei are usually more pleomorphic, and immunostains can help in difficult cases (Table 28.3). Follicle-like areas of granulosa cell tumors in infants may resemble the solid and cystic pattern of yolk sac tumor, and the enteric pattern may appear similar to glandular areas in teratoma. Usually, the former problem can be resolved with immunohistochemical stains for AFP and inhibin.

f. **Trophoblastic tumors** are almost always choriocarcinoma. Pure choriocarcinoma is extremely rare; instead, choriocarcinoma most commonly occurs as a component of mixed germ cell tumors. Grossly, necrotic and hemorrhagic nodules may be observed. Microscopically, the more viable peripheral areas show randomly admixed syncytiotrophoblasts, cytotrophoblasts, and intermediate trophoblasts, although one component may predominate, giving rise to monophasic tumors (e-**Fig. 28.18**). Very rare tumors composed of intermediate trophoblastic cells resembling placental site trophoblastic tumor have also been reported. There is a propensity for vascular invasion (e-**Fig. 28.18**). The syncytiotrophoblasts are positive for hCG, alpha subunit of inhibin, and EMA, and the intermediate trophoblasts are reactive for human placental lactogen (HPL); all cell types are positive for cytokeratin. The differential diagnosis includes syncytiotrophoblast-rich seminoma, and isolated syncytiotrophoblasts found in nonseminomatous germ cell tumors.

g. **Teratomas** include mature and immature teratoma, dermoid cyst, monodermal teratoma, and teratoma with somatic-type malignancies. The age distribution is bimodal. Teratomas occurring in children are benign whereas those in young adults have significant rates of metastases despite their histologic appearance. Grossly, there are cystic and solid areas, and cartilage (e-**Fig. 28.19**) and bone may be evident. Microscopically, teratomas may show well-differentiated elements derived from one (monodermal) or all three germ layers (ectoderm, mesoderm, and endoderm), or may be immature with fetal type tissue. Skin and its appendages, respiratory and intestinal-type epithelium, cartilage, and muscular tissue are common (e-Fig. 28.20, A and B); neural-type tissue is less frequent. Immature tissues can resemble renal blastema or embryonic neural tube (e-Fig. 20.21). Foci with the appearance of a primitive neuroectodermal tumor (PNET) have been classified as such if present. Pure teratomas are much less common than the finding of teratoma as an element of a mixed malignant germ cell tumor.

Dermoid cysts, which harbor keratinizing squamous epithelium and skin appendages, are very rare and are benign. Epidermoid cysts lack skin appendages and are possibly monodermal teratomas; grossly, epidermoid cysts are distinctive with a ringlike "onion-skin" cut surface (e-Figs. 28.22, 28.23).

Several nongerm cell malignant tumors, characterized by expansile growth of at least a 4× field, including adenocarcinoma, squamous cell carcinoma, neuroendocrine tumors, sarcomas, and PNETs have been known to arise in primary or metastatic teratomas.

Immunostains are not usually necessary for the diagnosis of teratoma, but it is noteworthy that AFP immunopositivity can be present in intestinal-type areas of teratomas.

  h. **Tumors of more than one histologic type** (mixed forms), termed **mixed malignant germ cell tumor,** are germ cell neoplasms composed of more than one type of tumor. They comprise approximately 30% of all germ cell tumors, and the most frequently encountered components include embryonal carcinoma (in about one half of the cases), yolk sac tumor (one half), and teratoma (about 40%). About 40% of mixed malignant germ cell tumors also contain scattered syncytiotrophoblasts. A rare subtype of mixed germ cell tumor is the polyembryoma with characteristic embryoid bodies with central cores of embryonal carcinoma (forming the dorsal amnionlike cavity) and a surrounding (ventral) yolk sac component. Mixed germ cell tumors with an embryonal component are predictive of a higher stage than tumors with a large seminomatous component, so for mixed tumors it is very important to quantitate, on a percentage basis, the amount of embryonal carcinoma, as well as all other components. Tumors with a yolk sac or teratoma component show a lower incidence of metastatic disease.

  i. **Burnt out (regressed) germ cell tumors** are germ cell tumors in which the primary tumor in the testis has undergone necrosis and fibrosis. This most commonly occurs with seminoma (*Am J Surg Pathol* 30:858, 2006) and choriocarcinoma. The most specific histologic finding of a regressed germ cell tumor is a distinct scar (e-Fig. 28.24) in association with either IGCNU or coarse intratubular calcifications; however, many cases lack these latter two features (*Am J Surg Pathol* 30:858, 2006). Some patients may present with metastatic disease, the only evidence of the testicular primary being a scar, with or without IGCNU.

  j. **Molecular genetics** are not currently used to diagnose germ cell tumors. The one possible exception is detection of isochromosome 12p, the most common structural chromosomal alteration in invasive germ cell neoplasms, by fluorescence in situ hybridization, to identify a metastatic neoplasm as being of germ cell type (*Mod Pathol* 17:1309, 2004).

B. **Sex cord/gonadal stromal tumors** comprise 4% to 6% of all testicular tumors in adults and include Leydig cell tumor, Sertoli cell tumor, granulosa cell tumor, thecoma, and fibroma.

  1. **Leydig cell tumors** are the most common and are known to occur in patients with gynecomastia, Klinefelter's syndrome, and cryptorchidism. Grossly, the tumor cut surface is homogeneous, solid, and brown to yellow. The tumor cells are large and polygonal, and have abundant, eosinophilic, lipid-laden cytoplasm (e-Fig. 28.25). The characteristic Reinke's crystals are found in only 30% of cases. The main differential diagnoses are with Leydig cell hyperplasia and tumors in patients with

adrenogenital syndrome. Leydig cell tumors form a nodule without seminiferous tubules, whereas in Leydig cell hyperplasia the foci are bilateral and multifocal, and wrap around and extend between the tubules (e-**Fig. 28.26**). Adrenogenital tumors are bilateral and dark brown, with pigmentation and fibrous stroma. About 90% of Leydig cell tumors are benign; a constellation of features, including size >5 cm, cytologic atypia, increased mitotic activity, necrosis, and vascular invasion, favors malignancy.

2. **Sertoli cell tumors** account for only 1% of all testicular tumors. Grossly, the mass is usually well-circumscribed, with tan-yellow to white, sometimes hemorrhagic cut surfaces (e-**Fig. 28.27**). The pathologic subtypes are the lipid rich, large cell calcifying (e-**Fig. 28.28**), and sclerosing variants. The known clinical associations are with Carney's syndrome, Peutz–Jeghers syndrome (which can be associated with bilateral tumors), and androgen insensitivity syndrome. Histologically, the cytologically bland cells are arranged in tubules, potentially with retiform, tubular-glandular, and solid nodular areas. The tubules can be closed (solid) (e-**Fig. 28.29**) and are surrounded by a basement membrane. Intratubular growth can be present. Sertoli cell tumors should be distinguished from small incidental Sertoli cell nodules (benign and thought to be nonneoplastic) as can be seen in cryptorchid testes. The tumor cells are cytokeratin and sometimes inhibin positive, but PLAP and OCT4 negative, by immunohistochemistry. Malignant Sertoli cell tumors are rare.

3. **Granulosa cell tumors and thecoma/fibroma tumors** are similar in appearance to those in the ovary. There are two variants: adult and juvenile types. All are rare in the testis.

C. **Mixed germ cell and sex cord/gonadal stromal tumors** include gonadoblastoma, most commonly seen in the setting of mixed gonadal dysgenesis, ambiguous genitalia, and 45X/46XY mosaicism. Microscopic examination shows a two-cell population: a germ cell component resembling seminoma and a component resembling immature Sertoli cells (e-**Fig. 28.30**). Round deposits of basement membrane-like material and coarse calcification are common features. A large number of patients develop invasive germ cell tumors, particularly seminoma, and are therefore treated with bilateral orchiectomy.

D. **Miscellaneous tumors** of the testis include carcinoid tumors, tumors of ovarian epithelial types (serous borderline tumor, serous carcinoma, mucinous cystadenomas and cystadenocarcinomas, Brenner tumor, and endometrioid carcinoma), nephroblastoma, and paraganglioma.

E. **Hematolymphoid neoplasms,** of which the most common is malignant lymphoma, comprise 5% of all testicular malignancies. These are the most common bilateral tumors of the testis, and their incidence is higher in elderly men. The most common subtype is diffuse large B-cell lymphoma. The growth pattern is typically intertubular (e-**Fig. 28.31**), and the main differential diagnosis is with seminoma, especially the spermatocytic type. Immunostains can be helpful in establishing the diagnosis (Table 28.3). The prognosis is generally poor. Young age, low stage, and presence of sclerosis are indicators of a good prognosis. Isolated plasmacytoma of testis is rare.

F. **Tumors of the collecting ducts and rete.** Benign tumors of the rete include adenoma, cystadenoma, and adenofibroma. Adenocarcinomas of the rete are rare, and their diagnosis is subject to strict histologic criteria that include tumor centered on testicular hilum, morphology distinct from any other testicular/paratesticular tumor, solid growth pattern, transition between tumor and normal tissue, and absence of histologically similar extratesticular malignancy (especially lung and prostate). The main histologic patterns are tubular, papillary, and solid. The main differential diagnoses are extratesticular adenocarcinomas and mesothelioma. The tumor shows extensive regional spread and distant metastasis, and the overall prognosis is poor.

G. **Tumors of the paratesticular organs.** The most common benign neoplasm of the testicular adnexa is the adenomatoid tumor, representing almost 60% of all cases. These are of mesothelial origin (*Semin Diagn Pathol* 17:294, 2000) and arise in the upper or lower pole of the epididymis as solitary, round to oval nodules invariably <5 cm in size. Histologically, the tumor shows round to oval or slitlike tubules in a fibrous, and hyalinized and/or muscular stroma (e-**Fig. 28.32**). The lining cells are columnar or flat with vacuolated cytoplasm. Adenomatoid tumors show immunoreactivity for cytokeratin, EMA, and mesothelial markers including calretinin and WT-1. The tumor should be differentiated from signet-ring-cell carcinoma and mesothelioma; tumors with a more diffuse growth pattern simulate Sertoli or Leydig cell tumors (inhibin positivity, lipofuscin pigment, and presence of Reinke's crystals favor Leydig cell tumor).

Another benign paratesticular tumor is papillary cystadenoma of epididymis; about two thirds are seen in patients with von Hippel–Lindau syndrome, and in this setting they tend to be bilateral. A much rarer entity is the retinal anlage tumor or the melanotic neuroectodermal tumor, which is composed of two cell populations: larger melanin-containing cells and smaller neuroblastlike cells.

Malignant tumors of the testicular adnexa include malignant mesothelioma. The microscopic appearance and immunophenotypic profile are similar to those of mesothelioma of the pleura. The main differential diagnoses are with adenomatoid tumor, which is better circumscribed, and with carcinoma of the rete testis.

Primary adenocarcinoma of the epididymis is rare, and may histologically and cytologically simulate a cystadenoma due to the presence of columnar cells with clear cytoplasm containing glycogen. Metastatic adenocarcinoma from other organs should also be excluded.

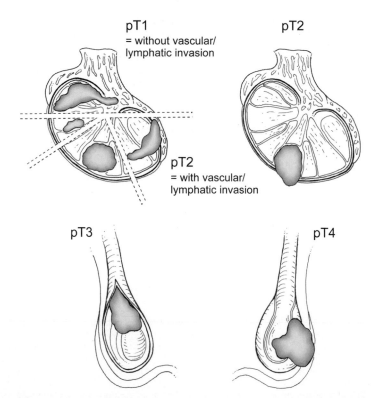

Figure 28.1. Pathologic staging of germ cell tumors of the testis. (Modified from Greene FL, Compton CC, Fritz AG, Shah JP, Winchester DP, eds. *AJCC Cancer Staging Atlas.* New York: Springer; 2006).

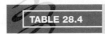

TABLE 28.4	Tumor, Node, Metastasis (TNM) Staging Scheme for Germ Cell Tumors of the Testes

PRIMARY TUMOR (T)

pTX	Primary tumor cannot be assessed
pT0	No evidence of primary tumor (e.g., histologic scar in the testes)
pTis	Intratubular germ cell neoplasia (carcinoma in situ)
pT1	Tumor limited to the testis and epididymis without vascular/lymphatic invasion, tumor may invade into the tunica albuginea but not the tunica vaginalis
pT2	Tumor limited to the testis and epididymis with vascular/lymphatic invasion, or tumor extending through the tunica albuginea with the involvement of the tunica vaginalis
pT3	Tumor invades the spermatic cord with or without vascular/lymphatic invasion
pT4	Tumor invades the scrotum with or without vascular/lymphatic invasion

Note: Except for pTis and pT4, extent of primary tumor is classified by radical orchiectomy. TX may be used for other categories in the absence of radical orchiectomy.

REGIONAL LYMPH NODES (N)
Clinical

NX	Regional lymph nodes cannot be assessed
N0	No regional lymph node metastasis
N1	Metastasis with a lymph node mass of ≤2 cm in greatest dimension or multiple lymph nodes, none >2 cm in greatest dimension
N2	Metastasis with a lymph node mass of >2 cm but not >5 cm in greatest dimension; or multiple lymph nodes, any one mass >2 cm but not >5 cm in greatest dimension
N3	Metastasis with a lymph node mass >5 cm in greatest dimension

PATHOLOGIC (PN)

pNx	Regional lymph nodes cannot be assessed
pN0	No regional lymph node metastasis
pN1	Metastasis with a lymph node mass of ≤2 cm in greatest dimension or multiple lymph nodes, none >2 cm in greatest dimension
pN2	Metastasis with a lymph node mass of >2 cm but not >5 cm in greatest dimension; or multiple lymph nodes, any one mass >2 cm but not >5 cm in greatest dimension
N3	Metastasis with a lymph node mass >5 cm in greatest dimension

DISTANT METASTASIS (M)

MX	Distant metastasis cannot be assessed
M0	No distant metastasis
M1	Distant metastasis
M1a	Nonregional nodal or pulmonary metastasis
M1b	Distant metastasis other than nonregional lymph nodes and lungs

SERUM TUMOR MARKERS (S)

SX	Marker studies not available or not performed
S0	Marker study levels within normal limits
S1	LDH < 1.5 × N* AND hCG (mIu/mL) < 5000 AND AFP (ng/mL) < 1000
S2	LDH 1.5–10 × N OR hCG (mIu/mL) < 5000–50,000 OR AFP (ng/mL) < 1000–10,000
S3	LDH >10 × N OR hCG (mIu/mL) > 50,000 OR AFP (ng/mL) >10,000

STAGE GROUPING

Stage 0 pTis	N0	M0	S0
Stage I pT1-4	N0	M0	SX
Stage1A pT1	N0	M0	S0
Stage1B pT2	N0	M0	S0
pT3	N0	M0	S0
pT4	N0	M0	S0
Stage IS Any pT/Tx	N0	M0	S1–3
Stage II Any pT/Tx	N1–3	M0	SX
Stage IIA Any pT/Tx	N1	M0	S0
Any pT/Tx	N1	M0	S1
Stage IIB Any pT/Tx	N2	M0	S0
Any pT/Tx	N2	M0	S1
Stage IIC Any pT/Tx	N3	M0	S0
Any pT/Tx	N3	M0	S1

(Continued)

TABLE 28.4	Tumor, Node, Metastasis (TNM) Staging Scheme for Germ Cell Tumors of the Testes (*Continued*)			
Stage III Any pT/Tx	Any N	M1	SX
Stage III A Any pT/Tx	Any N	M1a	S0
Any pT/Tx	Any N	M1a	S1
Stage III B Any pT/Tx	N1–3	M0	S2
Any pT/Tx	Any N	M1a	S2
Stage III C Any pT/Tx	N1–3	M0	S3
Any pT/Tx	Any N	M1a	S3
Any pT/Tx	Any N	M1b	S3

Abbreviations: LDH = low-density lipoprotein; hCG = human chorionic gonadotropin; AFP = alpha-fetoprotein. N* = upper limit of normal
From: Greene FL, Page DL, Fleming ID, Fritz AG, Balch CM, Haller DG, Morrow M, eds. *AJCC Cancer Staging Manual.* 6th edition. New York: Springer; 2002. Used with permission. (A new AJCC TNM staging system is scheduled for release in 2009; after its publication, the new staging scheme will appear on the website for this book.)

Desmoplastic small round cell tumor occurs in the epididymis of young adults. Molecular, genetic, histologic, and immunohistochemical features are similar to those of tumor when it occurs at more conventional sites such as the peritoneum. The tumor should be differentiated from other small blue cell tumors such as malignant lymphoma and embryonal rhabdomyosarcoma.

Mesenchymal tumors of the scrotum, paratesticular organs, and spermatic cord include benign neoplasms such as lipoma, leiomyoma, neurofibroma, and granular cell tumor and malignant tumors such as liposarcoma, leiomyosarcoma, malignant fibrous histiocytoma, and rhabdomyosarcoma (e-**Figs. 28.33, 28.34**).

H. Secondary malignancies include metastatic adenocarcinomas from the prostate (e-**Fig. 28.35**), lung, and colon, and melanoma.

V. PATHOLOGIC STAGING applies only to germ cell neoplasms of the testis (Fig. 28.1). The 2002 Tumor, Node, Metastasis (TNM) American Joint Committee on Cancer/International Union Against Cancer (AJCC/UICC) staging classification is given in Table 28.4. Clinical staging should be distinguished from pathologic staging.

VI. REPORTING OF GERM CELL NEOPLASMS. The basic elements that need to be included for the primary tumor are primary tumor size, multifocality, and presence or absence of involvement of extratesticular tissues including the epididymis, tunica vaginalis (via penetration through the tunica albuginea), spermatic cord, and scrotum (if present). Note that the rete testis does not count as an extratesticular structure. Histologic typing should follow the WHO classification (Table 28.2) and, for mixed tumors, the percentage of each component should be provided; it is particularly critical to assess for the presence and amount of embryonal carcinoma. It is also vital to report on the presence or absence of lymphovascular invasion. Spermatic cord margin status should be given. For metastatic deposits, the histological components and tumor viability should be reported. Postchemotherapy, the report should indicate whether the viable tumor is teratoma or another germ cell component.

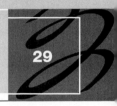

I. **NORMAL ANATOMY.** The normal weight of the prostate is 20 grams for ages 20 to 50, and 30 grams for ages 60 to 80. Anatomically, the prostate gland is comprised of three zones: central zone, transition zone (where benign prostatic hyperplasia [BPH] occurs), and peripheral zone (e-**Fig. 29.1**),* where most carcinomas originate. Microscopically, the normal adult prostate is a branching duct-acinar glandular system embedded in a dense fibromuscular stroma (e-**Fig. 29.2**). The epithelium has two layers: a luminal or secretory cell layer and a basal cell layer. Central zone epithelium can normally have architectures such as cribriform and Roman bridgelike structures.

II. **GROSS EXAMINATION, TISSUE SAMPLING, AND HISTOLOGIC SLIDE PREPARA-TION.** The most common prostatic parenchymal tissue samples examined in surgical pathology laboratories in the United States are, in order, 18-gauge needle cores, transurethral resection of prostate (TURP) chips, radical prostatectomy specimens, and fine needle aspirates.

   A. **Needle cores.** Needle core biopsy sample handling and processing begins in the office or room where the procedure is performed. The needle biopsy tissue should be immediately placed into a container with fixative, which is usually 10% neutral buffered formalin although a few laboratories prefer Bouin's solution, Hollande's solution, or IBF fixative. Bouin's and Hollande's solutions are picric acid–based fixatives that provide superior nuclear detail, but these strong oxidizing agents can react violently with combustible materials and reducing agents. Fixation in formalin should be at least for 6 hours. The number of cores received per container is highly variable, from 1 to >20. If the urologist and treating physician desire site-specific diagnosis, the core(s) should be placed in a separate site-designated container. Inking of cores to indicate site, with placement of cores marked with different colors into the same container, should not be performed because fragmentation renders site assignment impossible. Gross examination of prostate needle core tissue is not diagnostic, but is important for correlation with amount of tissue seen in histologic sections. It is vital to record, for each container, size and number of tissue cores or fragments. It is recommended that no more than two cores be submitted per cassette for processing and embedding; some laboratories submit one core per cassette. Prostate cores can be marked with ink, which facilitates identification during embedding and the ability to see the cores in the paraffin blocks. The cores should be placed into a cassette after being put into a fine mesh envelope, wrapped in lens paper, sandwiched between sponge pads, or double-embedded in agar–paraffin wax. After processing, the cores should be embedded in the same plane, in the same direction, with even spacing. From each paraffin block one should prepare three hematoxylin and eosin (H&E)-stained slides, each with three to four serial sections on each slide. Some laboratories cut interval, unstained sections on coated slides in case special studies such as immunohistochemistry are needed. Clinical requests for frozen section diagnosis of prostate needle cores are rare and should be restricted to patients with clinical evidence of metastatic cancer who are to undergo immediate treatment (usually orchiectomy) for pain relief.

   B. **TURP chips.** The amount of prostate tissue resected in TURP is variable, ranging from 5 g to >75 g of tissue, with a mean of about 25 g. The gross description should

---

*All e-figures are available online via the Solution Site Image Bank.

include the weight of all chips. Recognizable gross features such as yellow coloration and induration can be recorded, but it has not been proven that chip color, size, or induration is linked to cancer presence, such that gross selection of specific chips is not required. Although gross TURP chip-sampling procedures are not standardized, one initial approach is to submit 12 g of chips or 6 to 8 blocks of tissue (with 1 to 2 g per cassette). For specimens >12 g, the initial 12 g are submitted, with one cassette for every additional 5 g. (*Arch Pathol Lab Med* 130:936, 2006). If the patient is younger than 60 years, submit all tissue. All chip tissue should be submitted if microscopic examination of partially submitted chips reveals carcinoma in <5% of tissue. Consideration should be given to submitting all chips if high-grade prostatic intraepithelial neoplasia (PIN) or atypical glands (atypical small acinar proliferation) is found in sections of partially submitted chips. One H&E-stained slide, with one or two sections, is typically generated from each paraffin block of TURP chips.

C. **Open suprapubic or retropubic simple prostatectomy (enucleation) tissue.** The prostatic tissue from simple prostatectomies may be submitted to the pathology laboratory as a single mass or as pieces. The prostatectomy tissue should be weighed and sectioned at 3-mm to 5-mm intervals. The gross description for each piece should include size in three dimensions, weight in grams, firmness, and coloration. One should sample any hard nodules and submit a total of eight cassettes or one cassette of tissue for each 5 grams of tissue. One should submit additional tissue if carcinoma is histologically detected in initial sections of partially submitted tissue, although no rules or recommendations exist on how many additional sections. One H&E-stained slide should be made per block.

D. **Radical prostatectomy.** The entire prostate gland is excised in prostate cancer surgery using open retropubic or perineal approaches, and using laparoscopic (including robotic) approaches. The prostate gland is also resected *in toto* in radical cystoprostatectomy for bladder cancer.

1. **Pelvic lymph nodes.** Pelvic lymphadenectomy may be performed as a separate procedure, often laparoscopic, or during the radical prostatectomy operation. Sentinel lymph node sampling is not routinely done. Frozen section analysis of the sampled lymph nodes may be requested for patients at risk for nodal metastasis, based on serum prostate-specific antigen (PSA) level, needle biopsy Gleason score, and clinical stage. All grossly recognizable lymph nodes should be examined by frozen section; cytologic touch imprints can be made at the same time. Frozen section diagnosis of metastatic carcinoma in lymph nodes is highly specific, but fairly insensitive. The low sensitivity rate of 58% to 73% is due to sampling error. Gross sampling of tissue after frozen section should entail submission of all grossly identifiable lymph node tissue and wide sampling of associated adipose tissue. The gross description of pelvic lymph nodes should include number, location, and size. One H&E-stained slide is made per paraffin block. Special studies to detect occult lymph node markers, such as immunohistochemistry for cytokeratins or PSA, or reverse transcription–polymerase chain reaction (RT–PCR) for PSA RNA, are currently experimental.

2. **Prostate gland and seminal vesicles.** The prostate gland and seminal vesicles from radical prostatectomy may be received fresh or in fixative. Frozen section requests on fresh specimens are uncommon, and are usually made to evaluate margin status. This procedure has a high false-negative rate and is not typical practice. Fresh specimens are also used for tissue-banking protocols: After inking of the entire outside of the specimen, and incision into the gland, tissue may be harvested from inside the gland, while preserving the inked periphery. Alternatively, after inking, margin sampling and seminal vesicle amputation (discussed later in this paragraph), the whole unfixed gland is sectioned with a large, sharp knife from apex to base at 4-mm intervals, perpendicular to the prostatic urethra. Areas suspicious for carcinoma, as judged by palpation or visual inspection, may be sampled by imprints, scrapes, core biopsy, or small wedge sections. Fixation of the inked radical prostatectomy specimens (sectioned or unsectioned) is accomplished by at least overnight (or 24 to 48 hour) room temperature immersion in 10% neutral buffered formalin at 10 times the volume of the specimen. The

following procedure is for unsectioned glands: After inking and weighing the entire specimen, distal apical (urethral) and bladder neck margins should be taken, if not already submitted separately. The distal apical margin is evaluated by amputating the distal 5 to 10 mm, dividing it into the right and left sides, and submitting radial sections (like a cervical cone). The bladder neck margin can be assessed by a thin 2-mm shave margin or by conization. Ink on tumor cells is indicative of a positive margin for cone sections and the peripheral margin, whereas tumor anywhere in shave margin tissue indicates a positive margin. The seminal vesicles are amputated with soft tissue and prostatic tissue at the base of the seminal vesicles and submitted separately as right and left seminal vesicles. Vasa deferentia stumps may be sampled using *en face* sections, but this is not routine. The prostate gland is serially sectioned in a plane perpendicular to the urethra at 3- to 5-mm intervals using a long knife. The cut surfaces should be evaluated for gross evidence of BPH and carcinoma. One can take photographs or digital images to document location and gross appearance of tissue in submitted cassettes. Diagrams (Fig. 29.1) or pictorial maps can also be used to indicate location of sections and any gross abnormality. Most pathology laboratories in the United States partially submit the prostate gland, with complete embedding of all prostate tissue done in only a minority of cases. For partial sampling, all lesions grossly suspicious for carcinoma should be submitted. Several protocols for partial submission exist (*Scand J Urol Nephrol Suppl* 216:34, 2005; *Arch Pathol Lab Med* 130:936, 2006). For cases with no evident tumor, one can submit either alternate sections or the posterior aspect of each transverse slice along with a mid-anterior block from each side. Sections should be submitted as quarters or halves of the prostate, depending on gland size. Whole-amount sections are rarely made and do not provide additional morphological information. If no or minimal tumor is seen in initial section of a partially submitted gland, all tissue should be embedded (including any frozen tissue sent to a tissue bank).

E. **Cystoprostatectomy.** The prostate gland in radical cystoprostatectomies performed for bladder cancer can be sampled by taking several sections of prostatic urethra and surrounding prostate tissue, any gross lesions, one block from the periphery of each side, and both seminal vesicles. The distal urethral shave margin is important in urothelial carcinoma cases.

III. **DIAGNOSTIC FEATURES OF COMMON DISEASES OF THE PROSTATE**

A. **Inflammation and infection.** Histopathologic identification of inflammatory cells in the prostate is common, but histologic identification of specific infectious agents is rare.

1. **Asymptomatic inflammatory prostatitis,** including acute, neutrophilic inflammation and chronic lymphocytic, lymphoplasmacytic, or lymphohistiocytic inflammatory cells, is common in all prostate tissue samples. Reporting this inflammation is optional; it may be useful to report if the inflammation is extensive or persistent in several needle core samples taken over time, because prostatic inflammation can raise the serum PSA. Inflammation can be associated with prostatic glandular atrophy, and reactive nuclear changes, including prominent nucleoli. Inflammation is more commonly associated with benign epithelial conditions, especially atrophy and BPH, compared to high-grade PIN and carcinoma, where only a small percentage of foci (around 10%) are inflamed.

2. **Granulomatous prostatitis** can clinically elevate the serum PSA and/or present as a palpable abnormality. The most common type is nonspecific granulomatous prostatitis, which is thought to be a response to prostatic secretions released into stroma by duct-acinar rupture. Microscopically, this is a lobulocentric noncaseating granulomatous inflammatory cell infiltrate with giant cells (e-Fig. 29.3). Variants include xanthogranulomatous prostatitis and prostatic "xanthoma." Other types of granulomatous prostatitis include infectious and postbiopsy/postresection cases. Infectious granulomatous prostatitis is most often bacille Calmette–Guérin (BCG)-related in patients treated for bladder urothelial carcinoma. Fungal prostatitis is rare and usually seen in immunosuppressed patients. Postbiopsy/resection granulomas are most often identified in TURP chip

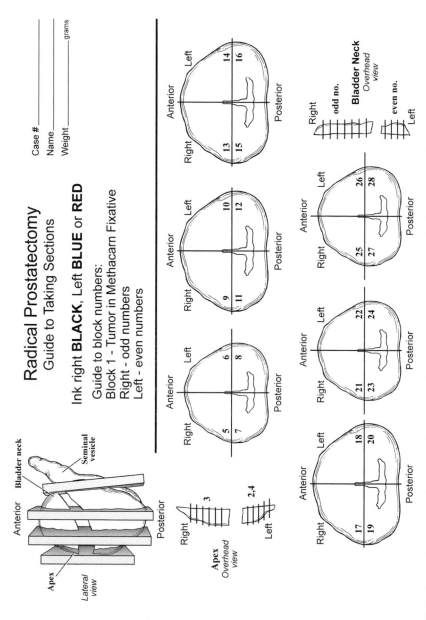

Figure 29.1. Diagram depicting guide to taking sections from a radical prostatectomy specimen. (Modified from True LD. Surgical pathology examination of the prostate gland. Practice survey by American Society of Clinical Pathologists. *Am J Clin Pathol.* 1995;103:376.)

tissue, and are characterized by a fibrinoid central zone surrounded by palisading histiocytes.

B. Atrophy of prostatic glands is the benign condition most likely to be misdiagnosed as prostatic carcinoma by light microscopy. It is a common, age-related process that could be related to inflammation, hormones, obstruction, or ischemia. It can also be caused by treatment, including radiotherapy and hormonal therapy. Histologically, atrophy is defined as cytoplasmic volume loss. It is not necessary to subtype atrophy, but it is important to recognize the existence of different histomorphological patterns including simple atrophy (with or without cystic change), sclerotic atrophy, partial atrophy, and postatrophic hyperplasia (or hyperplastic atrophy) (e-Figs. 29.4, 29.5). Atrophy can be confused with carcinoma because it is usually a small gland lesion that can show a pseudoinfiltrative pattern of growth, stromal sclerosis, nuclear atypia, and closely packed acini (in postatrophic hyperplasia). Atrophy can also be noted in cystically dilated peripheral zone glands and in cystic change in BPH nodules. Another diagnostic pitfall is that atrophic glands can show a fragmented basal cell layer and even loss of basal cells in a few glands, using immunohistochemical stains for basal cells (such as 34betaE12 and p63) (*Semin Diagn Pathol* 22:88, 2005). Also, the selective but not specific marker for neoplastic epithelial cells, alpha-methylacyl coenzyme A racemase (AMACR), can be focally positive in atrophy by immunostaining.

C. Metaplasia or change in cell type in benign prostatic epithelium can be squamous, transitional cell (urothelial), mucinous, and Paneth cell-like. These metaplasias are usually secondary to inflammation, therapy, or injury. They are not preneoplastic.

1. **Squamous cell metaplasia** is most often an incidental finding associated with inflammation and infarction in BPH nodules. Microscopically, small, solid nests or partially involved glands, with a retained lumen, are common. Squamoid cytoplasm and intercellular bridges may be evident, but keratin pearls are rare. Nuclear atypia, including prominent nuclei, and mitoses may be present in squamous metaplasia adjacent to infarcts. Squamous metaplasia postradiation or hormonal therapy can be more diffuse and is frequently immature with less cytoplasm and absence of keratinization.

2. **Transitional cell or urothelial metaplasia** should be distinguished from urothelial cells that normally line the prostatic urethra and central ducts of the prostate. This is usually a focal, incidental finding with small, solid nests or partial gland involvement by cytologically bland and uniform elongated cells, with some cells exhibiting nuclear grooves and cytoplasmic clearing.

3. **Mucinous metaplasia** is replacement of benign luminal epithelium by benign mucin-secretory cells. This is a focal, incidental microscopic finding in which the constituent cells have a granular blue cytoplasmic appearance. Goblet cells and luminal secretion of the mucin are uncommon.

4. **Paneth cell-like metaplasia** is a microscopic, cellular alteration characterized by large, cytoplasmic, eosinophilic granules. This alteration can be due to lysosomelike granules, neuroendocrine differentiation, or even true Paneth cell differentiation.

D. Hyperplasia. The diagnosis of BPH is a clinical one. Histologically, BPH can be diagnosed in TURP chips and simple and radical prostatectomy specimens, but it should not be diagnosed in needle biopsy tissue.

1. **Usual nodular epithelial and stromal hyperplasia** is the most common morphologic presentation of BPH. Grossly, these nodules, which characteristically arise in the transition zone and periurethral area, are multiple and vary from solid white to spongy with cystic change.

   a. **Pure stromal nodules (nodular stromal hyperplasia)** exist. Microscopically, the nodules can appear myxoid, hyalinized, or leiomyomatous, with spindled, ovoid, or stellate cells. Prominent thick-walled blood vessels and lymphocytes may be noted.

   b. **Mixed epithelial and stromal hyperplasia** is most common, with variable admixtures of spindled stromal cells and complex benign glands with complex

papillary and branching architecture (e-**Fig. 29.6**). Cystic change, inflammation, and basal cell hyperplasia are commonly detected in BPH nodules.
   c. Epithelial predominant BPH nodules are unusual.
   d. Infarcts can be identified in larger BPH nodules and can elevate the serum PSA.
2. **Basal cell hyperplasia** is usually discovered in BPH nodules, but can also be found in peripheral zone needle biopsy tissue, often associated with inflammation. Microscopically, there are two or more layers of basal cells arranged in acinar, cribriform, and solid growth patterns (e-**Fig. 29.7**). In usual basal cell hyperplasia, the basal cells are uniform and cytologically bland, whereas in so-called "atypical" basal cell hyperplasia prominent nucleoli are discerned. The term atypical should be avoided because no form of basal cell hyperplasia is a known risk factor for neoplasia.
3. **Cribriform hyperplasia,** which is completely benign and not a risk factor for neoplasia, is an infrequently seen variant of BPH.
4. **Mesonephric remnant hyperplasia** is a very rare prostatic proliferation displaying a vaguely lobular or infiltrative growth of small tubules with cuboidal epithelium and intraluminal, eosinophilic secretions. A negative high-molecular-weight cytokeratin (34betaE12) immunostain may raise concern for prostatic adenocarcinoma, but a helpful clue is negative PSA and prostate-specific acid phosphatase (PSAP) immunostains.
5. **Verumontanum gland hyperplasia** is a benign, small gland proliferation of the verumontanum and adjacent posterior urethra. The closely packed glands could be confused with carcinoma, but lack of nuclei atypia and basal cell presence will rule out carcinoma.
   E. **Atypical adenomatous hyperplasia (adenosis)** is a nodular proliferation of closely packed small acini (e-**Fig. 29.8**). It is invariably an incidental histologic finding, most often found in transition zone tissue in TURP chips or prostatectomy specimens. The densely packed small pale acini are sometimes intermingled with larger, more complex glands. Nuclear atypia is absent to minimal. The basal cell layer is fragmented, and, on average, 50% of glands completely lack basal cells. Of note, AMACR is diffusely positive in about 8% of cases. Adenosis can be mistaken for well-differentiated Gleason score 2 to 4 adenocarcinoma. It does not have known premalignant potential.
   F. **Prostatic intraepithelial neoplasia (PIN)** is a proliferation of atypical epithelial cells in pre-existing ducts and acini (synonyms used in the past include atypical hyperplasia and dysplasia). Currently, PIN is graded as low-grade PIN and high-grade PIN (HG-PIN), although only HG-PIN has potential clinical significance and merits reporting. Isolated HG-PIN is diagnosed in about 5% to 10% of needle biopsies (*J Urol* 175: 820, 2006). It is found in the vast majority of radical prostatectomy specimens with prostatic carcinoma. Microscopically, there are four major structural patterns of HG-PIN growth: tufting, micropapillary, cribriform, and flat (*Mod Pathol* 17:360, 2004) (**Fig. 29.2**; e-**Fig. 29.9**). These patterns are often admixed. At high-power magnification, HG-PIN shows basal cells (which are typically reduced in number) and atypical luminal cells. Nuclear abnormalities that should be present to diagnose HG-PIN include increased nuclear size, increased chromatin clumping and content, and prominent nucleoli. The diagnosis can usually be made on H&E-stained sections. Immunostains for basal cells (34betaE12 and p63) and AMACR can be useful when the differential diagnosis is HG-PIN with outpouching versus HG-PIN with associated invasive adenocarcinoma (*Am J Surg Pathol* 29:529, 2005). Isolated HG-PIN in needle biopsy and TURP chips has been considered a risk factor for subsequent detection of carcinoma on rebiopsy, although the level of risk has decreased with increased 10- to 12-core sampling of the prostate (*Urology* 65: 538, 2005; *Am J Surg Pathol* 29: 1201, 2005), such that not all patients necessarily need to undergo rebiopsy in the first year following diagnosis of isolated HG-PIN (*J Urol* 175: 820, 2006). Patients with four or more cores with HG-PIN do appear to be at increased risk for subsequent detection of carcinoma and should be considered candidates for rebiopsy (*Am J Surg Pathol* 30: 1184, 2006).

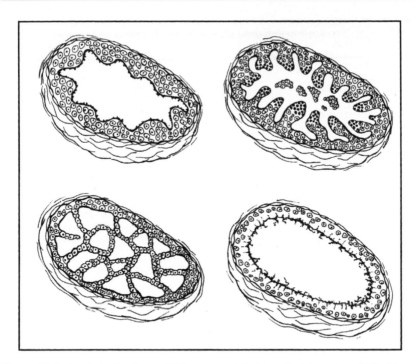

Figure 29.2. Architectural patterns of high-grade prostatic intraepithelial neoplasia (PIN). (Reproduced with permission from Humphrey PA. *Prostate Pathology.* Chicago: ASCP Press; 2003. © 2003 American Society for Clinical Pathology. Used with permission.)

G. **Focal glandular atypia (atypical small acinar proliferation)** is a descriptive diagnosis for a gland or group of glands with architectural or cytologic atypia that does not allow for a definitive diagnosis of reactive atypia, atypical adenomatous hyperplasia, PIN, or carcinoma. If there is significant concern for malignancy, a diagnosis of focal glandular atypia suspicious for carcinoma may be rendered. A diagnosis of atypia is applied in about 3% (range 1% to 9%) of needle biopsies (*J Urol* 175: 820, 2006). Distortion artifact, section thickness, and overstaining can contribute to difficulty in interpretation. Immunostains for basal cells (34betaE12 and p63) and AMACR can be very useful in establishing a definitive diagnosis when atypia is the initial diagnosis in H&E-stained sections. Patients with a diagnosis of atypia or atypical small acinar proliferation (ASAP) in needle biopsy should be clinically followed and rebiopsied, because about 43% of men are diagnosed with carcinoma on rebiopsy (*J Urol* 175: 820, 2006).

H. **Prostate cancer,** which is adenocarcinoma in the vast majority of cases, is a common malignancy in North America, Europe, and Australia, whereas it is less common in Asia.

1. **Risk factors.** Proven risk factors for adenocarcinoma include age, family history, and race. Prostatic adenocarcinoma is uncommonly diagnosed clinically before the age of 50, whereas a significant minority of men (around 31%) in their 30s and 40s have small adenocarcinoma detectable at autopsy (*In Vivo* 8: 1459, 1994). Hereditary prostatic adenocarcinoma accounts for about 10% of prostatic adenocarcinomas. Several candidate genes involved in hereditary transmission have been identified (*Mod Pathol* 17: 380, 2004), but currently genetic testing for predisposition to prostatic adenocarcinoma is not performed. Probable risk

TABLE 29.1	WHO Histological Classification of Tumors of Prostate

Epithelial tumors
Glandular neoplasms
Adenocarcinoma (acinar)
  Atrophic
  Pseudohyperplastic
  Foamy
  Colloid
  Signet ring
  Oncocytic
  Lymphoepithelioma-like
  Carcinoma with spindle cell differentiation
    (carcinosarcoma, sarcomatoid carcinoma)
Prostatic intraepithelial neoplasia (PIN)
Ductal adenocarcinoma
  Cribriform
  Papillary
  Solid
Urothelial tumors
Urothelial carcinoma
Squamous tumors
Adenosquamous carcinoma
Squamous cell carcinoma
Basal cell tumors
Basal cell adenoma
Basal cell carcinoma

Neuroendocrine tumors
Endocrine differentiation within adenocarcinoma
Carcinoid tumor
Small cell carcinoma
Paraganglioma
Neuroblastoma

Prostatic stromal tumors
Stromal tumor of uncertain malignant potential
Stromal sarcoma

Mesenchymal tumors
Leiomyosarcoma
Rhabdomyosarcoma
Chondrosarcoma
Angiosarcoma
Malignant fibrous histiocytoma
Malignant peripheral nerve sheath tumor
Hemangioma
Chondroma
Leiomyoma
Granular cell tumor
Hemangiopericytoma
Solitary fibrous tumor

Hematolymphoid tumors
Lymphoma
Leukemia

Miscellaneous tumors
Cystadenoma
Nephroblastoma (Wilms tumor)
Rhabdoid tumor
Germ cell tumors
  Yolk sac tumor
  Seminoma
  Embryonal carcinoma and teratoma
  Choriocarcinoma
Clear cell adenocarcinoma
Melanoma

Metastatic tumors

Tumors of the seminal vesicles

Epithelial tumors
Adenocarcinoma
Cystadenoma

Mixed epithelial and stromal tumors
Malignant
Benign

Mesenchymal tumors
Leiomyosarcoma
Angiosarcoma
Liposarcoma
Malignant fibrous histiocytoma
Solitary fibrous tumor
Hemangiopericytoma
Leiomyoma

Miscellaneous tumors
Choriocarcinoma
Male adnexal tumor of probably Wolffian
  origin

Metastatic tumors

From: Ebele JN, Sauter G, Epstein JI, Sesterhenn IA, eds. *World Health Organization Classification of Tumours. Pathology and Genetics. Tumours of the Urinary System and Male Genital Organs.* Lyon: IARC Press; 2004. Used with permission.

factors include dietary fat and androgens; potential risk factors are cadmium, low vitamin D, low vitamin E, low selenium, herbicides, and sedentary lifestyle.

2. **Clinical diagnosis** of clinically localized prostate cancer is based on serum PSA and digital rectal examination (DRE). Serum PSA is widely used for early detection in the United States, although its use for screening is controversial. Serum PSA level is clearly related to risk for histologic diagnosis of carcinoma, but risk exists below the most often used 4.0 ng/mL prompt for biopsy (*N Engl J Med* 347: 215, 2003). The DRE is neither particularly sensitive nor specific for a diagnosis of prostatic carcinoma. Thus, histopathological tissue diagnosis is the standard to establish a diagnosis of malignancy in the prostate. Prostatic carcinoma generally does not cause symptoms until late in the course of the disease. Local growth into the urethra and bladder neck can cause increase in frequency and difficulty in urination. Metastatic spread to bone can produce pain in the lower back, chest, hip, legs, and shoulders. Response to treatment is followed by serum PSA and in some cases, radiological studies.

3. **Histologic typing and diagnosis** of prostate cancer are accomplished by examination of H&E-stained sections. The 2004 World Health Organization (WHO) classification of neoplasms of the prostate is given in Table 29.1.

4. **Acinar adenocarcinoma** of the prostate is by far the most common type of prostate cancer.

   a. **Gross diagnosis** of prostatic carcinoma is possible in radical prostatectomy tissues but not in needle biopsy or TURP chip tissues. Impalpable prostatic carcinomas detected due to an elevated serum PSA (clinical stage T1c) are difficult to impossible to visualize on cut sections of radical prostatectomy specimens. When visible, the carcinoma can appear nodular and white to irregular and gray or white-yellow (e-Fig. 29.10).

   b. **Microscopic diagnosis** is based on a synthesis of a constellation of histologic attributes (Table 29.2) (*J Clin Pathol* 60:35, 2007). Major criteria are architecture (pattern of growth), absence of basal cells, and nuclear atypia. The architectural patterns of cellular arrangement are well-depicted in the Gleason grading picture (Fig. 29.3). Well-differentiated prostatic adenocarcinoma of Gleason patterns 1 and 2 displays abnormal glandular arrangements in the form of well-circumscribed nodules of closely packed small acini (e-Fig. 29.11). Gleason pattern 3 usually presents as single, small, infiltrating glands, with wide stromal separation (e-Fig. 29.12). High-grade Gleason pattern 4 is cribriform (e-Fig. 29.13), fused small acinar, or hypernephromatoid, whereas high-grade Gleason pattern 5 is composed of sheets, single cells, or comedocarcinoma (e-Fig. 29.14) (*Am J Surg Pathol* 29:1228, 2005). Basal cell absence, the second major criterion, can sometimes be difficult to evaluate in H&E-stained sections, so in difficult cases and for small foci of adenocarcinoma (minimal

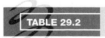

TABLE 29.2   **Criteria for Diagnosis of Prostatic Adenocarcinoma**

Major criteria

Architectural: Infiltrative small glands or cribriform glands too large or irregular to represent high-grade prostatic intraepithelial neoplasia (PIN)

Single cell layer (absence of basal cells)

Nuclear atypia: Nuclear and nucleolar enlargement

Minor criteria

Intraluminal wispy blue mucin (blue-tinged or basophilic mucinous secretions)

Pink amorphous secretions

Mitotic figures

Intraluminal crystalloids

Adjacent high-grade PIN

Amphophilic cytoplasm

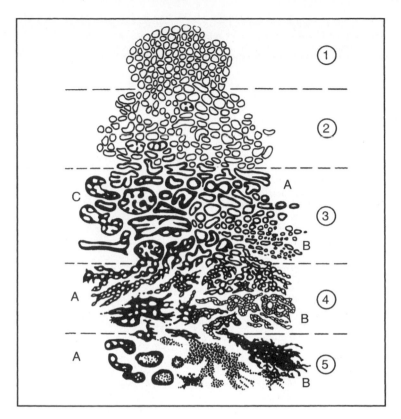

Figure 29.3. Gleason grades 1 to 5.

or limited adenocarcinoma), immunohistochemical staining for basal cells using antibodies against high-molecular-weight cytokeratins (such as 34betaE12, also known as CK903) and p63 may be performed (**e-Fig. 29.15**). While a positive basal cell immunostain effectively rules out invasive adenocarcinoma, benign glands can focally lack a basal cell layer, so basal cell immunostains should be interpreted in the context of the H&E histological findings (*Semin Diagn Pathol* 22:88, 2005). Nuclear atypia in the form of nuclear enlargement and nucleolar enlargement is the third of the major criteria. The minor criteria (Table 29.2) tend to be found more often in adenocarcinoma, but are not specific for adenocarcinoma. Features considered specific for a diagnosis of prostatic adenocarcinoma include extraprostatic spread of prostatic glands, collagenous micronodules, glomeruloid intraglandular projections, and perineural invasion (**e-Fig. 29.16**). Of note, benign glands can abut intraprostatic nerves (*Am J Surg Pathol* 29:1159,2005).

   c. **Immunohistochemical studies** are helpful in a minority of cases. The most commonly used immunostains are those for basal cells and an immunostain for a neoplastic cell-selective marker (alpha-methylacyl coenzyme A racemase [AMACR or P504S]), usually to assess a few atypical glands in needle biopsy. AMACR is fairly sensitive for neoplastic prostatic epithelial cells (in both PIN and invasive carcinoma), staining 80% to 100% of adenocarcinomas, but is not specific as it can be found focally in benign glands (*Semin Diagn Pathol* 22:88, 2005). Cocktails using p63 and AMACR or p63/34betaE12/AMACR antibodies are useful when a limited amount of

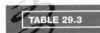

TABLE 29.3	Immunophenotype of Prostatic vs. Urothelial (Transitional Cell) Carcinoma	
	Prostatic carcinoma	**Urothelial carcinoma**
Marker	**(percentage of cases positive)**	
PSA	94% to 100%	0%
PSAP	89% to 100%	0%
Thrombomodulin	0%	69% to 91%
Uroplakin III	0%	57%
High molecular weight cytokeratin[1]	0% to 10%[2]	65% to 100%

PSAP = Prostate-specific acid phosphatase
[1] Detected by antibody 34betaE12.
[2] Mean = 3% prostatic carcinoma cases positive. Up to 20% of cases of metastatic prostatic carcinoma can be positive.

tissue is available for staining (e-**Fig. 29.15**) (*Am J Surg Pathol* 29:579, 2005; *Semin Diagn Pathol* 22:88, 2005). PSAP, PSA, thrombomodulin, and high-molecular-weight cytokeratin immunostains should be used for poorly differentiated carcinomas when the differential diagnosis is poorly differentiated prostatic adenocarcinoma versus poorly differentiated urothelial (transitional cell carcinoma) (Table 29.3) (*Semin Diagn Pathol* 22:88, 2005). PSA and PSAP immunostains should always be performed when one is confronted with a metastatic adenocarcinoma of unknown primary origin in a man.

    d. Molecular studies are not currently used to diagnose prostatic carcinoma.

  5. Variants of acinar adenocarcinoma include atrophic, pseudohyperplastic, foamy, colloid (mucinous), signet ring, oncocytic, lymphoepithelioma-like, and sarcomatoid carcinoma (carcinosarcoma) (Table 29.1). Atrophic pattern adenocarcinoma displays decreased cytoplasm and can thereby mimic benign atrophy. Such cytoplasmic volume loss can be seen with or without a history of hormonal or radiation therapy. Most cases are Gleason pattern 3. Pseudohyperplastic carcinoma is another malignancy that can resemble benign glands (*Am J Surg Pathol* 22:1139, 1998). Here, the malignant glands simulate BPH glands—they are complex with intraluminal papillary projections, undulating luminal surfaces, branching patterns, and/or cystic dilatation. Foamy gland carcinoma is characterized by xanthomatous cytoplasm and bland nuclei; these carcinomas range in Gleason score from 5 to 7. Mucinous carcinoma of the prostate is defined as adenocarcinoma with at least 25% of the tumor composed of lakes of extracellular mucin. This is an aggressive, rare variant, with Gleason grade patterns of 4 (usually) or 3. Signet-ring carcinoma of the prostate is also rare and clinically aggressive. The Gleason grade is 5. Only a few cases of oncocytic and lymphoepithelioma-like carcinoma have been reported. Sarcomatoid carcinoma of the prostate is rare (*Am J Surg Pathol* 30:1316, 2006) and may be a homologous spindle cell malignancy or heterologous, with an osteosarcomatous, chondrosarcomatous, or rhabdomyosarcomatous component. In one half of the men there was a history of prostatic adenocarcinoma treated by hormonal and/or radiation therapy. The outcome is poor.

  6. Ductal adenocarcinoma is the second most common subtype of prostatic adenocarcinoma (after acinar). Previously known as endometrioid adenocarcinoma, in pure form it accounts for about 1% of prostatic cancers and, when mixed with acinar adenocarcinoma, roughly 5% of prostatic cancers. Microscopically, these are usually papillary and/or cribriform adenocarcinomas (e-**Fig. 29.17**) that can arise centrally (causing urinary obstruction and hematuria), but can also be found peripherally. Cytologically, tall columnar neoplastic cells with cleared or amphophilic cytoplasm may be observed. Most patients present at a more advanced stage, and outcome is worse than that of acinar adenocarcinoma.

7. **Rare types of prostatic carcinoma** include urothelial carcinoma (arising from central prostatic ducts), squamous and adenosquamous carcinoma, basal cell carcinoma, and neuroendocrine carcinomas, including small cell and large cell neuroendocrine carcinomas (*Mod Pathol* 17:316, 2004). It is important to exclude primary urethral and urinary bladder urothelial carcinoma before diagnosing primary prostatic urothelial carcinoma. An in situ component can be extensive in the prostate, with solid plugs of cytologically pleomorphic tumor cells, often with comedo necrosis, and stromal inflammation. Prostatic stromal invasion is typified by irregular solid nests and cords. Squamous cell and adenosquamous carcinomas of the prostate comprise less than 1% of all prostatic carcinomas, and in about two thirds of cases there is a history of hormonal and or radiation treatment (*Am J Surg Pathol* 28:651, 2004). Average survival is 2 years. Basal cell carcinoma of the prostate includes malignant basaloid proliferations (basaloid or basal cell carcinomas) and also neoplasms that resemble, to a certain degree, adenoid cystic carcinomas of the salivary glands (*Am J Surg Pathol* 27:1523, 2003). For basal cell carcinomas there are several growth arrangements, including large basaloid nests with peripheral palisading and necrosis, a florid basal cell hyperplasia-like pattern, and an adenoid basal cell hyperplasia-like pattern (adenoid cystic carcinoma pattern). Small cell carcinoma of the prostate is quite rare and in one half of cases is admixed with adenocarcinoma. The histological appearance is similar to that of small cell carcinoma of the lung. In one third of cases there is a history of prostatic adenocarcinoma, followed by hormonal therapy. A similar history is obtained in most cases of large cell neuroendocrine carcinoma of the prostate (*Am J Surg Pathol* 30:684, 2006). Outcome is very poor for neuroendocrine carcinomas of the prostate.

8. **Mesenchymal neoplasms** are rare. The most common benign mesenchymal neoplasm is the leiomyoma, and the most common malignant mesenchymal neoplasms are rhabdomyosarcoma in children and leiomyosarcoma in adults.

9. **Hematolymphoid neoplasms** may involve the prostate, including leukemia, lymphoma, Hodgkin disease, and multiple myeloma. Leukemic infiltrates almost always indicate secondary spread, and are usually chronic lymphocytic leukemia. About one third of prostatic lymphomas are felt to be primary. The most common histologic type is diffuse large B cell lymphoma.

10. **Miscellaneous neoplasms** rarely encountered in the prostate include paragangliomas, melanocytic neoplasms, and germ cell tumors.

11. **Secondary malignancy** in the prostate is overall uncommon, but can be seen in a substantial minority of patients with urothelial carcinoma of the bladder, leukemia, and non-Hodgkin lymphoma.

12. **Treatment effects** can substantially alter the morphology of prostatic carcinoma, resulting in difficulty in diagnosis.
    a. **Hormonal androgen deprivation therapy** can cause a decrease in number of glands, glandular atrophy, single tumor cells, nuclear pyknosis, and cytoplasmic vacuolization (e-**Fig. 29.18**). Carcinoma cells may then resemble lymphocytes or histiocytes. PSA and pan-cytokeratin immunostains can be useful.
    b. **Radiation therapy** can induce striking nuclear atypia in benign glands. Positive basal cell and negative AMACR immunostains support a diagnosis of benign atypia. Adenocarcinoma postradiotherapy shows a decrease in number of neoplastic glands, poorly formed glands and single cells, cytoplasmic vacuolization, and nuclear pyknosis.

I. **Seminal vesicles** are rarely the site of origin of primary disease, including inflammation and neoplasia. Amyloid can be identified in about 10% of seminal vesicles, as a function of aging. Its presence does not indicate systemic amyloidosis unless there is also co-existing vascular amyloid deposition, which is rare. Seminal vesicles are usually examined for prostatic carcinoma as a part of pathologic staging.

J. **Prostatic urethra** urothelium is subject to the same diseases as urothelium in urinary bladder, namely inflammation, metaplasia (squamous metaplasia, urethritis cystica and glandularis, and nephrogenic metaplasia [adenoma]), hyperplasia, and neoplasms such as papilloma and carcinoma. However, primary, isolated malignancies of the prostatic urethra are exceedingly rare, and malignancy in the prostatic urethra is most often due to secondary synchronous involvement by urothelial (transitional cell carcinoma) of the urinary bladder.

IV. **HISTOLOGIC GRADING OF PROSTATIC ADENOCARCINOMA.** Grading should be performed using the Gleason system (Fig. 29.3). All adenocarcinomas of the prostate should be graded, except those posthormonal therapy or postradiotherapy (when radiation effect is evident). Grading is based solely on architecture and does not incorporate cytologic atypia or mitotic counting. At low magnification (40 to 100×), the most common pattern and the second most common pattern are summed to yield a score (on a scale of 2 to 10). Recent recommendations in application of the Gleason system include the following (*Am J Surg Pathol* 29:1228, 2005):

   A. Do not (or rarely) assign a well-differentiated Gleason score 2 to 4 to carcinoma in needle biopsy. This almost always represents undergrading.

   B. When three grades are present, in needle biopsy give most common grade and worst grade. So if 3 + 4 + 5 are present, the Gleason grade is 3 + 5 = score of 8. In radical prostatectomy, give the most common and second most common grades, but if there is a minor tertiary high-grade 4 or 5 pattern, this should be noted in a comment.

   C. If there is 95% high-grade pattern 4 or 5 and 5% or less of 2 or 3, one should ignore the lower grade component. Any high-grade tissue (pattern 4 or 5) should be incorporated into a needle biopsy Gleason score. So 98% pattern 3 and 2% pattern 4 in needle is Gleason grade 3 + 4 = score of 7.

   D. Variants of prostatic adenocarcinoma can be graded. Most ductal adenocarcinomas are pattern 4 (4 + 4 = score of 8), but comedocarcinoma (pattern 5) can also be seen.

   E. The vast majority of cribriform adenocarcinomas are high-grade pattern 4.

   F. For needle biopsies, provide grade by clinically submitted container, even if several cores are within the container. One can also provide the Gleason grade for the core with highest Gleason score, if different from the overall Gleason score for cores from that container.

      Gleason grade is critical for patient prognosis. It is commonly used clinically along with serum PSA level and clinical or pathological stage in tables (Partin tables) (http://urology.jhu.edu/Partin_tables/index.html) and nomograms (*J Urol* 165:1562, 2001) to predict pathological stage and response to treatment and outcome.

V. **PATHOLOGIC STAGING.** Staging applies only to adenocarcinomas of the prostate and not to sarcomas and prostatic carcinoma variants that are not adenocarcinomas. The 2002 Tumor, Node, Metastasis (TNM) American Joint Committee on Cancer/International Union Against Cancer (AJCC/UICC) staging classification is given in Table 29.4. Clinical staging should be distinguished from pathologic staging. Note that a new TNM AJCC staging scheme is expected to be released in 2009.

   A. Needle biopsy. Pathologic staging is not performed. However, extraprostatic spread should be diagnosed if carcinoma is seen in fat (rare) or in seminal vesicle tissue.

   B. TURP chips and open prostatectomy. Pathologic staging is not done, but for incidental carcinoma, the amount of carcinoma determined by visual, light microscopic inspection of tissue involved will place the patient into clinical stage T1a or T1b.

   C. Radical prostatectomy and pelvic lymphadenectomy are used for pathologic staging (Table 29.4) (*Arch Pathol Lab Med* 130:936, 2006).

      1. pT2: Organ-confined prostatic carcinoma, subdivided into a, b, and c.

      2. pT3: Extraprostatic extension (EPE) by carcinoma, diagnosed if carcinoma extends into posterolateral periprostatic adipose tissue (e-**Fig. 29.19**) or beyond the outer boundary of normal prostatic glands at the anterior or apical prostate. Note that carcinoma in skeletal muscle at apex does not always mean EPE. Site(s) and extent of EPE should be specified. EPE extent should be given as focal (only a few glands outside the prostate) or nonfocal. Capsular invasion is not part of the staging scheme. pT3b is seminal vesicle wall invasion (e-**Fig. 29.20**).

      3. pT4: Gross bladder neck or rectal involvement by carcinoma. Microscopic involvement of bladder neck should not be equated with pT4 (*Urology* 64:551, 2004).

      4. pN: Number of involved and total number of examined lymph nodes should be given.

      5. pM: At time of radical prostatectomy, patients are clinical M0 (cM0).

TABLE 29.4 | **Tumor, Node, Metastasis (TNM) Staging Scheme for Prostatic Carcinoma**

Primary tumor, clinical (T)

TX	Primary tumor cannot be assessed
T0	No evidence of primary tumor
T1	Clinically inapparent tumor neither palpable nor visible by imaging
T1a	Tumor incidental histologic finding in $\leq$5% of tissue resected
T1b	Tumor incidental histologic finding in >5% of tissue resected
T1c	Tumor identified by needle biopsy (e.g., because of elevated prostate-specific antigen)
T2	Tumor confined within prostate[1]
T2a	Tumor involves one half of one lobe or less
T2b	Tumor involves more than one half of one lobe but not both lobes
T2c	Tumor involves both lobes
T3	Tumor extends through the prostate capsule[2]
T3a	Extracapsular extension (unilateral or bilateral)
T3b	Tumor invades seminal vesicle(s)
T4	Tumor is fixed or invades adjacent structures other than seminal vesicles; bladder neck, external sphincter, rectum, levator muscles, and/or pelvic wall

Primary tumor, pathologic (pT)

pT2[3]	Organ confined
pT2a	Unilateral, involving one half of one lobe or less
pT2b	Unilateral, involving more than one half of one lobe but not both lobes
pT2c	Bilateral
pT3	Extraprostatic extension
pT3a	Extraprostatic extension
pT3b	Seminal vesicle invasion
pT4	Invasion of bladder, rectum

Regional lymph nodes (N)

NX	Regional lymph nodes cannot be assessed
N0	No regional lymph node metastasis
N1	Metastasis in regional lymph node or nodes

Distant metastasis[5] (M)

MX	Distant metastasis cannot be assessed
M0	No distant metastasis
M1	Distant metastasis
M1a	Nonregional lymph node(s)
M1b	Bone(s)
M1c	Other site(s)

Stage grouping

Stage I	T1a	N0	M0	G1	(Gleason score 2 to 4)
Stage II	T1a	N0	M0	G2,3-4	(Gleason score 5 to 10)
	T1b	N0	M0	Any G	
	T1c	N0	M0	Any G	
	T1	N0	M0	Any G	
	T2	N0	M0	Any G	
Stage III	T3	N0	M0	Any G	
Stage IV	T4	N0	M0	Any G	
	Any T	N1	M0	Any G	
	Any T	Any N	M1	Any G	

[1]Note: Tumor found in one or both lobes by needle biopsy, but not palpable or reliably visible by imaging, is classified as T1c.
[2]Note: Invasion into the prostatic apex or into (but not beyond) the prostatic capsule is not classified as T3, but as T2.
[3]Note: There is no pathologic T1 classification.
[4]Note: Positive surgical margin should be indicated by an R1 descriptor (residual microscopic disease).
[5]Note: When more than one site of metastasis is present, the most advanced category is used. pM1c is most advanced.
From: Greene FL, Page DL, Fleming ID, Fritz AG, Balch CM, Haller DG, Morrow M, eds. *AJCC Cancer Staging Manual.* 6th edition. New York: Springer; 2002. Used with permission. (A new AJCC TNM staging system is scheduled for release in 2009; after its publication, the new staging scheme will appear on the website for this book.)

VI. REPORTING PROSTATE CANCER (*Arch Pathol Lab Med* 130:303, 2006; *Arch Pathol Lab Med* 130: 936, 2006).

For fine needle aspiration biopsy samples with carcinoma identified, grade should be given as well, moderately, or poorly differentiated.

For needle core biopsy samples, histologic type, Gleason grade, and amount of tumor should be provided. Amount of tumor can be quantitated as number of positive cores/total number of cores, percentage of tissue involved by carcinoma (by visual inspection), and linear millimeters of carcinoma per total millimeters of tissue. If present, report periprostatic fat invasion, seminal vesicle invasion, perineural invasion, and lymphovascular space invasion.

For TURP and simple (enucleation) prostatectomy specimens, report histologic type, Gleason grade, and amount of tumor. For Gleason grade, if three patterns are present, use predominant and worst pattern of remaining two. Amount of tumor should always include percentage of tissue involved by tumor (by visual inspection); number of positive chips per total number of chips is also recommended. If present, report periprostatic fat invasion, seminal vesicle invasion, perineural invasion, and lymphovascular space invasion.

For radical prostatectomy specimens, report histologic type, Gleason grade, amount of tumor, pathologic stage, and margin status. Amount of tumor can be reported as percentage of tissue involved by carcinoma (by visual inspection). Another option is greatest dimension of dominant nodule (if present). For margins involved by carcinoma, specify number and location of positive sites. (Note: If margin is positive for carcinoma without EPE, designate as pT2+). Additional findings worth reporting: lymphovascular space invasion by carcinoma, inflammation, BPH, PIN, and adenosis.

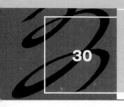

30 PENIS AND SCROTUM

Peter A. Humphrey

I. **NORMAL ANATOMY.** The penis is anatomically composed of three parts: posterior (root); central body or shaft; and anterior portion, composed of glans, coronal sulcus, and foreskin (prepuce). In the shaft there are three cylinders of erectile tissues: a ventral corpus spongiosum surrounding the urethra, and two corpora cavernosa. Histologically, the erectile tissues are characterized by numerous vascular spaces with surrounding smooth muscle fibers (e-Fig. 30.1).* The tunica albuginea, a sheath of hyalinized collagen, encases the corpora cavernosa. All three corpora are surrounded by Buck's fascia, adipose tissue, dartos muscle, dermis, and a thin epidermis. Distally, the corpus spongiosum forms the conical glans, which is also composed of a stratified squamous epithelium, lamina propria, tunica albuginea, and corpora cavernosa. The coronal sulcus is a cul de sac just below the glans corona. The foreskin is a double membrane that has five layers: mucosal epithelium similar to glans epithelium, lamina propria, dartos smooth muscle, dermis, and epidermis (Young RH, Srigley JR, Amin MB, Ulbright TM, Cubilla AL, eds. *Tumors of Prostate Gland, Seminal Vesicles, Male Urethra, and Penis.* AFIP Third Series, Fascicle 28, Washington DC: American Registry of Pathology 1998:, pp. 403–488).

The scrotum contains the testes and lower spermatic cords. It consists of skin that covers the dartos smooth muscle, fibers of the cremasteric muscle, and several layers of fascia. The skin is pigmented, hair-bearing, and loose, with numerous sebaceous and sweat glands. Lymphatic drainage is to the superficial inguinal lymph nodes.

II. **GROSS EXAMINATION AND TISSUE SAMPLING.** Tissue samples include mucosal or skin biopsies, penile urethral biopsies, foreskin resection specimens, and partial and total penectomy specimens.

A. **Punch and shave biopsies** of penile glans and skin should be handled like skin biopsies from other sites (see Chapter 38).

B. **Foreskin resection** is indicated for primary carcinomas of this site. The entire periphery of the mucosal margin should be submitted as shave resection margins (usually in three to four sections). The foreskin should then be pinned and fixed overnight in 10% formalin. Several full-thickness sections should allow for identification of all five layers.

C. For **partial penectomy specimens,** the surgical division of the penis is made 2 cm proximal to gross tumor extent. Three to four frozen sections are typically necessary to sample the cut surface of this margin. Permanent sections are taken as described below.

D. For **total penectomy specimens,** only proximal urethral and periurethral margin tissues should be submitted for frozen section, unless the mass is grossly close to or involves the skin, which should also then be sampled. For permanent sections of both partial and total penectomy specimens, the foreskin (except for a 2- to 3-mm remnant), when present, should be removed and handled as noted above. A thin 2-mm shave of all the structures in the shaft margin should be taken, if not already sampled at frozen section. One to three additional transverse sections should be taken from the glans. Any mass or masses should be sampled to demonstrate pattern of growth, depth of extension, and relationship to normal anatomic structures.

---

*All e-figures are available online via the Solution Site Image Bank.

E. Lymph nodes. There may be a clinical request for frozen section(s) of enlarged inguinal lymph nodes; if positive for carcinoma, a more extended ilioinguinal lymph node dissection may follow. Bilateral inguinal lymphadenectomy specimens may also be received after removal of the primary tumor and a course of antibiotics, or in patients with T2, high-grade tumors or with vascular invasion (*Critical Rev Oncol-Hematol* 53:165, 2005).

A nomogram has been developed to predict nodal metastases using the presence of clinically palpable groin lymph nodes and histologic lymphovascular invasion in the primary tumor (*J Urol* 175:1700, 2006). The utility of sentinel lymph node sampling is not yet settled.

III. DIAGNOSTIC FEATURES OF COMMON DISEASES OF THE PENIS AND SCROTUM

A. Inflammation and infection. Three categories may be defined: inflammatory conditions specific to penis and scrotum, systematic dermatoses (not considered here), and sexually transmitted diseases. (Murphy WM (ed). *Urological Pathology* (2nd ed). Philadelphia: WB Sanders Co., 1999; BJU Int 90:498, 2002).

1. **Phimosis,** the clinical condition in which the foreskin cannot be retracted behind the glans penis, is associated with fibrosis, inflammation, and edema of the prepuce.

2. **Paraphimosis** is diagnosed clinically when the foreskin cannot be advanced back over the glans secondary to fibrosis and inflammation.

3. **Balanoposthitis** is inflammation of the glans penis and prepuce, usually in uncircumcised men with poor hygiene.

4. **Balanatis,** or inflammation of the glans, may occur in several forms.

   a. **Plasma cell balanitis (Zoon's balanitis)** can clinically and grossly mimic carcinoma in situ, with presentation as brown or red patches or plaques. The histologic appearance can vary with time, and the inflammatory cell infiltrate can vary from patchy and lymphoplasmacytic (early) to dense and plasmacytic (later) (*Am J Dermatopathol* 24:459, 2002).

   b. **Balanitis xerotica obliterans (BXO)** is lichen sclerosus of the glans and prepuce that macroscopically appears as a white patch or plaque. Histologically, the squamous epithelium is typically atrophic and hyperkeratotic, with a band of pale homogenous collagen in the upper dermis and an underlying lymphocytic infiltrate (e-**Fig. 30.2**). Complications include meatal stenosis (urethral stricture), and very uncommonly, squamous cell carcinoma.

   c. **Balanitis circinata** microscopically looks like pustular psoriasis and is seen in Reiter's syndrome, which includes nongonococcal urethritis, conjunctivitis, and arthritis.

5. **Human papillomavirus (HPV) infection** can lead to condyloma acuminata. The growth is typically papillary or warty, and histologically papillomatosis, acanthosis, parakeratosis, and hyperkeratosis are found. Koilocytes, with wrinkled nuclear membranes, nucleomegaly, cytoplasmic halos, and binucleation, may be prominent or inconspicuous. The causal HPV types are usually 6 and 11, but it is not necessary to verify the presence of HPV. Bowenoid papulosis is also an HPV-related proliferation that presents with multiple 2- 10-mm papules than can coalesce to form plaques; it is usually caused by types 16, 18, and/or 35. Microscopically, while the image is similar to carcinoma in situ, the clinical course is typically self-limited and benign.

6. **Herpes simplex virus (HSV) infection** of the male genitalia is usually caused by subtype 2, which produces multiple vesicles. The diagnosis may be confirmed by scraping and performance of a Tzanck smear, which reveals multinucleated giant cells with intranuclear inclusions.

7. **Scabies** is an infestation by a mite that burrows into the keratin layer of the epidermis, with generation of erythematous papules and nodules. Detection of the mites may be accomplished via scrapes or biopsy. In tissue sections, the 400-micron mite, eggs, or egg walls, are diagnostic. Dermal eosinophils and epidermal spongiosis are characteristic responses.

8. **Pediculosis pubis** is infection by *Pediculus pubis*, also known as the crab louse. Biopsy is not necessary; the lice may be seen by a magnifying lens.

9. **Syphilis** is caused by *Treponema pallidum*, a Gram-negative spirochete. The primary lesion, the chancre, is a single, round, craterlike painless ulcer most often located on the glans or prepuce. Biopsy is not usually necessary, but if done (for example, when syphilis is not clinically suspected), it will show a perivascular lymphoplasmacytic infiltrate. The spirochetes may be identified in the epidermis or in dermal perivascular regions by silver stains (Steiner, Dieterle, or Warthin–Starry). The secondary and tertiary stages of syphilis are characterized by condyloma latum and gumma, respectively. Smears from the gray maculopapules of condyloma latum should be examined by dark-field microscopy for spirochetes. Biopsy may yield nonspecific findings. The gumma is a necrotic mass with surrounding granulomatous inflammation, and associated obliterative endarteritis with perivascular plasma cells.

10. **Gonorrhea** is caused by *Neisseria gonorrhoeae*, a Gram-negative diplococcus. Urethritis, with urethral discharge, may lead to urethral stricture. Biopsies are hardly ever performed.

11. **Lymphogranuloma venereum** is due to *Chlamydia trachomatis*. Vesicles, then ulcers, develop in the primary genital phase; biopsies are not useful. In the secondary stage, patients develop painful inguinal lymphadenopathy (bubo). Histologically, the lymph nodes demonstrate stellate necrosis surrounded by palisaded histiocytes. This histologic picture can also be seen in cat scratch fever, tularemia, bubonic plague, and fungal and atypical mycobacterial infections.

12. **Granuloma inguinale** is caused by *Calymmatobacterium granulomatis*, a Gram-negative intracellular bacillus, resulting in ulcers. Smears or biopsy sections reveal histiocytes with inclusions (Donovan bodies), best visualized by Warthin–Starry or Giemsa stains.

13. **Chancroid** is caused by *Haemophilus ducreyi*, a Gram-negative rod, and is typified by painful nonindurated penile ulcers and lymphadenopathy. The organisms can be found in smears or histologic sections stained with Giemsa, Gram, or methylene blue stains.

14. **Molluscum contagiosum** is caused by a DNA pox virus and produces multiple small dome-shaped papules with a central umbilication. Biopsy sections show a crater with an acanthotic epidermis and the diagnostic intracytoplasmic viral inclusions (molluscum bodies).

15. **Penile infections in acquired immunodeficiency syndrome (AIDS)** potentially include almost all sexually transmitted infections including gonorrhea, syphilis, herpes, candidiasis, chancroid, molluscum contagiosum, HPV, scabies, and Reiter's syndrome.

16. **Lipogranulomas** in the scrotum or penis are secondary to injections of oil-based chemicals. Sections show a foreign-body, lymphoplasmacytic, and histiocytic reaction to lipid droplets that appear as cleared spaces.

17. **Hidradenitis suppurativa,** more typical of the sweat glands in the axilla, can also involve the scrotum. Acute and chronic inflammation, fibrosis, and even sinus tract formation can occur.

18. **Gangrene,** as a necroinflammatory process, can involve the scrotum due to many insults. Fournier gangrene is an extreme fulminant infection of the genitals, perineum, or abdominal wall (*Int J Urol* 13:960, 2006).

19. **Idiopathic scrotal calcinosis** can occur due to calcification of dermal connective tissue (idiopathic) or in association with keratinous cysts. Multiple firm nodules are found, measuring several millimeters to several centimeters in greatest dimension, typically in the scrotum of younger men. Microscopically, calcific material is present with or without granulomatous inflammation and/or cyst wall remnants.

20. **Elephantiasis** or massive scrotal lymphedema is usually secondary to filariasis.

B. **Miscellaneous benign nonneoplastic conditions**

1. **Peyronie's disease** presents with a painful bending of the erect penis. Histologically, there is fibrosis or fibromatosis of the tunica albuginea (e-**Fig. 30.3**). Rarely, calcification and ossification may occur in these fibrous plaques.

2. Penile cysts

    a. Median raphe cyst is most commonly located in the midline on the ventral aspect of the shaft. It is lined by pseudostratified, columnar, mucinous epithelial cells.

    b. Mucoid cysts are thought to arise from ectopic urethral mucosa, can be seen on the prepuce or glans, and are lined by stratified columnar epithelium with mucinous cells.

    c. Epidermal inclusion cysts are usually found on the penile shaft. They are also common in scrotal skin. They have the appearance as they do elsewhere in the skin.

C. Benign epithelial neoplasms include squamous papilloma, common condyloma, and the very rare giant condyloma of Buscke–Lowenstein. Most reported giant condylomas likely represent warty or verrucous carcinomas. Grossly, giant condylomas are 5 cm in average diameter, and microscopically look like a regular condyloma except for exuberant surface papillomatosis and pushing bulbous growth at the base. When carefully defined, they may be locally destructive but do not show malignant cytologic features or metastasize. (Eble JN, Sauter G, Epstein JI, Sesterhenn IA, eds. *Tumors of the Urinary System and Male Genital Organs.* Lyon, France: IARC Press, 2004).

D. Penile intraepithelial neoplasia. Carcinoma in situ or high-grade squamous intraepithelial lesion (grade III) includes erythroplasia of Queyrat (on glans) and Bowen disease (on penile shaft or prepuce). These are HPV-related (usually type 16 and 18) intraepithelial proliferations. Lower grade intraepithelial neoplasias (dysplasia) can be graded as I or II. It should be noted that condylomas can also exhibit intraepithelial neoplasia. Grossly, erythroplasia of Queyrat appears as a sharply demarcated patch on the glans, whereas Bowen disease is a solitary, brownish-red plaque on the shaft or foreskin. Microscopically, the two lesions are similar and are composed of a full-thickness proliferation of pleomorphic basaloid cells that exhibit loss of polarity (e-**Fig. 30.4**).

E. Penile cancer

    1. Risk factors for penile cancer are phimosis, chronic inflammation, lichen sclerosus, smoking, ultraviolet (UV) radiation, condyloma, HPV infections (usually type 18, less commonly type 18), and lack of circumcision (*J Am Acad Dermatol* 54:364, 2006). This latter factor is an extremely strong risk factor.

    2. Clinical diagnosis. Patients are typically 50 to 70 years of age and present with an exophytic or flat ulcerative mass of the glans, prepuce, or coronal sulcus. Patients with advanced disease may present with pubic or scrotal skin nodules and inguinal lymph node metastasis. Magnetic resonance imaging of primary penile cancer can help define local tumor extent and any shaft involvement (*Radiographics* 25: 1629, 2005).

    3. Histologic typing and diagnosis of penile cancer are accomplished via examination of hematoxylin and eosin (H&E)-stained sections. The 2004 World Health Organization (WHO) classification of penile neoplasms is provided in Table 30.1.

    4. Squamous cell carcinoma of the penis accounts for the vast majority of penile cancers.

        a. Gross diagnosis is readily done in penectomy specimens, because most masses are several centimeters, usually solitary, firm, and ulcerated (e-**Fig. 30.5**). Multicentric tumors are more frequently in the foreskin.

        b. Microscopic diagnosis is usually straightforward, but small superficial biopsies can be problematic in the differential distinction from pseudoepitheliomatous squamous cell hyperplasia. There are three major prognostically important growth patterns: superficial spreading, with horizontal growth and only superficial invasion; vertical growth, which is deeply invasive (e-**Fig. 30.6**); and multicentric. Histologically, most usual squamous cell carcinomas are moderately differentiated with some keratinization (e-**Fig. 30.7**). Small nests, cords, and single neoplastic cells infiltrate into the lamina propria, corpus spongiosum, and uncommonly, the corpus cavernosum (e-**Fig. 30.8**). Poorly differentiated carcinoma may grow as sheets, with necrosis and a high mitotic rate.

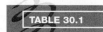

TABLE 30.1   WHO Histological Classification of Tumors of the Penis

Malignant epithelial tumors of the penis
Squamous cell carcinoma
  Basaloid carcinoma
  Warty (condylomatous) carcinoma
  Verrucous carcinoma
  Papillary carcinoma
  Sarcomatous carcinoma
  Mixed carcinoma
  Adenosquamous carcinoma
Merkel cell carcinoma
Small cell carcinoma
Sebaceous carcinoma
Clear cell carcinoma
Basal cell carcinoma

Precursor lesions
Penile intraepithelial neoplasia
Paget disease

Melanocytic tumors
Melanocytic nevus
Melanoma

Mesenchymal tumors

Hematopoietic tumors

Secondary tumors

From: Ebele JN, Sauter G, Epstein JI, Sesterhenn IA, eds. *World Health Organization Classification of Tumours. Pathology and Genetics. Tumours of the Urinary System and Male Genital Organs.* Lyon: IARC Press; 2004. Used with permission.

Giant cells and sarcomatoid features may be found in these high-grade tumors. Local extension into several compartments may occur. For example, a carcinoma originating on the glans may spread to the foreskin, to skin of the shaft, and to the urethra. In very advanced cases, direct spread to inguinal, pubic, or scrotal skin can occur.

  c. Immunohistochemical studies are useful the small minority of cases when uncertainty exists after examination of the H&E-stained slides, mainly for the distinction of a poorly differentiated squamous cell carcinoma from another malignant neoplasm such as a sarcoma, melanoma, or lymphoma. Immuno-histochemical detection of carcinoma cells in lymph nodes is of uncertain significance (*BJU Int* 98:70, 2006).

  d. Molecular studies are not currently used to diagnose penile carcinoma. HPV DNA typing is not necessary.

5. Variants of squamous cell carcinoma include basaloid, warty (condylomatous), verrucous, papillary, sarcomatoid, mixed, and adenosquamous (Table 30.1). Basaloid carcinoma is an uncommon, aggressive, HPV-related variant that is comprised of small, uniform, basaloid cells with high nuclear/cytoplasmic ratios and numerous mitoses (e-**Fig. 30.9**). Warty (condylomatous) carcinoma is one of the verruciform carcinomas (the others being verrucous carcinoma and papillary carcinoma) (**Fig. 30.1**). (Young RH, Srigley JR, Amin MB, Ulbright TM, Cubilla AL, eds. *Tumors of the Prostate Gland, Seminal Vesicles, Male Urethra, and Penis.* Washington DC: Armed Forces Institute of Pathology, 2005, p. 424); microscopically, it is hyperkeratotic and papillomatous, with cells of low to intermediate

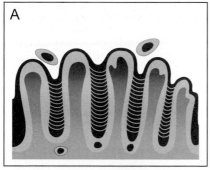
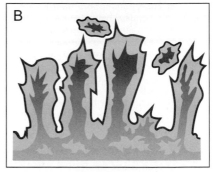
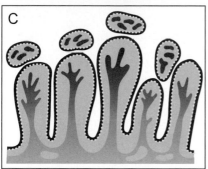
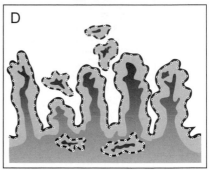

Figure 30.1. Verruciform tumors of the penis. **A.** Verrucous carcinoma with regular papillae, broad pushing base, and hyperkeratosis. **B.** Papillary carcinoma with irregular papillae and cores, and ragged infiltration at base. **C.** Giant condyloma, with branching cores and koilocytosis. **D.** Warty (condylomatous) carcinoma with irregular papillae and koilocytosis. (Modified from Young RH, Srigley JR, Amin MB, Ulbright TM, Cubilla AL, eds. *Tumors of the Prostate Gland, Seminal Vesicles, Male Urethra, and Penis.* Washington DC: Armed Forces Institute of Pathology; 2005:424).

nuclear grade. Koilocytic atypia may be prominent. Verrucous carcinoma is a very well-differentiated papillary neoplasm with hyperkeratosis, papillomatosis, and a broad pushing base. Papillary carcinoma is well-differentiated, hyperkeratotic, with complex papillae and an irregular infiltrative base. Sarcomatoid (spindle cell) carcinoma is an aggressive, high-grade, deeply invasive spindle cell malignancy with or without heterologous elements such as muscle, bone, and cartilage. Co-existing carcinoma in situ or invasive carcinoma is usually evident (*Am J Surg Pathol* 29:1152, 2005). In one quarter of cases the carcinoma can be mixed, such as warty–basaloid, adenocarcinoma–basaloid, and squamous–neuroendocrine. In adenosquamous carcinoma the glandular component is a minority component. Rare, recently recognized patterns include pseudohyperplastic squamous cell carcinoma (*Am J Surg Pathol* 28:895, 2004), and carcinoma cuniculatum (*Am J Surg Pathol* 31:71, 2007). The former can resemble pseudoepitheliomatous hyperplasia, and the latter is another verruciform squamous cell carcinoma that is low grade and has deeply-penetrating and burrowing patterns of growth.

6. **Rare types of primary penile carcinoma** include Merkel cell carcinoma, small cell carcinoma, sebaceous carcinoma, and clear cell carcinoma.

7. **Mesenchymal neoplasms** are rare and comprise 5% of all penile tumors. The most common benign soft tissue tumors are vascular (hemangioma and lymphangioma), followed by neural, myxoid, and fibrous tumors. The most frequent malignant soft tissue tumors are Kaposi's sarcoma and leiomyosarcoma (*Anal Quant Cytol Histol* 28:193, 2005).

8. **Hematolymphoid neoplasms** include very rare primary penile lymphomas and secondary lymphomas.
9. **Miscellaneous neoplasms** rarely encountered include melanoma (*J Urol* 173:1958, 2005).
10. **Secondary malignancies** are rare, with prostatic and urinary bladder carcinomas predominating. The corpus cavernosum is the most common site of metastasis, but spongiosum, skin, and glans may also be involved.
F. **Scrotal cancer** is most commonly squamous cell carcinoma.
   1. Squamous cell carcinoma of the scrotum is usually detected as invasive disease, but some examples of squamous cell carcinoma in situ have been reported.

TABLE 30.2	Tumor, Node, Metastasis (TNM) Staging Scheme for Penile Carcinoma

PRIMARY TUMOR (T)

TX	Primary tumor cannot be assessed
T0	No evidence of primary tumor
Tis	Carcinoma in situ
Ta	Noninvasive verrucous carcinoma
T1	Tumor invades subepithelial connective tissue
T2	Tumor invades corpus spongiosum or cavernosum
T3	Tumor invades urethra or prostate
T4	Tumor invades other adjacent structures

REGIONAL LYMPH NODES (N)

NX	Regional lymph nodes cannot be assessed
N0	No regional lymph node metastasis
N1	Metastasis in a single superficial, inguinal lymph node
N2	Metastasis in multiple or bilateral superficial inguinal lymph nodes
N3	Metastasis in deep inguinal or pelvic lymph nodes(s) unilateral or bilateral

DISTANT METASTASIS (M)

MX	Distant metastasis cannot be assessed
M0	No distant metastasis
M1	Distant metastasis

ADDITIONAL DESCRIPTOR

The m suffix indicates the presence of multiple primary tumors and is recorded in parentheses, e.g., pTa(m)N0M0.

STAGE GROUPING

Stage 0	Tis	N0	M0
	Ta	N0	M0
Stage I	T1	N0	M0
Stage II	T1	N1	M0
	T2	N0	M0
	T2	N1	M0
Stage III	T1	N2	M0
	T2	N2	M0
	T3	N0	M0
	T3	N1	M0
	T3	N2	M0
Stage IV	T4	Any N	M0
	Any T	N3	M0
	Any T	Any N	M1

From: Greene FL, Page DL, Fleming ID, Fritz AG, Balch CM, Haller DG, Morrow M, eds. *AJCC Cancer Staging Manual*. 6th edition. New York: Springer; 2002. Used with permission. (A new AJCC TNM staging system is scheduled for release in 2009; after its publication, the new staging scheme will appear on the website for this book.)

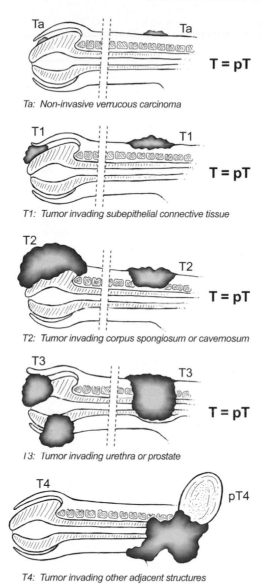

Ta: Non-invasive verrucous carcinoma

T = pT

T1: Tumor invading subepithelial connective tissue

T = pT

T2: Tumor invading corpus spongiosum or cavernosum

T = pT

T3: Tumor invading urethra or prostate

T = pT

pT4

T4: Tumor invading other adjacent structures

Figure 30.2. pT staging of penile carcinoma. (Modified from Greene FL, Compton CC, Fritz AG, Shah JP, Winchester DP, eds. *AJCC Cancer Staging Atlas.* New York: Springer; 2006.)

Associations exist with exposure to soot (in chimney sweeps, described in 1775 by Sir Percival Pott), machine oil, psoriasis treated with coal tar, arsenic, psoarelens / UV radiation, and HPV infection. Grossly, scrotal squamous cell carcinomas initially appear as a solitary nodule, followed by ulceration and induration. Microscopically, most are well to moderately differentiated (e-**Fig. 30.10**). They invade the scrotal wall, and larger cancers can involve the testis, spermatic cord, penis,

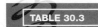

TABLE 30.3	Staging System for Scrotal Carcinoma

Stage	Description
A1	Localized to scrotal wall
A2	Local extension with involvement of adjacent structures (testis, spermatic cord, penis, pubis, perineum)
B	Metastasis to inguinal lymph nodes
C	Metastasis to pelvic lymph nodes
D	Metastasis to distant organs

From: Lowe FC. *J Urol.* 1983;130:423.

and perineum. Initial metastatic spread is to ipsilateral inguinal lymph nodes. Outcome is related to tumor size and pathological stage.

2. **Basal cell carcinomas** of scrotal skin are rare and have the same appearance as they do elsewhere in the skin.

3. **Paget's disease** of the scrotum can be associated with underlying carcinoma of the urinary bladder, urethra, prostate, or eccrine sweat glands.

4. **Sarcomas** of the scrotal wall are rare and should be distinguished from paratesticular, intrascrotal sarcomas. By far the most common histologic type of scrotal wall sarcoma is leiomyosarcoma, which likely arises from the dartos muscle.

IV. **HISTOLOGIC GRADING OF PENILE AND SCROTAL SQUAMOUS CELL CARCINOMAS** is done in three tiers as well differentiated, moderately differentiated, or poorly differentiated. Histologic grade of penile squamous cell carcinoma is linked to depth of infiltration, inguinal lymph metastasis, and survival.

V. **PATHOLOGIC STAGING OF PENILE CANCER** applies to carcinomas only. Pathologic primary tumor (pT) 2002 Tumor, Node, Metastasis (TNM) American Joint Committee on Cancer (AJCC) stage categories are given in Table 30.2 and are illustrated in Fig. 30.2. pN and pM groupings are also indicated in Table 30.2. An AJCC staging scheme for scrotal carcinoma does not exist; the currently used system is provided in Table 30.3.

VI. **REPORTING PENILE CARCINOMA** (*Eur Urol* 46:434, 2004). For circumcision and penectomy specimens, the following should be reported for the primary tumor: tumor size, histological type, histologic grade (G1, G2, or G3), origin, depth of invasion (mm) and structures involved, vascular and perineural invasion (if present), and margins of resection. For regional lymph nodes, the report should include the number identified and their location, number involved by tumor, size of metastatic deposit (if present), and extracapsular extension (if present). Additional pathological findings that can be noted (if present) are penile intraepithelial neoplasia and therapy-related changes.

Jamie K. Donnelly, John D. Pfeifer, and Phyllis C. Huettner

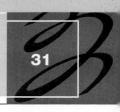

I. **NORMAL GROSS AND MICROSCOPIC ANATOMY.** The ovaries lie on either side of the uterus along the posterior surface of the broad ligament, inferior to the fallopian tubes. The gross measurement of the ovary varies depending on age and reproductive status. The average ovary, from a reproductive age woman, measures about 4 × 2.5 × 1.5 cm, whereas postmenopausal ovaries are about half that size. The outer surface is white-tan and smooth during early reproductive life, becoming more bosselated with age. The cut surface shows three ill-defined zones: a cortex, medulla, and hilus. Cystic follicles, yellow corpora lutea, and white corpora albicantia may be visualized grossly in the cortex and medulla.

Histologic sections of the ovary show a simple cuboidal to columnar surface epithelial layer, derived from mesothelium. The ovarian parenchyma consists of stroma composed of closely-packed, s-shaped spindled cells and collagen with interspersed follicular structures in varying phases of development. Bright yellow, centrally hemorrhagic corpora lutea and white, gritty acellular corpora albicantia (e-**Fig. 31.1**)* may also be seen. The hilus is composed of abundant blood vessels, nerves, and interspersed eosinophilic hilus cells that are histologically identical to the Leydig cells of the testis. The rete ovarii, the developmental analogue of the rete testis, is also present in the hilum.

II. **GROSS EXAMINATION AND TISSUE SAMPLING.** The most common ovarian specimens encountered in surgical pathology are oophorectomies (with or without hysterectomy) and cystectomies. The weight and gross measurements of all three dimensions should be recorded. The capsule should be inspected for areas of rupture, adhesions, tumor involvement, or other lesions. The ovary should then be bivalved along the long axis, and any lesions on the cut surface should be noted. Solid, cystic, and papillary lesions should be thoroughly sampled (one section per cm). If no lesions are identified, one section for every 2 cm is adequate. If cysts are present, the color and consistency of the cyst fluid should be noted, and any areas of nodularity or papillary excrescences should be sampled. Prophylactic oophorectomy specimens from excisions performed for a family history of a hereditary cancer syndrome should be cut perpendicular to the long axis and entirely submitted.

The surgical management of malignant primary ovarian tumors includes a staging procedure, so an ovary excised for a primary malignancy will usually be accompanied by multiple abdominal peritoneal biopsies, omentectomy, and regional lymph nodes. The small peritoneal biopsies are submitted entirely. The omentum sample must be serially sectioned. If grossly visible tumor is present, only one section need be submitted; when no tumor is identified, at least five sections should be submitted. All identified lymph nodes should be submitted from lymph node dissections.

III. **DIAGNOSTIC FEATURES OF COMMON BENIGN DISEASES OF THE OVARY**
   A. **Inflammatory disease**
      1. **Infection** of the ovaries is most commonly due to ascending pelvic inflammatory disease (PID). Concurrent fallopian tube infection is usually seen, leading to tubo-ovarian abscesses. These infections are typically polymicrobial. PID caused by *Actinomyces* is classically associated with intrauterine contraceptive devices. Tubo-ovarian infections may resolve completely, leave scarring and fibrous adhesions, or form complex tubo-ovarian masses.

*All e-figures are available online via the Solution Site Image Bank.

2. **Autoimmune oophoritis** is often associated with premature ovarian failure and infertility. These patients often have other autoimmune disorders, and microscopic examination of their ovaries shows a lymphoplasmacytic infiltrate.

B. Cysts

1. **Epithelial inclusion cysts** are thought to arise from invaginations of the surface epithelium associated with episodes of ovulation; consequently, they are most numerous in postmenopausal women, although they can occur at any age. They are lined by a single layer of flattened, cuboidal, or columnar epithelium that is often ciliated (e-**Fig. 31.2**). By convention, inclusion cysts >1 cm in diameter are diagnosed as serous cystadenomas.

2. **Follicular cysts** are common lesions, measuring 2.5 to 10 cm in diameter. They may be asymptomatic or present as an adnexal mass. Follicular cysts are unilocular with a smooth lining, and contain clear or blood-tinged fluid. Microscopically, the cysts are lined by an inner layer of granulosa cells and an outer layer of theca cells.

3. **Corpus luteum cysts** are seen in women of reproductive age and measure 2.5 to 5 cm. Grossly, they are yellow with a wavy border, and are filled with thick, bloody fluid. Microscopically the lining is composed of large luteinized granulosa cells (e-**Fig. 31.3**). Corpus luteum cysts of pregnancy often contain intra- and extracellular hyaline globules and foci of calcification.

4. **Paraovarian or paratubal cysts** are often found in the hilar region. Mesonephric cysts are remnants of the Wolffian ducts and are lined by simple cuboidal epithelium with smooth muscle in the cyst wall. Paramesonephric cysts are derived from Müllerian epithelium and are lined by columnar epithelium with or without cilia. Paraovarian cysts may also be lined by mesothelium.

5. **Polycystic ovarian (Stein–Leventhal) syndrome** has an unknown etiology and often presents with hirsutism and infertility. The ovaries are usually slightly enlarged, with numerous subcortical follicles of similar sizes. The ovarian capsule is thick and collagenized, and the ovarian stroma is often hyperplastic, and may be luteinized.

6. **Endometriosis** is characterized by the presence of endometrial glands and stroma outside of the endometrium. The ovary is the most commonly involved site. Endometriotic or "chocolate" cysts are filled with thick, clotted brown blood. Microscopic examination will show endometrial glands or epithelium and endometrial stroma, with associated hemosiderin-laden macrophages and chronic inflammation (e-**Fig. 31.4**).

C. Lesions of pregnancy

1. **Solitary luteinized follicle cysts** can reach enormous sizes (up to 25 cm).

2. **Hyperreactio luteinalis** is characterized by the presence of multiple luteinized cysts that are usually bilateral and are usually associated with conditions resulting in high human chorionic gonadotropin (hCG) levels (e.g., multiple gestations, molar pregnancy). Microscopically, the follicular cysts are lined by luteinized granulosa and theca cells, often with stromal edema and luteinization.

3. **Pregnancy luteoma** is a nodular proliferation of luteinized cells, typically found in multiparous black women, which may be associated with virilization in a subset of patients. These are frequently bilateral (33%) and multifocal (50%).

IV. OVARIAN NEOPLASMS. Table 31.1 presents a (simplified) version of the World Health Organization (WHO) histological classification of tumors of the ovary.

A. Surface epithelial tumors. Tumors of ovarian surface epithelium represent approximately two thirds of all ovarian tumors. Ovarian surface epithelium may differentiate into any Müllerian-type epithelium, accounting for the various subtypes of ovarian epithelial tumors: serous (resembling fallopian tube), endometrioid (resembling endometrium), and mucinous (resembling endocervix).

1. **Serous tumors** represent the most common type of surface epithelial tumor. The majority of serous tumors are benign and occur in women ages 30 to 40 years. Up to 25% of serous tumors are malignant, and these occur in a slightly older population. About 15% of serous tumors are borderline tumors (also known as low malignant potential [LMP] or atypically proliferating tumors). Serous lesions

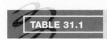

TABLE 31.1	WHO Histological Classification of Tumors of the Ovary

Surface epithelial–stromal tumors
Serous tumors
  Malignant
    Adenocarcinoma
  Borderline tumor
  Benign
    Cystadenoma, adenofibroma, cystadenofibroma
Mucinous tumors
  Malignant
    Adenocarcinoma
  Borderline tumor
  Benign
    Cystadenoma, adenofibroma, cystadenofibroma
  Mucinous cystic tumor with pseudomxoma peritonei
Endometrioid tumors including variants with squamous differentiation
  Malignant
    Adenocarcinoma
    Malignant mixed müllerian tumor (carcinosarcoma)
    Endometrioid stromal sarcoma (low grade)
    Undifferentiated ovarian sarcoma
  Borderline tumor
  Benign
    Cystadenoma, adenofibroma, cystadenofibroma
Clear cell tumors
  Malignant
    Adenocarcinofibroma
  Borderline tumor
  Benign
    Cystadenoma, adenofibroma, cystadenofibroma
Transitional cell tumors
  Malignant
    Transitional cell carcinoma (non-Brenner type)
    Malignant Brenner tumor
  Borderline
  Benign
    Brenner tumor
Squamous cell tumors
  Squamous cell carcinoma
Mixed epithelial tumors (specify components)
  Malignant
  Borderline
  Benign
Undifferentiated and unclassified tumors
  Undifferentiated carcinoma
  Adenocarcinoma, not otherwise specified

Sex-cord stromal tumors
Granulosa-stromal cell tumors
  Granulosa cell tumor group
    Adult granulosa cell tumor
    Juvenile granulosa cell tumor

(Continued)

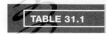

| TABLE 31.1 | WHO Histological Classification of Tumors of the Ovary (Continued) |

Thecoma-fibroma group
  Thecoma, not otherwise specified
    Typical
    Luteinized
  Fibroma
  Cellular fibroma
  Fibrosarcoma
  Stromal tumor with minor sex cord elements
  Sclerosing stromal tumor
  Signet-ring stromal tumor
  Unclassified (fibrothecoma)
Sertoli-stromal cell tumors
  Sertoli-Leydig cell tumor group
    Well differentiated
    Of intermediate differentiation
      Variant with heterologous elements (specify type)
    Poorly differentiated (sarcomatoid)
      Variant with heterologous elements (specify type)
    Retiform
      Variant with heterologous elements (specify type)
  Sertoli cell tumor
  Stromal-Leydig cell tumor
  Sex cord-stromal tumors of mixed or unclassified cell types
  Sex cord tumor with annular tubules
  Gynandroblastoma (specify components)
  Sex cord-stromal tumor, unclassified
Steroid cell tumors
  Stromal luteoma
  Leydig cell tumor group
    Hilus cell tumor
    Leydig cell tumor, nonhilar type
    Leydig cell tumors, not otherwise specified
  Steroid cell tumor, not otherwise specified
    Well differentiated
    Malignant

Germ cell tumors
Primitive germ cell tumors
Dysgerminoma
Yolk sac tumor
Embryonal carcinoma
Polyembryoma
Nongestational choriocarcinoma
Mixed germ cell tumor (specify components)
Biphasic or triphasic teratoma
Immature teratoma
Mature teratoma
  Solid
  Cystic
  Fetiform teratoma (homunculus)
Monodermal teratoma and somatic-type tumors associated with dermoid cysts
Thyroid tumor group
  Struma ovarii
    Benign
    Malignant (specify type)

(Continued)

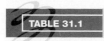

| TABLE 31.1 | **WHO Histological Classification of Tumors of the Ovary (Continued)** |

Cardinoid group
Neuroectodermal tumor group
Carcinoma group
Melanocytic group
  Malignant melanoma
  Melanocytic nevus
Sarcoma group (specify type)
Sebaceous tumor group
Pituitary-type tumor group
Retinal anlage tumor group
Others

Germ cell sex cord-stromal tumors
Gonadoblastoma
  Variant with malignant germ cell tumor
Mixed germ cell-sex cord-stromal tumor
  Variant with malignant germ cell tumor

Tumors of the rete ovarii
Adenocarcinoma
Adenoma
Cystadenoma
Cystadenofibroma

Miscellaneous tumors
Small cell carcinoma, hypercalcemic type
Small cell carcinoma, pulmonary type
Large cell neuroendocrine carcinoma
Hepatoid carcinoma
Primary ovarian mesothelioma
Wilms tumor
Gestational choriocarcinoma
Hydatidiform mole
Adenoid cystic carcinoma
Basal cell tumor
Ovarian Wolffian tumor
Paraganglioma
Myxoma
Soft tissue tumors not specific to the ovary
Others

Tumorlike conditions
Luteoma of pregnancy
Stromal hyperthecosis
Stromal hyperplasia
Fibromatosis
Massive ovarian edema
Others

Lymphoid and hematopoetic tumors
Malignant lymphoma (specify type)
Leukemia (specify type)
Plasmacytoma

Secondary tumors

From: Tavassoli FA, Devilee P, eds. *World Health Organization Classification of Tumours. Pathology and Genetics. Tumours of the Breast and Female Genital Organs.* Lyon: IARC Press; 2001. Used with permission.

often contain clear to yellow fluid, although the consistency may be gelatinous, and higher grade tumors may have hemorrhagic fluid.

a. Serous cystadenoma. On gross examination, serous cystadenomas present as a cystic lesion. When the cystadenoma shows a prominent stromal component, it is termed a cystadenofibroma. Microscopically, benign serous tumors are lined by a single layer of eosinophilic ciliated columnar cells closely resembling tubal epithelium (e-**Fig. 31.5**). This lining may be attenuated in long-standing lesions. Adenofibromas and cystadenofibromas show broad stromal papillae lined by simple columnar epithelium.

b. Borderline or LMP tumors. These tumors have papillary excrescences lined by an architecturally complex epithelium that demonstrates branching and tufting. The lining epithelium is often stratified with accompanying mild to moderate cytologic atypia, and sections show detached papillary clusters of epithelium (e-**Fig. 31.6**). Tangential sectioning of complex papillae may show invagination into the stroma. However, by definition, borderline tumors do not show destructive stromal invasion, the criterion used to differentiate borderline tumors from serous adenocarcinomas.

Most borderline serous tumors are confined to the ovary, but they may present with extraovarian disease such as peritoneal implants and even lymph node metastases. The classification of these tumors is based on features of the primary ovarian tumor, not the metastases. Peritoneal implants associated with borderline tumors are classified as invasive or noninvasive (*Cancer* 62:2212, 1988). Noninvasive implants show papillary proliferations that have a smooth interface with the surrounding tissue without destructive invasion. Noninvasive implants are subclassified as epithelial, if there is an epithelial proliferation with no stromal response, or desmoplastic, if there is a stromal response that distorts or compresses the epithelial cells. In contrast, invasive implants irregularly infiltrate and efface the underlying tissue.

c. Occasional serious borderline tumors exhibit individual cells or small clusters of cells with eosinophilic cytoplasm in the stroma, surrounded by a clefted space. Even less common are small cribriform masses, solid nests, or papillae. Small foci of microinvasion are not thought to portend a worse prognosis, but the upper limit for microinvasion (whether 3 mm, 5 mm, or a volume of 10 mm^2) is not well established (*Hum Pathol* 35:934, 2004).

d. Serous adenocarcinomas grossly consist of large masses of multiloculated cysts, friable papillary areas, and solid areas, often with foci of hemorrhage and/or necrosis. Serous adenocarcinomas are usually bilateral. Microscopically, serous adenocarcinomas may show a surface papillary pattern similar to borderline tumors, but by definition also show destructive stromal invasion by irregularly shaped glands, or single cells with an associated desmoplastic stromal response (e-**Fig. 31.7**). Psammoma bodies (concentric lamellated calcifications) are often present in more well-differentiated tumors.

   i. A rare form of serous adenocarcinoma known as psammocarcinoma is characterized by invasive stromal growth, abundant psammoma bodies in at least 75% of the papillae, and no areas of solid growth >15 cells across (*Gynecol Pathol* 9:110, 1990). This tumor generally has a good prognosis.

   ii. Micropapillary serous adenocarcinoma shows many minute micropapillae arising from large thick cores or cysts. The lining shows more architectural complexity and cytologic atypia than is typical of borderline serous tumors, with which it is often confused, and may be associated with a more aggressive clinical course.

2. **Mucinous tumors.** The majority of mucinous tumors are cystadenomas. The remaining mucinous tumors are equally divided between borderline (LMP) and adenocarcinomas.

   a. Benign mucinous tumors, or cystadenomas, show a smooth external surface, and are often multiloculated. These tumors may grow to be quite large, often >20 cm in maximal dimension. Mucinous tumors are filled with thick viscous secretions, although in some cases the cyst fluid is more watery.

Microscopically, they are lined by a single layer of tall columnar cells with apical mucin and no cilia, similar to normal endocervical glandular epithelium (e-**Fig. 31.**8), intestinal-type epithelium with goblet cells, or epithelium resembling gastric foveolar epithelium. If there is a prominent stromal component, the lesion is termed a mucinous cystadenofibroma.

b. Mucinous borderline or LMP tumors present grossly as multiloculated cysts with papillary excrescences and thick cyst walls. Microscopically, most borderline tumors have an intestinal-type lining which may be several layers thick; mild to moderate nuclear atypia is present. Glandular stromal invaginations may be seen, but destructive stromal invasion with an associated desmoplastic stromal response is, by definition, not present (e-**Fig. 31.**9).

Twenty percent of mucinous borderline tumors with an endocervical-type lining are associated with endometriosis. These endocervical lined tumors are more likely to be bilateral and have associated peritoneal implants than are borderline tumors with intestinal type lining.

c. Mucinous borderline tumor with intraepithelial carcinoma. These tumors resemble borderline tumors on gross examination and microscopically, except some areas have the cytologic features of carcinoma with pleomorphism and prominent nucleoli. No destructive stromal invasion is present. Intraepithelial carcinoma probably does not portend a worse prognosis.

d. Mucinous adenocarcinomas. As with mucinous borderline tumors, adenocarcinomas present as multiloculated cysts with papillary excrescences. These tumors often show solid areas, hemorrhage, and necrosis. A diagnosis of adenocarcinoma can be made when destructive stromal invasion is present or when complex back-to-back epithelium without intervening stroma involves 10 mm^2, or measures 3 mm in 2 linear dimensions (*Hum Pathol* 35:949, 2004). The lining epithelium of mucinous adenocarcinomas may be intestinal, endocervical, or of so-called indifferent type (large polygonal cells with eosinophilic cytoplasm and nuclear atypia).

Approximately 5% of women with a mucinous ovarian tumor will present with pseudomyxoma peritonei, a condition in which pools of mucin fill the peritoneal cavity. The vast majority of these patients have a synchronous primary appendiceal tumor (*Int J Gynecol Pathol* 16:1, 1997). Ovarian involvement is characterized by pools of mucin that dissect through the ovarian tissue without a desmoplastic response; small glands and groups of mucinous epithelial cells will often be found floating freely in the mucin pools. Another group of patients with pseudomyxoma peritonei have a synchronous cervical mucinous adenocarcinoma, often in the context of Peutz–Jeghers syndrome.

When trying to distinguish a primary from a metastatic ovarian mucinous adenocarcinoma, both histologic and immunohistochemical features are helpful. Features seen more commonly in metastatic disease include a concomitant extraovarian neoplasm, involvement of the external surface of the ovary, pools of mucin dissecting ovarian stroma, and extensive tumoral lymphovascular space invasion. Metastatic adenocarcinoma from the colorectum will show abundant luminal karyorrhectic debris ("dirty necrosis"), a garland pattern of glands lining cystic spaces, an abrupt transition between viable and necrotic epithelium, and immunopositivity for cytokeratin (CK) 20 and carcinoembryogenic antigen (CEA) but immunonegativity for CK7 and cancer antigen (CA) 125.

3. **Endometrioid tumors.** The majority of endometrioid tumors of the ovary are carcinomas, of which 10% to 20% are associated with endometriosis. Squamous differentiation may be seen in all types of endometrioid tumors.

a. Endometrioid adenofibromas and cystadenofibromas are benign lesions lined by tubulovillous glands similar to those seen in the normal endometrium. The glands are embedded in a fibroblastic stroma.

b. Endometrioid tumors that show cytologic atypia and areas of confluent epithelial proliferation without stromal support up to 5 mm in maximal dimension are commonly referred to as borderline endometrioid tumors, although there

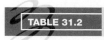

TABLE 31.2	Gynecologic Oncology Group (GOG) Grading Guidelines for Endometrioid Adenocarcinoma
Grade 1 or well differentiated	Well-formed glands resembling villoglandular carcinoma of the uterine corpus* ≤5% solid tumor growth
Grade 2 or moderately differentiated	More complex glandular architecture Increased nuclear stratification 6% to 50% solid tumor growth
Grade 3 or poorly differentiated	Poorly formed glands, large sheets of cells >50% solid tumor growth

*Areas of squamous differentiation are not included when assessing the amount of solid tumor growth.

is disagreement as to diagnostic criteria and nomenclature (*Am J Surg Pathol* 24:1465, 2000). Criteria for microinvasion within these tumors are not well established.

    c. Endometrioid adenocarcinomas show villous papillary structures and/or tubular glands composed of a stratified layer of epithelial cells with smooth luminal borders. By definition, destructive stromal invasion is present with an associated desmoplastic response (e-**Fig. 31.10**). The International Federation of Gynecology and Obstetrics (FIGO) scheme grading for endometrioid adenocarcinomas is listed in Table 31.2.

4. Clear cell tumors. The majority of clear cell tumors are frank adenocarcinomas, often associated with endometriosis. Clear cell adenocarcinomas present grossly as white-tan to yellow mixed solid and cystic masses, often associated with hemorrhage and necrosis. Microscopically, clear cell carcinoma shows many growth patterns including solid, tubulocystic, and papillary. As the tumor's name suggests, cytologically the tumor cells are large with abundant clear cytoplasm that may contain hyaline globules. These cells exhibit a high degree of nuclear atypia, with nuclei that jut into the lumen, giving the cells a "hobnail" appearance (e-**Fig. 31.11**). The stromal cores are characteristically densely hyalinized and eosinophilic. Clear cell carcinomas are always high grade.

5. Brenner and transitional cell tumors

    a. Benign Brenner tumors are usually unilateral and often incidental. Grossly, these tumors have a white to tan-yellow whorled cut surface, but may show cystic spaces and calcification. Histologic sections show small solid to cystic nests of bland transitional epithelial cells with longitudinal nuclear grooves, surrounded by abundant fibrous stroma, often with areas of calcification. The cystic spaces may be filled with eosinophilic material (e-**Fig. 31.12**). Brenner tumors have an associated benign mucinous cystic component in 25% of cases.

    b. Borderline or LMP Brenner tumors are grossly cystic with papillary excrescences. Microscopically, the cysts and papillae are lined by stratified transitional cells resembling the cells of noninvasive papillary urothelial carcinoma. Stromal invasion is not present by definition.

    c. Malignant Brenner tumors are grossly solid or cystic. The epithelium of these tumors shows desmoplastic stromal invasion, although areas of benign or borderline Brenner tumor are still identifiable.

    d. Transitional cell carcinomas (TCCs) of the ovary resemble other epithelial carcinomas with solid and cystic areas. Microscopically, they are composed of papillary cores lined by stratified, cytologically atypical epithelium, and they closely resemble TCC of the bladder. By definition, no Brenner tumor component is present. Ovarian TCC is graded using the criteria for TCC of the urothelial tract.

6. **Carcinosarcoma.** Also known as malignant mixed Müllerian tumor (MMMT), carcinosarcoma occasionally presents as a primary tumor of the ovary. The tumor usually occurs in postmenopausal women and has a poor prognosis.

As with their endometrial counterparts, carcinosarcomas contain both malignant epithelial and malignant mesenchymal elements. Numerous genetic studies have demonstrated that both elements are derived from the same precursor, proving that the neoplasm does not represent a collision tumor; the tumor is now considered to represent a poorly differentiated carcinoma with metaplastic sarcomatous elements. The epithelial component is often serous carcinoma, but may be endometrioid, mucinous, clear cell, or even squamous. The mesenchymal elements may be homologous to the female genital tract (e.g., smooth muscle, endometrial stroma) or may be heterologous elements not normally found in the female genital tract (e.g., bone, cartilage, skeletal muscle).

B. **Sex cord-stromal tumors**
1. **Granulosa cell tumors**
   a. Adult granulosa cell tumors (AGCT) are low-grade neoplasms that occur most commonly in postmenopausal women. The tumors may secrete estrogen with resulting endocrine manifestations, such as endometrial hyperplasia or carcinoma. The tumors are usually large (>10 cm) and unilateral. The cut surface is soft and yellow-tan with cysts and hemorrhage.

   A number of different histologic patterns occur, including microfollicular, macrofollicular, "watered-silk," gyriform, and diffuse. However, all are composed of round to oval granulosa cells that have little cytoplasm and round to angular nuclei with longitudinal nuclear grooves (e-**Fig. 31.13**). There is minimal cytologic atypia or karyorrhexis, and the mitotic rate is low. The microfollicular and diffuse variants often contain characteristic Call–Exner bodies consisting of a very small collection of eosinophilic material lined by well-differentiated granulosa cells.

   b. Juvenile granulosa cell tumors (JGCTs) are also low-grade tumors. They occur in children and young adults, and usually present with a palpable mass and symptoms of hyperestrogenism. Gross findings are similar to those of the adult form.

   JGCTs are characterized histologically by solid sheets of cells mixed with small immature follicles with basophilic or eosinophilic secretions lined by more mature-appearing granulosa cells. Areas of luteinization are frequently present. JGCTs exhibit more cytologic atypia and a higher mitotic rate than do AGCTs.

   Both adult and juvenile granulosa cell tumors are positive for inhibin expression by immunohistochemistry, a helpful feature in difficult cases.

2. **Thecoma-fibroma**
   a. Fibromas represent the most common of the sex cord-stromal tumors. Fibromas are not hormonally functional, are usually bilateral, and measure an average of 5 cm in diameter. Grossly, they are solid and lobulated with a firm, white-gray cut surface. Histologically, they are characterized by interlacing bundles and storiform areas of spindle cells that show no atypia and few mitoses (e-**Fig. 31.14**). Immunohistochemically, the tumor is diffusely positive for vimentin.
   b. Thecomas occur in postmenopausal women, with the luteinized variant occurring in a younger population. The tumor often presents with symptoms of hyperestrogenism. Most are unilateral and can measure up to 10 cm in diameter. Grossly, the tumor is lobulated, solid and yellow-tan, and may contain areas of hemorrhage, cystic change, necrosis, and/or calcification. Histologically, typical thecomas show sheets of lipid-laden theca cells with varying amounts of a fibrous stromal component that may show calcification. Cytologically, theca cells show rounded to spindled nuclei with only mild atypia and rare mitoses. Immunohistochemically, the tumor is positive for inhibin expression. Oil Red O fat stains (which require fresh tissue) highlight the intracellular lipid.

Luteinized thecomas show thecalike cells with abundant clear to eosinophilic cytoplasm and central rounded nuclei.

3. **Sertoli and Sertoli–Leydig cell tumors**
   a. Sertoli cell tumors are rare, low grade, nonfunctioning tumors that occur in women of childbearing age. Grossly, they are yellow-tan, solid, lobulated tumors. Microscopically, they are composed of closely packed tubules separated by fibrous stroma. The tubules are lined by cuboidal to columnar cells with abundant pale eosinophilic cytoplasm, with little atypia or mitotic activity.
   b. Sertoli-Leydig cell tumors (SLCT) are androgen-secreting tumors that occur in young women. Grossly, these tumors average 10 cm in diameter, are yellow to red-brown, and may show cystic degeneration. Well differentiated SLCTs show tubules (similar to those seen in Sertoli cell tumors), with interspersed clusters of Leydig cells that have abundant eosinophilic cytoplasm (e-Fig. 31.15). SLCTs of intermediate differentiation show dense cellularity, fewer well-formed tubules, and more immature hyperchromatic Sertoli cells. Poorly differentiated SLCTs show densely packed atypical spindled cells. Heterologous elements (most often gastrointestinal or neuroendocrine epithelium) are identified in 20% of SLCTs.

      The retiform variant of SLCT shows a histology similar to the rete testis with cystic structures and tubules lined by cells with round regular nuclei.

      Both Sertoli cell tumors and SLCTs show immunoreactivity for inhibin.

4. **Steroid cell tumors** are a family of tumors composed of large cells with intracellular lipid that resemble Leydig cells or luteinized stromal cells.
   a. Stromal luteomas occur in postmenopausal women and are often associated with hyperestrogenism. Grossly, they are yellow-tan, measure <3 cm in maximal dimension, and are confined to the ovarian stroma. Histologically, they consist of sheets of large cells with abundant eosinophilic cytoplasm and bland cytologic features. Concomitant stromal hyperplasia may be present. Focal degenerative changes produce irregular spaces that resemble vessels or glands in a subset of tumors.
   b. Leydig cell tumors are commonly androgen secreting, and occur in postmenopausal women. Most are well circumscribed and show a yellow-brown cut surface. They may also show areas of hemorrhage. Microscopically, the tumor is composed of large polygonal cells with abundant granular to foamy eosinophilic cytoplasm. The cells exhibit central round nuclei with prominent nucleoli (e-Fig. 31.16). Reinke crystalloids (slender rod-shaped crystals) must be present for diagnosis.
   c. Hilus cell tumors are composed of the same cell population, but as the name implies, originate in the hilus of the ovary from hilar Leydig cells. Hilus cell tumors are also usually associated with virilization or hirsutism.
   d. Steroid cell tumor, not otherwise specified (NOS), is a steroid cell tumor that does not meet the criteria for any of the types above. The tumor is the most common of the steroid cell tumors, and may occur at any age. The tumor is usually androgenic, but varies in size and location. It has a similar gross morphology to the other two types of steroid cell tumor. Histologically, steroid cell tumor, NOS is composed of large cells with abundant granular cytoplasm separated by a vascular stroma. A poorer prognosis is seen in tumors >7 cm in maximal dimension, with necrosis, hemorrhage, or an increased mitotic rate.

5. **Other sex cord stromal tumors**
   a. Sclerosing stromal tumor is a rare tumor that occurs in young women and girls. Grossly, the tumor is firm and white with areas of cystic degeneration and edema. Microscopically, lobules of spindled cells and vacuolated cells are separated by dense collagen or edematous connective tissue.
   b. Sex cord tumor with annular tubules (SCTAT) occurs in women of childbearing age. In some women, the tumor occurs as a component of Peutz–Jeghers syndrome, in which case the SCTATs are usually small and incidental. Those unassociated with Peutz–Jeghers syndrome form a large, solid, yellow

mass. Histologically, the tumor is composed of well-circumscribed ring-shaped tubules that contain central hyalinized material. The tubules are lined by cells with pale cytoplasm oriented toward the center of the tubule, with peripheral elongated nuclei.

C. Germ cell tumors

1. Teratomas

a. Mature teratomas are the most common ovarian tumor. They occur most often in adult women of reproductive age. Grossly, they are solid or cystic and may grow quite large. The cysts may contain hair, soft yellow keratinous debris, teeth, and many other tissue types. Mature tissue from all three germ layers (ectoderm: skin or neural elements; mesoderm: smooth muscle, teeth, bone; endoderm: respiratory epithelium, gastrointestinal epithelium, thyroid) may be present. The term "dermoid cyst" is commonly used to refer to mature cystic teratomas lined by squamous epithelium that contains skin appendages (e-**Fig. 31.17**). Mature cystic teratomas should be thoroughly sampled (one section per cm) to exclude an immature component, and to exclude malignant transformation of one of the mature components (a rare occurrence).

b. Immature teratomas are rapidly growing malignant tumors that occur in childhood and early adulthood. They are usually unilateral and may be solid or cystic. Microscopically, they contain immature or primitive tissue (derived from any or all three germ cell layers) that is usually mixed with areas of mature tissue (e-**Fig. 31.18**). The most common immature element is neuroectodermal and consists of rosettes, masses, or tubules of primitive neural cells.

Immature teratomas are graded based on the relative amount of immature tissue present (*Int J Gynecol Pathol* 13:283, 1994). Tumors with more than one low-power field of immature neuroepithelium on any given slide are considered high grade, and require adjuvant chemotherapy.

c. Struma ovarii is a unique type of monodermal (tissue from only one germ cell layer) teratoma. Microscopically, the tumor is composed predominantly of mature thyroid tissue, with follicles and colloid (e-**Fig. 31.19**). Secondary changes such as hyperplasia, adenoma, and even carcinoma may be seen.

2. Primary carcinoid tumors of the ovary usually have an insular or islet histology consisting of islands of small uniform epithelial cells with abundant cytoplasm and round nuclei with coarse chromatin. The tumor most often arises in association with respiratory or gastrointestinal epithelium in a mature cystic teratoma, but it has also been reported in association with other primary ovarian neoplasms, and in pure form. Metastasis from a primary site outside the ovary must always be excluded.

3. Dysgerminoma is the most common malignant germ cell tumor. It occurs as pure dysgerminoma or as a component of mixed germ cell tumor. Dysgerminoma develops most commonly in young women, and is frequent in patients with ovarian dysgenesis. Occasionally, the tumor produces hCG. Pure dysgerminomas have an excellent prognosis when treated by current therapeutic regimens.

Grossly, dysgeminomas are usually large and solid with a smooth external surface and a lobulated gray-tan cut surface. The tumor should be thoroughly sampled (one section per cm) for microscopic examination; special attention should be directed to hemorrhagic and cystic areas to exclude other germ cell tumor types.

Dysgerminomas are analogous to testicular seminomas and have an identical histologic appearance. They are composed of nests and sheets of uniform large round cells with abundant clear cytoplasm. Tumor cells are separated by a lymphocyte-rich fibrous stroma (e-**Fig. 31.20**). Often a histiocytic or granulomatous infiltrate is present, and multinucleated syncytiotrophoblastic cells may also be identified. Dysgerminomas are immunopositive for placental alkaline phosphatase (PLAP) and c-kit (CD117), but are immunonegative for epithelial membrane antigen (EMA).

4. Yolk sac tumor, also known as endodermal sinus tumor, occurs in young women, usually with an associated elevated serum alpha fetoprotein (AFP) level. Yolk sac

tumor is a rapidly growing tumor that has often spread outside the ovary at the time of diagnosis. It is often a component of mixed germ cell tumors.

Grossly, yolk sac tumor is usually unilateral and large, with a smooth external surface and a variegated solid and cystic yellow to tan cut surface. Hemorrhage and necrosis are often present.

Many different histologic variants occur, including the reticular, endodermal sinus (papillary), polyvesicular–vitelline, hepatoid, and glandular patterns. The reticular pattern is the most common variant, and is composed of small cystic spaces lined by cuboidal to columnar cells with clear cytoplasm and large hyperchromatic nuclei. The endodermal sinus pattern is the second most common pattern; this pattern features characteristic Schiller–Duvall bodies (rounded papillae containing a single central vessel and lined by columnar tumor cells) (e-**Fig. 31.21**). The polyvesicular–vitelline pattern is composed of abundant cystic structures lined by tumor cells that are embedded in a dense cellular stroma. For all histologic variants, AFP immunohistochemical staining highlights the tumor cell cytoplasm; EMA immunostaining is negative.

5. **Embryonal carcinoma** is rare and usually presents in adolescents as a painful mass with or without hormonal symptoms. It is often a component of a mixed germ cell tumor.

   Grossly, the tumor has a smooth external surface and a solid yellow to gray-tan cut surface with frequent areas of hemorrhage and necrosis. Histologically, the tumor is composed of sheets or nests of large anaplastic cells with pale, often vacuolated cytoplasm (e-**Fig. 31.22**). The tumor cell nuclei are large, and may be hyperchromatic or vesicular and contain prominent nucleoli. Mitoses are invariably present and may be atypical. Syncytiotrophoblast-like tumor giant cells may be present. Embryonal carcinoma is immunopositive for CD30 and cytokeratin expression.

6. **Polyembryoma** is a very rare, highly malignant neoplasm that usually is a component of a mixed germ cell tumor. Grossly, it presents a unilateral solid mass with areas of hemorrhage and necrosis. Microscopically, the tumor is composed of embryoid bodies (embryonic disks lined by endoderm on one side, ectoderm on the opposite side, and associated yolk sac and amniotic cavities).

7. **Choriocarcinoma.** Pure choriocarcinoma of the ovary is rare. Choriocarcinoma is most often seen as a component of a mixed germ cell tumor, or as a metastasis from gestational trophoblastic disease. Primary choriocarcinoma presents in children and adolescents. Elevated hCG levels are invariably present.

   Grossly, the tumor mass is hemorrhagic, soft, and tan. Microscopically, both cytotrophoblast and syncytiotrophoblast are present. Cytotrophoblast have centrally located hyperchromatic nuclei, prominent nucleoli, clear cytoplasm, and well-defined cytoplasmic borders; syncytiotrophoblast are multinucleated and are immunopositive for hCG. Whereas syncytiotrophoblast may be seen as components of other germ cell tumors, cytotrophoblast are only seen in choriocarcinoma.

8. **Malignant mixed germ cell tumor.** Ten percent of germ cell tumors contain a mixture of histologic tumor types. The most common combination is dysgerminoma and yolk sac tumor, although any combination may occur. The relative composition of the various histologic subtypes should be included in the final report because it can impact therapy and prognosis.

D. **Other**

1. **Gonadoblastoma** is a rare tumor that contains both germ cell and sex cord-stromal components. Most patients have gonadal dysgenesis, and >90% have a Y chromosome. Approximately half of all cases harbor a malignant germ cell component, most often dysgerminoma. Gonadoblastoma is benign unless a malignant germ cell component is present.

   Grossly, the tumor is usually small with a yellow to gray cut surface and areas of calcification. Histologically, the tumor consists of admixed primitive germ cells and sex cord-stromal derivatives (that resemble immature granulosa cells and Sertoli cells) surrounded by abundant basement membrane-like material, often with calcification.

2. **Hypercalcemic small cell carcinoma** is a highly malignant tumor with a poor prognosis that presents in young women. Approximately two thirds of patients manifest hypercalcemia.

   This tumor is generally large and unilateral, with a soft white-tan lobulated cut surface that shows areas of hemorrhage and necrosis. Histologic examination demonstrates sheets of small cells with scant cytoplasm, admixed with follicle-like spaces filled with eosinophilic fluid. The tumor nuclei are round with coarse chromatin and prominent nucleoli (e-Fig. 31.23). Some tumor cells have globular hyaline inclusions producing a vague rhabdoid morphology. The tumor cells are immunopositive for CK, EMA, vimentin, nuron specific enolave (NSE), and chromogranin and show neuroendocrine differentiation by electron microscopy.

   Conventional small cell carcinoma (high-grade neuroendocrine carcinoma) occasionally presents as an ovarian primary, but unlike the hypercalcemic type, primarily occurs in older women and does not manifest hypercalcemia.

3. **Hematopoetic malignancies.** Primary ovarian lymphoma or leukemia is extremely rare. However, ovarian involvement by disseminated hematopoietic disease may be seen in up to one half of all lymphomas, and in up to one quarter of all leukemias. Bilateral ovarian involvement by lymphoma is usually a sign of widespread disease.

   Ovaries involved by hematopoietic malignancy usually show a smooth tan cut surface, and if the tumor burden is large, there may be areas of hemorrhage and necrosis. Microscopically, the tumors resemble their nodal or marrow counterparts. Immunohistochemical stains such as CD45 (leukocyte common antigen), as well as B and T cell markers may, be used to demonstrate a hematopoietic origin in difficult cases.

4. **Primary ovarian tumors of mesenchymal origin.** A wide variety of primary ovarian tumors of mesenchymal origin, although rare, have been reported.
   a. Vascular tumors, including hemangioma, lymphangioma, and hemangioendothelioma (low-grade angiosarcoma) have all been described as primary ovarian neoplasms.
   b. Tumors of striated muscle origin also rarely occur, including rhabdomyoma and rhabdomyosarcoma. Primary osteosarcomas and chondrosarcomas have also been rarely reported. For all of these neoplasms, generous sampling of the tumor is required to exclude the presence of an epithelial component, which if present, would indicate that the mesenchymal neoplasm was merely the sarcomatous component of a carcinosarcoma (see section IV.A.6).
   c. Neural tumors, including neurofibromas, schwannomas, and ganglioneuromas, have been reported, and may present in association with neurofibromatosis.
   d. Primary ovarian myxomas are rare tumors; they are usually unilateral, and are composed of stellate and spindled cells in an abundant myxoid stroma. Primary ovarian myxomas must be distinguished from pseudomyxoma ovarii, which is characterized by the presence of strips of mucin-secreting epithelial cells floating in pools of mucin.

5. **Metastases.** Five to ten percent of ovarian tumors represent metastases. The most common sources of ovarian metastases are the gastrointestinal tract (especially the large intestine, stomach, and appendix), breast, uterine corpus, and cervix. In young girls, ovarian metastases are represented by neuroblastoma, rhabdomyosarcoma, Ewing sarcoma/peripheral neuroectodermal tumor, and malignant rhabdoid tumor of kidney.

V. STAGING OF OVARIAN MALIGNANCIES
   A. **Pathologic staging.** Ovarian cancer is staged surgically. The staging procedure includes bilateral salpingo-oophorectomy, hysterectomy, and omental biopsy, biopsies of multiple pelvic and abdominal peritoneal surfaces, and regional lymph node dissections (as noted in section II). Cytologic examination of peritoneal washings is also

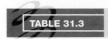

TABLE 31.3	Tumor, Node, Metastasis (TNM) Staging Scheme for Ovarian Carcinoma

PRIMARY TUMOR (T)

TNM categories	International Federation of Gynecology and Obstetrics (FIGO) Stages
TX	Primary tumor cannot be assessed
T0	No evidence of primary tumor
T1 I	Tumor limited to ovaries (one or both)
T1a IA	Tumor limited to one ovary; capsule intact, no tumor on ovarian surface. No malignant cells in ascites or peritoneal washings
T1b IB	Tumor limited to both ovaries; capsules intact, no tumor on ovarian surface. No malignant cells in ascites or peritoneal washings
T1c IC	Tumor limited to one or both ovaries with any of the following: capsule ruptured, tumor on ovarian surface, malignant cells in ascites or peritoneal washings
T2 II	Tumor involves one or both ovaries with pelvic extension and/or implants
T2a IIA	Extension and/or implants on uterus and/or tube(s). No malignant cells in ascites or peritoneal washings
T2b IIB	Extension to and/or implants on other pelvic tissues. No malignant cells in ascites of peritoneal washings
T2c IIC	Pelvic extension and/or implants (T2a or T2b) with malignant cells in ascites or peritoneal washings
T3 and/or N1 III	Tumor involves one or both ovaries with microscopically confirmed peritoneal metastasis outside the pelvis
T3a IIIA	Microscopic peritoneal metastasis beyond pelvis (no macroscopic tumor)
T3b IIIB	Macroscopic peritoneal metastasis beyond pelvis $\leq$2 cm in greatest dimension
T3c and/or N1 IIIC	Peritoneal metastasis beyond pelvis >2 cm in greatest dimension and/or regional lymph node metastasis
M1 IV	Distant metastasis (excludes peritoneal metastasis)

REGIONAL LYMPH NODES (N)

NX	regional lymph nodes cannot be assessed
N0	No regional lymph node metastasis
NI	Regional lymph node metastasis

DISTANT METASTASIS (M)

MX	Distant metastasis cannot be assessed
M0	No distant metastasis
M1	Distant metastasis (excludes peritoneal metastasis)

STAGE GROUPING

Stage IA	T1a	N0	M0
Stage 1B	T1b	N0	M0
Stage 1C	T1c	N0	M0
Stage IIA	T2a	N0	M0
Stage IIB	T2b	N0	M0
Stage IIC	T2c	N0	M0
Stage IIIA	T3a	N0	M0
Stage IIIB	T3b	N0	M0
Stage IIIC	T3c	N0	M0
	Any T	N1	M0
Stage IV	Any T	Any N	M1

From: Greene FL, Page DL, Fleming ID, Fritz AG, Balch CM, Haller DG, Morrow M, eds. *AJCC Cancer Staging Manual.* 6th edition. New York: Springer; 2002. Used with permission. (A new AJCC TNM staging system is scheduled for release in 2009; after its publication, the new staging scheme will appear on the website for this book.)

performed. The 2002 American Joint Committee on Cancer/International Union Against Cancer/FIGO (AJCC/UICC/FIGO) staging classification is given in Table 31.3.

B. Items to include in the pathology report. Tumor histologic subtype and grade can have therapeutic and prognostic significance and should therefore always be included in the final report.

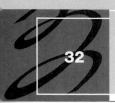

FALLOPIAN TUBE

32

Jamie K. Donnelly, John D. Pfeifer, and Phyllis C. Huettner

I. **NORMAL ANATOMY.** The fallopian tubes, or oviducts, conduct eggs from the surface of the ovary to the uterine cavity. They are also the usual site of fertilization. Each fallopian tube is shaped like an elongated funnel and is divided into four parts (from lateral to medial: infundibulum, ampulla, isthmus, interstitium). The infundibulum contains fingerlike fimbriae distally.

The fallopian tube mucosa is branched and folded into plicae and lined by a single layer of elongated ciliated and nonciliated cells. The wall of the fallopian tube contains smooth muscle to aid in moving the fertilized egg into the uterus. The serosa contains abundant blood vessels and is continuous with the broad ligament.

II. **GROSS EXAMINATION, TISSUE SAMPLING, AND HISTOLOGIC SLIDE PREPA-RATION.** Fallopian tubes are usually received as a portion of a total abdominal hysterectomy–bilateral salpingo-oophorectomy specimen. Short cross-sections of fallopian tube are received after tubal ligation procedures. Ectopic pregnancy specimens also usually contain a portion of fallopian tube. Rarely, specimens are received for primary fallopian tube tumors.

At the grossing station, the length and diameter of the fallopian tube should be documented, as well as the presence or absence of a fimbriated end, or evidence of prior ligation. The serosal surface should also be assessed for the presence of adhesions, cysts, exudates, rupture, or metastatic tumor. The tube is then serially sectioned.

A. **Benign specimens.** Three sections are submitted from a normal fallopian tube, specifically from the fimbriated end, mid-section, and cornual end. Additional sections of any gross lesions are also submitted. Complete cross-sections must be identified from a tubal ligation specimen.

When examining an ectopic pregnancy specimen, an embryo and/or placental villi will often be grossly evident. Hemorrhagic areas, along with obvious villous or embryonic tissue, should be submitted for histologic examination.

B. **Neoplastic specimens.** Primary tubal carcinoma specimens will show a dilated lumen filled with a papillary or solid tumor. An ovarian tumor secondarily involving the fallopian tube is more common than a primary fallopian tube tumor, and careful sectioning can help distinguish the two. Grossly papillary and solid areas should be sampled thoroughly (at least one section per centimeter of tumor), along with uninvolved areas. If possible, a section showing the tumor's relationship to the ovary should be submitted.

C. **Prophylactic excision specimens.** Fallopian tube specimens received as part of a prophylactic hysterectomy–oophorectomy from patients with hereditary cancer syndromes (for example, BRCA1 syndrome) should be, together with the ovaries, entirely submitted for histologic examination. In addition, the distal 2 cm of the fimbriated end should be transected, opened, then sectioned longitudinally (Fig. 32.1) (*Am J Surg Path* 30:230, 2006).

III. **DIAGNOSTIC FEATURES OF COMMON DISEASES**

A. **Inflammatory and nonneoplastic lesions of the fallopian tube**

1. **Cystic lesions.** Embryologic remnants may be found in the fallopian tube, usually as an incidental finding (e-**Fig. 32.1**).* Paratubal cysts of Müllerian origin (ciliated lining), or Wolffian origin (stratified transitional lining) may be encountered.

---

*All e-figures are available online via the Solution Site Image Bank.

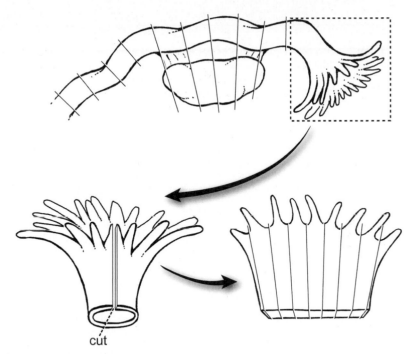

Figure 32.1. Approach to sectioning fallopian tube specimens received as part of a prophylactic hysterectomy–oophorectomy from patients with a hereditary cancer syndrome. Each tube and ovary should be entirely submitted for histologic examination; note that the fimbriated end of the tube should be transected, opened longitudinally, serially sectioned longitudinally, and then entirely submitted for microscopic examination.

If the lining is atrophic secondary to compression, they can be difficult to differentiate microscopically. Pedunculated paratubal cysts with a Müllerian epithelium present along the fimbriae are termed Hydatids of Morgagni.

2. **Inflammatory lesions**
   a. Acute salpingitis usually presents in young to middle-aged women, is generally an ascending infection initiated by *Chlamydia* or *Neisseria gonorrhoea,* and is often followed by polymicrobial infection (pelvic inflammatory disease). The damage to the tube that results from acute salpingitis may lead to infertility and/or ectopic pregnancy. Grossly, the tubal lumen may be distended by pus, blood, or secretions. Histologic sections show marked acute inflammation in the plicae and the tubal wall, often severely distorting the normal architecture (e-**Fig. 32.2**).
   b. Chronic salpingitis is usually due to resolving acute salpingitis. Grossly, the tubal wall is fibrotic with adhesions. Microscopically, a lymphoplasmacytic infiltrate is seen in the plicae. Fusion of the tubal plicae after resolution of acute salpingitis may lead to formation of folliclelike spaces, a histologic pattern known as salpingitis follicularis. Hydrosalpinx may be seen in end-stage chronic salpingitis, microscopically characterized by a dramatically thinned wall with few plicae and a lumen filled with clear fluid.
   c. Granulomatous salpingitis may be caused by tuberculosis, fungal infection, Crohn's disease, or sarcoidosis.
   d. Salpingitis isthmica nodosum (SIN) typically presents in young women. It is associated with ectopic pregnancy and infertility, and has an unclear

pathogenesis. Grossly, it presents as 1- to 2-cm nodules in the wall of the fallopian tube isthmus. The lesions consist of outpouchings of tubal epithelium surrounded by a thickened wall of smooth muscle (e-**Fig. 32.3**).

3. **Other nonneoplastic lesions of the fallopian tube**
   a. The fallopian tube is a frequent site of involvement of endometriosis, primarily in women of reproductive age. It is associated with infertility. Grossly, tubal endometriosis consists of dark brown serosal nodules; the microscopic findings include endometrial glands surrounded by a cuff of endometrial stroma with associated hemosiderin-laden macrophages and chronic inflammatory cells (e-**Fig. 32.4**).
   b. Ectopic pregnancy affects 1% to 2% of all conceptions, and the fallopian tube is the most common site; the most commonly involved region of the tube is the ampulla. Risk factors include salpingitis, congenital tubal anomalies, SIN, and endometriosis. Patients may present with tubal rupture and shock. Grossly, the fallopian tube is dilated and hemorrhagic, with identifiable chorionic villi, with or without an identifiable embryo. Histologic sections should show chorionic villi or trophoblast in the tubal mucosa or wall.

B. **Neoplastic lesions of the fallopian tube.** The World Health Organization (WHO) histologic classification of tumors of the fallopian tube is presented in Table 32.1.
   1. **Benign tumors**
      a. Adenomatoid tumors are the most common benign tumor of the fallopian tube. They are usually incidental and unilateral, and present grossly as a well-circumscribed white-tan lesion in the tubal wall. They are derived from mesothelium, and the usual histologic pattern shows slitlike or glandular spaces lined by a single layer of flattened cuboidal cells (e-**Fig. 32.5**). The cells are positive for cytokeratin, calretinin, and vimentin expression immunohistochemically, but are negative for expression of factor VIII–related antigen and CD31, a profile that indicates a mesothelial rather than a vascular origin.
      b. Other benign tumors include epithelial papillomas, adenomas, cystadenomas, adenofibromas, and leiomyomas. Epithelial papillomas are usually incidental and show a branched pattern with a central fibrovascular core lined by a single layer of eosinophilic cells. Adenomas, cystadenomas, adenofibromas, and leiomyomas all resemble their ovarian and uterine counterparts.
   2. **Malignant tumors**
      a. Primary fallopian tube carcinoma is quite rare. Carcinomas typically occur in elderly women, and are usually widespread at the time of diagnosis, with a correspondingly poor prognosis. Serum CA125 levels may be elevated. Grossly, the fallopian tube is distended by a papillary or solid tumor. Serous adenocarcinoma, which microscopically is identical to ovarian serous adenocarcinoma (e-**Fig. 32.6**), is the most common subtype of carcinoma. The pathologic staging of primary fallopian tube malignancies is presented in Table 32.2.

      Carcinoma in situ, characterized by a papillary proliferation with cellular stratification, loss of polarity, and high-grade nuclear atypia, is distinguished from carcinoma by the lack of stromal invasion.
      b. Other primary malignant tumors of the fallopian tube include leiomyosarcoma, which may affect the fallopian tube or broad ligament, and carcinosarcoma (malignant mixed Müllerian tumor). Both tumors microscopically resemble their ovarian counterparts.
      c. Metastatic tumors are the most common category of malignancies involving the fallopian tube. Consequently, metastasis from a primary tumor at another site must always be excluded before making the diagnosis of a primary fallopian tube malignancy. Other primary tumors of the female reproductive tract, especially the ovary and endometrium, are the most frequent sources of metastases. Recently, it has been proposed that small serous carcinomas of the fallopian tube, particularly the fimbria in women with *BRCA* mutations, are the primary source for peritoneal, and possibly ovarian, serous carcinomas (*Am J Surg Pathol* 31:161, 2007).

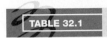

TABLE 32.1	WHO Histological Classification of Tumors of the Fallopian Tube

Epithelial tumors
Malignant
   Serous adenocarcinoma
   Mucinous adenocarcinoma
   Endometrioid adenocarcinoma
   Clear cell adenocarcinoma
   Transitional cell carcinoma
   Squamous cell carcinoma
   Undifferentiated carcinoma
   Others
Borderline tumor (of low malignant potential)
   Serous borderline tumor
   Mucinous borderline tumor
   Others
Carcinoma in situ (specify type)
Benign tumors
   Cystadenoma (specify type)
   Adenofibroma
   Cystadenofibroma
   Endometrioid polyp
   Papilloma (specify type)
   Metaplastic papillary tumor
   Others
Tumorlike epithelial lesions
   Tubal epithelial hyperplasia
   Salpingitis isthmica nodosa
   Endosalpingiosis
Mixed epithelial-mesenchymal tumors
Malignant mixed müllerian tumor (carcinosarcoma)
Adenosarcoma
Soft tissue tumors
Leiomyosarcoma
Leiomyoma
Others
Mesothelial tumors
Adenomatoid tumor
Germ cell tumors
Teratoma
   Mature
   Immature
   Others
Trophoblastic disease
Choriocarcinoma
Placental site trophoblastic tumor
Hydatidiform mole
Placental site nodule
Others
Lymphoid and hematopoetic tumors
Malignant lymphoma
Leukemia
Secondary tumors

From: Tavassoli FA, Devilee P, eds. *World Health Organization Classification of Tumours. Pathology and Genetics. Tumours of the Breast and Female Genital Organs.* Lyon: IARC Press; 2001. Used with permission.

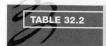

TABLE 32.2	Tumor, Node, Metastasis (TNM) Staging Scheme and International Federation of Gynecology and Obstetrics (FIGO) Classification of Carcinomas of the Fallopian Tube

PRIMARY TUMOR (T)

TNM Categories	FIGO Stages	
TX		Primary tumor cannot be assessed
T0		No evidence of primary tumor
Tis	0	Carcinoma in situ (previnvasive carcinoma)
T1	I	Tumor confined to fallopian tube(s)
T1a	IA	Tumor limited to one tube, without penetrating the serosal surface
T1b	IB	Tumor limited to both tubes, without penetrating the serosal surface
T1c	IC	Tumor limited to one or both tube(s) with extension onto or through the tubal serosa, or with malignant cells in ascites or peritoneal washings
T2	II	Tumor involves one or both fallopian tube(s) with pelvic extension
T2a	IIA	Extension and / or metastasis to uterus and / or ovaries
T2b	IIB	Extension to other pelvic structures
T2c	IIC	Pelvic extension (2a or 2b) with malignant cells in ascites or peritoneal washings
T3 and/or N1	III	Tumor involves one or both fallopian tube(s) with peritoneal implants outside the pelvis and / or positive regional lymph nodes
T3a	IIIA	Microscopic peritoneal metastasis outside the pelvis
T3b	IIIB	Macroscopic peritoneal metastasis outside the pelvis ≤2 cm in greatest dimension
T3c and/or N1	IIIC	Peritoneal metastasis >2 cm in greatest dimension and / or positive regional lymph nodes
M1	IV	Distant metastasis (excludes peritoneal metastasis)

Note: Liver capsule metastasis is T3 / stage III, liver parenchymal metastasis, M1 / stage IV. Pleural effusion must have positive cytology for M1 / stage IV.

REGIONAL LYMPH NODES (N)

NX	Regional lymph nodes cannot be assessed
N0	No regional lymph node metastasis
N1	Regional lymph node metastasis

DISTANT METASTASIS (M)

MX	Distant metastasis cannot be assessed
M0	No distant metastasis
M1	Distant metastasis

STAGE GROUPING

Stage 0	Tis	N0	M0
Stage IA	T1a	N0	M0
Stage IB	T1b	N0	M0
Stage IC	T1c	N0	M0
Stage IIA	T1c	N0	M0
Stage IIB	T2b	N0	M0
Stage IIC	T2c	N0	M0
Stage IIIA	T3a	N0	M0
Stage IIIB	T3b	N0	M0
Stage IIIC	T3c	N0	M0
	Any T	N1	M0
Stage IV	Any T	Any N	M1

From: Greene FL, Page DL, Fleming ID, Fritz AG, Balch CM, Haller DG, Morrow M, eds. *AJCC Cancer Staging Manual.* 6th edition. New York: Springer; 2002. Used with permission. (A new AJCC TNM staging system is scheduled for release in 2009; after its publication, the new staging scheme will appear on the website for this book.)

C. Reporting. The final report in any case of malignancy should include the histologic type and grade of the malignancy; the presence or absence of a precursor lesion (i.e., carcinoma in situ); tumor size, including depth and width; whether the malignancy is unifocal or multifocal; and the presence or absence of lymphovascular space invasion. In addition, the report should explicitly include all of the information required for assigning a stage, as well as other information of clinical interest not required for staging.

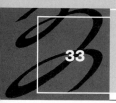

UTERUS (CORPUS)
Anahit Nowrouzi, John D. Pfeifer, and Phyllis C. Huettner

33

I. **NORMAL ANATOMY.** The uterus is a pear-shaped hollow organ with normal weight of between 40 and 80 g in adults. It is divided into the corpus, the lower uterine segment, and the cervix. The uterine cavity is triangular, measuring, on average, 6 cm in length. It is composed of the inner endometrial lining and the myometrium or muscular wall, with a serosal covering that extends to the peritoneal reflection. The peritoneal reflection is shorter anteriorly than posteriorly and so can be used for orienting hysterectomy specimens.

II. **GROSS EXAMINATION, TISSUE SAMPLING, AND HISTOLOGIC SLIDE PREPARATION**
   A. **Endometrial biopsy and curettage specimens.** The most common endometrial tissue samplings examined in surgical pathology are endometrial biopsy and curettage specimens, obtained from cervical dilation and curettage procedures. Endometrial biopsy samples are obtained from a relatively painless and limited office sampling procedure in which no cervical dilation is required. The dimension (size range of the largest tissue fragments or the dimensions of the tissue in aggregate) and/or volume of the specimen should be documented. The entire specimen should be submitted for microscopic examination, and three hematoxylin and eosin (H&E)-stained levels are prepared for microscopic examination.
   B. **Hysterectomy specimens.** The type of the hysterectomy (abdominal or vagina, with or without salpingoophorectomy) should be determined, and the size, weight, and shape of the uterus recorded (the processing of radical hysterectomy specimens, which differs substantially, is discussed in Chap. 34). The uterine serosa should be carefully examined for any abnormalities, which should be sampled. The uterus is next bivalved in the coronal plane to show the endometrial cavity and endocervical canal, which are examined and measured. The maximum thickness of the endometrium and myometrium should also be noted. Both halves of the uterus are then serially sectioned parallel to the long axis of the uterus.
      1. For specimens excised for benign disease, sections of the anterior cervix, posterior cervix, anterior endomyometrium, and posterior endomyometrium are submitted. Additional sections of any identified lesions must also be submitted.
      2. For specimens excised for malignancies, contiguous sections of both anterior and posterior endomyometrium, lower uterine segment, and cervix (including the serosa from the deepest area of myometrial invasion by the tumor) are submitted. Representative sections from any other lesions must also be submitted (Fig. 33.1).

III. **ENDOMETRIUM**
   A. **Dating**
      1. The endometrial mucosa is composed of glands and stroma. It is divided into the functional (luminal) layer and the basal (inner) layer. The basal cell layer acts as a reserve cell layer and is responsible for the regeneration of the endometrium. The stroma is composed of endometrial stromal cells and blood vessels.
      2. The menstrual cycle is divided into menstrual phase, proliferative phase, and secretory phase. Menstrual endometrium, present for the first 4 days of the 28-day cycle, is characterized by glandular and stromal breakdown,

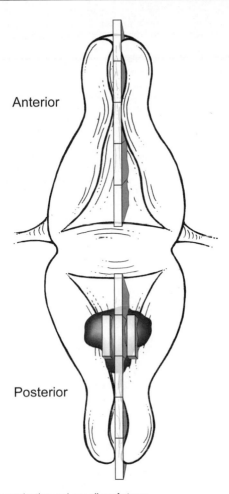

Anterior

Posterior

Figure 33.1. Gross examination and sampling of uterus.

glandular secretory exhaustion, and background inflammation (**e-Figs. 33.1** and **33.2**).*

Day 1 of menstrual bleeding is defined as day 1 of the cycle; the menstrual phase lasts for 3 to 4 days. The proliferative phase begins on day 4, and in an idealized situation lasts until day 14. Although it usually lasts about 11 days, it may greatly vary. During the early proliferative phase, the endometrium is thin and composed of straight glands in a loose stroma (**e-Fig. 33.3**). By days 8 to 10, stromal edema due to estrogen causes increased endometrial thickening, and the glands become more coiled as the gland–stroma growth rate increases. Throughout the proliferative phase, the epithelial lining the glands shows nuclear stratification, with a high mitotic rate in both glands and stroma.

The secretory phase begins with ovulation. In an idealized 28-day cycle, the secretory phase begins at day 14 and lasts 14 days, although it may range from 11 to 18 days. Following an interval phase from day 14 to day 15 (during which there are no dateable changes), the first dateable change of secretory

*All e-figures are available online via the Solution Site Image Bank.

phase is the appearance of subnuclear vacuoles (early day 16, secretory phase), as a clear zone between the basement membrane and the nucleus pushing the nucleus toward the glandular lumen. The vacuoles then move to the supranuclear position (day 18) and eventually are secreted into the glandular lumen (e-**Fig. 33.4**). Maximal stromal edema occurs during the midsecretory phase, around day 22. At day 23, the stroma begins to condense, and the first signs of periarteriolar predecidualization become apparent. Prominent glandular sawtoothing and maximal stromal decidualization occur at day 26 to 27 (e-**Fig. 33.5**). Numerous granular lymphocytes, marked stromal decidual change, and glandular breakdown are the features of day 28 of the late secretory phase.

B. Pregnancy

1. The earliest gestation-related changes occur following the implantation of the blastocyst. These changes are characterized by decidualization of the stroma with edema; the glands exhibit distension with increased secretion and a serrated architecture. By 4 to 8 weeks postimplantation, the endometrial epithelium often exhibits a physiologic response known as the Arias–Stella reaction, characterized by atypical cells lining hypersecretory-pattern endometrial glands (e-**Fig. 33.6**).

2. The placental implantation site, often seen in curettage specimens obtained because of a missed spontaneous abortion, is characterized by decidualized stroma infiltrated by intermediate trophoblast. Intermediate trophoblast may also infiltrate maternal spiral arteries, causing dilatation and fibrinoid deposition in the vessel wall. Intermediate trophoblast also normally infiltrates myometrium, which may occasionally be present in curettage specimens (e-**Fig. 33.7**).

3. Placental site nodules are incidental, usually microscopic findings that are characterized by small foci of hyalinized material with entrapped intermediate trophoblast cells, often with vacuolated cytoplasm. Placental site nodules are occasionally encountered in endometrial biopsies and curettage specimens but may also be seen in cervical specimens.

4. Abnormalities of implantation. Placenta accreta occurs when an intervening layer of decidua is not present between the placental villi and the myometrium at the implantation site. Placenta increta is present when villi penetrate into the myometrium, and transmural extension of villi with perforation is termed placenta percreta.

    Risk factors for abnormalities of implantation include prior Cesarean section, placenta previa, and prior instrumentation, among others. All forms of accreta may be associated with life-threatening hemorrhage, which may require hysterectomy.

C. Exogenous hormone therapy

1. Estrogen causes proliferation of endometrial glands and stroma. Persistent exposure to exogenous estrogen (as well as persistent exposure to endogenous estrogen as occurs with anovulatory cycles, obesity, or an estrogen-secreting tumor) causes endometrial proliferation with subsequent glandular and stromal breakdown, often clinically interpreted as irregular menstrual bleeding. Microscopically, the findings include stromal condensation with formation of so-called 'exodus bodies' or 'stromal blue-balls,' glandular degeneration and apoptosis of the glandular epithelial cells, and fibrin thrombi in stromal vessels.

2. Prolonged exposure to progestogens results in atrophic endometrium with a characteristic pattern that includes underdeveloped, inactive glands in a background of a stroma that shows marked decidual change.

3. Tamoxifen is primarily used for treatment of breast cancer. In the endometrium, tamoxifen competitively binds to estrogen receptors, and acts as an agonist. Tamoxifen increases the risk of endometrial hyperplasia and adenocarcinomas (*Ann N Y Acad Sci.* 2001;949:237), and up to 20% of women on tamoxifen develop endometrial polyps (*Cancer.* 2001;92:1151).

IV. COMMON BENIGN DISEASES OF THE ENDOMETRIUM

A. Endometritis

1. Acute endometritis is defined by the presence of acute neutrophilic inflammation in the stroma of the nonmenstruating endometrium. In severe cases, the

neutrophils are present throughout the stroma, the endometrial epithelium, and the glandular lumina (e-**Fig. 33.8**). Acute inflammation present during the menstrual phase of the endometrium should not be misdiagnosed as active infection. Acute endometritis is uncommon and is usually only seen in postpartum or postabortive endometrium.

2. Chronic endometritis is defined by the presence of plasma cells in the endometrial stroma. Associated features include glandular and stromal breakdown, and dyssynchronous glandular and stromal development (e-**Fig. 33.9**). The most common causes of chronic endometritis include *Chlamydia trachomatis, Ureaplasma urealyticum,* cytomegalovirus, and herpesvirus infection. Infection by *Actinomyces israelii* or *Neisseria gonorrheae* usually causes a mixed acute and chronic pattern of inflammation.

    Granulomatous inflammation is rare. Common causes include *Mycobacterium tuberculosis* infection, fungal infection, sarcoidosis, and hysteroscopic ablation therapy.

B. **Atrophy** most commonly is seen in postmenopausal women. Premenopausal causes include treatment with oral contraceptives or gonadotropin agonists. Patients with premature menopause also show an atrophic pattern. Microscopically, the endometrium is composed of a thin layer of endometrial glands lined by an attenuated layer of inactive epithelial cells, surrounded by thin stroma. No mitotic activity is present (e-**Fig. 33.10**).

C. **Metaplasia.** The presence of any type of glandular epithelium other than the normal columnar type is called metaplasia. Metaplasia is a common finding in menopausal and postmenopausal women, and is often associated with abnormal uterine bleeding or recent use of exogenous hormonal therapy.

1. Tubal metaplasia consists of foci of normal tubal epithelium within the endometrial glands, including ciliated, nonciliated secretory, and intercalated cells. The ratio of the ciliated to nonciliated cells is cyclical and depends on hormonal influences.

2. Ciliated cell metaplasia is the most common form of metaplasia. It is composed of a layer of ciliated columnar cells with round to oval nuclei and abundant pale eosinophilic cytoplasm. Ciliated cell metaplasia is a normal response of endometrial epithelium to various hormonal exposures. It is most commonly found around menopause and is associated with endometrial polyps, anovulatory cycles, and exogenous hormonal therapy.

3. Squamous metaplasia is often caused by chronic irritation, and often takes the form of squamous morules or rounded, swirling nests of squamous cells. Squamous metaplasia must not be confused with endometrial hyperplasia or malignancy, although it can occur as a secondary change in both of the latter.

4. Eosinophilic metaplasia or eosinophilic change refers to glandular epithelium with abundant eosinophilic cytoplasm and central round to oval nuclei. It is often associated with a neutrophilic infiltrate, the formation of small epithelial papilla, and mild nuclear atypia.

5. Mucinous metaplasia is rare. It is morphologically similar to endocervical mucinous epithelium in that it consists of columnar epithelium with basally located oval nuclei and abundant apical mucin.

6. Clear cell metaplasia is also rare. It is characterized by columnar cells with round nuclei and clear cytoplasm.

D. **Endometrial polyps.** A local overgrowth of endometrial glands and stroma that protrudes into the endometrial cavity forms an endometrial polyp. Polyps are present in about 20%–25% of women, and are frequently found in the menopausal and postmenopausal period. Grossly, polyps appear as broad based to pedunculated lesions; some pedunculated polyps can extend into the endocervical canal, and even through the os. Microscopically, polyps are composed of endometrial glands within a fibrous stroma; the presence of thick-walled blood vessels within the fibrous stroma is the most common key to the diagnosis (e-**Fig. 33.11**). Frequently, the glands are variably shaped and irregularly distributed.

Although endometrial polyps in postmenopausal women usually contain dilated glands lined by one layer of atrophic epithelium, foci of metaplastic or hyperplastic epithelium, as well as frank adenocarcinoma, may be present. Consequently, endometrial polyps should be entirely submitted for microscopic examination.

1. Polyps with stromal smooth muscle are referred to as adenomyomatous polyps.
2. Atypical polypoid adenomyoma is a polypoid lesion characterized histologically by crowded irregular endometrial glands with a complex architecture and cytologic atypia in stroma that is predominantly composed of smooth muscle. The lesion has a high rate of recurrence upon incomplete surgical removal, and mainly occurs in premenopausal nulliparous women. It is associated with a clinical history of infertility.

E. **Disordered proliferative endometrium** predominantly exhibits a normal proliferative pattern, with mild irregular branching and budding and some cystic dilation. However, the gland-to-stroma ratio is not increased, the main factor that helps to differentiate a disordered proliferative pattern from simple hyperplasia. The epithelium lining the glands is composed of stratified and columnar cells with no atypia. Mitotic activity is similar to that of normal proliferative endometrium (e-Fig. 33.12).

V. **ENDOMETRIAL HYPERPLASIA AND ENDOMETRIAL INTRAEPITHELIAL CARCINOMA.** Endometrial hyperplasia is thought to develop as a result of unopposed estrogenic stimulation. Any disorder that causes an increase in endogenous or exogenous estrogenic stimulation such as polycystic ovarian disease, obesity, or ovarian neoplasms (e.g., thecomas, granulosa cell tumors) can therefore cause endometrial hyperplasia. Abnormal bleeding is the major clinical symptom.

A. **Endometrial hyperplasia.** Hyperplasia is subclassified into simple or complex, with or without cytologic atypia. Numerous studies have demonstrated that the risk of progression to adenocarcinoma (specifically, endometrioid adenocarcinoma and its variants) is more highly correlated with the presence of cytologic atypia than with the degree of glandular crowding.

1. Simple hyperplasia shows a gland-to-stroma ratio that is slightly increased ($>1:1$) with prominent variability in size of the glands, glandular budding, and cystic glandular dilatation (e-Fig. 33.13).
2. Complex hyperplasia is composed of crowded, architecturally complex glands with little intervening stroma. The gland-to-stroma ratio is elevated (at least 3:1) (e-Fig. 33.14).
3. Cytologic atypia, which may be a feature of simple or complex hyperplasia, is based on the nuclear cytology of the glandular epithelium. The most reliable indicators of cytologic atypia are an enlarged nucleus that is round rather than oval, that has coarse clumped chromatin, and that has a prominent nucleolus. A diagnosis of hyperplasia should be made with extreme caution during the secretory phase of the endometrium because of the usual crowding of the glands in this phase of the menstrual cycle. The presence of cytologic atypia must be distinguished from the cellular changes that accompany metaplasias and from an Arias–Stella reaction.

B. **Endometrial intraepithelial neoplasia (EIN)** is defined as a proliferation of islands of endometrial glands that have cytological and architectural abnormalities and are considered to be premalignant. The EIN scheme has been proposed both as an approach to simplify the diagnosis of premalignant changes and as a classification more closely linked to the genetic changes in premalignant endometrial epithelium (*Gynecol Oncol.* 2000;76:287). These glands genetically have the potential of transforming into endometrioid adenocarcinoma. Studies have shown that some of these lesions harbor *PTEN* tumor suppressor gene inactivation, mutation of *k-ras*, and microsatellite instability. EIN is considered to be a monoclonal proliferation composed of cells in early stages of carcinogenesis.

Diagnostic criteria for EIN (http://www.endometrium.org) are based on size of the lesion, nuclear cytology, and glandular architecture (including glandular crowding with an increased gland-to-stroma ratio, cytologic differences between the neoplastic glands and the adjacent normal glands, and an area of glandular crowding that is >1 mm in greatest dimension). EIN can have squamous, mucinous, or clear cell differentiation. The treatment of these lesions is similar to the clinical management of atypical endometrial hyperplasia.

C. Endometrial intraepithelial carcinoma (EIC) is thought to represent the precursor lesion to serous carcinoma. Microscopically, EIC is composed of glands lined by cells with the same cytologic abnormalities as serous carcinoma, but without evidence of myometrial stromal invasion. The development of EIC is independent of prior unopposed estrogenic stimulation.

VI. EPITHELIAL MALIGNANCIES. Epithelial malignancies are the most common gynecological malignancy in women in developed countries. Endometrial cancer can be divided into two broad categories that have differences in their clinical and pathologic features as well as in their underlying genetic abnormalities.

Type I tumors consist of endometrioid adenocarcinoma and its variants. They account for >80% of endometrial tumors, and usually develop in postmenopausal women in their fifth and sixth decades in the background of long-term estrogen stimulation. Type 1 tumors are strongly associated with diabetes and obesity, and have a relatively good prognosis. The endometrial glands and stroma in Type I tumors are strongly positive for estrogen and progesterone receptors. In addition, the stromal cells show diffuse strong immunopositivity for CD10 (CALLA) antigen. Genetically, they show microsatellite instability and mutations in the *PTEN* tumor suppressor gene, *k-ras*, and *CTNNB1*, but assessment for these genetic abnormalities is not necessary for diagnosis.

Type II tumors (for example, serous papillary carcinoma) usually occur in women in their sixth and seventh decades and are not associated with estrogen stimulation; therefore, they do not occur in a background of complex atypical hyperplasia. They tend to be at an advanced stage at the time of presentation, so they have a relatively poor prognosis. Genetically they are characterized by *TP53* mutations. The World Health Organization (WHO) classification of uterine corpus malignancies is presented in Table 33.1, and the pathologic staging of uterine corpus malignancies is shown in Table 33.2.

A. Endometrioid adenocarcinoma usually arises in the uterine corpus and grossly usually consists of a raised to exophytic, pink tan, hemorrhagic mass that projects into the endometrial cavity. Microscopically, the tumor consists of irregular, confluent, complex, glandular, or villoglandular structures lined by pleomorphic stratified columnar cells with pleomorphic nuclei. The presence of areas of definitive cribriform architecture is a microscopic feature that can be used to distinguish well-differentiated endometrioid adenocarcinoma from complex hyperplasia with cytologic atypia. Foci of squamous differentiation, which should not be mistaken as solid component of the tumor, are often encountered.

Myometrial invasion is recognized by the presence of an irregular endometrial–myometrial border or by an associated desmoplastic and inflammatory stromal response. The depth of myometrial invasion and the presence or absence of lymphovascular space invasion should be noted.

The International Federation of Gynecology and Obstetrics (FIGO) grading system for endometrioid adenocarcinoma is based on the degree of differentiation as defined by the percentage of glandular and solid components (areas of squamous differentiation are not considered regions of solid growth). Tumors with 0–5% solid growth are grade 1, with 6–50% solid growth are grade 2, and with >50% solid growth are grade 3 (e-**Figs. 33.15–33.18**). Notable nuclear pleomorphism inappropriate for the tumor architecture increases the tumor grade by one step.

Variants of endometrioid adenocarcinoma include villoglandular, secretory, mucinous, and squamous. The villoglandular pattern is diagnosed by the presence of a predominantly branching glandular architecture with central fibrovascular cores lined by stratified columnar cells containing elongated pleomorphic nuclei. The secretory pattern is characterized by glands composed of cells with supra- or subnuclear vacuoles resembling secretory endometrium. The mucinous pattern is defined by the presence of foci of endometrial glands lined by columnar cells with

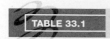

TABLE 33.1   WHO Histological Classification of Tumors of the Uterine Corpus

Epithelial Tumors and Related Lesions
Endometrial carcinoma
Endometrioid adenocarcinoma
Variant with squamous differentiation
Villoglandular variant
Secretory variant
Ciliated cell variant
Mucinous adenocarcinoma
Serous adenocarcinoma
Clear cell adenocarcinoma
Mixed cell adenocarcinoma
Squamous cell carcinoma
Transitional cell carcinoma
Small cell carcinoma
Undifferentiated carcinoma
Others
Endometrial hyperplasia
  Nonatypical hyperplasia
    Simple
    Complex
  Atypical hyperplasia
    Simple
    Complex
Endometrial polyp
Tamoxifen-related lesions

Mesenchymal Tumors
Endometrial stromal and related tumors
  Endometrial stromal nodule
  Endometrial stromal sarcoma, low grade
  Undifferentiated endometrial sarcoma
Smooth muscle tumors
  Leiomyosarcoma
    Epithelioid variant
    Myxoid variant
  Smooth muscle tumors of uncertain
    malignant potential
  Leiomyoma, not otherwise specified
    Histological variants
      Mitotically active variant
      Cellular variant
      Hemorrhagic cellular variant
      Epithelioid variant
      Myxoid variant
      Atypical variant
      Lipoleiomyoma variant

    Growth pattern variants
      Diffuse leiomyomatosis
      Dissecting leiomyoma
      Intravenous leiomyomatosis
      Metastasizing leiomyomatosis
Miscellaneous mesenchymal tumors
  Mixed endometrial stromal and smooth
    muscle tumors
  Perivascular epithelioid cell tumor
  Adenomatoid tumor
  Other malignant mesenchymal tumors
  Other benign mesenchymal tumors

Mixed Epithelial and Mesenchymal Tumors
  Carcinosarcoma (malignant mixed
    Müllerian tumor)
  Adenosarcoma
  Carcinofibroma
  Adenofibroma
  Adenomyoma
    Atypical polypoid variant

Gestational Trophoblastic Disease
Trophoblastic neoplasms
  Choriocarcinoma
  Placental site trophoblastic tumor
  Epithelioid trophoblastic tumor
Molar pregnancies
  Hydatidiform mole
    Complete
    Partial
    Invasive
    Metastatic
Nonneoplastic, nonmolar trophoblastic lesions
  Placental site nodule and plaque
  Exaggerated placental site

Miscellaneous Tumors
  Sex cord-like tumors
  Neuroectodermal tumors
  Melanotic paraganglioma
  Tumors of germ cell type
  Others

Lymphoid and Hematopoietic Tumors
  Malignant lymphoma
  Leukemia

Secondary Tumors

WHO, World Health Organization.
From: Tavassoli FA, Devilee P, eds. *World Health Organization Classification of Tumours. Pathology and Genetics. Tumours of the Breast and Female Genital Organs.* Lyon: IARC Press; 2001. Used with permission.

TABLE 33.2	Tumor, Node, Metastasis (TNM) Staging Scheme and FIGO of Nontrophoblastic Tumors of the Uterine Corpus

TNM and FIGO classification
PRIMARY TUMOR (T)

TNM categories	FIGO stages	
TX		Primary tumor cannot be assessed
T0		No evidence of primary tumor
Tis	0	Carcinoma in situ (preinvasive carcinoma)
TI	I*	Tumor confined to corpus uteri
T1a	IA	Tumor limited to endometrium
T1b	IB	Tumor invades less than one half of myometrium
T1c	1C	Tumor invades one half or more of myometrium
T2	II	Tumor invades cervix but does not extend beyond uterus
T2a	IIA	Endocervical glandular involvement only
T2b	IIB	Cervical stromal invasion
T3 and/or N1	III	Local and/or regional spread as specified in T3a, b, N1, and FIGO IIIA, B, C below
T3a	IIIA	Tumor involves serosa and/or adnexa (direct extension or metastasis) and/or cancer cells in ascites or peritoneal washings
T3b	IIIB	Vaginal involvement (direct extension or metastasis)
T3c	IIIC	Metastasis to pelvic and/or para-aortic lymph nodes
T4	IVA	Tumor invades bladder mucosa and/or bowel mucosa
M1	IVB	Distant metastasis (*excluding* metastasis to vagina, pelvic serosa, or adnexa)

REGIONAL LYMPH NODES (N)

NX	Regional lymph nodes cannot be assessed
N0	No regional lymph node metastasis
N1	Regional lymph node metastasis

DISTANT METASTASIS (M)

MX	Distant metastasis cannot be assessed
M0	No distant metastasis
M1	Distant metastasis

STAGE GROUPING

Stage 0	Tis	N0	M0
Stage IA	T1a	N0	M0
Stage IB	T1b	N0	M0
Stage IC	T1c	N0	M0
Stage IIA	T2a	N0	M0
Stage IIB	T2b	N0	M0
Stage IIIA	T3a	N0	M0
Stage IIIB	T3b	N0	M0
Stage IIIC	T1, T2, T3	N1	M0
Stage IVA	T4	Any N	M0
Stage IVB	Any T	Any N	M1

TNM, Tumor, Node, Metastasis; FIGO, International Federation of Gynecology and Obstetrics.
From: Greene FL, Page DL, Fleming ID, Fritz AG, Balch CM, Haller DG, Morrow M, eds. *AJCC Cancer Staging Manual.* 6th edition. New York: Springer; 2002. Used with permission. (A new AJCC TNM staging system is scheduled for release in 2009; after its publication, the new staging scheme will appear on the website for this book.)

abundant intracytoplasmic mucin, often with a papillary architecture (e-**Fig. 33.19**). Squamous differentiation is defined as the presence of sheets of squamous cells that are usually, but not always, nonkeratinizing.

B. **Serous adenocarcinoma** is a high-grade tumor characterized by cells with a high nuclear-to-cytoplasmic ratio, a high mitotic rate, and complex papillary architecture. Deep myometrial and lymphovascular invasion are often present (e-**Fig. 33.20**).

C. **Clear cell adenocarcinoma** is a high-grade tumor composed of pleomorphic cells with hobnail nuclei (nuclei that jut into the gland lumen), abundant clear cytoplasm, and distinct cell borders arranged in papillary, solid, and tubular structures, often admixed (e-**Fig. 33.21**). Clear cell adenocarcinoma is often at an advanced clinical stage at the time of presentation.

D. **Mixed adenocarcinoma** is defined as a tumor demonstrating a mixture of endometrioid adenocarcinoma (or its variants) together with serous, mucinous, or clear cell adenocarcinoma. By convention, the minor component must comprise at least 10% of the tumor.

E. **Carcinosarcoma** (malignant mixed Müllerian tumor or MMMT) comprises approximately 10% of all the uterine malignancies. The diagnostic criteria are based on the presence of malignant epithelial and mesenchymal (sarcomatous) elements. Numerous genetic studies have demonstrated that both elements are derived from the same precursor, proving that the neoplasm does not represent a collision tumor (*Cancer Res.* 2000;60:114). Consequently, the tumor is now considered to represent a poorly differentiated endometrial carcinoma with metaplastic differentiation.

Grossly, carcinosarcomas appear to be larger and fleshier than typical adenocarcinomas. Microscopically, they consist of areas of adenocarcinoma intermixed with a wide range of malignant mesenchymal elements such as smooth muscle, undifferentiated sarcoma, cartilage, or skeletal muscle (e-**Figs. 33.22** and **33.23**). Foci of poorly differentiated cells with marked pleomorphism and a high mitotic rate with no distinct pattern are not uncommon. Extensive areas of necrosis are often present. Carcinosarcomas can be divided into homologous or heterologous tumors depending on whether the stromal component is normally found in the uterus; this distinction is now recognized to have no clinical significance.

Carcinosarcoma generally has a poor prognosis. Specific adverse prognostic factors include the presence of epithelial component with foci of serous or clear cell differentiation, deep myometrial invasion, cervical involvement, and lymphovascular space involvement; the grade of tumor, type of the mesenchymal element, and mitotic rate have no correlation with the outcome.

F. **Squamous cell carcinoma** of the endometrium is rare and usually occurs in postmenopausal women in association with pyometria and cervical stenosis. Microscopically, it is identical to squamous cell carcinoma of the cervix, and so must be distinguished from a cervical primary that has extended into the endometrium.

G. **Other primary malignant tumors.** Transitional cell carcinoma is extremely rare and occurs in postmenopausal women. Microscopically, it consists of sheets of urothelial cells admixed with another type of the endometrial adenocarcinoma, and must be distinguished from metastatic transitional cell carcinoma from the urinary bladder or ovary. Small cell carcinoma of endometrium is extremely rare and comprises >1% of the primary endometrial malignancies. Microscopically, the tumor has the same cytomorphology as high-grade neuroendocrine tumors arising at other sites. Undifferentiated carcinomas do not show differentiation toward any defined tumor pattern.

VII. **ENDOMETRIAL STROMAL TUMORS.** Endometrial stromal tumors are composed of small cells with scant cytoplasm that morphologically resemble endometrial stromal cells of proliferative phase endometrium. A subset of tumors exhibit variant morphologic patterns including smooth muscle differentiation, a fibromyxoid component, and sex cord-like/epithelioid patterns. The t(7;17)(p15;q21) translocation that produces a JAZF1-JJAZ1 fusion protein is a recurring feature of all classes of endometrial stromal tumors, but demonstration of its presence is not required for diagnosis.

A. **Endometrial stromal nodules** are grossly tan to yellow, well-circumscribed lesions with a smooth border, and range from 0.5 to 12 cm in greatest dimension. They are primarily located in the myometrium, and an obvious connection to the endometrium is not necessary for diagnosis. Histologically, these tumors are composed of sheets of small cells with scant cytoplasm and an accompanying vascular pattern reminiscent of the spiral arterioles present in the stroma of proliferative phase endometrium. These tumors are strongly and diffusely positive with CD10 (although a minority of cases may show weak positivity) and are desmin negative. Because cellular leiomyomas and leiomyosarcomas are usually negative for CD10 but are desmin positive, immunohistochemistry can be helpful in difficult cases. Endometrial stromal nodules are benign, and total abdominal hysterectomy is curative.

B. **Endometrial stromal sarcomas** predominantly occur in middle-age women, and do not share the same risk factors as endometrial carcinoma. On gross examination, endometrial stromal sarcomas exhibit a tan to yellow cut surface with an infiltrative margin into the surrounding myometrium, often with foci of hemorrhage and necrosis. Microscopically, the tumor consists of fingerlike projections into the myometrium of cells with similar cytomorphology as those seen in endometrial stromal nodules, but with a higher rate of mitosis, greater nuclear pleomorphism, prominent stromal vascularity, and areas of collagenized stroma (e-**Fig. 33.24**). Extensive lymphatic invasion is the hallmark of the tumor. Hysterectomy is the treatment of choice. Because some of the tumor cells are positive for progesterone receptors, hormonal therapy following excision is a treatment option. Patients with early-stage disease have 5-year survival rates of 90%; recurrence may occur in up to 25% of the patients, often several years to a decade or more following the primary diagnosis.

C. **Undifferentiated endometrial sarcoma** is composed of sheets of pleomorphic undifferentiated cells with a moderate volume of cytoplasm and a high mitotic rate with frequent atypical forms. This tumor lacks the plexiform vasculature reminiscent of proliferative phase endometrium. These tumors have an aggressive course usually resulting in death within 3 years of diagnosis.

VIII. SMOOTH MUSCLE NEOPLASMS

A. **Leiomyoma** is the most common neoplasm of the uterus and can occur as a submucosal, intramural, or subserosal lesion. Leiomyomas predominantly affect women of reproductive age; they can be found in 20%–30% of women in their fourth decade, and >40% of women in their fifth decade. They tend to enlarge during pregnancy because they express estrogen and progesterone receptors. Grossly, leiomyomas are well-circumscribed lesions; they have a white-tan cut surface and are sharply demarcated from the adjacent myometrium. Microscopically, leiomyomas are composed of interlacing fascicles of closely packed cells with uniform elongated nuclei and eosinophilic cytoplasm (e-**Fig. 33.25**). Degenerative changes including hyaline change, coagulative necrosis, and hydropic degeneration are often present.

1. Cellular leiomyomas have the same gross features as ordinary leiomyomas but microscopically demonstrate an increased cellularity with sheets of spindle cells with hyperchromatic elongated nuclei and a scant amount of eosinophilic cytoplasm. There is no pleomorphism or increased mitotic activity. These lesions behave as classic leiomyoma.

2. Epithelioid leiomyomas are composed of predominantly epithelioid cells with eosinophilic to clear cytoplasm and fine nuclear chromatin. The cells are arranged in clusters and single cells, with no pleomorphism. The mitotic rate is not elevated, and necrosis is absent. They behave the same as classic leiomyoma.

3. Symplastic leiomyoma contains scattered enlarged, markedly atypical cells, often with multiple nuclei. However, the mitotic count is still <10 mitotic figures/10 high-power field, and no necrosis is present. These have the same benign behavior as classic leiomyoma.

4. Lipoleiomyoma refers to a classic leiomyoma that contains islands of mature adipocytes. This variant has no clinical significance.

   5. Myxoid leiomyoma consists of fascicles of uniform spindle cells surrounded by pools of myxoid edematous stroma. Large vessels are not uncommonly present.

B. Benign metastasizing leiomyoma. Many patients who have benign metastasizing leiomyoma have a prior history of hysteroscopy with dilatation and curettage, or other procedures such as myomectomy or hysterectomy. Microscopically, benign metastasizing leiomyomas have the same histologic features as ordinary leiomyomas, although they may extend into adjacent vessels. The tumor can migrate to the lung, and lymph node involvement may be present. The differential diagnosis includes low-grade leiomyosarcoma, and a smooth muscle tumor of another site (such as gastrointestinal tract or retroperitoneum) must be excluded. Some cases may respond to hormonal therapy.

C. Intravascular leiomyomatosis refers to classic leiomyomas that grow into the lumen of the uterine or pelvic veins. The tumor may migrate or extend into the inferior vena cava and even into the right heart. The tumor is composed of sheets of spindle to round cells with minimum atypia and rare mitosis, for which the differential diagnosis often includes low-grade endometrial stromal sarcoma. With local control, the tumor has an excellent long-term prognosis.

D. Leiomyosarcoma is the malignant counterpart of leiomyoma. It is the most common sarcoma of the uterus, with an incidence of 2 to 3 for every 1000 women with leiomyomata. Leiomyosarcoma usually occurs in women older than 50 years and has a higher rate of occurrence in African Americans. Some studies have suggested unopposed estrogen exposure as one of the underlying etiologies. The genetics of leiomyosarcomas have confirmed that they do not arise from leiomyomas.

   Grossly, leiomyosarcoma consists of an irregular, soft, and fleshy mass with a pink-tan cut surface with obvious foci of hemorrhage and necrosis. This tumor almost always demonstrates an ill-defined and infiltrating border. Microscopically, leiomyosarcoma is composed of sheets of pleomorphic spindle cells with elongated nuclei, high-grade cytologic atypia, and a high mitotic rate with frequent atypical mitotic figures (e-**Fig. 33.26**). A comprehensive study (*Am J Surg Pathol.* 1994;18:535) recommended that the diagnostic approach for leiomyosarcoma include evaluation of the degree of cytologic atypia (graded as mild, moderate, or severe), assessment of the presence or absence of coagulative tumor cell necrosis (CTCN, defined as an abrupt transition from viable cells to necrotic cells without a transition zone of hyalinized tissue or granulation tissue), and determination of the mitotic index (MI), as outlined in Table 33.3.

   Leiomyosarcoma has a poor prognosis. The patient's age, tumor MI, and clinical stage of the disease at the time of presentation are among the important prognostic factors. Surgical intervention including total abdominal hysterectomy with bilateral salpingo-oophorectomy is the treatment of choice. Variants include epithelioid (clear cell) leiomyosarcoma and myxoid leiomyosarcoma; both are relatively rare.

E. Smooth muscle tumor of uncertain malignant potential (STUMP) is the nomenclature used to designate problematic uterine smooth muscle neoplasms that fall between benign leiomyoma and leiomyosarcoma. Cases of STUMP represent tumors for which the classification by established criteria is uncertain, and for which the alternative diagnostic possibilities vary in their clinical implications.

IX. OTHER MYOMETRIAL DISEASES

A. Adenomyosis is defined as the presence of benign endometrial glands surrounded by endometrial stroma within the myometrium (conventionally at least 2.5 mm below the endomyometrial junction). Grossly, the myometrial wall can show a thick trabeculated pattern with punctate hemorrhage. Microscopically, the glands usually show an inactive pattern or a pattern that is dyssynchronous with the endometrium (e-**Fig. 33.27**). In some cases, only the stromal component is present and the glands are sparse or completely absent. Endometrial adenocarcinoma occasionally involves adenomyosis, but this occurrence is not considered myometrial invasion for staging purposes.

TABLE 33.3	Strategy for Diagnosis of Uterine Smooth Muscle Tumors

Morphologic features to be evaluated
  Degree of cytologic atypia; none to mild (insignificant) or moderate to severe (significant)
Presence or absence of coagulative tumor cell necrosis
Mitotic index (MI)
Tumors with usual differentiation
  MI <20 per 10 high-power field (hpf), no coagulative tumor cell necrosis, no atypia or no more
  than mild cytologic atypia - leiomyoma or leiomyoma with increased MI (MI <5 per 10 hpf -
  leiomyoma; MI ≥5 per 10 hpf - leiomyoma with increased mitotic index)
  MI ≥20 per hpf, no coagulative tumor cell necrosis, no atypia or no more than mild cytologic
  atypia - leiomyoma with increased MI, but experience limited
  MI <10 per hpf, no coagulative tumor cell necrosis but with diffuse moderate to severe
  cytologic atypia - atypical leiomyoma with low risk of recurrence
  MI ≥10 per 10 hpf, no coagulative tumor cell necrosis but with diffuse moderate to severe
  cytologic atypia - leiomyosarcoma
  MI <20 per 10 hpf, no coagulative tumor cell necrosis but with focal moderate to severe
  cytologic atypia - atypical leiomyoma, but experience limited
  Any MI, with diffuse moderate-to-severe atypia and with coagulative tumor cell necrosis -
  leiomyosarcoma
  MI ≥10 per 10 hpf, no to mild atypia but with coagulative tumor cell necrosis - leiomyosarcoma
  MI <10, no to mild atypia but with coagulative tumor cell necrosis - smooth muscle tumor of
  low malignant potential, but experience limited.

Modified from *Am J Surg Pathol.* 1994;18:535.

B. Postoperative spindle cell nodule is a benign lesion that usually occurs within a
few weeks following endometrial instrumentation or other surgical procedure. It is
grossly pink-tan and friable. Microscopically, it consists of granulation tissue with
surface ulceration, accompanied by a hypercellular proliferation of spindle cells
with elongated nuclei, moderate amounts of pink cytoplasm, and a high mitotic rate
arranged in fascicles. Numerous extravasated red blood cells are usually present.
Postoperative spindle cell nodule must be distinguished from leiomyosarcoma; the
distinct fascicular pattern of growth, lack of pleomorphism, and characteristic clinical presentation of the former are clues to the correct diagnosis.

C. Adenofibroma is a rare entity that usually occurs in postmenopausal women who
present with abnormal bleeding. Microscopically, it is composed of a layer of epithelium with bland nuclear cytology that overlies a cellular fibrous stroma composed
of fibroblasts and endometrial stromal cells. Adenofibroma is a benign entity, and
hysterectomy is curative.

D. Adenosarcoma is characteristically a tumor of postmenopausal women. It is a
rare tumor that arises most commonly from the endometrium and forms a large,
polypoid, lobulated mass that may fill the entire endometrial cavity and prolapse
through the cervical os. Microscopically, adenosarcomas are composed of benign
glandular elements in a malignant stroma that shows increased cellularity, pleomorphism, and a high mitotic rate. The stroma is often condensed and hypercellular in
periglandular areas.

Adenosarcoma is best considered a tumor of low malignant potential, and
has a better outcome compared with other uterine sarcomas. However, recurrence
(which occurs in up to 25% of patients) is associated with very poor prognosis.
Treatment includes hysterectomy with bilateral salpingo-oophorectomy.

X. GESTATIONAL TROPHOBLASTIC DISEASE. Gestational trophoblastic disease is a
group of tumors that arise from gestational trophoblast, from normal diploid as well
as molar pregnancies. In western populations, about 0.1% of pregnancies are affected;
patients are often at the extremes of reproductive age, and women with previous gestational trophoblastic disease are at higher risk.

A. Hydatidiform mole

1. Complete molar pregnancies develop from fertilization of an empty ovum. Complete moles are diploid, but may be either heterozygous (15% of cases, due to fertilization of an empty ovum by two sperm) or homozygous (85% of cases due to fertilization of an empty ovum by a single sperm with subsequent duplication). Complete moles classically present as a larger uterus than expected for gestational age that, on ultrasound examination, shows a so-called 'snow storm' pattern without fetal parts; the patient's serum human chorionic gonadotropin (hCG) is usually elevated for gestational age. Histopathologically, complete moles are composed of markedly enlarged villi with central villous cavitation and circumferential villous surface trophoblastic proliferation. They carry an increased risk of subsequent development of choriocarcinoma (up to 10% in Asian populations).

2. **Partial molar pregnancies** develop from fertilization of a normal ovum by two sperm, and so has a triploid karyotype. Patients may have a normal, elevated, or even low serum hCG for gestational age; fetal parts are sometimes present by ultrasound imaging. Histologically, partial moles are composed of two populations of villi; one population is essentially normal, and one population exhibits enlargement with at least focal cavitation, irregular villous outlines, trophoblast inclusions, and subtle circumferential trophoblast in the form of buds or lacy mounds. Partial moles also carry a very small but increased risk of subsequent development of choriocarcinoma.

3. **Invasive mole** refers to a molar pregnancy (either complete or partial) in which the villi and associated trophoblast invade the myometrium and blood vessels or are exported to extrauterine sites.

B. Trophoblastic tumors

1. **Choriocarcinoma.** Although molar pregnancies have a much increased risk of subsequently developing gestational choriocarcinoma, the tumor can also develop following any type of pregnancy. Microscopically, the tumor is composed of sheets of highly atypical trophoblast with prominent foci of hemorrhage and necrosis. The pleomorphic trophoblast consists of admixture of cytotrophoblast, syncytiotrophoblast, and intermediate trophoblast, and often forms alternating collections of syncytiotrophoblast and mononucleate trophoblast. Choriocarcinoma spreads hematogenously, and the most common metastatic sites are the lung, pelvis, vagina, liver, and brain. Choriocarcinoma is strongly positive for cytokeratin, hCG, melanoma cell adhesion molecule (Mel-CAM), human placental lactogen (hPL), and placental alkaline phosphatase expression by immunohistochemistry.

2. **Placental site trophoblastic tumor** is composed of intermediate trophoblast and cytotrophoblast. Characteristic features include abundant eosinophilic fibrinoid deposition and dissection of individual smooth muscle cells by the neoplastic cells. Placental site trophoblastic tumor typically presents as a mass that may be deeply invasive; serum hCG levels are usually elevated. About 15% of cases exhibit malignant behavior; unlike most forms of gestational trophoblastic disease, the tumor is not very responsive to chemotherapy.

3. **Epithelioid trophoblastic tumor** is composed of chorionic-type intermediate trophoblast. It is a very rare form of trophoblastic disease that has only recently been recognized as a distinct disease entity. Morphologically, the tumor resembles a carcinoma in that it is composed of a relatively uniform population of atypical mononucleate cells arranged in sheets and nests with abundant eosinophilic cytoplasm.

XI. SEROSAL TUMORS

A. Endometriosis affects 5%–10% of women of childbearing age. Patients usually present with symptoms of pelvic pain, dyspareunia, secondary dysmenorrhea, and in some cases, infertility. Many cases remain asymptomatic. The three most common accepted theories regarding its etiology are retrograde spillage of menstrual tissue into the pelvic cavity, serosal metaplasia, and a developmental abnormality. The most commonly involved sites include the ovary, uterine serosa, fallopian tube, peritoneum, and cul-de-sac. Oral contraceptives have been shown to have a protective role. Histologically, endometriosis is defined as the presence of endometrial glands surrounded by endometrial stroma; associated hemosiderin deposition and chronic inflammation are usually present.

B. Adenomatoid tumor is a benign peritoneal tumor that originates from mesothelium. It most commonly involves the serosal surfaces of the uterus and fallopian tubes. Grossly, the tumor usually forms a tan 1- to 2-cm well-circumscribed nodule. Microscopically, the tumor is composed of tubular and slitlike spaces lined by a single layer of flattened cuboidal cells with bland cytology. The cells are immunopositive for cytokeratin, calretinin, and vimentin expression, but are immunonegative for factor VIII–related antigen and CD31 expression, a profile that can be used to distinguish the tumor from metastatic carcinoma and vascular tumors. Adenomatoid tumor is clinically asymptomatic and usually found incidentally.

XII. OTHER MISCELLANEOUS NEOPLASMS

A. Lymphoid neoplasms involving the uterine corpus (of which the most frequent is large B-cell lymphoma) most commonly represent a manifestation of disseminated disease. Primary disease of the uterus is extremely rare.

B. Metastatic tumors only rarely involve the uterus. The most common primary tumors that spread to the uterus are those of breast, lung, stomach, gallbladder, and thyroid, and melanoma. In most instances, uterine involvement by primary tumors of the ovary, cervix, bladder, and rectum/colon represents direct extension rather than hematogenous spread.

Suggested Readings

Manzur MT, Kurman RJ. *Diagnosis of Endometrial Biopsies and Curettings. A Practical Approach.* 2nd ed. New York, New York: Springer; 2005.

Tavassoli FA, Devilee P, eds. *Tumours of the Breast and Female Genital Organs.* 1st ed. Lyon, France: International Agency for Research on Cancer; 2003.

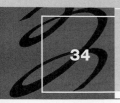

UTERINE CERVIX

34

Michael E. Hull, John D. Pfeifer, and Phyllis C. Huettner

I. NORMAL GROSS AND MICROSCOPIC ANATOMY

A. Gross. The cervix is the tubular distal portion of the uterus, divided into the ectocervix and endocervix. The smooth tan-white ectocervix is covered by a reflection of the vaginal mucosa, and the anterior and posterior fornices are formed by the protrusion of the cervix into the vaginal vault. The tan, rugous endocervix is a narrow canal that begins at the external os. The external os is round and small in the nulliparous state and becomes slitlike with parity. An internal os, or isthmus, marks the transition from the endocervix to the endometrium. The parametrial soft tissue, which attaches to the lateral aspects of the cervix, contains the uterine vessels and the ureters. The posterior cervix is the anterior border of the pouch of Douglas, the space between the uterus and the rectum; the anterior cervix is immediately posterior and inferior to the bladder.

B. Microscopic. The ectocervix is generally covered by squamous epithelium in continuity with the vaginal epithelium, whereas the endocervix is lined by columnar mucinous epithelium. The transition from columnar to squamous epithelium through the process of squamous metaplasia occurs over a region of the cervical epithelium called the transformation zone. In states of low estrogenization, the transition to columnar epithelium occurs approximately at the external os. With higher levels of estrogen, the transition is observed on the portion of cervix in the vaginal vault. The transformation zone is important diagnostically because it is the site of the majority of cervical epithelial neoplasms and their precursors (e-**Fig. 34.1**).*

1. Squamous epithelium. The squamous epithelium is composed of a basal layer, intermediate layer, and superficial layer. The basal layer is one cell thick and has a relatively high nuclear/cytoplasmic (N/C) ratio. The N/C ratio decreases progressively from the basal layer to the superficial layer during normal maturation, and the superficial squamous cells tend to align with their longest axis parallel to the basement membrane. Directly sampled normal squamous epithelium in cytologic preparations shows individual and clustered superficial polygonal squamous cells with pyknotic nuclei, intermediate cells with somewhat larger nuclei, and more rounded parabasal cells with the highest N/C ratio. In the estrogenized state, superficial cells predominate.

2. Columnar epithelium. The mucinous columnar epithelium of the endocervix is one cell layer thick, with basal polarization of the cells' nuclei, little, if any, mitotic activity, and an N/C ratio of about 1:4. Mucinous columnar epithelium also lines the endocervical glands, which represent infoldings of the surface epithelium rather than true glands. Directly sampled endocervical columnar epithelium is seen in cytologic preparations either as sheets of uniform round nuclei in a "honeycomb" arrangement or as single-layered strips of epithelium with basally oriented nuclei, depending on the plane of section. If the cells are exfoliated, they appear in smears as singly dispersed, rounded cells with central nuclei.

3. Squamous metaplastic epithelium. This is an expected finding in the transformation zone of cervical specimens. Histologically, in the immature form, the squamous epithelium underlies a layer of superficial residual columnar epithelium (e-**Fig. 34.1**). Mature squamous metaplastic epithelium may appear very similar

---

*All e-figures are available online via the Solution Site Image Bank.

to native squamous epithelium. Metaplastic squamous cells in cytologic smears are present either dispersed singly or in small sheets; they show cyanophilic cytoplasm with a nuclear size and N/C ratio between those of normal intermediate and basal cells.

II. GROSS EXAMINATION, TISSUE SAMPLING, AND HISTOLOGIC SLIDE PREPARATION. Diagnostic cervical cytologic and tissue specimens are obtained in several ways.

A. Biopsy. Colposcopic cervical biopsy specimens are small pieces of mucosa and superficial stroma that are taken, most often, from acetowhite areas identified visually. Documentation of the number and size of tissue fragments is important to ensure that the biopsies are adequately represented on the slides. If a tissue fragment exceeds 4 mm in diameter, it should be bisected prior to histologic processing. The tissue should be wrapped in lens paper or placed between sponges to avoid loss during processing, and the biopsies should be embedded such that the microscopic sections are perpendicular to the mucosal surface. Three hematoxylin and eosin (H&E)-stained levels are prepared for microscopic examination.

B. Curettage. Curettage specimens consist of numerous and often miniscule tissue fragments in mucus, so it is imperative to filter the contents of the container and to collect any tissue that may be adherent to the pad or paper that is within the specimen container. It is necessary to wrap curettings in lens paper to avoid loss in processing. Materials from curettage procedures should be submitted in their entirety. Three H&E-stained levels are prepared for microscopic examination.

C. Conization. Ideal cold knife cone biopsy specimens consist of a single tube of ectocervix and cervical canal surrounded by stroma. Marking sutures attached by the surgeon enable the sections to be designated using the hours of the clock; by convention, the midanterior location is the 12 o'clock position. The endocervical margin must be identified and inked differentially from the ectocervical and stromal margins. After fixation, the specimen should be radially sectioned, with each section encompassing the endocervical margin, the mucosal surface of the endocervical canal with the transformation zone, and ectocervical margin, as shown in Figure 34.1.

D. Loop electrosurgical excision procedure (LEEP). The key to the correct processing of these specimens is identification of the endocervical margin (which may be inked by the surgeon to facilitate identification); the ectocervix is smooth and gray-white, whereas the endocervix is tan and more rugated. The endocervical margin should be differentially inked from the ectocervical and stromal margins. Radial sections should be taken perpendicular to the mucosa, encompassing the endocervical margin, transformation zone, and ectocervical margin in the same manner as for conization specimens.

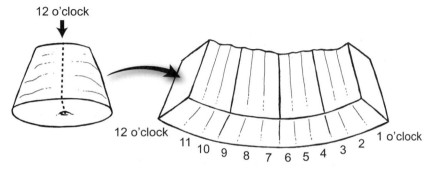

Figure 34.1. Gross processing of conization specimens. After the endocervical and stromal margins are inked, the specimen is radially sectioned so that each tissue slice includes the endocervical margin, the mucosal surface of the endocervical canal, and the ectocervix.

E. Radical hysterectomy

1. **Uterus.** Prior to opening, the parametrial soft tissue is inked as this represents soft tissue margins of interest. The vaginal margin is also inked. The uterus is then bivalved (as in Fig. 33.1). If no tumor is visible or the tumor does not appear to extend into the parametrial soft tissue, the parametrial soft tissue is removed, sectioned, and completely submitted. If the vagina appears free of tumor, shave margins are submitted. If tumor appears to extend into the parametrial soft tissue or vagina, radial sections of that area from tumor to margin are submitted. If a cervical mass is present, at least one section per centimeter of tumor, including the deepest extension into the cervical wall, is submitted. If no tumor is visible, the cervix is amputated and processed as a conization specimen.

2. **Lymph nodes.** Separate packets of pelvic and para-aortic lymph nodes are typically submitted with radical hysterectomy specimens. The lymph nodes should be separated from the soft tissue and entirely submitted.

III. DIAGNOSTIC FEATURES OF COMMON NON-NEOPLASTIC DISEASES

A. Inflammation and infection. Acute cervicitis is a pattern of inflammation marked by a stromal and epithelial neutrophilic infiltrate, with associated stromal edema, and, often, reactive epithelial atypia. Reactive epithelium shows enlarged nuclei and prominent nucleoli in a pattern that may be confused with neoplasia. Acute cervicitis is usually a nonspecific diagnosis, as the inciting agent can be any of a wide variety of bacterial, fungal, or protozoan organisms. Chronic cervicitis consists of a lymphoplasmacytic infiltrate that is also nonspecific. Inflamed endocervical mucosa may form papillary structures and is referred to as papillary endocervicitis.

1. **Noninfectious cervicitis.** Cervicitis can be due to irritation from chemical exposure, foreign materials (e.g., pessary, tampons), or surgical trauma. The cervix may also be a site of involvement in systemic inflammatory conditions such as collagen vascular disease. The type of inflammatory response may be neutrophilic, lymphoplasmacytic, or granulomatous.

2. **Infectious cervicitis**

   a. **Bacterial cervicitis.** *Neisseria gonorrhea* and *Chlamydia trachomatis* both produce mucopurulent cervicitis that requires additional nonhistologic methods for specific diagnosis. With chronicity, *C. trachomatis* infection can result in follicular cervicitis, a pattern of intense lymphocytic infiltration that characteristically includes lymphoid aggregates with germinal centers (e-**Fig. 34.2**). Although often associated with *C. trachomatis* infection, follicular cervicitis is not specific for this disease.

   Actinomyces spp. infection is associated with intrauterine device (IUD) use and is often asymptomatic. The pattern of inflammation is distinctive in that clusters of the purple-red filamentous organism are seen on smears, with associated "sulfur granules" consisting of clusters of neutrophils with a basophilic center.

   Bacterial vaginosis is characterized by "clue cells," which are squamous cells coated with bacterial organisms. *Gardnerella vaginalis* and *Mobiluncus* spp. are both implicated in the disease.

   b. **Viral cervicitis.** Herpes simplex virus (HSV; primarily HSV type 2) infection is characterized by ulceration with enlarged epithelial nuclei, nuclear molding, multinucleation, and margination of the chromatin in virally infected cells at the edge of the ulcer. Cytomegalovirus is distinctive for its nuclear and cytoplasmic inclusions. Adenovirus is notable for its smudged nuclear inclusions. The poxvirus *Molluscum contagiosum* generates large, round, intensely eosinophilic cytoplasmic inclusions, as it does in its cutaneous sites. Human papillomavirus (HPV) infection is closely tied to cervical neoplasia; its features are discussed in the sections below on preinvasive and invasive squamous neoplasia and in the section on cervical cytology.

   c. **Granulomatous cervicitis.** Infectious causes of granulomatous cervicitis include *Mycobacterium tuberculosis* and *Treponema pallidum* infections. As noted above, the differential diagnosis of non-necrotizing granulomas includes noninfectious etiologies.

d. Fungal. *Candida* spp. are commonly encountered in smears and are not necessarily always pathogenic. They cannot be speciated reliably on their morphology in either tissue sections or cervical smears.

e. Parasitic. *Trichomonas vaginalis* is one of the most common sexually transmitted infections of women. Many infections are asymptomatic. In Papanicolaou-stained smears or liquid-based preparations, an ovoid organism with an eccentric nucleus is observed; in liquid-based preparations, squamous cells may be coated with the organism.

B. Atrophy. Epithelial atrophy is seen in the postmenopausal state when estrogen levels are decreased. As noted above in the discussion of normal histology and cytology, high estrogen states are associated with large numbers of superficial squamous cells; however, when the epithelium is thinned, the histologic picture is dominated by small cells with an increased N/C ratio and nuclei at least as large or larger than those of normal intermediate cells. The overall epithelial architecture and lack of nuclear atypia distinguish epithelial atrophy from high-grade squamous intraepithelial lesions (HSIL).

C. Metaplasia. Tubal metaplasia occurs most frequently in the upper endocervix. Transitional cell metaplasia is rare and recapitulates urothelium; it is not associated with a specific insult and must not be confused with neoplasia. Intestinal metaplasia is another uncommon metaplasia; it features columnar epithelium with goblet and Paneth cells.

D. Hyperplasia

1. **Squamous hyperplasia** consists of thickening of the epithelium with normal maturation. It occurs in situations of prolapse and chronic irritation.

2. **Squamous papilloma** is a benign squamous proliferation that covers fibrovascular cores. Squamous papilloma may be associated with HPV infection but it does not show classic koilocytic atypia.

3. **Microglandular hyperplasia** is an increase in glandular elements in the cervical stroma. Seen in histologic sections, the exuberant proliferation sometimes has cribriform architecture that can raise the question of neoplasia. However, microglandular hyperplasia shows no cytologic atypia, does not infiltrate the stroma, and is not associated with a desmoplastic reaction.

4. **Lobular endocervical glandular hyperplasia** is a benign proliferation of bland glands surrounding a central dilated gland forming a well-circumscribed lobule.

E. Nabothian cysts are pronounced dilatations of endocervical glands. They are extremely common.

F. Endocervical tunnel clusters are superficial collections of endocervical gland ductal spaces.

G. Mesonephric remnants are developmental remnants of the mesonephric (Wolffian) duct that are occasionally identified in the deep stroma. Mesonephric remnants must not be confused with adenocarcinoma; helpful distinguishing features include the bland cytology of the lining epithelium, a lack of atypia in the overlying endocervical glands, and the absence of a desmoplastic stromal response.

H. Postoperative spindle cell nodule is a benign proliferation of fibroblasts that usually occurs following surgical manipulation.

I. Endocervical polyps are often identified colposcopically. They consist of an exophytic configuration of benign glands and stroma usually with thick-walled vessels. They must be carefully examined microscopically to exclude coexisting squamous dysplasia or a glandular neoplasm.

J. Inclusion cysts are benign. Microscopically, they are filled with keratinizing debris and are related to surgical manipulation. Similar inclusions occur in the vagina following episiotomies.

K. Endometriosis can involve any layer of the cervical stroma, as well as the parametrial/paracervical soft tissue.

L. Decidual change occurs in the cervical stroma during pregnancy. The nests of cells that show abundant amphophilic cytoplasm, a prominent cell border, and a single, centrally placed nucleus are usually not visible grossly, but sometimes form polyps (e-Fig. 34.3).

M. The Arias–Stella reaction, characterized by epithelial cells with nuclear enlargement and clear cytoplasm in response to progesterone, is most commonly seen in the uterine corpus in pregnancy, but may also occur in the cervix. The significance of the Arias–Stella reaction lies in the fact that it can easily be confused with a glandular neoplasm.

IV. CERVICAL NEOPLASIA. The World Health Organization (WHO) classification of cervical tumors is shown in Table 34.1.

A. Benign

1. **Submucosal and stromal neoplasms.** Leiomyomas identical to those of the uterine corpus are also seen in the cervix.

2. **Blue nevus.** This benign melanocytic proliferation is common, noted clinically as a bluish discoloration of the cervical epithelium. Microscopic examination shows hyperpigmented spindle cells infiltrating the stroma in a haphazard pattern.

B. Malignant and premalignant squamous lesions. Worldwide, cervical cancer is the third most common malignancy and the fifth most common cause of cancer mortality in women. Effective screening programs have dramatically reduced deaths due to cervical cancer in the developed world, but such gains have not been seen elsewhere.

The major risk factor for cervical cancer is sexually transmitted HPV infection. Although there are >40 different HPV serotypes that infect the female genital tract, high-risk serotypes (including 16, 18, 31, 35, 39, 45, 51, 52, 56, and 58) are associated with a markedly increased risk of high-grade squamous dysplasia and subsequent cervical squamous cell carcinoma. Immunodeficiency may increase the likelihood of persistent infection and may increase the risk of subsequent epithelial malignant transformation. Host factors such as smoking, concomitant sexually transmitted diseases, high parity, and oral contraceptive use may also increase the risk of malignant transformation among already infected women. For example, among women with HPV infection, smoking doubles to quadruples the odds in favor of malignant transformation (*Cancer Causes Control.* 2003;14:805 and *J Natl Cancer Inst.* 2002;94:1406).

1. **HPV infection.** The viral cytopathic effect that results from HPV infection is termed koilocytosis and consists of nuclear enlargement with irregular nuclear borders, condensed chromatin, occasional binucleation or multinucleation, and a perinuclear halo. Flat lesions that exhibit koilocytosis are usually associated with low-risk HPV types 6 and 11. High risk HPV types such as HPV 16 and 18 encode proteins that have the capacity to immortalize keratinocytes by enhancing the ubiquitin-mediated degradation of the tumor suppressors TP53 and pRb. Malignant transformation is not a committed endpoint of HPV infection, but its likelihood may be enhanced by environmental and host factors as discussed above.

2. **Cervical intraepithelial neoplasia-1 (CIN1)** is defined by disordered maturation and cytologic abnormalities of the lower one third of the squamous epithelium, often with koilocytic changes in the upper two thirds of the epithelium (**e-Fig. 34.4**). Most cases of CIN1 regress; those that progress rarely lead to invasive cancer (*Int J Gynecol Pathol.* 1993;12:186).

3. **Cervical intraepithelial neoplasia-2 and -3 (CIN2 and CIN3)** are defined by cytologic abnormalities of the lower two thirds and full thickness of the epithelium, respectively (**e-Fig. 34.5**). CIN2 and CIN3 are often combined into the diagnostic category of high-grade dysplasia because of considerable interobserver variability between the categories, and because the treatment is identical for both. Spontaneous regression occurs at lower rates than in CIN1, ranging from 33% for CIN3 to 40% for CIN2. A more aggressive approach to the management of these lesions is warranted, because progression to invasive carcinoma occurs in a higher percentage of these lesions (*Int J Gynecol Pathol.* 1993;12:186).

4. **Invasive squamous cell carcinoma** is recognized by penetration of the epithelial basement membrane by neoplastic squamous cells with an associated desmoplastic stromal response (**e-Fig. 34.6**). Keratinizing and nonkeratinizing types are encountered. In contrast to the atypical cells characteristic of

TABLE 34.1	WHO Histological Classification of Tumors of the Uterine Cervix

Epithelial Tumors
Squamous tumors and precursors
  Squamous cell carcinoma, not otherwise specified
    Keratinizing
    Nonkeratinizing
    Basaloid
    Verrucous
    Warty
    Papillary
    Lymphoepitheliomalike
    Squamotransitional
  Early invasive (microinvasive) squamous cell carcinoma
  Squamous intraepithelial neoplasia
    Cervical intraepithelial neoplasia-3 (CIN3) squamous cell carcinoma in situ
  Benign squamous cell lesions
    Condyloma acuminatum
    Squamous papilloma
    Fibroepithelial polyp
Glandular tumors and precursors
  Adenocarcinoma
    Mucinous adenocarcinoma
      Endocervical
      Intestinal
      Signet-ring cell
      Minimal deviation
      Villoglandular
    Endometrioid adenocarcinoma
    Clear cell adenocarcinoma
    Serous adenocarcinoma
    Mesonephric adenocarcinoma
  Early invasive adenocarcinoma
  Adenocarcinoma in situ
  Glandular dysplasia
  Benign glandular lesions
    Müllerian papilloma
    Endocervical polyp
Other epithelial tumors
  Adenosquamous carcinoma
    Glassy cell carcinoma variant
  Adenoid cystic carcinoma
  Adenoid basal carcinoma
  Neuroendocrine tumors
    Carcinoid
    Atypical carcinoid
    Small cell carcinoma
    Large cell neuroendocrine carcinoma
  Undifferentiated carcinoma

Mesenchymal Tumors and Tumorlike Conditions
Leiomyosarcoma
Endometrioid stromal sarcoma, low grade
Undifferentiated endocervical sarcoma
Sarcoma botryoides

(Continued)

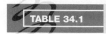

TABLE 34.1	WHO Histological Classification of Tumors of the Uterine Cervix (*Continued*)

Alveolar soft part sarcoma
Angiosarcoma
  Malignant peripheral nerve sheath tumor
  Leiomyoma
  Genital rhabdomyoma
  Postoperative spindle cell nodule

Mixed Epithelial and Mesenchymal Tumors
  Carcinosarcoma (malignant mixed Müllerian tumor)
  Adenosarcoma
  Wilms tumor
  Adenofibroma
  Adenomyoma

Melanocytic Tumors
  Malignant melanoma
  Blue nevus

Miscellaneous Tumors
Tumors of germ cell type
  Yolk sac tumor
  Dermoid cyst
  Mature cystic teratoma

Lymphoid and Hematopoetic Tumors
  Malignant lymphoma (specify type)
  Leukemia (specify type)

Secondary Tumors

From: Tavassoli FA, Devilee P, eds. *World Health Organization Classification of Tumours. Pathology and Genetics. Tumours of the Breast and Female Genital Organs.* Lyon: IARC Press; 2001. Used with permission.

high-grade squamous dysplasia in which the N/C ratio is markedly increased, the invasive tumor cells often exhibit paradoxical maturation characterized by abundant, eosinophilic cytoplasm.

  a. Microinvasive squamous cell carcinoma is defined as a tumor that is not recognized as such clinically, that invades ≤3 mm from the basement membrane of the adjacent surface epithelium or endocervical gland from which it arises, and that extends ≤7 mm in greatest lateral extent. When no lymphatic or vascular involvement is present, when the entire lesion is excised, and when no dysplasia is present at the margins of excision, the potential for lymph node metastasis or recurrence is very low. Long-term follow-up studies have shown that the portion of patients harboring residual invasive carcinoma in a hysterectomy specimen after conization for microinvasive squamous cell carcinoma with maximum invasion of ≤1 mm is 0%; when invasion is ≤3 mm, the recurrence and lymph node metastasis rates are <1%. For lesions between 3 and 5 mm in depth, the recurrence rate increases to 2% and the lymph node metastasis rate increases to 4% (*Pathol Ann.* 1995;30:103).

  b. Squamous cell carcinoma variants

    i. Keratinizing tumors contain keratin pearls and nests of tumor cells with central keratin; cytoplasmic keratinization and keratohyaline granules are also present. Intercellular bridges can be identified.

    ii. Nonkeratinizing tumors show cytoplasmic keratinization of individual cells and intercellular bridges, but keratin pearls and nests of tumor cells with central keratin are not present.

    iii. Basaloid carcinoma features cells with scanty cytoplasm that resemble basal type squamous cells. Only rare nests of tumor cells show central keratin. This variant has an aggressive behavior.

    iv. Verrucous carcinoma is a very well-differentiated squamous cell carcinoma that betrays its malignant character only in its invasion of the stroma along broad pushing borders. There is minimal cytologic atypia, and viral cytopathic effect is absent. Aggressive local invasion and recurrence after excision are common. Metastasis is uncommon.

    v. Warty carcinoma is a rare squamous malignancy that shows definitive stromal invasion but also abundant cytologic features of HPV infection. It may behave less aggressively than other well-differentiated squamous cell carcinomas.

    vi. Papillary squamous cell carcinoma is an exophytic tumor in which epithelium resembling CIN2 or CIN3 covers fibrovascular cores. Koilocytosis is not characteristic. Although much of the tumor may have the appearance of a precursor lesion, definitive stromal invasion is present in the deep aspects of the lesion. Therefore, superficial biopsies of papillary lesions should be interpreted with caution.

    vii. Lymphoepithelial-like carcinoma resembles the nasopharyngeal tumor of the same name. The tumor consists of syncytial sheets and islands of undifferentiated epithelioid cells that have eosinophilic cytoplasm and large vesicular nuclei with prominent nucleoli in a background that contains an intense lymphocytic infiltrate.

C. Glandular neoplasms

    1. Adenocarcinoma in situ (AIS) is an HPV-associated glandular lesion (most strongly associated with HPV serotypes 16 and 18) that is a precursor to invasive adenocarcinoma. Cytologically, AIS is characterized by loss of cytoplasmic mucin, cellular stratification, cellular crowding, nuclear enlargement and atypia, mitotic activity, and epithelial apoptotic debris. The various subtypes can mimic endocervical, endometrial, or intestinal epithelium, and can have a papillary or cribriform architectural pattern. AIS is often seen in conjunction with CIN.

        In contrast to in situ squamous epithelial lesions, AIS of the cervix is less common than its invasive counterpart. Because of this, follow-up studies are sparse. However, a number of series do show that a positive margin for AIS in a cone biopsy predicts the presence of either an invasive adenocarcinoma or the recurrence of AIS (*Gynecol Oncol.* 2000;79:207), therefore, AIS requires complete excision.

    2. Microinvasive adenocarcinoma. The existence and treatment of microinvasive adenocarcinoma remains controversial. Microscopically, it can be extremely challenging to identify this class of lesions because the glandular irregularities and stromal response indicative of invasion may be quite subtle. Although lymph node involvement is identified in 5–9% of patients with microinvasive carcinoma, lymph node metastases virtually never occurs when the definition is narrowed to lesions of depth ≤ 2 mm (*Obstet Gynecol.* 1985;65:46; *Obstet Gynecol.* 1997;89:88; *Int J Gynecol Pathol.* 2000;19:29).

    3. Invasive adenocarcinoma. Infiltrating glands with cribriform and papillary structures are the architectural characteristics of invasive adenocarcinoma. A desmoplastic stromal reaction, a feature that helps to distinguish adenocarcinoma from both AIS and the hyperplastic entities described above, is present.

    a. Mucinous adenocarcinoma. Most primary mucinous adenocarcinomas have cytologic features resembling endocervical glands (e-Fig. 34.7). The cells are cuboidal to columnar and show nuclear pleomorphism, nuclear atypia, and many mitoses. The relatively abundant cytoplasm stains positively for mucin. Mucinous adenocarcinomas with goblet cells that have an overall morphology more similar to intestinal epithelium are termed intestinal variants.

    b. Minimal deviation adenocarcinoma (adenoma malignum). This rare entity comprises only 1% of primary adenocarcinomas of the cervix. The glandular epithelium is so bland in appearance that these lesions may not be recognized as malignant on biopsy or curettage specimens; increased mitotic activity and cytologic atypia may be present focally, but these findings are not prominent. The diagnosis rests on the presence of deep infiltration, aggregation of glands around vessels or nerves, and a stromal reaction—features that are easiest to assess on cone biopsy or hysterectomy. Because of the difficulty in making this diagnosis, patients present at advanced stage and have a worse prognosis than do patients with other forms of adenocarcinoma. The incidence of this lesion is increased in Peutz–Jeghers syndrome.

   c. Endometrioid adenocarcinoma. Comprising 30% of cervical adenocarcinomas, endometrioid adenocarcinoma of the cervix is identical in appearance to its counterpart in the endometrium. When well differentiated, the lesion shows tall columnar cells without mucin. It may be very difficult to distinguish a cervical primary lesion from direct extension into the cervix from a lesion tumor originating in the uterine corpus.

   d. Well-differentiated villoglandular adenocarcinoma is considered to be a subtype of endometrioid adenocarcinoma. It shows an exophytic growth pattern with glandular and villous elements, little nuclear pleomorphism, and a low mitotic rate, quite similar to an intestinal villous adenoma. There is value in the distinction, as this is a tumor of young women and has a favorable prognosis (*Gynecol Oncol.* 1997;64:147).

   e. Clear cell adenocarcinoma. This tumor's association with in utero diethylstilbestrol (DES) exposure has made it widely recognized. Although rare, the tumor can occur as well in patients without a history of DES exposure. Clear cells with hobnail morphology are observed in solid, papillary, and tubular arrangements. The presence of this tumor in the cervix should prompt a search for a primary tumor of the ovary, endometrium, or vagina—sites where this entity is much more common.

   f. Serous adenocarcinoma is another adenocarcinoma that only rarely occurs as a cervical primary tumor; it is more common as a primary lesion of the ovaries, endometrium, or peritoneum. The tumor's morphology is identical to that of serous adenocarcinomas that occur at other sites in the female reproductive tract.

   g. Mesonephric adenocarcinoma. This lesion differs from the mesonephric remnants from which it arises in its cytologic atypia, crowding, and increased mitotic activity. A variety of architectural patterns are characteristic, including tubular, papillary, solid, and retiform. Knowledge of the immunophenotypic profile may assist in the separation of this tumor from other adenocarcinomas, especially endometrioid adenocarcinoma. CD10 expression is seen in both benign mesonephric remnants and in mesonephric adenocarcinoma, as is immunoreactivity for cytokeratin 7 (CK7); however, mesonephric adenocarcinoma does not express CK20, estrogen or progesterone receptors, or monoclonal carcinoembryogenic antigen (CEA).

D. Other carcinomas

   1. Adenosquamous carcinoma. Both squamous and glandular differentiation are observed in this lesion; the presence of cytoplasmic mucin alone is not sufficient for diagnosis. The epidemiologic profile is similar to that of squamous cell carcinoma and adenocarcinoma.

   2. Glassy cell carcinoma is considered a subtype of adenosquamous carcinoma (see above) that occurs in young women. It carries a poor prognosis because it is unresponsive to radiotherapy; progression is rapid, and distant metastases are common. Microscopically, the tumor consists of sheets of pleomorphic cells with granular eosinophilic cytoplasm, nucleoli, and brisk mitotic activity. The tumor is usually infiltrated by eosinophils and plasma cells. An in situ precursor lesion is not typically found in association with this tumor.

   3. Adenoid cystic carcinoma is a rare cervical tumor found mostly in postmenopausal African-American women who present with abnormal bleeding and a pelvic mass. This tumor shows cystic spaces filled with eosinophilic hyaline material or basophilic mucin surrounded by palisades of epithelial cells. The tumor architecture may be tubular, cribriform, or solid. Adenoid cystic carcinoma of the cervix typically shows more cytologic atypia than is present in its salivary gland counterpart, but displays the same tendency for perineural invasion and local aggressiveness.

4. **Adenoid basal carcinoma.** This tumor occurs in a population similar to that of adenoid cystic carcinoma. It also shows a nested cribriform architecture. The epithelium, however, is composed of more uniform, round to oval, basophilic cells often with central squamous differentiation, without significant atypia or increased mitotic activity. There is often an associated CIN. Correct identification of this lesion is important because it is low grade and does not have aggressive behavior; in fact, the tumor's bland behavior has led some investigators to suggest that the tumor is more appropriately termed adenoid basal epithelioma (*Am J Surg Pathol.* 1998;22:965).

E. **Neuroendocrine neoplasms.** A variety of neuroendocrine neoplasms may occur in the cervix, although rarely. The classification of these tumors is identical to that of neuroendocrine tumors of the lung.

1. **Carcinoid.** These benign tumors are organoid in their architecture and are composed of small, oval to spindled cells with granular cytoplasm. Mitoses are rare in typical carcinoid tumors. Immunoreactivity with neuroendocrine markers synaptophysin, chromogranin A, and neuron-specific enolase is the rule.

2. **Atypical carcinoid.** Moderate cytologic atypia and mitotic counts of 5 to 10 mitotic figures/10 high-power fields are sufficient to classify a carcinoid as atypical; at least small foci of necrosis are often present (*Arch Pathol Lab Med.* 1997;121:34). These tumors generally retain the organoid architecture of typical carcinoids. Their biologic behavior is difficult to assess systematically due to the subjectivity involved in separating atypical carcinoids from typical carcinoids and large cell neuroendocrine carcinomas (see below).

3. **Large cell neuroendocrine carcinoma.** These tumors show frequent vascular invasion, have higher mitotic activity than atypical carcinoids (>10 mitotic figures/10 high-power fields), and show loss of the organoid architecture seen in less aggressive neuroendocrine tumors. There may be focal adenocarcinomalike areas with abundant cytoplasm and large nucleoli. Necrosis is frequent. The prognosis is poor, similar to that of small cell carcinoma.

4. **Small cell carcinoma.** Identical to its counterpart in the lung, small cell carcinoma (also known as high-grade neuroendocrine carcinoma) is a tumor of variably sized, round to oval to spindled cells with scanty cytoplasm, high mitotic activity, nuclear molding, and frequent crush artifact (**e-Fig. 34.8**). Necrosis may be extensive. Clinical series are small due to the rarity of the tumor, but the prognosis is uniformly poor.

F. **Mesenchymal neoplasms.** A wide variety of sarcomas may be primary to the cervix, including leiomyosarcoma, embryonal rhabdomyosarcoma, endometrioid stromal sarcoma, and alveolar soft part sarcoma.

G. **Mixed epithelial and mesenchymal neoplasms**

1. **Adenosarcomas** are polypoid lesions that microscopically consist of large papillae of malignant stroma covered with benign endocervical epithelium. The stroma can have many different appearances; it can consist of plump, mitotically active spindle cells or more undifferentiated round cells similar to those of small cell carcinoma. Heterologous sarcomatous elements may be present showing skeletal muscle, cartilage, adipose, or bone differentiation. Prognosis after excision is apparently good, although only small numbers of cases have been reported.

2. **Malignant mixed Müllerian tumor (MMMT),** also known as carcinosarcoma, also presents as a polypoid mass. In contrast to its more common counterpart in the uterine corpus, the malignant epithelial component is more often squamous or basaloid as opposed to glandular. The sarcomatous component is usually homologous, with a spindle-cell morphology similar to that of fibrosarcoma. In limited series of MMMT of the cervix, it appears that the prognosis is better than that of MMMT of the uterine corpus.

TABLE 34.2 Tumor, Node, Metastasis (TNM) Staging Scheme and International Federation of Gynecology and Obstetrics (FIGO) Classification of Carcinomas of the Uterine Cervix

TNM Classification
PRIMARY TUMOR (T)

TNM Categories	FIGO Stages	
TX		Primary tumor cannot be assessed
T0		No evidence of primary tumor
Tis	0	Carcinoma in situ (preinvasive carcinoma)
T1	I	Cervical carcinoma confined to uterus (extension to corpus should be disregarded)
T1a	IA1	Invasive carcinoma diagnosed only by microscopy All macroscopically visible lesions—even with superficial invasion—are T1b/Stage 1B
T1a1	IA1	Stromal invasion no greater than 3.0 mm in depth and ≤7.0 mm in horizontal spread
T1a2	IA2	Stromal invasion >3.0 mm and not >5.0 mm with a horizontal spread ≤7.0 mm
T1b	IB	Clinically visible lesion confined to the cervix or microscopic lesion greater than T1a2/1A2
T1b1	IB1	Clinically visible lesion ≤4.0 cm in greatest dimension
T1b2	IB2	Clinically visible lesion >4 cm in greatest dimension
T2	II	Tumor invades beyond uterus but not to pelvic wall or to lower third of the vagina
T2a	IIA	Without parametrial invasion
T2b	IIB	With parametrial invasion
T3	III	Tumor extends to pelvic wall, involves lower third of vagina, or causes hydronephrosis or nonfunctioning kidney
T3a	IIIA	Tumor involves lower third of vagina, no extension to pelvic wall
T3b	IIIB	Tumor extends to pelvic wall or causes hydronephrosis or nonfunctioning kidney
T4	IVA	Tumor invades mucosa of bladder or rectum or extends beyond true pelvis
M1	IVB	Distant metastasis

REGIONAL LYMPH NODES (N)

NX	Regional lymph nodes cannot be assessed
N0	No regional lymph node metastasis
N1	Regional lymph node metastasis

DISTANT METASTASIS (M)

MX	Distant metastasis cannot be assessed
M0	No distant metastasis
M1	Distant metastasis

STAGE GROUPING

Stage 0	Tis	N0	M0
Stage IA	T1a	N0	M0
Stage IA1	T1a1	N0	M0
Stage IA2	T1a2	N0	M0
Stage IB	T1b	N0	M0
Stage IB1	T1b1	N0	M0
Stage IB2	T1b2	N0	M0
Stage IIA	T2a	N0	M0
Stage IIB	T2b	N0	M0
Stage IIIA	T3a	N0	M0
Stage IIIB	T1, T2, T3a	N1	M0
	T3b	Any N	M0
Stage IVA	T4	Any N	M0
Stage IVB	Any T	Any N	M1

From: Greene FL, Page DL, Fleming ID, Fritz AG, Balch CM, Haller DG, Morrow M, eds. *AJCC Cancer Staging Manual.* 6th edition. New York: Springer; 2002. Used with permission. (A new AJCC TNM staging system is scheduled for release in 2009; after its publication, the new staging scheme will appear on the website for this book.)

H. Hematolymphoid neoplasms. Lymphoma of the cervix is usually a part of systemic disease.

I. Melanoma. Primary melanoma of the cervix is rare, and its description is confined to case reports (*Gynecol Oncol.* 1999;75:170). Vaginal bleeding due to a cervical mass is a common presentation. The tumor is usually low stage at presentation, but the prognosis is dismal. Morphologically, the tumor is similar to melanomas of other sites, although cervical melanomas have been noted for a tendency toward a spindle-cell morphology. Melanin pigment is variable from tumor to tumor. It is important to identify a junctional component in a tumor if it is to be classified as primary to the cervix; otherwise, a thorough search for another primary site is warranted.

J. Secondary malignancies. Most metastases to the cervix arise from tumors at other sites in the female reproductive tract. Similarly, because most female genital tract carcinomas, sarcomas, and germ cell tumors may have a primary site in the cervix, there must be a careful examination of all components of a hysterectomy specimen performed for a presumed cervical malignancy. Correlation with radiographic studies and clinical history is also important for clarifying a tumor's primary site.

V. PATHOLOGIC AND CLINICAL STAGING OF MALIGNANCIES. The clinical stage of cervical neoplasms is the basis for treatment decisions in gynecological oncology, and data on the effectiveness of the various treatment modalities accrued over decades are based on this standard of practice. The pathologic stage may be more advanced than the clinical stage in an individual case, yet the clinical stage drives the therapy.

A. American Joint Committee on Cancer (AJCC) and International Federation of Gynecology and Obstetrics (FIGO) criteria. The AJCC criteria for the staging of cervical cancer with the corresponding FIGO clinical staging categories are outlined in Table 34.2.

B. Additional information. The final report in any case of malignancy should explicitly include all of the information required for assigning a stage, as well as other information of clinical interest not required for staging. For the cervix, the pathology report should include the histologic type and grade of the malignancy; the presence or absence of precursor lesions (either CIN or AIS); tumor size, including depth and width; whether the malignancy is unifocal or multifocal; presence or absence of lymphovascular space invasion; presence or absence of vaginal, paracervical/parametrial, or uterine extension; margin status; and presence or absence of lymph node or distant metastases.

CYTOLOGY OF THE UTERINE CERVIX
Rosa M. Dávila

I. SPECIMEN TYPES

A. Conventional smears are made by using a spatula and/or brush to sample the cervix, smearing the endo- and ectocervical samples on a glass slide, and then immediately fixing the sample (usually with a spray fixative). The slides are usually not stained until they arrive in the cytology laboratory; the Papanicolaou stain is the most widely used stain.

B. Liquid-based preparations are made by using a brush to sample the cervix and then rinsing the brush in transport fluid; the resulting slides are stained with Papanicolaou stain. Two systems are commercially available for processing liquid-based cervical samples: SurePath (TriPath Imaging, Inc., Burlington, NC) and ThinPrep (Cytyc Corporation, Boxborough, MA). Some advantages of liquid-based preparations include the presence of a clean background, a monolayer of cells, increased sensitivity for preneoplastic lesions, and ability to perform HPV testing on the unused sample.

II. ANCILLARY TESTING

A. HPV testing has been recommended for patients with atypical squamous cells of undetermined significance (ASCUS) by cervical cytology (*Arch Pathol Lab Med.* 2003;127:950). The testing is usually performed on liquid-based cytology preparations. Three HPV testing methods are currently available: the Digene Hybrid Capture 2 assay (Digene Corporation, Gaithersburg, MD), the Ventana Inform HPV assay

(Ventana Medical Systems, Inc., Tucson, AZ), and polymerase chain reaction–based assays (*Arch Pathol Lab Med.* 2003;127:984).

B. Automated screening of cervical cytology specimens can be performed. When compared with manual screening, its performance is similar for detecting HSIL (*Int J Cancer.* 2005;115:307). Laboratories choose between methods according to their needs, demands, and cost.

III. THE BETHESDA SYSTEM was developed in 1988, with the help of the National Cancer Institute, with the objective of standardizing and optimizing the terminology of cervical cytology to promote communication between the laboratory and clinicians. The 2001 Bethesda System is in current use (*The Bethesda System for Reporting Cervical Cytology*, 2nd ed. New York: Springer; 2004).

A. Adequacy. A statement of adequacy should be included in all reports of cervical cytologic samples. The absence of endocervical cells is no longer considered a reason for calling a sample inadequate. Reasons for inadequate samples include, among other things, broken slides, leaky samples, improper labeling, sparse cellularity, and obscuring factors like blood, inflammation, and air drying.

B. Negative for intraepithelial lesion or malignancy

1. Microorganisms identified in cervical samples should be reported. Various causes of vaginitis can be detected cytologically. The protozoan *T. vaginalis* is seen as a degenerated, pear-shaped structure, approximately 30 μm in diameter. It has a small nucleus and small eosinophilic cytoplasmic granules; its flagella are difficult to visualize in cytologic preparations.

Patients can suffer alterations in the normal vaginal flora resulting in bacterial vaginosis. Cervical samples from these patients can reveal abundant coccobacilli that cover some squamous cells resulting in what have been called "clue cells" (**e-Fig. 34.9**). Detection of *Actinomyces*, presenting as small colonies of filamentous bacteria, is particularly important in patients with IUDs because the presence of the bacteria is an indication for removal of the device.

Candida albicans is responsible for most cases of vulvovaginal candidiasis. Although the fungus can be a commensal microorganism, when it is accompanied by acute inflammation it is usually symptomatic (*N Engl J Med.* 2006;355:1244). The fungus can be seen as budding yeast and/or as pseudohyphae (**e-Fig. 34.10**).

Herpes genitalis is usually caused by HSV type 2. Early after infection, the squamous cells have enlarged nuclei with a ground glass appearance; formation of multinucleated cells and nuclear inclusions surrounded by a clear halo follow (**e-Fig. 34.11**).

2. Other non-neoplastic findings

a. Reactive changes of squamous cells include nuclear enlargement (up to 2 times the nuclear diameter of an intermediate cell) with or without multinucleation, with an associated smooth nuclear contour, small nucleoli, and mild nuclear hyperchromasia. Reactive cells can be arranged as a sheet and display elongated cellular and nuclear profiles (**e-Fig. 34.12**). Reactive endocervical cells may show even greater nuclear enlargement, multinucleation, mild hyperchromasia, and prominent nucleoli (**e-Fig. 34.13**).

b. The presence of normal-appearing glandular cells in samples from posthysterectomy patients should not be interpreted as an abnormal finding (*Acta Cytol.* 1997;41:1701).

C. Epithelial cell abnormality

1. Squamous cell

a. Atypical squamous cells of undetermined significance (ASCUS) have nuclear enlargement (21/2 to 3 times the nuclear diameter of a normal intermediate cell), minimal nuclear hyperchromasia, and a normal or mildly increased N/C ratio. In most laboratories, the residual liquid sample of cases diagnosed as ASCUS is processed for HPV testing.

b. Atypical squamous cells cannot exclude HSIL are approximately the size of squamous metaplastic cells, with associated nuclear enlargement resulting in an appearance resembling that of HSIL. However, they usually lack significant nuclear hyperchromasia, irregularly clumped chromatin, and abnormal nuclear contours. Patients with this diagnosis usually undergo colposcopy because approximately 30% have a high-grade epithelial lesion (*Am J Obstet Gynecol.* 2003;183:1383).

c. **Low grade squamous intraepithelial lesion (LSIL)** is diagnosed when koilocytes are present and/or when squamous cells have enlarged nuclei (>3 times the diameter of a normal intermediate cell), chromatin abnormality, and a normal N/C ratio (e-**Fig. 34.14**).

d. **High grade squamous intraepithelial lesion (HSIL)** displays cells with severe nuclear abnormalities but that are smaller than the cells typical of LSIL (e-**Fig. 34.15**). Cells of HSIL can be arranged singly or in syncytial groups. The nuclear abnormalities of HSIL include irregular contours, hyperchromasia, clumped chromatin, and pleomorphism. In cases of keratinizing dysplasia, it is often difficult to exclude an invasive carcinoma, and in this setting it is recommended to use the category "HSIL with features suspicious for invasion" (*The Bethesda System for Reporting Cervical Cytology,* 2nd ed. New York: Springer; 2004).

e. **Squamous cell carcinoma** has nuclear abnormalities that are either the same or more severe than those seen in HSIL; the tumor cells tend to exhibit a prominent nucleolus (e-**Fig. 34.16**). The cell size and the amount of cytoplasm vary according to the type of squamous cell carcinoma, e.g., keratinization is more prevalent in the keratinizing type. An inflammatory/proteinaceous background (also known as a tumor diathesis) favors the presence of invasion; this background may not be evident in liquid cytology samples.

2. **Endocervical cell**

a. **Atypical endocervical, endometrial, and glandular cells** show nuclear enlargement, mild nuclear hyperchromasia, variable pleomorphism, and an increased N/C ratio. When some morphologic features of adenocarcinoma are present, the term "atypical endocervical or glandular cells, favor neoplastic" is recommended (*The Bethesda System for Reporting Cervical Cytology,* 2nd ed. New York: Springer; 2004).

b. **Endocervical adenocarcinoma in situ** has glandular groups with nuclear pseudostratification, feathering, nuclear crowding, nuclear overlap, and/or a "bird tail-like" cell arrangement (*The Bethesda System for Reporting Cervical Cytology,* 2nd ed. New York: Springer; 2004). The neoplastic nuclei are often elongated and lack prominent nucleoli (e-**Fig. 34.17**).

c. **Adenocarcinoma of the endocervix** can be detected by cervical cytology in approximately 80% of cases. However, only 22% of endometrial adenocarcinoma cases show abnormal cells in cervical cytology specimens (*Acta Cytol.* 2007;51:47). The cells of endocervical carcinoma can be arranged singly or in tridimensional clusters, and exhibit malignant nuclear features of pleomorphism, clumped chromatin, hyperchromasia, and irregular nuclear contours. Large nucleoli are also present. The presence of columnar neoplastic cells and/or cytoplasmic vacuoles is evidence of glandular differentiation (e-**Fig. 34.18**).

D. **Other.** The 2001 Bethesda System recommends the use of this category in cases with endometrial cells when the patients are ≥40 years old. The endometrial component can be epithelial or stromal, and a statement regarding the absence of a squamous intraepithelial lesion should be included in the report.

Suggested Readings

American College of Obstetricians and Gynecologists. Evaluation and management of abnormal cervical cytology and histology in the adolescent. ACOG Committee Opinion no. 330. *Obstet Gynecol.* 2006;107:965.

Davey DD, Zarbo RJ. Human papillomavirus testing-are you ready for a new era in cervical cancer screening? *Arch Pathol Lab Med.* 2003;127:927.

Giuliano AR, Harris R, Sedjo RL, et al. Incidence, prevalence, and clearance of type-specific human papillomavirus infections: The Young Women's Health Study. *J Infect Dis.* 2002;186:462.

Wright TC Jr, Cox FT, Massad LS, et al. 2001 Consensus guidelines for the management of women with cervical cytological abnormalities. *JAMA.* 2002;287:2120.

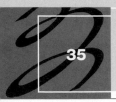

VAGINA

Anahit Nowrouzi, John D. Pfeifer,
and Phyllis C. Huettner

I. NORMAL STRUCTURE. The vagina is derived from the Müllerian ducts and is composed of three layers: the mucosa, muscularis propria, and adventitia. The mucosa is composed of squamous epithelium overlying a lamina propria that contains a rich vascular and lymphatic network with scattered stromal cells that may show multinucleation.

II. BENIGN CONDITIONS

A. Infectious diseases

1. **Vulvovaginal candidiasis** is a common condition that predominantly affects adult women in their 2nd and 3rd decades. Up to 70% of women will experience at least one episode in their lifetime. Common predisposing factors include antibiotic use, steroid use, oral contraceptive use, immunosuppression, and uncontrolled diabetes. Pruritus, erythema, and thick white vaginal discharge are the most common symptoms. Histologically, squamous epithelial hyperplasia with hyperkeratosis and/or parakeratosis is seen. Foci of neutrophilic infiltration of the squamous epithelium are commonly present. *Candida* can be present in the form of budding yeasts as well as pseudohyphae.

2. **Bacterial vaginosis** is most commonly found among adult women. It is caused by *Gardnerella vaginalis*, a bacillus which usually grows when the vaginal flora shifts toward a more acidic environment. A watery malodorous discharge without significant inflammation is a common symptom. Microscopically, the bacteria overgrow and cover the squamous cells producing so-called clue cells.

3. **Trichomoniasis,** a sexually transmitted disease, is caused by *Trichomonas vaginalis*, an oval protozoon with flagella. Microscopically, the organisms are identified by their blue-pink–stained body, elongated nuclei, and flagella.

4. **Herpes simplex infection** is a sexually transmitted disease caused by herpes simplex virus (HSV). Grossly, the virus causes a mucosal ulceration within a few days to 2 weeks following the exposure. These lesions are highly infectious until crusting, with final scarring within 2 to 3 weeks of initial symptoms. The majority of cases are caused by HSV-2, and recurrence is higher with infection by HSV-2 than by HSV-1.

   Microscopically, the ulcerated lesions are characterized by epithelial necrosis with associated degenerated cells containing viral inclusions best identified at the periphery of the ulcer. The cells with viral inclusions have characteristic features including multinucleation and ground glass nuclei with a rim of chromatin condensation at the nuclear border surrounded by a cytoplasmic halo.

5. **Actinomyces-like organisms** are most commonly seen in women having noncopper intrauterine contraceptive devices.

B. Inflammatory diseases

1. **Atrophic vaginitis** occurs most commonly in postmenopausal women, but can also occur during the postpartum period. Grossly, the primary finding is punctate hemorrhage of the vaginal mucosa. Microscopically, the squamous cells show decreased glycogen due to lower estrogen levels. Atrophy can be distinguished from vaginal intraepithelial neoplasia (VAIN) by the monotomy of the cell population and the lack of cytologic atypia and mitotic activity.

2. **Crohn disease** can result in rectovaginal fistula formation. Vaginal fistulas can also form as a result of radiation therapy to this region, from a perforated colonic diverticulum, or as a complication of hysterectomy.

3. **Stenosis,** ulceration, and necrosis are well-described sequelae of radiation therapy. Stenosis can also follow severe bullous erythema multiforme (Stevens–Johnson syndrome).

C. Cysts

1. **Müllerian cyst** is the most common type of vaginal cyst, and may be lined by endocervical, endometrial, or endosalpingeal type epithelium.

2. **Epithelial inclusion cysts** are lined by keratinizing squamous epithelium and filled with white sebaceous and keratinous debris. They most commonly arise in areas of previous trauma such as episiotomy sites.

3. **Mesonephric cyst.** Also known as Gartner's duct cysts, they are usually located along the anterolateral wall of the vagina (along the path of the mesonephric duct). This type of cyst is lined by low cuboidal, nonmucinous epithelium.

4. **Bartholin gland cysts** are thought to develop from obstruction of ducts of Bartholin glands, which normally open into the vestibule. The cyst lining varies from squamous to transitional to mucin secreting.

D. Adenosis occurs in about 30% of women who were exposed to diethylstilbestrol (DES) in utero, and is associated with an increased risk of clear cell adenocarcinoma (see section on clear cell adenocarcinoma below). Adenosis usually involves the upper third of the vagina, but the middle third or lower third are affected in about 10% of the cases. Grossly, it presents as a red erythematous granular lesion. Microscopically, adenosis is defined by the presence of columnar epithelium of endometrial or endocervical type in the vaginal mucosa or underlying submucosa (e-Fig. 35.1).*

E. Endometriosis of the vagina comprises <10% of cases of pelvic endometriosis. The presence of endometrial stroma is required for a diagnosis of endometriosis, and can be used to distinguish endometriosis from adenosis.

III. BENIGN NEOPLASMS. The WHO classification of vaginal tumors is given in Table 35.1.

A. Epithelial

1. **Squamous papilloma** is usually asymptomatic and can occur at any age. Grossly, it usually presents as a cluster of papillary lesions. Microscopically, squamous papillomas have a fibrovascular core and are lined by benign squamous epithelium.

2. **Fibroepithelial polyps** most commonly occur in adult women during their reproductive years. They occur in the lower third of the vagina and grossly have a soft and papillary surface. Microscopically, they are composed of squamous epithelium with underlying hypocellular fibrovascular stroma. Atypical myofibroblasts are common in the stroma, and scattered multinucleated cells with bizarre atypical nuclei may also be seen. However, rhabdomyoblasts and a cambium layer are not present and mitotic figures are rare, features that distinguish fibroepithelial polyp from sarcoma botryoides.

3. **Condyloma acuminatum** is caused by human papilloma virus (HPV) serotypes 6 and 11. Microscopically, it is composed of papillary fibrovascular cores lined by squamous epithelium with acanthosis, hyperkeratosis, and parakeratosis, with associated viral cytopathic effect or koilocytosis characterized by nuclear enlargement and irregularity, chromatin clumping and hyperchromasia, occasional bi- or multinucleation, and perinuclear clearing.

B. Mesenchymal

1. **Leiomyoma** is the most common benign mesenchymal tumor of the vagina in adults, with a mean age at presentation of 40 years. Leiomyomas rarely affect children. The tumor most commonly develops in the submucosa. Grossly, it consists of a well-circumscribed firm mass with a white-tan cut surface. Microscopically, the tumor is composed of fascicles of spindle cells with elongated uniform nuclei, fine chromatin, smooth nuclear membranes, and a moderate amount of eosinophilic cytoplasm. Mitotic figures are rare.

2. **Genital rhabdomyoma** is a rare tumor of the vagina that shows skeletal muscle differentiation. It affects middle-aged women, and patients usually present with

---

*All e-figures are available online via the Solution Site Image Bank.

TABLE 35.1   WHO Histological Classification of Tumors of the Vagina

Epithelial Tumors
Squamous tumors and precursors
   Squamous cell carcinoma, not otherwise specified
     Keratinizing
     Nonkeratinizing
     Basaloid
     Verrucous
     Warty
   Squamous intraepithelial neoplasia
   Benign squamous lesions
     Condyloma acuminatum
     Squamous papilloma (vaginal micropapillomatosis)
     Fibroepithelial polyp
Glandular tumors
   Clear cell adenocarcinoma
   Endometrioid adenocarcinoma
   Mucinous adenocarcinoma
   Müllerian papilloma
   Adenoma
Other epithelial tumors
   Adenosquamous carcinoma
   Adenoid cystic carcinoma
   Adenoid basal carcinoma
   Carcinoid
   Small cell carcinoma
   Undifferentiated carcinoma

Mesenchymal Tumors and Tumorlike Conditions
Sarcoma botryoides
Leiomyosarcoma
Endomentrioid stromal sarcoma, low grade
Undifferentiated vaginal sarcoma
Leiomyoma
Genital rhabdomyoma
Deep angiomyxoma
Postoperative spindle cell nodule

Mixed Epithelial and Mesenchymal Tumors
Carcinosarcoma (malignant mixed Müllerian tumor)
Adenosarcoma
Malignant mixed tumor resembling synovial sarcoma
Benign mixed tumor

Melanocytic Tumors
Malignant melanoma
Blue nevus
Melanocytic nevus

Miscellaneous Tumors
Tumors of germ cell type
   Yolk sac tumor
   Dermoid cyst
Others
   Peripheral primitive neuroectodermal tumor/Ewing tumor
   Adenomatoid tumor

Lymphoid and Hematopoetic Tumors
Malignant lymphoma
Leukemia

Secondary Tumors

From: Tavassoli FA, Devilee P, eds. *World Health Organization Classification of Tumours. Pathology and Genetics. Tumours of the Breast and Female Genital Organs.* Lyon: IARC Press; 2001. Used with permission.

vaginal bleeding or dyspareunia. Grossly, it is a solid polypoid to nodular lesion that creates a bulging mass under the mucosa. Microscopically, rhabdomyoma is composed of loosely interweaving bundles of spindle cells with oval nuclei, abundant eosinophilic cytoplasm, and occasional cross-striations. Nuclear pleomorphism and mitotic activity are absent. Immunohistochemical stains for skeletal muscle markers such as desmin, myogenin, and myo-D1 are positive. Rhabdomyoma can be distinguished from rhabdomyosarcoma based on the absence of a dense layer of atypical neoplastic cells beneath the epithelium, cytologic atypia, and mitotic activity.

3. **Angiomyofibroblastoma** is a benign tumor that occurs in the vagina and vulva. Grossly, it has a well-circumscribed outline with a white-tan cut surface, and can range from 0.5 cm to 14 cm in maximal dimension. Microscopically, it is composed of fascicles of spindle cells that have abundant eosinophilic cytoplasm, elongated nuclei, and minimal to no atypia, although scattered multinucleated cells may be present. Architecturally, the cells form alternating hyper- and hypocellular areas, although the hypercellular areas are accentuated around vessels. The absence of red blood cell extravasation and stromal mucin distinguishes this entity from aggressive angiomyxoma. Surgical excision is the treatment of choice.

4. **Deep "aggressive" angiomyxoma** predominantly affects the sacroiliac soft tissue and perineum of women in their 5th decade. Grossly, it presents as a large mass with a gelatinous, soft cut surface. Microscopically, it is composed of bland spindle cells with delicate eosinophilic cytoplasmic processes scattered throughout a hypocellular myxoid stroma. Medium to large thick-walled hyalinized vessels are commonly present; loose fibrillar arrangements of collagen fibers (so-called myoid bundles) are typically found around the thick-walled vessels (**e-Fig. 35.2**). The stromal cells are usually immunopositive for smooth muscle actin (SMA) and desmin.

5. **Postoperative spindle cell nodule** is a pseudosarcomatous vaginal lesion that most commonly appears at the site of an excision, a few weeks to months after the surgery. Grossly, it presents as a small friable reddish mass in the vaginal vault. Microscopically, it is composed of fascicles of spindle cells with stromal granulation tissue and extravasated red blood cells. Although atypical mitotic figures can be seen, atypical nuclear cytology is not present.

   The differential diagnosis of postoperative spindle cell nodule includes vaginal leiomyosarcoma. A clinical history of a recent surgery can aid diagnosis.

6. **Müllerian papilloma** is a benign papillary tumor of childhood. It typically occurs in the upper vaginal wall of children with a mean age of 5 years. Microscopically, it is composed of a complex branching fibrovascular core surrounded by hypocellular stroma covered by bland cuboidal to columnar epithelial cells that show no atypia. Mitotic figures are not seen.

IV. MALIGNANT NEOPLASMS

A. **Epithelial.** The AJCC staging guidelines for vaginal carcinomas are given in Table 35.2.

1. **Vaginal intraepithelial neoplasia (VAIN)** is a premalignant, HPV-associated lesion that primarily affects women 20 to 40 years old. The risk factors for VAIN are the same as for cervical intraepithelial neoplasia (CIN) and include a low age at first intercourse and an increased number of sexual partners. HPV serotypes 6 and 11 are associated with low-grade VAIN (VAIN1), and HPV serotypes 31, 33, 35, and 39 are associated with most high-grade VAIN (VAIN2 and 3). The majority of low-grade lesions regress spontaneously, although about 5% of cases of low-grade VAIN progress to higher grades of dysplasia and invasive carcinoma. Progression into higher grades may take several years to a decade.

   Grossly, VAIN appears as an exophytic to verrucopapillary lesion. Microscopically, the squamous epithelium shows nuclear atypia (nuclear enlargement, hyperchromasia, and an irregular nuclear membrane) with koilocytosis and an increased number of mitotic figures. Grading is based on the extent to which the thickness of the squamous epithelium shows atypia; VAIN1, 2, and 3 are defined as the involvement of the lower third (**e-Fig. 35.3**), lower two thirds (**e-Fig. 35.4**),

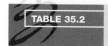

TABLE 35.2	Tumor, Node, Metastasis (TNM) Staging Scheme and American Joint Committee on Cancer Staging Guidelines for Carcinomas of the Vagina

PRIMARY TUMOR (T)

TNM Categories	FIGO* Stages	
TX		Primary tumor cannot be assessed
T0		No evidence of primary tumor
Tis	0	Carcinoma in situ (preinvasive carcinoma)
T1	I	Tumor confined to vagina
T2	II	Tumor invades paravaginal tissues but does not extend to pelvic wall
T3	III	Tumor invades to pelvic wall
T4	IVA	Tumor invades mucosa of bladder or rectum, and/or extends beyond the true pelvis; note that the presence of bullous edema is not sufficient evidence to classify a tumor as T4
M1	IVB	Distant metastasis

REGIONAL LYMPH NODES (N)

NX	Regional lymph nodes cannot be assessed
N0	No regional lymph node metastasis
N1	Regional lymph node metastasis

DISTANT METASTASIS (M)

MX	Distant metastasis cannot be assessed
M0	No distant metastasis
M1	Distant metastasis

STAGE GROUPING

Stage 0	Tis	N0	M0
Stage 1	T1	N0	M0
Stage II	T2	N0	M0
Stage III	T3	N0	M0
	T1,T2,T3	N1	M0
Stage IVA	T4	N0	M0
Stage IVB	Any T	Any N	M1

*International Federation of Gynecology and Obstetrics Classification
From: Greene FL, Page DL, Fleming ID, Fritz AG, Balch CM, Haller DG, Morrow M, eds. *AJCC Cancer Staging Manual.* 6th edition. New York: Springer; 2002. Used with permission. (A new AJCC TNM staging system is scheduled for release in 2009; after its publication, the new staging scheme will appear on the website for this book.)

and full thickness (**e-Fig. 35.5**) of the squamous epithelium with loss of maturation, respectively. Clinical management of VAIN1 is simple observation of the patient; the preferred treatment of VAIN2 or 3 is local excision or laser ablation.

2. **Squamous cell carcinoma** of the vagina accounts for 85% of vaginal carcinomas and occurs most commonly in women between the ages of 60 and 80 years. In younger women, squamous cell carcinoma is usually associated with HPV infection. Squamous cell carcinoma often metastasizes to the regional lymph nodes, and has a predilection for distant metastasis to lung and bone.

3. **Verrucous carcinoma** is a variant of squamous cell carcinoma. It is a slowly growing, well-differentiated tumor with a warty gross appearance. Microscopically, it demonstrates verruciform architecture with minimal nuclear epithelial atypia, and a pushing rather than infiltrative margin. Local excision is the treatment of choice. Local or distant metastasis is extremely rare.

4. **Clear cell adenocarcinoma** rarely occurs in women who do not have a history of DES exposure. The lifetime risk of developing clear cell carcinoma in women exposed to DES is about 0.1%, with a mean age of 20 years. In women who have not been exposed to DES, clear cell adenocarcinoma develops in the postmenopausal years around the age of 60. Patients typically present with bleeding or a grossly visible mass of the cervix or the vagina.

Histologically, clear cell carcinoma is composed of cells with pleomorphic and hyperchromatic nuclei with abundant clear cytoplasm; hobnailing is often a prominent feature. The malignant cells may form papillary or tubulocystic structures. The most common metastatic sites are the regional lymph nodes and lung.

5. **Other epithelial malignancies.** Primary adenocarcinoma of the vagina of non–clear cell type is rare; most non–clear cell adenocarcinomas represent metastasis from the endocervix or endometrium, or other sites such as the ovary, colon, or breast. The non–clear cell types of adenocarcinoma that most frequently involve the vagina include mucinous, papillary serous, endometrioid, and adenosquamous.

B. **Mesenchymal**

1. **Sarcoma botryoides** (a subtype of embryonal rhabdomyosarcoma) is the most common malignant vaginal tumor in children, usually affecting girls younger than 5 years. It is commonly located submucosally and grossly appears as grapelike clusters of tumor that fill (and in some cases protrude from) the vagina. Microscopically, the tumor is composed of cells with elongated small nuclei and a moderate amount of bright eosinophilic cytoplasm. For diagnosis, at least one microscopic field must show the malignant cells forming a condensed layer (a so-called cambium layer) beneath an intact epithelium (*Pediatr Dev Pathol*. 1998;1:550). The tumor cells are immunopositive for skeletal muscle markers such as actin, desmin, myo-D1, and myogenin. Surgical excision with radiation and chemotherapy is the treatment of choice, and the prognosis is usually excellent.

2. **Leiomyosarcoma** is the most common malignant vaginal sarcoma of adults. Grossly, the tumor is typically a mass of about 3 to 5 cm in maximal dimension. Microscopically, the tumor is identical to its counterparts at other sites in the female reproductive tract.

The criteria for distinguishing leiomyosarcoma from smooth muscle tumors of uncertain biologic potential are not as well defined for vaginal tumors as for tumors of the myometrium; current recommendations are that tumors larger than 3 cm in maximal dimension with an infiltrating margin, moderate to marked cytologic atypia, and ≥5 mitoses per 10 high-power fields be diagnosed as leiomyosarcoma (*Obstet Gynecol*. 1979;53:689).

C. **Other tumors**

1. **Malignant melanoma** of the vagina is a rare tumor. It most commonly occurs in postmenopausal women in lower third of the vagina. Grossly, it can present as a bulky palpable mass, with or without pigmentation. Microscopically, the cells have same cytomorphology as the cells of cutaneous malignant melanoma. Immunohistochemical stains for S-100, HMB45, MelanA and vimentin are positive in the malignant cells; immunostains for cytokeratin are negative. Vaginal melanomas are treated surgically; radiation and chemotherapy have not proven effective. The prognosis is very poor and the recurrence rate is high.

2. **Metastasis** to the vagina from primary tumors of other sites is uncommon. As noted above, metastasis usually originates from malignancies of the cervix, endometrium, ovary, colon, and breast.

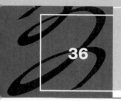

VULVA

36

John D. Pfeifer and Phyllis C. Huettner

I. **NORMAL ANATOMY.** The vulva or external female genital region encompasses the mons pubis, the labia majora, labia minora, clitoris, and vestibule. The entire vulva except for the vestibule is covered by keratinized, stratified squamous epithelium. The epithelium of the vestibule is glycogenated squamous epithelium. The lateral aspects of the labia majora and the mons pubis contain hair follicles. Sebaceous glands are present in the labia majora and the perineum. The clitoris is lined by keratinizing stratified squamous epithelium overlying paired corpora cavernosa that contain vascular spaces surrounded by nerves.

The urethral meatus, major vestibular glands (Bartholin glands), minor vestibular glands, paraurethral glands (Skene's glands), and vagina all open onto the vulva. The Bartholin's glands are paired glands that open posterolaterally on the hymenal ring; they are composed of acini lined by cuboidal mucus-secreting epithelium that drain into a duct that may be lined by mucus-secreting, transitional, or squamous epithelium depending on the location from deep to surface. Skene's glands open on either side of the urethral meatus and are composed of acini lined by mucus-secreting epithelium that opens into ducts lined by transitional epithelium.

II. **GROSS EXAMINATION, TISSUE SAMPLING, AND HISTOLOGIC SLIDE PREPARA-TION**

A. **Vulvar biopsies.** Vulvar biopsies should be oriented as for skin biopsies (see Chapter 38) and three hematoxylin and eosin (H&E)-stained levels examined.

B. **Vulvar resections.** It is helpful to ask the surgeon to orient the specimen with a diagram or labeled sutures so that orientation can be maintained during processing. The margins of resection should be inked and, depending on the location of the resection, the periurethral, vaginal, and perianal margins need to be noted. In cases with an obvious malignant neoplasm, one section per centimeter of tumor, including the areas closest to the deep margin and closest to the nearest lateral or other margins, are recommended. In cases where no tumor is observed grossly, the entire specimen is submitted. Because many gynecologic oncologists consider resection for squamous cancer in this area to be adequate if tumor is >8 mm from the margin (*Cancer.* 2002;95:2331), radial rather than shave margins should be taken so that the distance from tumor to margin can be measured.

III. **DIAGNOSTIC FEATURES OF COMMON DISEASES OF THE VULVA.** Many inflammatory and neoplastic conditions that affect the skin will also affect the vulva. These are discussed in the skin chapters (Chapters 38 and 39). This section only covers those conditions for which the vulva is a common site of disease.

A. **Inflammation**

1. **Bartholin abscess** presents as a painful swelling in the area of the Bartholin gland. Microscopically, there is acute inflammation of the Bartholin duct glands and connective tissue, with purulent luminal contents. The etiology includes *Neisseria gonorrhea*, *Staphylococcus*, or other aerobic or anaerobic organisms. Treatment includes excision, drainage, and appropriate antibiotics.

2. **Hidradenitis suppurativa** presents as painful, subcutaneous nodules in areas containing apocrine glands, particularly the vulva and axilla. Initial changes include acute and chronic inflammation around hair follicles, which progresses to abscess formation, sinus tract formation, and dermal scarring. Treatment may include total excision of the involved area or laser ablation.

3. **Crohn disease** may present as vulvar or perianal erythema, ulceration, abscesses, or fistulas between bowel and vulva or between two different areas of vulva. Microscopically, there is acute and chronic inflammation of the deep dermis, often with associated noncaseating granulomas, fistulas, or sinus tracts.

B. **Infection**

1. ***Candida*** infection is often a chronic inflammatory condition of the vulva that may be associated with diabetes. It may present as pruritus and clinically may show areas of redness with thickened, edematous skin. Microscopically, there is acanthosis with acute and chronic inflammatory cells in the epithelium, and parakeratosis with neutrophils. Often fungal organisms are visible on H&E stain in the keratin layer; they are easily identified by silver stains.

2. **Syphilis** is a sexually transmitted disease caused by the spirochete *Treponema pallidum.* The primary lesion of syphilis, the chancre, develops in about half of women within 3 weeks of infection, and is characterized by a single or sometimes multiple painless ulcers. The ulcer heals in 2 to 6 weeks without a scar. Secondary syphilis develops within 6 weeks to 6 months and is characterized by the development of a rash on the palms, soles, and mucosal surfaces, as well as elevated plaques and papules, termed condyloma lata, on the vulva and mucosal surfaces. On microscopic sections, the chancre shows epidermal ulceration, dermal acute and chronic inflammation with numerous plasma cells, and severe arteritis. Condyloma lata are characterized by marked epidermal acanthosis and hyperkeratosis, dermal inflammation with numerous plasma cells, and arteritis. The organisms may be detected on Warthin–Starry, Steiner, or Dieterle stain; no organisms are seen in some cases of active infection.

3. **Human papilloma virus (HPV) infection.** Condyloma acuminatum, also referred to as genital warts, is the result of sexually transmitted infection caused by HPV types 11 (75% of cases) or 6 (25% of cases). They present as asymptomatic, usually multiple or confluent, papillary or papular lesions, and may occur anywhere on the vulva or perianal region.

   Microscopically, condylomata of the vulva typically have a fibrovascular stalk. The epithelium exhibits acanthosis, papillomatosis, hyperkeratosis, dyskeratosis, and an accentuated granular cell layer. Viral cytopathic effect, termed koilocytosis, takes the form of cytoplasmic clearing around enlarged nuclei with irregular nuclear outlines and clumped chromatin. Vulvar condylomata usually follow a protracted course. They may grow rapidly during pregnancy and then regress after delivery. Small condylomas may be treated with topical agents, whereas large ones are excised or treated with laser ablation or cryotherapy.

4. **Herpes simplex virus (HSV).** Infection with HSV type 2, or less commonly type 1, is typically heralded by fever, dysuria, and severe pain. Painless vesicles then appear and progress to an intensely painful ulcer. The ulcer typically heals in about 2 weeks. Microscopically, epithelial ulceration is surrounded by virally infected keratinocytes that exhibit multinucleation, "ground glass" nuclear chromatin, or eosinophilic nuclear inclusions (e-**Fig. 36.1**).*

5. **Molluscum contagiosum** is a sexually transmitted disease in adults caused by infection with the *Molluscum contagiosum* poxvirus. The lesions are small, 3- to 6-mm diameter papules with a characteristic central depression or umbilication, and are usually asymptomatic although perianal lesions may be pruritic. Microscopic features (e-**Fig. 36.2**) include formation of a cup-shaped papule with marked epidermal acanthosis, and intracytoplasmic inclusions that are initially eosinophilic but become more basophilic as the lesion ages. Most lesions regress spontaneously.

C. **Noninfectious squamous lesions**

1. **Lichen sclerosus** presents as symmetric plaque-like areas of white, thinned epithelium that may be superficially ulcerated. In advanced cases there may be scarring of involved areas and stenosis of the introitus.

---

*All e-figures are available online via the Solution Site Image Bank.

Microscopically, there is thinning of the epidermis with flattening of the rete, a zone of collagenous connective tissue (that may be edematous and that does not contain vessels) immediately beneath the epidermis, and an underlying zone of chronically inflamed connective tissue (e-**Fig. 36.3**). The epidermis often contains a spongiotic basal layer with loss of melanocytes. Treatment involves high dose corticosteroids. Postmenopausal women with lichen sclerosus have a small risk of developing vulvar intraepithelial neoplasia (VIN) and squamous cell carcinoma.

2. **Squamous cell hyperplasia** typically occurs in adults and presents as a localized area of pruritus. It is thought to be a nonspecific response triggered by a variety of irritants. Clinically, the area is white or red, with accentuated skin markings and sometimes areas of excoriation. The characteristic feature on microscopy is marked acanthosis without atypia, increased mitotic activity, inflammation, or the features of other specific dermatoses. Hyperkeratosis may be present. The dermis is normal. Treatment includes limiting exposure to irritants, with topical corticosteroids and antipruritic agents.

D. Cystic lesions

1. **Bartholin cyst.** Obstruction of the Bartholin duct leads to the accumulation of secretions and the formation of a cystic dilatation of the duct. The epithelium lining these cysts may be squamous, transitional, or mucinous. Cysts can be treated by drainage, marsupialization, or excision of the gland.

2. **Keratinous cysts** occur at any age and typically affect the labia majora. They are small, measuring just a few millimeters in maximal dimension, and are filled with white cheesy material without hair. Microscopically, they are lined by stratified squamous or flattened epithelium. They can be excised if symptomatic.

3. **Mucous cysts** occur in the vestibule and are lined by mucinous epithelium with or without squamous metaplasia. They probably result from occlusion of minor vestibular glands.

IV. TUMORS. The World Health Organization (WHO) classification of tumors of the vulva is presented in Table 36.1.

A. Benign tumors and tumor-like lesions

1. **Fibroepithelial polyps** are also known as acrochordons or skin tags. They may be hyperpigmented, hypopigmented, or flesh-colored, and typically occur on hair-bearing skin. They usually have a papillomatous or pedunculated growth pattern and a soft cut surface. Microscopically, the epithelium may be thickened with hyperkeratosis, or may be flattened. The stroma contains loose bundles of collagen and may be edematous. Fibroepithelial polyps are clinically insignificant but can be excised if they are cosmetically unacceptable.

2. **Papillary hidradenoma** is a benign tumor that originates from apocrine sweat glands. It presents as a dome-shaped mass, usually <2 cm in diameter, arising between the labium majus and labium minus. The mass may ulcerate and bleed, but is usually asymptomatic. Microscopically, papillary hidradenoma forms tubules and acini lined by a luminal layer of epithelial cells and an outer layer of myoepithelial cells (e-**Fig. 36.4**). Cytologic atypia and mitotic activity are rare. These lesions exhibit a pseudocapsule, and caution should be exercised before interpreting compression of glandular epithelium at the periphery as invasion. Local excision is curative.

3. **Granular cell tumors** may be seen in many sites, but about 7% involve the vulva. They usually present as a painless, slowly growing subcutaneous mass involving the labial majora, clitoris, or mons pubis. On gross examination, they are not encapsulated. Microscopically, they are composed of sheets of large cells with abundant, eosinophilic, granular cytoplasm and relatively small uniform nuclei separated by hyalinized stroma. The epithelium overlying a granular cell tumor often exhibits pseudoepitheliomatous hyperplasia (e-**Fig. 36.5**). It is important not to interpret this finding as squamous cell carcinoma on a superficial biopsy. The cytoplasm of the neoplastic cells is PAS positive and diastase resistant; immunohistochemically, the cytoplasm is positive for S-100 and myelin basic protein.

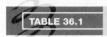

TABLE 36.1	WHO Histological Classification of Tumors of the Vulva

Epithelial tumors
Squamous and related tumors and precursors
  Squamous cell carcinoma, not otherwise specified
    Keratinizing
    Nonkeratinizing
    Basaloid
    Warty
    Verrucous
    Keratoacanthoma-like
    Variant with tumor giant cells
    Others
  Basal cell carcinoma
  Squamous intraepithelial neoplasia
    Vulvar intraepithelial neoplasia (VIN) 3/squamous cell carcinoma in situ
  Benign squamous cell lesions
    Condyloma acuminatum
    Vestibular papilloma (micropapillomatosis)
    Fibroepithelial polyp
    Seborrheic and inverted follicular keratosis
    Keratoacanthoma
Glandular tumors
  Paget disease
  Bartholin gland tumors
    Adenocarcinoma
    Squamous cell carcinoma
    Adenoid cystic carcinoma
    Adenosquamous carcinoma
    Transitional cell carcinoma
    Small cell carcinoma
    Adenoma
    Adenomyoma
    Others
Tumors arising from specialized anogenital mammary-like glands
  Adenocarcinoma of mammary gland type
  Papillary hidradenoma
  Others
Adenocarcinoma of Skene gland origin
Adenocarcinoma of other types
Adenoma of minor vestibular glands
Mixed tumor of the vulva
Tumors of skin appendage origin
  Malignant sweat glad tumors
  Sebaceous carcinoma
  Syringoma
  Nodular hidradenoma
  Trichoepithelioma
  Trichilemmoma
  Others

(Continued)

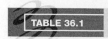

TABLE 36.1	WHO Histological Classification of Tumors of the Vulva (*Continued*)

Soft tissue tumors
Sarcoma botryoides
Leiomyosarcoma
Proximal epithelioid sarcoma
Alveolar soft part sarcoma
Liposarcoma
Dermatofibrosarcoma protuberans
Deep angiomyxoma
Superficial angiomyxoma
Angiomyofibroblastoma
Cellular angiofibroma
Leiomyoma
Granular cell tumor
Others

Melanocytic tumors
Malignant melanoma
Congenital melanocytic nevus
Acquired melanocytic nevus
Blue nevus
Atypical melanocytic nevus of the genital type
Dysplastic melanocytic nevus

Miscellaneous tumors
Yolk sac tumor
Merkel cell tumor
Ewing sarcoma/primitive neuroectodermal tumor

Hematopoetic and lymphoid tumors
Malignant lymphoma (specify type)
Leukemia (specify type)

Secondary tumors

From: Tavassoli FA, Devilee P, eds. *World Health Organization Classification of Tumours. Pathology and Genetics. Tumours of the Breast and Female Genital Organs.* Lyon: IARC Press; 2001. Used with permission.

Granular cell tumor is treated with wide local excision; margins should be assessed carefully as the tumor may recur if not completely excised. Malignant granular cell tumors of the vulva are very rare and are best diagnosed in the presence of distant metastases.

4. **Leiomyomas** are the most common soft tissue tumors of the vulva. They present as painless masses. Like leiomyomata elsewhere, they are grossly well circumscribed with a firm, whorled cut surface. Microscopically, they are identical to leiomyomata in the uterus, composed of interlacing fascicles of smooth muscle cells with no atypia or necrosis, and only occasional mitotic figures. The criteria for distinguishing benign from malignant smooth muscle tumors in the vulva are not as well established as they are in the uterus. Excision is the treatment of choice.

B. **Malignant neoplasms and their precursors**

1. **Vulvar intraepithelial neoplasia** (VIN). Although most cases of VIN are associated with HPV infection, the correlation is not as strong as with cervical intraepithelial neoplasia (CIN). It is generally agreed that there are two broad types of VIN, VIN of the usual type (u-VIN) and differentiated VIN (d-VIN). u-VIN is strongly HPV associated and occurs in younger women of reproductive age; it can be further subclassified into warty, basaloid, and mixed types, and is graded as with CIN into grade 1, 2, or 3. d-VIN affects mostly postmenopausal women,

is not HPV-related, and has a high likelihood of progressing to well-differentiated squamous cell carcinoma (*J Med Virol.* 2005;77:102 and *Int J Gynecol Pathol.* 2007;26:248).

  a. u-VIN is analogous to CIN. It is usually caused by HPV infection, most commonly serotype 16. The gross appearance is variable; it usually forms discrete plaques that may be flat, hyperkeratotic, or pigmented.

     Microscopically, u-VIN shows nuclear enlargement, irregularity, and hyperchromasia. Mitotic figures are common and are frequently atypical. Warty type u-VIN has a growth pattern similar to a condyloma and microscopically exhibits acanthosis, hyperkeratosis, and parakeratosis; koilocytotic atypia and multinucleation are common. Basaloid type u-VIN is usually flat without hyperkeratosis or parakeratosis; the cells are small, resembling the cells of the basal epithelium, and features of viral cytopathic effect are not prominent. Mixed types with both warty and basaloid features are also seen. VIN 1 is diagnosed when the dysplastic cells involve the lower third of the epithelium; in VIN 2 the dysplastic cells involve the lower two thirds of the epithelium, and in VIN 3 the dysplastic cells involve the full thickness of the epithelium (e-**Fig. 36.6**). The treatment for u-VIN is excision.

  b. d-VIN is characterized by acanthosis with elongation of the rete ridges and parakeratosis. The atypia is frequently confined to the basal layers, and the tips of the rete often exhibit keratinization. The cells do not show viral cytopathic effect; rather, they have enlarged nuclei with prominent nucleoli and abundant eosinophilic cytoplasm (e-**Fig. 36.7**). Frequently there is edema between keratinocytes with prominence of the intercellular bridges. Because of the high risk of squamous cell carcinoma, excision is the treatment of choice.

2. Squamous cell carcinoma may be an incidental finding in a resection for VIN, may develop in the background of lichen sclerosus or an inflammatory dermatosis, or may develop in women with no history of VIN. Tumors may be exophytic, endophytic, or plaque-like and may be located anywhere on the vulva.

     On microscopic examination, nests of invasive carcinoma will exhibit nuclear atypia and increased mitotic activity, and will be associated with a reactive and desmoplastic stroma. A characteristic feature is keratinization in nests deep in the stroma (e-**Fig. 36.8**). Tumors may show warty, keratinizing, verrucous, basaloid, or mixed features.

     In addition to the size of the tumor, the thickness of invasive tumor (as measured from the top of the granular cell layer to the point of deepest invasion) as well as the depth of invasion (as measured from the top of the nearest normal dermal–epidermal junction to the point of deepest invasion) should be recorded. Lymphovascular space invasion is also an important prognostic feature and should be noted if found. The staging scheme for vulvar carcinomas is presented in Table 36.2.

     The role of sentinel lymph node biopsy in the management of patients with vulvar squamous cell carcinoma continues to be evaluated (*Curr Opin Obstet Gynecol.* 2004;16:65). One theme that is emerging, however, is that the intensity of the histopathologic evaluation determines the frequency at which metastases are identified (*Anticancer Res.* 2004;24:1281), as is true for sentinel lymph node biopsy in other clinical settings.

3. Melanoma, although rare, is the second most common malignancy of the vulva after squamous cell carcinoma. Common presenting symptoms include bleeding, a mass, and pain. Vulvar melanomas may be flat or polypoid, and are usually pigmented, often with satellite lesions. Vulvar melanomas very uncommonly arise from a nevus.

     The features of vulvar melanoma are the same as those of melanomas arising elsewhere, and are covered in detail in Chapter 40. Important features to note are the thickness, presence or absence of ulceration, histologic pattern, degree of inflammation, presence of vascular or perineural invasion, and the presence of satellitosis. Most vulvar melanomas exhibit an acral–lentiginous pattern; however, those arising on vulvar skin are more likely to be superficial spreading.

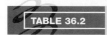

TABLE 36.2	Tumor, Node, Metastasis (TNM) Staging Scheme for Carcinomas of the Vulva

PRIMARY TUMOR (T)

TX	Primary tumor cannot be assessed
T0	No evidence of primary tumor
Tis	Carcinoma in situ (pre-invasive carcinoma)
T1	Tumor confined to vulva or vulva and perineum, ≤2 cm in greatest dimension
T1a	Tumor confined to vulva or vulva and perineum, ≤2 cm in greatest dimension and with stromal invasion no greater than 1 mm
T1b	Tumor confined to vulva or vulva and perineum, ≤2 cm in greatest dimension and with stromal invasion >1 mm
T2	Tumor confined to vulva or vulva and perineum, >2 cm in greatest dimension
T3	Tumor invades any of the following: lower urethra, vagina, anus
T4	Tumor invades any of the following: bladder mucosa, rectal mucosa, upper urethra; or is fixed to pubic bone

REGIONAL LYMPH NODES (N)

NX	Regional lymph nodes cannot be assessed
N0	No regional lymph node metastasis
N1	Unilateral regional lymph node metastasis
N2	Bilateral regional lymph node metastasis

DISTANT METASTASIS (M)

MX	Distant metastasis cannot be assessed
M0	No distant metastasis
M1	Distant metastasis (including pelvic lymph node metastasis)

STAGE GROUPINGS (TNM and International Federation of Gynecology and Obstetrics [FIGO])

Stage 0	Tis	N0	M0
Stage I	T1	N0	M0
Stage IA	T1a	N0	M0
Stage IB	T1b	N0	M0
Stage II	T2	N0	M0
Stage III	T1, T2	N1	M0
	T3	N0, M1	M0
Stage IVA	T1, T2, T3	N2	M0
	T4	Any N	M0
Stage IVB	Any T	Any N	M1

From: Greene FL, Page DL, Fleming ID, Fritz AG, Balch CM, Haller DG, Morrow M, eds. *AJCC Cancer Staging Manual*. 6th edition. New York: Springer; 2002. Used with permission. (A new AJCC TNM staging system is scheduled for release in 2009; after its publication, the new staging scheme will appear on the website for this book.)

Treatment is wide local excision aiming for 1- to 2-cm margins (which can be difficult to obtain in the vulva). The prognosis for vulvar melanoma is poorer than for melanoma of other skin sites.

4. **Paget disease** tends to affect elderly women and presents with patchy, erythematous, excoriated areas of vulvar skin and epithelium. Microscopically, the squamous epithelium is infiltrated by enlarged cells, either individually or in clusters, that hug the epidermal–dermal junction (e-**Fig. 36.9**). These cells have abundant mucinous cytoplasm, large nuclei with small nucleoli, and often form small glands within the epithelium. These Paget cells may also involve the adnexal structures. Invasion of the stroma needs to be excluded.

Immunohistochemistry is very helpful in distinguishing Paget disease from melanoma, which may appear morphologically similar. The neoplastic cells of

Paget disease will be positive for cytokeratin and carcinoembryogenic antigen, but negative for HMB-45, melanoma has the opposite staining pattern.

Cases of Paget disease associated with underlying carcinoma (usually vulvar adnexal adenocarcinoma, rectal adenocarcinoma, or bladder carcinoma) have a significantly worse prognosis, so careful gross and microscopic examination of excision specimens is warranted. In cases that lack an associated invasive malignancy, radical surgical excision does not seem to provide any benefit compared with wide local excision (*Gynecol Oncol.* 2000;77:183).

Suggested Readings

de Hullu JA, van der Zee AG. Surgery and radiotherapy in vulvar cancer. *Crit Rev Oncol Hematol.* 2006;60:38.

Tavassoli FA, Devilee P, eds. *Tumours of the Breast and Female Genital Organs.* 1st ed. Lyon, France: International Agency for Research on Cancer; 2003;313–334.

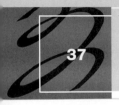

PLACENTA
37
Phyllis C. Huettner

I. **NORMAL ANATOMY.** The normal, unfixed term placenta weighs 350 to 550 grams, trimmed of membranes and cord. The placenta consists of three parts: fetal membranes, umbilical cord, and placental disk. The fetal membranes insert at the edge of the disk and envelop the fetus and amniotic fluid. Microscopically, they are composed of a cuboidal amniotic epithelium with underlying connective tissue, a chorionic layer (composed of connective tissue, intermediate trophoblast, and degenerated villi), and sometimes a layer of decidua (gestational endometrium).

The umbilical cord is composed of two umbilical arteries and one umbilical vein surrounded by Wharton's jelly, a paucicellular connective tissue matrix. Its outer surface is lined by a layer of cuboidal amniotic epithelium.

The placental disk is typically oval and microscopically composed of chorionic villi surrounded by maternal blood in the intervillous space. The chorionic villi contain vessels of the fetal circulatory tree embedded in mesenchymal stroma. A layer of cytotrophoblast encompasses the villous stroma, and this is surrounded by a layer of syncytiotrophoblast that is in contact with the intervillous space. The maternal surface of the placental disk, which is adjacent to the uterine wall, contains variable amounts of fibrin, intermediate trophoblast, and decidua. The umbilical cord inserts near the center of the placental disk, and branches of the umbilical cord vessels arborize over the shiny fetal surface of the disk. Microscopically, the fetal surface of the disk is lined by amnion and chorion.

II. **GROSS EXAMINATION, TISSUE SAMPLING, AND HISTOLOGIC SLIDE PREPARATION**
   A. **Fetal membranes.** The fetal membranes should be assessed for completeness. The presence of green, blue, or brown staining, indicating meconium or hemosiderin staining, should be noted. The membranes should be inspected for amniotic bands, nodules of amnion nodosum or squamous metaplasia, and hemorrhage. A strip of membranes should be cut from the rupture site to the disk insertion site, one end grasped by a forceps and the strip rolled around the forceps. This membrane roll should be eased off the forceps into formalin. At least one cross-section of this membrane roll should be examined.
   B. **Umbilical cord.** The length of the cord is measured, including any detached segments. The distance from the insertion to the disk edge should be measured. Note should be made of marginal insertion (at the disk edge), or velamentous/membranous insertion (into the membranes). Abnormalities of cord color (meconium staining) should be noted. Focal abnormalities such as stricture, hematoma, knots, nodules, plaques, or amniotic bands should be noted and measured. Cross-sections should be made at regular intervals throughout the cord length. The number of vessels and the presence of thrombi should be noted. At least two cross-sections of cord should be examined microscopically, avoiding the area just above the insertion site where the two umbilical arteries fuse.
   C. **Disk.** The disk should be assessed for completeness and measured in three dimensions. After examining and removing the membranes and cord, the unfixed disk should be weighed. The fetal surface of the disk, which is covered by amnion and chorion, is examined for the same abnormalities as the membranes. The branches of the umbilical cord vessels are examined for lacerations, calcifications, and thrombi. The maternal surface of the disk is examined for retroplacental hematomas,

indentations, or other focal abnormalities. The disk is then sliced at 1-cm intervals, and each slice is examined and palpated. The color, location (central vs. peripheral), size, texture (firm vs. spongy), demarcation (whether well-circumscribed or ill-defined), and number of all focal lesions are recorded. An estimate of the percentage of the placental parenchyma involved by each type of process is made and noted. Any organized blood clot in the container is measured. At least two sections of central placenta that include fetal and maternal surfaces should be examined microscopically. Additional sections of focal lesions should be submitted.

D. **Multiple gestation.** Placentas from twin gestations may have completely separate disks, a fused disk with two gestational sacs, or a fused disk and just one gestational sac (monoamniotic). If present, the dividing membranes should be inspected. The percentage of placental parenchyma associated with each twin should be determined. A roll of the dividing membranes should be made as for the fetal membranes, and at least one cross-section of the roll should be examined microscopically to confirm the gross and ultrasound impression of chorionicity. The chorionic plate vessels should be inspected for anastomoses. The type of anastomoses (artery to artery, artery to vein, vein to vein) should be recorded, keeping in mind that arteries cross over veins. Note should be made of large vessels that do not have a pair in the other placental vascular territory as these likely represent areas of physiologically important deep artery-to-vein anastomoses.

III. DIAGNOSTIC FEATURES OF COMMON DISORDERS OF THE PLACENTA
A. Fetal membranes
1. **Meconium.** With recent meconium passage the fetal plate and membranes will be green or blue. The membranes are often slimy. With longstanding meconium passage, the membranes, fetal plate, and even the umbilical cord will be dull brown. Microscopically, the amniotic epithelium is stratified and tufted with pyknotic nuclei. There is marked edema between the amnion and chorion. Macrophages in this area are filled with yellow-brown, waxy, meconium pigment (e-Fig. 37.1).* Pigmented macrophages may also be seen in the chorion and decidua.
2. **Hemosiderin deposition** may stain the fetal plate and membranes brown or green. Often there is old blood clot where the disk meets the fetal membranes. Circumvallation (see section on implantation disorders below) may also be present. Microscopically, the membranes do not show the epithelial stratification, tufting, and edema seen with meconium. Membrane macrophages contain refractile pigment that is positive with an iron stain. Diffuse chorioamniotic hemosiderosis is an indication of chronic peripheral separation and is associated with oligohydramnios in the absence of membrane rupture, preterm delivery, and chronic lung disease.
3. **Amnion nodosum** forms small, gray-white, discrete nodules or plaques that may be anywhere on the cord or fetal membranes but are most common on the fetal plate near the cord insertion. These nodules, which represent vernix caseous, are easy to remove with a cotton swab. Microscopically they consist of fetal squamous cells, amniotic epithelial cells, and sometimes fetal hair (e-Fig. 37.2). Sometimes nodules of amnion nodosum become re-epithelialized by contiguous amniotic epithelium.

    Amnion nodosum is the result of oligohydramnios. It therefore serves as a marker of conditions such as renal agenesis that may cause decreased fluid production, and can also alert to possible complications of oligohydramnios such as pulmonary hypoplasia.
4. **Squamous metaplasia.** Plaques or nodules of squamous metaplasia are present in nearly every placenta. Squamous metaplasia is not clinically significant.
5. **Amniotic bands** may appear as shredded amnion on the fetal surface of the placenta or as thin adhesionlike threads connecting one part of the fetal plate to another, connecting the fetal plate to the umbilical cord, or attached to the fetal digits or other fetal parts. Microscopically they are composed of fibrous tissue often with no attached amnion. Amniotic bands are associated with a wide variety

---

*All e-figures are available online via the Solution Site Image Bank.

of abnormalities in the fetus including digital amputations (e-**Fig. 37.**3), cleft lip and palate, and body-wall defects. Characteristically, the defects are asymmetric, no two cases are identical, and the spectrum of defects in any given case does not fit into a recognizable genetic syndrome.

   6. Fetus papyraceous. Occasionally a mummified remnant of an embryo from much earlier in gestation will be compressed on the fetal membranes. This is referred to as fetus papyraceous. It may represent an unrecognized twin gestation or may be the result of selective termination of a higher order gestation.

B. Umbilical cord

   1. Length abnormalities. The normal umbilical cord is 55 to 60 cm long. Short cords (<35 to 40 cm) make up about 5% of cords; they are usually associated with conditions of decreased fetal movement such as amniotic bands, oligohydramnios, body-wall defects, fetal neuromuscular disorders, and arthrogryposis. Long cords (>80 cm) occur in about 5% of cords; long cords are associated with an increased likelihood for encirclement around the fetal neck or other body part, knots, cord prolapse, and marked cord twisting.

   2. Single umbilical artery (SUA). The incidence of SUA (e-**Fig. 37.4**) is about 1%, and SUA is about 4 times more common in twins. There is a strong association between SUA and congenital malformations, mortality, and low birth weight. SUA is likely an acquired defect as the incidence is lower earlier in gestation; in fact, the absence of the artery may be the cause of associated malformations. In some cases of SUA, a small, atrophic remnant of the second artery can be seen. SUA is also strongly associated with other cord and placental abnormalities such as velamentous insertion, marginal insertion, extrachorialis, and shape abnormalities.

   3. Abnormal cord insertion

      a. Marginal insertion. In marginal insertion, the umbilical cord inserts at the edge of the disk. This occurs in from 6% to 18% of placentas and is not clinically significant.

      b. Velamentous insertion. In velamentous insertion, the umbilical cord inserts into the fetal membranes. This insertion abnormality is seen in about 1% of placentas. In about 75% of cases, the vessels branch within the membranes before the branches insert into the placental disk; in 25% of cases the cord vessels run through the membranes without branching. Because the branches of the umbilical cord are not protected by Wharton's jelly, they are at risk for compression, thrombosis, and laceration.

   4. Umbilical cord knots. About 1% of umbilical cords have a true knot (e-**Fig. 37.5**), which may be loose or tight. Differences in the diameter and color of the cord on either side of the knot should be noted. Cords with size differences, particularly with a dusky appearance between the knot and the fetus, are likely to be associated with an adverse outcome. The cord on either side of the knot should be examined microscopically for thrombi, a feature that suggests a clinically important knot. The knot should be untied in the fresh state to look for persistent grooving of Wharton's jelly, a feature that suggests chronic tightening. The fetal mortality rate for umbilical cord knots is between 5% and 11%.

   5. Umbilical cord coiling. The normal cord has a left-handed twist, a feature that is thought to increase turgor, preventing compression of cord vessels. A coiling index can be determined by counting the number of complete turns divided by the length of the cord and comparing this to a standard reference. About 5% of cords will have no twist, a finding that has been correlated with increased fetal mortality, operative delivery for fetal distress, abnormal karyotype, preterm delivery, and fetal heart rate abnormalities. Hypocoiled cords, with a coiling index below the 10th percentile, and hypercoiled cords, with a coiling index above than 90th percentile, have also been associated with a variety of adverse outcomes.

   6. Umbilical cord stricture is a focal area of cord that is markedly narrowed with a depletion of Wharton's jelly, fibrosis, and often thrombosis of the umbilical cord vessels. The most common location for a stricture is the area adjacent to the umbilicus. There is a high association between cord stricture and stillbirth, especially early in gestation. Most cases also show excess twisting.

7. **Umbilical cord hematomas** occur once in every 5,500 deliveries, although recently small hematomas have been documented in 1.5% of cases following ultrasound-guided cord blood sampling. Hematomas nearly always occur in the portion of cord closest to the fetus and present as a fusiform swelling with a dark, hemorrhagic color. It is important not to confuse a true hematoma, which will be obvious at the time of delivery, with blood accumulation in the cord as a result of clamping, blood drawing, or other manipulation during or after delivery. Large hematomas have a perinatal mortality rate of 50%, whereas small ones have very low fetal morbidity or mortality.

C. Circulatory disorders

1. **Infarcts** are firm and well circumscribed, with one edge usually abutting the maternal surface of the disk (e-Fig. 37.6). Early infarcts are red whereas older ones are white. Sometimes there is central hemorrhage. Microscopically, there is collapse of the intervillous space, which crowds the villi together (e-Fig. 37.7). Depending on the age, the trophoblast may be pale and degenerative (recent) or there may be little staining at all with only ghost outlines of villi (longstanding).

   Infarcts are common, occurring in 10%–25% of term placentas from normal pregnancies, typically at the periphery. Extensive infarction, infarcts >3 cm, infarcts that occur in the central placenta, and infarcts in the first or second trimester of pregnancy are clinically significant and often indicate significant underlying maternal disease such as pre-eclampsia, collagen vascular disease, or a hereditary thrombophilic condition. Infarcts are caused by an interruption in the maternal blood supplied by a given spiral artery to an area of placental tissue.

   The normal placenta can lose 15%–20% of the parenchyma without adversely affecting the fetus. However, in placentas that are chronically underperfused, such as in pre-eclampsia, a lesser degree of infarction may be clinically significant. Extensive infarction may cause fetal hypoxia, intrauterine growth restriction, periventricular leukomalacia in preterm infants, or fetal death.

2. **Massive perivillous fibrin deposition.** When large amounts of fibrin are deposited in the placenta, a firm, white or yellow, slightly gritty, ill-defined mass forms (e-Fig. 37.8). Often small pockets of red, villous tissue are interspersed within strands of white fibrin. Microscopically there is expansion of the intervillous space by eosinophilic fibrinoid material pushing the villi away from each other (e-Fig. 37.9). Often clusters of cytotrophoblast proliferate in the fibrinoid material. The villi entrapped in this fibrinoid material become ischemic. The amount of fibrin deposition needed to make this diagnosis or to be associated with an adverse outcome for the fetus is not well established. Massive perivillous fibrin is associated with intrauterine growth retardation, periventricular leukomalacia in preterm infants, and fetal death, and may recur in subsequent pregnancies.

3. **Maternal floor infarct.** The term maternal floor infarct is a misnomer in that it is a form of fibrin deposition, not infarction. It is defined as perivillous fibrin deposition surrounding at least one third of the villi adjacent to the basal plate, often with extension of fibrin into the underlying decidua. An alternative definition is that basal villi of the entire maternal floor be encased in fibrin at least 3 mm thick on at least one slide. As in massive perivillous fibrin deposition, the villi in maternal floor infarct that are surrounded by fibrin undergo ischemic changes.

   Maternal floor infarct is quite uncommon, seen in far fewer than 1% of placentas. It is associated with stillbirth, intrauterine growth retardation, preterm delivery, and neurodevelopmental impairment. It may recur in subsequent pregnancies.

4. **Subchorionic fibrin deposition** is common and appears as firm, oval, tan-white, slightly raised plaques of the fetal surface of the placenta, beneath the amnion and chorion. On cut section, it is laminated and clearly beneath the

membranes but above the villous tissue (e-**Fig. 37.10**). Microscopically, sections show layers of blood and fibrin beneath the chorion. Subchorionic fibrin plaques are not clinically significant.

5. **Retroplacental thrombohematomas** occur in about 4.5% of placentas. They are organized blood clots beneath the maternal surface of the placenta that indent that surface. Recent retroplacental hematomas are soft, red, and easily dislodged, and are often seen in the specimen container rather than adherent to the placenta by the time the placenta arrives in the laboratory. Older hematomas are firm, brown, and densely adherent with definite indentation (e-**Fig. 37.11**). Microscopically, retroplacental hematomas consist of organized blood clot and fibrin. The underlying placental parenchyma may be infarcted depending on how long the hematoma has been present. Sometimes the villi immediately beneath the thrombohematoma exhibit villous stromal hemorrhage in which the vessels are disrupted and the stroma contains extensive red cells.

Retroplacental hematoma is an important cause of stillbirth. Although retroplacental hematoma and the clinical syndrome of placental abruption share many of the same risk factors, in only a third of cases with clinically identified abruption will a retroplacental hematoma be found on placental examination, and in only a third of cases where retroplacental hematoma is identified on placental examination will there be a history of placental abruption.

6. **Intervillous thrombohematomas** are very common lesions, seen in up to 50% of normal placentas and 78% of placentas from complicated pregnancies. They are well-circumscribed, round to oval, very firm lesions with a laminated cut surface (e-**Fig. 37.12**). Recent intervillous thrombohematomas are red, whereas older ones are white. They are located midway between the fetal and maternal surfaces. Microscopically they are composed of layers of red cells and fibrin devoid of villi. A thin rim of infarcted villous tissue may be present at the periphery.

The blood in intervillous thrombohematomas is of both maternal and fetal origin, and so they serve as markers of fetomaternal hemorrhage. There is a very good correlation between the number of intervillous thrombohematomas in the placenta and the degree of fetomaternal hemorrhage as measured by the Kleihauer–Betke test on maternal blood. Fetomaternal hemorrhage may be associated with fetal anemia, fetal thrombocytopenia, fetal death, and maternal sensitization to fetal antigens that she does not express.

7. **Subamniotic hematomas** are liquid collections of blood that pool between the amnion and chorion of the fetal plate. Microscopically they may be difficult to demonstrate as the blood drains out once a cut is made. Subamniotic hematomas are thought to result from trauma to chorionic plate vessels when traction is placed on the cord during delivery of the placenta. Because this occurs after delivery of the infant it is not usually clinically significant.

8. **Marginal hematomas** occur in about 2% of placentas. They are wedge-shaped collections of blood at the margin of the placenta where the fetal membranes meet the placental disk. Often there is blood clot beneath the free membranes in this area. Sometimes a thin layer of blood forms on the adjacent maternal surface of the placenta, but it does not indent or infarct the placenta and therefore it is not clinically significant.

9. **Massive subchorial thrombosis** (Breus' mole) is a very rare condition, occurring in fewer than 1 in 1000 placentas. It is defined as a red thrombus measuring at least 1 cm in thickness immediately beneath the chorionic plate. Microscopically, sections show an organizing blood clot. The pathogenesis of this rare condition is uncertain.

10. **Fetal thrombotic vasculopathy.** Occlusion of vessels in the fetal circulatory system can involve the large umbilical cord vessels, the chorionic plate vessels, or the smaller fetal vessels within the chorionic villi. Because during gestation there is one continuous circulation between the fetus and the placenta, thrombotic lesions in the placenta, particularly when extensive, may serve as a marker for thrombotic or embolic lesions in the circulation of the fetus itself.

The prevalence of fetal thrombotic vasculopathy is not known. On gross examination, collections of avascular terminal villi appear as well-circumscribed pale areas of parenchyma of varying sizes that retain the same spongy consistency as the surrounding placental tissue (e-Fig. 37.13). Microscopically, these areas appear as villi with dense, eosinophilic, nearly acellular stroma with an absence of vessels (e-Fig. 37.14). The villi are normally spaced without collapse of the intervillous space. A second pattern, formerly termed hemorrhagic endovasculitis but now referred to as villous stromal-vascular karyorrhexis, is characterized by karyorrhexis of fetal cells such as endothelium, stromal cells, or blood cell elements. In this pattern, the villi are more cellular than in avascular terminal villi, with degenerating fetal capillaries and fragmented red cells. Fetal vascular obstruction in the placenta is usually related to stasis, hypercoagulability, or vascular damage.

11. **Chorangiomas** are placental hemangiomas. They are found in about 1% of placentas and are usually small. Typical chorangiomas are well circumscribed, red or gray, with a firmer consistency than the surrounding parenchyma (e-Fig. 37.15). Sometimes fibrous septae form lobules within the chorangioma. Microscopically, chorangiomas are composed of small capillary-type vessels with a few intermixed larger vessels (e-Fig. 37.16). Occasional cases may be more cellular, show calcification or degeneration, or exhibit some cytologic atypia. They do not undergo malignant transformation. Most chorangiomas are incidental findings with no clinical consequences. Large or multiple chorangiomas may cause polyhydramnios, preterm delivery, antepartum bleeding, hydrops fetalis, fetal anemia or thrombocytopenia, fetal growth restriction, and cardiomegaly. Infants with placentas containing chorangiomas have a higher than expected incidence of hemangiomas elsewhere.

12. **Chorangiosis** is defined as the presence of ≥10 capillaries per terminal villus in 10 terminal villi in at least three different regions of the placenta (e-Fig. 37.17). Care should be taken to distinguish chorangiosis from congestion that makes the vessels appear more prominent.

D. Implantation disorders

1. In **placenta accreta**, the placenta is abnormally adherent. On gross examination, the placenta is often severely disrupted or fragmented due to attempts to remove it manually. Sometimes thick areas of gray myometrial tissue will be visible on the maternal surface. Microscopically, the key feature is an absence of decidua between villi and myometrium.

2. **Placenta extrachorialis.** Usually the fetal membranes insert at the edge of the disk. In placenta extrachorialis the membranes insert away from the disk edge, leaving a portion of the disk uncovered by fetal membranes. There are two types of extrachorialis, and they are best distinguished on gross examination. In circummarginate placentation, the junction between the membranes and the disk is relatively smooth and flat. In circumvallate placentation this junction forms a thick, rolled ridge. A given placenta may exhibit partial or complete extrachorial placentation and may exhibit a combination of circummarginate and circumvallate placentation. The percentage of the disk circumference involved by each type should be recorded.

Circummarginate placentation is not clinically significant. Complete circumvallate placentation is thought to be caused by chronic abruption or peripheral separation at the disk edge.

3. **Shape abnormalities.** The placental disk is usually oval or round. A wide variety of shape abnormalities may be seen, the most common or important of which follow.

   a. **Succenturiate (accessory) lobe.** In about 3%–5% of placentas, a small portion of placenta (the succenturiate lobe) is completely separated from the main disk by membranes devoid of underlying villi. The umbilical cord almost always inserts into the main disk; the branches of the main vessels that supply the succenturiate lobe are at an increased risk of thrombotic events.

b. **Bilobed placenta.** Occasionally the placenta will form two distinct lobes of approximately equal size, usually connected at one edge by villous tissue. The umbilical cord usually inserts between the lobes. The clinical significance of bilobed placenta, if any, has not been established.

E. **Maternal disease.** Many of the most common and clinically important maternal diseases affecting women during pregnancy have the shared feature of low uteroplacental blood flow, which results in a characteristic set of changes in the placenta and a growth-retarded fetus.

1. **Pre-eclampsia** is the most common maternal disease to occur in pregnancy, complicating from 2%–7% of all pregnancies. It is defined as the development of hypertension with proteinuria or generalized edema after 20 weeks' gestation. Eclampsia is diagnosed when seizures occur in the setting of pre-eclampsia. Pre-eclampsia is a leading cause of maternal and fetal morbidity and mortality.

On gross examination, the placentas of pre-eclamptic women are often small. Decidual vasculopathy may be present. (In the placentas of normal women, intermediate trophoblast remodels the intramyometrial segments of the spiral arteries late in the first trimester or early in the second trimester by replacing smooth muscle and elastic tissue with fibrinoid material, converting these vessels into flaccid tubes and thereby dramatically increasing the blood flow to the placenta. In pre-eclampsia, the remodeling of these intramyometrial segments of spiral arteries does not occur.) One form of decidual vasculopathy is absence of this physiologic transformation; this condition can only be diagnosed in the decidual tissue adherent to the maternal surface of the placenta. A second form of decidual vasculopathy is acute atherosis; in this condition the spiral arteries exhibit fibrinoid necrosis, infiltration by lipid-laden macrophages, and often a chronic inflammatory infiltrate (e-Fig. 37.18). Vessels with acute atherosis, while already narrow, often have superimposed thrombi further reducing the blood flow through them. Acute atherosis can be diagnosed in the decidual tissue adherent to the maternal surface of the placenta but is most frequently seen in decidual spiral arteries in the membrane roll.

The villi exhibit changes related to low uteroplacental blood flow. They are small with an increased number of syncytial knots, and exhibit a prominent cytotrophoblast layer, increased villous stroma, and a thickened trophoblastic membrane (e-Fig. 37.19). Placentas from pre-eclamptic women are more likely to have infarcts, and the infarcts are more likely to be larger and/or more numerous. Retroplacental hematomas also have an increased incidence in the placentas of pre-eclamptic women.

The HELLP syndrome (*h*emolysis, *e*levated *l*iver enzyme levels, *l*ow *p*latelet count) and acute fatty liver of pregnancy complicate a subset of pregnancies with pre-eclampsia. Although there is a much higher rate of preterm delivery, fetal mortality, maternal complications, and maternal mortality with these two syndromes compared with pre-eclampsia, the placental findings are not significantly different.

2. **Diabetes.** The placental findings in diabetes are variable because the duration and severity of the disease are highly variable. Women with longstanding diabetes and significant vascular disease may show placental changes similar to those seen in pre-eclampsia. The placentas in the majority of cases, however, are larger and heavier than normal. The microscopic findings are not specific but are characteristic. The villi are often edematous and immature for gestational age. The cytotrophoblast is prominent. There is irregular thickening of the trophoblastic basement membrane. Chorangiosis, avascular terminal villi, and SUA are more common in placentas from diabetic women.

Women with diabetes are more likely to deliver stillborn infants or infants with malformations and/or macrosomia. There is no relationship between these adverse outcomes and the severity of the placental findings.

3. **Maternal thrombophilic disorders.** There is increased interest in the relationship between hereditary thrombophilic disorders (such as protein C and S deficiency, factor V Leiden, and hyperhomocysteinemia) and pregnancy

complications. Although controversial, it appears that various hereditary thrombophilic conditions, alone and in combination, are associated with an increased number and larger infarcts, acute atherosis, spiral artery thrombi, retroplacental hematoma, and fetal thrombotic vasculopathy.

4. **Sickle cell disease.** The placentas from women with sickle cell disease may be small and may have an increased number of infarcts. A characteristic finding is the presence of sickled maternal erythrocytes in the intervillous space (e-**Fig. 37.20**). Sickled maternal red cells may also be seen in the placentas of women with sickle cell trait.

F. **Multiple gestations**
   1. **Types of placentation**
      a. **Diamniotic dichorionic.** In this type of placentation, the placental disks may be completely separate or fused. Each fetus is enveloped by its own gestational sac composed of amnion and chorion. The dividing membranes are thick. Sections show amniotic epithelium from each twin on the outer surfaces with fused chorion from both twins in the middle (e-**Fig. 37.21**).

      Dizygous (fraternal) twins exhibit diamniotic dichorionic placentation, but about 25% of monozygous (identical) twins also exhibit this type of placentation if the blastocyst splits within the first 3 days postfertilization. Because diamniotic dichorionic twins do not share vascular anastomoses, these twins are the least likely to have complications such as fetal loss, preterm delivery, and twin–twin transfusion syndrome (TTTS).

      b. **Diamniotic monochorionic placentation.** In this type of placentation, the placental disks are typically fused. Each fetus is enveloped by its own gestational sac lined by amnion. A chorionic layer surrounds both sacs so that the dividing membranes are composed of only fused amnion from each sac with no chorion in between (e-**Fig. 37.22**).

      Twins with monochorionic placentation are monozygous. This type of placentation is seen in about 75% of monozygous twins and results when the blastocyst splits between 4 and 7 days after fertilization. Twins with monochorionic placentation usually share vascular anastomoses and are therefore at risk for complications such as fetal loss, preterm delivery, and TTTS.

      c. **Monoamniotic placentation.** In monoamniotic placentation, the twins share a gestational sac; therefore, there are no dividing membranes. Twins with monoamniotic placentation are monozygous, but only 1% of twins are monoamniotic. This type of placentation results when the blastocyst splits between 8 and 13 days after fertilization. Monoamniotic twins have a very high rate of complications, with only 50% surviving to term. They share vascular anastomoses, so are at risk for the associated complications noted above for monochorionic twins. In addition, because they share the same gestational sac, these twins have a high rate of umbilical cord accidents.

   2. **TTTS** complicates about 15% of monochorionic twin gestations. It is the result of a chronic imbalance of blood flow across the two placental circulations. The vascular anastomoses normally seen in monochorionic placentas may be artery-to-artery, vein-to-vein, or artery-to-vein. The artery-to-vein anastomoses are usually at the capillary level and are not visible on gross examination, but are the most important physiologically as they allow blood to flow in only one direction and therefore can result in a chronic imbalance of blood flow. Twins with artery-to-artery anastomoses are much less likely to develop TTTS because these anastomoses tend to cancel any circulatory imbalances that occur. Hemodynamic imbalance may also be affected by the type of cord insertion, especially a velamentous cord in the donor twin, and extensive infarction or other abnormalities of the placenta in one twin, with resultant increased placental resistance.

      Often the twins are discrepant in size. The donor twin supplies blood for both twins and is hypovolemic, oliguric, and oligohydramnic. The donor twin may be anemic and hypoglycemic, with small and pale organs. The placental territory of this twin is usually large, bulky, and pale with edematous villi and increased nucleated red cells in fetal vessels. The recipient twin experiences circulatory overload resulting in polyuria, polyhydramnios, and eventually hydrops fetalis; this twin develops heart failure, hemolytic jaundice, and kernicterus, with heavy and congested organs. The placental territory of this twin is small, firm, and congested.

G. Infection. Intrauterine infections can have important consequences for the fetus including abortion, stillbirth, active infection after birth, and long-term sequelae such as cerebral palsy, blindness, deafness, and learning disabilities. There are two patterns of placental infection: ascending and transplacental. Ascending infections are the most common and are typically caused by bacteria. They result in inflammation of the fetal membranes, chorioamnionitis, and inflammation of the umbilical cord (funisitis). Transplacental infections are much less common and may be caused by viruses, protozoa, and some bacteria. The placenta usually shows chronic and sometimes acute inflammation within the villi (villitis). Most villitis, however, does not have an infectious etiology but is rather villitis of unknown etiology (VUE).

1. Ascending infections are caused by aerobic or anaerobic organisms that travel through the cervix or uterine soft tissues to the amniotic cavity. Ascending infections complicate about 4% of term deliveries but a much higher percentage of preterm deliveries. Both the mother and the fetus (after about 20 weeks) respond to the infection. Maternal neutrophils emigrate from vessels in the decidua through the chorion and eventually into the amnion (e-Fig. 37.23). They also marginate from the intervillous space to the subchorionic fibrin under the fetal plate of the placenta, and eventually emigrate through the chorion and amnion of the fetal plate. Fetal neutrophils emigrate from chorionic plate vessels toward the amnion. They also emigrate from the umbilical cord vessels, a process termed funisitis (e-Fig. 37.24). A staging and grading system has been developed to assess the extent and severity of both the maternal and fetal inflammatory response (*Pediatr Dev Pathol.* 2003;6:435–448).

In term gestations there is a relationship between the time elapsed since membrane rupture and the likelihood of developing chorioamnionitis. In preterm gestations it is thought that the chorioamnionitis precedes and contributes to the development of membrane rupture. There is also a relationship between acute chorioamnionitis and adverse fetal outcome such as neonatal sepsis, neonatal pneumonia, cerebral palsy, chronic lung disease, and necrotizing enterocolitis. Some of these complications may be directly related to infection and others to the effect of prematurity, but the fetal response to infection, with release of cytokines and other molecules, also likely plays a role in pathogenesis.

2. Transplacental infections reach the placenta by hematogenous spread from the mother. They are usually caused by viruses or protozoa such as those of TORCH infections (Toxoplasma gondii, rubella, cytomegalovirus, and herpes simplex virus), but some bacteria, most notably *Treponema pallidum* and *Listeria monocytogenes*, may also be spread transplacentally.

The tissue response pattern to infections spread transplacentally is villitis. There are usually no findings on gross examination although occasionally small yellow nodules may be seen. Microscopically, the villi contain an inflammatory infiltrate, usually lymphocytes and histiocytes but occasionally plasma cells and neutrophils (e-Fig. 37.25). Sometimes multinucleated giant cells are seen. Villitis may be necrotizing or nonnecrotizing; necrotizing villitis, in which there is destruction of the trophoblastic membranes with fibrin deposition causing affected villi to agglutinate is most common. This abnormal agglutination, rather than inflammation, is the feature that is most easily recognized on low-power examination. Usually villitis is randomly distributed throughout the placenta, but sometimes villitis only involves the basal villi. There are subtle features that suggest a specific etiology in some cases; some of the most common of these are detailed below.

a. Cytomegalovirus (CMV). On gross examination, the placenta may be small, normal, or enlarged and pale. The characteristic microscopic features are necrotizing lymphoplasmacytic villitis, stromal hemosiderin, necrotizing vasculitis, and areas of villous vessel sclerosis. Cases often show areas of active villitis as well as areas of scarred villi. In about 20% of cases, viral inclusions are seen involving the fetal capillaries, villous stromal cells, or trophoblast (e-**Fig. 37.26**). Immunohistochemistry, in situ hybridization, and polymerase chain reaction (PCR) may all be used to confirm a diagnosis of CMV in cases with a clinical suspicion or suggestive microscopic features.

CMV infections are usually acquired in utero and are more commonly the result of a primary infection rather than reactivation of latent viral infection. Infected women are usually asymptomatic.

b. **Herpes simplex virus** (HSV) infections are typically acquired during delivery through an infected birth canal and therefore usually do not cause abnormalities in the placenta. Occasionally, however, the virus may be transmitted as an ascending infection, causing acute necrotizing lymphoplasmacytic chorioamnionitis with viral inclusions in the amniotic epithelium or acute funisitis. The virus may also be transmitted hematogenously, giving rise to necrotizing or nonnecrotizing villitis. Immunohistochemistry and in situ hybridization may be helpful in confirming infection. Disseminated HSV infection may cause severe disease or death of a newborn.

c. **Parvovirus B19.** On gross examination, the placenta is often large for gestational age and pale, as would be expected in any condition causing fetal anemia. Microscopically, the villi are edematous and there are numerous nucleated fetal red cells in the villous vessels. Many of the red cell precursors contain eosinophilic intranuclear glassy inclusions with peripheral margination of the chromatin (e-**Fig. 37.27**). Immunohistochemistry or in situ hybridization may be useful in confirming the diagnosis.

Parvovirus causes a mild disease with a rash in children and is usually asymptomatic in adults. Pregnant women are more severely affected with a flulike syndrome and polyarthralgia; most fetuses are unaffected by maternal infection. Because red cell precursors, endothelial cells, and cardiac myocytes are specific targets for parvovirus, fetal anemia and eventual hydrops fetalis are the usual causes of death.

d. **Human immunodeficiency virus** (HIV) is usually transmitted from mother to child at delivery or through breastfeeding in the postnatal period. Transplacental transmission is the least common method of spread. The role of the placenta in promoting or preventing the spread of HIV is unclear. There are typically no gross abnormalities. The microscopic features are not specific and are controversial.

e. **Syphilis** is caused by the spirochete *T. pallidum*. Placentas from cases of syphilis may be normal but are often markedly enlarged, bulky, and edematous. Microscopically, many cases show a classic triad of large, hypercellular, immature villi; villous vascular proliferation with perivascular fibroblastic proliferation and medial hypertrophy; and villitis that is usually chronic but may be acute, plasmacytic, or granulomatous. However, this triad is seen in only 43% of cases, although two of the three features is seen in another 47% of cases. In addition to the triad, some cases show necrotizing funisitis or lymphoplasmacytic deciduitis. Special stains for spirochetes may identify organisms although often the number of organisms is very low (e.g., one per slide). PCR identifies cases even when staining is negative.

f. **Toxoplasmosis** is caused by the protozoal organism *Toxoplasma gondii*, and the placental findings in congenital toxoplasmosis are highly variable. The placenta may be normal but is often very large and edematous. Microscopically, the villitis is subtle and nonnecrotizing or results in fibrotic villi. The inflammatory infiltrate is lymphohistiocytic. Occasionally, true granulomas are present in the inflammatory infiltrate. In addition to villitis, some cases show a plasmacytic infiltrate in the decidua, chronic chorioamnionitis and funisitis, and thrombosis and calcification of the large vessels of the chorionic plate. The encysted organism may be identified in the cord, membranes, decidua, or villi but it is not associated with inflammation and is very difficult to identify. Tachyzoites released from the cysts cause marked inflammation and necrosis. Immunohistochemistry, immunofluorescence, and PCR may all aid in the diagnosis.

   g. _Listeria monocytogenes._ The pathologic features of listerial infections differ in several respects from those of other transplacental infections. The placenta is typically normal on gross examination but occasional small, yellow-white microabscesses can be seen. Microabscesses, which feature an abundance of neutrophils between the villous stroma and the trophoblast as well as extensive necrosis, are present microscopically. Occasionally palisaded histiocytes and multinucleated giant cells will be seen. Usually acute chorioamnionitis is also present. The organism is a small rod-shaped or curved gram-positive coccus that can be found in amniotic epithelial cells, and immunohistochemistry may be more sensitive than routine special stains for its identification.

   Listeria can have devastating consequences for the fetus. It may cause spontaneous abortion prematurity, neonatal sepsis, meningitis, and death. Infections at birth are typically associated with sepsis and death.

3. VUE. In most cases of villitis, an infectious etiology is not identified; serologic studies of both the infant and mother can be used to exclude many infectious causes if clinically indicated. These cases are referred to as VUE. Most cases of VUE are seen in the third trimester. The placenta is normal on gross examination. Microscopically about 85% of cases are very mild or mild; most are necrotizing and have a lymphohistiocytic inflammatory infiltrate. Sometimes there is vasculitis of the stem villus vessels with associated downstream avascular terminal villi. The inflammatory cells in VUE are of maternal origin.

   There are two theories about the pathogenesis of VUE. One theory proposes that VUE is a response to an unrecognized infectious agent, although many cases have been studied with increasingly sophisticated techniques and no agent has been identified. The other theory proposes that VUE is an immunologic phenomenon, specifically a host-versus-graft reaction; the maternal origin of the inflammatory cells, the tendency of VUE to recur, and the increased incidence of autoimmune diseases in the mother all support this theory.

   In most cases of VUE, the fetus is unaffected. Adverse fetal outcomes in the form of intrauterine growth restriction, oligohydramnios, and perinatal mortality are related to the severity of the villitis.

SKIN: NONNEOPLASTIC DERMATOPATHOLOGY 38

Kimberley G. Crone and Anne C. Lind

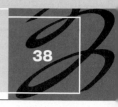

I. NORMAL MICROANATOMY. Microscopically, the skin is composed of three compartments: the epidermis (a keratinizing epithelium), the dermis (a connective tissue matrix), and the subcutis (a layer of adipose tissue). Specific features and the relative size of each of these compartments vary with body site and age and reflect the many functions of the skin.

The epidermis, a stratified squamous epithelium, rests on a normally invisible basement membrane. The keratinocytes of the basal layer (stratum basale) have a generative function and are anchored to the basement membrane by hemidesmosomes. Immediately above the basal layer is the variably thick "prickle" or "spinous" cell layer (stratum spinosum). This name refers to the slender eosinophilic processes that extend between adjacent keratinocytes as seen by light microscopy. These processes correspond to the desmosomes or cytoplasmic attachment plaques. Above the spinous layer is the granular layer (stratum granulosum), which features fine intracytoplasmic basophilic keratohyaline granules. The granular cell layer is 1 to 3 cells thick and forms a water-tight barrier. The most mature and outermost cell layer of the epidermis, the cornified layer (stratum corneum), is composed of flat keratinocytes without nuclei.

Cells other than keratinocytes are also present in the epidermis. Melanocytes are located beneath the basal keratinocytes. They are histologically distinct, having a rounded, hyperchromatic nucleus as compared to the more elongated nucleus of the basal keratinocyte. Melanocytes produce melanin, which has an ultraviolet light–protective function. Melanin is packaged in melanosomes that are exported via slender, elongated, dendritic processes that extend between keratinocytes. Langerhans cells, usually histologically invisible, function as antigen presenting cells. Merkel cells, located along the stratum basale and also histologically unrecognized, are likely derivatives of the neuroendocrine system.

Small, slender, regularly spaced downward extensions of the epidermis (rete) divide the superficial dermis into papillae. The papillary dermis, located immediately beneath the basement membrane, is composed of fine collagen and elastic tissue fibers and contains the capillary loops of the vascular plexus. The reticular dermis, with its haphazardly arranged thick collagen bundles and elastic tissue fibers, is separated from the papillary dermis by the superficial vascular plexus. Elastic tissue, a component of both the papillary and reticular dermis, is usually visible only with the aid of special stains. The dermis provides structural support and flexibility to the skin. Adnexal structures (hair follicles, sebaceous glands, eccrine and apocrine glands, and ducts), arrector pili muscles, nerves, and blood vessels are based here.

The subcutis is composed of mature adipose tissue separated into lobules by fibrous septae. The deep vascular plexus separates the subcutis from the reticular dermis.

II. COMMON DESCRIPTIVE TERMS
  A. Acantholysis—Loss of attachment(s) between keratinocytes (e-Fig. 38.1)*
  B. Acanthosis—Thickening of the epidermis (e-Fig. 38.2)
  C. Dyskeratosis—Abnormal keratinization that results in altered eosinophilic cytoplasm; individual dyskeratotic cells may be referred to as Civatte or colloid bodies (e-Fig. 38.3)
  D. Epidermotropism—Migration of malignant cells into the epidermis

---

*All e-figures are available online via the Solution Site Image Bank.

E. Exocytosis—Migration of benign, nonepithelial cells into the epidermis
F. Hypergranulosis—Thickening (increased number of layers) of the granular layer (e-**Fig. 38.4**)
G. Hyperkeratosis—Thickening of the stratum corneum
H. Orthokeratosis—Appropriately mature stratum corneum composed of superficial keratinocytes without nuclei. Seen in a characteristic loose "woven" pattern on nonacral skin, and densely compact on the acral skin of the palms and soles (e-**Fig. 38.5**)
I. Parakeratosis—Abnormally retained keratinocyte nuclei in the stratum corneum (e-**Fig. 38.6**)
J. Spongiosis—Fluid/edema creating a space between adjacent cells in the stratum spinosum, which makes the desmosomes appear prominent (e-**Fig. 38.7**)
K. Vacuolar change—Clearing of basal keratinocyte cytoplasm secondary to inflammation at the epidermal-dermal junction (e-**Fig. 38.8**)

III. GROSS EXAMINATION AND TISSUE SAMPLING. The skin biopsy/excision is generally received in the laboratory in a fixative such as 10% formalin. If special studies are required, a nonfixative preservative (for example, Michel's medium) is required. The gross description should include all pertinent information, including tissue size (length × width × thickness), presence or absence of epidermis, color, presence or absence of hair (especially if from the scalp), and alterations to the epidermal surface (including documentation of the dimensions, color, and distance to the nearest margin of discrete lesions). All surfaces, except the epidermis, must be inked prior to sectioning. Avoiding the use of black ink facilitates interpretation of commonly used special stains and immunostains, natural pigments, and some exogenous pigments. If the clinician has provided orientation for specific margin identification, inking with two or more colors is required.

Shave or punch biopsies with a greatest epidermal dimension < 0.3 cm are submitted for processing without sectioning. Specimens with a greatest epidermal measurement of at least 0.4 cm are sectioned vertically through the epidermis resulting in pieces of relatively uniform thickness (~0.2 to 0.3 cm thick) (Figs. 38.1; 38.2). As seen in Figure 38.1, if an epidermal lesion is present, sectioning that will best represent the lesion and its relationship to the nearest margin is optimal. Biopsy tissue is otherwise sectioned along the longest epidermal axis, thus maximizing microscopic visualization (which is particularly important when incisional/wedge biopsies are performed). Punch biopsies of the scalp for evaluation of alopecia are sectioned horizontally (every 0.2 to

Punch Biopsy

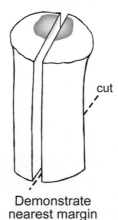

cut

Demonstrate
nearest margin

Figure 38.1. Gross processing of a punch biopsy.

Shave Biopsy

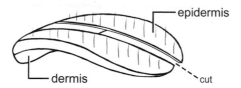

Figure 38.2. Gross processing of a shave biopsy.

0.3 cm) to permit evaluation of follicular density and architecture at various tissue levels (Fig. 38.3). Elliptical biopsies and excisions are approached, in general, in a similar fashion. If an ellipse is oriented by a suture or any other means, inks of different colors are applied to the two long margins to allow specific margin identification under the microscope. Sections of an ellipse should be taken at regular intervals of 2 to 3 mm. Laboratories vary in their handling of the tip ends of ellipses; the recommended method is illustrated in Figure 38.4. To prevent embedding errors, cassettes should never be overcrowded. Sponges can help prevent distortion of the tissue during processing; for example, submit punch biopsies on one sponge, and lay the pieces of a shave biopsy flat between two sponges. If alternative embedding is required, as for alopecia biopsies, clear instructions to the histology technicians are helpful in ensuring appropriate sections.

Frozen sections may be helpful in evaluating margins of cutaneous carcinomas and may (rarely) be requested if a life-threatening condition (such as toxic epidermal necrolysis) requires tissue diagnosis prior to treatment. Frozen sections for diagnosis or margin examination of melanocytic neoplasms are never indicated and may compromise diagnosis based on subsequent permanent sections. The majority of dermatopathology diagnoses are best made on adequately processed, fixed tissue.

IV. **INFLAMMATORY DERMATOSES**
  A. **Lichenoid/interface:** Characterized by basal keratinocyte damage.
    1. **Lichen planus**
      a. **Clinical:** Multiple, flat topped papules and plaques, pruritic, sometimes featuring superficial white lines (Wickham's striae), most common in adults, can involve skin, hair, nails, and mucous membranes.

Punch Biopsy
for Alopecia

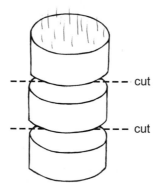

Figure 38.3. Gross processing of an alopecia biopsy.

Unoriented Ellipse   ## Oriented Ellipse

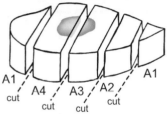 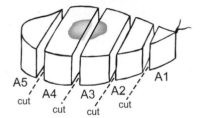

Figure 38.4. Gross processing of an elliptical excision specimen.

   b. Microscopic: Compact hyperkeratosis, acanthosis, band of lymphocytes at the dermal–epidermal junction, dyskeratotic keratinocytes in (Civatte bodies) and under (colloid bodies) the epidermis, rete with a "saw-tooth" pattern, melanophages (e-Fig. 38.9).

2. **Lichen planus-like keratosis**
   a. Clinical: A single red, scaly plaque on sun-damaged skin (arms and chest/shoulders).
   b. Microscopic: Basketweave orthokeratosis with patchy parakeratosis, obscuring band of lymphocytes at the dermal–epidermal junction, flattened/atrophic epidermis sometimes, vacuolar alteration, dyskeratosis, melanophages.

3. **Erythema multiforme/Stevens–Johnson syndrome/toxic epidermal necrolysis**
   a. Clinical: Erythema multiforme is characterized by symmetric, targetoid lesions usually on flexor surfaces and often associated with infection (most commonly herpes simplex virus). Stevens–Johnson syndrome features mucocutaneous erosions. Toxic epidermal necrolysis is a life-threatening mucocutaneous disease, causing sloughing of the epidermis from the dermis over >30% of the body surface area.
   b. Microscopic: Vacuolar alteration of basal keratinocytes, aggregates of dyskeratotic keratinocytes throughout the epidermis, possible subepidermal bulla with full-thickness epidermal necrosis, lymphocytes present in the epidermis and around the superficial vessels (e-Fig. 38.10).

4. **Lupus erythematosus**
   a. Clinical: Lupus can involve the skin only or involve multiple organ systems. Skin findings, which vary with the clinical disease, include a "butterfly"-shaped erythematous rash on the cheeks and nose, scaly erythematous lesions on sun-exposed skin and/or scarring, and alopecic plaques.
   b. Microscopic: The spectrum of changes includes epidermal atrophy, follicular plugging, vacuolar alteration of basal keratinocytes, scattered dyskeratotic keratinocytes, thickened basement membrane, superficial and deep perivascular and periadnexal infiltrate of lymphocytes, some extravasated erythrocytes, and interstitial dermal mucin (e-Fig. 38.11). Direct immunofluorescence usually shows linear–granular immunoglobulin G (IgG), IgM, and/or complement deposition at the basement membrane.

5. **Graft versus host disease (GVHD)**
   a. Clinical: GVHD may be acute (≤90 days after transplantation) or chronic (>90 days after transplantation). Acute GVHD is often a maculopapular rash (palms, soles, head, and neck) and may occur before gastrointestinal or hepatic manifestations. Chronic GVHD may clinically resemble lichen planus (lichenoid GVHD) or morphea (sclerodermoid GVHD).
   b. Microscopic: Acute GVHD shows epidermal atrophy with a spectrum of changes at the basement membrane zone (see grading below). Because the

process is mediated by lymphocytes, lymphocytes in the epidermis and superficial dermis are required for the diagnosis. The histologic changes of acute GVHD are indistinguishable from those seen in response to marrow engraftment (cutaneous eruption of lymphocyte recovery). Grading of acute GVHD is:

Grade 0: No histologic alteration by skin biopsy
Grade 1: Vacuolar alteration
Grade 2: Dyskeratotic keratinocytes
Grade 3: Clefting of the epidermis from the dermis
Grade 4: Complete separation of the epidermis from the dermis

B. Psoriasiform: Characterized by regular elongation of the rete.
  1. Psoriasis
    a. Clinical: Psoriasis has diverse clinical forms (pustular, erythrodermic, guttate), the most common being psoriasis vulgaris, which presents as erythematous plaques with a thick scale on the extensor surfaces (knees, elbows).
    b. Microscopic: Confluent parakeratosis, absent granular cell layer, regular elongation of the rete, neutrophils in the stratum corneum (Munro's microabscess) and stratum spinosum (spongiform pustule of Kogoj), widely dilated papillary dermal vessels, increased mitoses, and a lymphocytic infiltrate in the dermis (e-**Fig. 38.12**).
  2. Lichen simplex chronicus
    a. Clinical: Thick, hyperkeratotic (and sometimes hyperpigmented) plaques, commonly on the back of the neck, extensor forearms, and legs or genital region, caused by chronic rubbing or scratching.
    b. Microscopic: Compact orthokeratosis, a thickened stratum granulosum, thick and elongated rete. The papillary dermis characteristically has collagen fibers that run toward the skin surface ("vertical streaks") (e-**Fig. 38.13**).
  3. Other. Other entities with a psoriasiform pattern include dermatophytosis, pityriasis rubra pilaris, mycosis fungoides, and chronic spongiotic dermatitis.
C. Spongiotic: Characterized by expanded space between adjacent keratinocytes of the spinous layer.
  1. Eczema/atopic dermatitis
    a. Clinical: Erythematous scaly patches or plaques, variable distribution, any age/gender.
    b. Microscopic: Parakeratosis, spongiosis, variable acanthosis, and a superficial perivascular inflammatory infiltrate that may be lymphocytic or mixed with other inflammatory cells such as eosinophils.
  2. Pityriasis rosea
    a. Clinical: Scaly erythematous patches/plaques; classically distributed in a "Christmas tree-like" pattern on the back.
    b. Microscopic: Mounds of parakeratosis, irregular acanthosis, patchy spongiosis, and a mild superficial perivascular lymphocytic infiltrate with extravasated erythrocytes. Prominent exocytosis of lymphocytes is occasionally present (e-**Fig. 38.14**).
  3. Eosinophilic spongiosis
    a. Clinical: Varied, depending on etiology. Etiologies include allergic contact dermatitis, arthropod bite reactions, urticarial phase of pemphigus or pemphigoid, and incontinentia pigmenti.
    b. Microscopic: Spongiosis with exocytosis of eosinophils; the degree of either may vary, and the epidermis may be acanthotic.
  4. Other. Other entities that have a spongiotic tissue pattern include allergic contact dermatitis, irritant contact dermatitis, early and partially treated psoriasis, and mycosis fungoides.
D. Vesiculobullous: Characterized by a vesicle or bullae.
  1. Bullous pemphigoid
    a. Clinical: Tense blisters on an erythematous base, may be pruritic, may be generalized, usually in the elderly. Variants include pemphigoid gestationis,

which occurs in pregnancy, and cicatricial pemphigoid, which has mucosal involvement and resolves with mucosal scarring.

  b. **Microscopic:** Subepidermal vesicle/bulla with a dermal infiltrate of eosinophils. A variant without significant inflammation also occurs. Direct immunofluorescence shows linear deposition of IgG and C3 at the basement membrane zone. Collagen IV can be demonstrated at the floor of the blister by immunoperoxidase or immunofluorescence stains (e-**Fig. 38.15**).

2. **Pemphigus vulgaris**
  a. **Clinical:** Painful oral erosions and flaccid cutaneous blisters that extend easily with lateral pressure (Nikolsky's sign).
  b. **Microscopic:** Suprabasilar acantholysis without dyskeratosis. Direct immunofluorescence shows intercellular IgG and complement. Indirect immunofluorescence may also be useful for diagnosis and to follow response to therapy.

3. **Porphyria cutanea tarda**
  a. **Clinical:** Blistering of sun-exposed skin, especially hands and face; milia (small subepidermal cysts) may develop. Patients may have hypertrichosis.
  b. **Microscopic:** Subepidermal blisters with minimal inflammation. The dermal papillae extend into the blister floor ("festooning"). The thickened vascular basement membrane(s) can be highlighted by periodic acid-Schiff (PAS) stain (e-**Fig. 38.16**).

4. **Epidermolysis bullosa acquisita**
  a. **Clinical:** Blister formation at sites of trauma, generally in adults.
  b. **Microscopic:** Subepidermal bulla with a sparse inflammatory infiltrate. Direct immunofluorescence shows basement membrane linear deposition of IgG and complement as in bullous pemphigoid, however, collagen IV will be seen at the roof of the blister by immunoperoxidase or immunofluorescence stains.

5. **Dermatitis herpetiformis**
  a. **Clinical:** Highly pruritic, small vesicles and/or excoriations on the extensor surfaces (elbows, knees, and buttocks/sacrum) associated with gluten sensitivity.
  b. **Microscopic:** Neutrophils in the dermal papillae with a small subepidermal cleft. Direct immunofluorescence shows granular IgA at the dermal papillae (e-**Fig. 38.17**).

E. **Granulomatous:** Characterized by a variable number and arrangement of epithelioid histiocytes.
  1. **Necrobiotic granuloma**
    a. **Granuloma annulare**
      i. **Clinical:** Clinically variable, may present as annular erythematous lesions, papules, or plaques.
      ii. **Microscopic:** Epithelioid histiocytes palisade around dermal collagen with nuclear drop-out; may be an associated lymphocytic infiltrate, and interstitial mucin may be increased in the center. The interstitial variant has less definitive architectural features. Subcutaneous granuloma annulare has a tumorlike presentation with central necrosis with mucin, palisaded histiocytes, and a hypervascular rim containing chronic inflammatory cells (e-**Fig. 38.18**).
    b. **Necrobiosis lipoidica**
      i. **Clinical:** Depressed, erythematous or yellow plaques with a raised rim/border, usually pretibial; female predilection.
      ii. **Microscopic:** Dermal collagen is fibrotic; alternating layers of fibrosis and histiocytes with plasma cells replace the dermal collagen (e-**Fig. 38.19**).
  2. **Sarcoidal granuloma (sarcoidosis)**
    a. **Clinical:** Highly variable, but with a predilection to areas of cutaneous injury/scars.
    b. **Microscopic:** Naked, noncaseating granulomata are classic. The type of dermal granulomatous inflammation is highly variable in patients with documented systemic sarcoidosis.

F. Vasculopathic: Characterized by damaged/incompetent endothelial cells.
   1. **Acute vasculitis** (leukocytoclastic vasculitis)
      a. Clinical: Palpable purpura, generally on the extremities.
      b. Microscopic: Involves the vessels at the interface of the papillary and reticular dermis (the superficial vascular plexus) with perivascular neutrophils, nuclear debris, fibrinoid necrosis of the vessel walls, and extravasation of erythrocytes. Direct immunofluorescence may be positive (e.g., Henoch–Schoenlein purpura) for IgA and complement (e-Fig. 38.20).
   2. **Neutrophilic dermatosis (Sweet's syndrome)**
      a. Clinical: Erythematous plaques, generally on the upper body.
      b. Microscopic: Diffuse superficial dermal infiltrate of neutrophils; presence or absence of vasculitis and/or folliculitis is controversial.
   3. **Urticaria**
      a. Clinical: Wheals that generally last <24 hours, any body site.
      b. Microscopic: At low power may appear histologically normal; sparse perivascular and interstitial infiltrate of neutrophils, eosinophils, lymphocytes, mast cells, and plasma cells without extravasation of erythrocytes or necrosis. Dermal edema may be noted, and there may be neutrophils in the vascular lumina (e-Fig. 38.21).
   4. **Pigmented purpuric dermatosis/capillaritis**
      a. Clinical: Multiple clinical variants
         i. Schamberg's disease—multiple, small, "cayenne-pepper"-like macules sprinkled on the lower extremities, usually transient and self-limited. Most common in young adults.
         ii. Lichen aureus—solitary or multiple, golden-brown plaques on trunk or extremities, most common in young adults, may persist for years.
      b. Microscopic: Lymphocytes surround the capillaries of the papillary dermis, with scattered extravasated erythrocytes; an iron stain will highlight siderophages. Some vacuolar alteration, as seen in a lichenoid dermatitis, may be present. All variants have similar histology and are distinguishable only by clinical presentation (e-Fig. 38.22).
   5. **Noninflammatory purpura**
      a. Clinical: Purplish/erythematous discoloration of a small (petechia) or large (purpura/ecchymosis) area of skin at any body site. No age/gender predilection.
      b. Microscopic: Erythrocytes in the dermis without associated inflammation; amount/degree varies. In senile purpura, there are telangiectatic blood vessels and, generally severe, solar elastosis (e-Fig. 38.23).

G. Panniculitis: Characterized by inflammatory changes to the septa or lobules of the subcutaneous adipose tissue.
   1. **Erythema nodosum**
      a. Clinical: Single or multiple, painful, erythematous nodules on the anterior lower leg/shin, other sites can be involved; predilection for young adults. This is a cutaneous reaction that is associated with multiple systemic diseases and medications, including inflammatory bowel disease, sarcoidosis, infections (viral, bacterial, and rickettsial), leukemia/lymphoma, antibiotics, salicylates, and oral contraceptives.
      b. Microscopic: Adipose tissue septa are affected, and the lobules are relatively spared; early lesions have neutrophils in the septa, and late lesions have variable numbers of lymphocytes, multinucleate giant cells, histiocytes, and eosinophils; septa become fibrotic over time (e-Fig. 38.24).
   2. **Erythema induratum/nodular vasculitis**
      a. Clinical: Single or multiple erythematous nodules on the posterior lower leg/calf; any age/gender may be affected.
      b. Microscopic: Adipose tissue lobules are infiltrated by histiocytes in well- to poorly-formed granulomata; there may be lymphocytes, neutrophils, and plasma cells. A mixed cellularity vasculitis is usually seen, and some vessels of the subcutis can have the classic alterations of an acute/necrotizing vasculitis.

3. **Subcutaneous fat necrosis of the newborn**
   a. **Clinical:** Firm, sometimes nodular areas in body sites associated with increased adipose tissue (shoulders/buttocks/cheeks) of an otherwise healthy newborn infant. Some infants develop hypercalcemia.
   b. **Microscopic:** Adipose tissue lobules with numerous multinucleate histiocytes that contain classic, radiating, needlelike inclusions; lymphocytes and histiocytes may also be present (e-Fig. 38.25).
4. **Calcifying panniculitis**
   a. **Clinical:** Highly varied depending on the underlying systemic pathology including disorders of coagulation, peripheral vascular disease, localized trauma/inflammation, and calciphylaxis of renal failure.
   b. **Microscopic:** Stippled basophilic calcium deposits in and around vessels that range in size from capillaries to arterioles, with lipophages, variable inflammation, and variable erythrocyte extravasation.
5. **Membranous lipodystrophy**
   a. **Clinical:** Varied pathologic processes/alterations are associated with this histologic alteration.
   b. **Microscopic:** Small cysts in the lobules of the subcutis that have a complex eosinophilic cuticle with frondlike excrescences (arabesque); minimal/no inflammatory response (e-Fig. 38.26).
6. **Other.** Inflammatory and/or structural alterations with varied clinical and histologic presentations can also be seen in the subcutaneous adipose tissue as a result of primary inflammatory dermatoses such as lupus (profundus), human immunodeficiency virus (HIV) infection, pancreatitis, alpha-1 anti-trypsin deficiency, or in response to venous insufficiency, trauma, or infection.

V. COMMON CUTANEOUS INFECTIONS
A. Viral
1. **Molluscum contagiosum**
   a. **Clinical:** Single to multiple, small (1 to 2 mm), umbilicated papules, most common in children and young adults, no site or gender predilection. In immunosuppressed persons, lesions may be numerous and large (>1 cm).
   b. **Microscopic:** Exo-/endophytic, acanthotic, and papillomatous epidermis, with classic homogeneous eosinophilic cytoplasmic inclusions (Henderson–Patterson bodies) that displace and compress keratinocyte nuclei into small peripheral crescents; keratinocyte cytoplasm has a violaceous hue (e-Fig. 38.27).
2. **Verruca vulgaris**
   a. **Clinical:** Single to multiple, hyperkeratotic (verrucous) lesions, no age or gender predilection, occurs most commonly on exposed skin.
   b. **Microscopic:** Compact orthokeratosis with parakeratosis at the peaks of a papillomatous epidermis, hypergranulosis due to increased number and size of irregular keratohyaline granules (viral keratohyaline), keratinocytes with large, irregular hyperchromatic nuclei with a conspicuous perinuclear halo (koilocytes), and elongated rete that bow inward toward the center of the lesion. Any of these alterations can be lost over time (e-Fig. 38.28).
3. **Verruca plana**
   a. **Clinical:** Usually multiple, small, flat-topped, flesh-colored to pink papules; most common on the face and hands, any age/gender; may spread to adjacent skin by trauma such as scratching or shaving.
   b. **Microscopic:** Hyperorthokeratosis (basketweave), hypergranulosis/viral keratohyaline, some scattered koilocytes, epidermal acanthosis with a relatively flat surface and base (e-Fig. 38.29).
4. **Condyloma accuminatum**
   a. **Clinical:** Single or multiple, flesh-colored, papillomatous papules/plaques; external genitalia, perineum, and anus.
   b. **Microscopic:** Variable parakeratosis with compact orthokeratosis, acanthosis with mild papillomatosus, viral keratohyaline, and koilocytes in varying

amounts. If dysplasia/dysmaturation of the keratinocytes is noted, testing for high risk human papilloma virus (HPV) serotypes (e.g., serotypes 16 and 18) can be performed. Striking cytologic atypia can also be incited by topical treatment with agents such as podophyllin (e-**Fig. 38.30**).

5. **Myrmecia/deep palmoplantar wart**
   a. **Clinical:** Single to multiple, small, hyperkeratotic, variably papillomatous; restricted to acral or periungual skin (hands/feet).
   b. **Microscopic:** Exo-/endophytic, compact hyperortho- and parakeratosis, viral keratohyaline, prominent basophilic nuclei, koilocytes, multiple large irregular eosinophilic cytoplasmic inclusions; nuclear size is not affected by the viral inclusions, and the nucleus is not displaced by the inclusions (e-**Fig. 38.31**).

6. **Herpes (herpes simplex virus/varicella zoster virus)**
   a. **Clinical:** Variable.
      i. Primary varicella—Vesicles on an erythematous base with eventual crusting; highly pruritic, lesions appear in crops, most commonly seen in children.
      ii. Primary herpes simplex—Grouped vesicles on a hemorrhagic base with ulceration/crusting; painful.
      iii. Recurrent varicella (zoster)—Most commonly restricted to a dermatome (an area innervated by one nerve); may otherwise appear similar to herpes simplex infection.
      iv. Herpes folliculitis—Painful, erythematous nodules.
   b. **Microscopic:** Acantholysis, dyskeratosis, multinucleate keratinocytes with irregularly shaped nuclei, chromatin displaced to the nuclear membrane by central homogeneous basophilic material that corresponds to the viral protein. Neutrophils, hemorrhage, and necrosis are invariably present, but variable in amount. In herpes folliculitis, similar changes are restricted to some portion of the hair follicle epithelium, and the epidermis is usually spared (e-**Fig. 38.32**).

B. **Fungal.** The most common fungal organism present on the surface of the skin is the yeast form of *Malassezia* sp. (*pityrosporum*). These small, ovoid forms in the stratum corneum are incidental findings and, unless seen deep in the hair follicle and associated with inflammation, are usually not reported.

1. **Dermatophytosis**
   a. **Clinical:** Variable.
      i. Tinea corporis—Annular, erythematous plaques with scale; any site/age/gender.
      ii. Tinea capitis/tinea barbae—Folliculitis of scalp or face.
      iii. Tinea faciei—Facial erythema and scaling.
      iv. Tinea pedis/athlete's foot—Erythematous pustules on feet.
      v. Onychomycosis—Thickened and/or discolored nails.
   b. **Microscopic:** Fungal hyphae are present in the stratum corneum, usually/often visible without the use of special stains such as Gomori methenamine silver (GMS)/PAS. All other changes are highly variable, including parakeratosis, intracorneal neutrophils, and dermal inflammation. Clippings of nails for the evaluation of fungal nail infections/onychomycosis are processed after softening in a phenol solution (such as a depilatory) and should always be stained for organisms because the hyphae are usually invisible without special stains (e-**Fig. 38.33**).

2. **Angioinvasive fungus**
   a. **Clinical:** Necrotic papules/plaques in severely immunosuppressed persons; frequent, but not invariable, systemic symptoms.
   b. **Microscopic:** Ischemic necrosis of the epidermis and superficial dermis; extravasation of erythrocytes; fungal hyphae present in mid to deep dermal blood vessels of all sizes with extension through the vascular wall; inflammation type and amount highly variable and may be absent (e-**Fig. 38.34**).

3. Dematiaceous fungus

a. Clinical: Variable from scaly and erythematous to nodular and verrucous; often at sites of trauma or implantation of vegetable matter, such as a wood splinter.

b. Microscopic: Pseudocarcinomatous epidermal hyperplasia and/or ulceration; mixed acute, chronic, and granulomatous inflammation; brown/golden hyphae and spore forms (Medlar bodies/"copper pennies") readily apparent (e-**Fig. 38.35**).

VI. DERMAL DEPOSITS

A. Myxoid

1. Myxoma

a. Clinical: Usually solitary, flesh-colored, papule or nodule; most common in adults, with no site predilection.

b. Microscopic: Pools of acellular, hypovascular, wispy blue material in the papillary and/or reticular dermis; usually moderately well circumscribed but not encapsulated. Stains such as colloidal iron or alcian blue at low pH can be used to confirm the presence of interstitial mucin (e-**Fig. 38.36**).

2. Digital mucous cyst

a. Clinical: Solitary dome-shaped papule or nodule that may appear cystic, on the distal finger/toe in proximity to joint or nail; middle-aged to elderly adults, slightly more common in women.

b. Microscopic: Compact hyperorthokeratosis with variable other epidermal change(s); acellular, wispy blue material in the papillary dermis; there may be cystic degeneration.

3. Calcinosis cutis

a. Clinical: Varied, ranging from small firm papules, to plaques, to tumor nodules.

b. Microscopic: Basophilic deposits usually in the dermis, varying from small areas with a cracked geographic appearance, to large, well-circumscribed pools with less intense basophilia and a homogeneous appearance (e-**Fig. 38.37**).

4. Osteoma cutis

a. Clinical: Highly varied. One common variant presents as multiple, firm papules, most common on the face at the sites of acne scars; may be seen as a secondary change in cysts, benign cutaneous neoplasms, or malignant cutaneous neoplasms.

b. Microscopic: Trabecular bone with fatty replacement of the marrow cavity and/or hematopoiesis; osteoblasts in Haversian canals; sometimes osteoclasts (e-**Fig. 38.38**).

VII. KERATINOUS CYSTS. Keratinous cysts are epithelial-lined cystic structures in the dermis and/or subcutis. They vary in manner of keratinization and/or cyst contents.

A. Infundibular type

1. Clinical: Solitary, slow growing, dome-shaped, mobile nodule with a small opening to the skin (punctum); most common on the face, neck, and trunk.

2. Microscopic: Lined by stratified squamous epithelium with orthokeratotic (basketweave) keratin and an intact granular layer, but devoid of rete. The cyst contains laminated loose keratin (e-**Fig. 38.39**).

B. Trichilemmal type (pilar)

1. Clinical: Solitary or multiple, smooth, mobile, firm nodule(s); most common on the scalp of females.

2. Microscopic: Lined by stratified squamous epithelium with an abrupt transition to compact orthokeratotic keratin; granular layer is absent or minimally present; keratinocytes grow larger towards the lumen. The cyst contains compact eosinophilic keratin, which may be focally calcified (e-**Fig. 38.40**).

C. Steatocystoma

1. Clinical: Uncommon, solitary (simplex) or multiple (multiplex) smooth, firm, yellow or skin-colored cystic papules and nodules; most common on the trunk and proximal extremities.

2. **Microscopic:** An undulating cyst lined by a thin, stratified squamous epithelium that is covered by a homogeneous eosinophilic cuticle; sebaceous glands may communicate with the cyst cavity, which is usually devoid of contents (e-Fig. 38.41).

D. **Vellus hair cyst**
   1. **Clinical:** Multiple, small, asymptomatic skin-colored papules; most common on the chest and axillae of children or young adults.
   2. **Microscopic:** Small cyst lined by stratified squamous epithelium showing either epidermal or trichilemmal keratinization; contains multiple small vellus hairs intermixed with keratin (e-Fig. 38.42).

VIII. **DISORDERS OF COLLAGEN AND ELASTIN**
   A. **Morphea/localized scleroderma**
      1. **Clinical:** One or more depressed, firm, slightly erythematous, or violaceous plaques; most common on the trunk or extremities in children or young adults, slight female predominance.
      2. **Microscopic:** Thick hypocellular collagen bundles replace the usual haphazardly arranged reticular dermal collagen; adipose tissue around eccrine coils may be absent, arrector pili muscles may hypertrophy, dermal–subcutaneous interface is flattened; plasma cells may be present and, in early-stage/inflammatory-stage morphea, deep interstitial plasma cells may be the only alteration (e-Fig. 38.43).
   B. **Lichen sclerosus et atrophicus**
      1. **Clinical:** Slightly depressed, pale patches/plaques with a tissue paper-like surface; preferentially involves the female genitalia; more common past middle age; extragenital lesions most common on hair-bearing skin. Called *balanitis xerotica obliterans* when the glans penis/prepuce is affected.
      2. **Microscopic:** Compact hyperkeratosis, epidermal atrophy, homogenization/pallor of the papillary dermal collagen, which is acellular but contains prominent dilated vessels. Evidence of a pre-existing lichenoid infiltrate may be seen as a band of lymphocytes with melanophages beneath the altered collagen (e-Fig. 38.44).
   C. **Pseudoxanthoma elasticum**
      1. **Clinical:** Small, flesh-colored papules with the appearance of plucked chicken skin, most common on the neck/axillae; may be associated with retinal changes (angioid streaks) and incompetence of blood vessels manifested by hypertension, cerebrovascular accidents, and sudden cardiac death. Involvement of the vessels of the gastrointestinal system may result in bleeding/hemorrhage. Hereditary, with both autosomal dominant and recessive forms that map to chromosome 16. A nonhereditary, acquired variant affects only the skin and is most common in the periumbilical region of obese multigravida women.
      2. **Microscopic:** Short, coiled, beaded basophilic/amphophilic elastic tissue fibers are present in the superficial reticular dermis (e-Fig. 38.45).
   D. **Solar elastosis**
      1. **Clinical:** Wrinkled skin at sites of extensive sun exposure, usually seen in the elderly or in persons with excess exposure to ultraviolet light.
      2. **Microscopic:** Amorphous, acellular basophilic material replaces the papillary and superficial reticular dermis (e-Fig. 38.46).

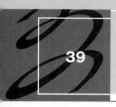

39 NONMELANOCYTIC TUMORS OF THE SKIN
Nathan C. Walk, Anne C. Lind, and Dongsi Lu

I. BENIGN TUMORS OF THE EPIDERMIS
A. Seborrheic keratosis
1. **Clinical:** Single or multiple discrete papules or plaques, typically measuring 0.5 to 1.0 cm, variably pigmented and with a "stuck-on" appearance, only on hair-bearing skin; most commonly found in people >30 years of age.
2. **Microscopic:** Endophytic or exophytic lesion sharply demarcated from adjacent epidermis, composed of basaloid and often homogeneous cells mixed with squamoid cells. Intraepidermal pseudocysts filled with loose orthokeratotic keratin are usually present. There are many microscopic patterns of seborrheic keratoses, the most common being hyperkeratotic, acanthotic, reticulated, clonal, and irritated (e-Fig. 39.1).*

B. Clear cell acanthoma
1. **Clinical:** Uncommon slow-growing, pink to brown, dome-shaped nodule or small plaque, most frequently on the leg of middle-aged and elderly individuals.
2. **Microscopic:** Acanthotic epidermis with a sharply demarcated proliferation of keratinocytes with pale/clear cytoplasm with associated parakeratosis, agranulosis, and neutrophils in the stratum corneum and spinosum (e-Fig. 39.2).

C. Large cell acanthoma
1. **Clinical:** A sharply demarcated, scaly patch on the sun-exposed skin of middle-aged and elderly individuals.
2. **Microscopic:** Sharply demarcated acanthosis, keratinocyte nuclear and cytoplasmic enlargement (about 2× normal), hypergranulosis and hyperorthokeratosis (e-Fig. 39.3).

II. PREMALIGNANT AND MALIGNANT TUMORS OF THE EPIDERMIS
A. Actinic keratosis
1. **Clinical:** Scaly, erythematous papules or nodules on sun-exposed skin of the head and neck, upper and lower extremities; more common in fair-skinned individuals.
2. **Microscopic:** Patchy parakeratosis and agranulosis that often spares adnexal ostia, irregular downward buds of atypical (dysplastic) basal keratinocytes. Dyskeratotic cells are sometimes present. Dysplasia does not involve the full thickness of the epidermis, and solar elastosis is frequently seen (e-Fig. 39.4).
3. **Genetics:** Genetic information is not currently used in the diagnosis of actinic keratoses, and the following is provided for interest only. Approximately 50% of actinic keratoses show *TP53* mutations and overexpression of cyclin D1, whereas 16% have independent activation of *ras*. Loss of heterozygosity at several chromosome arms, including 17p, 17q, 9p, 9q, 3p, and 13q, is noted in many cases.

B. Squamous cell carcinoma in situ (Bowen's disease)
1. **Clinical:** Sharply demarcated, scaly, often hyperkeratotic macule, papule, or plaque; most common in sun-exposed areas (particularly the face and legs); more common in fair-skinned, older individuals.
2. **Microscopic:** Keratinocytes with enlarged, hyperchromatic nuclei and minimal cytoplasm occupy the full thickness of the epidermis, variable acanthosis, hyperparakeratosis, agranulosis, dyskeratosis, mitoses above the basal layer and loss of maturation; the neoplastic cells populate adnexal structures (e-Fig. 39.5).

---

*All e-figures are available online via the Solution Site Image Bank.

3. **Genetics:** Genetic information is not currently used in the diagnosis of squamous cell carcinoma in situ, and the following is provided for interest only. Increased expression and mutation of *TP53* have been observed. Allelic deletion of one or more chromosome 9q markers has also been detected in occasional lesions of Bowen's disease.

C. **Invasive squamous cell carcinoma**
   1. **Clinical:** Early lesions are firm, skin-colored or erythematous nodules; later lesions are shallow ulcers with firm, elevated or indurated surroundings, sometimes with crust or scale; most common in fair-skinned, older individuals in sun-exposed areas and in immunocompromised persons. Metastatic potential depends on location, histology, and precursor lesions/etiology.
   2. **Microscopic:** Acanthosis, invasion of the dermis by individual or nested keratinocytes with variable amounts of cytoplasm and nuclear pleomorphism, dyskeratosis, and swirls of parakeratotic keratin (keratin pearls); there may be dermal desmoplasia and variable inflammation; acantholysis, perineural invasion, and sarcomatoid change predict more aggressive behavior (e-Fig. 39.6).

D. **Basal cell carcinoma**
   1. **Clinical:** Variable presentation; most commonly a dome-shaped, firm papule with a pearly, telangiectatic surface, slow growing, majority on the head, neck, and trunk. The most common skin cancer in Caucasians; rarely metastasizes unless neglected.
   2. **Microscopic:** Variable histology. Common features include basaloid cells with hyperchromatic nuclei and scant cytoplasm, usually connected to an unremarkable or ulcerated epidermis. Basaloid islands show peripheral palisading, mitoses, and apoptosis; a retraction artifact separates the basaloid cells from the surrounding basophilic, variably mucinous, stroma (e-Fig. 39.7).
   3. **Genetics:** Genetic information is not currently used in the diagnosis of basal cell carcinoma, and the following is provided for interest only. Mutations of genes *PTCH1* on chromosome 9q22.3 and *SMD* on chromosome 7q31–32 involved in activating hedgehog signaling pathway have been identified in both sporadic basal cell carcinomas and basal cell nevus syndrome, a rare autosomal dominant disorder.

III. **TUMORS OF THE CUTANEOUS APPENDAGES.** Tumors of the cutaneous appendages have a somewhat nebulous nomenclature. A traditional system organizes the tumors based on their origin from one of the normal cutaneous appendages: hair follicle, sebaceous gland, eccrine gland, or apocrine gland. There are also complex adnexal tumors with abnormalities of two or more of the normal skin constituents, including the epidermis itself. There is sometimes controversy as to a tumor's precise histogenesis (i.e., eccrine versus apocrine, etc.). The following is a succinct review of the major tumors derived from the skin appendages.

A. **Benign appendage tumors.** Benign adnexal tumors have architectural symmetry when viewed at low power and, usually, a distinctive cleft between the stroma of the tumor and the native dermal collagen.
   1. **Hair follicle tumors**
      a. **Trichofolliculoma**
         i. **Clinical:** Rare, solitary, small (<1 cm), skin-colored papule on the face. A tuft of fine hairs protrudes from the center.
         ii. **Microscopic:** One or more cystically dilated hair follicles with radiating follicles that project into a relatively cellular stroma. The secondary hair follicles are of variable maturity and may give rise to more hair follicles (e-Fig. 39.8).
      b. **Trichoepithelioma**
         i. **Clinical:** Usually solitary, skin-colored papule, most common on the central face; if multiple, associated with autosomal dominant (AD) inheritance. The desmoplastic variant is a solitary, firm annular lesion with a raised border and central depression exclusively on the face.

ii. Microscopic: A relatively well-circumscribed dermal tumor composed of islands of basaloid cells with pilar differentiation in a cellular stroma; papillary mesenchymal bodies are characteristic. Small keratinous cysts and foci of calcification are often present. The tumor epithelium may mimic basal cell carcinoma, but there is no retraction artifact or mucinous stroma (e-**Fig. 39.9**). The desmoplastic variant shows a well-circumscribed lesion in the upper and mid-dermis composed of cords or small nests of basaloid cells in a sclerotic stroma (e-**Fig. 39.10**). It may be confused with a syringoma or an infiltrative basal cell carcinoma.

c. Trichoadenoma (of Nikolowski)

    i. Clinical: Rare nodule on the face or buttocks.

    ii. Microscopic: A well-demarcated dermal tumor composed of multiple cyst-like structures lined by multilayered keratinizing pilar-type squamous epithelium. The cysts contain keratinous debris and no hair shafts (e-**Fig. 39.11**).

d. Dilated pore of Winer

    i. Clinical: Common, usually solitary, comedo-like lesion on the head and neck or trunk.

    ii. Microscopic: A cystically dilated hair follicle, filled with loose keratin and lined by acanthotic stratified squamous epithelium with irregular budding (e-**Fig. 39.12**).

e. Trichilemmoma

    i. Clinical: A solitary, small, skin-colored/pink or brown papule on the face and neck; multiple lesions are associated with Cowden's syndrome.

    ii. Microscopic: A well-circumscribed, endo-/exophytic tumor composed of clear squamoid cells with glycogenated cytoplasm. The tumor extends from the epidermis with a lobular configuration. There is a thin, peripheral rim of palisading columnar cells and variable, thick, eosinophilic basement membrane (e-**Fig. 39.13**).

f. Pilomatrixoma (calcifying epithelioma of Malherbe)

    i. Clinical: Firm, deeply located nodule, most common on the face and upper extremities; onset frequently in childhood.

    ii. Microscopic: A sharply demarcated tumor in the lower dermis and, often, the subcutis. The tumor is composed of large, irregularly shaped tumor islands and intervening stroma. Two basic cell types are present: basaloid cells and "shadow" or "ghost" cells. The basaloid cells resemble the cells in basal cell carcinoma and are present at the periphery of the tumor islands. The shadow cells, which have eosinophilic cytoplasm, distinct cell borders, and no nuclear staining, occupy the center of tumor islands. Several layers of transitional cells with intermediate features may be present. In addition, dystrophic calcification, a mixed inflammatory infiltrate, hemosiderin, melanin, bone, and foreign body giant cells can be seen (e-**Fig. 39.14**).

2. Eccrine tumors

a. Syringoma

    i. Clinical: Usually multiple, skin-colored, small, firm papules on the lower eyelids and cheeks, more common in women; onset is often at puberty.

    ii. Microscopic: Multiple small ducts in a dense fibrous stroma in the dermis. The ducts are lined by two layers of cuboidal epithelium, and sometimes are "tadpole" or "commalike." Solid nests and strands of tumor cells can be present (e-**Fig. 39.15**).

b. Eccrine (or apocrine) mixed tumor (chondroid syringoma—eccrine/apocrine type)

    i. Clinical: Solitary, firm, dermal or subcutaneous nodule on the head and neck.

    ii. Microscopic: Well-circumscribed dermal tumor of small epithelial cells in solid nests, small clusters, and ducts in a prominent myxoid, cartilaginous, and/or fibrous stroma (e-**Fig. 39.16**).

c. **Cylindroma**
   i. **Clinical:** Solitary, small nodule on the head and neck of a middle-aged to elderly woman; if multiple, associated with autosomal dominant inheritance, occurring as "turban tumors" on the scalp.
   ii. **Microscopic:** A poorly circumscribed dermal tumor composed of irregularly shaped nests of basaloid cells, surrounded by a thick eosinophilic basement membrane. The cellular nests fit together in a "jigsaw" pattern (e-Fig. 39.17).
d. **Spiradenoma**
   i. **Clinical:** Usually solitary, firm, tender or painful dermal nodule. There is no characteristic distribution; they occur primarily in young adults.
   ii. **Microscopic:** One or more sharply demarcated dermal nodule(s) of basaloid cells. Two types of cells are present: small lymphocyte-like cells with hyperchromatic nuclei and larger basaloid cells with paler nuclei. There may be a thin pseudocapsule, and a few duct-like structures are present (e-Fig. 39.18).
e. **Poroma group (including eccrine poroma, dermal duct tumor, hidroacanthoma simplex)**
   i. **Clinical:**
      a. Poroma—solitary, sessile or slightly pedunculated, pink nodule often on the plantar or palmar skin, or other locations with sweat glands.
      b. Dermal duct tumor—a solitary, firm nodule on the head, neck, and extremities.
      c. Hidroacanthoma simplex—a solitary plaque or nodule on the extremities and trunk; resembles seborrheic keratosis or basal cell carcinoma.
   ii. **Microscopic:**
      a. Poroma—a circumscribed tumor composed of columns of basaloid cells extending from the epidermis into the dermis, with a loose, vascular stroma. Ducts and, rarely, small cysts may be seen in the tumor columns. There is a sharp demarcation from the epidermis (e-Fig. 39.19).
      b. Dermal duct tumor—similar islands of basaloid cells entirely within the dermis. An epidermal connection may be found if multiple sections are examined.
      c. Hidroacanthoma simplex—similar islands of basaloid cells confined to the epidermis.
f. **Acrospiroma (e.g., solid-cystic hidradenoma, apocrine/eccrine hidradenoma, clear cell hidradenoma)**
   i. **Clinical:** Solitary nodule, 0.5 to 2.0 cm or more; no site predilection; disputed histogenesis, so nomenclature for this entity is confusing.
   ii. **Microscopic:** Variable histologic appearance, as reflected by the nosology; usually a circumscribed, nonencapsulated, multilobular, central dermal tumor with variable proportions of cystic and solid areas; tumor cells have variable clear or eosinophilic cytoplasm and are round, fusiform, or polygonal. Ductlike structures are typically present and may have a squamous appearance. The stroma varies from rather fine fibrous tissue to dense hyalinized collagen (e-Fig. 39.20).
3. **Sebaceous hyperplasia and tumors**
   a. **Sebaceous hyperplasia**
      i. **Clinical:** Yellow to whitish papules with central umbilication, typically on the face of older individuals. It may mimic a basal cell carcinoma.
      ii. **Microscopic:** Multiple large, but otherwise normal, sebaceous lobules centered on a large central orifice; solar elastosis is frequently present (e-Fig. 39.21).
   b. **Sebaceous adenoma**
      i. **Clinical:** Rare, solitary or multiple, pink or flesh-colored, usually <1 cm nodule(s) on the face or scalp of adults; may be associated with Muir–Torre syndrome (visceral carcinoma).

ii. **Microscopic:** Multiple, circumscribed sebaceous lobules usually centered in the mid-dermis; composed of peripheral basaloid germinative cells, central mature sebaceous cells, and a variable zone of transitional forms. Mature cells usually outnumber the basaloid cells (e-**Fig. 39.22**).

4. **Apocrine tumors**
   a. **Apocrine hidrocystoma (apocrine cystadenoma)**
      i. **Clinical:** Solitary, translucent to bluish nodule predominantly on the face.
      ii. **Microscopic:** Several large cysts in the dermis; the cyst wall is composed of an outer myoepithelial layer and an inner layer of cuboidal to columnar cells with apocrine decapitation secretion; pseudopapillary projections may be present (e-**Fig. 39.23**).
   b. **Syringocystadenoma papilliferum**
      i. **Clinical:** Varied; most commonly a raised, warty plaque on the scalp; associated with nevus sebaceus in approximately 1/3 of cases.
      ii. **Microscopic:** Deep invaginations of ductlike structures extend from an acanthotic, variably papillomatous epidermis into the dermis; they are lined by squamous epithelium in the upper portion and by two-layered, sweat duct-like epithelium in the lower portion; numerous plasma cells are present in the connective tissue stroma of the papillae (e-**Fig. 39.24**).
      iii. **Genetics:** Genetic information is not currently used in the diagnosis of syringocystadenoma papilliferum, and the following is provided for interest only. Allelic deletions of the patched gene on chromosome 9q22 and loss of heterozygosity of chromosome 9p21 have been reported in syringocystadenoma papilliferum.

5. **Complex adnexal tumors: Nevus sebaceus of Jadassohn (organoid nevus)**
   a. **Clinical:** Solitary, yellow or waxy patch or plaque with alopecia on the scalp (most common), face, neck, or trunk; present at birth or early childhood.
   b. **Microscopic:** A complex hamartoma involving the epidermis, pilosebaceous unit, and ducts/glands. There is variable epidermal acanthosis, papillomatosis, and abnormally formed/abortive hair follicles with bulbs that do not extend into the subcutis; increased numbers of large sebaceous glands are present around and after puberty; dilated apocrine glands are found in up to 50% of cases. Secondary tumors may develop, such as syringocystadenoma papilliferum (e-**Fig. 39.25**).

B. **Malignant tumors of the cutaneous appendages** are rare and far less common than their benign counterparts. As with the benign tumors discussed above, a malignant neoplasm can arise from any of the normal skin appendages, and there may be more than one component to a particular tumor. Only extramammary Paget's disease will be discussed.

1. **Clinical:** A red, scaly plaque, typically in areas rich in apocrine glands such as the anogenital region and, less commonly, the axilla; usually pruritic and slowly spreading. An underlying adnexal carcinoma is present in approximately 20% to 25% of cases; visceral carcinoma (rectal, prostate, bladder, cervix, or urethra) is present in 10% to 15% of cases.

2. **Microscopic:** Similar to mammary Paget's disease, there are large, predominantly intraepidermal, epithelioid tumor cells with large, pleomorphic nuclei and abundant pale cytoplasm that may or may not contain mucin. The tumor cells are concentrated in the lower epidermis and randomly dispersed throughout the epidermis; they may also be seen in the dermis. Special stains may be needed to distinguish extramammary Paget's disease from melanoma in situ and squamous cell carcinoma in situ with pagetoid features. The tumor cells are positive for mucicarmine and periodic acid–Schiff (PAS); immunoreactive for carcinoembryonic antigen (CEA), epithelial membrane antigen (EMA), and low-molecular-weight keratin; and negative for Melan-A/Mart-1 and S-100 (e-**Fig. 39.26**).

IV. **BENIGN AND MALIGNANT TUMORS OF MESENCHYMAL ORIGIN.** Classification of mesenchymal neoplasms is based on the mature, nonneoplastic tissue from which they are believed to derive: blood vessel, nerve, smooth muscle, skeletal muscle, bone, cartilage, fibrous tissue, neuroendocrine tissue, or hematopoietic elements. Many of these tumors are discussed elsewhere in this text (see Chapters 43, 44, and 46 covering soft tissue and hematolymphoid malignancies, respectively), and only the most common entities will be discussed.

A. Vascular tumors

1. **Lobular capillary hemangioma (pyogenic granuloma)**
   a. **Clinical:** Common, rapidly developing polypoid or pedunculated, red, eroded papules or nodules that bleed easily; seen on mucous membranes and skin.
   b. **Microscopic:** An exophytic, frequently ulcerated, proliferation of capillaries divided into lobules by fibrous tissue septae; variably cellular, often surrounded by a collarette of epidermis (e-**Fig. 39.27**).

2. **Arteriovenous hemangioma (acral arteriovenous tumor)**
   a. **Clinical:** A solitary, usually asymptomatic, red or purple, enlarging or bleeding papule, averaging 4 mm in diameter; most common on the lips, perioral skin, nose, and eyelids of middle-aged to elderly men.
   b. **Microscopic:** Well circumscribed, nonencapsulated vascular tumor in the upper to mid-dermis, composed of closely packed, large caliber, thick-walled, and thin-walled vessels (e-**Fig. 39.28**).

3. **"Cherry" angioma (senile angioma, Campbell de Morgan spot)**
   a. **Clinical:** Solitary or multiple tiny, bright red papules, predominantly on the trunk and proximal extremities; common in adults, almost universal in the elderly.
   b. **Microscopic:** Early lesions with one or more dilated interconnecting thin-walled vessels in the papillary dermis. Established lesions are polypoid with an epidermal collarette and are composed of dilated and congested vascular channels in the papillary dermis (e-**Fig. 39.29**).

4. **Angiokeratoma**
   a. **Clinical:** Single to multiple red to black papule(s) or plaque(s) that may be warty or hyperkeratotic; multiple variants exist with characteristic clinical presentations and carrying various eponyms.
   b. **Microscopic:** Markedly dilated and congested papillary dermal vessels form cavernous channels that have an intimate association with the epidermis; irregular acanthosis and variable hyperkeratosis (e-**Fig. 39.30**).

5. **Lymphangioma (cystic lymphatic malformation)**
   a. **Superficial lymphangioma (lymphangioma circumscriptum)**
      i. **Clinical:** Multiple, localized scattered or grouped translucent vesicles or papulovesicles; may be red or purple due to intralesional hemorrhage and thrombus formation; usually congenital, sometimes presents later in childhood and is rare in adults. There may be a deeper component.
      ii. **Microscopic:** Multiple dilated, thin-walled lymphatic channels in the papillary and upper reticular dermis; epidermis is sometimes acanthotic and forms a collarette (e-**Fig. 39.31**).
   b. **Deep lymphangioma (including cavernous lymphangioma and cystic hygroma)**
      i. **Clinical:** Usually solitary, rubbery, skin-colored nodules that may result in swelling of the soft tissue; most common on the face, trunk, and extremities; varies from spongy to a large cystic tumor. Most are present at birth or the first few years of life.
      ii. **Microscopic:** Variable. In general, there are irregularly dilated vascular channels with variable size in the dermis, the subcutis, and deeper tissue. The vessels are thin- or thick-walled, and contain proteinaceous fluid or lymphocytes in the lumen. There is no endothelial atypia or mitosis. The intervening stroma is unremarkable or fibrotic (e-**Fig. 39.32**).

6. **Glomus tumor and glomangioma**
   a. **Clinical:** Painful, solitary or multiple, red to purple subungual macule(s), may be a nodule at other sites. Glomangioma is less painful.
   b. **Microscopic:** Well-circumscribed or encapsulated dermal tumor composed of sheets of glomus cells surrounding blood vessels. The glomus cells are

homogeneous with eosinophilic cytoplasm and dense, round nuclei. The tumor stroma is fibrous and often pale staining (e-**Fig. 39.33**). A glomangioma is predominantly vascular and has fewer glomus cells. The glomus cells are positive for smooth muscle actin and negative for endothelial markers such as CD31.

7. **Kaposi's sarcoma**
   a. **Clinical:** Early lesions are ecchymotic macules or patches; later lesions are bluish or purple papules, nodules, plaques, and tumors; all are palpable. There are four clinical subtypes with similar cutaneous findings: Classic, African (endemic), Epidemic (human immunodeficiency virus [HIV]-associated), and Iatrogenic (immunosuppressive therapy related). Regardless of type, it is a borderline malignancy that is slowly progressive, but may involve internal organs. Etiologic agent is human herpesvirus type 8 (HHV-8) in all types.
   b. **Microscopic:** Early lesions show a dermal proliferation of irregular slitlike vascular channels with extravasated erythrocytes, hemosiderin, and plasma cells. The endothelial cells are plump or inconspicuous; there is no significant cytological atypia. The vascular channels infiltrate between collagen bundles and surround existing blood vessels (promontory sign) and appendages (e-**Fig. 39.34**). As the lesions evolve into papules, plaques, and nodules, there are increased spindle cells between the poorly defined slitlike vessels. Intracytoplasmic eosinophilic hyaline globules (PAS positive) can be identified within the tumor cells (e-**Fig. 39.35**).

8. **Epithelioid hemangioendothelioma**
   a. **Clinical:** Firm, tan-pink subcutaneous nodules and plaques, uncommonly involving the dermis, measuring several centimeters in maximal diameter; common sites are the trunk and extremities. The lesion is seen primarily in adults and has a slight female predilection; 40% of tumors recur, and approximately 15% develop distant metastasis.
   b. **Microscopic:** Sheets and cords of large polyhedral tumor cells in the subcutis/dermis. The tumor cells have amphophilic cytoplasm, prominent cytoplasmic vacuoles, and round nuclei often with small nucleoli, and have a tendency to grow around pre-existing large vessels. The stroma is variably fibrous or myxoid. Mitotic figures and necrosis may be seen and may indicate worse behavior. The tumor cells are immunoreactive for endothelial cell markers CD31, CD34, von Willebrand factor, and thrombomodulin (e-**Fig. 39.36**).

9. **Angiosarcoma**
   a. **Clinical:** Single or multifocal, purpuric or black plaque(s) on the head and neck of elderly patients or purplish-red papules or polypoid tumors in the chronically edematous skin associated with lymphedema and/or prior radiation.
   b. **Microscopic:** Poorly circumscribed and often multifocal proliferation of anastomosing, infiltrative vascular channels in the dermis and subcutis with prominent extravasation of erythrocytes and hemosiderin. The vascular channels are lined by crowded, variably plump, and atypical endothelial cells; papillary processes sometimes extend into the lumens of the vessels. Poorly differentiated tumors with an epithelioid cellular morphology may resemble carcinoma or melanoma. The tumor cells are positive for endothelial cell markers, such as CD31, CD34, Factor VIII-related antigen and Ulex europaeus (e-**Fig. 39.37**).

B. **Neural and neuroendocrine tumors**
   1. **Traumatic neuroma**
      a. **Clinical:** Usually firm, pea-sized nodules in the subcutis and deep soft tissue at sites of previous injury. They may be painful.
      b. **Microscopic:** Irregularly arranged nerve fascicles embedded in fibrous scar tissue. Each fascicle is surrounded by fibrous tissue and perineural cells. There are scattered mast cells (e-**Fig. 39.38**).

2. **Solitary circumscribed neuroma (palisaded and encapsulated neuroma)**
   a. **Clinical:** Uncommon, usually solitary, skin-colored or pink papule, most common on the face of middle-aged adults; slow-growing, painless, and <6 mm in diameter.
   b. **Microscopic:** Well-circumscribed and partially encapsulated dermal nodule composed of fascicles of bland spindle cells with amphophilic cytoplasm and serpiginous nuclei that appear parallel to each other within a single fascicle. No intervening collagen is present (e-Fig. 39.39).
3. **Neurofibroma**
   a. **Clinical:** Soft, skin-colored, pedunculated papules or nodules. Multiple lesions in a segmental or widespread distribution are related to neurofibromatosis.
   b. **Microscopic:** A nonencapsulated dermal or subcutaneous tumor characterized by loosely arranged wavy spindle cells in a pale-staining stroma. There are increased small caliber vessels and mast cells in the stroma. The spindle cells tend to surround adnexal structures, rather than displacing them (e-Fig. 39.40).
4. **Cutaneous Schwannoma (neurilemmoma)**
   a. **Clinical:** Uncommon, slow-growing, usually solitary tumor/nodule with a predilection for the limbs of adults. The neoplasm can be either sporadic or associated with neurofibromatosis 2 (NF-2) or schwannomatosis. Schwannomas are more commonly seen in the deep soft tissue, intracranially, or intraspinally.
   b. **Microscopic:** Similar to their soft tissue counterpart; a circumscribed and encapsulated subcutaneous/dermal nodule. The tumor cells are spindled Schwann cells with indistinct cytoplasmic borders arranged in interlacing fascicles. There are hypercellular areas (Antoni A) containing rows or palisades of nuclei aligned around eosinophilic cellular processes (Verocay bodies) and hypocellular (Antoni B) areas. No axons are present (e-Fig. 39.41).
5. **Merkel cell carcinoma**
   a. **Clinical:** A rapidly growing, often ulcerated, red nodule or plaque usually arising on the sun-exposed skin of the elderly, particularly on the head, neck, and extremities.
   b. **Microscopic:** Trabeculae, nests, and sheets of small cells with scant cytoplasm, indistinct cytoplasmic borders, vesicular nuclei with nuclear molding, and multiple small nucleoli, infiltrating the entire dermis and sometimes the subcutis. There are numerous apoptotic forms and mitoses. Local intralymphatic spread is commonly seen. The tumor cells are positive for neuron-specific enolase, chromogranin, and synaptophysin and have a characteristic "paranuclear dot-like" staining pattern for low-molecular-weight keratin, such as CK20. The tumor cells are negative for CD45, S-100, and TTF-1, allowing distinction from hematopoietic and melanocytic neoplasms, as well as metastatic small cell carcinoma of the lung (e-Fig. 39.42, A and B).
   c. **Genetics:** Genetic information is not currently used in the diagnosis of Merkel cell carcinoma, and the following is provided for interest only. Deletion of chromosome 1p36 is commonly seen; numerous other chromosomal abnormalities have been described, of which trisomy 6 is the most common (present in almost 50% of tumors).
6. **Granular cell tumor**
   a. **Clinical:** Asymptomatic, solitary, skin-colored nodule <3 cm in diameter. Multiple lesions in ~10% of cases. Most common in black adults and women. Malignant counterpart is exceedingly rare.
   b. **Microscopic:** A nonencapsulated, dermal based tumor composed exclusively of large polyhedral cells with abundant fine to coarsely granular eosinophilic cytoplasm, and small oval, centrally located nuclei. The granular cells infiltrate between collagen bundles and surround adnexa. The epidermis may be markedly acanthotic as in pseudocarcinomatous hyperplasia (e-Fig. 39.43).

C. Fibrous and fibrohistiocytic tumors
  1. Keloid
   a. Clinical: Firm, pink to purple, mildly tender, bosselated tumors that develop at sites of previous injury; most common on the upper back, shoulders, presternal area, and ear lobes of dark skinned individuals.
   b. Microscopic: A nodule of haphazardly arranged, broad, homogenous, brightly eosinophilic collagen bundles outlined by large, pale-staining fibroblasts in the superficial dermis (e-**Fig. 39.44**).
  2. Dermatofibroma
   a. Clinical: Brownish, round, firm dermal nodules, usually <1 cm in diameter; most common on the legs of young adults.
   b. Microscopic: Poorly circumscribed dermal proliferation of spindled fibroblasts, histiocytes, and blood vessels. Fibroblasts at the periphery surround the collagen bundles ("collagen-trapping"). Dermatofibromas are histologically varied, and there are, correspondingly, many named variants such as cellular, aneurysmal, "Monster" cell, etc. The epidermis typically shows acanthosis, basal keratinocyte hyperpigmentation, and broad flattened rete or a basaloid proliferation, which can be mistaken for basal cell carcinoma in a shave biopsy (e-**Fig. 39.45**).
  3. Dermatofibrosarcoma protuberans
   a. Clinical: Solitary or multiple polypoid nodules arising in an indurated plaque on the trunk or extremities of adults; slow growing, locally aggressive tumor, which rarely metastasizes.
   b. Microscopic: A cellular dermal tumor composed of homogeneous spindle cells arranged in a storiform or cartwheel pattern. The tumor cells infiltrate between adnexa, and there is characteristically extension into the subcutis with fat trapping. Occasional mitotic figures can be found, and atypia is mild. The epidermis is normal, atrophic, or ulcerated (e-**Fig. 39.46**).
   c. Genetics: Genetic information is not currently used in the diagnosis of dermatofibrosarcoma protuberans, and the following is provided for interest only. The tumor characteristically exhibits the translocation t(17;22)(q22;q13), which results in production of a COLIA1-PDGFB fusion protein.
  4. Giant cell fibroblastoma: A histological variant of dermatofibrosarcoma protuberans, primarily affecting children, with a strong male predominance. It has a similar anatomic distribution and the same translocation as dermatofibrosarcoma protuberans.
   a. Clinical: Grossly, it is a firm yellow or gray tumor with a gelatinous or rubbery consistency without hemorrhage or necrosis.
   b. Microscopic: The tumor is usually hypocellular and composed of wavy spindle cells and scattered giant cells with hyperchromatic and angulated nuclei. The stroma is variable from myxoid to collagenous to sclerotic. Scattered mast cells are seen within the stroma. Irregular branching "angiectoid" spaces resembling dilated lymphatics may be seen, and these are lined by spindle or multinucleated cells with morphology identical to those of the surrounding stroma. The lining and stromal cells are positive for CD34 and negative for CD31, S-100, actin, desmin, and EMA.
  5. Angiofibromas
   a. Clinical
    i. Fibrous papule of the face: A solitary, firm, dome-shaped, often flesh-colored lesion on the nose or central face.
    ii. Pearly penile papules: Tiny white papules, 1 to 3 mm in diameter, arranged in groups or rows on the coronal margin of the penis.
    iii. Angiofibroma of tuberous sclerosis: Multiple papules or nodules with a predilection for the butterfly area of the face.
    iv. Digital fibrokeratoma: A solitary, thin, tall horn on the digit.
   b. Microscopic: Dermal fibrosis, dilated small vessels, and variably enlarged, angulated or stellate fibroblasts. Vascular proliferation can be seen in angiofibromas associated with tuberous sclerosis (adenoma sebaceum). Fibrous papule

of the face is often dome-shaped on low power (e-**Fig. 39.47**). The epidermis of digital fibrokeratomas shows the hyperkeratosis and acanthosis of acral skin.

    c. **Genetics:** Genetic information is not currently used in the diagnosis of angiofibromata, and the following is provided for interest only. Mutations of two different genes, *TSC1* on chromosome 9 and *TSC2* on chromosome 16, have been identified in digital fibrokeratoma of patients with tuberous sclerosis.

6. Acrochordon (skin tag, soft fibroma, fibroepithelial polyp, etc.)

    a. **Clinical:** Flesh-colored, pedunculated papules or nodules with irregular or smooth surfaces. Most common on the axilla, neck, groin, and eyelids; incidence increases with age, more common in obese females.

    b. **Microscopic:** Polypoid, variable epidermal change, well vascularized, loose dermal connective tissue. A variable amount of fat can be seen in the dermis of larger lesions (soft fibroma). There are no appendages present (e-**Fig. 39.48**).

7. Epithelioid sarcoma

    a. **Clinical:** One or more slow growing, firm, painless, tan-white subcutaneous nodules with an indistinct infiltrating margin. The tumor occurs most commonly on the distal extremities, particularly the hands of young men. Ulceration and sinus formation may be present weeks or months after the lesion is first noted. The local recurrence rate is near 80%, and distant metastasis occurs in 30% to 45% of cases, most commonly to the lymph nodes and lung.

    b. **Microscopic:** Deep seated tumor (subcutaneous or soft tissue, rarely dermal) with nodular arrangement of tumor cells that tend to palisade around geographic central degeneration/necrosis. A lymphohistiocytic infiltrate often surrounds the tumor nodules. The tumor cells are large and polygonal, with abundant, deeply eosinophilic cytoplasm, round to oval nuclei, and prominent nucleoli. Plump spindled tumor cells are sometimes present. Mitoses are frequent. The tumor cells are positive by immunohistochemistry for both low- and high-molecular-weight keratins, EMA, and vimentin, and are also positive for CD34 in 60% to 70% of cases. The architectural features are similar to those seen in deep granulomatous processes such as deep granuloma annulare.

    c. **Genetics:** Genetic information is not currently used in the diagnosis of epithelioid sarcoma, and the following is provided for interest only. Loss of heterozygosity on chromosome 22q has been reported in some cases.

D. Fatty and muscular tumors

  1. Lipoma

    a. **Clinical:** Common, asymptomatic, soft subcutaneous nodules.

    b. **Microscopic:** Unremarkable adipocytes are surrounded by a thin fibrous capsule; there is a paucity of fibrous septae.

  2. Angiolipoma

    a. **Clinical:** Often multiple, painful, subcutaneous nodules of the extremities or trunk; first tumor usually appears after puberty.

    b. **Microscopic:** Varying proportions of mature adipose tissue and small-caliber blood vessels with fibrin thrombi, surrounded by a thin fibrous capsule, and arranged vaguely into lobules by fine incomplete fibrous septae (e-**Fig. 39.49**).

  3. Leiomyoma

    a. **Clinical:** Solitary or multiple red nodules, often painful.

    b. **Microscopic:** Pilar leiomyoma is a circumscribed, nonencapsulated tumor composed of interlacing smooth muscle bundles (e-**Fig. 39.50**). Scrotal leiomyomas are similar but often have ill-defined or focally infiltrative margins. Angioleiomyoma is a deep dermal/subcutaneous, well-circumscribed nodule of interlacing smooth muscle bundles between multiple thick walled vessels.

  4. Leiomyosarcoma

    a. **Clinical:** Rare, dermal or subcutaneous nodule or plaque, most common on the extremities. Dermal leiomyosarcomas frequently extend into the subcutaneous tissue; there are no confirmed cases of metastases from dermal tumors. Subcutaneous leiomyosarcomas have greater tendency for local recurrence and metastasis.

    b. Microscopic: Interlacing, hypercellular smooth muscle bundles with pleomorphic and hyperchromatic nuclei, and occasional mitoses (at lease one per 10 high-power field).

V. CUTANEOUS LYMPHOID INFILTRATES. These infiltrates are highly varied and encompass reactive lymphoid infiltrates, primary cutaneous lymphoma, and cutaneous involvement by systemic disease/nodal lymphoma. With the exception of mycosis fungoides, determination of whether the skin is the primary or a secondary site of a lymphoma requires a complete clinical examination for appearance and distribution of cutaneous lesions, presence or absence of lymphadenopathy and/or organomegaly, systemic symptoms, and peripheral blood smear abnormalities. The two most common primary cutaneous T-cell lymphoproliferative disorders will be discussed below.

A. Mycosis fungoides

  1. Clinical: Patches, plaques, and/or tumors with a wide anatomic distribution; most common in middle-aged to elderly persons, but documented in children. Usually pruritic, may present with or develop erythroderma, clinical course usually indolent.

  2. Microscopic: Histologic features vary with clinical morphology. Epidermal changes range from atrophic to psoriasiform. Spongiosis may be disproportionately decreased compared to the number of intraepidermal lymphocytes.

    a. Patch stage/early mycosis fungoides is histologically subtle: A patchy, paucicellular band of lymphocytes is present in a fibrotic papillary dermis; lymphocytes extend into the epidermis (epidermotropism); intraepidermal lymphocytes are larger than the dermal lymphocytes and have hyperchromatic, cerebriform nuclei; they are separated from keratinocytes by a halo and file along the basal layer of the epidermis ("string of beads"). Aggregates of atypical intraepidermal lymphocytes (Pautrier's microabscesses) are rare. Dermal lymphocytes align along collagen bundles (e-**Fig. 39.51**).

    b. Plaque stage has a more prominent band of lymphocytes in the upper dermis and easily identifiable Pautrier's microabscesses in the epidermis (e-**Fig. 39.52**).

    c. Tumoral stage shows a dense nodular or diffuse infiltrate filling the dermis and extending into the subcutis. Epidermotropism may be lost. There may be transformation to a large cell phenotype. The infiltrate is characteristically CD3+, CD5+, CD 4+, and CD8−. A minority of cases are CD3+, CD5+, CD4−, and CD8+. CD2 and CD7 may be lost in the neoplastic lymphocytes.

  3. Genetics: Some human leukocyte antigen (HLA) class II alleles (specifically HLA-B8, Aw31, and Aw32) are more prevalent among patients with mycosis fungoides. Studies of T-cell receptor genes have shown that the infiltrate is clonal. There is also an increased rate of aberrations involving multiple chromosomes, including chromosomes 1, 6, 11, 8, 17, 13, 15, and 9, in advanced stage disease.

B. Primary cutaneous CD30+ lymphoproliferative disorders include primary cutaneous anaplastic large cell lymphoma (ALCL), lymphomatoid papulosis (LyP), and borderline cases with overlapping features of these two conditions. Primary cutaneous ALCL and LyP show considerable histologic overlap and are best separated on the basis of clinical presentation and course.

  1. Primary cutaneous anaplastic large cell lymphoma (ALCL)

    a. Clinical: Solitary or localized, large (>2 cm), often ulcerated, red/brown tumors; mostly in adults. Partial regression is common, complete spontaneous regression is rare; extracutaneous involvement is possible.

    b. Microscopic: Nodular or diffuse dermal infiltrate composed of sheets of cohesive CD30+ atypical cells, frequently involving the superficial subcutis. The atypical cells have large rounded or irregular vesicular nuclei; prominent, centrally placed nucleoli; and ample clear to amphophilic cytoplasm. A nonneoplastic mixed inflammatory infiltrate is present (e-**Fig. 39.53**). The large lymphocytes in cutaneous ALCL are negative for anaplastic lymphoma kinase-1 (ALK-1), which is frequently positive in systemic ALCL.

    c. Genetics: Clonal rearrangement of T-cell receptor genes is detected in >90% of cases of primary cutaneous ALCL. However, the translocation t(2;5)(p23;q35) characteristic of systemic ALCL is rarely, if ever, found in primary cutaneous ALCL.

2. Lymphomatoid papulosis (LyP)

  a. Clinical: Recurrent crops of papules, nodules, and plaques at different stages of evolution, mainly on the trunk and extremities of young adults. Spontaneous regression occurs within a few weeks or months; the course may last for decades. Correlation with clinical lesion size, behavior, and distribution is required for diagnosis.

  b. Microscopic: There are three histologic subtypes:

    i. Type A: Wedge-shaped, mixed cellular infiltrate of small lymphocytes, eosinophils, neutrophils, histiocytes, and variable numbers of large atypical lymphocytes; some have hyperchromatic nuclei and others are ALCL-like.

    ii. Type B: Histology similar to plaque stage mycosis fungoides.

    iii. Type C: Histology similar to ALCL.

    The characteristic immunophenotype of the tumor cells is CD 30+/CD 3+/CD 4+ and CD 8/EMA negative.

  c. Genetics: Clonal rearrangement of T-cell receptor gene can be found in at least 40% of LyP lesions. Chromosome deletions and rearrangements of chromosomes 1, 7, 9, and 10 have also been demonstrated.

VI. CUTANEOUS METASTASIS (FROM VISCERAL CARCINOMA). Skin is an uncommon site for metastasis from visceral malignancies. Carcinoma may reach the skin by direct extension from an underlying tumor, by lymphatic and/or hematogenous spread as part of systemic involvement, or by accidental implantation during a diagnostic or surgical procedure. Metastases tend to occur on the skin near the primary malignancy. Sites distant from the primary tumor are more common in tumors that demonstrate angioinvasion (such as kidney and lung).

Cutaneous metastases most commonly develop subsequent to 'or at the time of' primary diagnosis of a visceral malignancy. Rarely, a cutaneous metastasis is the first indication of a visceral malignancy. The umbilicus, and less frequently the scalp, is particularly involved. Adenocarcinoma is more frequently observed as a cutaneous metastasis than is squamous cell carcinoma or urothelial carcinoma. Cutaneous metastases are variable in clinical appearance, appearing either as solitary or multiple papules/nodules, or mimicking inflammatory/infectious conditions.

A. Sister Mary Joseph nodule

  1. Clinical: This condition was named after Sister Mary Joseph (1856–1939), a surgical assistant for Dr. William Mayo, who noted the association between paraumbilical nodules observed during skin preparation for surgery and metastatic intra-abdominal cancer confirmed at surgery. Usually a solitary, firm, indurated nodule, sometimes with surface fissuring or ulceration; variable in size, can be painful. Common underlying tumors include gastrointestinal malignancy (>55%, male predominance) and ovarian malignancies (34%).

    Sister Mary Joseph nodules account for 60% of all malignant umbilical tumors (primary or secondary). Most patients die within months after the appearance of the umbilical tumor.

  2. Microscopic: Most commonly, the histology is a dermal based adenocarcinoma with histology resembling the primary malignancy. Signet-ring-cell morphology may be present, especially in a gastric primary (**e-Fig. 39.54**).

B. Metastatic breast carcinoma

  1. Clinical: Typically small papules, ranging from 1 to 2 mm in diameter to large tumor masses, on the anterior chest wall. Intralymphatic spread of tumor cells (inflammatory carcinoma) can manifest as a diffuse, warm, indurated plaque (carcinoma erysipeloides). Scalp metastasis can present as alopecia (alopecia neoplastica), also seen in metastases from the lung and kidney.

  2. Microscopic: Usually a poorly differentiated adenocarcinoma. Ductal and sometimes lobular arrangements are present. The proportion of intravascular tumor varies (**e-Fig. 39.55**).

C. Metastatic renal cell carcinoma
1. **Clinical:** Typically erythematous, vascular papule or nodule, may be misdiagnosed as lobular capillary hemangioma or Kaposi's sarcoma. Solitary in 15% to 20% of cases. The scalp is a common site.
2. **Microscopic:** Usually well circumscribed, dermal nodule(s), composed of sheets and nests of polygonal tumor cells with clear cytoplasm, distinct cytoplasmic borders, and enlarged hyperchromatic nuclei, associated with a delicate rich vascular stroma, red blood cell extravasation, and hemosiderin deposition. The histologic features can be bland, and the differential diagnosis may include primary and metastatic tumors with clear cell morphology (**e-Fig. 39.56**).

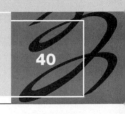

SKIN: MELANOCYTIC LESIONS

Anne C. Lind, Emily A. Bantle, and Louis P. Dehner

40

I. NORMAL ANATOMY. Melanocytes migrate to the skin from the neural crest during the first 3 months of gestation. They normally occupy a space slightly beneath the basal keratinocytes. A melanocyte nucleus is rounded and slightly hyperchromatic as compared to the more elongated or ovoid basal keratinocyte nucleus with evenly dispersed chromatin. A pale, often eccentric, rim of eosinophilic cytoplasm is usually noted, and a clear space or halo separates the melanocyte from the neighboring basal keratinocytes and/or basement membrane (e-Fig. 40.1).* Occasionally, dendritic processes can be seen as they extend between the keratinocytes. On the trunk and extremities there is approximately one melanocyte to every 7 to 10 basal keratinocytes. On the face and external genitalia, the ratio is approximately one melanocyte to three basal keratinocytes.

Melanocytes produce and export melanosomes, which are membrane-bound and have an internal latticelike structure. Melanin granules are deposited on the lattice, eventually obscuring this architectural feature. Melanin pigment can be classified as eumelanin (brown–black pigment) or pheomelanin, which is rich in sulfur and results in yellow–red pigment.

In addition to considerations for gross examination of skin specimens as already discussed in the chapter on nonneoplastic dermatopathology (Chapter 38), when performing the gross examination of a biopsy or excision of a pigmented lesion, a complete description of the background skin color and the clinical "ABCDs" (see melanoma section below) is required. Therefore, the size of the surface lesion, presence of the lesion at the margin, color regularity or irregularity and border, should all be included in the gross description.

Diagnosis of a melanocytic lesion is based on multiple architectural and cytologic criteria that usually allow for a specific diagnosis, and therefore, prediction of biologic behavior. In most cases, these microscopic qualities result in a specific diagnosis that reliably correlates with the anticipated biologic behavior of the melanocytic proliferation. Features associated with benignancy include symmetry, circumscription, maturation, predominance of nested melanocytes, cohesive nests of melanocytes, and melanocytes with regular nuclear borders and without nucleoli or atypical mitoses. These histologic criteria as compared with those that support a diagnosis of melanoma can be found in Table 40.1. Because there are numerous criteria, there are instances in which the histologic features that support a benign diagnosis (nevus) and those that support a malignant diagnosis (melanoma) seem to be equally represented. In some cases, even among "experts," there is not a consensus regarding the benign or malignant nature of the melanocytic lesion. Clearly, in these cases, a complete excision is necessary, and consultation with a pathologist or dermatopathologist either within the department or from an outside institution should be sought. In some cases the ultimate "true" diagnosis can be elusive. Chromosomal studies are sometimes helpful. For example, Spitz nevi have either a normal genotype or an isolated amplification in 11p. Melanomas, by comparison, have variable gains and losses across multiple genes when studied by comparative genomic hybridization and/or fluorescence in situ hybridization (FISH).

The status of the margins should be included routinely on all pathology reports of melanocytic nevi, even in punch biopsy specimens. Although there admittedly is no

---

*All e-figures are available online via the Solution Site Image Bank.

TABLE 40.1	Histopathologic Features in the Differential Diagnosis of Benign and Malignant Melanocytic Proliferations	

Microscopic feature	Nevus	Melanoma
Symmetry	+	– or ±
Circumscription	+	– or ±
Nested melanocytes	+	±
Cohesive nests	+	±
Regular nuclear border	+	–
Absence of nucleoli	+	–
Atypical mitotes	–	±
"Deep" mitoses	–	+

consensus on this point, the margin status provides additional information that is often clinically useful.

II. **NONMELANOCYTIC PIGMENTED LESIONS.** The pathologist is sometimes presented with a biopsy or excision of skin for a clinically pigmented lesion, often with the clinical description of "atypical pigmented lesion; rule out melanoma." Clinical lesions that are not composed of melanocytes microscopically, but can mimic a nevus or melanoma clinically, include: a pigmented seborrheic keratosis, pigmented basal cell carcinoma, pigmented actinic keratosis, solar lentigo, dermatofibroma, postinflammatory pigmentary alteration, intracorneal hemorrhage (calcaneal petechiae), and tinea nigra.

III. **CLINICAL AND MICROSCOPIC FEATURES OF BENIGN MELANOCYTIC PROLIFERATIONS.** Any nevus, by definition, is benign. A melanocytic nevus, when the histologic diagnosis is given without modifiers such as "with severe atypia," is a benign proliferation/hamartoma of melanocytes in the epidermis, epidermis and dermis, or dermis alone. In general, a melanocytic nevus is a small (<6 mm), symmetric, well-circumscribed proliferation of nested melanocytes, and the melanocytes that are deepest in the dermis are smaller than superficial melanocytes, a process known as maturation. The basic histologic criteria stated above, and shown in Table 40.1, apply to most nevi. However, there are multiple histologic subtypes of nevi, some with exceptions to these criteria. Therefore, knowledge of the histologic subtypes, and the exceptions they present, is helpful. A summary of these variants is provided in Table 40.2, and the World Health Organization (WHO) classification of melanocytic tumors is given in Table 40.3. Both compound and intradermal melanocytic nevi may have a variety of configurations from polypoid to papillomatous, reflecting, in part, the appearance of the epidermis.

A. **Lentigo simplex**
   1. **Clinical:** An acquired pigmented lesion; small, flat, evenly colored, usually on sun-exposed skin, seen in persons <40 years of age.
   2. **Microscopic:** Long slender rete with increased numbers of cytologically unremarkable melanocytes; aggregates (nests) of melanocytes are not seen; melanin pigment is increased in the basal keratinocytes (**e-Fig. 40.2**).

B. **Junctional melanocytic nevus**
   1. **Clinical:** An acquired pigmented lesion; small, flat, evenly colored, usually on sun-exposed sites.
   2. **Microscopic:** Nests/aggregates of melanocytes are present at the tips of the rete; there may be increased numbers of cytologically unremarkable melanocytes along the sides of the rete, but there is no confluent growth of melanocytes (**e-Fig. 40.3**). The presence of a purely junctional nevus should be viewed with some concern in an individual >50 years. In these cases, it is helpful to take into consideration the size of the lesion and also to determine whether the junctional population of melanocytes has a confluent or nonconfluent pattern of proliferation. Immunohistochemical staining for Melan-A and/or HMB-45 is helpful in the demonstration of confluence or nonconfluence. The latter is reassuring that the junctional proliferation is more likely a junctional nevus.

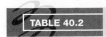

TABLE 40.2	Histologic Types of Melanocytic Nevus and their Borderline or Malignant Counterpart
Benign	**Borderline or malignant**
Junctional melanocytic nevus with or without AD	Melanoma in situ, lentiginous or superficial spreading type
Compound melanocytic nevus with or without AD	Melanoma of nevoid type, melanoma arising in nevus or malignant melanoma
Dermal melanocytic nevus	Metastatic or recurrent melanoma
Spitz nevus	"Spitzoid" melanoma or "borderline" atypical Spitz tumor
Pigmented spindle cell nevus of Reed	Spindle cell melanoma
Deep penetrating nevus	Spindle cell melanoma
Halo nevus	Melanoma with intense host reaction
Balloon cell nevus	Melanoma with balloon cell features
Congenital nevus with proliferative nodule(s)	Melanoma arising in congenital nevus
Blue nevus	Melanoma with regression
Cellular blue nevus	Spindle cell melanoma or malignant cellular blue nevus

AD, architectural disorder.

C. Compound melanocytic nevus
  1. **Clinical:** An acquired pigmented lesion; small, slightly raised, evenly colored, usually on sun-exposed skin.
  2. **Microscopic:** Nests/aggregates of melanocytes are present at the tips of the rete, and nests/aggregates of melanocytes are present in the dermis. The proportion of epidermal melanocytes to dermal melanocytes is variable. Dermal melanocytes generally are smaller than epidermal melanocytes and appear progressively smaller with increasing distance from the epidermis. This is known as maturation (**e-Fig. 40.4**). Care should always be taken to make certain that the deep dermal melanocytes are smaller, do not have nucleoli, and lack mitotic figures. A second population or clone of nevoid cells should be viewed with concern. There is no more diagnostically treacherous lesion than the nevoid or nevus-like melanoma.
D. Intradermal melanocytic nevus
  1. **Clinical:** A raised (papular), nonpigmented lesion that may be mistaken clinically for a skin tag (fibroepithelial polyp) or a basal cell carcinoma.
  2. **Microscopic:** Nested and individual melanocytes are found only in the dermis (**e-Fig. 40.5**). The dermal component of compound or intradermal nevi can show so-called neurotization with a resemblance to a neurofibroma, contain spaces with a pseudovascular appearance, and have scattered multinucleated cells as a feature of presumed senescence.
E. Spitz nevus (spindle and/or epithelioid cell nevus)
  1. **Clinical:** Most common on the head and neck or extremities of children and adolescents, with decreasing incidence with increasing age. It may arise suddenly, and may rarely be multiple. It frequently is not pigmented; consequently, the clinical differential diagnosis might include a vascular lesion (angioma) or juvenile xanthogranuloma.
  2. **Microscopic:** Compact hyperkeratosis, hypergranulosis, and acanthosis of the epidermis are common. The melanocytes are spindled, epithelioid, or a mixed population that are arranged in vertically oriented nests (mimicking clusters of bananas) at the epidermal–dermal junction; often a cleft/space between the epidermis and nested melanocytes is present (**e-Fig. 40.6**). Epithelioid melanocytes have large nuclei and abundant eosinophilic cytoplasm. Numerous ectatic,

TABLE 40.3	WHO Histological Classification of Melanocytic Tumors

Malignant melanoma
Superficial spreading melanoma
Nodular melanoma
Lentigo maligna
Acral–lentiginous melanoma
Desmoplastic melanoma
Melanoma arising from blue nevus
Melanoma arising in a giant congenital nevus
Melanoma of childhood
Nevoid melanoma
Persistent melanoma

Benign melanocytic tumors
Congenital melanocytic nevi
  Superficial type
  Proliferative nodules in congenital melanocytic nevi
Dermal melanocytic lesions
  Mongolian spot
  Nevus of Ito and Ota
Blue nevus
  Cellular blue nevus
Combined nevus
Melanotic macules, simple lentigo, and lentiginous nevus
Dysplastic nevus
Site-specific nevi
Acral
Genital
Myerson nevus
Persistent (recurrent) melanocytic nevus
Spitz nevus
Pigmented spindle cell nevus (Reed)
Halo nevus

From: Weedon D, LeBoit P, Burg G, Sarasin A, eds. *World Health Organization Classification of Tumours. Pathology and Genetics. Skin Tumours.* Lyon: IARC Press; 2005. Used with permission.

thin-walled vascular spaces may be seen in the papillary dermis (which accounts for the clinical impression of a vascular lesion). Superficial mitoses may be seen; however, atypical mitoses, clustered mitoses, or deep mitoses should raise the possibility of a Spitz-like or spitzoid melanoma, regardless of age or site. Pagetoid spread may be seen in an otherwise typical Spitz nevus. Caution is required when considering the diagnosis of an epithelioid Spitz nevus in a person past middle age and/or on sun-damaged skin. The designation of 'Spitz tumor' has been suggested for the Spitz nevus with atypical features or even all Spitz nevi. Although we acknowledge that the melanocytic lesion with Spitz features is a diagnostic challenge, the overwhelming majority of Spitz nevi occurring in children and adolescents have benign behavior.

F. Pigmented spindle cell nevus of Reed
1. **Clinical:** Heavily but evenly pigmented, small, acquired lesion in the shoulder/pelvic girdle region; most common in women in their second and third decades.
2. **Microscopic:** Symmetric and well-circumscribed proliferation of spindled melanocytes in the epidermis and superficial dermis with a pattern reminiscent of a woven basket. Fascicles of spindled cells are oriented vertically, horizontally, and tangentially. A broad zone of melanophages in the superficial dermis is

invariably present beneath the melanocytes (e-**Fig. 40.7**). The relationship of the Reed nevus to the Spitz nevus is uncertain except for the fact that both are melanocytic proliferations.

G. Blue nevus

1. **Clinical:** Flat to slightly raised, small lesion that is blue rather than black or brown; may be congenital or acquired, most common on the head, neck and extremities.

2. **Microscopic:** Superficial dermal, lentil-shaped, variably cellular proliferation of spindled and dendritic melanocytes that interdigitate between collagen bundles. Melanophages are frequently admixed. The epithelioid variant has, as the name implies, melanocytes with a more epithelioid appearance (e-**Fig. 40.8**). The differential diagnosis includes dermal melanocytosis.

H. Cellular blue nevus

1. **Clinical:** Large (1 to 2 cm) heavily pigmented, blue to blue–black, raised lesion most common on the scalp or buttocks.

2. **Microscopic:** This lesion is characterized as a mid- to deep dermal multinodular biphasic proliferation the nodular centers of which are composed of small epithelioid melanocytes, with pale to amphophilic cytoplasm. The nodules are surrounded by a rim of pigmented spindled melanocytes and melanophages. There may be extension of the nodules into the contiguous subcutis in some cases. Despite the striking tumorlike appearance, consideration of malignancy should not be entertained in the absence of necrosis, atypical mitosis, and prominent nucleoli (e-**Fig. 40.9**).

I. Dermal melanocytic lesions (Nevus of Ota, Nevus of Ito, Mongolian spot)

1. **Clinical:** Flat, slate-gray patch on the face, shoulder, sacrum, or bilateral temples; it predominantly occurs in people of Asian descent, more commonly in females.

2. **Microscopic:** Mid- to deep dermal, ill-defined, paucicellular infiltrate consists of pigmented, spindled, and/or dendritic melanocytes. There are some overlapping features with the blue nevus.

J. Congenital and congenital-pattern nevi

1. **Clinical:** Congenital nevi are pigmented lesions that are present at birth or appear during infancy and can be classified as small (< 2 cm), intermediate (2 to 20 cm), or large (>20 cm). They are frequently varied in pigmentation and have irregular borders; they may be hairy and/or become progressively more hairy, and may cover large areas of the body. Involvement of the leptomeninges by benign or malignant melanocytes in a child with a large or giant congenital nevus is known as neurocutaneous melanosis.

2. **Microscopic:** A junctional component exists in these lesions in early infancy, but the melanocytes are predominantly dermal with time. Individual nevoid to small epithelioid melanocytes in the dermis extend along or into dermal structures such as the adnexa, arrector pili muscles, and small peripheral nerves and into lymphovascular spaces. The subcutis and deeper structures may be infiltrated by nevus cells. The epidermal melanocytic pattern is highly variable, ranging from no significant melanocytic proliferation, to nested melanocytes, to confluent lentiginous hyperplasia. Mitotic figures, but not atypical forms, may be present at any level. Proliferative nodules of monomorphous melanocytes and brisk mitotic activity may be present and might lead to an erroneous interpretation of melanoma.

An apparent congenital nevus, especially from the scalp, with a more complex pattern of spindle cells, perivascular pseudorosettes, and tactoid bodies likely represents a so-called neurocristic hamartoma.

A congenital-pattern nevus is regarded as an acquired lesion, but it has similarities to the dermal growth pattern of a congenital nevus, including a predominance of individual cells rather than nests, and preferential growth in or along adnexal structures (e-**Fig. 40.10**).

K. Deep penetrating nevus

1. **Clinical:** Small, pigmented lesion most common on the upper half of the body; may resemble a blue nevus, usually acquired during early adulthood.

2. **Microscopic:** Dermal fascicles and nodules of epithelioid to spindled melanocytes with conspicuous granular, gray–brown cytoplasm admixed with melanophages and some nevoid melanocytes. It may extend to the subcutis in a mixed pushing and infiltrative pattern; nuclear pleomorphism, mitotic figures, and nucleoli may be noted. The lesion may be seen as one component of a combined nevus. The combination of the cytologic and architectural features may lead to a concern for melanoma (e-Fig. 40.11).

L. **Halo nevus**
1. **Clinical:** Central zone of pigment, raised or flat, with a circumferential rim of hypo-/depigmentation; may be noted as a recent change in a pre-existing pigmented lesion.
2. **Microscopic:** A junctional, compound, or intradermal melanocytic nevus has been obscured or nearly obscured by a dense band of lymphocytes. Regressive changes (immature fibroplasia, neovascularization, paucicellular lymphocytic infiltrate, melanophages) may be seen at the perimeter. The lymphocytic infiltrate should not impart a sense of asymmetry, and the epidermal melanocytes, if present, should be predominantly nested (e-Fig. 40.12).

M. **Nevus with architectural disorder/Clark's nevus/dysplastic nevus**
1. **Clinical:** Highly variable, ranging from small, symmetric, and evenly pigmented to large (>6 mm), irregularly shaped, and irregularly pigmented, seen in the setting of familial melanoma and multiple (>100) clinically atypical nevi. It is a cutaneous marker for the dysplastic nevus syndrome, but is a controversial entity of uncertain significance outside of this syndrome. The lack of uniformity in diagnostic terms is one sign of this controversy.
2. **Microscopic:** This junctional or compound melanocytic proliferation has its diagnostic features centered on the dermal–epidermal junction. The nested melanocytes bridge between adjacent rete, nested melanocytes arise between or from the sides of rete (rather than the tips), eosinophilic collagenous tissue drapes beneath the epidermis in a festoon-like pattern (lamellar fibroplasia), and there is nonconfluent lentiginous melanocytic hyperplasia. The melanocytes may have a bland, nevoid appearance; have a size greater than that of the basal keratinocytes (mild cytologic atypia); have increased size and variable chromatin patterns (moderate cytologic atypia); or have increased size, variable chromatin patterns, pleomorphism, and nucleoli (severe cytologic atypia). A nevus with architectural disorder and severe cytologic atypia should be considered a borderline melanocytic proliferation; a conservative but complete excision should be encouraged (e-Fig. 40.13).

N. **Nevi on special sites**
1. **Clinical:** Varies with site. Special sites include mucocutaneous sites such as the conjunctiva, anus, external genitalia, umbilicus, acral skin (palms/soles), and areola.
2. **Microscopic:** In addition to the features associated with junctional and/or compound nevi, the junctional melanocytic proliferations at these sites may have an increase in the number of individual melanocytes with either a lentiginous or pagetoid pattern, loss of cohesion, and asymmetry.

O. **Combined melanocytic nevus**
1. **Clinical:** Varied; may be flat, raised, or both; may be variably pigmented; most common in the first three decades, but may come to attention at any age. The combination of features in these lesions (asymmetry, color variations, and possible border irregularities) often raises concern for melanoma.
2. **Microscopic:** May have any of the features of the previously described nevi in a side-by-side arrangement or top-to-bottom arrangement. One of the more common combinations is a compound melanocytic nevus and a blue nevus; the most worrisome combinations include a compound melanocytic nevus with a deep penetrating nevus, or a side-by-side Spitz nevus and compound nevus.

P. **Recurrent melanocytic proliferations**
1. **Clinical:** Sudden appearance or reappearance of pigment in a scar from a previously biopsied or excised nevus and/or melanoma. In some instances, the patient

may not be able to provide reliable information regarding the biologic nature and/or diagnosis of the previous lesion.

2. **Microscopic:** Lentiginous melanocytic hyperplasia and randomly scattered, irregular nests of melanocytes are present above an immature or mature dermal scar. The features of a recurrent nevus may be indistinguishable from a recurrent melanoma and have been referred to as "pseudomelanoma." Adjacent lesional tissue outside of the scar and/or knowledge of the initial biopsy or excision findings is imperative for arriving at the correct diagnosis (e-**Fig. 40.14**).

Q. Nevus ambiguous. This category could include any/all melanocytic lesions that have some of the classic features of a distinctive subtype (such as a Spitz nevus) but are variant in others.

IV. MELANOMA is a malignant melanocytic neoplasm that can occur in any tissue at any body site. Ninety percent of all melanomas arise in the skin, and only cutaneous melanoma will be considered in this section.

Melanoma accounts for only a small percentage (3–5%) of primary cutaneous malignancies; basal cell carcinoma and squamous cell carcinoma are far more prevalent (95–97%). However, melanoma accounts for ≥50% of cancer deaths from a primary cutaneous malignancy. The incidence of melanoma has increased over the past 25 years, but the recognition and diagnosis of lower stage lesions account for a substantial proportion of this increased incidence. As expected, the overall survival has shown improvement as pathologically lower stage lesions are diagnosed. Melanoma is most common in individuals >50 years of age, but affects persons of all ages, including infants. It is slightly more common in males, in whom the pattern of distribution is slightly different. In males, melanoma is more common on the trunk/head and neck; in females, melanomas on the lower extremities are more common. There are numerous histologic types (see Table 40.3), and early study results suggest that the genetic signature of melanoma is different depending on its association with sun exposure (chronic, intermittent, or none; *N Engl J Med.* 2005;353:2135). While the majority of melanomas have easily recognized histologic patterns, some subtypes, such as nevoid and spitzoid, are unsettlingly similar to benign melanocytic lesions.

Clinical features may vary slightly with anatomic site and/or histologic subtype; however, in general, a melanoma is Asymmetric and has an irregular Border, its Color is uneven, and it has a Diameter that is >6 mm. These clinical features have been described as the ABCDs of pigmented lesions. The patient may report a change in a pre-existing pigmented lesion and/or complain of pruritus. A clinical description of a worrisome pigmented lesion can be helpful, especially in the case of a biopsy with borderline atypical histologic features. A biopsy may or may not be representative of the overall pathology.

A. Melanoma in situ

1. **Microscopic:** There is an increase in the number of atypical, enlarged melanocytes found only in the epidermis. These cells have a range in the degree of nuclear enlargement and hyperchromatism. There may be prominent pagetoid spread (i.e., melanocytes are present above the suprapapillary plate) in the superficial spreading pattern, or confluent spread of melanocytes at the level of the basal keratinocytes in the lentiginous pattern. Nests may or may not be present, but if present are randomly distributed and vary in size and shape. Melanocytes are not seen in the dermis, although features of regression may be seen and should be commented on because invasion may have been present earlier (e-**Fig. 40.15**).

2. **Differential diagnosis:** Sun-induced melanocytic hyperplasia, recurrent melanocytic proliferations, lentiginous dysplastic melanocytic nevus, pagetoid Spitz nevus, and psoralen and ultraviolet A light (PUVA) lentigo.

B. Malignant melanoma–superficial spreading type

1. **Microscopic:** Increased numbers of melanocytes with enlarged nuclei and increased amounts of cytoplasm are present at all levels of the epidermis, pagetoid spread is easily identified, and melanocytes with similar cytologic features are present in the dermis. In the dermis, melanocytes may be seen as individual cells, in small clusters, and/or in sheets (e-**Fig. 40.16**).

    2. Differential diagnosis: Compound melanocytic nevus.

C. Malignant melanoma–lentiginous type (lentigo maligna melanoma)

    1. Microscopic: Increased numbers of melanocytes with enlarged nuclei and a mild increase in cytoplasm are present in a confluent pattern at the level of the basal keratinocytes. Poorly, formed and randomly, scattered nests of melanocytes may be present; pagetoid cells are not seen. An artifactual subepidermal cleft might be noted, and melanocytes might extend along the adnexal epithelium. In this variant, cytologic atypia might not be prominent. Melanocytes are present in the dermis (e-**Fig. 40.17**).

    2. Differential diagnosis: Sun-induced melanocytic hyperplasia, recurrent melanocytic proliferations (benign or malignant), and lentiginous dysplastic melanocytic nevus.

D. Malignant melanoma–nodular type

    1. Microscopic: Melanocytes with atypical, but often monotonous, nuclear and cytoplasmic features including enlarged nuclei, irregular nuclear borders, increased amounts of cytoplasm, and abundant mitotic activity (including atypical forms) are present in the dermis in a large nodule or sheet. There may be no apparent intraepidermal melanocytic proliferation, and if malignant melanocytes are present in the epidermis, they do not span the entire dermal tumor. Ulceration is frequently noted (e-**Fig. 40.18**).

E. Malignant melanoma–desmoplastic-neurotropic type

    1. Microscopic: Predominantly dermal proliferation of individual, large spindled melanocytes with prominent nuclear pleomorphism. Melanocytes are noted between collagen bundles and along nerves. The lesion may be poorly defined and variably cellular. Unlike most types of cutaneous melanoma, the desmoplastic melanoma may be S-100 negative and generally is nonreactive with other markers of melanocytic differentiation such as Melan-A/Mart-1/A-103 and/or HMB-45. Apparent expression of smooth muscle actin (SMA) has been noted (e-**Fig. 40.19**).

    2. Differential diagnosis: Malignant fibrous histiocytoma, scar, dermatofibroma, sclerotic dermatofibrosarcoma protuberans, and leiomyosarcoma.

F. Malignant melanoma–nevoid type

    1. Microscopic: Symmetric, well-circumscribed, nested proliferation of small, nevoid melanocytes with dermal maturation. At low power, it may be indistinguishable from a compound melanocytic nevus. At higher power, deep dermal melanocytes have prominent nucleoli and mitoses (e-**Fig. 40.20**).

    2. Differential diagnosis: Melanocytic nevus.

G. Malignant melanoma–spitzoid type

    1. Microscopic: Epithelioid and spindled melanocytes in a predominantly nested pattern are seen in an acanthotic and hyperkeratotic epidermis. The epidermal architectural features are strikingly similar to a Spitz nevus. Dermal melanocytes may be preferentially present in sheets or in large confluent nests, and lack maturation. There is a degree of nuclear pleomorphism that exceeds the atypia seen in the usual Spitz nevus. Mitotic figures, including atypical forms, may be present at all levels of the dermis and may be asymmetrically distributed. A lymphocytic response, if present, may abut the deep aspect of the lesion and provide a suggestion of asymmetry. Frequently the nuclear to cytoplasmic ratio is greater than that of a Spitz nevus, and there is no apparent decrease in nuclear size between the superficial and deep dermal melanocytes.

    2. Differential diagnosis: Spitz nevus.

V. MICROSCOPIC STAGING OF MELANOMA. The Tumor, Node, Metastasis (TNM) classification of malignant melanoma is provided in Table 40.4.

A. Breslow thickness is the single most important prognostic parameter associated with an invasive melanoma. An optical micrometer, calibrated to the microscope, is aligned perpendicularly to the epidermis, and the melanoma is measured from the top of the granular cell layer through the dermal melanocytes at the thickest portion of the melanoma, avoiding the adventitial dermis along adnexal structures. Measurements of the clinical lesion (width and breadth) together with the measured Breslow thickness provide an estimate of tumor volume.

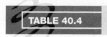

TABLE 40.4	Pathologic Tumor, Node, Metastasis (TNM) Classification of Malignant Melanoma

PRIMARY TUMOR (T)

TX	Primary tumor cannot be assessed (includes shave biopsies and regressed melanoma); pTX includes shave biopsies and regressed melanomas
T0	No evidence of primary tumor
Tis	Melanoma in situ (Clark level I) (atypical melanocytic hyperplasia, melanocytic
Tis	dysplasia, not an invasive malignant lesion)
T1	Tumor ≤1 mm in thickness
	T1a: Clark level II or III, without ulceration
	T1b: Clark level IV or V, or with ulceration
T2	Tumor >1 mm but not >2 mm in thickness
	T2a: Without ulceration
	T2b: With ulceration
T3	Tumor >2 mm but not >4 mm in thickness
	T3a: Without ulceration
	T3b: With ulceration
T4	Tumor >4 mm in thickness
	T4a: Without ulceration
	T4b: With ulceration

REGIONAL LYMPH NODES (N)

NX	Regional lymph nodes cannot be assessed
N0	No regional lymph node metastasis
N1	Metastasis in one regional lymph node
	N1a: Only microscopic metastasis (clinically occult)
	N1b: Macroscopic metastasis (clinically apparent)
N2	Metastasis in two or three regional lymph nodes or intralymphatic regional metastasis
	N2a: Only microscopic nodal metastasis
	N2b: Macroscopic nodal metastasis
	N2c: Satellite or in-transit metastasis without regional nodal metastasis
N3	Metastasis in four or more regional lymph nodes, or matted metastatic regional lymph nodes, or satellite* or in-transit metastasis with metastasis in regional lymph node(s).

DISTANT METASTASIS (M)

MX	Distant metastasis cannot be assessed
M0	No distant metastasis
M1	Distant metastasis
	M1a: Skin, subcutaneous tissue, or lymph nodes beyond the regional lymph nodes
	M1b: Lung
	M1c: Other sites, or any site with elevated serum lactate dehydrogenase (LDH)

STAGE GROUPING

Stage 0	Tis	N0	M0
Stage I	T1	N0	M0
Stage IA	T1a	N0	M0
Stage IB	T1b	N0	M0
	T2a	N0	M0
Stage IIA	T2b	N0	M0
	T3a	N0	M0
Stage IIB	T3b	N0	M0
	T4a	N0	M0
Stage IIC	T4	N0	M0
Stage IIIA	T1a-4a	N1a,2a	M0

(Continued)

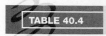

TABLE 40.4	Pathologic Tumor, Node, Metastasis (TNM) Classification of Malignant Melanoma (Continued)		
Stage IIIB	T1a-4a	N1b,2b,2c	M0
	T1b-4b	N1a,2a,2c	M0
Stage IIIC	T1b-4b	N1b,2b	M0
	Any pT	N3	M0
Stage IV	Any T	Any N	M1

*Satellites are tumor nests or nodules within 2 cm of the primary tumor. In-transit metastasis involves skin or subcutaneous tissue >2 cm from the primary tumor but not beyond the regional lymph nodes. From: Greene FL, Page DL, Fleming ID, Fritz AG, Balch CM, Haller DG, Morrow M, eds. *AJCC Cancer Staging Manual.* 6th edition. New York: Springer; 2002. Used with permission. (A new AJCC TNM staging system is scheduled for release in 2009; after its publication, the new staging scheme will appear on the website for this book.)

B. Ulceration. The presence or absence of ulceration is documented on all gross and microscopic examinations. Ulceration may correlate with proliferative activity and predicts more aggressive clinical behavior. The presence of ulceration modifies the T stage of a melanoma. Ta melanomas are not ulcerated; Tb indicates ulceration and predicts a biologic behavior closer to the next T category.

C. Clark level. The Clark level documents the extension of the melanoma to its deepest microscopic compartment. A melanoma in situ, where melanoma is confined to the epidermis, has a Clark level of 1. This Clark level is not routinely reported. Clark level 2 indicates extension of malignant melanocytes into the papillary dermis, and Clark level 3 indicates that malignant melanocytes fill the papillary dermis and extend superficially into the reticular dermis. Clark level 4 refers to melanomas with significant extension into the reticular dermis, and Clark level 5 melanomas extend into the subcutis. By current American Joint Committee on Cancer (AJCC) guidelines, Clark level is reported only for melanomas with a measured Breslow thickness of ≤1.0 mm.

D. Satellite and/or in-transit metastasis. The presence of a focus of melanoma in the field of the primary melanoma, but separated from the main tumor nodule by uninvolved dermis and/or subcutis, is reported as a satellite metastasis. The presence of a focus of metastatic melanoma in the skin between the primary melanoma and the first draining lymph node basin is considered an in-transit metastasis. Either of these events affects staging adversely and has a biologic impact that is comparable to that of nodal metastases.

E. Sentinel lymph node examination. This is a controversial aspect of melanoma prognosis. There are varying protocols and varying attitudes regarding this procedure; a common approach involves the following steps.
1. Nodes are grossly identified, and each is submitted in a separate cassette.
2. All nodes are bivalved through the hilum.
3. The cut faces of the bivalved node are placed face down in a tissue cassette.
4. Histotechs are requested to waste as little tissue as possible when cutting from the face of the paraffin block.
5. Slides are cut at 4 to 5 μm. Slides representing levels 1, 10, and 20 are stained with hematoxylin and eosin (H&E). Slides representing levels 2, 11, and 21 are saved on charged slides for potential immunoperoxidase studies.
6. The H&E-stained slides are examined; if there is diagnostic melanoma present, a diagnosis is rendered and stains are not performed.
7. If there is no obvious melanoma, or if there are suspicious areas that could represent melanoma, Melan-A immunostains are performed on the reserved slides. Final diagnosis is given only after these studies are completed.

Suggested Readings

Baneriee SS, Harris M. Morphological and immunophenotypic variations in malignant melanoma. *Histopathology.* 2000;36:387–402.

Barnhill RL, Piepkorn M, Busam KJ. *Pathology of Melanocytic Nevi and Malignant Melanoma*. 2nd ed. New York: Springer; 2004.

Crowson AN, Magro CM, Mihm MC. *The Melanocytic Proliferations. A Comprehensive Textbook of Pigmented Lesions*. New York: Wiley-Liss; 2001.

Culpepper KS, Granter SR, McKee PH. My approach to atypical melanocytic lesions. *J Clin Pathol*. 2004;57:1121–1131.

Elder D, van den Oord J. Pathology and pathophysiology of melanocytic disorder. *Histopathology*. 2002;41(Suppl. 2):120–146.

Massi G, Leboit PE. *Histological Diagnosis of Nevi and Melanoma*. Darmstadt: Steinkopff Berlin: Springer; 2004.

Thompson JF, Morton DL, Kroon BBR. *Textbook of Melanoma*. New York: Martin Dunitz; 2004.

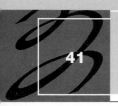

41 CENTRAL NERVOUS SYSTEM: BRAIN, SPINAL CORD, AND MENINGES

Sushama Patil and Arie Perry

I. INTRODUCTION. The task of evaluating a neuropathological specimen often seems daunting, given the enormity and the complex nature of this organ system and the ever enlarging list of the diseases. However, when a methodical approach is applied using clinical and radiologic, as well as histologic information, the chances of error can be significantly reduced. This chapter provides a baseline approach to common neuropathologic entities that are encountered in the daily practice of surgical pathology.

II. ANATOMY AND HISTOLOGY. The central nervous system (CNS) consists of: (1) cerebrum, cerebellum, and the brain stem, which continues distally as the spinal cord; (2) the meninges; (3) 12 pair of cranial nerves; and (4) the blood vessels supplying these structures. The brain and spinal cord are enclosed within the skeletal confines of the cranium and vertebral canal. The mature (adult) brain weighs around 1200 to 1400 grams. The meninges covering the brain and spinal cord are of two principle types: (1) the dense fibrous dura mater and (2) the more delicate leptomeninges (pia and arachnoid mater). The cerebrum is divided into a right and left hemisphere by a thick dural fold: the falx cerebri. A second dural fold between the cerebrum and cerebellum (tentorium cerebelli) divides the brain into supra and infratentorial compartments. The brain stem is composed of midbrain, pons, and medulla oblongata (cranial to caudal), and the cerebellum is connected to the brain stem by means of three (superior, middle, and inferior) cerebellar peduncles. The supratentorial compartment consists of cerebral cortex (frontal, temporal, parietal, and occipital lobes), white matter, and deep gray nuclei, such as basal ganglia, thalamus, and hypothalamus. The infratentorial compartment contains the cerebellum and most of the brain stem structures (pons and medulla). The term "neuraxis" is sometimes used to refer to brain and spinal cord parenchyma; thus lesions that involve brain parenchyma are said to be "intra-axial" (e.g., astrocytoma, central neurocytoma, ependymoma), and those located outside of the parenchyma are referred to as "extra-axial" (meningioma, hemangiopericytoma [HPC], solitary fibrous tumor, and schwannoma of cranial nerve VIII). Similarly, in the spinal cord region, the term "intramedullary" and "extramedullary" are used to denote lesions within or adjacent to the spinal cord parenchyma, respectively.

The CNS is composed of two distinct regions both on gross and microscopic examination, namely gray and white matter. The neurons reside mostly in the gray matter (cortex and deep gray nuclei), whereas glial cells (oligodendroglia and astrocytes) are more abundant in the white matter. The eosinophilic, finely granular to fibrillary material between cells is often referred to as "neuropil" and consists predominantly of neuronal processes (axons and dendrites). Neuronal morphology varies significantly, with size ranging from <15 μm (e.g., small neocortical granular stellate neurons) to 100 μm (Betz cells of the primary motor cortex). For descriptive purposes, pyramidal neurons are often considered the morphologic prototype and contain abundant amphophilic cytoplasm, dark clumpy Nissl substance, a large central nucleus with a prominent nucleolus, and coarse cytoplasmic processes. Neocortical neurons exhibit a prominent apical dendrite oriented perpendicular to the cortical surface, a feature often lost in cortical dysplasias and ganglion cell tumors. Ependymal cells are cuboidal-shaped glial cells with epithelium-like features. They line the ventricular surface and focally transition with the choroid plexus, which is composed of papillary fronds with fibrovascular cores lined by specialized true epithelial cells that produce cerebrospinal fluid (CSF).

III. INTRAOPERATIVE EVALUATION, GROSS EXAMINATION, AND TISSUE SAMPLING. Evaluation of a surgical neuropathology specimen often begins with intraoperative consultations, which are requested: (1) to confirm the presence of lesional tissue, (2) to provide a preliminary diagnosis that will guide the surgical management (e.g., aggressive surgery for ependymoma, limited biopsy for lymphoma, culture sample to microbiology for abscess), and (3) to sample fresh or frozen tissue for ancillary studies (e.g., Western blot for Creutzfeldt–Jakob disease [CJD], molecular pathology, tumor banking, karyotyping). For optimal evaluation, the specimens should ideally be submitted on Telfa non-stick gauze pads in normal saline. Fresh brain tissue is very fragile, and improper handling can introduce cellular "touch" artifacts. Fresh brain tissue, especially small biopsy specimens, *should not* be placed on a piece of gauze or tissue paper, because subsequent tissue retrieval from these materials is almost impossible.

For intraoperative diagnosis, a small portion of fresh brain tissue, part of which is also used for smear preparation, should be chosen for freezing. Freezing the entire specimen for intraoperative diagnosis should be avoided because the tissue accrues freezing artifacts (ice crystals, clumping of nuclear chromatin; e.g., permanent sections of frozen tissue of an oligodendroglioma appear artificially irregular or astrocytic) that can easily compromise the accuracy of the final diagnosis. In addition, some ancillary studies are not optimal on tissues frozen before formalin fixation. Lastly, a small tissue fragment (1 mm^3) should also be submitted in glutaraldehyde for potential electron microscopic studies, particularly if the intraoperative diagnosis is unclear. Cytological evaluation by smear preparation is also extremely helpful, because it preserves nuclear cytology without freezing artifacts. This can be accomplished by gently compressing a representative tissue fragment between two glass slides, gently pulling them apart, and immediately fixing the smear in 95% alcohol (e-Fig. 41.1).* For frozen section preparations, the tissue is first placed at the center of a partially frozen (soft central region) block of embedding medium such as OCT; a cooled metallic weight is then placed (for a few seconds) over the partially frozen medium to complete the freezing process, typically within a cryostat. This procedure is sometimes referred to as the 'heat extraction' method (e-Fig. 41.2). By using this method of rapid freezing, the chance of formation of ice crystal artifacts is reduced. Once the tissue is frozen, two 5-μm-thick sections (20 sections apart) are cut and stained with hematoxylin and eosin (H&E) for intraoperative diagnosis.

Gross examination and tissue sampling for permanent sections is less complicated with neuropathologic specimens when compared to other body sites. This is in part due to the fact that most tissues submitted for histopathologic analysis are either small or fragmented and thus appreciation of meaningful gross features is limited. In fact, radiographs are commonly considered the 'gross pathology' for CNS biopsies; therefore, it is often important to review the imaging features at the time of intraoperative consultation. Even when intact large resection specimens are submitted, the gross abnormalities are sometimes subtle, and thus the entire tissue often gets submitted. Therefore, on a routine basis, small resection specimens and stereotactic needle biopsy cores are entirely submitted for histopathologic analysis after adequate formalin fixation (a few hours for smaller specimens and overnight fixation for large specimens). Cavitronic ultrasound aspirator (CUSA) material may be somewhat less preserved than resected tissue due to partial autolysis and other artifacts, but often aids in the final diagnosis nonetheless. When evaluating large resections, sampling should be extensive if the intraoperative diagnosis was inconclusive; even when the diagnosis is relatively clear, however, the one section per centimeter rule should be applied because heterogeneity is common and additional sampling may reveal features that were not evident on frozen section or on a prior small biopsy.

A. CNS biopsy for special circumstances. Brain and sometimes meningeal biopsies for nonneoplastic indications are occasionally performed (e.g., nonresolving chronic meningitis, neurosarcoidosis). Similarly, a 'blind' frontal lobe biopsy is sometimes obtained for neurodegenerative disorders that do not have a clearly defined etiology, particularly in younger patients. When a prion protein disease like

---

*All e-figures are available online via the Solution Site Image Bank.

CJD is suspected, a neuropathologist should be involved from the outset; a piece of cortex from the biopsy should be snap frozen for Western blot analysis by a reference lab (special shipping procedures must be followed), and the remaining tissue fixed in 10% neutral buffered formalin overnight followed by immersion in 100% formic acid (nondiluted stock solution) prior to routine processing. It is recommended that, after formalin fixation, suspected CJD tissues be treated with formic acid for 2 to 4 hours for small to medium-sized specimens, and overnight for larger tissue slices. Lab equipment (gloves, instruments, etc.) are decontaminated with 2N sodium hydroxide solution for a minimum of 1 hour or, alternatively, in 5% bleach solution for 1 hour. Frozen tissue diagnosis *should not* be attempted on tissues suspected of prion protein diseases.

B. Ancillary studies

1. Electron microscopy (EM). The utilization of EM for diagnosis of CNS lesions has declined over the last several decades. It is labor intensive, time consuming, and expensive, and it is mainly used by neuropathologists to evaluate nerve and muscle biopsies. EM applications in tumor neuropathology however, are still valuable, particularly in proving ependymal differentiation, a task for which it remains the gold standard.

2. Immunohistochemistry as an ancillary diagnostic test is now routinely used in evaluation of complex surgical neuropathology cases, especially in the area of tumor neuropathology. Frequently utilized antibodies and their immunoreactivity for common tumor types are summarized in Table 41.1.

a. Glial markers. The most commonly used glial marker in neuropathology practice is glial fibrillary acid protein (GFAP). This intermediate filament is fairly (but not completely) specific for glial lineage. However, it does not reliably distinguish astrocytic, oligodendroglial, and ependymal tumors from one another. Apart from the gliomas, GFAP expression may also be encountered in other tumors with glial differentiation, such as choroid plexus tumors, medulloblastomas and/or primitive neuroectodermal tumors (PNETs), gangliogliomas (GGs), and even to some extent in nonglial neoplasms, such as nerve sheath and cartilaginous tumors. Lastly, when GFAP expression is absent (due to technical reasons or minimal cytoplasmic synthesis of intermediate filaments), glial lineage is supported by S-100 immunoreactivity (although less specific).

b. Neuronal markers. Some of the most commonly used neuronal markers include neurofilament (NF) protein, synaptophysin, chromogranin, and Neu-N. NF is a heteropolymer composed of three subunits that are unique to neurons and axons. Normal neurons and mature neuronal tumors, such as GGs, stain for NF; however, more primitive neuronal tumors such as medulloblastomas are often negative. Additionally, NF also stains normal axons, a property that is of great utility for highlighting infiltrative growth via entrapped axons (**e-Fig. 41.3**).

Synaptophysin is another neuronal marker present as a component of presynaptic vesicle membranes. It is a relatively reliable marker of neuronal differentiation and is typically found even in the most primitive neuronal tumors (medulloblastomas and PNETs). The major disadvantage of synaptophysin is that it fails to differentiate native (entrapped) neuropil from tumor neuropil. Along with chromogranin, it is useful in highlighting neoplastic ganglion cells, as well as neuroendocrine tumors such as pituitary adenomas, carcinoids, and paragangliomas.

Neu-N is another neuronal marker that highlights mostly advanced neuronal differentiation; it has the advantage of clearly marking tumor nuclei rather than surrounding neuropil. Surprisingly, most neoplastic ganglion cells in GGs are negative for Neu-N, although this can also be useful because entrapped cortical neurons are virtually always strongly positive. Purkinje cells (cerebellum), however, are Neu-N negative.

c. Epithelial markers. The commonly used epithelial markers in surgical neuropathology include cytokeratin (CK; AE1/AE3), epithelial membrane

TABLE 41.1 | Typical Immunoprofiles of Common CNS Neoplasms*

Tumor	Positive (+)	Positive or negative (±)	Negative (−)
Astrocytoma	S-100, GFAP		CK,[1] LCA, SYN, HMB-45
Oligodendroglioma	S-100, GFAP[2]		CK,[1] LCA, SYN
Ependymoma	S-100, GFAP, CD99 (lumens)	EMA (luminal), CK	LCA, SYN
Choroid plexus tumors	S-100, CK, VIM, transthyretin[3]	GFAP	EMA, CEA
Metastatic carcinoma	EMA and CK, CK7 (lung), CK20 (colon), TTF1 (lung)	CEA, S-100, SYN	GFAP, LCA, HMB-45
Melanoma	S-100, HMB-45, Melan-A (MART-1)		GFAP, CK, LCA
Lymphoma	LCA, CD20 (L26), CD79a	EMA[4]	CK, GFAP, HMB-45, SYN, CD3
Meningioma	EMA, VIM	S-100, CD34, CK[5]	GFAP, HMB-45
Hemangiopericytoma	VIM, CD99, bcl-2, Factor XIIIa[6]	CD34	EMA, CK, GFAP, S-100
Medulloblastoma	SYN	S-100, GFAP	CK, LCA, EMA
Atypical teratoid/rhabdoid tumor	VIM, EMA, CK, actin	SYN, GFAP, desmin, AFP	PLAP, β-hCG, LCA
Ganglioglioma	SYN, NF, CG, GFAP	Neu-N	CK, EMA, PLAP
Central neurocytoma	SYN, Neu-N	GFAP, S-100	NF, CG, CK, LCA
Schwannoma	S-100,[7] CD34, Coll IV[7]	GFAP, HMB-45[8]	EMA, NF, CK
Paraganglioma	SYN, CG, S-100[9]	NF	GFAP, CK, HMB-45
Hemangioblastoma	S-100, NSE, inhibin	GFAP	CK, EMA
Germinoma	PLAP, c-kit (CD117)	β-hCG,[10] CK	AFP, EMA, HMB-45, LCA
Yolk sac tumor	AFP, CK	PLAP, EMA	β-hCG, GFAP
Choriocarcinoma	β-hCG, CK, EMA	PLAP	AFP, GFAP, HMB-45, LCA
Embryonal carcinoma	CK, PLAP, CD30		β-hCG, AFP, EMA, LCA, HMB-45
Teratoma	CK, PLAP, EMA	AFP	β-hCG

*Modified from short course syllabus #37, USCAP, 2006.
[1] CAM 5.2 recommended, because CK (AE1/AE3) AE1/AE3 frequently stains gliomas.
[2] Strongly positive in microgemistiocytes and gliofibrillary oligodendrocytes.
[3] Not specific for choroid plexus.
[4] Positive in myeloma.
[5] Positive in secretory variant.
[6] Characteristic pattern of scattered, individual immunoreactive cells.
[7] Diffuse, strong expression.
[8] Positive in melanocytic variant.
[9] Positive in sustentacular cells.
[10] Positive in syncytiotrophoblasts.

GFAP, glial fibrillary acid protein; CK, cytokeratin; TTF1, thyroid transcription factor 1; LCA, leukocyte common antigen; SYN, synaptophysin; EMA, epithelial membrane antigen; VIM, vimentin; CEA, carcinoembryonic antigen; PLAP, placental alkaline phosphatase; AFP, α-fetoprotein; β-hCG, β-human chorionic gonadotrophin; CG, chromogranin; Coll IV, collagen type IV; NSE, neuron-specific enolase; NF, neurofilament.

antigen (EMA), and CAM 5.2. CKs are used predominantly in the diagnosis of metastatic carcinomas, but are also used to identify craniopharyngiomas, chordomas, and choroid plexus tumors. Due to cross-reactivity with GFAP, gliomas may show CK reactivity, a major pitfall in the differential between glioblastoma (GBM) and metastatic carcinoma. In such instances, CAM 5.2 is recommended, because gliomas are virtually always negative. EMA is frequently used in the identification of meningiomas, which unlike true epithelial tumors usually display minimal to no CK expression (except secretory meningioma). EMA is also useful in the diagnosis of some ependymomas, along with CD99, for highlighting rounded intracytoplasmic lumina, which show dot-like intracytoplasmic reactivity.

d. S-100 protein is another commonly used marker in surgical neuropathology and is composed of three antigenically distinct portions. It is common to neuroectodermal cells, including melanocytes, glia, Schwann cells, chondrocytes, and the sustentacular cells in tumors such as paraganglioma, pheochromocytoma, and olfactory neuroblastoma. S-100 protein as a glial marker typically has higher sensitivity and considerably lower specificity than GFAP.

S-100 protein stains, along with basement membrane stains (collagen IV), are particularly helpful for demonstrating Schwann cell differentiation in benign and malignant peripheral nerve sheath tumors.

e. Proliferation markers are commonly used as ancillary aids to mitotic counts in brain tumors, and are popular as an ancillary marker for tumor grading and prognosis. The murine monoclonal antibody Ki-67 (MIB-1) binds to a human nuclear protein in the growth fraction (G_1, S, G_2, and M phases of the cell cycle), but not in the G_0 phase.

3. Molecular diagnostics (modified from short course syllabus #37, USCAP, 2006). Molecular changes can be detected at the genomic DNA, messenger RNA (mRNA), or protein levels. In situ hybridization (ISH) and genome expression profiling techniques can be used to detect tumor-related mRNAs (e.g., hormone-specific mRNAs in pituitary adenomas), and the same techniques can be useful in other CNS tumors. Other gene products, such as proliferation antigens, growth factors, and growth factor receptors, are similarly identifiable by RNA probes; however, the drawback of this technique is the degradation of RNA in paraffin-embedded tissue, thus making it inapplicable to routinely processed tissue specimens.

The most common and practical approaches to detect deletions of chromosomal regions or specific tumor suppressor genes include loss of heterozygosity (LOH), fluorescence in situ hybridization (FISH), and quantitative polymerase chain reaction (PCR) techniques. For detection of oncogene amplification, FISH, Southern blot, and quantitative PCR are most practical.

A few molecular diagnostic tests have become routinely utilized for standard of care in neuropathology. The most notable is the use of chromosome 1p and 19q testing as a prognostic and/or management tool for adult patients with oligodendroglial tumors (*Adv Anat Pathol.* 2005;12:180). FISH has the advantage of simplicity, morphologic preservation, and minimal tissue and purity requirements; however, accurate interpretation requires experience, especially in cases with aneuploid populations of tumor cells. A drawback of FISH is that it utilizes large probes (100 to 300 Kb) and is therefore insensitive to very small deletions. This disadvantage is overcome by LOH studies, which utilize smaller probes capable of detecting losses even in the presence of mitotic recombination (e.g., loss of wild-type allele and duplication of mutant allele). However, LOH has its own disadvantage in that it requires normal blood or microdissected tissue for reference DNA. Other clinical applications of FISH in surgical neuropathology include detection of *EGFR* amplification and/or 10q deletions to distinguish the small cell variant of GBM from anaplastic oligodendroglioma, 22q deletion to distinguish atypical teratoid rhabdoid tumor (AT/RT) from variants of medulloblastoma, i17q in medulloblastomas, *NMYC* or *CMYC* amplifications in large cell/ anaplastic medulloblastomas and other aggressive forms of CNS-PNET, and meningioma-associated deletions (*NF2, DAL1,* 1p, 14q) to distinguish anaplastic meningiomas from other malignancies or benign meningiomas from foci of meningothelial hyperplasia.

IV. BASIC CELLULAR PROCESSES

  A. Neuronal changes. Neurons may display several different cytologic abnormalities, some of which are specific, but many of which are nonspecific and thus should be interpreted in the correct clinicopathologic context. Acute neuronal necrosis (anoxic and/or ischemic neural change) contains two essential components: (1) shrunken pyknotic angulated nuclei and (2) intense cytoplasmic eosinophilia accounting for the name "red neurons" (e-Fig. 41.4). Although red neurons are commonly caused by ischemia, any process that causes acute neuronal death also results in red neurons (hypoxia, hypoglycemia, epilepsy, herpes simplex virus [HSV] infection, carbon monoxide poisoning, etc.). Red neurons are often confused with "dark neurons" or otherwise known as "dark cell change," a common histological artifact produced as a result of manual handling of fresh unfixed brain tissue; dark neurons most often are more basophilic, and the neuronal nucleus is shrunken or indistinct within the cell body because it blends into the compacted perikaryal cytoplasm (e-Fig. 41.5). Occasionally, damaged neurons around the edge of an infarct or traumatic injury become encrusted with basophilic mineral deposits, chiefly iron and calcium salts — a condition often referred to as mineralization or ferrugination of neurons. Binucleation of neurons is another abnormal feature, infrequently noted in dysplastic/malformative processes (e.g., tuberous sclerosis) or in certain neoplasms such as GGs.

  B. Intraneuronal inclusion bodies

    1. Pick bodies are rounded homogeneous intracytoplasmic neuronal silver (Bielschowsky)-positive, tau-positive inclusions encountered in Pick disease; they are found commonly in pyramidal neurons and dentate granule cells of the hippocampus, as well as in cortical neurons.

    2. Lewy bodies. Classic (brain stem) Lewy bodies are roughly spherical, with an eosinophilic core surrounded by a paler halo (e-Fig. 41.6). One or more may be present in the cytoplasm of a single neuron. Cortical Lewy bodies are less clearly defined and consist of a homogeneous zone of hypereosinophilia with no surrounding halo. Lewy bodies show immunoreactivity for ubiquitin, $\alpha\beta$-crystalline and α-synuclein. Brain stem Lewy bodies are seen in Parkinson disease, and cortical Lewy bodies are noted in dementia with Lewy body disease.

    3. Hirano bodies are brightly eosinophilic rod-shaped or elliptical cytoplasmic inclusions that may appear to overlap the edge of a neuron. They are commonly seen in the hippocampus and are particularly numerous in Alzheimer disease (AD).

    4. Bunina bodies are eosinophilic nonviral intracytoplasmic inclusions commonly observed in motor neurons in cases of familial and sporadic amyotropic lateral sclerosis.

    5. Marinesco bodies are small, eosinophilic, strongly ubiquitin-positive intranuclear inclusions located chiefly in melanin containing brain stem neurons (e-Fig. 41.7). These have no known pathologic significance.

    6. Lafora bodies are rounded structures composed of polyglucosan and are similar to corpora amylacea in composition and staining characteristics. They are found in large numbers in myoclonic epilepsy, particularly in the dentate nucleus. They usually have a dense, strongly periodic acid–Schiff (PAS)-positive core surrounded by a filamentous, less PAS-positive region.

  C. General reactions to injury

    1. Gliosis. Astrocytes undergo proliferation and hypertrophy in response to all forms of brain injury. This response is termed gliosis. Gliosis can be of different forms including acute or subacute, chronic, and piloid types. In acute gliosis, astrocytes undergo hypertrophy with prominent, radially oriented stellate processes; they often have plump eccentric cytoplasm (gemistocytes). The reactive astrocytes are evenly dispersed with no mitotic activity, and they immunostain strongly with GFAP. In chronic gliosis, these hyperplastic processes retract and become less obvious on routine staining, although their nuclei remain in increased numbers and continue to mark areas of prior damage. The regions affected by chronic gliosis are usually firm and appear fibrillary on histology. Gliosis resulting from Purkinje cell loss (cerebellum) is termed Bergmann's gliosis and is characterized by parallel fibrillary processes radiating through the molecular layer toward the pial surface, with the accumulation of astrocytic nuclei within the Purkinje cell layer. Piloid gliosis is a form of chronic gliosis with deposition of Rosenthal fibers; this form of gliosis is commonly seen adjacent to cyst walls and slowly growing neoplasms, especially craniopharyngioma, pineal cyst, ependymoma, meningioma, and syrinx. Piloid gliosis can occasionally cause diagnostic confusion with pilocytic astrocytoma (PA) on small suprasellar, posterior fossa, or spinal cord biopsies. However, the regions affected with piloid gliosis are often paucicellular and lack microcystic components, thus helping to differentiate PA from piloid gliosis.

2. **Rosenthal fibers** are beaded structures (round, oval, or elongated) measuring 10 to 40 μm in diameter and appear as homogeneous, brightly eosinophilic structures. Ultrastructurally, they represent swollen astrocytic processes filled with electron-dense amorphous granular material and glial filaments. A GFAP immunostain shows peripheral staining.

3. **Eosinophilic granular bodies (EGBs)** are found in slowly growing tumors and appear as clusters of rounded hyaline droplets that appear mostly extracellular on H&E stains. EGBs are frequently observed in PA, GG, and pleomorphic xanthoastrocytoma (PXA).

4. **Alzheimer type II glia** are seen in hyperammonemic states such as liver failure. They are metabolically active cells engaged in detoxification of ammonia and contain numerous mitochondria. Histologically, AD type II glia are astrocytes with enlarged nuclei (15 to 20 μm) that are generally pale and empty-looking because of the disappearance of chromatin granules. AD type II glia typically occur in deep gray nuclei (pallidum and dentate nuclei) and, to a lesser extent, in the cerebral cortex.

5. **Microphage/microglial reaction.** Microglial cells are of monocytic lineage and have vital phagocytic functions. They are recruited from the systemic circulation in response to injuries. Large accumulations are noted in infarcts, viral infections, and demyelinating diseases where they exhibit wide ranging morphologies. Occasional brisk mitotic activity in large accumulations causes diagnostic confusion with gliomas. Under antigenic stimulation, microglial cells become elongated rod cells; when surrounding a dying neuron, the process is known as neuronophagia. Microglial clusters form microglial nodules, which are particularly prominent in viral encephalitis.

6. **Cerebral edema** is an increase in brain volume due to increased water content. Depending on its pathogenesis, cerebral edema can be classified as vasogenic or cytotoxic. However, combinations of different edema types often coexist. In vasogenic edema (more common type), the fluid collection is predominantly extracellular and results from breakdown of the blood–brain barrier. In cytotoxic edema, the fluid accumulation is intracellular or generally ischemic, or has a metabolic etiology.

7. **Hydrocephalus** is an abnormal increase in the intracranial volume of CSF associated with dilatation of all or part of the ventricular system. Acute hydrocephalus often results from intraventricular hemorrhage or meningitis and is often life threatening. Chronic hydrocephalus often results from obstruction to flow of CSF (e.g., tumor, increased CSF production, and choroid plexus papilloma), whereas nonobstructive hydrocephalus occurs from extraventricular obstruction (e.g., inflammation or hemorrhage involving the arachnoid granulations). When the ventricles expand due to loss of adjacent parenchyma or generalized cerebral atrophy, it is referred to as hydrocephalus ex vacuo.

8. **Intracranial pressure (ICP) and brain herniation.** Despite changes in systemic blood pressure, the cerebral blood flow is kept constant through the process of autoregulation. Under normal circumstances, the cranial cavity contents (blood,

brain, and CSF) are contained within the rigid confines of the skull and dura. Increased ICP results from expansions of cerebral volume due to diffuse brain edema, increased cerebral blood flow and blood volume, or development of space-occupying lesions such as tumors, abscesses, hematomas, or large infarcts accompanied by edema. Elevated ICP, if not treated early and adequately, will lead to herniation syndromes, wherein portions of expanded brain are compressed by rigid dural reflections or bony structures. They include subfalcine (cingulate gyrus), transtentorial (uncal), and cerebellar tonsillar herniations. Tonsillar herniation is often fatal and results in death due to compression of nearby cardiorespiratory centers in the medulla. In contrast, uncal herniation causes compression of vessels and nerves adjacent to the tentorium, leading to posterior cerebral artery infarcts and "blown" pupils from involvement of sympathetic fibers at the periphery of cranial nerve III.

9. **Duret (secondary brain stem) hemorrhage** results from the downward herniation of the brain stem, which in turn results in kinking of the penetrating arteries (perpendicular branches of basilar artery) with acute hemorrhagic infarction of the pons. They are typically seen in association with severe uncal herniation; this is often fatal.

V. **NEOPLASMS OF THE CNS** occur both in adult and pediatric populations. Although adult and children may experience similar tumors, their incidences vary greatly with age. Among adults, metastases to the CNS, GBMs, and meningiomas are the most common neoplasms, whereas in the pediatric age group, PAs, medulloblastomas, and ependymomas are far more common.

In addition to the importance of patient age, tumor location, and radiographic features in narrowing the differential diagnosis in the brain or spinal cord biopsy, there are roughly eight major histopathologic patterns that may be encountered. The most common entities associated with these patterns are listed in Table 41.2.

The World Health Organization (WHO) currently lists more than 100 types of nervous system tumors and their variants (see Tables 41.3 and 41.4). Consideration of preclinical and imaging characteristics usually narrows the differential diagnosis to a few common possibilities. Table 41.5 depicts common CNS tumor diagnosis based on location, patient age, and imaging characteristics.

Microscopic evaluation of a CNS lesion (tumors in particular) is incomplete without considering the neuroradiologic findings. Particularly helpful for evaluating a CNS neoplasm are the magnetic resonance imaging (MRI) characteristics. T1-weighted MRIs with gadolinium enhancement and T2-weighted fluid-attenuated inversion recovery (FLAIR) studies allow assessment of vascular integrity and edema and/or invasion patterns, respectively. Imaging studies are particularly helpful when evaluating small biopsy samples. For example, an undersampled ring-enhancing mass (e.g., GBM) may show only features of low-grade astrocytoma. Thus, considering the radiologic findings along with histologic features helps to answer questions of biopsy adequacy and reduces the risk of misdiagnosis.

A. **Gliomas**

1. **Diffuse (infiltrating) astrocytomas (DA), WHO grade II.** Diffuse gliomas are the most frequent primary CNS neoplasms, and as their name indicates, they are diffusely infiltrative with complete resection being nearly impossible. On MRI imaging, DAs present as nonenhancing, ill-defined intra-axial masses (hypointense on T1 and hyperintense on T2 and FLAIR images). They occur throughout the neuraxis, but commonly involve the cerebral hemispheres and present clinically with new-onset seizures (most common symptom), headaches, or functional neurologic deficits. Grossly, these lesions appear gray-tan to gelatinous, and obscure the native gray-white junction. Microscopically, tumor cells invade adjacent cortex along white matter tracts. They aggregate around neurons and blood vessels and beneath pial and ependymal surfaces to produce the so-called secondary structures of Scherer. The histology of astrocytic tumor cells can vary widely from being uniform and minimally atypical to highly pleomorphic in terms of both the cytoplasmic and nuclear features (e-**Fig. 41.8**). Cells with elongate, irregular, hyperchromatic nuclei

| TABLE 41.2 | Major Histopathologic Patterns in Surgical Neuropathology* |

I. Parenchymal Infiltrate with Hypercellularity
- Diffuse glioma
- Central nervous system lymphoma
- Infections
- Inflammatory demyelinating disease
- Organizing infarct
- Reactive gliosis

II. Discrete Mass (Pure)
- Metastasis
- Ependymoma
- Subependymoma
- Subependymal giant cell astrocytoma
- Central neurocytoma
- Pineocytoma
- Primitive/embryonal tumor (e.g., atypical teratoid rhabdoid tumor)
- Choroid plexus papilloma
- Hemangioblastoma

III. Solid and Infiltrative Process
- Pilocytic astrocytoma
- Pleomorphic xanthoastrocytoma
- Glioblastoma/gliosarcoma
- Ganglioglioma
- Dysembryoplastic neuroepithelial tumor
- Primitive/embryonal tumor (e.g., medulloblastoma/ primitive neuroectodermal tumors)
- Choroid plexus carcinoma
- Germ cell tumors
- Craniopharyngioma
- Central nervous system lymphoma
- Sarcoma
- Abscess and other forms of infection

IV. Vasculocentric Process
- Central nervous system lymphoma
- Intravascular lymphoma
- Vasculitis
- Meningioangiomatosis
- Acute demyelinating encephalomyelitis
- Amyloid angiopathy and lobar hemorrhage
- Arteriolosclerosis
- Cerebral autosomal dominant arteriopathy with subcortical infarcts and leukoencephalopathy
- Vascular malformation
- Infection (e.g., aspergillus)
- Neurosarcoidosis
- Thromboembolic disease

(continued)

with minimal cytoplasm are seen in fibrillary astrocytomas, whereas cells with eccentrically located nuclei and abundant eosinophilic cytoplasm characterize the gemistocytic variant. Tumor cells are often, but not invariably, immunoreactive to GFAP. Mitotic activity is very low or nonexistent in DAs.

2. **Anaplastic astrocytoma (AA), WHO grade III,** is a diffusely infiltrating glioma that primarily affects adults in their 5th decade. AA may arise from progression of a DA (WHO grade II) or *de novo*, and preferentially involves the

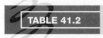

TABLE 41.2	Major Histopathologic Patterns in Surgical Neuropathology* (Continued)

V. Extra-axial Mass
- Meningioma
- Hemangiopericytoma
- Solitary fibrous tumor
- Hemangioblastoma
- Sarcomas
- Schwannoma
- Metastasis
- Melanoma/melanocytoma
- Secondary lymphoma/leukemia/plasmacytoma
- Paraganglioma
- Sarcoidosis/granulomatous diseases
- Inflammatory pseudotumors
- Calcifying pseudotumor of neuraxis
- Histiocytosis (e.g., Rosai–Dorfman disease)

VI. Meningeal Infiltrate
- Meningeal carcinomatosis (or lymphomatosis, gliomatosis, melanomatosis, meningiomatosis, etc.)
- Meningitis
- Sarcoidosis/granulomatous diseases
- Collagen vascular disease
- Inflammatory disorder (e.g., Castleman disease)

VII. Destructive/Necrotic Process
- Cerebral infarct
- Tumor with treatment effect
- Infection
- Vasculitis
- Severe demyelinating disease

VIII. Subtle Pathology or Near Normal Biopsy
- Hypothalamic hamartoma
- Low-grade glioma
- Cortical dysplasia/tuber
- Mesial temporal sclerosis
- Heterotopia
- Ischemic disease
- Neurodegenerative disease
- Benign cysts
- Reactive gliosis
- Cerebral edema

*Modified from short course syllabus #37, USCAP, 2006.

cerebral hemispheres. On MRI, they appear similar to DA, but may show focal enhancement. Histologically, AA is characterized by increased cellularity, pleomorphism, and an associated increase in proliferation. The defining feature that distinguishes DA from AA is mitotic activity, and it should be evaluated in the context of sample size. In a stereotactic biopsy, a single mitosis is sufficient to designate a glioma as anaplastic. However, in large resections there should be at least a few mitoses before the tumor is considered anaplastic. By definition, AAs do not have microvascular proliferation or necrosis.

3. **GBM, WHO grade IV,** is the most malignant form of astrocytoma and also the most common glioma subtype. GBMs occur mostly in adults with a peak age of onset in the 6th to 7th decades. On imaging, GBMs show heterogeneous or

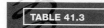

TABLE 41.3	WHO Histological Classification of Central Nervous System (CNS) Tumors

Tumors of neuroepithelial tissue
Astrocytic Tumors
Pilocytic astrocytoma
   Pilomyxoid astrocytoma
Subependymal giant cell astrocytoma
Pleomorphic xanthoastrocytoma
Diffuse astrocytoma
   Fibrillary astrocytoma
   Gemistocytic astrocytoma
   Protoplasmic astrocytoma
Anaplastic astrocytoma
Glioblastoma
   Giant cell glioblastoma
   Gliosarcoma
Gliomatosis cerebri

Oligodendroglial Tumors
Oligodendroglioma
Anaplastic oligodendroglioma

Oligoastrocytic Tumors
Oligoastrocytoma
Anaplastic oligoastrocytoma

Ependymal Tumors
Subependymoma
Myxopapillary ependymoma
Ependymoma
   Cellular
   Papillary
   Clear cell
   Tanycytic
Anaplastic ependymoma

Choroid Plexus Tumors
Choroid plexus papilloma
Atypical choroid plexus papilloma
Choroid plexus carcinoma

Other Neuroepithelial Tumors
Astroblastoma
Chordoid gliomas of the 3rd ventricle
Angiocentric gliomas
Neuronal and Mixed Neuronal-Glial Tumors
Dysplastic gangliocytoma of cerebellum
   (Lhermitte–Duclos)
Desmoplastic infantile astrocytoma/ganglioglioma
Dysembryoplastic neuroepithelial tumor
Gangliocytoma
Ganglioglioma
Anaplastic ganglioglioma
Central neurocytoma
Extraventricular neurocytoma
Cerebellar liponeurocytoma
Papillary glioneuronal tumor
Rosette-forming glioneuronal tumor of the 4th ventricle
Paraganglioma

(*continued*)

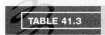

TABLE 41.3	WHO Histological Classification of Central Nervous System (CNS) Tumors *(Continued)*

Tumors of the Pineal Region
Pineocytoma
Pineal parenchymal tumor of intermediate differentiation
Pineoblastoma
Papillary tumor of the pineal region

Embryonal Tumors
Medulloblastoma
   Desmoplastic/nodular medulloblastoma
   Medulloblastoma with extensive nodularity
   Anaplastic medulloblastoma
   Large cell medulloblastoma
CNS primitive neuroectodermal tumor
   CNS neuroblastoma
   CNS ganglioneuroblastoma
   Medulloeplthelloma
   Ependymoblastoma
Atypical teratoid/rhabdoid tumor

Tumors of cranial and paraspinal nerves
Schwannoma (neurilemoma, neurinomas)
   Cellular
   Plexiform
   Melanotic
Neurofibroma
   Plexiform
Perineurioma
   Perineurioma, NOS
   Malignant perineurioma
Malignant peripheral nerve sheath tumor (MPNST)
   Epithelioid MPNST
   MPNST with mesenchymal differentiation
   Melanotic MPNST
   MPNST with glandular differentiation

Tumors of the meninges
Tumors of meningothelial cells
Meningioma
   Meningothelial
   Fibrous (fibroblastic)
   Transitional (mixed)
   Psammomatous
   Angiomatous
   Microcystic
   Secretory
   Lymphoplasmacyte rich
   Metaplastic
   Chordoid
   Clear cell
   Atypical
   Papillary
   Rhabdoid
   Anaplastic (malignant)

(continued)

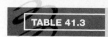

Mesenchymal tumors
Lipoma
Angiolipoma
Hibernoma
Liposarcoma
Solitary fibrous tumor
Fibrosarcoma
Malignant fibrous histiocytoma
Leiomyoma
Leiomyosarcoma
Rhabdomyoma
Rhabdomyosarcoma
Chondroma
Chondrosarcoma
Osteoma
Osteosarcoma
Osteochondroma
Hemangioma
Epithelioid hemangioendothelioma
Hemangiopericytoma
Anaplastic hemangiopericytoma
Angiosarcoma
Kaposi sarcoma
Ewing sarcoma–PNET

Primary melanocytic lesions
Diffuse melanocytosis
Melanocytoma
Malignant melanoma
Meningeal melanomatosis

Other neoplasms related to the meninges
Hemangioblastoma

Lymphomas and hematopoietic neoplasms
Malignant lymphomas
Plasmacytoma
Granulocytic sarcoma

Germ cell tumors
Germinoma
Embryonal carcinoma
Yolk sac tumor
Choriocarcinoma
Teratoma
   Mature
   Immature
   Teratoma with malignant transformation
Mixed germ cell tumor

Tumors of the sellar region
Craniopharyngioma
   Adamantinomatous
   Papillary
Granular cell tumor
Pituicytoma
Spindle cell oncocytoma of the adenohypophysis

Metastatic tumors

From: *WHO Classification of the Tumors of the Central Nervous System.* Lyon, France: IARC Press; 2007.

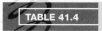

TABLE 41.4   WHO Grades of Central Nervous System (CNS) Tumors

	I	II	III	IV
Astrocytic Tumors				
Subependymal giant cell astrocytoma	•			
Pilocytic astrocytoma	•			
Pilomyxoid astrocytoma		•		
Diffuse astrocytoma		•		
Pleomorphic xanthoastrocytoma		•		
Anaplastic astrocytoma			•	
Glioblastoma				•
Giant cell glioblastoma				•
Gliosarcoma				•
Oligodendroglial Tumors				
Oligodendroglioma		•		
Anaplastic oligodendroglioma			•	
Oligoastrocytic Tumors				
Oligoastrocytoma		•		
Anaplastic oligoastrocytoma			•	
Ependymal Tumors				
Subependymoma	•			
Myxopapillary ependymoma	•			
Ependymoma		•		
Anaplastic ependymoma			•	
Choroid Plexus Tumors				
Choroid plexus papilloma	•			
Atypical choroid plexus papilloma		•		
Choroid plexus carcinoma			•	
Other Neuroepithelial Tumors				
Angiocentric gliomas	•			
Chordoid gliomas of the 3rd ventricle		•		
Neuronal and Mixed Neuronal–Gglial Tumors				
Gangliocytoma	•			
Ganglioglioma	•			
Anaplastic ganglioglioma			•	
Desmoplastic infantile astrocytoma and ganglioglioma	•			
Dysembryoplastic neuroepithelial tumor	•			
Central neurocytoma		•		
Extraventricular neurocytoma		•		
Cerebellar liponeurocytoma		•		
Paraganglioma of the spinal cord	•			
Papillary glioneuronal tumor	•			
Rosette-forming glioneuronal tumor of the 4th ventricle	•			
Pineal Tumors				
Pineocytoma	•			
Pineal parenchymal tumor of intermediate differentiation		•	•	
Pineoblastoma				•
Papillary tumor of the pineal region		•	•	
Embryonal Tumors				
Medulloblastoma				•
CNS primitive neuroectodermal tumor (PNET)				•
Atypical teratoid/rhabdoid tumor				•

(continued)

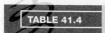

TABLE 41.4	WHO Grades of Central Nervous System (CNS) Tumors *(Continued)*			
		I	II	III	IV
Tumors of the Cranial and Paraspinal Nerves					
Schwannoma		•			
Neurofibroma		•			
Perineurioma		•	•	•	
Malignant peripheral nerve sheath tumor (MPNST)			•	•	•
Meningeal Tumors					
Meningioma		•			
Atypical meningioma			•		
Anaplastic/malignant meningioma				•	
Hemangiopericytoma			•		
Anaplastic hemangiopericytoma				•	
Hemangioblastoma		•			
Tumors of the Sella Region					
Craniopharyngioma		•			
Granular cell tumor of the neurohypophysis		•			
Pituicytoma		•			
Spindle cell oncocytoma of the adenohypophysis		•			

From: *WHO Classification of Tumors of the Central Nervous System.* Lyon, France: IARC Press; 2007.

ring enhancement, and are differentiated from AA histologically by endothelial hyperplasia (EH) and/or necrosis, the latter most often characterized as pseudopalisading (palisading) (hypercellular tumor lining around a zone of central necrosis). EH, also referred as microvascular proliferation or endothelial proliferation, is defined by the presence of multilayered vessels with enlarged, often cytologically atypical and mitotically active endothelial (and smooth muscle/pericytic) cells, often forming glomeruloid structures with multiple lumina (e-**Fig. 41.9**). There are several morphologic variants of GBM.

a. **Small cell GBM** has distinct histologic features that include the presence of deceptively bland appearing tumor cells that are slightly oval or elongate and often possess features mimicking oligodendroglioma, such as perinuclear halos, microcalcifications, and "chicken-wire"-like branching capillaries. Small cell GBM usually presents *de novo* rather than progressing from a lower grade astrocytoma. Contrasting with the bland chromatin pattern, there are usually numerous mitotic figures (e-**Fig. 41.10**). This disconnect (bland cytology and elevated mitotic counts) is often the first clue to the diagnosis of a small cell GBM rather than a high-grade oligodendroglial neoplasm (*Adv Anat Pathol.* 2005;12:180). Other helpful clues include the presence of a ring-enhancing cerebral mass and foci of pseudopalisading necrosis, although neither is absolutely specific for GBM.

Small cell GBM also has certain immunohistochemical and molecular characteristics that differentiate it from oligodendroglioma. The tumor cells in a small cell GBM often contain thin, GFAP-positive cytoplasmic processes, and the MIB-1 (Ki-67) labeling index is typically very high. FISH studies have shown *EGFR* amplifications in roughly 70% and deletions of chromosome 10q in >90% (e-**Fig. 41.11**). In contrast to high-grade oligodendrogliomas, there is no evidence of 1p and 19q codeletion (see oligodendroglioma section).

b. **Gliosarcoma, WHO grade IV,** a variant of GBM, consists of both astrocytic and sarcomatous elements. It is believed that the latter arises from mesenchymal metaplasia of the glial malignancy. The sarcoma usually is in the form of fibrosarcoma or malignant fibrous histiocytoma, but may

TABLE 41.5	Common CNS Tumor Diagnosis by Location, Age, and Imaging Characteristics	

Location	Child/young adult	Older adult
Cerebral/supratentorial	Ganglioglioma (TL, cyst-MEN) DNT (TL, intracortical nodules) PNET (solid, E) AT/RT (infant)	Grade II–III glioma (NE) GBM (ring E, butterfly) Mets (grey-white junctions, E) Lymphoma (periventricular, E)
Cerebellar/infratentorial	Pilocytic astrocytoma (cyst-MEN) Medulloblastoma (vermis, E) Ependymoma (4th v., E) Choroid plexus papilloma (4th v.) AT/RT (infant)	Mets (multiple, E) Hemangioblastoma (cyst-MEN) Choroid plexus papilloma (4th v.)
Brain stem	"brain stem glioma" (pons) Pilocytic astrocytoma (dorsal brain stem)	Gliomatosis cerebri (multifocal)
Spinal cord (intra-axial)	Ependymoma Pilocytic astrocytoma (cystic)	Ependymoma Diffuse astrocytoma (ill-defined) Paraganglioma (filum terminale)
Extra-axial/dural	Secondary lymphoma/leukemia	Meningioma Metastases Secondary lymphoma/leukemia
Intrasellar	Pituitary adenoma Craniopharyngioma Rathke's cleft cyst	Pituitary adenoma Rathke's cleft cyst
Suprasellar/hypothalamic/ optic pathway/3rd v.	Germinoma/germ cell tumor Craniopharyngioma Pilocytic astrocytoma	Colloid cyst (3rd v.)
Pineal	Germinoma/germ cell tumor Pineocytoma Pineoblastoma Pineal cyst	Pineocytoma Pineal cyst
Thalamus	Pilocytic astrocytoma AA/GBM	AA/GBM Lymphoma
Cerebellopontine angle	Vestibular schwannoma (NF2)	Vestibular schwannoma Meningioma
Lateral ventricle	Central neurocytoma SEGA (tuberous sclerosis) Choroid plexus papilloma Choroid plexus carcinoma (infant)	Central neurocytoma SEGA (tuberous sclerosis) Choroid plexus papilloma Subependymoma
Nerve root/paraspinal	Neurofibroma (NF1) MPNST (NF1)	Schwannoma Meningioma Secondary lymphoma Neurofibroma (NF1) MPNST

CNS, central nervous system; MEN, mural enhancing nodule; NE, nonenhancing; E, enhancing; DNT, dysembryoplastic neuroepithelial tumor; MPNST, malignant peripheral nerve sheath tumor; SEGA, subependymal giant cell astrocytoma; TL, temporal lobe; PNET, primitive neuroectodermal tumor; AT/RT, atypical teratoid rhabdoid tumor; GBM, glioblastoma; v., ventricle; AA, anaplastic astrocytoma; NF, neurofilament.

include bone, cartilage, muscle, and even epithelial lines of aberrant differentiation, the latter referred to as adenoid GBM. Gliosarcomas are often superficially located and appear deceptively circumscribed. Molecular studies have demonstrated similar genetic abnormalities within both elements, suggesting a monoclonal process rather than a collision tumor. The sarcomatous elements in a gliosarcoma are typically negative for GFAP but positive for vimentin, smooth muscle actin, muscle specific action (MSA), etc., based on the sarcomatous differentiation pattern. In contrast, the mesenchymal regions are reticulin rich, whereas the gliomatous portion is reticulin poor.

4. **Gliomatosis cerebri** is an extensively infiltrative glioma, often of astrocytic type, that involves three or more lobes of the cerebrum, often extending into brain stem, cerebellum, and/or spinal cord as well. Microscopically, gliomatosis most often has features of AA but is associated with a poor prognosis regardless of the grade impression. Foci of progression to GBM are not uncommon.

5. **Circumscribed astrocytomas**
   a. **PA, WHO grade I,** is a slowly growing, circumscribed neoplasm frequently occurring in children and young adults, with a predilection for cerebellum. It also occurs in the optic pathway, hypothalamus, dorsal brain stem, spinal cord, and rarely, cerebral hemispheres. On imaging, these tumors are often cystic with an enhancing mural nodule. In the brain stem region, they occur as exophytic lesions. Histologically, these tumors are characterized by a biphasic pattern of growth with compact pilocytic areas interspersed with microcystic loose and/or spongy areas. The tumor is variably cellular and populated by bipolar cells with long hair-like (piloid) processes. Rosenthal fibers and EGBs commonly occur within the compact (dense) regions. Mitotic activity is low. PAs are highly vascular neoplasms, and often the vascularity resembles the EH of a high-grade glioma. The vessels are more often lined by bland appearing endothelial cells without multilayers, although even when true EH is found, it has no prognostic significance. Infrequently the tumor cells bear a striking resemblance to oligodendroglioma. In longstanding cases, degenerative atypia along with prominent vasculature can be confused for high-grade glioma. PAs usually follow a benign clinical course.
   b. **Pilomyxoid astrocytoma (PMA), WHO grade II,** also known as infantile PA, is a piloid neoplasm closely related to PA. PMA typically presents in infants at a median age of 10 months, with favored locations being hypothalamus and optic chiasm. On imaging, PMA appears circumscribed, hypointense on T1 and hyperintense on T2, with homogenous contrast enhancement. The histologic hallmark of PMA is the presence of monomorphous bipolar cells in a markedly mucoid matrix and with a prominent angiocentric arrangement resembling the perivascular pseudorosettes of ependymoma (e-Fig. 41.12). By definition, PMA does not show Rosenthal fibers or EGBs. Mitoses can be present. The tumor cells show strong and diffuse immunoreactivity to GFAP, S-100, and vimentin. A subset of tumor cells is also positive for synaptophysin. Clinically, PMAs behave more aggressively than PAs, with frequent local recurrences as well as CSF seeding at the time of diagnosis in many cases.

6. **PXA, WHO grade II,** is an epileptogenic neoplasm commonly located in the cortical regions of the temporal lobe, often with meningeal attachment. Histologically, this tumor is composed of large pleomorphic, variably GFAP-positive astrocytes (e-Fig. 41.13). Some of the tumor cells have bizarre nuclei and nuclear cytoplasmic pseudoinclusions, with multinucleated giant cells being common. EGBs are often evident. Xanthomatous tumor cells are also helpful, but only encountered in about 25% of cases. Other features include perivascular lymphocytic cuffing and scant mitoses. Endothelial proliferation and necrosis are not evident in grade II examples. PXAs have a relatively favorable prognosis (81% 5-year survival). Anaplastic (WHO grade III) transformation occurs in 15% of PXAs, and ironically the tumor cells become less pleomorphic with

increased proliferative activity, necrosis, and/or microvascular proliferation. The tumor cells often appear more like those of conventional fibrillary astrocytoma.

7. **Subependymal giant cell astrocytoma (SEGA), WHO grade I,** is a variant of astrocytoma that occurs in children and young adults, most often presenting with obstructive hydrocephalus. SEGA is nearly exclusively found in patients with tuberous sclerosis. These intraventricular tumors usually occur near the foramen of Monro. Imaging studies reveal contrast enhancement and calcification. Histologically the tumor cells contain abundant glassy "astrocyte-like" eosinophilic cytoplasm and, despite their name, are more aptly considered large than "giant." Spindle cells and epithelioid to gemistocyte-like forms are seen forming occasional perivascular pseudorosettes. The tumor cells contain prominent nucleoli and fine granular chromatin resulting in ganglion-like nuclei. The hybrid astrocytic and neuronal features are also depicted in the immunohistochemical profile, which sometimes reveals both GFAP and neuronal marker positivity. Mitoses, microvascular proliferation, and necrosis are typically absent.

8. **Oligodendrogliomas, WHO grade II,** comprise 10–25% of all adult gliomas, behave less aggressively than astrocytomas, and show slower progression and longer patient survival. The distinction of oligodendroglial neoplasms from astrocytic tumors is subjective, the main distinction resting solely on nuclear cytology. To confuse the matter further, subsets of oligodendroglioma cells show strong GFAP immunoreactivity (gliofibrillary oligodendrocytes and minigemistocytes). Clear perinuclear haloes impart a "fried egg" or "honeycomb" appearance, but represent a formalin fixation artifact that is not seen in frozen sections or in rapidly fixed specimens. Other common features that are less specific include rich, branching "chicken-wire"-like capillary networks, microcalcifications, extensive cortical involvement, mucin-rich microcystic spaces, and secondary structuring, especially perineuronal satellitosis. Cortical involvement often results in seizures, which is the most common clinical manifestation.

The nuclear features in oligodendrogliomas consist of uniform, rounded nuclei with bland chromatin, sharp nuclear membranes, and small to inconspicuous nucleoli (e-**Fig. 41.14**). Other histologic features sometimes noted are minigemistocytes. Minigemistocytes have classic oligodendroglioma nuclear cytology with small bellies of eccentrically placed eosinophilic cytoplasm that stains strongly with GFAP. Gliofibrillary oligodendrocytes look identical to conventional oligodendroglioma cells on H&E stain, but display a thin rim of strong perinuclear GFAP immunoreactivity, sometimes with a tadpole-like tail of cytoplasmic extension.

In addition to oligodendrogliomas, several other tumors exhibit the so-called "fried egg" appearance with rounded nuclei and clear perinuclear haloes. Thus, the differential diagnosis for an oligodendroglioma is relatively broad and is shown in Table 41.6.

Genetic profiling of oligodendrogliomas (*Adv Anat Pathol.* 2005;12:180) is now a routine practice in surgical neuropathology. Several studies utilizing LOH and FISH techniques have established the presence of codeletions involving chromosomes 1p and 19q in 60–90% of oligodendrogliomas. Additionally, those tumors that harbor codeletions of 1p and 19q typically behave in a less aggressive fashion and are more sensitive to PCV (procarbazine, CCNU, vincristine) chemotherapy, as well as radiation and less toxic chemotherapeutic agents such as temozolomide. Oligodendrogliomas with 1p and 19q codeletions (e-**Fig. 41.15**) are thus designated as "genetically favorable." Apart from the obvious prognostic implications, identification of 1p and 19q codeletions also helps to differentiate "oligodendroglioma-like" mimics (Table 41.6) from true oligodendrogliomas.

Pediatric oligodendrogliomas as a group share similar histomorphologic features with the adult counterpart, but most lack the signature codeletions (1p and 19q); those tumors that do harbor the codeletions (1p and 19q) frequently

TABLE 41.6 Differential Diagnoses for Oligodendrogliomas

Diagnosis	Clinical	Helpful distinguishing features Gross/Radiology	Histopathology
Diffuse astrocytoma (WHO grade II)	None	Deeper epicenter	Long, dark nuclei Pleomorphism GFAP+ process
Pilocytic astrocytoma (WHO grade I)	Child	Location (see text) Cyst with enhancing mural nodule Discrete borders	Rosenthal fibers Eosinophilic granular Bodies (EGBs) GFAP+ processes
DNT (WHO grade I)	Long seizure history	Temporal lobe Limited to cortex Nodular	Mucin-rich nodules Floating neurons
Central neurocytoma (WHO grade II)	Hydrocephalus-type symptoms	Lateral ventricle/ septum pellucidum Enhancing	Rosette formation Neuropil formation Synaptophysin +
Clear-cell ependymoma (WHO grade II)	Child	Discrete borders Enhancing Cystic	Non-infiltrative Perivascular pseudorosettes

WHO, World Health Organization; GFAP, glial fibrillary acid protein; EGB, eosinophilic granular bodies.
From: Kleihues P, Cavenee WK, eds. *World Health Organization Classification of Tumors. Pathology and Genetics. Tumors of the Nervous System.* Lyon: IARC Press; 2000. Used with permission.

occur in teenagers and older children and likely represent the "adult type" oligodendroglioma (*J Neuropathol Exp Neurol*. 2003;62:53).

9. **Anaplastic oligodendroglioma, WHO grade III.** Based on the criteria defined by the WHO, anaplastic oligodendroglioma must have "significant mitotic activity, endothelial hyperplasia, or necrosis" along with increased cellularity and marked atypia (*WHO Classification of Tumors of the Central Nervous System.* Lyon, France: IARC Press; 2007). The exact number of mitoses has not been universally accepted, but a mitotic index of 6 or more per 10 high-power fields (40×) is often used to assign anaplastic grade III (based on *J Neuropathol Exp Neurol*. 2001;60:248) in the absence of EH or necrosis. Anaplastic transformation can be focal or diffuse. Focal anaplasia sometimes presents as hypercellular nodules with increased mitotic activity in an otherwise low-grade tumor; such cases are designated as oligodendroglioma with focal anaplasia, WHO grade III. Neuroimaging studies of an anaplastic oligodendroglioma often, but not invariably, show patchy or homogeneous contrast enhancement. Ring enhancement, however, is uncommon and predicts poor prognosis.

10. **Mixed oligoastrocytoma (MOA).** Although the majority of gliomas, when adequately sampled and well fixed, show classical features of either oligodendroglioma or astrocytoma, a significant subset show ambiguous or intermixed features and are therefore included in the category of MOA. MOAs exhibit low diagnostic concordance rates even among expert neuropathologists (*J Neuropathol Exp Neurol*. 2003;62:1118). This is largely due to the absence of specific markers for either astrocytic or oligodendroglial differentiation. Histologically, MOAs are a subset of gliomas that exhibit both oligodendroglial and astrocytic tumor components. These two components manifest either as geographically separate or more often intermingled forms. Unlike the classical oligodendroglioma, only a small subset of MOAs exhibits 1p and 19q codeletions. When MOAs exhibit an increased mitotic index, EH, or

palisading necrosis, they are designated as anaplastic (WHO grade III). MOAs with necrosis are sometimes referred to as GBM with oligodendroglial features, WHO grade IV (*J Clin Oncol.* 2006;24:5419). They have a better prognosis than classic GBMs, but worse than anaplastic MOAs lacking necrosis.

B. Ependymomas, WHO grade II. Ependymomas occur as discrete enhancing masses by CT and MRI studies. These tumors commonly occur in children and young adults, and favor a 4th ventricular location in children and spinal cord locations in young adults. Supratentorial examples are often unassociated with the ventricles and can present in either age group. CSF dissemination occurs in <5% of the cases. Calcification in ependymoma is common when the lesion is located intracranially, whereas cyst formation is common in supratentorial cases. Smear preparations of ependymoma show uniform round to oval nuclei, distinct nucleoli, and spindled to epithelioid cytoplasm often within a fibrillary background; histologically, ependymomas show similar cytology, and the tumor cells form both true ependymal rosettes and perivascular pseudorosettes. True rosettes (or ependymal canals) have central lumens reminiscent of the central canal of the spinal cord, whereas perivascular pseudorosettes have vessels at the center surrounded radially by the tumor cells with a nucleus-free zone in between. True rosettes are more specific, but are only seen in 5–10% of cases, whereas pseudorosettes are nearly universal. Ependymal canals are elongate versions of true rosettes and resemble ventricular linings. They are typically seen in only the most differentiated examples.

1. Anaplastic ependymoma, WHO grade III. Several grading systems have been proposed for ependymomas, but no consensus has been achieved. According to the WHO 2007 criteria, anaplastic ependymomas are characterized by increased cellularity, brisk mitotic activity, pseudopalisading necrosis, and microvascular proliferation (*WHO Classification of Tumors of the Central Nervous System.* Lyon, France: IARC Press; 2007). Necrosis by itself in the absence of pseudopalisading does not warrant the diagnosis of anaplasia, because lower grade ependymomas also show degenerative changes. Ependymomas are usually treated with surgery and, in many cases, radiation. Gross total resection (GTR) favors better prognosis. Poor prognostic indicators include age <3 years, posterior fossa location, and anaplastic tumor grade. Grade II ependymomas have a 5-year progression-free survival rate of 60–80% as compared to 25–50% in anaplastic ependymomas.

Ependymomas are glial neoplasms and thus exhibit GFAP positivity in the majority of cases. GFAP also highlights the perivascular pseudorosettes (positive cell processes radiating toward the central blood vessel). EMA staining is variable but, when present, is seen along the luminal surface of the ependymal canals or as intracytoplasmic "dot-like" reactivity. This dot-like staining pattern is thought to represent intracytoplasmic lumina. The majority of ependymomas also show membranous and dot-like immunoreactivity for CD99, although the specificity of this pattern is unclear. In difficult cases, EM studies are helpful in establishing ependymal ontogeny by demonstrating long zipper-like intercellular junctions, microvilli, cilia, and/or intracytoplasmic lumina.

2. Myxopapillary ependymoma, WHO grade I, is a slowly growing tumor in young adults with a distinctive histological pattern that almost exclusively occurs in the cauda equina region, where it arises from the filum terminale. Grossly, these tumors present as encapsulated, intradural, sausage-shaped gelatinous masses. Histologically, the tumors are composed of cuboidal-to-columnar cells that surround an often hyalinized central vessel and fibrous stroma, giving a distinct papillary appearance in partially discohesive regions. A fairly consistent feature is the presence of a rim of basophilic mucin surrounding the blood vessels and separating them from the ependymal tumor cells (e-**Fig. 41.16**). The tumor cells are immunoreactive for GFAP, S-100 protein, and vimentin, with variable staining for EMA and CD99. These tumors have a favorable prognosis following complete resection. Other variants of WHO grade II or III ependymoma include the clear cell (mimic oligodendroglioma), cellular (mimic medulloblastoma or PNET), tanycytic (mimic schwannoma or PA), and papillary (mimic choroid plexus tumors) subtypes. Rare subtypes include ependymomas with lipidized, signet ring, giant cell, or neuronal features.

3. **Subependymomas, WHO grade I,** are benign, slow growing tumors related to ependymomas. They are solid and intraventricular. They are often asymptomatic, incidental lesions discovered on CT and MRI studies. Occasionally, they undergo intratumoral hemorrhage and become life threatening. Grossly, they are sessile or pedunculated masses within the ventricles (lateral > 4th > 3rd). Histologically, these tumors are lobulated and well demarcated. The tumor nuclei are cytologically similar to those noted in ependymomas and (sometimes) show prominent clustering and low mitotic index. However, the tumor background is fibrillar and rich with processes, reminiscent of astrocytoma. Occasional pseudorosettes are not unusual. Secondary degenerative changes include cyst formation, hemosiderin deposition, vascular hyalinization, myxoid change, and calcification. The prognosis is excellent following resection.

C. **Choroid plexus tumors**
1. **Choroid plexus papillomas, WHO grade I,** are benign lesions that often present with hydrocephalus and are commonly located in lateral ventricles in children, and in the 4th ventricle in adults. Histologically, they closely resemble normal choroid plexus. However, the fibrovascular cores are lined by cuboidal-to-columnar epithelium that lacks the superficial intercellular spaces that impart a "cobblestone" appearance to normal choroid plexus. Mitotic activity is low. Clear cytoplasmic vacuoles are noted in some cases. Overall, choroid plexus papillomas have limited architectural complexity. Occasionally, infarct-like necrosis may be present, but it is of no prognostic significance. Focal ependymal differentiation is common. Tumor cells show immunoreactivity for S-100, CAM 5.2, transthyretin, and often focal GFAP. EMA and carcinoembryonic antigen (CEA) are both negative in most cases. The differential diagnosis includes normal choroid plexus versus papillary ependymoma; the latter lesion can be distinguished based on immunohistochemical studies.

2. **Choroid plexus carcinomas, WHO grade III,** usually present before 3 years of age. These tumors are highly aggressive and nearly uniformly fatal. Patients experience high rates of metastasis, mainly through CSF dissemination. Radiologically, they are often intraventricular and enhancing. Histologically, the tumors are more solid and complex than papillomas. High-grade cytology and frequent mitoses are the rule. Foci of necrosis are characteristic, and microvascular proliferation may be seen. Focal small cell features may mimic embryonal tumors (e.g., PNET). There is immunoreactivity for S-100, CAM 5.2, and transthyretin. GFAP expression is variable. However, EMA and CEA are typically negative. The differential diagnosis includes anaplastic ependymoma (GFAP+, CK−, EMA+/−), GBM (GFAP+, CK−), medulloblastoma/PNET (synaptophysin+, CK−), and metastatic carcinoma (in older patients, EMA+, CEA+/−, S-100 +/−).

D. **Neuronal and glioneuronal neoplasms**
1. **GG or gangliocytoma, WHO grade I.** GGs are epileptogenic tumors that occur preferentially in the temporal lobes. On imaging, they commonly enhance and appear solid, cystic, or both. An enhancing mural nodule is common. Microscopically, they are usually cortically based, microcystic, variably fibrotic, and calcified, and they often show perivascular lymphocytic cuffing (e-**Fig. 41.17**). The defining feature of GG is the presence of dysmorphic neurons, including those with cytomegaly, coarse Nissl substance, coarse irregular processes, and nuclear abnormalities. Binucleate ganglion cells are helpful, but infrequent. Architecturally, the ganglion cells are often clumped or haphazardly arranged in comparison to the laminar well-ordered arrangement of the normal cortex. GGs have a variable glial component, typically astrocytic. Glial predominant GGs may resemble DAs or PAs. Other features commonly noted include EGBs and Rosenthal fibers. Cortical dysplasia may be seen adjacent to GG. High-grade glial transformation is exceedingly rare and difficult to define. The glial component is highlighted by GFAP immunoreactivity, whereas the neuronal component is variably immunoreactive for synaptophysin, NF, and chromogranin,

but is usually negative or minimally positive for Neu-N. A subset of cells both within and adjacent to the tumor often shows immunoreactivity for CD34. These CD34+ cells are characterized by the presence of long, stellate "spider-like" processes and are thought to represent progenitor cells. GGs have a favorable prognosis after surgical resection.

2. **Desmoplastic infantile GG (DIGG), WHO grade I,** is a pediatric variant of GG (typically occurring in children younger than 3 years) and is located superficially within the cerebral hemispheres. Grossly DIG is firm, massive, cystic, and attached to the dura; and it shows contrast enhancement on imaging studies. Histologically, DIGGs are reticulin-rich spindle cell tumors with storiform or fascicular architecture, often resembling a fibrous histiocytoma. The astrocytic cells resemble fibrillary and gemistocytic elements, but are often inconspicuous within the desmoplastic background; thus GFAP immunostaining is required for their demonstration. The neuronal component is often equally subtle because the tumor cells are often considerably smaller than the neurons of conventional GG. There is usually minimal mitotic activity, but occasionally PNET-like foci are seen. Nonetheless, the presence of such hyperproliferative foci, along with EH or necrosis, has no impact on the otherwise favorable prognosis.

3. **Dysplastic cerebellar gangliocytoma (DCG) (Lhermitte–Duclos disease), WHO grade I.** This unique cerebellar neoplasm is often associated with Cowden's syndrome. Patients with DCG often present with cerebellar dysfunction and obstructive hydrocephalus. The tumors have a characteristic striped appearance on MRI. Microscopically, DCGs present as mostly unilateral expansions of cerebellar folia with replacement of the internal granular layer by dysmorphic ganglion cells. Abnormal vascular proliferation is sometimes noted, and white matter is occasionally vacuolated. A work-up for other features of Cowden's syndrome (breast and gastrointestinal lesions) is warranted in patients presenting with DCG.

4. **Central neurocytomas, WHO grade II,** occur in young and middle-aged patients. Commonly located in the lateral ventricles near the foramen of Monro, they present with signs and symptoms of obstructive hydrocephalus. On imaging studies, they are large, globular, and often calcified masses. Moderate contrast enhancement is also noted. Histologically, the tumors are composed of solid sheets of round, uniform cells with salt and pepper nuclear chromatin. Typically, neurocytic rosettes (large, exaggerated Homer Wright rosettes) with central neuropil are also noted. In most cases, the neoplastic cells show diffuse and strong immunoreactivity with synaptophysin and variable Neu-N positivity. Occasionally, extraventricular neurocytomas occur within the parenchyma of the cerebral hemispheres, cerebellum, or spinal cord. In these locations, the tumors are generally circumscribed and the histology is similar with the exception of more common ganglion cell and astrocytic differentiation. The differential diagnosis of central neurocytoma includes oligodendroglioma and cellular or clear cell ependymoma.

E. **Pineal parenchymal tumors**
1. **Pineocytoma, WHO grade I,** is a well-differentiated neoplasm that commonly occurs in adults. Clinical signs and symptoms are variable and often relate to increased ICP and upward gaze palsy (Parinaud's syndrome). Imaging studies show a globular, discrete, contrast enhancing, often calcified mass in the region of the pineal gland. Histologically, the tumors are composed of uniform tumor cells arranged in sheets, with round nuclei and salt and pepper nuclear chromatin (identical to neurocytomas). Mitotic activity is very low. Variable amounts of neuropil are seen, often forming pineocytic rosettes (large, exaggerated Homer Wright rosettes; i.e., identical to neurocytic rosettes) (e-Fig. 41.18). The tumor cells are positive for synaptophysin and Neu-N in most instances. Pineocytomas may be difficult to distinguish from normal pineal tissue in a small biopsy, although a lobular pattern with gliovascular septae favors the latter.
2. **Pineoblastoma, WHO grade IV,** is a rapidly growing malignant tumor that predominantly occurs in children and young adults. CSF dissemination is common

at the time of diagnosis. Occasionally, pineoblastomas occur in association with bilateral retinoblastoma (trilateral retinoblastoma). On T1-weighted MRI scan, pineoblastomas are hypo- to isodense and contrast enhancing. Grossly, they are soft, friable, and poorly demarcated. Hemorrhage and necrosis may be present, but calcification is rare. These tumors are extensively infiltrative and often involve the leptomeninges. Histologically, they are densely cellular and composed of cells with oval hyperchromatic nuclei and little cytoplasm, with resulting molding of nuclear contours. The cells are arranged in patternless sheets interrupted by occasional Homer Wright rosettes. Flexner–Wintersteiner rosettes have a central lumen and indicate retinoblastic differentiation. Mitotic activity varies but is generally high, and necrosis is common. The immunophenotype is similar to that of pineocytomas and includes variable reactivity for synaptophysin, chromogranin, neuron-specific enolase, and NFs. Occasionally, these tumor cells may additionally show retinal S-antigen, rhodopsin, and melatonin expression.

3. **Pineal parenchymal tumor of intermediate differentiation PPTID, WHO grade II–III,** is a recently recognized entity that occurs both in children and adults. Histologically, the tumor is moderately cellular and has a sheet-like growth pattern, with more pronounced cytologic atypia and mitoses than those of pineocytomas. Pineocytic rosettes are lacking. Recurrence and survival rates are intermediate between those of pineoblastoma and pineocytoma.

4. **Dysembryoplastic neuroepithelial tumor (DNT), WHO grade I,** is a benign, slowly growing neoplasm that most commonly occurs in children and young adults. The tumor is commonly localized to supratentorial regions and is characterized by the presence of longstanding, drug-resistant partial seizures. A first seizure before the age of 20 years is almost universal. On imaging, DNT is a cortically based neoplasm with nodularity (in some cases), occasional cystic change, and calcification. Peritumoral edema and mass effect are typically absent. Microscopically, DNT demonstrates mucin-rich, patterned (usually in ribbons) intracortical nodules. The histologic hallmark of classical DNT is the glioneuronal component, which is characterized by oligodendroglioma-like cells; instead of prominent perineuronal satellitosis, however, neurons with relatively normal cytology appear to float in a mucin-rich space (so-called floating neurons) (e-**Fig. 41.19**). Cortical dysplasia may be seen adjacent to DNTs. DNTs are commonly misdiagnosed as oligodendrogliomas, but they have a benign course and postsurgical seizure resolution is common.

F. **Embryonal tumors** are malignant neoplasms most common to the pediatric age group; they are composed of primitive appearing "small blue cells." These tumors are typically bulky, grow rapidly, and seed the CSF pathways. By definition, all embryonal tumors are WHO grade IV.

1. **Medulloblastomas, WHO grade IV,** are the prototype and the most common form of embryonal CNS tumor. They are thought to originate from either remnants of the external granular layer or the 4th ventricular germinal matrix. On imaging, they are often homogeneously contrast-enhancing cerebellar masses. Those that seed the CSF commonly give rise to "drop metastases" in the lumbosacral spinal cord. Although distant metastases are rare, they most often involve bone and lymph nodes. Several histological subtypes have been described, the most common among these include the "classic/undifferentiated" medulloblastoma; "desmoplastic and nodular" medulloblastoma; "medulloblastoma with extensive nodularity." The "anaplastic" and the "large cell" variants. Classic medulloblastomas contain patternless sheets of tumor cells with high nuclear/cytoplasmic ratios, with or without Homer Wright rosettes (tumor cells surrounding islands of delicate fibrillary neuropil). These tumors have high mitotic counts and karyorrhexis.

The desmoplastic and/or nodular variant (e-**Fig. 41.20**) has a characteristic low-power appearance of rounded, pale islands of tumor separated by darker internodular tumor. The pale islands (reticulin free) are less cell dense and are composed of more mature appearing round to oval cells with neurocyte-like chromatin and less mitotic activity. These cells are embedded within a neuropil-like stroma and represent regions of neuronal maturation. The tumor cells in the internodular region are more dense and primitive appearing with high mitotic rates. The desmoplastic and/or nodular medulloblastomas compose a genetically distinct subset of medulloblastomas and have a slightly more favorable prognosis than do the other subtypes (*Acta Neuropathol.* 2006;112:5).

Anaplastic medulloblastomas are characterized by tumor cells that are highly pleomorphic with cytomegaly, nuclear atypia, hyperchromasia, and increased apoptosis. Anaplasia is also characterized by the presence of cell wrapping, apoptotic lakes, and markedly elevated mitotic counts.

Large cell medulloblastoma is the least common subtype and accounts for 2%–4% of all medulloblastomas. Histologically, in keeping with the large cell designation, the tumor cells are large and round, and contain vesicular nuclei with prominent nucleoli and moderate cytoplasm. Mitotic and apoptotic figures are very common. The cytologic features overlap with the anaplastic variant, and the two are often intermingled, leading to the use of the term "anaplastic/large cell" by some.

Medulloblastomas are generally positive for synaptophysin and variably positive for GFAP, and have high MIB-1 (Ki-67) labeling indices. Recent attempts at grading medulloblastomas have concluded that anaplastic and/or large cell medulloblastomas are associated with a worse clinical outcome and lower likelihood of therapeutic responsiveness. Cytogenetic studies of medulloblastomas often show losses involving chromosome 17p, with associated duplication of its long arm resulting in isochromosome 17q (i17q); i17q is encountered in about 30% of medulloblastomas and the majority of anaplastic and/or large cell examples. Losses of 17p and amplifications of *MYC* oncogenes, either *c-* or *N-myc*, are associated with aggressive behavior and shortened survival times. The 5-year survival rate for classic medulloblastomas has improved and now stands at 70–80%, although the side effects of craniospinal irradiation can be devastating in young patients, particularly those younger than 3 years.

2. **CNS-PNET, WHO grade IV,** is a malignant tumor that is essentially identical to medulloblastoma histologically, but occurs outside the cerebellum (e.g., cerebrum, brain stem, spinal cord). On imaging, the tumor is contrast enhancing and may exhibit calcification, hemorrhage, and/or necrosis. Tumors with evidence of extensive neuronal differentiation have been alternatively termed "cerebral neuroblastomas." Other variants include ganglioneuroblastoma (with ganglion cell differentiation), ependymoblastoma (containing ependymoblastic rosettes with central lumens), and medulloepithelioma (containing neoplastic neuroepithelium resembling the developing neural tube).

3. **AT/RT, WHO grade IV** (e-Fig. 41.21), is a densely cellular tumor of infants and young children (most patients are <3 years old). The tumor is usually large, cystic, hemorrhagic, and enhancing on imaging studies; it can occur anywhere in the neuraxis, but is commonly seen in the cerebellum. Histologically, these tumors are defined by the presence of rhabdoid cells with eccentrically placed vesicular nuclei, prominent nucleoli, and globular eosinophilic paranuclear inclusions corresponding to whorled bundles of intermediate filaments ultrastructurally. Ironically, rhabdoid cells may only be a focal finding, so a high index of suspicion is sometimes needed to arrive at the correct diagnosis. A small blue cell component is seen in 65% of cases, which helps to explain why AT/RTs are often confused with medulloblastoma or CNS-PNET. An epithelioid component that often resembles carcinoma, and sarcoma-like features, are also possible. The tumor cells are typically immunopositive for vimentin, EMA, CK, and smooth muscle actin in the majority of the cases. A subset of cells is also positive for synaptophysin and GFAP. A highly sensitive and specific immunohistochemical stain that differentiates AT/RT from other embryonal tumors is the BAF47/INI1 protein, the product of the *INI1/BAF47/hSNF5* tumor suppressor gene on chromosome 22q11. AT/RT results from biallelic inactivation of this gene, and hence virtually all AT/RTs are immunonegative for BAF47/INI1 with intratumoral endothelial cells providing an internal positive control. These are highly aggressive tumors; most patients die in less than a year.

G. Tumors of the meninges

1. **Meningiomas** are tumors thought to arise from the arachnoidal cap cells that are normally loosely attached to the inner surface of the dura. They account for 13%–25% of primary intracranial tumors and ~25% of intraspinal tumors. Most meningiomas occur in adults between the ages of 20 to 60 years, with a peak incidence around 45 years. Most benign meningiomas are asymptomatic and are often discovered incidentally by neuroimaging studies. In general, meningiomas show a slight female preponderance (male/female = 2:3). Spinal meningiomas in particular show marked female preponderance, with the female to male ratio being as high as 9:1 in some series. Radiation-induced meningiomas are also well recognized and represent a minority of cases. Meningiomas generally grow slowly; however, atypical and malignant forms are often aggressive. The vast majority of meningiomas are intracranial, including cerebral convexities and parasagittal locations. Other common sites include olfactory groove, sphenoid ridge, parasuprasellar regions, optic nerve sheath, tentorium, and posterior fossa. Occasionally, they also occur within a ventricle, presumably arising from the leptomeningeal invagination at the base of the choroid plexus known as the tela choroidea. In the spinal region, thoracic segments are favored. Neurologic symptoms are produced by compression of adjacent structures. Headache and seizures are common, but nonspecific. On imaging, meningiomas are extra-axial enhancing lesions, and trailing of the enhancement into adjacent dura is a useful radiologic sign (the so-called dural tail). Hyperostosis of the adjacent skull is most commonly associated with bone invasion. Smear preparations show cellular three-dimensional clusters, and the tumor cells have variable morphologies ranging from epithelioid to spindled. Tumor cells commonly show intranuclear pseudoinclusions (cytoplasmic invaginations) and nuclear clearings or holes (empty chromatin), although neither finding is specific. Fibrous meningiomas usually smear poorly due to increased collagen.

   Grossly, meningiomas are spherical to lobulated, firm or rubbery, usually well circumscribed, and firmly attached to the inner surface of the dura. Most invade the underlying dura or dural sinuses. Meningiomas that occur along the sphenoid wing may grow as flat, carpet-like masses termed "en plaque meningioma." The microscopic features of meningioma are highly variable as evidenced by the 13 WHO-sanctioned variants; however, features common to most meningiomas include epithelioid to elongated tumor cells with variable amounts of collagenous or mucinous stroma, concentric microcalcifications (psammoma bodies), and hyalinized blood vessels. Meningothelial whorls are most common in transitional meningiomas. Most meningiomas display patchy or weak membranous EMA positivity. Immunostains for progesterone receptor are variable but often positive in benign meningiomas. The secretory variant of meningiomas is positive for CK and CEA. A GFAP stain is useful to confirm brain invasion (e-Fig. 41.22).

   a. **Brain invasion and metastases.** Brain invasion by meningioma is characterized by irregular, tongue-like protrusions of tumor tissue into underlying brain parenchyma. This results in reactive astrocytosis, with entrapped islands of brain parenchyma at the periphery of the tumor. Brain invasion may occur in otherwise histologically benign, atypical, or anaplastic meningiomas. However, the presence of brain invasion increases the likelihood of recurrence; therefore, brain-invasive meningiomas are considered WHO grade II even when appearing otherwise benign.

   b. **Grading of meningiomas.** Most meningiomas follow a benign clinical course, but a subset disfigure the patient, cause neurologic deficits, relentlessly recur, or may even kill the patient. Roughly 80% of meningiomas are considered WHO grade I (benign) tumors and have a low risk of recurrence with GTR. WHO grade II (atypical) meningiomas constitute 15%–20% and have a high risk of recurrence even after GTR, whereas WHO grade III (anaplastic) meningiomas account for 1%–2% of cases and are associated with high mortality rates. The recurrence rates are about 7%–25% for benign

(WHO grade I), 29%–52% for atypical (WHO grade II), and 50%–94% for anaplastic (WHO grade III) meningiomas.

Meningothelial, fibrous, transitional, psammomatous, angiomatous, microcystic, secretory, and metaplastic variants are considered WHO grade I unless they have additional features qualifying for atypical or anaplastic meningiomas as listed above. Included in WHO grade II are chordoid and clear cell variants, whereas the papillary and rhabdoid variants are considered WHO grade III. Often more than one histologic subtype is observed in the same tumor. Some of the common differential diagnoses for meningioma subtypes are provided in Table 41.7.

c. **Genetic changes in meningioma.** To date several cytogenetic abnormalities have been reported in meningiomas. In general, most meningiomas show deletions of chromosome 22; approximately half of all meningiomas have allelic losses that involve chromosome 22q12. Other cytogenetic alterations include deletions of chromosome 1p, 6, 10, 14, and 19. In addition, atypical meningiomas often show allelic losses of chromosomal arms 1p, 6q, 9q, 10q, 14q, 17p, and 18q, suggesting progression-associated tumor suppressor genes at these foci. Another genetic alteration with prognostic implications is loss (deletion) of the 9p21 ($p16$ ^{NK4a}) region in anaplastic meningioma, which is associated with decreased survival.

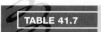

TABLE 41.7 Common Differential Diagnosis for Meningioma Subtypes*

Variant	Differential diagnoses
Meningothelial/transitional	Metastatic carcinoma
Fibroblastic	Schwannoma
Psammomatous	Reactive process
Angiomatous (vascular)	Hemangioblastoma
	Atypical meningioma (degenerative atypia)
Microcystic	Diffuse or pilocytic astrocytoma
	Clear-cell meningioma
Secretory	Metastatic adenocarcinoma
Lymphoplasmacyte rich	Inflammatory process
Metaplastic (bone, cartilage, xanthomatous, myxoid, fat, etc.)	Soft tissue tumors
Clear cell (WHO grade II)	Metastatic renal cell carcinoma
	Microcystic meningioma
	Hemangioblastoma
Chordoid (WHO grade II)	Chordoma
	Chordoid glioma of 3rd ventricle
	Epithelioid hemangioendothelioma
Papillary (WHO grade III)	Papillary ependymoma
	Astroblastoma
	Hemangiopericytoma
	Metastatic malignancy
Rhabdoid (WHO grade III)	Metastatic malignancy
	Atypical teratoid rhabdoid tumor
	GBM/gliosarcoma

*Modified from short course syllabus #37, USCAP, 2006.
WHO, World Health Organization; GBM, glioblastoma.
From: Kleihues P, Cavenee WK, eds. *World Health Organization Classification of Tumours. Pathology and Genetics. Tumours of the Nervous System.* Lyon: IARC Press; 2000. Used with Permission.

    d. Other prognostic indicators. The two most important prognostic variables include histologic grade and extent of surgical resection. Subtotally resected meningiomas have a 39% recurrence rate, which drops to 12% for tumors that have complete or GTR. Young age and male gender are less powerful predictors of recurrences. Other histologic parameters such as absence of progesterone receptors and elevated Ki-67 index are associated with increased risk of recurrence.

    e. Atypical meningioma, WHO grade II. Meningiomas with increased mitotic activity or three or more of the following histologic features are included in this category: (1) increased cellularity; (2) "small cells" with high nuclear/cytoplasmic ratio resembling clusters of lymphocytes on low magnification; (3) prominent nucleoli; (4) uninterrupted patternless or sheet-like growth; and (5) foci of spontaneous or geographic necrosis (not induced by embolization or radiation). Increased mitotic activity is defined as four or more mitoses per 10 high-power fields (*Am J Surg Pathol.* 1997;21:1455). Atypical meningiomas also have moderately elevated MIB-1 labeling indices (typically >4%). Dural and bone invasion do not alter the histologic grade.

    f. Anaplastic (malignant) meningioma, WHO grade III, typically exhibit histologic features of frank malignancy far in excess of those observed in atypical meningiomas. These histologic features include cytology resembling carcinoma, melanoma, or a high-grade sarcoma or a markedly elevated mitotic index of 20 or more mitoses per 10 high-power fields (*Cancer.* 1999;85:2046) (e-Fig. 41.23). Meningiomas that meet the above criteria are often fatal. Invasion of the brain alone is not sufficient for a diagnosis of anaplastic meningioma.

2. **HPC, WHO grade II–III.** Meningeal HPCs are much less frequent than meningiomas, although they have similar gross and imaging features, with the exceptions of a general lack of calcifications and hyperostosis in HPC. They are also highly vascular on angiogram. Microscopically, these monomorphous tumors are composed of closely packed, randomly oriented tumor cells with little intervening stroma. HPC's have reticulin fibers in their stroma. These fibers surround both "individual" as well as "small groups" of tumor cells. These tumors are highly vascular and contain slit-like vascular channels lined by flattened endothelial cells and frequent ectatic, thin walled, and branching vascular spaces known as staghorn sinusoids. The distinction between WHO grade II and III tumors is based mainly on the degree of cellular anaplasia and mitotic activity. Grade III (anaplastic) tumors tend to have more numerous mitoses (five or more per 10 high-powered fields) along with features of anaplasia, such as nuclear pleomorphism, necrosis, and foci of hemorrhage. Brain invasion may be observed. The tumor cells are positive for vimentin, bcl-2, and CD99, with variable immunoreactivity for CD34. Scattered factor XIIIa–positive cells can be present, which may represent recruited dendritic cells. The tumor is usually negative for EMA, CD31, progesterone, and S-100.

3. **Solitary fibrous tumor (SFT)** is an uncommon benign neoplasm that involves both cranial and spinal meninges. Occasionally, it also occurs in the lateral ventricles of adults and closely mimics meningiomas. Microscopically, the tumor is composed of elongated spindle cells arranged in fascicles and separated by prominent collagen bundles. The tumor cells show strong diffuse positivity for vimentin and CD34, but are negative for EMA. Some of these tumors overlap with HPC, suggesting a possible histogenetic relationship between these two entities.

4. **Hemangioblastomas, WHO grade I,** are slowly growing, highly vascular neoplasms that occur in the cerebellum, brain stem, or spinal cord region of adults. They occur both sporadically and in association with von Hippel–Lindau disease. Sporadic lesions are usually single; however, multiple lesions, supratentorial location, and location outside the CNS all favor von Hippel–Lindau disease. These tumors usually follow a benign course. On imaging studies, they are intra-axial and often cystic with an enhancing mural nodule. Microscopically, hemangioblastomas have two main components: stromal cells and a vascular

component. Stromal cells vary in their content and morphology, but typically are large and polygonal with vacuolated (lipid laden) cytoplasm (e-**Fig. 41.24**). Based on the prominence of stromal cells, two histologic variants are described: the cellular and reticular types. The vascular component is characterized by the presence of thin walled channels lined by flattened endothelial cells. In about 10% of cases, foci of extramedullary erythropoiesis are seen. The stromal cells are positive for inhibin, neuron-specific enolase, and S-100; GFAP staining is variable, and EMA is negative. Occasionally, these tumors produce brisk piloid gliosis in the adjacent brain parenchyma. The differential diagnosis includes PA and metastatic renal cell carcinoma (EMA and/or CK positive, CD10 positive, inhibin negative).

H. **Tumors of sellar and/or suprasellar region (other than pituitary adenomas).** Craniopharyngiomas, WHO grade I, are partly cystic, histologically benign epithelial tumors, thought to be derived from Rathke's pouch epithelium. Two morphologically distinct subtypes are identified: adamantinomatous and papillary.

Adamantinomatous craniopharyngiomas usually present in children, but occasionally in adults. Grossly, the cyst contents have the appearance of "motor oil." Calcifications are frequently noted. Microscopically, this variant resembles adamantinoma of the bone (tibia) and ameloblastoma of the jaw. The cyst wall is lined by complex squamous epithelium with peripheral basal palisading, loosely disposed cells with processes (stellate reticulum), a Malpighian-like layer, and a keratin-producing layer. Nodules of "wet keratin" represent islands of pale, ghost-like anucleate squames (e-**Fig. 41.25**). Rupture of the cyst contents produces granulomatous inflammation associated with cholesterol clefts and giant cells. Surrounding the cyst wall, abundant piloid gliosis with Rosenthal fibers is often noted. Finger-like projections of tumor often infiltrate the adjoining brain and/or hypothalamus and make complete resection difficult or impossible. Therefore, despite the benign grade, such tumors often recur and cause considerable morbidity due to, for example, hypopituitarism or vision loss. The differential diagnosis includes Rathke's cleft cysts.

The papillary variant typically occurs in adults and is less common. Most are in the third ventricle or suprasellar region. This variant is solid and/or cystic, although calcification is uncommon. The cysts usually contain clear fluid. Histologically, these are well-demarcated lesions composed of solid sheets with papillary dehiscence. The squamous epithelium is nonkeratinizing with no granular layers. Mucin-secreting goblet cells are commonly present focally.

I. **Germ cell tumors.** Included in this category are germinoma, teratoma, yolk sac tumor, embryonal carcinoma, and choriocarcinoma. The tumors are morphologically and immunophenotypically homologous to their gonadal and mediastinal counterparts. Typically, these tumors are seen in children or young adults. They occur in the pineal and/or suprasellar regions. Most germinomas are solid, whereas teratomas are cystic. Calcification is a common feature in teratomas. Occasionally, germinomas show marked lymphocytic inflammation and a granulomatous response, which sometimes mask the underlying tumor cells leading to misdiagnosis. Pure germinomas are radiosensitive and have an excellent prognosis. Likewise, mature teratomas follow a benign clinical course. The presence of other elements imparts the potential for more aggressive disease.

J. **Lymphoma and/or leukemia.** Primary CNS lymphomas (PCNSLs) are malignant lymphomas that occur in the absence of systemic lymphoma at the time of diagnosis. These tumors typically occur in elderly or immunosuppressed patients. On imaging, PCNSLs occur as single or multiple, homogeneously enhancing lesions. A periventricular location is common. These lesions often respond to steroid therapy, at least during the initial presentation. Surgery is often restricted to stereotactic biopsy to establish histologic diagnosis, and unless indicated, corticosteroids should be withheld before biopsy.

Microscopically, PCNSLs present as both infiltrative and angiocentric lesions composed of highly atypical lymphocytes (e-**Fig. 41.26**), the majority of which are of B-cell lineage. A minor to brisk component of reactive CD3+ T cells is a universal feature. Necrosis and Epstein–Barr virus immunopositivity are features associated with acquired immunodeficiency syndrome (AIDS) or immunosuppression-associated PCNSL. Lymphomas metastasizing to the CNS (i.e., secondary lymphomas) typically occur in epidural, dural, or leptomeningeal locations.

K. **Metastatic tumors to the CNS.** As a group, metastatic tumors are the most common CNS neoplasms; up to 30% of adult patients and 6%–10% of pediatric cancer patients experience CNS metastases. Tumors metastatic to the CNS in adults commonly include carcinomas of lung, breast, kidney, and colon, as well as melanomas. In children, leukemia, lymphoma, osteogenic sarcoma, rhabdomyosarcoma, and Ewing sarcoma are the most common primaries. Prostate, breast, lung, and kidney carcinomas are the most common primaries that metastasize to the spinal cord. The majority of CNS metastases are located in the cerebral hemispheres at the junction of cortex and white matter. Histologically, metastases resemble their primary (parent) tumors.

VI. INFLAMMATORY AND INFECTIOUS DISORDERS

A. Inflammatory demyelinating disorders are characterized by the unifying histomorphologic feature of myelin loss, often accompanied by sheets of macrophages and perivascular lymphocytes. Although myelin disorders are not classically surgical disorders, they are occasionally subjected to biopsy due to unusual clinical or radiologic manifestations. Such disorders require careful consideration of clinical and radiologic features. Some of the commonly encountered demyelinating disorders include multiple sclerosis (MS; Marburg's variant), acute disseminated encephalomyelitis (ADEM)/perivenous encephalomyelitis, and demyelinating viral infections such as progressive multifocal leukoencephalopathy (PML).

1. **MS** is an idiopathic demyelinating disorder probably with multifactorial genetic and environmental components. It typically affects young adults (especially women) and is classically multifocal with a remitting–relapsing course. Several variants have been described; however, the tumefactive variant most often mimics a glioma and is thus the type most likely to be biopsied. Imaging studies show a white matter–based T2 bright lesion, often with a peripheral rim of enhancement that may be incomplete at the cortical side, forming a "horseshoe-shaped" profile. Other locations of MS plaques include the periventricular, optic pathway, brain stem, or spinal cord regions. Perilesional edema is variable, but more often is noted around rapidly evolving lesions. Microscopically, MS shows a triad of histomorphologic features (numerous macrophages, perivascular lymphocytes, and gliosis). The demyelinated regions are best visualized on a Luxol fast blue and PAS (LFB–PAS) stain for myelin, with Bielschowsky (silver) or NF immunostains showing relative preservation of axons (e-**Fig. 41.27**). Often, PAS-positive myelin debris is noted within the macrophages. MS plaques may also mimic an infarct; a feature that helps to distinguish it from an infarct includes the presence of intact axons in the former.

2. **ADEM/perivenous encephalomyelitis** is a spectrum of disorders that includes postinfectious or postvaccination encephalomyelitis and acute hemorrhagic encephalomyelitis. Demyelinating lesions typically develop after a viral infection or a vaccination. ADEM is thought to result from an autoimmune mediated attack against CNS myelin or related antigen due to cross-reactivity with viral epitopes. Widespread perivenous demyelination, inflammation, and/or hemorrhage are noted. Brain stem and spinal cord involvement is common and sometimes predominant.

3. **Demyelinating viral infections.** Viral infections that commonly cause CNS demyelination include human immunodeficiency virus, human T-cell lymphotropic virus-1, JC virus, and measles virus (subacute sclerosing panencephalitis). PML is caused by the JC papovavirus (named after the patient John Cunningham and so has no association with CJD). PML typically occurs in immunocompromised individuals, particularly AIDS patients, and is believed to be a "reactivation disease" because ~70% of the population is seropositive. The hallmark feature of this disease is the presence of demyelinating or necrotizing white matter lesion(s), that contain viral inclusions within the enlarged nuclei of oligodendrocytes (e-**Fig. 41.28**). Also noted within and around these lesions are bizarre astrocytes that can mimic astrocytoma on a small biopsy specimen. Occasionally,

perivascular inflammation is noted and, if significant, may indicate immune reconstitution. EM studies or ISH studies are useful to demonstrate the virus.

B. Infections

  1. Herpes encephalitis. Herpes virus is a common cause of viral encephalitis; most cases are due to HSV-1 subtype, whereas type 2 infections typically occur in infants exposed during vaginal delivery. Asymmetric, bilateral involvement of the temporal lobes is common. Histologically, the regions involved show areas of hemorrhage and necrosis, along with the typical features of encephalitis in general: microglial activation, microglial nodules, perivascular lymphocytic cuffing, and neuronophagia (dying neurons surrounded by activated microglia). Characteristic neuronal and glial nuclear inclusions of the Cowdry A and B types when present are helpful; however, they are often difficult to find in a biopsy specimen. In such instances, immunostains for herpes virus are very helpful. Currently, biopsy diagnosis for herpes encephalitis is rarely performed due to the availability of less invasive studies such as CSF detection of herpes through PCR tests. Most cases are fatal unless treated early.

  2. Toxoplasmosis is an opportunistic infection commonly seen in AIDS patients and neonates (one of the TORCH infections: toxoplasma, other, rubella, cytomegalovirus, herpes). Adult infections result from reactivation. Toxoplasma infections may mimic lymphoma clinically and radiologically, and because it is a treatable disorder in AIDS patients, it is not uncommon for patients to be treated empirically with subsequent biopsy only if treatment is unsuccessful. Toxoplasmosis usually presents with multiple, enhancing, deep seated, and/or cortical lesions. Histologically (e-**Fig. 41.29**), necrotizing encephalitis with microglial nodules is the dominant feature; sometimes macrophages and secondary vasculitis are also noted. Toxoplasma organisms (encysted and free forms), when present, are seen at the periphery of the necrotic foci. Immunostains for toxoplasma are helpful and confirm the diagnosis when in doubt. Healed lesions often show abundant, lipid-laden macrophages with dystrophic calcification.

C. Granulomatous inflammation: Neurosarcoidosis. Sarcoidosis commonly involves the basal meninges. Approximately 5% of all patients with sarcoidosis have CNS involvement; often, the associated systemic disease is not obvious. The inflammation also affects cranial nerves, the optic pathway, and hypothalamus. Parenchymal lesions are rare, although granulomatous inflammation typically spreads along the leptomeninges to involve the Virchow–Robin spaces. Grossly, the involved meninges appear nodular and thickened. Microscopically, the meninges show epithelioid granulomas with giant cells frequently targeting the blood vessels. Necrosis is not a usual feature of neurosarcoidosis, although it may be seen focally. The differential diagnosis for sarcoidosis is broad and includes fungal, tuberculous, and rheumatologic etiologies. Granulomatous inflammation in the suprasellar or the pineal regions, particularly in young patients, requires careful evaluation to rule out the possibility of germinoma, particularly in small biopsy specimens.

VII. SEIZURE DISORDERS. Surgically curable seizure disorders are broadly classified into neoplastic and nonneoplastic lesions. Distinct neoplastic entities that generate chronic seizures include DNT, GGs, and PXAs, and are discussed above. Common nonneoplastic entities are discussed below.

A. Hippocampal (mesial) sclerosis. Hippocampal sclerosis (HS) is a disorder characterized by neuronal loss and gliosis of the hippocampus and adjacent mesial temporal structures such as the amygdala. Patients with HS present with longstanding complex partial seizures, often beginning in early childhood. Radiologically, HS appears as an ill-defined area of increased signal within the white matter on T2-weighted MRIs. Often the hippocampus is atrophic. Histologically, there is variable neuronal loss and gliosis, most pronounced in the CA1 and CA4 sectors (cornu ammonis/Ammon's horn) (e-**Fig. 41.30**). Occasionally, there is also splitting of the granular layer neurons of dentate gyrus. Postsurgery, the vast majority of patients experience a significant reduction in seizure frequency or are cured altogether.

B. Cortical dysplasia is a malformative process commonly resulting in chronic seizures. Grossly, cortical dysplasias produce lesions that blur the underlying gray-white junction. On MRI, these lesions are seen as T2 bright signals and extend into the subcortical white matter. The most classic form of cortical dysplasia (type IIB or Taylor type) includes "balloon cells" (enlarged neurons with eccentric pink glassy cytoplasm) and dysmorphic cytomegalic neurons. Often the normal laminar architecture of the neurons with apical dendrites (normal cortex) is lost, with clusters of dysmorphic neurons showing multidirectional dendrites. Gliosis is also common, but nonspecific.

C. **Other seizure-associated disorders** encountered less often are hemimegalencephaly, hypothalamic hamartoma, and Sturge–Weber angiomatosis.

VIII. **VASCULAR DISORDERS**

A. **Arterial venous malformations (AVMs)** typically occur within the cerebral hemisphere and only rarely in the spinal cord. AVMs are often characterized by absence of a capillary bed between the arterial and venous circulation, which results in shunting of blood from the high-pressure arterial bed directly into the low-pressure venous system. These pressure changes remodel the vascular architecture, resulting in vascular channels with both venous and arterial morphologies (hybrid vessels). With time, most of these vessels develop ectasias and muscularization, and also entrap gliotic brain parenchyma with hemosiderin deposits indicative of prior microhemorrhages. Patients with AVM frequently present with hemorrhage (more than half of the cases), and a subset of these patients also develop seizures and headaches. Imaging studies are quite characteristic and include the presence of dark flow voids; angiography studies highlight the arterial–venous shunting. Microscopically, AVMs consist of tortuous vessels with mixed arterial and venous features. Chronic degenerative changes (hyalinization, calcification) are also noted. The vascular pathology is very well demonstrated by a trichrome stain. Large AVMs are often embolized prior to resection, and this results in varying degrees of thrombosis and secondary giant cell reactions. The presence of extensive fibrosis suggests prior radiation to these lesions.

B. **Cavernous angioma,** also called cavernoma, is a vascular malformation characterized by large, thin-walled ectatic vessels with minimal intervening brain parenchyma (e-**Fig. 41.31**). Cavernomas typically present with seizures and, unlike AVMs, rarely bleed. Due to their epileptogenic potential, cavernomas are often resected. MRI studies of cavernomas show small discrete lesions with calcification that appear as "popcorn" lesions on coronal images. Grossly, these lesions appear spongy and dark red with golden brown hues (hemosiderin deposition). Occasionally, longstanding cases show marked calcification. Microscopically, they are composed of patternless, thin-walled, sometimes hyalinized vascular channels. Most often, the vascular channels are arranged back to back without much intervening brain parenchyma. The brain parenchyma in the immediate vicinity of cavernous angiomas is often gliotic.

C. **Vasculitis.** Inflammation of the CNS vasculature is often secondary to meningitis or other inflammatory and/or infectious processes. However, a subset of vasculitides occurs as primary afflictions of the CNS vessels and histologically shows granulomatous inflammation. These are thought to result from autoimmune system–mediated inflammation that is confined to the vessel walls. Primary CNS vasculitis often causes secondary infarcts in young and middle-aged patients, and has a poor prognosis unless treated aggressively with immunosuppressants. Angiography is often helpful but is not entirely sensitive. Similarly, because vasculitis is often a patchy process, a negative biopsy does not exclude this possibility.

Granulomatous angiitis (also known as primary CNS vasculitis) typically produces granulomatous inflammation of the CNS blood vessels. Men are far more commonly affected than women, and these lesions occur in the absence of polymyalgia rheumatica syndrome. On angiography, these lesions appear as beaded shadows corresponding to patchy areas of vascular constriction. Leptomeningeal vessels are commonly involved. Epithelioid histiocytes often predominate, and well-formed granulomas are not always seen.

D. **Congophilic (or cerebral) amyloid angiopathy (CAA)** is a vascular disorder that commonly affects elderly persons and is characterized by amyloid deposition in leptomeningeal and superficial cortical vessels. Frequently, CAA produces superficial lobar hemorrhage. Patients with AD type dementia often show CAA pathology.

However, not all patients with CAA are demented. Superficial lobar hemorrhage resulting from cerebral amyloid angiopathy is often mistaken for an intratumoral hemorrhage, and thus patients are subjected to surgical resection. Microscopically, involved vessels show amyloid deposits both on routine and special stains (Congo red and thioflavin S stains) (e-**Fig. 41.32**). The vessel lumen often appears "double-barreled." Inflammation is characteristically absent.

  E. Cerebral infarcts. Most often, biopsies for infarcts are performed in clinically atypical examples where the diagnosis of glioma enters into the differential diagnosis, particularly in young patients. Gross and microscopic features of a cerebral infarct vary with its age. In the acute stage (~1 to 3 days), red necrotic neurons, vacuolated neuropil, and variable neutrophilic infiltrates are present. Subacute infarcts (days to weeks) demonstrate capillary proliferation with prominent endothelial cells, pericytes, and numerous foamy macrophages that have engulfed the lipidic debris. Reactive astrocytes are common at the periphery. Large infarcts eventually evolve into cystic lesions that are traversed by delicate blood vessels forming a web-like network. Infarcts disrupt and destroy axons, a feature often helpful in distinguishing infarcts from a demyelinative process, particularly MS, in which the axons remain largely intact.

IX. **NEURODEGENERATIVE DISORDERS** mainly affect elderly patients. They are most often idiopathic, progressive, and fatal. Almost all of these disorders are characterized by neuronal loss and gliosis. Biopsy diagnosis is undertaken only when these disorders occur in unusual circumstances, such as with younger age of onset or rapid progression.

  A. AD is the most common neurodegenerative disorder. The incidence increases with age. It manifests early in patients with Down syndrome and inherited forms of the disease (approximately 10% of AD cases are familial). Microscopic hallmarks of AD include neuritic plaques and neurofibrillary tangles (e-**Fig. 41.33**) in the neocortex and hippocampus (temporal lobe). Neurofibrillary tangles are characterized by the presence of fine fibrillar (flame shaped or globular) aggregates in the neuronal perikarya. These are best demonstrated by Bielschowsky silver stain or immunostains for phosphorylated tau protein, a microtubule-associated protein. Varying degrees of glial and microglial activation are also common. Other microscopic changes associated with AD include the presence of granulovacuolar degeneration and Hirano bodies, found almost exclusively in hippocampal neurons. CAA often coexists with AD changes.

  B. CJD/spongiform encephalopathies. CJD is a rapidly progressive form of dementia, characterized clinically by a triad of myoclonus, periodic shortwave EEG activity, and rapidly progressive dementia. Most cases are sporadic, 10% are familial, and only rare examples are iatrogenic (inadvertent inoculation of contaminated tissues). CJD is transmitted by protease-resistant prion protein. Microscopically, CJD cases show neuronal loss, gliosis, and spongiform change localized to both deep gray nuclei (basal ganglia and thalamus) and superficial cortex. Spongiform change is characterized by the presence of small, sharply defined, punched out vacuoles. Cerebellar amyloid plaques are noted only in about 5% of cases.

  C. New variant CJD (nvCJD) is a rare form of CJD linked to bovine spongiform encephalopathy that occurs in patients younger than 40 years. Most reported cases are clustered primarily in the U.K. and other parts of Europe. Unlike CJD, nvCJD runs a prolonged clinical course characterized by behavioral changes; dementia is a less prominent feature. On MRI, nvCJD cases show hyperintense T2 signals in deep gray matter (basal ganglia and thalamus). Microscopically, the most characteristic feature is the presence of numerous amyloid plaques (florid plaques) in the cerebral and cerebellar cortices.

CYTOLOGY OF THE CENTRAL NERVOUS SYSTEM
Lourdes R. Ylagan

  I. **SPECIMEN TYPES.** The most common specimen type obtained for cytologic evaluation of pathologic conditions of the central nervous system (CNS) is cerebrospinal fluid. Rarely, stereotactic fine needle aspiration (FNA) of cysts or masses of the CNS is used to provide specimens for cytologic diagnosis.

A. Cerebrospinal fluid (CSF). Several methods have been developed in the last decade for concentration of samples obtained via lumbar puncture, including cytocentrifugation and membrane filtration. Slides prepared via the cytocentrifugation technique using a cytofunnel (http://www.shandon.com) are usually DiffQuik® stained since leukemic involvement of the CSF is the most common malignant diagnosis; the limited amount of material obtained (0.5.0 ml) usually precludes allocating material for Papanicolaou and other stains. Although the precise proportions vary by practice setting, most CSF specimens obtained for headaches and mental status changes show reactive (e-**Fig. 41.34**) or nonspecific features, and usually contain benign lymphocytes and monocytes (e-**Fig. 41.35**). Other normal cells which can be found in CSF specimens include ependymal and choroidal cells (e-**Fig. 41.36**).

   1. Traumatic tap. CSF samples that consist predominantly of peripheral blood are diagnosed as "negative for malignant cells" with a caveat to the clinician that the sample may represent traumatic tap (which occurs in about one quarter of cases). When a CSF sample shows leukemic involvement in the presence of peripheral blood, a repeat sample should be obtained to rule out the possibility of peripheral blood contamination.

   2. Infectious processes. Suspicion of an infectious process should always lead to culture of the CSF for bacterial, fungal, and viral patholgens. With the advent of highly active antiretroviral therapy (HAART), AIDS related CSF lesions have become rare in recent years (*J Neurovirol* 2005;11(Suppl 3):72).

   3. Lymphoma and leukemia. A primary diagnosis of lymphoma or leukemia should not be made in the absence of flow cytometric analysis of the cells to demonstrate a clonal process. A diagnosis of involvement by lymphoma or leukemia may be rendered if cells consistent with immunoblasts are present (e-**Fig. 41.37**) in a patient with a previously proven history of lymphoma or leukemia.

   4. Metastasis. Cytologic examination of CSF can be used to document CNS involvement in patients who have a known history of metastatic carcinoma (e-**Fig. 41.38**) or melanoma (e-**Fig. 41.39**), as well as leukemia or lymphoma (e-**Fig. 41.40**) as noted above. In cases of metastasis, the diagnosis should be confirmed by immunocytochemical stains or by comparison of the cytologic material with the patient's primary malignancy. The diagnostic approach to the rare metastatic tumors of unknown origin that present in the CSF is the same as for tumors of unknown origin presenting at other sites (*Semin Oncol* 1993;20:206).

B. Stereotactic brain FNA is an uncommon procedure, and the choice of the preparatory method is dependent upon the type of tissue aspirated. Involvement by a known primary brain lesion should be confirmed by comparison of the cytologic specimen with the prior diagnostic material. Fluid or purulent fine needle aspirates should be cultured as well as submitted for cytologic evaluation.

C. Diagnostic categories

   1. Negative for malignancy. This diagnosis is rendered for CSF specimens in which only peripheral blood elements are present, or in which mature lymphocytes and/or monocytes are present.

   2. Atypical cytology. This diagnosis is rendered when there are rare atypical cells but for which there is inadequate material for ancillary studies. This diagnosis should prompt the collection of additional material for either flow cytometric or immunocytochemical evaluation.

   3. Positive for malignancy. This diagnosis is rendered when there is both quantitative and qualitative evidence of a malignant neoplasm. Ancillary tests can be used to provide a definitive diagnosis as to the type of neoplasm.

D. Special techniques. Special techniques, such as confirmatory FISH, can be performed on CSF samples (e-**Fig. 41.41**).

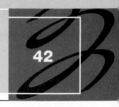

PERIPHERAL NERVE

Robert E. Schmidt

42

I. NORMAL PERIPHERAL NERVE AND METHODS OF ANALYSIS. Successful use of nerve biopsy requires a discussion between the clinician and neuropathologist because the clinical differential diagnosis may dictate an unusual sampling scheme, e.g., vasculitis in which multiple cross-sections may be required for diagnosis.

The sural nerve, a cutaneous sensory nerve to the lateral foot, is typically biopsied without stretching or use of intraneural anesthetic. The nerve is divided into portions for fixation in formalin for paraffin embedding and glutaraldehyde (Karnovsky's fixative) for plastic sections and possible electron microscopy. The entire nerve is typically used rather than dissected individual fascicles. A portion (~1 cm) of the nerve should be fixed in formalin, cut into 3-mm segments, and examined in cross-section with paraffin-embedded hematoxylin and eosin (H&E) sections, thioflavin-S histochemistry, and possible immunohistochemistry.

An H&E-stained cross-section of the sural nerve (e-**Fig. 42.1**)* contains 6 to 12 fascicles, each surrounded by flattened perineurial cells. Outside the perineurium is the epineurium, containing connective tissue and an anastomotic vascular network. The endoneurium (the space inside of the perineurial cell layer and outside the axon/Schwann cell units) contains fluid, collagen, capillaries, venules, fibroblasts, macrophages/monocytes, and scattered mast cells. Immunohistologic localization is useful for the demonstration of neurofilaments (a rough measure of axon number), amyloid, immunoglobulins, subtypes of inflammatory cells, and growth factors and their receptors.

One-micron-thick plastic-embedded sections (e-**Fig. 42.2**) provide a wealth of information. Myelinated axons range in diameter from 2 to 18 μm, coarsely separated into small (mean of 4 μm) and large (average 12 μm) myelinated axon populations with myelin thickness related directly to axonal diameter. The patterns of nerve damage visible in plastic sections may be characteristic (although rarely pathognomonic) of certain disease entities or pathogenetic processes. Qualitative information is provided on the degree of myelinated axon loss, the distribution of axon loss, the presence of active axonal degeneration or demyelination, regenerative clusters of axons, swollen axons, onion-bulb formation, the nature of cellular infiltrates, and/or amyloid deposition.

Ultrastructure provides additional detail and is the only definitive method to evaluate unmyelinated axons, which are 3- to 4-fold more numerous than myelinated axons in the sural nerve. For analysis, lengths of individual lightly fixed, osmicated myelinated axons are dissected or "teased" out of a fascicle with pins. Each myelin internode, maintained by a single Schwann cell, ranges from 0.2 to 1.8 mm in length, increasing linearly with axon diameter. Ongoing activity or residua of past episodes of demyelination or axonal degeneration are readily identified.

Morphometry provides quantitative data concerning axon number and axon size–frequency distribution. Large axons are lost in uremia, abetalipoproteinemia, thallium, arsenic poisoning, acute intermittent porphyria, cisplatin toxicity, vincristine toxicity, and Friedreich's ataxia. Small axons are selectively damaged (Fig. 42.1) in amyloidosis, some forms of diabetic neuropathy, acute pandysautonomia, Fabry disease, and hereditary sensory and autonomic neuropathies (HSANs).

---

*All e-figures are available online via the Solution Site Image Bank.

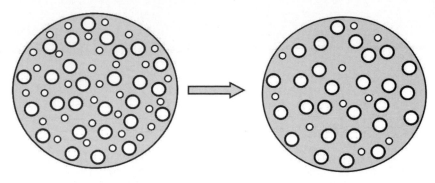

Figure 42.1. Selective loss of small myelinated axons. Normal fascicle is on the left.

II. THREE BASIC PATHOLOGIC MECHANISMS CHARACTERIZE NEUROPATHIES

A. Axonal degeneration is the most common pattern in biopsies, resulting in degeneration of the axon and its myelin sheath (e-**Fig. 42.3**). Often the distal portions of the longest axons are preferentially involved (i.e., "distal axonopathy" or "dying-back neuropathy"). Myelin destruction and its early catabolism occur in the Schwann cell, producing the myelin "ovoid" of teased fibers, and is subsequently continued in hematogenously and endogenously derived macrophages that engulf the debris. Early regenerative events begin immediately with the proliferation of Schwann cells and their processes, which accumulate within the original basal lamina of the axon–Schwann cell unit as "bands of Büngner," which are conduits for regenerating axonal sprouts. Schwann cells increase their synthesis of growth factors as trophic and tropic stimuli. Maturing axons form regenerative clusters of thinly myelinated axons within the original Schwann cell's basal lamina and, with time, one axon emerges and begins to function and the others regress. Such a regenerated axon characteristically has a myelin sheath relatively thin for its axon caliber. Teased fiber preparations show a distinctive and uniform internodal length regardless of axon diameter. The end stage of a chronic neuropathy may consist of rare preserved axons, scattered fibroblasts, and Schwann cells, and may provide little information concerning the process that preceded it.

Axonal degeneration shares mechanisms with Wallerian degeneration (WD), which is the reaction of axons and myelin distal to a crush injury. In WD, many axons show simultaneous involvement and are often at the same histologic stage; in AD it is typical to find degenerating, regenerating, and normal axons, some of which may have a distinctive pathologic signature (Fig. 42.2), together.

B. Segmental demyelination represents preferential damage to one or several internodes of the myelin sheath, directly to myelin or to its Schwann cell, with relative axonal sparing (e-**Fig. 42.4**). Schwann cell proliferation results in the replacement of each lost myelin internode by several shorter internodes resulting in variation in internodal length along individual teased fibers.

C. Secondary demyelination preferentially, nonrandomly involves selected axons, which may be atrophic or damaged, while entirely sparing others. It may reflect an abnormal axon–Schwann cell interaction resulting in secondary myelin loss. Uremic neuropathy is the prototype.

III. TOXIN-INDUCED NEUROPATHIES. A huge number of toxins and drugs (Table 42.1), including many the neuropathic toxicity of which limits their clinical usefulness, produce neuropathy, likely with different mechanisms. One group of axonal degenerations targets axonal transport; some selectively affect neurofilaments or microtubules. Acrylamide can result in distinctive neurofilament and tubulovesicular aggregates involving distal portions of axons. Zinc pyridinethione and bromophenylacetylurea preferentially target reversal of the polarity of axonal transport resulting in terminal swellings. Lead, diphtheria toxin, perhexiline, lysolecithin, and hexachlorophene are prominent

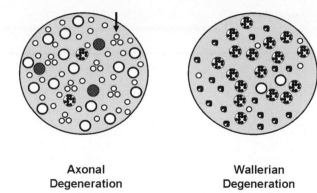

Axonal
Degeneration

Wallerian
Degeneration

Figure 42.2. Axonal degeneration versus Wallerian degeneration. Axonal degeneration is typically characterized by simultaneous axonal degeneration, regenerative clusters (*arrow*), and axons with pathologic signatures (*crosshatched*) as compared with synchronous degeneration of most axons in a fascicle in Wallerian degeneration.

toxins preferentially directed at the Schwann cell/myelin sheath, resulting in demyelination. Many therapeutic agents may induce peripheral nerve disease. Heavy metals (e.g., arsenic, mercury, thallium, gold) are well known for their toxic effects on peripheral nerves. Neuropathic industrial and environmental agents have resulted in epidemics of toxic neuropathy.

IV. **ISCHEMIC NEUROPATHIES.** The nerve vascular supply (i.e., vasa nervorum) is rich and anastomotic, requiring a substantial decrease in nerve blood flow to interrupt function. Vasculitis (i.e., vasculopathies with angionecrosis) is frequently patchy, resulting in asymmetric nerve involvement ("mononeuritis multiplex"), emphasizing the need for thorough sampling. Polyarteritis nodosa, the vasculitic prototype, is characterized by epineurial arteries damaged by polymorphonuclear leukocytes, macrophages, monocytes, and fibrin (e-**Fig. 42.5**), and by a range of axonopathy rarely culminating in infarction. There may be inter- or intrafascicular variability in axon loss (Fig. 42.3). Fibrotic recanalized vessels mark previous sites of vasculitic damage.

Patients with collagen vascular diseases may clinically present with mononeuritis multiplex histologically comparable to that of polyarteritis nodosa or a minimal epineurial perivascular mononuclear cell infiltrate (i.e., "microvasculitis") lacking angionecrosis. Epineurial perivascular collections of a few mononuclear cells are common, and some authors consider them, in isolation, to be of little pathologic importance in the absence of loss of vascular continuity or vasculopathy. Alternatively, they may represent an early or mild vascular injury or represent an area adjacent to more substantial vasculopathy. Immunoglobulins and complement deposition within the vascular wall in collagen vascular diseases may reflect the deposition of circulating immune complexes not specific for nerve.

V. **METABOLIC NEUROPATHIES** constitute a pathogenetically heterogeneous group.
A. **Diabetes.** There is a complex spectrum of neuropathies in diabetes that may have different pathogenetic mechanisms.
1. **Symmetrical sensori(motor)** polyneuropathy is the most well-known variety of diabetic neuropathy, presenting with distal sensory problems that may culminate in stocking-glove anesthesia. Patients may develop neuropathy after years of recognized diabetes or present de novo with neuropathic symptoms. Typically, distal axon loss is accompanied by vasculopathy (e-**Fig. 42.6**). Schwann, perineurial, and endothelial cells are enveloped by thickened basement membranes thought to reflect resistance to degradation because of the formation of advanced glycation end products (AGEs). Some patients with painful dysesthesias and a normal electrophysiologic exam show loss of intraepidermal axons in

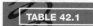

TABLE 42.1	Partial List of Agents Causing Toxic Neuropathies	

Metals	Toxins	Drugs
Aluminum	Acrylamide	Almitrine
Arsenic	Allyl chloride	Amiodarone
Cadmium	Buckthorn	Bortezomib
Gold	Carbon disulfide	Chloroquine
Lead	Dimethylaminopropionitrile	Cisplatin
Lithium	Dioxin	Clioquinol
Mercury	Ethanol	Colchicine
Tellurium	Ethylene oxide	Cyanide
Thallium	Hexacarbons and solvents	Dapsone
	Latrotoxin	Dichloroacetate
	Organophosphorus esters	Disulfiram
	Perchloroethylene	Doxorubicin
	Styrene	Ethambutol
	Toluene	Etoposide
	Toxic oil syndrome	Glutethimide
	Trichloroethylene	Hydralazine
	Vacor	Isoniazid
	Vinyl chloride	Metronidazole
	Xylene	Misonidazole
		Nitrofurantoin
		Nitrous oxide
		Nucleosides
		Perhexiline
		Phenytoin
		Podophyllin
		Polychloridyl biphenyls
		Procainamide
		Pyridoxine (vitamin B6)
		Sodium cyanate
		Statins
		Suramin
		Tacrolimus (FK506)
		Taxanes [paclitaxel (Taxol), docetaxel]
		Thalidomide
		Vinca alkaloids (vincristine, vinblastine)
		Zinc Pyridinethione

skin biopsies, a procedure becoming routine practice in some institutions. Multiple ischemic hits may summate to produce a symmetrical and uniform axon loss distally, but this mechanism has not been universally accepted. Diabetes-induced oxidative stress may reflect deranged metabolism and/or mitochondriopathy.

2. **Asymmetric neuropathies** include radiculoplexus neuropathy ("diabetic amyotrophy"), truncal radiculopathy, upper-limb mononeuropathy, and cranial nerve (chiefly III nerve) palsies characterized by an inflammatory microvasculitis and/or perineuritis, possible immune complex and complement deposition, and a mild to marked axonopathy.

3. **Diabetic autonomic neuropathy** produces a large range of symptoms contributed by the sympathetic and parasympathetic nervous systems (also enteric and visceral sensory). Autonomic axons may be involved in symmetrical sensorimotor polyneuropathy or in a more restricted pattern of autonomic fibers in the

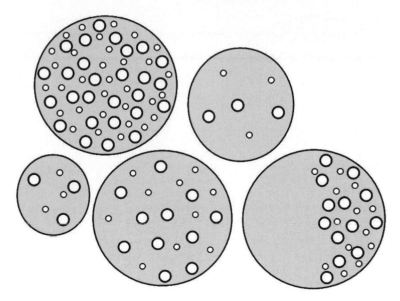

Figure 42.3. Ischemic pattern of axon loss. Intra- and interfascicular variability of axon loss is typical but not pathognomonic of a vasculitic/ischemic pathogenesis.

gut, bladder, penis, and other organs. Studies of human diabetics and rodents show markedly swollen dystrophic axons in prevertebral sympathetic ganglia (*J Neurocytol.* 1997;25:777).

B. Uremia results in demyelination of relatively atrophic axons (i.e., secondary demyelination).

C. Others. Deficiencies of pyridoxine, thiamine, vitamin E (found in abetalipoproteinemia, cystic fibrosis, and biliary atresia), niacin, and cobalamin and multiple nutritional deficiencies are associated with several forms of neuropathy. Hypothyroidism, acute intermittent porphyria, galactosemia, hepatic failure, acromegaly, chronic respiratory insufficiency, and critical illness may also be associated with neuropathy.

VI. NEUROPATHIES WITH AN IMMUNE-MEDIATED MECHANISM

A. Guillain–Barré syndrome (GBS)

1. **Acute inflammatory demyelinating polyneuropathy** (AIDP) results in a perivascular epineurial and endoneurial T-cell–rich infiltrate coupled with a distinctive macrophage-mediated stripping of layers of otherwise normal-appearing myelin (Fig. 42.4, e-Fig. 42.7). Circulating antibodies against endoneurial targets may secondarily gain access through a damaged blood nerve barrier or be locally synthesized. A similar experimental disease (experimental allergic neuritis) can be transferred into recipient naïve rats with CD4+ T cells, and is worsened with antibody against myelin (*J Neuropathol Exp Neurol.* 2001;60:637). Eventually, Schwann cells proliferate and remyelinate the denuded internode. Axonopathy and axon loss is seen, probably because of a noxious endoneurial environment (cytokines, oxidative mediators).

2. **Acute motor axonal neuropathy** (AMAN) and acute motor and sensory axonal neuropathy (AMSAN). In these "axonal" forms of GBS, the axon rather than myelin is the primary target and thus may produce AMAN or AMSAN. Macrophages may be found adjacent to nodes of Ranvier or entering the periaxonal space, possibly targeting axons with a resulting variable degree of axonal degeneration. Antibodies may target a constituent of the nodes of Ranvier, to

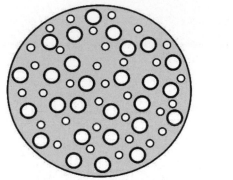 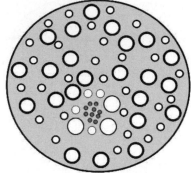

Figure 42.4. Acute inflammatory demyelinating polyneuropathy (AIDP). Patchy loss of myelin in large and small axons is accompanied by an inflammatory infiltrate (*solid dots*); normal fascicle is on the left.

which binding results in complement fixation, formation of a membrane attack complex, recruitment of macrophages, and eventual axonal degeneration. Axonal GBS may be associated with a more aggressive course with poorer outcome, electrophysiologic and pathologic evidence of prominent axonopathy, relatively increased incidence of enteric *Campylobacter jejuni* infection, and a role for antibody directed against GM1 ganglioside. Different patterns of nerve injury seen in GBS may reflect the strain of infecting organism or host human leukocyte antigen (HLA) alleles.

3. **Miller Fisher variant** of GBS is distinguished from AIDP/AMAN by a distinctive presentation of ataxia, areflexia, and ophthalmoplegia, and antibodies against the ganglioside GQ_{1b}, which is concentrated at the nodes of Ranvier, particularly those of the oculomotor nerves.

B. **Chronic inflammatory demyelinating polyradiculoneuropathy** (CIDP) is characterized by a symmetric progressive or relapsing/remitting, sensory and motor polyradiculoneuropathy, particularly involving proximal nerves. Perineurial inflammation and onion-bulbs reflect its chronicity, but do not occur in all cases. CIDP may be a chronic form of GBS in which there is failure of regulatory T cells to suppress the typically monophasic attack of GBS. Its autoimmune pathogenesis involves $CD4^+$ and $CD8^+$T cells and possibly anti-myelin antibodies. HLA subtype frequencies (e.g., HLA-DR2) differ between GBS and CIDP.

C. **Anti-myelin–associated glycoprotein** (MAG) neuropathy is a slowly progressive demyelinating neuropathy with an associated immunoglobulin M (IgM) monoclonal gammopathy ("monoclonal gammopathy of unknown significance"; MGUS) in which the M-protein is directed against MAG, a molecule which affects myelin integrity. Anti-MAG antibodies deposited on portions of the myelin sheaths of peripheral nerve axons result in altered myelin periodicity, demyelination, and axonal degeneration. Recent studies with rituximab, a mouse–human chimeric antibody against the B-cell surface marker CD20, are reported to benefit clinical status (*J Neurol Neurosurg Psychiatry.* 2003;74:485).

D. **Antiglycolipid, -sulfatide, and -ganglioside neuropathies** have been associated with a wide range of clinically identifiable acute and chronic neuropathy syndromes.

E. **Anti-Hu antibody neuropathy** is associated with paraneoplastic sensory neuropathy, which likely reflects development of antibodies against shared antigens of small cell lung carcinoma and dorsal root ganglion neurons and infiltration of $CD8^+$ T cells.

F. **Autoimmune autonomic neuropathy** resulting in autonomic failure following a viral illness may be mediated by circulating antibodies against the ganglionic nicotinic acetylcholine receptor.

VII. GENETIC NEUROPATHIES

A. Hypertrophic (onion-bulb) neuropathies. The concentric proliferation of Schwann cells in response to multiple episodes of demyelination and subsequent remyelination results in onion-bulbs, the defining pathologic hallmark (e-**Fig. 42.8**). Nerves may be palpably enlarged and conduction velocities markedly decreased. Genetic analysis has identified mutations in myelin constituents (P_o, PMP22, myelin basic protein), including those localized to noncompact myelin near the paranode (MAG, connexin-32, neurofascin 155) and axonal proteins (Caspr, contactin, kinesin) (for further information see http://www.molgen.ua.ac.be/ CMTMutations/).

1. **Hypertrophic Charcot–Marie–Tooth disease** (CMT1) is inherited as an autosomal dominant condition resulting from a duplication or point mutation in the *PMP-22* gene, a point mutation in P_o myelin protein (both needed for myelin compaction), a defect in the early growth response 2 gene (*EGR2*), or mutations of periaxin (a Schwann cell protein regulating its shape and axonal communication). $P_o^{+/-}$ transgenic mice have identified a role for macrophage and lymphocytic infiltration in disease pathogenesis. X-linked CMT demonstrates a defect in the gene for connexin-32 (*Science*. 1993;262:2039).

2. **Other types** (Table 42.2). Dejerine–Sottas disease (DSS, includes hereditary motor sensory neuropathy [HMSN-III+]) begins in early life, some cases of which have a demonstrable defect in the genes encoding PMP-22, periaxin, ganglioside-induced differentiation-associated protein 1 (GDAP1), EGR2 or myelin protein

TABLE 42.2	Forms of Hereditary Neuropathy with Onion-Bulbs (OB) and Tomaculi		
Designation	**Inheritance**	**Gene defect**	**Pathology**
CMT1A	AD	*PMP22*	OB
CMT1B	AD	*P_o*	OB
CMT1C	AD	*EGR2*	OB
		LITAF/SIMPLE	OB
CMT1X	XD	*Connexin 32*	Axonal/OB
CMT2A	AD	*Kif1b*	Axonal/±OB
CMT2B	AD	*RAB-7*	Axonal/±OB
CMT2D	AD	*Glycyl tRNA synthetase*	Axonal
CMT2E	AD	*Neurofilament-L*	Axonal
		PMP22, P_o, connexin 32	Axonal
CMT3 (DSS)	AD or AR (or de novo)	*PMP22, P_o, EGR2, Periaxin, GDAP1*	OB
CMT4A	AR	*GDAP1*	OB
CMT4B.1	AR	*Myotubularin-related protein 2*	Demyel +folds
CMT4B.2	AR	*Set binding factor-2*	OB + focal thickening
CMT4C	AR	*SH3 and tetratricopeptide repeat domain 2*	OB + focal thickening
CMT4D	AR	*N-myc downstream regulated gene 1 (NDRG1)*	OB
CMT4E	AR/AD	*EGR2, P_o*	Severe myelin loss
CMT4F	AR/AD	*Periaxin, PMP22, P_o, EGR2*	OB (+Tomaculi)
HNPP	AD	*PMP22*	Demyel + Tomaculi

CMT, Charcot–Marie–Tooth; AD, autosomal dominant; XD, X-linked dominant; AR, autosomal recursive; *EGR2*, early growth response 2 gene; LITAF/SIMPLE, lipopolysaccharide-induced tumor necrosis factor-α factor; Kif1b, kinesin family member IB; RAB-7, ras-related gtp binding protein 7; tRNA, transfer RNA; DSS, detorine sotias syndrome; GDAP1, ganglioside-induced differentiation-associated protein 1; HMSN, hereditary motor sensory neuropathy; HNPP, hereditary neuropathy with pressure palsies.

P_o (*Brain Pathol.* 1998;8:771). Refsum disease, caused by phytanic acid oxidase deficiency, also results in an onion-bulb neuropathy.

B. Hereditary neuropathy with pressure palsies (HNPP). Teased fiber preparations of this dominantly inherited neuropathy demonstrate marked focal hypermyelination (called "tomaculi" or sausages) characterized by redundant myelin folds, demyelination, and remyelination. Evidence suggests monosomy of the *PMP-22* locus due to loss of a portion of chromosome 17.

C. Hereditary giant axonal neuropathy results in axons distended by aggregates of neurofilaments and thinned myelin sheaths, a variety of central nervous system (CNS) symptoms, and "kinky hair." Schwann cells and endothelial cells may also have aggregates of intermediate filaments. Disruption of gigaxonin results in the accumulation of the microtubule-associated protein (MAP) 8 which that subsequently alters the microtubule network, trapping the dynein motor of retrograde axonal transport as an insoluble structure, and eventually leading to neuronal death.

D. HSANs. Included in this group with autonomic and sensory dysfunction are dominant and recessive forms of acral sensory neuropathy, familial dysautonomia, and congenital sensory neuropathy with anhidrosis, all of which are characterized by neuron loss in sensory and various sympathetic and parasympathetic ganglia.

VIII. AMYLOID AND RELATED NEUROPATHIES. Amyloid represents an extracellular deposit of proteins arranged in a β-pleated sheet conformation forming 10- to 20-nm unbranched filaments that stain with thioflavin-S fluorescence and Congo red (the latter polarizing an apple green color). Amyloid neuropathy occurs in primary (nonhereditary) amyloidosis, amyloidosis associated with dysglobulinemia (both composed of immunoglobulin-derived amyloid), and hereditary amyloidoses (e.g., Andrade disease) in which the deposited amyloid is derived from transthyretin or other materials. Amyloid may be deposited within the endoneurium, in the endoneurial and epineurial vasculature (e-**Fig. 42.9**), or within epineurial connective tissue. Axon loss, particularly small axons, is typical. Immunostains may identify the amyloid source, e.g., κ light chains in a myeloma patient.

IX. INFECTIOUS NEUROPATHIES

A. Herpes zoster ("shingles") presents as a painful cutaneous vesicular rash corresponding to a dermatome in which dorsal root ganglion varicella virus has emerged from latency, initially established at the time of childhood chickenpox infection. In response to immunologic cues or other stimuli, the virus activates, travels distally within axons forming a cutaneous eruption (rarely myelitis), and produces hemorrhagic ganglioradiculitis (e-**Fig. 42.10**), infecting satellite and Schwann cells as well as neurons in trigeminal ganglia and dorsal root ganglia.

B. Leprosy results in loss of cutaneous sensation and motor function as the result of direct infection (lepromatous form) or arising from a granulomatous response to the organism (tuberculoid form). The tuberculoid form involves the skin and adjacent nerves, in which few organisms are found (complicating distinction from sarcoid neuropathy). In patients with a compromised immune response to the organism, endoneurial fibrosis is accompanied by numerous organisms that can be demonstrated within Schwann cells (particularly those of unmyelinated axons) and endoneurial macrophages ("lepra cells"). The organism is particularly fond of Schwann cells, binding to laminin-α_2 (*Science.* 2002;296:927).

C. Acquired immunodeficiency syndromes (AIDS). Several different types of neuropathy may develop in patients infected with human immunodeficiency virus (HIV) (Table 42.3) including GBS, CIDP, and necrotizing vasculitis (*Muscle Nerve.* 2003;28:542). Distal sensory neuropathy (DSP) shows prominent activated HIV-infected macrophage activation and lymphocytic infiltration with local release of proinflammatory cytokines in the vicinity of degenerating axons and dorsal root ganglion (DRG) neurons. The viral product gp120 results in neuronal apoptosis and direct local toxicity to axons. Antiretroviral treatment may produce a clinical picture closely resembling DSP, possibly due to direct mitochondrial toxicity; gp-120 may also result in increased vulnerability to dideoxynucleoside-induced neurotoxicity. Skin biopsy is a sensitive and early monitor of the development of DSP,

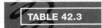

| TABLE 42.3 | Subtypes of Human Immunodeficiency Virus (HIV)-Associated Neuropathy (NP) |

Subtype of NP	Clinical stage	Mechanism
1. Distal sensory NP	Advanced HIV	Macrophage-mediated axonopathy
2. Toxic antiretroviral drug NP	Advanced HIV	Mitochondrial DNA synthesis
3. Mononeuritis multiplex		
Vasculitic form	Moderately advanced	Immune complex deposition
CMV multiple monoNP	Advanced HIV	CMV infection, Schwann cells,
4. Inflammatory demyelinating NP		vessels
GBS (demyelinating or axonal)	Early HIV	Immune dysfunction
CIDP	Early HIV	Immune dysfunction
5. Opportunistic infectious NP		
CMV polyradiculopathy	Advanced HIV	CMV necrotizing NP
Herpes zoster radiculopathy	Advanced HIV	Varicella zoster virus: Schwann cells and endothelium
6. Neoplastic (lymphoma)	Advanced HIV	Endoneurial infiltration
7. Autonomic NP	Advanced HIV	
8. Diffuse infiltrative lymphocytosis	Moderately advanced	CD8 lymphocytosis/vasculopathy

CMV, cytomegalovirus; GBS, Guillain–Barré syndrome; CIDP, chronic inflammatory demyelinating polyradiculoneuropathy.

demonstrating loss of epidermal axons and axonal swellings, often in the absence of neuropathic changes in the sural nerve.

D. Lyme disease. Cranial and peripheral nerves show an epineurial or perineurial perivascular lymphocytic/plasmacytic infiltrate ("perivasculitis") and axonal degeneration. Organisms are not typically seen in involved nerves.

X. TRAUMATIC NEUROPATHY. There are in many forms. Chronic nerve compression and entrapment are characterized by focal loss of myelin. More severe trauma with loss of nerve continuity may produce a traumatic neuroma, i.e., a combination of degenerative and regenerative responses resulting in a disorganized aggregate of collagen and axonal "minifascicles" (e-**Fig. 42.11**).

Suggested Readings

Kennedy WR. Opportunities afforded by the study of unmyelinated nerves in skin and other organs. *Muscle Nerve*. 2004;29:756–767.

Midroni G, Bilbao JM. *Biopsy Diagnosis of Peripheral Neuropathy*. Boston: Butterworth-Heinemann; 1995.

Pestronk A. Neuromuscular Disease Center. Washington University, St. Louis, MO. Available at: http://www.neuro.wustl.edu/neuromuscular/.

Spencer PS, Schaumburg HH, Ludolph AC. *Experimental and Clinical Neurotoxicology*. New York: Oxford University Press; 2000.

Zochodne DW. Diabetes mellitus and the peripheral nervous system: manifestations and mechanisms. *Muscle Nerve*. 2007;36:144–166.

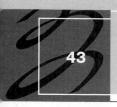

43 LYMPH NODES
Anjum Hassan and Friederike Kreisel

I. NORMAL ANATOMY. Lymph nodes are the most widely distributed collections of lymphoid tissue within the lymphoreticular system, which also includes the thymus, tonsils, adenoids, spleen, and Peyer patches. Due to their easy accessibility, lymph nodes are the most frequently examined lymphoid tissue for a lymphoreticular disorder. Microscopically, the lymph node shows four compartments: The most obvious are the primary and secondary follicles, which are usually found near the capsule. Surrounding the follicles and extending deeper into the node is the paracortex. The third and fourth compartments represent the medullary region and the sinuses, respectively (e-Fig. 43.1).*

II. GROSS EXAMINATION, TISSUE SAMPLING, AND HISTOLOGIC SLIDE PREPARATION. Fresh lymphoid tissue should be examined by gross inspection, touch preparation, or frozen section examination to assess whether the:
  A. Tissue represents adequate sampling, and
  B. Tissue needs allocation to various ancillary studies essential to a correct diagnosis. The fresh lymph node should be cut perpendicularly to the long axis, and material for ancillary studies procured as follows:
   1. Wet touch preparations fixed in 95% alcohol or formalin for hematoxylin and eosin or Papanicolaou staining
   2. Air-dried touch preparations for Giemsa or Wright–Giemsa staining, cytochemistry (myeloperoxidase, nonspecific esterase, etc.), or cytogenetics (i.e., fluorescence in situ hybridization [FISH])
   3. Rapidly frozen tissue for immunohistochemistry, cytochemistry, or genetic analysis
   4. Fresh tissue (in RPMI 1640 medium or saline) for flow cytometry
   5. Sterile fresh tissue for microbial cultures or cytogenetics (karyotyping or FISH)
   6. Thin-shaved tissue rapidly fixed in glutaraldehyde for electron microscopy
   7. Paraffin-embedded tissue after fixation for routine hematoxylin and eosin staining, immunohistochemistry, and special stains (e.g., Giemsa, periodic acid–Schiff [PAS], elastin, trichrome, Leder, etc.)
      Procuring tissue for histology takes priority over other studies. The most commonly used fixative for permanent sections is 10% neutral buffered formalin. B5 fixative is commonly used in addition to 10% neutral buffered formalin because of the sharp nuclear detail it produces. However, this mercuric chloride–based fixative is very expensive and poses an environmental hazard. Furthermore, molecular studies cannot be carried out on B5-fixed paraffin-embedded tissue, because it will generally yield poor polymerase chain reaction (PCR) amplification results.

III. DIAGNOSTIC FEATURES OF COMMON BENIGN DISEASES OF LYMPH NODES. In reactive lymphadenopathy there are five different architectural patterns to be recognized, with many showing a mixed pattern of response.
  A. Follicular hyperplasia (e-Fig. 43.2) is characterized by an increase in number and size of B-cell germinal centers and is common in lymph node–draining sites of chronic inflammation. This pattern is also present in syphilitic lymphadenitis where, in addition to the marked lymphoid hyperplasia, thickening of the capsule

---

*All e-figures are available online via the Solution Site Image Bank.

by chronic inflammation, fibrosis and neovascularization with arteritis and phlebitis, and a marked a plasma cell infiltrate in the medullary region predominate. Rheumatoid lymphadenopathy and acute human immunodeficiency virus (HIV) lymphadenitis are other examples of marked follicular hyperplasia.

B. **Diffuse (paracortical) hyperplasia** shows expansion of the T-cell paracortical areas. This pattern is commonly seen in viral lymphadenitis (Epstein–Barr virus [EBV], cytomegalovirus [CMV], herpes) and vaccinia lymphadenitis revealing an expansion of the paracortex with increased immunoblasts, imparting a "mottled" appearance. Follicular hyperplasia and sinus dilation are often concurrent findings in this entity resulting in a mixed pattern of lymphoid hyperplasia. Phenytoin lymphadenopathy represents a relatively pure diffuse hyperplasia showing an expanded paracortical T zone with numerous large immunoblasts, eosinophils, plasma cells, and neutrophils.

C. **Sinus hyperplasia** describes increased cellularity within the medullary sinuses of lymph nodes. Sinus histiocytosis is seen in numerous nonspecific responses to chronic inflammation, as well as in lymph node–draining cancer. Sinus histiocytosis with massive lymphadenopathy or Rosai-Dorfman disease, a disease entity initially described in 1969, is characterized by markedly dilated sinuses filled with CD68+, S100+ histiocytes showing emperipolesis. Lipophagic reactions causing sinus histiocytosis with accumulation of phagocytosed fat include mineral oil ingestion, Whipple disease, and lymphangiography procedures. Prominent vacuoles in the histiocytes can generate a signet-ring cell histiocytosis, a pattern that should not be confused with signet-ring-cell carcinoma. Finally, vascular transformation of lymph node sinuses (e-Fig. 43.3) shows a sinus pattern, and it is important to distinguish this entity from Kaposi sarcoma (e-Fig. 43.4). The latter can be distinguished from the former by the proliferation of spindle-shaped Kaposi sarcoma cells forming cleftlike vascular spaces that contain erythrocytes, many of which are extravasated.

D. **Granulomatous lymphadenopathy** describes formation of epithelioid granulomas in lymph nodes. Caseating granulomas are epithelioid granulomas that form central necrosis and caseation, and are typically seen in *Mycobacterium tuberculosis* lymphadenitis. Special stains for mycobacteria in paraffin-embedded tissue (Ziehl–Nelson, Fite–Faraco) will detect the bacilli as bright red, slender, beaded microorganisms (e-Figs. 43.5 and 43.6). *Mycobacterium leprae* lymphadenitis and histoplasma lymphadenitis are other examples of caseating granulomatous inflammation. Necrotizing, noncaseating granulomas are present in cat-scratch disease (e-Fig. 43.7) caused by *Bartonella henselae*, in which suppurative granulomas with stellate microabscesses surrounded by palisading histiocytes predominate. Kikuchi–Fujimoto lymphadenopathy is characterized by necrotizing granulomas containing karyorrhectic debris, but lacking neutrophils. This form of necrotizing lymphadenitis is characteristically present in young Asian women. Nonnecrotizing, noncaseating granulomas are pathognomotic for sarcoidosis lymphadenopathy (e-Fig. 43.8), composed primarily of epithelioid histiocytes with scattered multinucleated giant cells, lymphocytes, and plasma cells. This type of epithelioid granuloma can also be seen in draining lymph nodes of Crohn disease.

E. **Acute lymphadenitis** is an acute inflammation in lymph nodes draining an infected focus. Acute lymphadenitis is almost exclusively bacterial in nature, and morphologic features range from focal infiltration by neutrophils to necrosis and suppuration with abscess formation. It should be mentioned that in most cases of benign reactive lymphadenopathy, a combination of more than one architectural pattern is present in the same lymph node.

IV. **INCIDENCE AND EPIDEMIOLOGY OF NON-HODGKIN LYMPHOMAS**

A. **B-cell lymphomas.** B-cell lymphomas constitute the vast majority of lymphomas in North America and Europe, accounting for nearly 90% of all lymphomas. Diffuse large B-cell lymphoma (~31%) (e-Fig. 43.9) and follicular lymphoma (~22%) (e-Fig. 43.10) are the most common types (*WHO Classification of Tumors; Pathology and Genetics; Tumors of Hematopoietic and Lymphoid Tissues,* 1st ed.) Lyon, France: IARC Press; 2001:121–126). Immunosuppression, specifically due to HIV infection and immunosuppressive therapy to prevent graft versus host disease (GVHD), is associated with a markedly increased incidence of developing mature B-cell lymphomas, particularly diffuse large B-cell lymphoma and Burkitt's lymphoma (e-Fig. 43.11).

Some of the low-grade B-cell lymphoproliferative disorders include follicular lymphoma grades 1 and 2, chronic lymphocytic leukemia/small lymphocytic lymphoma (CLL/SLL) (e-Fig. 43.12), nodal and extranodal marginal zone B-cell lymphoma (e-Fig. 43.13), and lymphoplasmacytic lymphoma, which are generally indolent, but incurable and usually present in a disseminated stage with bone marrow involvement. Mantle cell lymphoma (e-Figs. 43.14 and 43.15) and diffuse large B-cell lymphoma represent "intermediate-grade" B-cell lymphomas that generally show a more aggressive clinical behavior, but are potentially curable. The same applies to high-grade B-cell lymphomas, which include Burkitt's lymphoma and precursor B-lymphoblastic leukemia/lymphoma.

B. T-cell lymphomas. Mature T-cell and natural killer (NK)-cell malignancies are rare, accounting for only 10% to 12% of all Non-Hodgkin lymphoma, and usually are more aggressive than B-cell lymphomas. The most common subtypes are peripheral T-cell lymphoma, unspecified (~4%) (e-Fig. 43.16) and anaplastic large cell lymphoma (~3%) (e-Fig. 43.17) (*WHO Classification of Tumors; Pathology and Genetics; Tumors of Hematopoietic and Lymphoid Tissues.* (1st ed.) Lyon, France: IARC Press; 2001:191–194). In general, T-cell and NK-cell malignancies are much more common in Asia and are linked to viral infection with EBV (NK-cell lymphomas) (e-Fig. 43.18) and human T-cell leukemia virus (HTLV-1) (adult T-cell leukemia/lymphoma) (e-Fig. 43.19). The current World Health Organization classification of lymphoid malignancies is summarized in Table 43.1.

V. PATHOPHYSIOLOGY OF NON-HODGKIN LYMPHOMAS

A. B-cell lymphomas. Mature B-cell malignancies mimic stages of normal B-cell differentiation; therefore, classification is generally based on their morphologic and immunophenotypic resemblance to the normal B-cell counterpart (Fig. 43.1) (*Best Pract Res Clin Haematol* 2005;18:11). Normal B-cell development begins in the bone marrow where precursor B lymphocytes undergo immunoglobulin VDJ gene rearrangement and develop into IgM+, IgD+ naïve B cells with surface immunoglobulin light chain and CD5 expression. These resting B cells circulate in the blood and occupy primary follicles and mantle zones of secondary follicles. Malignant counterparts of CD5+ naïve B-cells are believed to be CLL and mantle cell lymphoma. Upon antigen stimulation, naïve B cells undergo blastic transformation, migrate into the center of the primary follicle, and form the germinal center. These centroblasts are large lymphoid cells with vesicular chromatin and several eccentrically located nucleoli. They express BCL-6 and CD10 but switch off BCL-2 protein expression, therefore becoming susceptible to death through apoptosis. Centroblasts undergo intense proliferation that is accompanied by somatic hypermutation of their rearranged variable-region genes, giving rise to cells carrying receptors with high affinity for the stimulating antigen. This leads to a large pool of B-lymphoid cells with intraclonal diversity. Centroblasts then mature into centrocytes, representing intermediate-sized lymphoid cells with irregular, cleaved nuclei and inconspicuous nucleoli. Centrocytes with mutations resulting in decreased affinity for antigen die by apoptosis, whereas centrocytes with high affinity for antigen are rescued from apoptosis by re-expressing BCL-2. Malignant counterparts of germinal center–derived B cells are follicular lymphoma, a subset of diffuse large B-cell lymphoma, and Burkitt lymphoma. Via interactions with follicular dendritic cells through CD23 and with T lymphocytes through CD40 ligand (CD40L), centrocytes switch off BCL-6 expression and differentiate into either memory cells or plasma cells. Memory cells are found in the marginal zone of follicles; they typically express immunoglobulin M (IgM) and lack expression of IgD, CD5, CD10, or CD23. Plasma cells home to the bone marrow; they lack surface immunoglobulin and pan-B-cell expression, but express CD79a, CD138, and cytoplasmic IgG or IgA. Neither memory cells nor plasma cells undergo further somatic hypermutations. Marginal zone B-cell lymphoma corresponds to postgerminal center cells, possibly memory

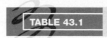

TABLE 43.1	WHO Classification of Lymphoid Neoplasms

Mature B-cell neoplasms
Chronic lymphocytic leukemia / small lymphocytic lymphoma
B-cell prolymphocytic leukemia
Lymphoplasmacytic lymphoma Waldenström macroglobulinemia
Splenic marginal zone lymphoma
Hairy cell leukemia
Plasma cell neoplasms
  Plasma cell myeloma
  Plasmacytoma
  Monoclonal immunoglobulin deposition diseases
  Heavy chain diseases
Extranodal marginal zone B-cell lymphoma (mucosa-associated lymphoid tissue [MALT]
  lymphoma)
Nodal marginal zone B cell lymphoma
Follicular lymphoma
Mantle cell lymphoma
Diffuse large B-cell lymphoma
Mediastinal (thymic) large B-cell lymphoma
Intravascular large B-cell lymphoma
Primary effusion lymphoma
Burkitt lymphoma / leukemia
Lymphomatoid granulomatosis

Mature T-cell and natural killer (NK)-cell neoplasms
T-cell prolymphocytic leukemia
T-cell large granular lymphocytic leukemia
Aggressive NK-cell leukemia
Adult T-cell leukemia / lymphoma
Extranodal NK-/T-cell lymphoma, nasal type
Enteropathy-type T-cell lymphoma
Hepatosplenic T-cell lymphoma
Subcutaneous panniculitislike T-cell lymphoma
Blastic NK-cell lymphoma
Mycosis fungoides / Sezary syndrome
Primary cutaneous CD30+ T-cell lymphoproliferative disorders
  Primary cutaneous anaplastic large cell lymphoma (C-ALCL)
  Lymphomatoid papulosis
  Borderline lesions
Angioimmunoblastic T-cell lymphoma
Peripheral T-cell lymphoma, unspecified
Anaplastic large cell lymphoma

From: Jaffee ES, Harris NL, Stein H, Vardiman JW, eds. *World Health Organization Classification of Tumours. Pathology and Genetics. Tumours of Haematopoietic and Lymphoid Tissues.* Lyon: IARC Press; 2001. Used with permission.

cells of marginal zone type. Plasma cell myeloma is the malignant counterpart of bone marrow–homing IgG- or IgA-producing plasma cells.

  B. T lymphocytes. Two major classes of T lymphocytes exist based on the structure of the T-cell receptor (TCR) (*Immunobiology,* (6th ed.) New York and London: Garland Publishing; 2005:149–153). Approximately 95% of all T cells are $\alpha\beta$ T-lymphocytes that can be subdivided into CD4+ helper T cells or CD8+ cytotoxic T cells. Only 5% of T cells are $\gamma\delta$ cells, which are primarily found in the splenic pulp and intestinal epithelium and are not MHC restricted in their function because they do not express CD4 or CD8. The TCR is composed of either the $\alpha\beta$ or $\gamma\delta$

Normal and Abnormal Counterparts of B Cell Progeny†

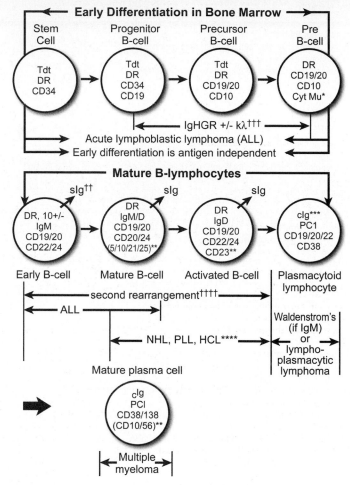

Figure 43.1. Brief overview of normal B-cell progeny and malignant counterparts.

† Only positive markers are noted;
  +/- indicates partial expression
†† Surface immunoglobin
††† Immunoglobulin heavy chain (VDJ) gene
  rearrangement with or without light chains
†††† Isotype switch, IgH and kλ rearrangements

* Cytoplasmic heavy chains
** Markers abnormally expressed in neoplastic B cells
  or plasma cells
*** Cytoplasmic immunoglobulin
**** Non-Hodgkin's lymphoma, prolymphocytic lymphoma,
  hairy cell leukemia, etc.

chains, each consisting of an external variable (V) and constant (C) domain. The TCR is complexed with CD3 that contains γ, δ, and ε chains. NK cells do not have a complete TCR, but usually express the ε chain of the CD3 in the cytoplasm; therefore, NK cells will stain positively with a polyclonal antibody to CD3. Malignant counterparts of $\gamma\delta$ T cells are believed to be hepatosplenic T-cell lymphoma (e-**Fig. 43.20**) and enteropathy-type T-cell lymphoma (e-**Fig. 43.21**). NK cells share some immunophenotypic markers and functions with cytotoxic CD8+ T cells; these include expression of CD2, CD7, CD8, CD56, CD57, granzyme B, perforin, and

T-cell intracellular antigen (TIA-1). Due to their broad cytologic spectrum, absence of immunophenotypic markers of monoclonality, and general lack of specific genetic abnormalities, clinical presentation plays a major role in the subclassification of T-cell and NK-cell malignancies (Fig. 43.2). For example, hypercalcemia is associated with adult T-cell leukemia; hemophagocytic syndrome occurs more frequently in cytotoxic T-cell or NK-cell malignancies; persistent severe neutropenia is a relatively common clinical feature in T-cell granular lymphocyte leukemia (e-Fig. 43.22); and systemic symptoms of edema, pleural effusion, ascites, arthritis combined with anemia, and polyclonal hypergammaglobulinemia are relatively specific for angioimmunoblastic T-cell lymphoma (e-Fig. 43.23).

VI. **A RATIONAL APPROACH TO GENERAL LYMPHOMA WORK-UP.** As follows, the classification of lymphomas may appear to be difficult; however, a systematic approach can be used to efficiently narrow the differential diagnosis for most cases. Needless to say, knowledge of clinical history and a basic complete blood count are required to guide the initial steps of the evaluation (for example, to direct the immunophenotypic work-up of the sample by flow cytometry), because tissue sections are often not available until the next day. The general algorithm (see Table 43.2) starts with the low-power appearance of the tissue section. Is the architecture nodular, follicular, diffuse, or mixed? What is the cell size; small (close to a normal lymphocyte), medium, or large (about three times the size of a normal lymphocyte)? What is the nuclear shape? Is the process high grade (necrosis, starry sky appearance, high mitotic rate)? The work-up continues with a determination of the lineage and stage of maturation (as mentioned above, flow cytometry is usually extremely helpful in delineating the lineage, provided care is taken to save fresh tissue in RPMI medium and order appropriate markers; alternatively, immunohistochemistry can be performed on formalin-fixed, paraffin-embedded tissue). The work-up concludes with evaluation of disease-specific markers (such as cyclin D1 and anaplastic large cell lymphoma kinase [Alk]-1, which can only be evaluated by immunohistochemistry in tissue sections).

Antigen markers useful in delineating and subclassifying lymphoid malignancies are the following:

A. **Leukocyte marker.** CD45 (also known as leukocyte common antigen [LCA]) is expressed on all leukocytes.

B. **Markers of immaturity**
   1. TdT (terminal deoxynucleotidyl transferase, a specialized DNA polymerase; nuclear expression present only in pre-B and pre-T lymphoblasts)
   2. CD34 (present on pluripotent hematopoietic stem cells and progenitor cells of many lineages)
   3. CD10 (CALLA [common acute lymphoblastic leukemia antigen]; expressed on marrow pre-B cells and mature follicular center B cells)
   4. CD22 (present on pre-B cells)
   5. cμ (cytoplasmic μ heavy chain)

C. **Primarily B-cell associated markers**
   1. CD19 (present on marrow pre-B cells, mature B cells, but not on plasma cells; no paraffin-reactive antibody available)
   2. CD20 (present on marrow pre-B cells, mature B cells, but not on normal plasma cells)
   3. CD79a (present on mature and pre-B cells, as well as on plasma cells)

D. **Markers helpful in subclassifying mature B-cell lymphomas**
   1. CD5 (expressed on all T cells and small subset of B cells, expressed on neoplastic CLL and mantle cell lymphoma cells)
   2. CD10
   3. CD11c (expressed in high levels on monocytes, macrophages, and NK cells, as well in moderate levels on granulocytes; expressed on subsets of T and B cells)
   4. CD23 (present on activated mature B cells)
   5. CD38 (primarily expressed on mature B cells and plasma cells)
   6. CD43 (leukosialin, expressed on the surface of all leukocytes except resting B cells; CD43 expression in B-cell lymphomas is highly correlated with CD5, therefore, is a sensitive indicator for aberrant B-cell populations)

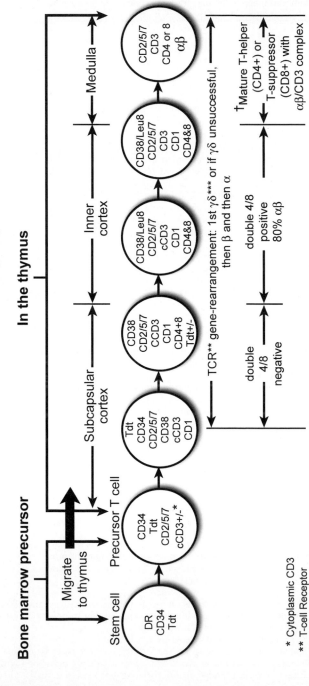

Normal T-Cell Progeny[††]

Bone marrow precursor

In the thymus

Stem cell
DR
CD34
Tdt

Migrate to thymus

Precursor T cell
CD34
Tdt
CD2/5/7
cCD3+/-*

Subcapsular cortex
Tdt
CD34
CD2/5/7
CD38
cCD3
CD1

Inner cortex
CD38
CD2/5/7
cCD3
CD1
CD4+8
Tdt+/-

CD38/Leu8
CD2/5/7
cCD3
CD1
CD4&8

Medulla
CD38/Leu8
CD2/5/7
CD3
CD1
CD4&8

CD2/5/7
CD3
CD4 or 8
αβ

TCR** gene-rearrangement: 1st γδ*** or if γδ unsuccessful, then β and then α

double 4/8 negative

double 4/8 positive 80% αβ

[†]Mature T-helper (CD4+) or T-suppressor (CD8+) with αβ/CD3 complex

* Cytoplasmic CD3
** T-cell Receptor
*** Gamma-Delta chains expressed on immature thymocytes and Natural Killers cells only
[†] Mature T-cells can circulate in peripheral blood and tissues
[††] Only positive markers are noted. Markers partially expressed or about to lose expression are noted by a "+/-".

Figure 43.2. Brief overview of normal T-cell progeny.

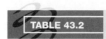

TABLE 43.2   An Algorithm for the Work-Up of Lymphomas

Cell type: Are the cells lymphoid?

In a tissue section, what is the low-power architecture?

Cell size
Are the majority of cells small (same size as a lymphocyte)? Or large (~3 times as big as a lymphocyte, or even bigger)?
Is there an even mixture of small and large cells? Are they anaplastic?

Nuclear shape
Do the cells have round nuclei with a smooth contour (noncleaved)? Or a round shape with a bumpy or notched contour (irregular)? Or a variable shape with deeply folded or grooved nuclei (cleaved)?

Histologic grade
Is necrosis present? Is there a "starry sky" appearance? Are mitoses easy to find?

Lineage (by flow cytometry or immunohistochemistry)
Are the cells of B lineage (generally CD20+) or T lineage (generally CD3+)?

Maturation
Are the cells at a precursor (TdT+) or a mature (TdT–) stage of maturation?
If mature and of B lineage, are they prefollicular, follicular, postfollicular, or effector cell stage?
If mature and of T lineage, are they at a thymic or postthymic / effector cell stage?

Disease specific markers
Do the cells express cyclin D1, bcl6, anaplastic large cell lymphoma kinase (ALK)-1, and so on?

7. BCL-6 (expressed normally in germinal center lymphocytes in the normal lymph node; it is distributed in a pattern reciprocal to that of BCL-2)
8. BCL-2 (present on T cells and normal mantle B lymphocytes; aberrantly expressed in majority of B-cell lymphomas)
9. Cyclin D1 (cell cycle regulatory protein identified through the t(11;14) of its gene in mantle cell lymphoma, also expressed weakly in hairy cell leukemia and plasma cell dyscrasias; nuclear protein detectable in paraffin-embedded sections)
10. CD138 (Syndecan-1, expressed on most cases of myeloma, but also present in carcinomas)
E. **Markers of clonality:** κ and λ immunoglobulin light chains
F. **Primarily T cell– and NK cell–associated markers:**
1. CD1 (expressed on cortical thymocytes and Langerhans cell histiocytes)
2. CD2 (present on all T cells [thymic and peripheral T cells] and NK cells)
3. CD3 (lineage-specific marker for T cells, also expressed in cytoplasmic forms in NK cells)
4. CD5 (expressed on all T cells and a small subset of B cells)
5. CD7 (expressed on all T cells and a small subset of myeloid precursor cells)
6. CD8 (present on cytotoxic subset of peripheral T cells and on a subset of thymocytes and NK cells)
7. CD16 (present on NK cells and granulocytes)
8. CD56 (present on NK cells and subset of T lymphocytes; also present on myeloma cells)
9. TIA-1 (cytotoxic granule-associated RNA binding protein), granzyme B, and perforin (proteins released by cytotoxic T cells, inducing apoptosis) are expressed in cytotoxic T cells and NK cells
G. **Flow cytometry** can easily detect clonality in B-cell malignancies (normal κ to λ light chain ratio ranges between 1:1 and 4:1), clonality for T-cell malignancies can only be detected by molecular or cytogenetic studies.

H. Southern blot analysis is considered the gold standard for identifying clonal immunoglobulin heavy chain (*IgH*) gene or *TCR* gene rearrangements. T lymphocytes normally rearrange four different *TCR* genes (*TCRα, β, γ*, and *δ*) to encode a unique antigen receptor expressed on their surface, and Southern blot analysis targets the *TCRβ* gene. In contrast to normal tissue, where only one band corresponding to the germline configuration is visible with this technique, both B-cell and T-cell malignancies will yield an additional band corresponding to the clonal population.

I. PCR. Because Southern blot analysis is labor intensive and expensive to perform, many laboratories have turned to PCR amplification methods to detect clonal *IgH* and *TCR* gene rearrangements.

The 200 variable segments of the *IgH* gene contain three highly variable and mutation-prone regions called complementary determining regions (CDR1, 2, and 3) that are interspersed between four conserved framework regions (FR1, 2, 3, and 4) that provide reliable targets for consensus primers. About 70% of B-cell malignancies harbor clonal rearrangements that are detectable with framework 3 primers, and about 15% to 20% of additional clonal rearrangements can be detected when framework 2 primers are used. Therefore, most laboratories use primers targeting frameworks 2 and 3 to detect at least 80% of all B-cell lymphomas.

The rearranged *TCRγ* gene is most suitable for clonal detection by PCR amplification in T-cell malignancies, because most T lymphocytes harbor rearrangements in 1 of the 11 *γ* segments. Because many of these segments are homologous to one another, they can be targeted by a single consensus primer set. *TCRδ* and *TCRα* cannot be targeted because *TCRδ* is deleted during *TCRα* gene rearrangement and *TCRα* has such a diversity of possible rearrangements that these cannot be covered by current probe technology.

J. Cytogenetic analysis is a morphologic study of chromosomes to assess changes in their number and structure.

1. Conventional karyotyping requires viable cells, and analysis of chromosomes is performed according to their size and banding pattern after chromosome staining. Although this study has become critical in the diagnosis and classification of acute leukemias, it is not frequently used as part of a routine diagnostic work-up for lymph node biopsies.

2. FISH uses one or more labeled probes directed toward specific portions of chromosomes. It is helpful in locating specific translocations, deletions, and additions of chromosome fragments. The advantage of this method is that it can be performed on nondividing nuclei (interphase nuclei), eliminating the need for cell cultures. Furthermore, interphase FISH can be performed on a wide range of specimen types, such as peripheral blood smears, cytospins, or paraffin-embedded tissue. Many of the classic chromosomal translocations that characterize specific lymphomas can be identified with interphase FISH techniques. Tables 43.3 and 43.4 summarize the characteristic morphologic, immunophenotypic, and genetic features of B-cell and T/NK-cell malignancies, respectively.

VII. PLASMA CELL DYSCRASIAS. Although plasma cell dyscrasias usually do not involve lymph nodes, this disease entity is appropriately covered in this chapter because plasma cells represent terminally differentiated B cells. They are characterized by secretion of a single homogenous immunoglobulin product known as the monoclonal or "M" component, which can be detected by serum and urine protein electrophoresis. The World Health Organization categorizes plasma cell dyscrasias into monoclonal gammopathy of undetermined significance (MGUS), plasma cell myeloma, plasmacytomas, monoclonal immunoglobulin deposition diseases, osteosclerotic myeloma (POEMS syndrome), and heavy chain diseases (*WHO Classification of Tumors; Pathology and Genetics; Tumors of Hematopoietic and Lymphoid Tissues.* (1st ed.) Lyon, France: IARC Press; 2001:142–166).

A. Patients with MGUS are usually asymptomatic with no evidence of lytic bone lesions, but reveal a clonal plasma cell population in the bone marrow of <10% and an associated small M component.

Disease	Clinical presentation	Morphology	Immunophenotype	Genetics
CLL / SLL	Mostly asymptomatic, may present with fatigue, autoimmune hemolytic anemia, hepatosplenomegaly, lymphadenopathy; peripheral absolute lymphocytosis	PB: Small cells with coarsely clumped chromatin and inconspicuous nucleoli LN: Proliferation centers composed of "paraimmunoblasts" and prolymphocytes	CD20 (weak), CD19, IgM, IgD, CD22 (weak), CD5, CD23, CD79a, CD43	Trisomy 12, deletions at 13q14, deletions at 11q22–23 50% to 60% have somatic hypermutations, IgH clonally rearranged
Prolymphocytic leukemia	Marked splenomegaly without lymphadenopathy, rapidly rising lymphocyte count (>100 × 10⁹/L)	PB: Medium-sized cells with round nucleus, moderately condensed chromatin, and prominent central nucleolus	CD20 (bright) CD19, IgM, CD22, CD79a, FMC7, CD23 typically absent, CD5 present in 1/3 of cases	t(11;14)(q13;q32) in 20% of cases (? leukemic mantle cell lymphoma), abnormalities of TP53, IgH clonally rearranged
Hairy cell leukemia	Predominantly middle-aged men, splenomegaly, pancytopenia with monocytopenia	PB: Small- to medium-sized cells with circumferential hairy projections Spleen: Red pulp infiltration (macroscopy: "bloody lakes")	CD19, CD20, CD22, CD79a, CD11c (bright), CD25 (bright), CD103, TRAP, DBA.44 in tissue sections	No specific cytogenetic abnormality, IgH clonally rearranged
Lymphoplasmacytic lymphoma/Waldenström macroglobulinemia	Monoclonal IgM serum paraprotein with associated hyperviscosity symptoms	Mixture of small lymphocytes, plasmacytoid lymphocytes, and plasma cells, Dutcher bodies	CD19, CD20, CD22, CD79a, CD38, surface and cytoplasmic IgM, no express on of CD5, CD23, or CD10	No specific cytogenetic abnormality, IgH clonally rearranged
Splenic marginal zone B-cell lymphoma	Splenomegaly, sometimes associated with autoimmune thrombocytopenia or anemia, peripheral lymphadenopathy uncommon	PB: Small- to medium-sized cells with polar villi (villous lymphocytes) Spleen: Both white pulp and red pulp infiltration	CD19, CD20, CD79a, IgM and IgD, no expression of CD5, CD23, CD10, or CD43	Allelic loss of chromosome 7q21–32 in 40% of cases, trisomy 3 in rare cases, IgH clonally rearranged

(Continued)

TABLE 43.3   Characteristic Features of Different B-Cell Malignancies (Continued)

Disease	Clinical Presentation	Morphology	Immunophenotype	Genetics
Extranodal marginal zone B-cell lymphoma (MALT lymphoma)	History of chronic inflammatory or autoimmune disorders (*Helicobacter pylori* gastritis, Hashimoto thyroiditis, Sjögren syndrome), GI tract most common site of involvement	Heterogenous infiltrate of centrocytelike cells, monocytoid cells, small lymphocytes, scattered immunoblasts and lymphoid cells with plasmacytic differentiation, "overrun follicles," lymphoepithelial lesions	CD19, CD20, CD79a, IgM, no expression of CD5, CD23, CD10	Trisomy 3 in 60% of cases, t(11;18)(q21;q21) in ~25% to 50% of cases, IgH clonally rearranged
Nodal marginal zone B-cell lymphoma	Localized or generalized lymphadenopathy	Marginal zone and interfollicular areas infiltrated by centrocytelike B cell, monocytoid B cells, or small lymphocytes; plasma cell differentiation may be present	CD19, CD20, CD79a, IgM, no expression of CD5, CD23, CD10	Cytogenetics not well studied; IgH clonally rearranged
Follicular lymphoma	Widespread peripheral and central lymphadenopathy, bone marrow involved in 40% of cases	Follicular pattern of closely packed neoplastic follicles composed of either small cleaved centrocytes or large centroblasts Grade 1: 0 to 5 centroblasts/hpf Grade 2: 6 to 15 centroblasts/hpf Grade 3: >15 centroblasts/hpf	CD19, CD20, CD22, CD79a, BCL-6, BCL-2, CD10	t(14;18)(q32;q21) → rearrangement of the BCL-2 gene leading to overexpression of the BCL-2 protein and survival advantage of malignant cells; IgH clonally rearranged
Mantle cell lymphoma	Lymphadenopathy, most common extranodal site is the GI tract (multiple lymphomatous polyposis)	May show vaguely nodular, diffuse or mantle zone pattern, medium-sized lymphoid cells with irregular nuclear contours, may be blastoid in appearance	CD19, CD20, CD5, FMC-7, CD43, cyclin-D1, lack of expression of CD23, CD10, BCL-6	t(11;14)(q13;q32), translocation between IgH and BCL-1 genes; IgH clonally rearranged

Diffuse large B-cell lymphoma	Rapidly enlarging, often symptomatic mass, often disseminated disease	Sheets of large cells with nuclear size equal or exceeding normal macrophage nucleus Morphologic variants: Centroblastic, immunoblastic, T cell / histiocyte rich, anaplastic	CD19, CD20, CD22, CD79a, CD10, and BCL-6 co-expression: germinal center B-like (better overall survival than activated B-type)	IgH clonally rearranged, ~30% with abnormalities of 3q27 region involving BCL6
Mediastinal (thymic) large B-cell lymphoma	Mostly women in their third to fifth decade, large anterior mediastinal mass, sometimes with impending superior vena cava syndrome	Large cells with associated delicate interstitial fibrosis causing compartmentalization, possible thymic remnants, biopsy samples often small and obscured by profuse sclerosis and crush artifact	CD19, CD20, CD30 (weak), Ig and HLA class I and II expression is often absent	IgH clonally rearranged; hyperdiploid karyotype, gains in chromosome 9p
Burkitt lymphoma	Highly aggressive lymphoma often presenting at extranodal sites or as acute leukemia, risk for central nervous system involvement, "endemic" Burkitt lymphoma with involvement of jaws and other facial structures, "sporadic" Burkitt lymphoma with abdominal masses	Medium-sized cells with basophilic vacuolated cytoplasm and regular nuclei with several small nucleoli, tangible-body macrophages imparting "starry-sky" appearance	CD19, CD20, CD22, CD10, CD79a, BCL-6, no expression of TdT, BCL-2, Ki-67 index of 100%	IgH clonally rearranged; t(8;14) in most cases, t(2;8) and t(8;22) rare

Abbreviations: CLL = chronic lymphocytic leukemia; SLL = small lymphocytic lymphoma; MALT = mucosa-associated lymphoid tissue; Ig = immunoglobulin; GI = gastrointestinal; PB =; LN =; hpf = high-powered field; TRAP = tartrate-resistant acid phosphatase; HLA = human leukocyte antigen; TdT = terminal deoxynucleotidyl transferase.

Disease	Clinical presentation	Morphology	Immunophenotype	Genetics
T-cell prolymphocytic leukemia	Aggressive disease with hepatosplenomegaly and generalized lymphadenopathy, marked lymphocytosis, usually >100 × 10⁹/L, anemia and thrombocytopenia	PB: Medium-sized cells with nongranular cytoplasm, visible nucleolus, and cytoplasmic protrusions or blebs	CD3, CD2, CD7, CD4+/CD8− in 60%, CD4+/CD8+ in 25%, CD4−/CD8+ in 15%	inv(14)(q11;q32) in 80%, t(14;14) (q11;q32) in 10% involving TCR-α/β and TCL-1, rearranged TCR
T-cell large granular lymphocyte leukemia	Indolent clinical course, severe neutropenia with/without anemia, mild to moderate lymphocytosis, moderate splenomegaly, rheumatoid arthritis, circulating immune complexes, hypergammaglobulinemia	PB: Large granular lymphocytes with abundant cytoplasm and fine or coarse azurophilic granules; BM: Interstitial infiltrate	CD3, TCR-α/β, CD8 in 80%, co-expression of TIA-1, CD57, perforin, granzyme B, Fas (CD95) and FasL	Rearranged TCR, no unique cytogenetic abnormality
Aggressive NK-cell leukemia	More prevalent among Asians; fever, leukemic blood picture, constitutional symptoms, cytopenias, hepatosplenomegaly, multiorgan failure due to ↑ serum soluble Fas ligand level	PB: Lymphoid cells larger than normal LGL with lightly basophilic cytoplasm containing granules, hyperchromatic nucleus	CD2, cCD3ε, CD56, TIA-1, granzyme B, perforin, EBV, no expression of surface CD3 or CD57	TCR not rearranged, EBV present in clonal episomal form
Adult T-cell leukemia	Endemic in Japan, the Caribbean basin, parts of Central Africa, linked to HTLV-1, hypercalcemia, hepatosplenomegaly, ↑ LDH, associated T-cell immunodeficiency with opportunistic infections	PB: Medium- to large-sized cells with polylobated nucleus ("flower cells")	CD2, CD3, CD5, CD4, CD25, lack CD7 expression	Clonally integrated HTLV-1, clonally rearranged TCR

Entity	Clinical features	Immunophenotype	Genetics
Extranodal NK-/T-cell lymphoma, nasal type	More prevalent in Asia, Mexico, Central and South America, extensive midfacial destructive lesions, other extranodal sites include skin, soft tissue, testis, GI tract	Extensive ulceration and necrosis, angiocentric and angiodestructive growth pattern, hyperchromatic nucleus, intermixed inflammatory cells	CD2, CD56, cCD3ε, granzyme B, TIA-1, perforin, surface CD3 not expressed	TCR not rearranged, EBV present in clonal episomal form
Enteropathy-type T-cell lymphoma	Increased in areas with celiac disease and ulcerative jejunitis	Ulcerating mucosal mass in jejunum or ileum, broad cytologic spectrum, intermixed inflammatory cells	CD3, CD8+/−, CD103, TIA-1, granzyme, perforin	Rearranged TCR, HLA DQA1*0501, DQB1*0201 genotype of celiac disease
Hepatosplenic T-cell lymphoma	Peak incidence in adolescents and young adults, marked hepatosplenomegaly with no peripheral lymphadenopathy, more common in patients with immunosuppression	Sinusoidal infiltration of liver, spleen, and bone marrow by monotonous small- to medium-sized cells	CD3, TCR-γ/δ, TIA-1, negative for CD4, CD8, TCR-α/β, and perforin	Rearranged TCR, isochromosome 7q, trisomy 8
Subcutaneous panniculitislike T-cell lymphoma	Multiple subcutaneous nodules, may be associated with hemophagocytic syndrome with pancytopenia, fever, and hepatosplenomegaly	Diffuse, lacelike infiltrate in subcutis without sparing septae; epidermis uninvolved; necrosis, karyorrhexis, rimming of fat cells	CD3, CD8, granzyme B, perforin, TIA-1	Rearranged TCR
Mycosis fungoides	Long natural history, multiple skin lesions, patch → plaque → tumor, frequently on trunk	Epidermotropic infiltrate of tumor cells with "cerebriform" nuclei. Pautrier's microabscesses	CD2, CD3, CD5, CD4, TCR-α/β, no expression of CD7	Rearranged TCR

(Continued)

Disease	Clinical presentation	Morphology	Immunophenotype	Genetics
Sezary syndrome	Aggressive variant of mycosis fungoides; erythroderma, lymphadenopathy, and circulating Sezary cells	PB: Minimum of 1000 Sezary cells per mm³, "ceribriform" nuclei	Increased CD4/CD8 ratio lacking expression of CD7	Rearranged TCR
Angioimmunoblastic T-cell lymphoma	Immunodeficiency secondary to lymphoma, skin rash, edema, pleural effusion, ascites, cytopenia, polyclonal hypergammaglobulinemia, + rheumatoid factor	Mixture of pleomorphic lymphocytes, plasma cells, eosinophils, clear cells, and immunoblasts; arborizing HEV; prominence of FDC meshwork outside follicles	CD2, CD3, CD4 with co-expression of CD10, follicular dendritic cells are highlighted by CD21, CD23, CD35, immunoblasts are CD20+ and EBV+	Rearranged TCR, trisomy 3, trisomy 5, additional X chromosome
Peripheral T-cell lymphoma, unspecified	Predominantly nodal based lymphomas that cannot be better classified, generalized disease	Broad cytologic spectrum, T-zone variant with preservation of follicles, Lennert variant with many epithelioid clusters	CD2, CD3, mostly CD4, may express CD30	Rearranged TCR
Anaplastic large cell lymphoma	10% to 30% of childhood lymphomas advanced stage (III or IV) with frequent extranodal involvement	Hallmark cells = large cells with abundant cytoplasm and horseshoe-shaped nuclei	CD30 (membrane and Golgi), Alk-1 (60–85%), EMA+, CD43, CD2, CD4	Rearranged TCR, t(2;5) involving nucleophosmin and ALK

Abbreviations: NK = natural killer; HTLV =; LDH =; GI = gastrointestinal; PB =; BM =; LGL =; HEV =; FDC =; TCR =; TIA =; FasL = Fas ligand; EBV = Epstein–Barr virus; Alk =; EMA = epithelial membrane antigen; TCL =; HLA = human leukocyte antigen.

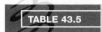

TABLE 43.5	Criteria for the Diagnosis of Multiple Myeloma

A. Major criteria
Plasmacytoma on tissue biopsy
Bone marrow plasmacytosis (>30% plasma cells)
Monoclonal immunoglobulin spike on serum electrophoresis: IgG > 3.5 g/dL or IgA > 2.0 g/dL;
  κ or λ light chain excretion > 1.0 g/d on 24-h urine electrophoresis

B. Minor criteria
Bone marrow plasmacytosis (10% to 30% plasma cells)
Monoclonal immunoglobulin spike present but of lesser magnitude than above
Lytic bone lesions
Reduced normal immunoglobulins (<50% of normal)

Diagnosis requires any two major criteria or a minimum of one major and one minor criterion or three minor criteria which must include the first two.
Abbreviations: Ig = immunoglobulin.

B. **Plasma cell myeloma** usually is characterized by multifocal bone marrow plasmacytosis causing osteolytic lesions, pathologic fractures, bone pain, hypercalcemia, and anemia (e-**Figs. 43.24** and **43.25**). The diagnostic criteria for the diagnosis of plasma cell myeloma are outlined in Table 43.5, requiring a minimum of one major and one minor criterion or three minor criteria. These criteria must be manifest in a symptomatic patient with progressive disease. Clinical variants include smoldering myeloma (patients fulfill the minimal criteria for the diagnosis of plasma cell myeloma, but are asymptomatic and have no lytic bone lesions), indolent myeloma (patients fulfill the minimal criteria for the diagnosis of plasma cell myeloma and have <3 lytic bone lesions, but are asymptomatic), and plasma cell leukemia (plasma cells constitute >20% of peripheral leukocytes) (Table 43.6).

C. **Plasmacytomas** manifest as a localized osseous or extraosseous lesion with no radiographic or morphologic evidence of bone marrow involvement (e-**Figs. 43.26** through **43.29**). The most common osseous location is the vertebral body, and the most common extraosseous location is the upper respiratory tract.

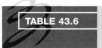

TABLE 43.6	Diagnostic Criteria of Monoclonal Gammopathy of Uncertain Significance (MGUS), Smoldering Multiple Myeloma (SMM), and Indolent Multiple Myeloma (IMM)

Type	Marrow plasmacytosis	Serum M component	Lytic bone lesions	Hemoglobin, serum calcium, and creatinine
MGUS	<10%	Less than myeloma levels (IgG < 3.5 g/dL; IgA < 2 g/dL)	None	Normal
SMM	10% to 30%	Myeloma levels (IgG > 3.5 g/dL; IgA > 2 g/dL)	None	Normal
IMM	>30%	Intermediate levels (IgG 3.5 to 7 g/dL, IgA 2 to 5 g/dL)	<3	Normal

Abbreviations: Ig = immunoglobulin.

D. Monoclonal immunoglobulin deposition diseases present with visceral and soft tissue deposits of immunoglobulin light chains, heavy chains, or both. An example of monoclonal light chain deposition is primary amyloidosis, a rare disease characterized by deposition of an abnormal immunoglobulin. These immunoglobulin light chains are predominantly λ, secreted by monoclonal plasma cells, ingested and processed by macrophages, and discharged into extracellular matrix as β-pleated sheets containing amyloid P component. The amyloidosis is visible as homogenous, pink deposits in tissue sections that are green birefringent by Congo Red staining. The clinical consequences are related to deposition of amyloid in organs, resulting in organomegaly.

E. POEMS syndrome represents a rare plasma cell dyscrasia with associated clinical features including polyneuropathy, organomegaly, endocrinology, monoclonal gammopathy, and skin changes. Bony lesions are usually sclerotic. Lymph node biopsies in these patients may demonstrate Castlemanlike features. The bone marrow shows plasmacytosis only in the vicinity of sclerotic lesions (*Blood and Bone Marrow Pathology*. (1st ed.) : Elsevier Science Ltd; 2003:437–469).

F. Immunophenotype. Neoplastic plasma cells typically express monotypic cytoplasmic immunoglobulin and lack surface immunoglobulin expression. Most cases lack CD19 and CD20 expression, whereas CD79a, CD38, and CD138 (syndecan-1) are found in the majority of cases. CD56 is usually expressed as well. Expression of cyclin D1 is also a feature of plasma cell dyscrasias, specifically multiple myeloma (see section G below), and diagnosis of mantle cell lymphoma must be avoided based on an isolated finding of cyclin D1 positivity.

G. Myeloma genetics. Plasma cell dyscrasias will demonstrate clonally rearranged immunoglobulin heavy and light chains by molecular studies. Cytogenetic methods to detect chromosomal abnormalities include cytokine-stimulated bone marrows for conventional karyotyping and FISH. Complex karyotypes with multiple chromosomal gains and losses are the most frequent abnormalities, the most common being gains in chromosomes 3, 5, 7, 9, 11, 15, and 19 and losses in chromosomes 8, 13, 14, and X (*Blood* 1995;85:2490). Monosomy or partial deletion of 13 (13q14) is the most common chromosomal loss. The most common translocation is t(11;14)(q13;q32) involving the *BCL1* locus on chromosome 11q13 and the immunoglobulin heavy (*IgH*) chain locus on 14q23, which leads to overexpression of cyclin-D1 (*J Clin Oncol* 2005;23:6333, *Brit J Hematol* 1998;101:189, *Blood* 2002;99:2185). Other translocation partners for the *IgH* locus are 4p16.3 (*FGFR-3* and *MMSET*), 6p21 (*CCND3*), 16q23 (*c-maf*), and 20q11 (*mafB*) (see Table 43.7).

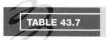

TABLE 43.7	Commonly Occurring Cytogenetic Abnormalities in Multiple Myeloma*	
Abnormality	**% Occurrence**	**Prognostic implications**
I. Numerical[†]		Good prognosis requiring standard therapeutic regimens
a. Hyperdiploidy	61% to 68%	
b. Pseudodiploidy	9% to 20%	
c. Hypodiploidy	10% to 30%	
II. Complex[‡] Partial or complete deletion of 13 and 11q, del 17q13	Ranging from 1% to 25%	Poor prognosis requiring vigorous pursuit of investigational drugs

*Up to 90% of cases show abnormalities using fluorescence in situ hybridization (FISH) techniques. By conventional cytogenetics, 30% to 50% of patients show an abnormal karyotype.
[†]Most common abnormalities are trisomy 3, 7, 9, and 11; monosomy 13; and, in females, monosomy X.
[‡]Including translocations and deletions involving chromosomes; t(4;14) and t(11;14) are the most common translocations.

VIII. HODGKIN LYMPHOMA. Hodgkin lymphoma typically presents as a primarily nodal disease characterized by a predominance of reactive cells and paucity of neoplastic Reed–Sternberg cells or variants. Hodgkin lymphoma comprises two distinct entities: classical Hodgkin lymphoma (CHL) and nodular lymphocyte–predominant Hodgkin lymphoma (NLPHL). These two entities differ in their clinical appearance, morphology, immunoglobulin transcription of the neoplastic cells, and immunophenotype.

    A. CHL accounts for ~95% of Hodgkin lymphoma and is subdivided into four categories: nodular sclerosis (~70%), mixed cellularity (~20% to 25%), lymphocyte rich (~5%), and lymphocyte depleted (<5%). The neoplastic cell is the classical Reed–Sternberg cell or variants (mononuclear forms, mummified forms, or lacunar cells).

        1. Nodular sclerosis CHL commonly presents with a mediastinal mass. Histology reveals scattered Reed–Sternberg cells embedded in a mixed inflammatory background of mostly T lymphocytes, plasma cells, eosinophils, neutrophils, and histiocytes, compartmentalized into nodules by thick strands of collagen fibrosis (e-**Figs.** 43.30 through 43.32).

        2. Mixed cellularity CHL presents with scattered Reed–Sternberg cells in a diffuse or vaguely nodular mixed inflammatory background without nodular sclerosing fibrosis.

        3. In lymphocyte-rich CHL, the nonneoplastic cellular background is composed predominantly of T lymphocytes. Other inflammatory cells are rare.

        4. Lymphocyte-depleted CHL is rare and occurs most commonly in association with HIV infection. Histologically, sheets of Reed–Sternberg cells predominate without a significant lymphocytic or mixed inflammatory infiltrate.

        The main clinical findings of CHL at diagnosis are painless peripheral lymphadenopathy, most commonly involving the cervical region, and constitutional symptoms, such as fever, night sweats, weight loss, and infections due to immunosuppression. Many of the pathologic and clinical features reflect an abnormal immune response due to the wide variety of cytokines and chemokines (Table 43.8) produced by the Reed–Sternberg cells (*Blood* 2002;99:4283). The

TABLE 43.8	Role of Cytokines in Classical Hodgkin Lymphoma	
Cytokine	**Biologic activity**	**Comments**
IL-1	Potent proinflammatory cytokine, induction of fever and acute phase proteins	Associated with B-symptoms
IL-5	Eosinophil differentiation, proliferation, and activation	Associated with blood and tissue eosinophilia
IL-6	Plasma cell differentiation, stimulation of IL-1 and TNF-α production	Associated with thrombocytosis and tissue plasmacytosis
IL-8	Neutrophil recruitment factor	Associated with tissue neutrophilia
IL-9	T-cell and mast cell growth factor	May be acting as a growth factor for Reed–Sternberg cells
IL-10	Impaired immune response	Associated with EBV+ cases
IL-13	B-cell proliferation and survival; Ig class switching to IgG4 and IgE	Autocrine growth factor for Reed–Sternberg cells
TGF-β	Inhibition of IL-2R upregulation and IL-2–dependent T- and B-cell proliferation, potent stimulator of fibroblast proliferation and collagen synthesis	Associated with tissue fibrosis

Abbreviations: IL = interleukin; IL-2R = interleukin 2 receptor; TGF = transforming growth factor; Ig = immunoglobulin; TNF-α = tumor necrosis factor-α; EBV = Epstein–Barr virus.

etiology of CHL is largely unknown. Studies based on the month of diagnosis have revealed peaks in February and March. The lymphoma appears to be more prevalent in adolescents and young adults with higher socioeconomic status (*Hematol Oncol* 2004;22:11). The association between EBV and CHL has been demonstrated in numerous seroepidemiological studies in which antibody titers to EBV and viral capsid antigens have been consistently found to be higher in the lymphoma cases compared to controls. There also have been reports of clustering of CHL within the same family, especially among siblings of same sex and close age. Certain human leukocyte antigen (HLA) types, such as A1, B5, and B18, appear also to be clearly associated with this lymphoma (*Hematol Oncol* 2004;22:11).

B. NLPHL is characterized by scattered large neoplastic L&H cells (lymphocytic and/or histiocytic cells, popcorn cells) residing in nodular meshworks of follicular dendritic processes, filled with nonneoplastic lymphocytes, mostly of B-cell lineage (e-Figs. 43.33 and 43.34). Clinically, patients present with localized peripheral lymphadenopathy. The disease develops slowly, with fairly frequent relapses, but remains responsive to chemotherapy and usually is not fatal.

C. Pathophysiology. The cellular origin of neoplastic cells in both CHL and NLPHL was finally determined when clonally rearranged immunoglobulin genes were amplified from purified Hodgkin cells obtained by microdissection (*Proc Natl Acad Sci U S A* 1994;91:10962). Additionally, the detection of somatic mutations within the rearranged immunoglobulin genes suggests a germinal center or postgerminal center B cell to be the precursor of Hodgkin cells. Although tumor cells of both CHL and NLPHL can rearrange immunoglobulin chains, these are not expressed in CHL due to lack of immunoglobulin messenger RNA (mRNA). Further studies have shown that the absence of immunoglobulin transcription is caused by inactivation of the immunoglobulin promoter through impaired or absent activation of the octamer-dependent transcription factor Oct2 and/or its coactivator BOB.1. Immunohistochemistry for Oct2 and BOB.1 usually is negative in classical Reed–Sternberg cells, unlike L&H cells in NLPHL that express these two markers (*Blood* 2001;91:496).

Normally, when B cells are no longer capable of expressing immunoglobulin they rapidly undergo apoptosis. However, although classical Reed–Sternberg cells do not express immunoglobulin chains due to the absence of immunoglobulin mRNA, they are resistant to apoptosis. One mechanism preventing apoptosis is believed to the persistent activation of the nuclear transcription factor nuclear factor kappa B (NFκB) in classical Reed–Sternberg cells caused by mutations within members of the IκB family, which are natural inhibitors of NFκB, or by aberrant activation of IκB kinase (*Lancet Oncol* 2004;5:11).

D. Immunophenotype studies. Immunohistochemistry markers important in the diagnosis of Hodgkin lymphoma are:

1. CD30 (expressed on classical Reed–Sternberg cells in ~98% of cases)
2. CD15 (expressed on classical Reed–Sternberg cells in ~80% of cases; also expressed in neutrophils)
3. CD20 (may be expressed in a small subset of classical Reed–Sternberg cells; strongly positive in L&H cells, positive in intermixed nonneoplastic small B lymphocytes)
4. CD45 (LCA) (negative in classical Reed–Sternberg cells, strongly positive in L&H cells, positive in accompanying nonneoplastic inflammatory cells)
5. CD79a (negative in classical Reed–Sternberg cells, strongly positive in L&H cells, positive in intermixed nonneoplastic small B lymphocytes)
6. Epithelial membrane antigen (EMA) negative in classical Reed–Sternberg cells, positive in L&H cells in ~50% of cases)
7. BCL-6 (positive in L&H cells in nearly all cases)
8. CD3 (positive in intermixed T lymphocytes, L&H cells are ringed by CD3+ T cells)
9. CD57 (positive in intermixed cytotoxic T cells, L&H cells are ringed by CD57+ T cells)

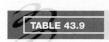

TABLE 43.9	Ann Arbor Staging for Hodgkin and Non-Hodgkin Lymphoma
Stage I	Involvement of single lymph node region or single extralymphatic site (IE)
Stage II	Involvement of two or more lymph node regions on same side of diaphragm; may include localized extralymphatic involvement on same side of diaphragm (IIE)
Stage III	Involvement of lymph node regions on both sides of the diaphragm; may include spleen (IIIS) or localized involvement of extralymphatic organ or site (IIIE), or spleen (IIIS), or both (IIISE)
Stage IV	Diffuse or disseminated extralymphatic disease (e.g., in liver, bone marrow, lung, skin) with or without lymph node involvement

10. BSAP (B cell–specific activator protein and product of the *PAX 5* gene; positive in both classical Reed–Sternberg cells and L&H cells)

11. EBV (positive in classical Reed–Sternberg cells in ~40% of cases)

IX. STAGING OF LYMPHOMAS AND PLASMA CELL MYELOMA

A. Hodgkin and non-Hodgkin lymphomas. Formal documentation of anatomic extent of disease is required in all patients newly diagnosed with lymphoma, prior to therapeutic intervention. Clinical staging takes into account variables such as history and physical examination, imaging studies, blood chemistry determination, complete blood count, and bone marrow biopsy. If a patient presents with relapsed disease, determination of anatomic extent of the disease is recommended but a new clinical stage is usually not assigned. The most widely used anatomic staging classification for Hodgkin and non-Hodgkin lymphomas is the Ann Arbor classification, which has been adapted by the American Joint Committee on Cancer (AJCC) as the official system for lymphoma staging (see Table 43.9).

1. Definition of lymph node regions is based on the definitions proposed by the Rye Symposium in 1965 and adapted both by the Ann Arbor and AJCC systems (*AJCC Cancer Staging Manual*, 6th edition. Eds: Frederick L. Greene FL, et al. Springer Verlag; 395). The currently accepted classification groups of lymph nodes are right cervical (includes cervical, supraclavicular, occipital, and preauricular nodes); left cervical; right axillary; left axillary; right infraclavicular; left infraclavicular; mediastinal; hilar; para-aortic; mesenteric; right pelvic; left pelvic; right inguinofemoral; and left inguinofemoral.

2. Definition of extranodal involvement (such as by direct extension into lung, thyroid, liver, etc.) is designated by an "E" alongside the anatomic stage. Involvement of bone marrow, cerebrospinal fluid, liver, or pleura equates to stage IV by convention.

B. Staging of multiple myeloma. The AJCC recommends the Durie–Salmon staging system for multiple myeloma (*AJCC Cancer Staging Manual*, 6th edition. Eds: Frederick L. Greene FL, et al. eds. et al. Springer-Verlag; :402). This system takes into account various complete blood count variables, blood chemistries, and imaging studies.

A newer, simpler, and more cost-effective alternative is the International Staging System (ISS), previously the International Prognostic Index. This system uses two simple blood parameters, specifically $\beta 2$ microglobulin ($\beta 2$-M) and albumin. The ISS has been proven to be useful for staging myeloma (*J Clin Oncol* 2005;23:3412) and is currently recommended for widespread use. A comparison of these myeloma staging systems is depicted in Table 43.10.

CYTOLOGY OF THE LYMPH NODE
Jing Zhai

I. INTRODUCTION. Diagnosis of non-Hodgkin lymphoma by fine needle aspiration (FNA) requires a multiparametric approach that combines cytomorphology with

TABLE 43.10 Staging Systems for Multiple Myeloma

			Durie–Salmon staging system					ISS criteria	
				Immunoglobulins					
Stage	Hb	Serum calcium	Bone x-ray or osteolytic lesion	IgG	IgA	Urine m-protein	Serum Cr	β₂M	Albumin
I	>10 g/dL	≤12 mg/dL	Normal or single lesion	<5 g/dL	<3 g/dL	<4 g/24 h	A <2.0 mg/dL B >2.0 mg/dL	<3.5 mg/dL	>3.5 g/dL
II	Neither I nor III							a) <3.5 mg/dL or b) 3.5 to 5.5 mg/dL	a) <3.5 g/dL b)–
III	<8.5 g/dL	>12 mg/dL	Advanced multiple lytic lesions	>7 g/dL	>5 g/dL	>12 g/24 h	>2.0 mg/dL	>5.5 mg/dL	–

Abbreviations: Hb = hemoglobulin; Cr = creatinine; β₂M = β2 microglobulin; Ig = immunoglobulin; – not required for staging.

ancillary studies. The multiparametric approach parallels the paradigm that is used for diagnosis of conventional excisional biopsy specimens, and includes flow cytometry, immunohistochemistry, FISH, cytogenetics, and molecular studies (*Diagn Cytopathol 2000;23:375, Cancer 2005;105:429*). Using a combined approach, diagnosis of non-Hodgkin lymphoma based on FNA specimens has >80% sensitivity and >90% specificity (*Diagn Cytopathol 2000;2:120*).

The lymphoid cells from FNA specimens are dyshesive, and the background frequently shows lymphoglandular bodies (cytoplasmic fragments of disrupted lymphocytes). In general, non-Hodgkin lymphoma exhibits a monotonous population of atypical lymphoid cells. Cytologically, non-Hodgkin lymphoma is classified as small cell lymphoma, intermediate cell lymphoma, and large cell lymphoma based on the cell size in comparison with histiocytes. Small cell lymphoma is further divided into SLL, lymphoplasmacytic lymphoma, follicular lymphoma (grade 1), mantle cell lymphoma, and marginal zone lymphoma. Intermediate cell lymphoma is further divided into lymphoblastic lymphoma and Burkitt lymphoma. Large cell lymphoma usually refers to diffuse large B-cell lymphoma, but also includes T- cell and NK-cell lymphoma.

II. REACTIVE LYMPHADENOPATHY. The aspirate is characterized by a polymorphous population of lymphoid cells with variable size and shape that predominantly contains small lymphoid cells with smooth nuclear contour and coarse chromatin, intermixed with scattered intermediate cells and large immunoblastlike cells. There are scattered plasma cells, histiocytes, and tingible body macrophages. Lymphohistiocytic aggregates are also present, consisting of collections of lymphoid cells and histiocytes held together by dendritic reticulum cells (e-**Fig. 43.35**) (*Acta Cytol 1987;31:8*). Clusters of neutrophils are indicative of suppurative lymphadenopathy. The presence of granulomas (collections of epithelioid histiocytes) is consistent with granulomatous lymphadenitis (e-**Fig. 43.36**) (*Sarcoidosis 1987;4:38*); special stains and culture are required for identification of fungi and mycobacteria. Fungal hyphae and yeast forms can occasionally be identified as negative images on Diff-Quik–stained smears (e-**Fig. 43.37**).

III. SLL. The aspirate contains a monotonous population of small lymphoid cells with round nuclear contours, characteristic checkerboardlike clumpy chromatin, and indistinct nucleoli (e-**Fig. 43.38**). Scattered large prolymphocytes/paraimmunoblasts with vesicular chromatin, prominent central nucleoli, and pale cytoplasm are present.

IV. LYMPHOPLASMACYTIC LYMPHOMA. The smear contains a mixed population of small lymphoid cells, plasmacytoid cells, and plasma cells.

V. FOLLICULAR LYMPHOMA. The aspirate is composed predominantly of small centrocytes (that have irregular and grooved nuclear membranes) intermixed with scattered centroblasts (that have large noncleaved nuclei with multiple small peripheral nucleoli) and immunoblasts (that have single prominent central nucleoli) (e-**Fig. 43.39**). Lymphoid aggregates without abundant histiocytes are not infrequently found (*Cancer 1999;87:216, Cancer 2006;108:1*). Although the cytological criteria for grading follicular lymphoma are not well-established, the percentage of centroblasts on smears has been proposed as a basis for grading by several groups (*Clin Pathol 2002;117:880, Am J Clin Pathol 1997;108:143*).

VI. MANTLE CELL LYMPHOMA. The aspirate is composed of a monotonous population of small to intermediate-sized lymphoid cells with variable nuclear membrane contour irregularity, more dispersed chromatin, and inconspicuous nucleoli (e-**Fig. 43.40**) (*Cancer 1999;87:216*).

VII. NODAL MARGINAL ZONE B-CELL LYMPHOMA. The aspirate contains a rather polymorphous lymphoid population, composed predominately of small lymphoid cells with round nuclei and clumpy chromatin, with scattered plasmacytoid cells and immunoblastlike large cells (*Diagn Cytopathol 1999;20:190*). Some intermediate lymphoid cells have a monocytoid appearance and exhibit a moderate amount of pale cytoplasm (e-**Fig. 43.41**). Lymphoepithelial lesions are not identified on smears. The diagnosis based on the cytologic findings alone is difficult without ancillary studies.

VIII. LYMPHOBLASTIC LYMPHOMA. The aspirate is composed of a monotonous population of intermediate-sized lymphoid cells with fine granular chromatin, irregular nuclear membrane contours, inconspicuous nucleoli, and scant basophilic cytoplasm (e-**Fig. 43.42**). Mitoses are frequently identified (*Acta Cytol* 1992;36:887).

In Burkitt lymphoma, the aspirate contains a monotonous population of intermediate-sized lymphoid cells with round nuclei, finely dispersed chromatin, and multiple distinct nucleoli. The cytoplasm is scant and blue with lipid-filled small vacuoles (e-**Fig. 43.43**). Tingible body macrophages and mitosis are prominent (*Cytopathology* 1995;12:201).

IX. **DIFFUSE LARGE B-CELL LYMPHOMA.** The aspirate shows a monotonous population of large atypical lymphoid cells. The centroblastic variant contains centroblasts with irregular nuclear membrane contours, coarse chromatin, and multiple small nucleoli (e-**Fig. 43.44**). The immunoblastic variant shows immunoblasts with irregular nuclear membrane contours, open chromatin, and single prominent nucleoli. The T cell–rich B-cell lymphoma variant is composed predominantly of small mature lymphocytes and scattered, large immature lymphoid cells with polymorphic nuclei and prominent nucleoli. The cytological diagnosis of this variant is challenging (*Diagn Cytopathol* 1998;18:1).

X. **PERIPHERAL T-CELL LYMPHOMA, UNSPECIFIED TYPE.** The aspirate is polymorphic. It contains scattered, large atypical lymphocytes with a convoluted nuclear membrane. There is a reactive lymphoid background composed of small mature lymphocytes, plasma cells, neutrophils, eosinophils, and macrophages. Ancillary studies are necessary for diagnosis (*Diagn Cytopathol* 2000;23:375).

XI. **ANAPLASTIC LARGE CELL LYMPHOMA.** The aspirate shows both singly dispersed and poorly cohesive groups of malignant cells with large and pleomorphic nuclei, prominent nucleoli, and a moderate amount of cytoplasm. Horseshoe- and donut-shaped nuclei, as well as binucleated and multinucleated Reed–Sternberglike tumor cells, are also present. Immunostains are necessary for diagnosis (*Acta Cytol* 1996;40:779).

XII. **HODGKIN LYMPHOMA.** The aspirate of CHL contains rare to scattered Reed–Sternberg cells. The classic binucleated Reed–Sternberg cells have markedly enlarged nuclei, macronucleoli, and a moderate amount of basophilic cytoplasm (e-**Fig. 43.45**). The mononuclear variant has cells with markedly enlarged, irregular, and multilobated nuclei and macronucleoli (e-**Fig. 43.46**). The characteristic reactive lymphoid background includes mainly mature lymphocytes, scattered eosinophils, neutrophils, plasma cells, and occasional epithelioid histiocytes (e-**Fig. 43.46**) (*J Clin Pathol* 1986;86:286). Diagnosis is challenging due to the scarcity of the Reed–Sternberg cells, and the cytological diagnosis of NLPHL from FNA specimens is very difficult if not impossible. Nonetheless, when FNA biopsy is used in conjunction with immunohistochemistry as a screening test for Hodgkin lymphoma, the approach has a positive predictive value that has been reported to be >90% in some studies (*Cytopathology* 1994;5:226, *Acta Cytol* 2001;45:300).

XIII. **METASTATIC MALIGNANCY.** The most common indication for lymph node FNA biopsy is metastatic malignancy. The reported sensitivity of diagnosis based on FNA specimens in this clinical setting is >90%, and specificity is >98% (*Diagn Cytopathol* 2003;28:175, *Cytopathology* 1996;15:382). The aspirate shows a nonlymphoid population of cells with malignant cytological features. Comparison with the primary malignancy will confirm the diagnosis. In case of an unknown primary malignancy, immunostains are helpful to identify the most likely site of tumor origin.

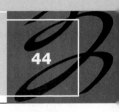

BONE MARROW PATHOLOGY
John L. Frater

44

I. NORMAL GROSS AND MICROSCOPIC ANATOMY. The bone marrow is generally considered the fourth largest organ in the human body, and is composed of cells derived from a variety of lineages including stromal cells, adipocytes, lymphocytes, and hematopoietic precursors. The most frequently sampled areas are the posterior superior iliac crest and, much less frequently, the sternum and long bones. The bone marrow has an orderly microscopic anatomy. The most superficial part consists of a layer of dense cortical bone with an adjacent cover of dense fibrous periosteum. Deep to the cortex are the bony trabeculae, which consist of thin trabecular bone and the marrow cavity itself. The marrow cavity contains islands of maturing hematopoietic cells with intervening areas of fat, the latter of which increase with age.

The cellularity of the bone marrow is defined as the percentage of the marrow cavity composed of hematopoietic cells. In biopsies from the posterior iliac crest, marrow cellularity decreases with age, and is expressed by the following formula:

$$\text{Marrow cellularity} = (100 - \text{patient age})\% \pm 20\%.$$

Thus a 50-year-old individual would be expected to have a marrow cellularity of approximately (100–50)% ± 20%, or 30% to 70%.

Under normal circumstances, maturing myeloid and erythroid elements occupy different regions of the marrow cavity. Myeloid precursors lie adjacent to the trabecular bone, and erythroid elements form "islands" of cells between trabeculae. The ratio of myeloid to erythroid elements is roughly 2:1. Megakaryocytes are irregularly distributed throughout the bone marrow. Under normal circumstances they are not present in clusters.

It is important to be cognizant of the multidisciplinary nature of hematopathology. Diagnoses in bone marrow pathology are not generally the product of morphologic analysis of the bone marrow core biopsy and peripheral blood and bone marrow aspirate smears alone. Clinical history may be extremely important in separating morphologically similar diseases and should be provided by the patient's physicians. Also, the pertinent features of the physical examination, such as lymphadenopathy, splenomegaly, or hepatomegaly, are of importance. Other clinical laboratory information, such as complete blood counts and serum and/or urine protein electrophoresis, are often of interest. Radiographic data are of importance, particularly in the evaluation of a monoclonal protein.

II. GROSS EXAMINATION AND TISSUE SAMPLING. The same pathologist should review both the bone marrow aspirate smears and core biopsies whenever possible to avoid ambiguities or outright contradictions. The bone marrow aspirate is generally performed before the biopsy. There are two kinds of aspirate smears: smears prepared directly from the specimen without pretreatment, and smears prepared from concentrated aspirate fluid. Concentrated bone marrow aspirate smears and touch preparations prepared from the bone marrow core biopsy are particularly useful in the evaluation of specimens diluted with peripheral blood. From three to five of the smears are stained using the Wright–Giemsa or similar technique, one is stained for iron using the Prussian blue technique, and additional unstained smears are reserved for ancillary techniques such as fluorescence in situ hybridization (FISH), if necessary. Although examination of bone marrow cells with enzyme cytochemistry is likely to be rendered obsolete in the coming years, its use is still highly recommended by the World Health Organization (WHO) committee for the diagnosis of acute myeloid leukemia, and high-quality aspirate smears should be reserved for this purpose when an acute myelogenous leukemia is suspected. Usually, a second bone marrow aspirate is obtained when flow cytometric and cytogenetic analyses of the specimen are desired. Aspirate smears are generally reviewed using high power ($600\times$ to $1000\times$) and are important for evaluating individual cell detail. However, because the process of aspiration disrupts cell cohesion, the relationship of the various cell types and the marrow cellularity cannot be reliably assessed. An adequate bone marrow core biopsy adds this important information.

III. **DIAGNOSTIC FEATURES OF COMMON BENIGN DISEASES.** The number and scope of nonneoplastic bone marrow disorders are vast. Emphasis is given to commonly encountered bone marrow diseases and conditions that may simulate neoplasia.

  A. **Megaloblastic anemia.** It is often not necessary to perform a bone marrow biopsy in patients who present with anemia, because the most common forms of anemia (iron deficiency, megaloblastic, and anemia of chronic disease) may be diagnosed by laboratory analysis of the peripheral blood, clinical history, and response to iron, vitamin B12, and/or folate replacement. Bone marrow biopsy is performed for patients with anemia that is unexplained or therapeutically resistant.

  It is important to note that megaloblastic anemia may simulate a neoplastic condition, particularly a myelodysplastic syndrome. Patients with megaloblastic anemia may present with marked cytopenias and pronounced dyspoiesis (e-**Figs. 44.1*** and **44.2**). Clues to discriminate this benign condition from a myelodysplastic syndrome include normal blast percentage, absence of karyotypic abnormalities, and improvement of cytopenias following administration of vitamin B12 / folate in megaloblastic anemia. Also, the degree of dyspoiesis in megaloblastic anemia often exceeds that encountered in most cases of neoplastic myelodysplasia.

  B. **Benign causes of lymphocytosis.** Numerous benign conditions may cause a transient increase in benign lymphocytes in the peripheral blood and may simulate chronic lymphocytic leukemia / small lymphocytic lymphoma (CLL/SLL), T-cell large granular lymphocytic leukemia, or other lymphoid leukemias. Stress lymphocytosis is a transient increase in morphologically normal peripheral blood lymphocytes encountered in individuals subjected to physiologic stresses, including individuals presenting to hospital emergency departments. An absolute increase in lymphocytes accompanied by "reactive" forms with increased basophilic cytoplasm and inconspicuous nucleoli may be seen in patients infected with Epstein–Barr virus (EBV, e.g., infectious mononucleosis) or, less commonly, cytomegalovirus or other viral pathogens. Interestingly, in cases of EBV infection the virus particles are present in morphologically normal lymphocytes, and the reactive lymphocytes represent cytotoxic T cells directed at the infected cells. Correlation with serum viral antibody titers is useful in arriving at the correct diagnosis and in avoiding unnecessary procedures such as bone marrow and lymph node biopsies. Many other infections are associated with lymphocytosis, including pertussis, in which the lymphocytes have characteristic clefted nuclei and thus may simulate peripheral blood involvement by a non-Hodgkin lymphoma. Persistent polyclonal B-cell hyperplasia, as its name implies, is often of longer duration than other benign forms of lymphocytes. It frequently affects women who smoke, and is associated with the human leukocyte antigen (HLA)-DR7 phenotype (*Hematopathology. Foundations in Diagnostic Pathology.* Philadelphia: Elsevier; 2007;55–66).

  C. **The granulocytic "left shift."** Other cases of leukocytosis represent a granulocytic shift to immaturity (colloquially known by the archaic term "left shift," referring to the traditional placement of immature myeloid cell percentages to the left of neutrophils in classical peripheral blood smear reports). Because many of these cases also demonstrate eosinophilia and/or basophilia, it is important to distinguish them from neoplastic conditions, in particular chronic myelogenous leukemia or other chronic myeloproliferative disorders. Most commonly, especially in hospitalized populations, a granulocytic shift to immaturity represents an acute response to

---

*All e-figures are available online via the Solution Site Image Bank.

bacterial or other infections. Transient increases in mature demarginated neutrophils may also follow surgery or other physical trauma. Unusual causes of increased peripheral blood neutrophils with or without immature granulocytes include chronic idiopathic neutrophilia, hereditary neutrophilia, and leukocyte adhesion factor deficiency.

D. Benign causes of erythrocytosis. Under normal conditions, the circulating red blood cell mass is maintained at a constant level by the actions of the cytokine erythropoietin, which is produced by renal peritubular cells. An absolute increase in circulating red blood cells (polycythemia) may be primary (most commonly due to the chronic myeloproliferative disorder polycythemia vera) or secondary (due to increased production of erythropoietin). Thus, in establishing a diagnosis of polycythemia vera, a number of conditions must be excluded that may cause secondary erythrocytosis, including smoking, living in a high-altitude environment, and high oxygen-affinity hemoglobins.

E. Benign causes of thrombocytosis. There are numerous causes of benign thrombocytosis (defined as a peripheral blood platelet count in excess of $450,000/\mu L$). Common reactive causes of peripheral thrombocytosis include childbirth, major hemorrhage, iron deficiency anemia, chronic inflammatory conditions, infection, and acute stress events (*Hematology: Clinical Principles and Applications*, (2nd ed.) Philadelphia: W.B. Saunders; 2002;696–698).

F. Aplastic anemia. Bone marrow aplasia is usually associated with bi- or pancytopenia rather than isolated anemia, and may be identified in a variety of clinical settings. It may occur secondary to a variety of drugs, most commonly chemotherapeutic agents, benzene, alcohol, and arsenic. It may also occur secondary to exposure to radiation, viral infection (e.g., viral hepatitis, EBV), or tuberculosis. An important cause of infection-mediated isolated anemia is infection with parvovirus B19. Other causes of bone marrow hypocellularity include paroxysmal nocturnal hemoglobinuria, Fanconi anemia, dyskeratosis congenital, and other very rare inherited bone marrow failure syndromes (*Int J Hematol* 2002;76 Suppl 1:207).

The common morphologic finding in bone marrow biopsies from patients with aplastic anemia is marked panhypoplasia; a notable exception is parvovirus infection in which there is selective suppression of erythroid precursors. These specimens should be carefully scrutinized for evidence of significant dyspoiesis or increased blasts, because a minority of myelodysplastic syndromes and acute myeloid leukemias present with markedly hypocellular bone marrow biopsies. These specimens should also be examined for evidence of infection as evidenced by granuloma formation in the case of tuberculosis, or intranuclear inclusions in the case of viral infection. The inclusions of parvovirus are ill-defined and are localized to the nuclei of proerythroblasts.

G. Serous degeneration (serous atrophy) is a pattern of bone marrow injury most often associated with acquired immunodeficiency syndrome (AIDS) and states of chronic nutritional deficiency such as starvation, chronic alcoholism, and anorexia nervosa (*Arch Pathol Lab Med* 1992;116:504). The primary morphologic finding in the bone marrow is stromal edema with associated microvesicular change. The bone marrow is hypocellular in these regions due to loss of normal hematopoietic elements. These findings may be focal, alternating with regions of relatively preserved normal hematopoiesis. It is important to recognize that the subcortical bone marrow is normally hypocellular and occasionally demonstrates edema, possibly related to trauma associated with the biopsy procedure, and thus may mimic serous degeneration.

H. Granulomas may be encountered in bone marrow core biopsies and are occasionally noted in aspirate smears. Granulomas may be quite subtle and are usually composed of admixed histiocytes, lymphocytes, and plasma cells. Some granulomas contain foci of necrosis and infiltrating neutrophils. The causes of granuloma formation in the bone marrow are similar to those in other sites: The most common etiologies are infectious, autoimmune, or idiopathic. In addition, granulomas are occasionally encountered in the bone marrow of patients with Hodgkin lymphoma, although their presence is not indicative of marrow involvement by disease. Because it is impossible to predict with certainty the etiology of bone marrow granulomas, their presence usually warrants the use of stains to aid in the identification of acid-fast bacilli or fungi. However, it should be noted that special stains are far less sensitive than microbiological culture in the detection of most infectious agents in the bone marrow, so microbiologic analysis of fresh bone marrow tissue is recommended when an infectious etiology is considered. An important item in the morphologic differential diagnosis of granulomas is the lipogranuloma, which is generally considered to be nonpathologic and consists of a collection of histiocytes and lymphocytes surrounding an area of fat demonstrating microvesicular change.

I. **Benign lymphoid aggregates** are present in the bone marrow of healthy individuals and at increased incidence in elderly individuals. Because they are common, it is important to recognize the attributes of benign aggregates and distinguish them from their malignant counterparts. Benign aggregates are often well-circumscribed and are small to medium-sized. They are composed of an admixture of cell types including small and mature-appearing lymphocytes, histiocytes, and granulocytes. They frequently contain a central small-caliber vessel. Although they occasionally abut bony trabeculae, they do not demonstrate the paratrabecular pattern of growth seen in follicular lymphoma and other non-Hodgkin lymphomas involving the marrow. In some cases, immunohistochemistry or in situ hybridization for κ and λ immunoglobulin light chains can be used to further evaluate aggregates.

J. **AIDS.** Since the first cases of AIDS were reported in 1981, a number of associated diseases have been identified in the bone marrow. Commonly encountered morphologic changes in the bone marrow of human immunodeficiency virus (HIV)-infected individuals include granulomas, lymphoid aggregates, plasma cell aggregates, and dysplasia in one or more hematopoietic lineages (*Haemophilia* 2001;7: 47). Since the development of combined drug therapy, the incidence of secondary infections has decreased. However, infectious agents are still encountered in the bone marrow of individuals infected with HIV and, because impaired inflammatory responses are a hallmark of HIV infection, it is recommended that all bone marrow biopsies from patients with HIV be examined with special stains for fungi and mycobacteria.

Lymphoid aggregates occur with increased frequency in the bone marrow of HIV-infected individuals, are sometimes large with ill-defined borders, and grow along bony trabeculae; these are all features suggestive of malignancy. They may be extremely difficult to evaluate, especially in view of the increased incidence of non-Hodgkin lymphomas in this population. Ancillary studies may be useful in monoclonal B-cell or phenotypically abnormal/monoclonal T-cell populations.

Dyspoiesis is a common finding in the bone marrow of patients with HIV infection. The significance of this finding may be difficult if not impossible to interpret because of the increased incidence of neoplastic myelodysplasia and acute leukemias in this population. Blasts are not typically increased in HIV-associated dysplasia, and clonal cytogenetic abnormalities are not present.

K. **Hemophagocytic syndrome** is a potentially deadly condition in which cytokine-stimulated benign histiocytes phagocytose other hematopoietic cells in an uncontrolled fashion. The most common causes of hemophagocytic syndrome are related to activation of benign macrophages by cytokines produced by malignant cells, and unregulated phagocytosis by macrophages following infection. Malignancy-related hemophagocytic syndrome is most commonly associated with peripheral T-cell lymphoma, although other hematopoietic and lymphoid malignancies are also rarely associated with this complication. The most common infectious cause of hemophagocytic syndrome is EBV. Regardless of the underlying cause, hemophagocytic syndrome presents with splenomegaly, fever, and wasting. Pancytopenia, elevated liver function tests, and coagulopathy are variably present. Evaluation of the bone marrow aspirate and core biopsy reveals variable numbers of macrophages containing phagocytosed hematopoietic cells (*Am J Surg Pathol* 2001;25:865).

L. **Chédiak–Higashi syndrome** is an autosomal recessive inherited disorder that is caused by a mutation in the *CHS1/LYST* gene located on chromosome 1q42. The clinical features of this syndrome are related to abnormal lysosomal trafficking and include recurrent infection, oculocutaneous albinism, neurologic disorders, and a

TABLE 44.1   Storage Diseases

A. MUCOPOLYSACCHARIDOSES

Disease	Enzyme deficiency
Hurler syndrome (mucopolysaccharidosis type I H)	α-L-iduronidase
Scheie syndrome (mucopolysaccharidosis type I S)	α-L-iduronidase
Hurler–Scheie syndrome (mucopolysaccharidosis type I H-S)	α-L-iduronidase
Hunter syndrome (mucopolysaccharidosis type II)	Iduronidate α-sulfatase
Sanfilippo syndrome type A (mucopolysaccharidosis type III A)	Heparin N-sulfatase
Sanfilippo syndrome type B (mucopolysaccharidosis type III B)	α-N-Acetylglucosaminidase
Sanfilippo syndrome type C (mucopolysaccharidosis type III C)	α-Glucosaminide transferase
Sanfilippo syndrome type D (mucopolysaccharidosis type III D)	N-Acetylglucosamine-6-sulfatase
Morquio syndrome type A (mucopolysaccharidosis type IV A)	N-Acetylgalactosamine, 6-sulfate sulfatase
Morquio syndrome type B (mucopolysaccharidosis type IV B)	β-Galactosidase
Maroteaux–Lamy syndrome (mucopolysaccharidosis type VI)	N-Acetylgalactosamine-4-sulfatase
Sly syndrome (mucopolysaccharidosis type VII)	β-Glucuronidase

B. LIPID STORAGE DISORDERS

Disease	Enzyme deficiency	Substance stored
Gaucher disease	β-Glucocerebrosidase	Glucocerebroside
Niemann–Pick disease	Sphingomyelinase	Sphingomyelin
Gangliosidosis	β-galactosidase	GM₁ ganglioside
Tay–Sachs disease	Hexosaminidase A	GM₂ ganglioside
Sandhoff disease	Hexosaminidase A	GM₂ ganglioside
Fabry disease	α-Galactosidase	Ceramide trihexalose

bleeding diathesis. Granulocytes, monocytes, and lymphocytes contain abnormal large granules derived from secondary or cytotoxic granules (**e-Fig. 44.3**) (*Platelets* 1998;9:21).

M. Mucopolysaccharidoses. Alder–Reilly anomaly is identified in the granulocytes of patients with a group of uncommon diseases characterized by X-linked or autosomal recessive transmitted defects in the enzymes involved in mucopolysaccharide metabolism (Table 44.1A) (*Clin Lab Haematol* 1996;18:39). Granulocytes in the peripheral blood and bone marrow have coarse azurophilic granules superficially resembling normal primary granules. Classification of cases of mucopolysaccharidosis requires chemical and/or molecular analysis.

N. Lipid storage disorders. There are numerous genetically mediated conditions related to defects in enzymes comprising the pathway of lipid metabolism (Table 44.1B). The most commonly encountered are Gaucher disease and Niemann–Pick disease. Gaucher disease demonstrates an autosomal recessive pattern of inheritance and is caused by a defect in the enzyme β-glucocerebrosidase. Clinically, patients present with bone pain and splenomegaly related to the proliferation of morphologically abnormal histiocytes at these sites. The cytoplasm of the macrophages has a "wrinkled tissue paper" appearance, which represents the accumulation of glucocerebroside in these cells (**e-Fig. 44.4**). Occasional cases are associated with

B-lineage malignancies (including plasma cell dyscrasias) and light chain amyloidosis (*J Intern Med* 1999;246:587).

Patients with Niemann–Pick disease typically present with organomegaly, neuropathy, and abnormal laboratory findings similar to those identified in Gaucher disease. The pathophysiology of Niemann–Pick disease is related to autosomal recessively inherited defects in the enzyme sphingomyelinase, with the presence of sphingomyelin in affected cells. Macrophages in this disorder have been described as "sea-blue" due to the cytoplasmic accumulation of periodic acid-Schiff–positive material representing the sphingomyelin (*Ann Hematol* 2001;80:620).

The remaining lipid storage diseases, which are somewhat less common, have clinical presentations similar to those of Gaucher and Niemann–Pick diseases. Some are associated with additional findings. For example, Hermansky–Pudlak syndrome is associated with platelet storage pool deficiencies and oculocutaneous albinism (*Platelets* 1998;9:21).

IV. DIAGNOSTIC FEATURES OF MALIGNANCIES

A. Myelodysplastic syndromes are clonal hematopoietic disorders characterized in most cases by peripheral cytopenias and increased bone marrow cellularity (*Hematology Am Soc Hematol Educ Program* 2006;199). The entities comprising this family of diseases are summarized in Table 44.2. Diagnosis is made by assessment of the bone marrow aspirate smear for significant dyspoiesis and correlation with the clinical history, including a failure to respond to iron, vitamin B_{12}, and folate replacement. Dyspoiesis is identified in one or more of the hematopoietic lineages. In the myeloid series this most commonly manifests as abnormal nuclear lobation, including cells with pseudo Pelger–Huët (hypolobate) nuclei, and cells with decreased cytoplasmic granules. Erythroid precursors demonstrate nuclear irregularities including budding, with occasional ringed sideroblasts (erythroid precursors with multiple punctate iron granules surrounding the nuclei that reflect iron abnormally trapped in mitochondria). Megakaryocytes contain multiple separate nuclei or are small with decreased nuclear lobation (e-**Figs. 44.5** through **44.8**).

Detection of a cytogenetic abnormality is helpful, although the majority of cases of "low-grade" myelodysplasia (refractory anemia, refractory anemia with ringed sideroblasts, refractory cytopenia with multilineage dysplasia, and refractory cytopenia with multilineage dysplasia and ringed sideroblasts) have normal karyotypes. Common cytogenetic abnormalities include partial or complete deletions of chromosomes 5 and 7, which are associated with an unfavorable clinical outcome, and del(17p) and del(20q). A special type of myelodysplastic syndrome is 5q–syndrome, in which dyspoiesis is most prominent in the megakaryocytic series, accompanied by thrombocytosis. This form of myelodysplasia is associated with long survival.

High-grade myelodysplasia (refractory anemia with excess blasts types 1 and 2) presents with a greater percentage of peripheral blood/bone marrow blasts compared to low-grade cases. In general, refractory anemia with excess blasts is more clinically aggressive than is refractory anemia with or without ringed sideroblasts, and has a variable propensity for progression to acute leukemia or bone marrow failure, both of which are essentially untreatable by any means short of a bone marrow transplant. Outcome in the myelodysplastic syndromes may be predicted using the International Prognostic Scoring System (IPSS), which takes into account blast percentage, karyotype, and the presence of cytopenias.

B. Chronic myeloproliferative disorders. The chronic myeloproliferative disorders are characterized by an expansion of one or more of the hematopoietic lineages as evidenced by increased bone marrow cellularity and increased circulating white blood cells (usually granulocytes), erythrocytes, and/or platelets. Initially, blasts are present in normal to slightly increased numbers in the marrow. Although these are malignant disorders, the affected cell line(s) are usually morphologically normal, and pronounced dyspoiesis is not a characteristic feature of the chronic myeloproliferative disorders. In contrast to myelodysplasia, organomegaly (splenomegaly and/or hepatomegaly) is a common feature of this disease, and becomes more pronounced with

TABLE 44.2 Myelodysplastic Syndromes

Disease	Blood	Bone marrow	Cytogenetics (percentage of cytogenetically abnormal cases)	Outcome (median survival)
Refractory anemia	Anemia No/rare blasts	Erythroid dysplasia <5% blasts <15% ringed sideroblasts	<25%	~6% progress to acute leukemia (66 mo)
Refractory anemia with ringed sideroblasts	Anemia No blasts	≥15% ringed sideroblasts Erythroid dysplasia <5% blasts	<10%	1% to 2% progress to acute leukemia (6 y)
Refractory cytopenia with multilineage dysplasia	Bi/pancytopenia No/rare blasts No Auer rods <1 × 10⁹/L monocytes	Dysplasia in ≥10% of cells in 2 or more myeloid cell lines <5% blasts No Auer rods <15% ringed sideroblasts	~50%	~11% progress to acute leukemia (33 mo)
Refractory cytopenia with multilineage dysplasia and ringed sideroblasts	Bi/pancytopenia No/rare blasts No Auer rods <1 × 10⁹/L monocytes	Dysplasia in ≥10% of cells in 2 or more myeloid cell lines ≥ ringed sideroblasts <5% blasts No Auer rods	Unknown; probably similar to refractory cytopenia with multilineage dysplasia	Unknown; probably similar to refractory cytopenia with multilineage dysplasia
Refractory anemia with excess blasts-1	Cytopenias <5% blasts No Auer rods <1 × 10⁹/L monocytes	Uni/multilineage dysplasia 5% to 9% blasts No Auer rods	~30% to 50%	~25%
Refractory anemia with excess blasts-2	Cytopenias 5% to 19% blasts ± Auer rods <1 × 10⁹/L monocytes	Uni/multilineage dysplasia 10% to 19% blasts ± Auer rods	~30% to 50%	~33%
Myelodysplastic syndrome – unclassifiable	Cytopenias No/rare blasts No Auer rods	Unilineage dysplasia <5% blasts No Auer rods	Unknown	Unknown
Myelodysplastic syndrome associated with isolated del(5q)	Anemia Normal/increased platelet count <5% blasts	Normal/increased megakaryocytes with hypolobate nuclei <5% blasts Isolated del(5q) cytogenetic abnormality No Auer rods	100% (isolated del(5q) cytogenetic abnormality; cases with additional abnormalities should not be classified under this diagnosis)	Unknown median survival – probably many years

From: Jaffee ES, Harris NL, Stein H, Vardiman JW, eds. *World Health Organization Classification of Tumours. Pathology and Genetics. Tumours of Haematopoietic and Lymphoid Tissues.* Lyon: IARC Press; 2001. Used with permission.

disease progression as the bone marrow becomes dysfunctional and extramedullary hematopoiesis is up-regulated.

Particularly in their early stages, it may be difficult to distinguish these diseases from reactive conditions affecting the marrow. Also, because the various chronic myeloproliferative disorders have overlapping morphologic features, distinguishing between them may be very difficult. However, it is important to recognize and distinguish between the various members of this family of disorders because the different malignancies have variable propensities for high-grade (i.e., acute leukemic) transformation and bone marrow failure. Accordingly, the identification of disease-specific molecular markers in this family of diseases is the subject of intense scrutiny, and important molecular lesions have been identified. The first, *BCR-ABL*, has been known for many years, and is largely limited to chronic myelogenous leukemia and occasional cases of acute myeloid leukemia, precursor B-lymphoblastic leukemia/lymphoma, and biphenotypic acute leukemia, at least some cases of which likely represent blast phases of clinically silent chronic myelogenous leukemia. This rearrangement is largely absent from the other classes of myeloproliferative disorders. *BCR-ABL* is most frequently encountered as the classic Philadelphia chromosome, t(9;22)(q34;q11), which juxtaposes the break cluster region gene (*BCR*) at chromosome 22q11 with the Abelson tyrosine kinase gene (*ABL*) at chromosome 9q34. The resultant BCR-ABL fusion protein is a constitutively activated tyrosine kinase directly responsible for the manifestations of disease in chronic myelogenous leukemia. In chronic myelogenous leukemia, BCR-ABL is typically of the 210 kd (p210) form, compared with BCR-ABL in precursor B-lymphoblastic leukemia/lymphoma, which is generally 190 kd (p190). The p230 (230 kd) form of BCR-ABL is identified in cases of chronic myelogenous leukemia with a predominance of mature neutrophils rather than immature granulocytes. Previously, cases of chronic myeloproliferative disorders with the p230 form of BCR-ABL and neutrophilia were classified as chronic neutrophilic leukemia; note that the WHO classification now recommends that such cases be classified as chronic myelogenous leukemia.

More recently, point mutations have been identified in the nonchronic myelogenous leukemia chronic myeloproliferative disorders, the most prominent of which is the point mutation *JAK2* V617F involving the Janus tyrosine kinase (*Am Soc Hematol Educ Program* 2006;240).

1. **Chronic myelogenous leukemia** is a well-characterized clinicopathologic entity, because essentially all cases have the characteristic Philadelphia chromosome t(9;22)(q34;q11) and corresponding rearrangement of BCR-ABL (*Br J Haematol* 1991;79 Suppl 1:34). This is a disorder derived from clonal expansion of an abnormal pluripotent hematopoietic stem cell. Affected individuals typically present with nonspecific constitutional symptoms and on physical examination are frequently found to have an enlarged spleen. Patients most often present in the chronic phase, characterized by a peripheral leukocytosis composed of granulocytes (in various stages of maturation) and peripheral and bone marrow basophilia and eosinophilia (e-**Fig. 44.9**). The blast percentage in chronic phase is usually <2% of white blood cells in the peripheral blood and <5% in the bone marrow. Untreated, cases of chronic myelogenous leukemia invariably acquire additional genetic lesions resulting in a maturation arrest in the malignant population and terminate in an acute leukemic (blast) phase. The blast phenotype is myeloid in ~80% of cases and lymphoid in most of the remaining cases, and has a biphenotypic or ambiguous phenotype in rare individuals. Chronic myelogenous leukemia in blast phase is essentially untreatable by any means short of a bone marrow transplant. Increasingly, patients presenting with chronic myelogenous leukemia in chronic phase are treated with small molecular inhibitors such as imatinib mesylate, a tyrosine kinase inhibitor with a high degree of specificity for the BCR-ABL–encoded tyrosine kinase. However, an increasing problem is the development of resistance to imatinib mesylate; new classes of drugs have been developed to treat such individuals.

2. **Polycythemia vera** is a clonal stem cell disorder in which the majority of disease manifestations are related to expansion of the cells of the erythroid

lineage as evidenced by increased hematocrit, blood volume, and blood viscosity (*Blood* 2002;100:4272). The clinical features of this disease are related to this phenomenon: The skin has a plethoric appearance, and there is an increased propensity for vascular thromboses, hemorrhage, and central nervous system phenomena including stroke, tinnitus, headache, and vertigo. The peripheral blood manifestations of disease are related to expansion of red blood cell mass. There is an increased red blood cell count (approximately 7,000,000 to 10,000,000/mm^3) and hemoglobin (usually 18 to 24 g/dL) without a corresponding increased reticulocyte count. Because polycythemia vera is related to expansion of a pluripotential hematopoietic stem cell, other cell lines are variably affected. Thus, some patients have an associated neutrophilic leukocytosis and/or thrombocytosis. Other clinical laboratory features of disease include an increased leukocyte alkaline phosphatase (LAP) score and increased serum vitamin B12 levels, the latter due to an increase in transcobalamin 1. Bone marrow analysis is performed to exclude other forms of myeloproliferative disorder and to assess baseline fibrosis. Usually, initial bone marrow analysis reveals increased bone marrow cellularity with multilineage expansion of hematopoiesis, and minimal fibrosis.

In establishing a diagnosis of polycythemia vera, nonneoplastic erythrocytosis and erythrocytosis due to cytokine production by nonhematopoietic malignancies must be excluded. Common causes of secondary erythrocytosis include pathologic conditions (such as chronic pulmonary disease and smoking) and physiologic conditions (such as living in high-altitude locations). Recently, a high percentage of cases of polycythemia vera have been shown to have the *JAK2* V617F mutation, which is important in distinguishing polycythemia vera from benign erythrocytosis.

In most cases, polycythemia vera is a clinically indolent condition. The treatment of choice for most patients is periodic phlebotomy to minimize the risks associated with increased blood viscosity. Less than 10% of patients develop bone marrow failure or acute leukemia.

3. **Essential thrombocythemia** is a clonal neoplasm, derived from a pluripotential hematopoietic stem cell, in which the majority of clinical and pathologic features are related to morphologically and physiologically abnormal megakaryocytes and platelets (*Haematologica* 1999;84:17). There is usually a marked peripheral thrombocytosis, generally in excess of 1,000,000/mm^3. The platelets are frequently morphologically abnormal, including forms with decreased granularity. There is occasionally an associated peripheral granulocytosis, which is sometimes associated with eosinophilia or basophilia and may simulate chronic myelogenous leukemia. The bone marrow is hypercellular with a variable degree of expansion of the granulocytic and erythroid lineages. The most prominent characteristic of the bone marrow is marked megakaryocytic hyperplasia. The megakaryocytes are frequently morphologically abnormal, with large overall size and large hyperlobate nuclei. The major pathophysiologic consequences of the thrombocytosis and proliferation of megakaryocytes are episodic bleeding and thrombosis, which are major causes of morbidity and mortality. Less than 1% of cases progress to acute leukemia.

4. **Chronic idiopathic myelofibrosis** (agnogenic myeloid metaplasia, myelofibrosis with myeloid metaplasia) is another chronic myeloproliferative disorder attributed to transformation of a pluripotential hematopoietic stem cell. Classically, there are two phases in the natural history of disease (*Hematol Oncol Clin North Am* 2003;17:1211). The first phase, referred to as the cellular phase, is characterized by a marked expansion of all hematopoietic lineages; it is followed by the spent phase, characterized by progressive bone marrow failure and fibrosis. Because the cellular phase is often clinically silent, the majority of clinical findings are related to increasing bone marrow fibrosis, and include fatigue (due to anemia), bleeding (due to thrombocytopenia), and infection (due to granulocytopenia). Hepatosplenomegaly due to extramedullary hematopoiesis is a common physical finding.

The cellular phase is often characterized by peripheral granulocytic leukocytosis and/or thrombocytosis. The former is sometimes accompanied by eosinophilia or basophilia clinically mimicking chronic myelogenous leukemia. In the cellular phase, the bone marrow is hypercellular due to a panhyperplasia of all hematopoietic lineages. Megakaryocytes cluster in the bone marrow and are characteristically quite large with hyperlobate nuclei. Fibrosis is minimal at this stage of disease. With time, the bone marrow becomes increasingly fibrotic and the patient becomes increasingly susceptible to the consequences of decreased peripheral white blood cells, red blood cells, and platelets. Death is most commonly due to infection or hemorrhage. Acute leukemia is an uncommon late sequela, occurring in <10% of individuals.

C. Acute leukemia. Compared with myelodysplastic and myeloproliferative disorders, acute leukemias frequently present with a greater tumor burden (i.e., with blast percentages of at least 20%) and are broadly categorized as myeloid or lymphoid according to their immunologic and enzyme cytochemical properties, the characteristic features of which are summarized in Table 44.3. There are two important exceptions to the requirement of at least 20% blasts in acute myeloid leukemia. In the WHO classification, the presence of t(8;21)(q22;q22) [*AML1/ETO*], inv(16)(p13;q22)/t(16;16)(p13;q22) [*CBFβ/MYH11*], and t(15;17)(q22;q12) [*PML/RARα*] are classified as acute myeloid leukemia regardless of the percentage of blasts (e-Figs. **44.10** through **44.14**). The second exception involves acute erythroid leukemia, for which blasts comprise at least 20% of the nonerythroid cell population, rather than at least 20% of all cells; because another requirement for acute erythroid leukemia is that at least 50% of all cells are erythroid precursors, cases with very high erythroid percentages may qualify as acute leukemia even in the presence of a very modest blast percentage. Immunophenotypic analysis of acute leukemia is discussed in Chap. 43.

Acute leukemias, particularly in children and the elderly, may present with isolated anemia and a lack of circulating blasts. Diagnosis requires detection of at least 20% blasts in the bone marrow and/or the presence of an acute myeloid leukemia–specific cytogenetic abnormality. Although replacement of the bone marrow by fibrosis, carcinoma, sarcoma, or other nonhematopoietic cell may result in anemia, it is generally accompanied by leukopenia and/or thrombocytopenia, reflecting indiscriminate displacement of normal marrow constituents.

Precursor B-lymphoblastic leukemia is arbitrarily separated from its tissue analogue, lymphoblastic lymphoma, by the presence of a tissue mass and ≤25% bone marrow blasts in the latter (e-Fig. **44.15**). Precursor B-lymphoblastic leukemia is most common in children <6 years old; patients with purely lymphomatous disease are somewhat younger on average. Precursor B-lymphoblastic leukemia/lymphoma is no longer subdivided on the basis of immunophenotype, because genetic features are more predictive of outcome. Most cases express HLA-DR, terminal deoxynucleotidyl transferase (TdT), CD10, CD19, CD24, and cytoplasmic CD79a. CD10-negative cases often demonstrate rearrangements of the mixed-lineage leukemia (*MLL*) gene and coexpress one or more myeloid-associated antigens. In the pediatric population, cytogenetic and molecular genetic findings are highly predictive of disease outcome. Predictors of good outcome include the following: age 4 to 10 years at diagnosis, hyperdiploidy (51 to 65 chromosomes) in the blast population, and presence of the translocation t(12;21)(p13;q22) [*TEL/AML1*]. Predictors of poor outcome include the following: age <4 years or >10 years, hypodiploidy, t(9;22)(q34;q11.2) [*BCR/ABL*], t(4;11)(q21;q23) [*AF4/MLL*], and t(1;19)(q23;q13.3) [*PBX/E2A*]. The prognostic significance of t(1;19) is controversial.

A special category of lymphoblastic leukemia is the leukemic analogue of Burkitt lymphoma. Patients with this disease commonly present with an abdominal mass (Western Europe and North America) or jaw lesion (Africa). The bone marrow is commonly involved, and the blasts have deeply basophilic cytoplasm with many lipid vacuoles that express CD10 and monoclonal surface immunoglobulin light chain, and are generally CD34 and TdT negative (e-Fig. **44.16**). Diagnosis requires demonstration of the translocation t(8;14)(q24;q32) [*MYC/IGH*] or, less commonly,

TABLE 44.3 WHO Classification of Acute Myeloid Leukemias

Disease	Clinical	Morphology	Immunophenotype	Prognosis
A. Acute myeloid leukemia with recurrent genetic abnormalities				
Acute myeloid leukemia with t(8;21)(q22;q22); (*AML1/ETO*)	Often presents with extramedullary disease	Blasts with long slender Auer rods, abnormal granulation	CD13+, CD33+, MPO+, CD19+, CD34+, CD56+	Favorable
Acute myeloid leukemia with abnormal bone marrow eosinophils inv(16)(p13q22) or t(16;16)(p13;q22) (*CBFβ/MYH11*)	Occasionally presents with extramedullary disease	Abnormal eosinophils with large basophilic granules, decreased lobation	CD13+, CD33+, MPO+; frequently CD4+, CD14+, CE11b+, CD11c+, CD64+, CD36+, lysozyme+	Favorable
Acute promyelocytic leukemia (acute myeloid leukemia with t(15;17)(q22;q12); (*PML/RARα* and variants)	Coagulopathy, normal/low WBC (hypergranular variant); high WBC (hypogranular variant)	Abnormal promyelocytes with multiple Auer rods predominate	CD13+ (heterogeneous), CD33+ (bright), HLA-DR–, CD34–	Favorable
Acute myeloid leukemia with 11q23 (*MLL*) abnormalities	Frequently occurs in children	Monocytic blasts predominate	Variable CD13 and CD33+, CD4+, CD14+, CD11b+, CD11c+, CD64+, CD36+, lysozyme+	Intermediate survival

B. Acute myeloid leukemia with multilineage dysplasia
- Following a myelodysplastic syndrome or myelodysplastic syndrome/myeloproliferative disorder
- Without antecedent myelodysplastic syndrome

C. Acute myeloid leukemia and myelodysplastic syndromes, therapy-related
- Alkylating agent-related
- Topoisomerase type II inhibitor–related (some may be lymphoid)
- Other types

(Continued)

TABLE 44.3 WHO Classification of Acute Myeloid Leukemias (Continued)

Disease	Clinical	Morphology/Cytochemistry	Immunophenotype	Prognosis
D. Acute myeloid leukemia not otherwise categorized				
Acute myeloid leukemia minimally differentiated	Usually presents in adulthood, cytopenias	<3% of blasts MPO+, <3% of blasts NBE+	Often CD13+, CD33+, CD117+, CD34+, CD38+, HLA-DR+	Unfavorable
Acute myeloid leukemia without maturation	Usually presents in adulthood, cytopenias, occasionally with markedly increased WBC	Blasts comprise ≥90% of nonerythroid cells; ≥3% of blasts MPO+, ≥3% of blasts NBE+	Often CD13+, CD33+, CD34+, CD117+, MPO+	Unfavorable
Acute myeloid leukemia with maturation	Variable age range and symptomatology	≥3% of blasts MPO+, ≤3% of blasts NBE+	Usually CD13+, CD33−, CD15+; variable CD117+, CD34+, HLA-DR+	Variable
Acute myelomonocytic leukemia	Anemia, fever, fatigue; WBC usually elevated	>20% blasts; ≥ monocytes and precursors; ≥ neutrophils and precursors; ≥3% of blasts MPO+, ≥3% of blasts usually NBE+*	Usually CD13+, CD33+; Often CD4+, CD14+, CD11b+, CD11c+, CD64+, CD36+, lysozyme+	Variable
Acute monoblastic leukemia	Most common in children, often presents with extramedullary disease, bleeding disorders	≥80% monocytic cells, of which ≥80% are monoblasts; <20% neutrophils and precursors; <3% of blasts MPO+, ≥3% of blasts NBE+	Variable CD13+, CD33+, CD117+; Often CD14+, CD4+, CD11b+, CD11c+, CD64+, CD68+, CD36+, lysozyme+	Unfavorable
Acute monocytic leukemia	Most common in adults, often presents with extramedullary disease, bleeding disorders	≥80% monocytic cells, of which the majority are promonocytes; <20% neutrophils and precursors; <3% of blasts MPO+, ≥3% of blasts NBE+	Variable CD13+, CD33+, CD117+; Often CD14+, CD4+, CD11b+, CD11c+, CD64+, CD68+, CD36+, lysozyme+	Unfavorable
Acute erythroid leukemia (erythroid/myeloid)	Adults; anemia	≥50% of entire nucleated population is erythroid and ≥20% myeloblasts in nonerythroid population; >3% of blasts may be MPO+	Erythroblasts are glycophorin A+ and hemoglobin A+; myeloblasts are CD13+, CD33+, CD117+, and MPO+	Unfavorable

Disease	Clinical features	Immunophenotype	Prognosis
Pure erythroid leukemia	Extremely rare	>80% of cells are immature erythroid cells; no significant myeloblast component; <3% of blasts MPO+, ≥3% of blasts NBE+	Blasts are sometimes glycophorin A+ and hemoglobin A+;	Unfavorable
Acute megakaryoblastic leukemia	Cytopenias	Dysplastic megakaryocytes, Blasts often have cytoplasmic pseudopods. Abnormal platelets and megakaryocyte fragments in peripheral blood; usually <3% of blasts MPO+ and <3% of blasts NBE+	Usually CD41+, CD61+; occasionally CD13+, CD33+; CD34−, CD45−, HLA-DR−	Poor
Acute basophilic leukemia	Very rare	Blasts are toluidine blue+; usually <3% of blasts MPO+, <3% of blasts NBE+	Usually CD13+, CD33+, CD34+, HLA-DR+, CD9+	Difficult to predict due to low number of reported cases, probably poor
Acute panmyelosis with myelofibrosis	Very rare, adults, pancytopenia with no/minimal splenomegaly	Panhyperplasia, dysplastic megakaryocytes; increased reticulin fibrosis	CD13+, CD33+, CD117+, MPO+; some cases express erythroid or megakaryocytic antigens	Poor

Abbreviations: MPO, myeloperoxidase; WBC, white blood count; NBE, naphthyl butyrate esterase; HLA, human leukocyte antigen.
* The World Health Organization allows the diagnosis of acute myelomonocytic leukemia in the absence of NBE reactivity if the "cells meet morphologic criteria for monocytes."
From: Jaffee ES, Harris NL, Stein H, Vardiman JW, eds. *World Health Organization Classification of Tumours. Pathology and Genetics. Tumours of Haematopoietic and Lymphoid Tissues*. Lyon: IARC Press; 2001. Used with permission.

the variant translocations t(2;8)(q11;q24) or t(8;22)(q24;q11) involving *MYC* and the κ and λ light chain genes, respectively. Precursor T-lymphoblastic leukemia/lymphoma is less common and involves an older demographic than its B-cell counterpart. Patients typically present with abundant blasts in the peripheral blood and a mediastinal mass. The blasts are generally TdT positive and demonstrate variable expression of other T-lineage antigens, most commonly CD3 and CD7. Genetic aberrations identified in this entity include translocations between the *TCRβ* and *TCRδ* genes and a variety of partners; microdeletions of *TAL1*; and del(9q), which results in deletion of the tumor suppressor gene *CDKN2A*. Although precursor T malignancies have historically had a poor prognosis, recent innovations in treatment have improved outcome.

D. **CLL / SLL and related disorders.** In patients (particularly elderly individuals) with unexplained lymphocytosis, an absolute increase in lymphocytes may represent peripheral blood involvement by low-grade non-Hodgkin lymphoma or leukemia such as CLL / SLL (Table 44.4). For most non-Hodgkin lymphomas, diagnosis is made following biopsy of an involved lymph node or extramedullary focus of disease, and bone marrow biopsy is performed for staging rather than precise classification. An exception to this is CLL/SLL, in which primary diagnosis is often made following flow cytometric analysis of the peripheral blood and demonstration of the characteristic immunophenotype (CD5+, CD10–, CD19 bright+, CD20 heterogeneously+, CD23+, FMC7–, CD79b–).

The various non-Hodgkin lymphomas have different patterns of marrow involvement. Because B-cell lymphomas are more common than T-cell tumors, the former are better characterized. For example, follicular lymphoma and mantle cell lymphoma have a paratrabecular pattern of marrow involvement, whereas CLL/SLL is never paratrabecular (e-Fig. 44.17). In the case of CLL/SLL, the pattern of involvement of the marrow may be predictive of prognosis: Cases with predominantly focal lesions are more indolent, whereas examples with a diffuse pattern of involvement are more aggressive. As in lymph nodes, the bone marrow infiltrate of CLL/SLL may contain proliferation (or growth) centers that represent aggregates of prolymphocytes (paraimmunoblasts) and presumably represent the proliferative component of the tumor mass (e-Figs. 44.18 and 44.19). Marginal zone lymphomas may demonstrate follicular colonization when they occur in bone marrows with lymphoid aggregates. Overall, the likelihood of marrow involvement by non-Hodgkin lymphoma is highly variable depending on type, ranging from very common (e.g., CLL/SLL) to rare (e.g., extranodal marginal zone lymphoma). Immunohistochemistry is typically not required in non-Hodgkin lymphoma staging biopsies, although it is occasionally helpful in delineating benign from malignant lymphoid aggregates.

E. **Hairy cell leukemia** is a rare form of chronic leukemia. Most commonly, the affected individual is a middle-aged man presenting with pancytopenia, including lymphopenia and monocytopenia, and an enlarged spleen. Occasionally, patients present with a leukemic blood picture mimicking CLL. The bone marrow is virtually always involved. Although identified in bone marrow aspirate preparations, hairy cells are more easily identified in the peripheral blood by the presence of cytoplasmic projections (hence the name "hairy cell leukemia," e-Fig. 44.20). The malignant cells frequently have an interstitial pattern of involvement of the bone marrow and for this reason are occasionally overlooked. Sometimes the pattern of marrow involvement recapitulates the pattern of splenic involvement by this malignancy with the collections of extravasated red blood cells surrounded by ill-defined collections of hairy cells (e-Figs. 44.21 and 44.22). The malignant cells are positive with tartrate-resistant acid phosphatase (TRAP) enzyme cytochemistry. Flow cytometry identifies a characteristic pattern of reactivity: The hairy cells are CD5, CD10, and CD23 negative, but positive for the pan B-cell antigens CD19 and CD20. In addition, they typically demonstrate bright coexpression of CD11c and CD25, and are also positive for CD103 and FMC7 (*Semin Oncol* 1998;25:6). Identification of this pattern of reactivity in the presence of appropriate cytomorphology essentially excludes other types of B-cell neoplasia, such as splenic marginal zone lymphoma and prolymphocytic

Disease	Phenotype	Morphology	Cytogenetics (significance)	Molecular genetics (impact on outcome)
Chronic lymphocytic leukemia/small lymphocytic lymphoma	CD5+, CD10–, CD19+ (bright), CD20+ (dim), CD23+, FMC7–, CD79b–, sIg light chain+ (dim) CD38 ± (unfavorable if +), Zap70 ± (unfavorable if +)	Usually small mature-appearing lymphocytes; diffuse, interstitial, or nodular patterns of marrow involvement (never paratrabecular)	13q14 deletions (favorable outcome), +12 (morphologically atypical, unfavorable outcome), 17p (TP53) deletions (unfavorable)	Presence of Ig heavy chain variable region mutation (favorable)
Mantle cell lymphoma	CD5+, CD10–, CD19+, CD20+ (bright), CD23–, FMC7+, CD79b+, sIg light chain+ (usually bright), cyclin D1+	Usually small lymphocytes with clefted/folded nuclei; diffuse, nodular, interstitial, or paratrabecular patterns of marrow involvement	t(11;14) [BCL1/IGH]	—
Follicular lymphoma	CD5–, CD10+, CD19+, CD20+, CD23–, sIg light chain+	Variable cytomorphology; diffuse, nodular, interstitial, or paratrabecular patterns of marrow involvement	t(14;18) [BCL2/IGH]	—
Marginal zone B-cell lymphoma	CD5–, CD10–, CD19+, CD20+, CD23–, sIg light chain+	Small lymphocytes, some with ample cytoplasm	t(11;18)(q21;q21) [API2/MALT1] identified in a subset of extranodal marginal zone lymphoma	—
Lymphoplasmacytic lymphoma/Waldenström macroglobulinemia	CD5–, CD10–, CD19+, CD20+, CD23–, sIg light chain+	Small lymphocytes, some with plasmacytoid features	t(9;14)(q13;q32) [PAX5/IGH] identified in ~50% of cases but is not limited to this type of lymphoma	—

Abbreviations: sIg, surface immunoglobulin; Ig, immunoglobulin.
From: Jaffee ES, Harris NL, Stein H, Vardiman JW, eds. *World Health Organization Classification of Tumours. Pathology and Genetics. Tumours of Haematopoietic and Lymphoid Tissues.* Lyon: IARC Press; 2001. Used with permission.

TABLE 44.5	WHO Criteria for Systemic Mastocytosis

Major criteria are as follows:
Multifocal infiltrates of mast cells ($\geq$15 mast cells constitute an aggregate) detected in sections of bone marrow and/or other extracutaneous organ(s), and confirmed by tryptase immunohistochemistry or other special stains.

Minor criteria are as follows:

a. In biopsy sections of bone marrow or other extracutaneous organs, >25% of the mast cells in the infiltrate are spindle-shaped or have atypical morphology, or, of all mast cells in the bone marrow aspirate smears, >25% are immature or atypical mast cells.

b. *Kit* point mutation at codon 816 in bone marrow, blood, or other extracutaneous organ(s)

c. Mast cells in bone marrow, blood, or other extracutaneous organs coexpress CD117 with CD2 and/or CD25.

d. Serum total tryptase persistently >20 ng/mL (unless there is an associated clonal myeloid disorder, in which case this parameter is not valid)

The diagnosis of systemic mastocytosis may be made if one major and one minor criterion are present, or if three minor criteria are fulfilled.

From: Jaffee ES, Harris NL, Stein H, Vardiman JW, eds. *World Health Organization Classification of Tumours. Pathology and Genetics. Tumours of Haematopoietic and Lymphoid Tissues.* Lyon: IARC Press; 2001. Used with permission.

lymphoma. Hairy cell leukemia is largely resistant to conventional chemotherapies but is associated with a prolonged median survival.

F. Systemic mastocytosis. Mastocytosis, the abnormal accumulation of mast cells in the skin and other tissues, has a wide range of clinical behavior. A benign form of disease is localized to the skin, occurs predominantly in younger individuals, and is characterized by spontaneous regression. In the systemic form of mastocytosis, mast cells are increased in many organs including the bone marrow (**e-Figs. 44.23** through **44.25**). The WHO criteria for systemic mastocytosis are summarized in Table 44.5. Systemic mastocytosis represents a clonal disorder in most cases: Mutations in the *kit* proto-oncogene (most commonly D816V) have been identified in many individuals, and presumably play a role in the pathophysiology of disease. In cases with associated eosinophilia, the *FIP1L1/PDGFRA* fusion gene has been identified. The same fusion gene has been identified in chronic eosinophilic leukemia/hypereosinophilic syndrome.

The clinical course of systemic mastocytosis is highly variable. Cases with cutaneous involvement (urticaria pigmentosa) are more likely to have a benign disease course, whereas individuals with peripheral blood involvement (mast cell leukemia) frequently die within weeks of diagnosis.

Suggested Readings

Foucar K. *Bone Marrow Pathology.* Chicago: ASCP Press; 2001.

Knowles DM, ed. *Neoplastic Hematopathology*, 2nd ed. Philadelphia: Lippincott Williams & Wilkins; 2001.

World Health Organization Classification of Tumors. Pathology and Genetics of Tumors of Haematopoietic and Lymphoid Tissues. Lyon: IARC Press; 2001.

SPLEEN

45

Michelle L. E. Powers and Anjum Hassan

I. NORMAL GROSS AND MICROSCOPIC ANATOMY. The spleen is the largest lymphatic organ. There is no agreement concerning the weight of normal adult human spleen, because it can range from 50 to 250 grams. Anatomically, the spleen is divided into two compartments—white pulp and red pulp—separated by an ill-defined interface known as the marginal zone (**e-Fig. 45.1A**).* A schematic version of spleen architecture is displayed in Figure 45.1.

A. The white pulp consists of the periarteriolar lymphoid sheets, which may contain lymphoid follicles. T lymphocytes are predominately located in periarteriolar lymphoid nodules and B lymphocytes in lymphoid follicles; the latter may contain germinal centers that can become extremely large and visible to the naked eye. These enlarged nodules are called splenic nodules or malphigian corpuscles. In routine hematoxylin and eosin–stained sections, the white pulp appears basophilic due to the dense heterochromatin in the nuclei of the numerous lymphocytes (**e-Fig. 45.1B**).

B. The red pulp has a red appearance in fresh specimens and in histologic sections because it contains a large number of red blood cells (**e-Fig. 45.1B**). Essentially, it consists of splenic sinuses separated by splenic cords (the cords of Billroth). These contain a loose network of reticular cells and fibers with a large number of erythrocytes, macrophages, lymphocytes, plasma cells, and granulocytes. The sinuses are lined by a special type of endothelial cell that expresses both endothelial and histiocytic markers (known as Littoral cells). The discontinuous wall of the sinusoidal lining epithelium allows the transport of blood cells between the splenic cords and sinuses).

II. GROSS EXAMINATION AND TISSUE SAMPLING

A. Biopsy and fine needle aspiration cytology. These procedures are rarely attempted because of the possibility of hemorrhage and the likelihood of undersampling. However, some studies have suggested that there is a better chance of a definitive diagnosis when fine needle biopsy data are combined with flow cytometry, with an overall accuracy of 91% and a reported incidence of major complications of <1% (*Am J Hematol* 2001;67:93).

B. Splenectomy. Trauma, staging procedures, and surgical convenience account for >50% of all splenectomies. Therapeutic splenectomy for known diagnoses [idiopathic thrombocytopenic purpura (ITP), chronic myeloproliferative disorders, lymphomas, etc.] accounts for the vast majority of the remaining cases (*Cancer* 2001;91:2001). The incidence of finding unexpected pathology in spleen specimens is extremely low; however, presence of significant splenomegaly (weight >300 g) and localizing lesions should prompt care in prosection and ancillary studies.

C. Processing of spleen. The spleen is weighed, and its outer dimensions are recorded. The fatty tissue at the hilum is removed and processed for lymph nodes. The capsule should be described, including texture and intactness. The spleen should be thinly sliced (every 2 to 3 mm), and any lesions and their distribution noted, followed by a description of the uninvolved spleen. Cassette-sized sections of any lesions (preferably following overnight formalin fixation of thin slices) and two additional noninvolved representative sections of spleen should be taken.

---

*All e-figures are available online via the Solution Site Image Bank.

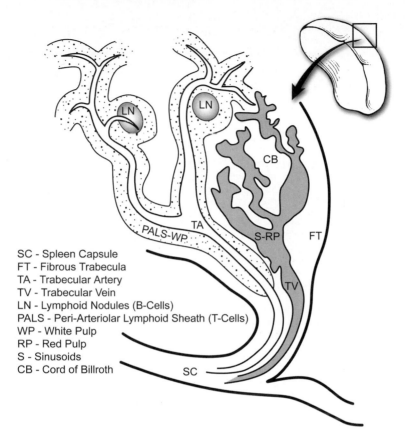

SC - Spleen Capsule
FT - Fibrous Trabecula
TA - Trabecular Artery
TV - Trabecular Vein
LN - Lymphoid Nodules (B-Cells)
PALS - Peri-Arteriolar Lymphoid Sheath (T-Cells)
WP - White Pulp
RP - Red Pulp
S - Sinusoids
CB - Cord of Billroth

Figure 45.1. Diagram of the spleen showing important anatomic landmarks and B- and T-cell distribution.

For ancillary flow cytometry studies, fresh lesional tissue in 1-mm pieces should be placed in RPMI medium and directed immediately to the flow cytometry lab with instructions regarding the appropriate protocol. Cytogenetic examination may be useful, especially for diagnosis of hematologic malignancies. Using a sterile technique, lesional material should be procured immediately after removal of the spleen in the operating room and directed to the cytogenetic lab. Samples can also be frozen or fixed for electron microscopy, although neither is routinely performed. Freezing preserves many of the antigens that can be used in immunohistochemical evaluation for hematopoietic malignancies (and enhances nucleic acid recovery for DNA- and RNA-based molecular diagnostic techniques). Most diagnostic molecular tests can be reliably performed with formalin-fixed, paraffin-embedded material.

III. GENERAL CONSIDERATIONS

    A. Hypersplenism refers to destruction of one or more of the peripheral blood cell lines by the spleen (*Eur J Gastroenterol Hepatol* 2001;13:317). It is the single most important clinical reason for elective splenectomy. The diagnostic criteria for hypersplenism include cytopenia of one or more peripheral blood cell lines, bone marrow hyperplasia, splenomegaly, and correction of cytopenias following splenectomy. A multitude of etiologies lead to hypersplenism (see Table 45.1), of which congenital disorders (such as hereditary spherocytosis; e-Fig. 45.2) and infiltrative disorders (such as leukemias, lymphomas, and autoimmune disorders) are the most common.

TABLE 45.1	Disorders Associated with Hypersplenism

I. Abnormal sequestration of intrinsically defective blood cells in a normal spleen
   A. Congenital disorders of erythrocytes
      (Hereditary spherocytosis, elliptocytosis; hemoglobinopathies, e.g., sickle cell disease,
      unstable hemoglobins)
   B. Acquired disorders of erythrocytes
      (Autoimmune hemolytic anemias, malaria, babesiosis)
      Autoimmune thrombocytopenia and/or neutropenia

II. Abnormal spleen causing sequestration of normal blood cells
   A. Disorders of the monocyte/macrophage system
      (Chronic congestion, storage diseases, parasitic infections, Langerhans cell histiocytosis,
      etc.)
   B. Malignant infiltrative disorders
      (Leukemias, lymphomas, plasma cell dyscrasias, metastatic carcinoma)
   C. Extramedullary hematopoiesis
      (Severe hemolytic states, chronic idiopathic myelofibrosis)
   D. Chronic infections, e.g., tuberculosis, brucellosis
   E. Vascular/stromal abnormalities
      (Vascular tumors, peliosis, splenic cysts, hamartomas)

III. Miscellaneous conditions
   A. Hyperthyroidism
   B. Hypogammaglobulinemia
   C. Progressive multifocal leukoencephalopathy

Histopathologic examination is facilitated by injection of formalin into the splenic pulp via the splenic artery. This ensures the sharp distinction of splenic sinusoids and cords in histologic sections.
   B. Hyposplenism is usually due to splenectomy; however, by definition, the term refers to any deficiency or absence of a functioning spleen. The adequacy of splenic function is usually judged by either radiologic imaging or morphologic techniques. Particularly useful is the examination of a peripheral blood smear in which findings suggesting the possibility of hyposplenism can occur in any of the blood cell lines, including erythrocytes (inclusions of Howell–Jolly bodies, poikilocytosis with target cells, acanthocytes, and nucleated red blood cells), platelets (thrombocytosis), and white blood cells (leukocytosis with either lymphocytosis or monocytosis and eosinophilia). Other possible causes of hyposplenism include congenital hypoplasia, as observed in cases of Fanconi anemia, sickle cell disease (e-**Fig. 45.3**), infiltrative disorders, and old age (see Table 45.2).
   C. Accessory spleens. Alternatively termed "spleniculi," these are most commonly located in the splenic hilum, tail of the pancreas, and the gastrohepatic ligament (*N Engl J Med* 1981;304:11). These are noted in up to one third of autopsy cases, and share the same histologic and pathologic features as native spleen (see e-**Fig. 45.4**). Accessory spleens are clinically significant in patients requiring splenectomy for hypersplenism.
   D. The term "splenosis" refers to spleen implants or the regrowth of splenic tissue after trauma or surgical splenectomy. When associated with trauma, the most common location is in the abdominal cavity, but splenosis has been reported at virtually all anatomic sites, including brain (*Am J Surg Pathol* 1998;22:894). The vast majority of cases are benign incidental findings; the clinical importance lies in their potential to mimic neoplastic and nonneoplastic lesions.
IV. REACTIVE SPLENIC DISORDERS. These can be divided into two broad categories: diffuse and localized processes. The diffuse category includes entities described as reactive lymphoid hyperplasia (e-**Fig. 45.5A**), follicular hyperplasia, and disorders such as

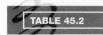

TABLE 45.2	Disorders Associated with Hyposplenism

I. Congenital
  A. Asplenia
  B. Hypoplasia
  C. Immunodeficiency disorders

II. Acquired
  A. Splenectomy
  B. Acquired atrophy and/or infarction
    1. Sickle cell disease
    2. Vascular disorders (vasculitides, thromboembolicconditions)
    3. Essential thrombocythemia
    4. Malabsorption syndromes
    5. Autoimmune diseases
    6. Irradiation
    7. Cytotoxic chemotherapy
    8. Chronic alcoholism
    9. Hypopituitarism
  C. Functional asplenia with normal-sized or enlarged spleen
    1. Infiltration by leukemia, lymphoma, multiple myeloma, mastocytosis
    2. Early (splenomegalic) sickle cell disease
    3. Amyloidosis
    4. Sarcoidosis
    5. Benign and malignant vascular tumors
    6. Malabsorption syndromes
  D. Depressed immune function
    1. Acquired immunodeficiency syndrome (AIDS)
    2. Status post:
      a. Irradiation
      b. Cytotoxic chemotherapy
      c. Immunosuppressive agents, including corticosteroids
    3. Endocrine disorders
      a. Hypothyroidism
      b. Hypopituitarism
      c. Diabetes mellitus
    4. Chronic alcoholism

Castleman disease (see Chapter 43). The more localized benign disorders of the spleen include granulomatous disorders and varieties of infectious processes similar to those noted in other locations (see Chapter 43).

A. Diffuse reactive processes. Reactive lymphoid hyperplasia in the spleen has been described with and without germinal center formation. Because of the reactive nature of the latter, and its histologic lack of maturing germinal centers, this entity is variably referred to as the "early activated immune reaction," "activated A," "reactive nonfollicular hyperplasia," and even "immunoblastic hyperplasia" (*Am J Surg Pathol* 1981;5:551). This nongerminal center hyperplasia is often associated with viral infections, especially the herpes simplex virus and Epstein–Barr virus (**e-Fig. 45.5B**), which explains the common occurrence of splenomegaly in patients with infectious mononucleosis.

Reactive lymphoid hyperplasia with germinal center formation (**e-Fig. 45.5C**) is more commonly referred to as "follicular" hyperplasia. This is the most common pattern of lymphoid hyperplasia in the spleen and is seen in both acute and chronic immune reactions. Follicular hyperplasia is frequently seen in the setting of bacterial infection; these patients usually present with other symptoms of bacteremia and are incidentally noted on exam to have splenomegaly. Splenomegaly is a characteristic finding in patients with subacute bacterial endocarditis that may alert the clinician to this process in the appropriate clinical context.

B. Focal reactive processes. Localized reactive splenic processes can also present with splenomegaly.

1. **Granulomas.** The most common form of focal splenic involvement by a benign process is granulomatous inflammation (e-**Fig. 45**.6), which may vary from lipogranulomatous inflammation (which has an unknown etiology), to caseating or noncaseating granulomatous inflammation. The cause of caseating granulomatous disease is primarily infectious, including tuberculosis and fungal infection; however, granulomas with purulent necrotic centers are also seen in X-linked childhood chronic granulomatous disease. Noncaseating granulomatous diseases are most frequently associated with sarcoidosis although, for some granulomas in the spleen, no known etiology can be found (*Arch Pathol Lab Med* 1974;98:261).

2. **Infarcts.** The spleen is a frequent site of systemic emboli, which commonly arise from cardiac valve lesions or mural thrombi of the heart. Infarcts are usually wedge-shaped lesions with a hemorrhagic to pale-tan to fibrotic appearance depending on the age of the lesion (e-**Fig. 45**.7). A variety of intrinsic hematopoietic and nonhematopoietic processes can lead to splenic infarcts that tend not to have a wedge shape. Essential thrombocythemia and chronic idiopathic myelofibrosis are the hematopoietic disorders most frequently associated with infarcts; the less common causes include paroxysmal nocturnal hemoglobinuria, sickle cell disease, and aplastic anemia. Among nonhematopoietic etiologies, vasculitides (polyarteritis nodosa, infections, thrombotic thrombocytopenic purpura (TTP)- or ITP-associated, etc.) and splenic artery aneurysms are commonly associated with infarcts.

V. NEOPLASTIC DISORDERS OF THE SPLEEN

A. Lymphoid neoplasms can present in the spleen as a primary site, or splenic involvement may be a part of a generalized lymphomatous processes. Splenomegaly is a nonspecific but classic component of many hematolymphoid disorders. A brief account of normal and neoplastic components of spleen follows in table 45.3 as a general work up guideline.

1. **Primary splenic lymphomas** account for <1% of all lymphomas and can be of B- or T-cell origin (see Chap. 43). Not unexpectedly, B-cell lymphomas are more common, with diffuse large B-cell lymphoma (which usually presents as single or multiple circumscribed nodules of varying sizes) accounting for the vast majority of cases (e-**Fig. 45**.8). The diagnostic approach to primary splenic lymphomas is identical to that to lymphomas presenting elsewhere.

2. **Secondary splenic lymphomas**

   a. **Hodgkin lymphoma (HL).** The spleen is the most common nonnodal site of involvement by HL, both classic (e-**Fig. 45.9A**) and lymphocyte predominant type (LPHD), although the latter is extremely rare (*Cancer* 1971;27:1277, *Cancer* 1987;59:99). Diagnostic Reed–Sternberg cells or variants (e-**Fig. 45.9B** and C) are a requirement for the diagnosis of classic HL, especially in cases without previously documented history. Immunohistochemical evaluation is often very helpful in the differential diagnosis of classic versus LPHD.

   b. **Non-Hodgkin lymphomas.** More than 50% of cases of low-grade lymphomas show splenic involvement either in the form of splenomegaly or splenic hilar lymph node involvement. Splenic involvement can be categorized as focal or diffuse; the latter is more common. Usually there is initial expansion of white pulp in a nodular pattern in cases of small B-cell lymphomas (e.g., small lymphocytic, mantle cell, follicular, or marginal zone) eventually evolving into a diffuse pattern. Often, both patterns can be seen in appropriately sampled splenectomy specimens. Intermediate- and high-grade lymphomas (large cell, Burkitt, lymphoblastic) tend to form single or multiple tumor masses. The general histopathologic considerations for the diagnosis of these lymphomas are similar to those occurring in lymph nodes (see Chapter 43).

3. **Lymphomas presenting with prominent splenomegaly**

   a. **Splenic marginal zone B-cell lymphoma.** This disease is an indolent process; splenectomy results in long remissions (*Semin Diagn Pathol* 2003;20:83).

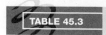

TABLE 45.3	Immunohistochemical Evaluation of Normal and Neoplastic Spleen: Critical Guidelines
General Guidelines To Evaluate The Stromal Compartment	Generally speaking, the stromal compartment consists of blood vessels, monocytes/macrophages, and dendritic cells. Together these comprise the "filtration unit" of spleen and are components of "cords of Billroth" in the red pulp.
a) Vascular endothelial cells	CD34, CD31, and factor VIII are useful to highlight both normal and neoplastic lesions.
Littoral cells	Share features of both endothelial cells and monocyte/macrophages; express CD8 uniformly
b) Monocytes/ macrophage	CD68, lysozyme, and antichymotrypsin are useful stains. When evaluation of intracellular material or infectious organisms is desired, PAS, Gram stain, AFB, and GMS stains can be used.
c) Dendritic cells	Two major types: IDC and FDC. CD68, S100, CD1A, lysozyme, alpha-1-antitrypsin may show variable positivity in dendritic cells. FDC are CD21+, CD35+; IDC are S100+
General Guidelines to Evaluate the B- and T- Cell Lymphoid Compartment	In general, most lymphomas involve the white pulp (nodular/follicular low-power appearance), but extensive disease may present as diffuse white pulp expansion.
a) Could this be a metastasis?	a) CD45, if lesion is not obviously lymphoid
b) Is it a B- or T-cell process?	b) B- (CD20, CD79a) and T- (CD3, CD45RO) cell markers are always used in concert to assess number and distribution of cells.
c) Are these malignant B cells?	c) CD43- (or CD5 by flow cytometry), aberrant T-cell markers, are often coexpressed in malignant B cells. By IHC, these must be evaluated with extreme care in B-cell distribution areas (normal T cells, most marrow derived [myeloid] cells, and macrophages can all express CD43 by IHC). CD43 stain also serves as a good T-cell marker in nonneoplastic spleen and is positive in myeloid, mast cell, and plasma cell neoplasms, in combination with other lineage-specific markers.
d) Are these follicles benign or reactive?	d) Bcl-2 is particularly helpful in differential diagnosis of follicular lymphoma and reactive follicular hyperplasia. Benign germinal centers retain the capacity to undergo apoptosis and do not express the anti-apoptosis protein BCL-2. About 80% of follicular lymphomas express BCL-2 in the follicles.
e) How should we subtype the lymphoid malignancies?	e) Additional B- and T-cell markers must be used to further characterize phenotypes of various lymphomas (see also Chap. 43, Tables 3 and 4).
Some Examples of Disorders with Predominantly Red Pulp Involvement	In general, disorders with large components of circulating cells have more extensive red pulp involvement.
a) Hairy cell leukemia	TRAP and DBA44+
b) Hepatosplenic T-celllymphoma	CD3+, CD4–, CD8–, often CD56+, markers of cytotoxic molecules (TIA, perforin, granzyme B)+
c) T-LGL	CD3+, CD8+
d) T-PLL	CD3+, usually CD4+
e) Acute leukemias and myeloproliferative disorders	For granulocytic or monocytic cells: MPO, CD34, CD117, CD68 For erythroid cells: Glycophorin and hemoglobin A For megakaryocytes: CD41, CD42b, CD61, factor VIII For precursor lymphoid leukemias: TdT, cyCD79a, cCD3, CD10

Abbreviations: T-LGL, T-large granular lymphocyte lymphoma; PAS, periodic acid-Schiff; AFB, acid-fast bacilli; GMS, Gomori methanamine silver; IDC, interdigitating dendritic cells; FDC, follicular dendritic cells; IHC, immunohistochemistry; TRAP, tartrate-resistant acid phosphatase; MPO, myeloperoxidase; TdT, terminal deoxynucleotidyl transferase; cy, cytoplasmic.

Splenic marginal zone B-cell lymphoma is sometimes accompanied by autoimmune thrombocytopenia or anemia, and villous lymphocytes (with polar projections) can sometimes be seen circulating in peripheral blood. Cytogenetically, allelic loss of chromosome 7q21-32 has been described in up to 40% of cases. Histologically, expanded periarteriolar lymphoid sheets are seen, composed of small lymphocytes and monocytoid lymphocytes (e-Fig. 45.10). Immunophenotypic studies by flow cytometry should demonstrate a clonal B-cell process (surface light chain restriction), usually lacking coexpression of CD5, CD10, and CD23. Alternatively, immunohistochemistry can be performed (to document B-cell phenotype and coexpression of CD43), coupled with in situ hybridization studies for κ and λ light chains; the latter is usually helpful in highlighting the clonal plasma cell population that forms part of the spectrum of B-cell differentiation in marginal zone B-cell lymphomas.

b. **Hepatosplenic T-cell lymphoma (HSTL).** This rare lymphoma has a clinically aggressive course and usually afflicts young men. It is characterized by a triad of peripheral cytopenias (anemia and thrombocytopenia), sinusoidal tropism, and hepatosplenomegaly. The disease tends to be somewhat more common in immunosuppressed/immunocompromised settings such as after solid organ transplantation, and the splenomegaly may exceed 3000 grams. The neoplastic process is red pulp based with conspicuous infiltration of sinuses (e-Fig. 45.11). The differential diagnosis includes other red pulp–based diseases, such as hairy cell leukemia. Immunophenotypic and genetic studies demonstrate clonal T cells, often double negative for CD4 and CD8, with the majority showing T-cell receptor γδ gene rearrangements. An isochromosome 7q10 is the strongest genetic association (*Am J Surg Pathol* 1997;21:781) in HSTL.

c. **In mantle cell lymphoma,** prominent splenomegaly usually represents the leukemic phase or stage III or IV disease. Consequently, the morphologic pattern of involvement can be diffuse, nodular, or both. Spleen involvement may sometimes occur in the absence of significant peripheral lymphadenopathy. (*Virchows Arch* 2000;437:591). The usual constellation of morphologic, immunophenotypic, and cytogenetic findings are required for diagnosis (see Chapter 43) (e-Fig. 45.12).

d. **Hairy cell leukemia.** Peripheral cytopenias, particularly monocytopenia (*Leuk Lymphoma* 1994;13:307) and splenomegaly in a young man with recurrent opportunistic infections are the classic clinical findings (*Am J Clin Pathol* 1977;67:415). In the spleen, hairy cell leukemia involves and expands the red pulp; the white pulp is usually inconspicuous (e-Fig. 45.13). The classic immunophenotype by flow cytometry (CD103+, CD11c+, CD25+), which can be easily demonstrated using peripheral blood in the presence of circulating "hairy cells," is required for diagnosis. This immunophenotype is also helpful in distinguishing hairy cell leukemia from HSTL, T-large granular lymphocyte lymphoma (T-LGL), other T-cell neoplasms, and mast cell disease (MSD), all of which can morphologically mimic hairy cell leukemia in spleen. By immunohistochemistry, DBA44 or tartrate-resistant acid phosphatase (TRAP) stains are helpful.

4. **Other B- and T-cell lymphomas.** Most commonly, T-prolymphocytic leukemia and T-LGL involve the spleen, as these neoplasms are usually leukemic at presentation (see Chap. 43). Likewise, B-cell lymphomas, presenting at stage III or IV (see Chap. 43) can also involve spleen. An example of stage IIIES follicular lymphoma involving spleen is shown in e-Fig. 45.14.

B. **Myeloid neoplasms**
1. **Chronic myelogenous leukemia (CML).** CML is classically associated with splenomegaly. The spleen is also the most common extranodal site of involvement in the blast crisis of CML (e-Fig. 45.15). Morphologic findings leading to the diagnosis of CML are best evaluated in touch preparations, although histologic sections are also easy to interpret. Enumeration of the blast count

mandates touch preparations; the blast count is especially helpful in diagnosing stable versus accelerated phase CML. Immunohistochemical and cytochemical stains (Leder, myeloperoxidase, CD34, c-kit) can also be useful in highlighting the blast population. CML blast crisis is usually obvious clinically and morphologically.

2. **Acute leukemias** cause diffuse involvement of the red pulp (e-**Fig. 45.16**). The spleen is rarely a primary site of myeloid disease; rather, involvement is part of the spectrum of systemic disease. Histopathologic and immunophenotypic considerations are similar to acute leukemias presenting with peripheral blood and bone marrow involvement (see Chap. 44). Evaluation for commonly occurring cytogenetic abnormalities, by conventional cytogenetics or fluorescence in situ hybridization (FISH), is a standard part of the work-up, although this work-up is generally not needed on spleen specimens from patients with a prior history of leukemia. However, care must be taken to appropriately evaluate for clonal evolution, morphologic progression, and aberrant phenotype changes (e.g., CD33 or CD20 expression) that may alter treatment course or effectiveness for targeted therapies, a scenario that can be observed postchemotherapy or posttransplantation.

3. **Mast cell disease (MSD) and/or systemic mastocytosis** frequently involve the spleen. The morphologic patterns of involvement vary from isolated white pulp accentuation with fibrosis, to red pulp involvement with diffuse infiltration, fibrosis, and/or nodular perivascular infiltrates. The presence of eosinophils, plasma cells, and fibrosis are all clues that point to the presence of mast cells. Flow cytometry is not readily available for MSD primarily because of technical difficulties in gating the desired population, although expression of CD2 and CD25 by flow cytometry is a feature specific to neoplastic mast cells (both benign and neoplastic mast cells are CD45+, CD33+, CD68+, and CD117+). In tissue sections, an immunohistochemical stain for CD117 is helpful in highlighting mast cells. Alternatively, a Leder stain (naphthol AS-D chloroacetate esterase) and tryptase cytochemistry are also helpful.

C. **Nonhematopoietic neoplasms and pseudoneoplasms.** A wide variety of mesenchymal cell types form the complex reticular support network of splenic pulp, and consequently a wide variety of mesenchymal tumors can occur as primary splenic neoplasms. These can generally be divided into stromal lesions, vascular lesions, and tumorlike lesions.

1. **Stromal lesions**
   a. **Dendritic cell tumors.** Two different kinds of dendritic cells exist in the normal lymphoid support network (see table 45.3): interdigitating dendritic cells (IDC; normally S-100 protein positive and major histocompatibility complex [MHC] II positive) and follicular dendritic cells (FDC; which express CD35 and CD21). Splenic involvement can be seen in neoplastic disorders of both IDC and FDC (*Cancer* 1997;79:294, *Am J Surg Pathol* 2002;26:530). Grossly, nodular involvement is usually present, although disseminated systemic disease may show diffuse splenic involvement. Dendritic cell tumors tend to behave in an aggressive manner despite their bland histologic appearance. In the absence of a preceding history, dendritic cell tumors are diagnoses of exclusion, mandating a thorough immunophenotypic work-up to exclude myeloid malignancies, lymphoid B- and T-cell malignancies, and nonhematopoietic malignancies. It is important to note that FDC neoplasia may be associated with the hyaline vascular type of Castleman disease.
   b. **Histiocytic lesions** range from Langerhans cell histiocytosis (LCH) to histiocytic sarcomas including Langerhans cell sarcoma. Splenic involvement usually is rare, occurring in the setting of disseminated disease and grossly presenting as single or multiple solid nodules.
      Expression of S-100 and CD1a by the neoplastic cells is consistent with a diagnosis of LCH. The sarcomatous forms may be less differentiated and may variably show expression of HLA-DR, CD45, CD68, placental alkaline phosphatase (PLAP), and vimentin.

2. **Vascular lesions.** Both benign and malignant vascular lesions may present in the spleen. Vascular tumors are not uncommon, which is not surprising given the rich vascular framework of the spleen (*Am J Surg Pathol* 1997;21:827).

   a. **Benign lesions**

   i. **Littoral cell angioma** is unique in its presentation in the spleen and grossly is characterized by multiple spongy, cystic nodules. The cystic spaces are lined by cuboidal epithelium with intracytoplasmic eosinophilic globules. The lumina often contain abundant desquamated cells. Vascular markers (CD31, VWF are characteristically expressed; expression of CD68 and CD21 is more variable. CD34 is uniformly negative.

   ii. **Peliosis,** characterized by ectatic sinusoids and blood-filled cysts, can involve the spleen. The location of the cysts (adjacent to periarteriolar lymphoid [PALS] and follicles) is helpful in establishing the diagnosis. The clinical importance of this lesion lies in its propensity to spontaneous rupture.

   iii. **Hemangiomas** are also common in the spleen and are frequently incidentally found at splenectomy (e-Fig. 45.17).

   b. **Malignant lesions**

   i. **Littoral cell hemangioendothelioma and angiosarcomas** rarely present in spleen. They are usually solid, often prompting a differential diagnosis that includes other spindle cell sarcomas. CD31 and VWF immunostains establish the vascular nature of these otherwise undifferentiated malignancies; some cases may also show CD34 expression.

   ii. **Kaposi sarcoma,** in the clinical setting of human immunodeficiency virus/acquired immunodeficiency syndrome (HIV/AIDS), must be considered in the differential diagnosis of any splenic vascular lesion. Kaposi sarcoma usually shows positive immunohistochemistry for human herpesvirus-8 (HHV-8) and vascular markers.

3. **Splenic pseudoneoplastic lesions** include splenic hamartoma (well-circumscribed lesions of angiomatoid lobular–nodular configuration resembling red pulp, usually CD8+ and CD68+), splenic cysts (with or without an epithelial cell lining; when an epithelial lining is present it is usually cytokeratin positive), angiomyolipoma (HMB-45 positive), and lymphangioma.

   Inflammatory pseudotumor is a reactive nodular process that shows a predominance of benign inflammatory cells and stromal cells with sclerosis (e-Fig. 45.18). Inflammatory pseudotumor must be distinguished from inflammatory pseudotumor-like FDC tumor (which is usually EBV associated and shows immunohistochemical expression of CD21 and CD35).

4. **Metastatic tumors.** A variety of carcinomas and sarcomas have been reported to metastasize to the spleen, although generally speaking, a lack of afferent lymphatics renders the spleen less amenable to metastatic disease. Metastases that do occur, therefore, commonly arise in the setting of disseminated disease. The most common epithelial metastatic tumors in the spleen are carcinomas of breast or lung origin. Sarcomas involving the spleen tend to be of dendritic/histiocytic or vascular lineage.

Suggested Readings

Jaffe ES, Harris NL, Stein H, Vardiman JW, eds. *Tumours of Haematopoietic and Lymphoid Tissues.* Lyon, France: International Agency for Research on Cancer; 2001:135.

Neiman RS, Orazi A, eds. *Disorders of Spleen*, 2nd ed. Philadelphia: W.B. Saunders; 1999.

Rosati S, Frizzera G. Pseudoneoplastic lesions of hematolymphoid system. In: Wick MR, Humphrey PA, Ritter JH, eds. *Pathology of Pseudoneoplastic Lesions.* Baltimore, MD: Lippincott-Raven; 1997:449.

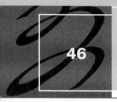

46

SOFT TISSUE
John D. Pfeifer and Louis P. Dehner

I. **INTRODUCTION.** If the term "soft tissue" were restricted to only mesodermally derived structures, then nerves and neural tumors would no longer be considered in the discussion. Similarly, there are any number of "soft tissue tumors" that present in organs not be derived from mesoderm. By convention, however, neural tumors, gastrointestinal stromal tumor, melanoma of soft parts, and so on, are all regarded as soft tissue neoplasms.

II. **TISSUE PROCESSING**
   A. **Biopsy specimens.** Incisional or core biopsy of a suspected soft tissue neoplasm is performed to determine the appropriate management based on the pathologic type. The biopsy tissue should be placed immediately into 10% formalin or other appropriate fixative. The number of biopsy fragments should be recorded, as well as their aggregate dimension, and all the submitted tissue should be processed. Three hematoxylin and eosin (H&E) levels should initially be prepared for microscopic examination. For very small specimens, to avoid wasting tissue when refacing the block, it is strongly recommended that additional unstained slides be cut from the block during initial sectioning in the event that additional studies such as immunohistochemistry are needed.

   B. **Resection specimens.** Excisional specimens are often complex and varied, and the macroscopic examination should be guided by tumor location, extent, and type. The margin of all intact specimens should be inked, and the distance from the tumor to the closest margin documented. The maximum dimension of the tumor should be recorded, as well as the color and consistency of the cut surface and presence of hemorrhage and necrosis. In general, it is recommended that one section per centimeter of tumor should be submitted for microscopic examination (scout sections can be used to evaluate whether such thorough sampling is required for definitive diagnosis). The closest surgical margin should be evaluated by either shave or radial sections, depending on the nature of the specimen.

   For those tumors in which a biopsy did not permit definitive diagnosis, tissue should be collected and processed for electron microscopy. Consideration should always be given to the need to send a sample of viable tumor for cytogenetic analysis. A sample of viable tumor should also be snap frozen and stored, in the event it is needed for subsequent molecular evaluation.

   Table 46.1 is a listing of the various soft tissue tumors and their characteristic chromosomal abnormalities.

III. **TERMINOLOGY REGARDING THE BIOLOGIC POTENTIAL OF SOFT TISSUE NEOPLASMS.** The current World Health Organization (WHO) classification of soft tissue tumors (Table 46.2) assigns each neoplasm to one of four categories: benign, intermediate (locally aggressive), intermediate (rarely metastasizing), or malignant. The four categories provide a standard nomenclature to indicate the biologic potential of the various soft tissue tumors. It is important to emphasize that the intermediate categories are not defined on the basis of histologic grade, but rather on biologic potential.

   A. **Benign.** Most tumors in this category do not locally recur. If recurrence does occur, it is typically nondestructive. Complete local excision is curative. The common lipoma is an example of this category.

   B. **Intermediate (locally aggressive).** Tumors in this category have a locally destructive and infiltrative growth pattern, and often locally recur. Wide excision is

Tumor type	Cytogenetic aberration	Loci involved
Lipoblastoma	Rearrangements of 8q12	Rearrangement of *PLAG1* gene
Lipoma	Rearrangements 12q14-q15 and 6p21-22; deletions of 13q12–14	*HMGA2* and *HMGA1* fusions
Well-differentiated liposarcoma	Supernumerary ring and/or marker chromosomes with amplification of 12q14-q15	Amplification of *MDM2, CDK4, HMGA2* genes
Myxoid/round cell liposarcoma	t(12;16)(q13;p11)	*TLS/FUS-CHOP* fusion
	t(12;22)(q13;q12)	*EWS-CHOP* fusion
Elastofibroma	1q abnormalities	Unknown
Desmoid fibromatosis	Trisomy 8 or 20; loss of 5q	Somatic *CTNNB1* or *APC* mutations (only in deep tumors)
Nasopharyngeal angiofibroma	Gains of 1p, 7q, 10q, 12q, 16p, 16q, 17q, 19p, 20q, 22c	Activating mutations in *CTNNB1*
Inflammatory myofibroblastic tumor	Translocations involving 2p23	*ALK* fusions with a variety of other genes
Congenital–infantile fibrosarcoma	t(12;15)(q13;q25)	*ETV6-NTRK3* fusions
Giant cell tumor of tendon sheath	Rearrangements of 1p13 in localized and diffuse types	Unknown
Leiomyosarcoma	Structural alterations of 1, 7, 10, 13, 14	Unknown
Embryonal rhabdomyosarcoma	Loss of heterozygosity at 11p15; gains of 2, 7, 8, 11, 12, 20, 21, 13q21, 20; losses of 1p35-36.3, 7, 6, 9q22, 14q21-32, 17	Unknown

(Continued)

TABLE 46.1 Recurring Cytogenetic Abnormalities Characteristic of Various Soft Tissue Neoplasms* (Continued)

Tumor type	Cytogenetic aberration	Loci involved
Alveolar rhabdomyosarcoma	t(2;13)(q35;q14)	PAX 3-FKHR fusion
	t(1;13)(p36;q14)	PAX 7-FKHR fusion
Epithelioid hemangioendothelioma	Losses or gains of 11q13–14 and 12q11–21	Unknown
Malignant peripheral nerve sheath tumor	Complex alterations including gains of 17q24-17 and losses of 7p22, 1p21, 7p11, 14q11, 17q11	Unknown
Angiomatoid fibrous histiocytoma	t(12;16)(q13;q11)	TLS/FUS-ATF1 fusion
	t(12;22)(q13;q12)	EWS-ATF1 fusion
Giant cell fibroblastoma	t(17;22)(q22;q13)	COL1A1-PDGFB fusion
Ewing sarcoma/ primitive neuroectodermal tumor	t(11;22)(q24;q12)	EWS-FLI1 fusion
	t(21;22)(q22;q12)	EWS-ERG fusion
Desmoplastic small round cell tumor	t(11;22)(p13;q12)	EWS-WT1 fusion
Synovial sarcoma	t(X;18)(p11;q11)	SYT-SSX1, -SSX2, -SSX4 fusions
Clear cell sarcoma (melanoma of soft parts)	t(12;22)(q13;q12)	EWS-ATF1 fusion
	t(2;22)(q32;q12)	EWS-CREB2 fusion
Alveolar soft part sarcoma	der(17)t(X;17)(p11.2;q25)	ASPL-TFE3 fusion
Extraskeletal myxoid chondrosarcoma	t(9;22)(q22;q12)	EWS-CHN/TEC fusion
	t(9;17)(q22;q11.2)	RBP56-CHN/TEC fusion
	t(9;15)(q22;q21)	TCF12-CHN/TEC fusion
Extrarenal malignant rhabdoid tumor	Alterations of 22q11.2	Biallelic inactivation of hSNF5/INI1
Epithelioid sarcoma (proximal type)	Alterations of 22q11.2	Biallelic inactivation of hSNF5/INI1

*Only the most common abnormalities are indicated. For more details, see Pfeifer JD. *Molecular Genetic Testing in Surgical Pathology*. Philadelphia, PA: Lippincott, Williams & Wilkins; 2006.

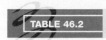

TABLE 46.2 WHO Classification of Soft Tissue Tumors

ADIPOCYTIC TUMORS
Benign
Lipoma
Lipomatosis
Lipomatosis of nerve
Lipoblastoma/lipoblastomatosis
Angiolipoma
Myolipoma
Chondroid lipoma
Extrarenal angiomyolipoma
Extra-adrenal myelolipoma
Spindle cell/pleomorphic lipoma
Hibernoma

Intermediate (locally aggressive)
Atypical lipomatous tumor/well-differentiated liposarcoma

Malignant
Dedifferentiated liposarcoma
Myxoid liposarcoma/round cell liposarcoma
Pleomorphic liposarcoma
Mixed-type liposarcoma
Liposarcoma, not otherwise specified

FIBROBLASTIC/MYOFIBROBLASTIC TUMORS
Benign
Nodular fasciitis
Proliferative fasciitis
Proliferative myositis
Myositis ossificans
   Fibro-osseous pseudotumor of digits
Ischemic fasciitis
Elastofibroma
Fibrous hamartoma of infancy
Myofibroma/myofibromatosis
Fibromatosis colli
Juvenile hyaline fibromatosis
Inclusion body fibromatosis
Fibroma of tendon sheath
Desmoplastic fibroblastoma
Mammary-type myofibroblastoma
Calcifying aponeurotic fibroma
Angiomyofibroblastoma
Cellular angiofibroma
Nuchal-type fibroma
Gardner fibroma
Calcifying fibrous tumor
Giant cell angiofibroma

Intermediate (locally aggressive)
Superficial fibromatosis (palmar/plantar)
Desmoid-type fibromatosis
Lipofibromatosis

(*Continued*)

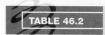

TABLE 46.2	WHO Classification of Soft Tissue Tumors (Continued)

Intermediate (rarely metastasizing)
Solitary fibrous tumor and hemangiopericytoma
Inflammatory myofibroblastic tumor
Low-grade myofibroblastic sarcoma
Myxoinflammatory fibroblastic sarcoma
Infantile fibrosarcoma

Malignant
Adult fibrosarcoma
Myxofibrosarcoma
Low-grade fibromyxoid sarcoma/hyalinizing spindle cell tumor
Sclerosing epithelioid fibrosarcoma

SO-CALLED FIBROHISTIOCYTIC TUMORS
Benign
Giant cell tumor of tendon sheath
Diffuse-type giant cell tumor
Deep benign fibrous histiocytoma

Intermediate (rarely metastasizing)
Plexiform fibrohistiocytic tumor
Giant cell tumor of soft tissues

Malignant
Pleomorphic malignant fibrous histiocytoma (MFH)/undifferentiated pleomorphic sarcoma
Giant cell MFH/undifferentiated pleomorphic sarcoma with giant cells
Inflammatory MFH/undifferentiated pleomorphic sarcoma with prominent inflammation

SMOOTH MUSCLE TUMORS
Angioleiomyoma
Deep leiomyoma
Genital leiomyoma
Leiomyosarcoma

PERICYTIC (PERIVASCULAR) TUMORS
Glomus tumor
    Malignant glomus tumor
Myopericytoma

SKELETAL MUSCLE TUMORS
Benign
Rhabdomyoma (adult type, fetal type, genital type)

Malignant
Embryonal rhabdomyosarcoma (including spindle cell, botryoid, anaplastic)
Alveolar rhabdomyosarcoma
Pleomorphic rhabdomyosarcoma

VASCULAR TUMORS
Benign
Hemangiomas of subcutaneous/deep soft tissue
    Capillary
    Cavernous
    Arteriovenous
    Venous
    Intramuscular
    Synovial
Epithelioid hemangioma
Angiomatosis
Lymphangioma

(Continued)

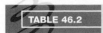

| TABLE 46.2 | WHO Classification of Soft Tissue Tumors (Continued) |

Intermediate (locally aggressive)
Kaposiform hemangioendothelioma

Intermediate (rarely metastasizing)
Retiform hemangioendothelioma
Papillary intralymphatic angioendothelioma
Composite hemangioendothelioma
Kaposi sarcoma

Malignant
Epithelioid hemangioendothelioma
Angiosarcoma of soft tissue

CHONDRO-OSSEOUS TUMORS
Soft tissue chondroma
Mesenchymal chondrosarcoma

TUMORS OF UNCERTAIN DIFFERENTIATION
Benign
Intramuscular myxoma
Juxta-articular myxoma
Deep (aggressive) angiomyxoma
Pleomorphic hyalinizing angiectatic tumor
Ectopic hamartomatous thymoma

Intermediate (rarely metastasizing)
Angiomatoid fibrous histiocytoma
Ossifying fibromyxoid tumor
Mixed tumor/myoepithelioma/parachordoma

Malignant
Synovial sarcoma
Epithelioid sarcoma
Alveolar soft part sarcoma
Clear cell sarcoma of soft tissue
Extraskeletal myxoid chondrosarcoma
Primitive neuroectodermal tumor (PNET)/extraskeletal Ewing tumor
Desmoplastic small round cell tumor
Extrarenal rhabdoid tumor
Malignant mesenchymoma
Neoplasms with perivascular epithelioid cell differentiation (PEComa)
   Clear cell myomelanocytic tumor
Intimal sarcoma

From: Fletcher CDM, Unni K, Mertens K, eds. *World Health Organization Classification of Tumours. Pathology and Genetics. Tumours of Soft Tissue and Bone.* Lyon: IARC Press; 2002. Used with permission.

required for local control. Tumors in this category do not metastasize. An example of this tumor type is desmoid fibromatosis.

C. **Intermediate (rarely metastasizing).** Tumors in this category also have a locally destructive and infiltrative growth pattern. However, they also may give rise to distant metastases in a small subset of cases (typically <2%), although the risk for metastasis of an individual tumor cannot be reliably predicted on the basis of morphologic features. Examples of this category include congenital–infantile fibrosarcoma, dermatofibrosarcoma protuberans, and angiomatoid fibrous histiocytoma.

D. Malignant. Tumors in this category also have a locally destructive and infiltrative growth pattern. However, they metastasize in a high percentage of cases; low-grade sarcomas have a metastatic rate of 2%–10%, and high-grade sarcomas metastasize in 20%–100% of cases.

IV. ADIPOCYTIC TUMORS

A. Benign

1. **Lipomas** are composed of mature adipocytes and are the most common soft tissue neoplasms in adults. Superficial lipomas arise in the subcutis; deep lipomas arise within the deep soft tissue; parosteal lipomas arise on the surface of bone; intramuscular and intermuscular lipomas arise within and between skeletal muscle; and lipoma arborescens arises in synovial membranes. Superficial tumors are generally <5 cm in maximum dimension, whereas deep tumors are often >5 cm. Lipomas are well circumscribed and have an oily light yellow cut surface, except in children whose tumors are pale white. Regardless of the anatomic site, the tumor is composed of mature adipocytes separated into complete and incomplete lobules. Numerous histologic subtypes have been described, but none have prognostic significance, including the following:

   a. **Angiolipoma** typically occurs in the subcutaneous tissue and consists of mature adipocytes with a variably prominent capillary network with scattered microthrombi (e-**Fig. 46.1**).*

   b. **Myolipoma** (intramuscular lipoma) is found in the deep soft tissues of the abdominal cavity, inguinal region, and retroperitoneum. Mature adipose tissue is intermixed with mature smooth muscle or skeletal muscle.

   c. **Chondrolipoma** occurs in the limb girdle and proximal extremities. Cords and nests of lipoblasts as well as mature adipocytes are present in a myxoid to hyalinized chondroid matrix. Despite the presence of immature fat cells, surgical excision is curative.

   d. **Spindle cell lipoma/pleomorphic lipoma** occurs predominantly on the posterior neck and shoulder area in middle aged and elderly men (only 10% of cases occur in women). Grossly, it is a mobile dermal or subcutaneous nodule, usually present for many years. The microscopic features are variable; at one end of the spectrum are tumors composed of bland spindled cells with associated dense collagen bundles between mature adipocytes; at the other end are tumors with small hyperchromatic cells admixed with multinucleated giant cells between mature adipocytes. The spindle cells are immunopositive for CD34, and in some cases also for S-100 protein.

2. **Lipomatosis** occurs in several different clinicopathologic settings, all of which are characterized by a diffuse overgrowth of mature adipose tissue. Regardless of the clinical subtype, the neoplastic cells are indistinguishable from those found in lipomas, which emphasizes the role of clinical history in arriving at the correct diagnosis.

   a. **Diffuse lipomatosis** preferentially occurs in children younger than 2 years, and primarily involves the majority of an extremity, trunk, head and neck, pelvis, abdomen, or intestinal tract. In this setting, Proteus syndrome, encephalocraniocutaneous lipomatosis, or Cowden disease should be considered.

   b. **Symmetric lipomatosis** occurs predominantly in middle-aged men of Mediterranean ancestry, and is characterized by symmetric deposition of fat in the upper body.

   c. **Pelvic lipomatosis,** which affects black males over a wide age range, usually manifests as an overgrowth of fat in perirectal and perivesical areas.

   d. **Steroid lipomatosis** occurs in the setting of adrenocortical hormonal therapy or with endogenous endocrine abnormalities, and characteristically involves accumulation of fat in the face, sternal region, or middle of the upper back (the so-called "buffalo hump").

---

*All e-figures are available online via the Solution Site Image Bank.

e. **Human immunodeficiency virus (HIV)-lipodystrophy** in patients with acquired immunodeficiency syndrome (AIDS) occurs in those undergoing treatment with protease inhibitors or other forms of antiviral therapy, and is characterized by the accumulation of visceral fat with fat wasting in the face and limbs.

3. **Lipomatosis of nerve** (neural fibrolipoma, fibrolipomatous hamartoma) is noted at birth or in early childhood, but is seen through the fourth decade. The median nerve and ulnar nerve are the most frequent sites of involvement, and a subset of cases is associated with macrodactyly. Perineurial and epineurial infiltration by a mixture of mature adipocytes and fibrous tissue typically separates individual nerve bundles.

4. **Lipoblastoma** occurs in children younger than 5 years, has a predilection for the lower extremities, but can also involve the neck, mediastinum, and abdomen. It is either a localized, well-circumscribed tumor (lipoblastoma) or has a diffuse infiltrating pattern (lipoblastomatosis). Like other fatty tumors, it has a lobulated architecture and is composed of a mixture of cell types including mature and immature adipocytes, a variable number of lipoblasts, and stellate mesenchymal cells (e-Fig. 46.2). Grayish myxoid areas seen grossly have microscopic features resembling myxoid liposarcoma. Despite the presence of immature fat cells, the neoplasm is benign and does not metastasize. These tumors may have the potential for maturation. Approximately 20% of cases recur (most are examples of lipoblastomatosis).

5. **Hibernoma** is a neoplasm composed of brown fat (adipocytes with multivacuolated granular cytoplasm) admixed with conventional adipose tissue. It occurs in young adults and is found in the thigh as well as the head and neck, trunk, and upper extremities. The cut surface ranges from yellow to brown; is usually greasy and spongy; may be lobulated but is well demarcated; and can measure >20 cm. Microscopically, lobules of brown fat are separated from conventional adipose tissue (e-Fig. 46.3).

B. **Intermediate (locally aggressive)**

1. **Atypical lipomatous** tumor/well-differentiated liposarcoma (ALT/WDLPS) occurs in adults in the fifth through eighth decade of life. The deep soft tissues of the lower extremity, retroperitoneum, paratesticular region, and mediastinum are the various primary sites. Those tumors arising in the retroperitoneum may attain sizes in excess of 20 cm. The tumor has a lobulated, yellow to white, soft to firm cut surface that varies in relation to its adipocytic, fibrous, and myxoid areas. Microscopically, the tumor is composed largely of cells with lipoma-like features except for the presence of scattered hyperchromatic, often multinucleated and vacuolated cells with features of atypical lipoblasts. Four histologic subtypes are designated, namely adipocytic (lipoma-like), sclerosing, inflammatory, and spindle cell types, but more than one morphologic pattern may be present in the same neoplasm. Sclerosing foci are helpful in diagnosis because the areas of collagen contain atypical stromal cells (e-Fig. 46.4).

   Prognosis is largely determined by anatomic site and size. Smaller, more superficial tumors can be locally resected with negative margins, but tumors in the retroperitoneum or mediastinum are likely to recur because of positive surgical margins. Recurrent tumors may show evidence of so-called dedifferentiation.

C. **Malignant**

1. **Dedifferentiated liposarcoma** shows a transition from ALT/WDLPS to a pleomorphic and/or high-grade spindle cell sarcoma (e-Fig. 46.5), either in the primary ALT/WDLPS (85%–90% of cases) or in a recurrence (10%–15% of cases). The change in pattern from ALT/WDLPS to high-grade sarcoma is usually abrupt. By convention, the focus of dedifferentiation should be at least several millimeters in greatest dimension. Because the area of dedifferentiation may be limited, thorough sampling and careful microscopic examination of all ALT/WDLPS is required to exclude the presence of dedifferentiation.

2. **Myxoid liposarcoma/round cell liposarcoma** peaks in incidence at age 30 to 40 years and occurs predominantly in the deep soft tissues of the extremities

(more than two thirds of cases arise in the musculature of the thigh). Occasional cases also arise in the retroperitoneum or subcutaneous tissue. Although liposarcoma is rare in children, myxoid liposarcoma is the most common type in the pediatric age group.

The cut surface of myxoid liposarcoma is tan, glistening, and gelatinous; the round cell morphology is associated with a fleshy and white cut surface. Myxoid tumors are composed of uniform, round to oval, primitive nonlipogenic mesenchymal cells and small lipoblasts embedded in a myxoid stroma with a delicate arborizing capillary network (e-**Fig. 46.6**). Sheets of high-grade primitive round cells are not accompanied by a myxoid stroma. Some tumors show a transition from myxoid to round cell areas. Round cell liposarcoma has a poorer prognosis than the more favorable pure myxoid liposarcoma. The same fusion transcripts are found in both tumor types and do not correlate with prognosis (*Cytogenet Genome Res.* 2007;118:138).

3. **Pleomorphic liposarcoma,** as the name implies, is by definition a high-grade sarcoma with a variable number of convincing pleomorphic lipoblasts. This tumor has a preference for the extremities, usually measures in excess of 10 cm, and primarily occurs in patients >40 years old. The tumor is usually a well circumscribed or infiltrative mass with a variable appearance on cut surface ranging from solid, to cystic, to overtly necrotic, to hemorrhagic, to myxoid. Pleomorphic lipoblasts with enlarged hyperchromatic nuclei that are scalloped by cytoplasmic lipid vacuoles are not always numerous in the background of highly atypical, even anaplastic round cells, spindle cells, and multinucleated tumor giant cells (e-**Fig. 46.7**). These tumors may have a prominent inflammatory infiltrate. Anaplastic mitotic figures are often present. In the absence of identifiable lipoblasts, these neoplasms are otherwise pleomorphic sarcomas.

V. FIBROBLASTIC/MYOFIBROBLASTIC TUMORS
A. Benign

1. **Nodular fasciitis** occurs in all age groups but has a predilection for young adults. It usually involves the subcutaneous tissue of the head and neck, trunk, or upper extremities (e-**Fig. 46.8**). Dermal involvement is uncommon, but deeper fascial or intramuscular tumors are other presentations. Similar lesions may involve small to medium-sized veins or the soft tissue of the outer table of the scalp, as intravascular and cranial fasciitis (e-**Fig. 46.9**), respectively.

These circumscribed, minimally infiltrative spindle cell proliferations have a fibrous to myxoid cut surface, and most are <2 cm in greatest dimension. Cystic degeneration is an uncommon gross feature, but one of the microscopic hallmarks is presence of microcysts among the more cellular foci. Collections of inflammatory cells, extravasated red cells, or osteoclast-like giant cells may be associated with the microcysts.

Compactly cellular foci with storiform profiles or interlacing fascicles may reside adjacent to cellular arrays with a myxoid background (e-**Figs. 46.8** and **46.9**). More collagenized foci can have a keloidal quality. Mitotic figures, but not atypical ones, are expected in variable numbers. As a myofibroblastic proliferation, the spindle cells are strongly reactive for smooth muscle actin (SMA).

2. **Proliferative fasciitis** and **proliferative myositis** primarily occur in middle aged and elderly patients. The subcutis in the upper extremity is the most common site of proliferative fasciitis, but some cases involve the trunk or lower extremity. Proliferative myositis is intramuscular, and primarily involves the trunk, shoulder girdle, and upper arm. Both lesions grow rapidly, measure between 3 and 5 cm, and are composed of similar plump fibroblastic and myofibroblastic spindled cells as in nodular fasciitis. However, the hallmark of proliferative fasciitis and proliferative myositis is the presence of large ganglion-like cells with an uneven distribution within the lesion. The ganglion-like cells may be mitotically active, but atypical mitotic figures are not present. In addition to SMA, CD68 may be expressed in ganglion-like cells.

3. **Ischemic fasciitis** occurs over bony prominences, usually due to impaired circulation and prolonged pressure in immobilized, often elderly individuals. A

zonal architecture consists of central areas of coagulative necrosis and myxoid change, with fibroblastic and vascular proliferation at the periphery.

4. **Myositis ossificans** and **fibro-osseous pseudotumor of digits** are related lesions that occur in a broad age range of patients, although young adults are most frequently affected. Myositis ossificans has a propensity for the extremities, trunk, and head and neck, whereas fibro-osseous pseudotumor primarily occurs, as its name indicates, in the subcutis of the proximal phalanx of the finger and toe. Both tumors are thought to be caused by soft tissue injury with resulting repair that initially consists of a cellular fibroblastic focus resembling nodular fasciitis, followed by development of an equally cellular osteoblastic proliferation and a peripheral rind of osseous metaplasia (e-**Fig. 46.10**). Biopsies from the fibroblastic and/or osteoblastic foci can be quite worrisome, but the mitotic activity is generally low and the mitotic figures are not atypical. The nuclei are not disproportionately large or hyperchromatic.

5. **Elastofibroma** is found predominantly in individuals older than 50 years in the connective tissues between the chest wall and the inferior region of the scapula, deep to the rhomboid major and latissimus dorsi muscles, usually with attachment to the periosteum of the ribs. The tumor can be unilateral or bilateral and has a gray-white, rubbery to fibrous cut surface with ill-defined margins. A paucicellular collagenized stroma (e-**Fig. 46.11**) contains elastic fibers with large, coarse, eosinophilic linear globules arranged in a so-called "beads on a string" pattern that is highlighted by a Weigert's elastic or pentachrome stain.

6. **Fibrous hamartoma of infancy** is one of the 'fibrous tumors of childhood' and is generally seen before 2 years of age. The anterior or posterior axillary fold, arm and shoulder, back, thigh, and groin are the preferred sites. The tumor forms an ill-defined mass in the subcutis; on cut sections, it has a white fibrocollagenous appearance with interspersed fat. Microscopically, intersecting fibrous bands of variable thickness radiate through the subcutis and are associated with discrete nodules of immature mesenchyme or so-called neuroid nodules. Without the latter nodules, there is a resemblance to another fibrous tumor of childhood, lipofibromatosis. When there is overgrowth of the fat by the fibrous component, the tumor acquires the features of fibromatosis or desmoid tumor. The distinction from the latter is important because of the low recurrence (only 10%–15%) of fibrous hamartoma.

7. **Myofibroma–myofibromatosis,** another fibrous tumor of childhood, although seen in adults on occasion, is a neoplasm composed of contractile myoid cells that seemingly originates within small vessels and extends into the surrounding dermis, soft tissues, various organs, and bone. A solitary mass in the head and neck in a young child (0 to 3 years) is the most common of three clinical presentations (Table 46.3). Individual tumors range from >1 to >7 cm in greatest dimension and have a cut surface that ranges from firm and fibrous, to cystic and hemorrhagic. Immature plump to spindled cells are arranged in whorls and fascicles within a fibromyxoid stroma; smaller nodules may be associated with a vessel to suggest an angiocentric origin. Hypercellular spindle cell foci are present in some cases with a resemblance to congenital–infantile fibrosarcoma.

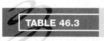

TABLE 46.3	The Three Clinical Presentations of Myofibroma-Myofibromatosis in Children		
	Solitary	**Multicentric**	**Generalized**
Sites	Skin, soft tissue, bone	Skin and soft tissue, and/or bone	Skin, soft tissue, bone plus organs (lung, heart, liver, intestinal tract, brain)
% of total cases	90%	3%–6%	1%–3%
Prognosis	Excellent	Excellent	Poor

Other findings include a hemangiopericytoma-like pattern centrally, often with ischemic or hemorrhagic regions, dystrophic calcifications, and hyalinization. The spindle cells express vimentin and SMA, whereas the hemangiopericytoma-like foci are CD34 positive.

8. **Angiomyofibroblastoma,** a rare tumor, occurs in women of reproductive age where it arises in the rises in the pelviperineal region (vulva and vagina) as a painless, well circumscribed, slowly enlarging mass. In men, the neoplasm usually involves the paratesticular soft tissues or scrotum. Microscopically, round to plump spindled myofibroblasts tend to cluster around blood vessels (**e-Fig. 46.12**); a subset of cases has a mature fatty component. Binucleate and multinucleate cells are common in the absence of mitotic activity. Some cases have an overlap with cellular angiofibroma and deep aggressive angiomyxoma.

9. **Cellular angiofibroma** involves the superficial soft tissues of the vulva or inguinoscrotal region as well as the perineum, retroperitoneum, and subcutis of the chest. Grossly, the tumor is a well-circumscribed mass that usually measures <3 cm in diameter in women and <10 cm in men. The cut surface of the tumor has a yellow to tan-brown, soft to rubbery appearance. The tumor is composed of plump spindled cells with minimal eosinophilic cytoplasm, little cytologic atypia, and few mitotic figures; a background of delicate collagen fibers is present in tumors in women. The vascular component of the tumor is composed of small to medium-sized vessels, with or without prominent hyaline walls, and is usually present throughout the entire lesion. Regressive and/or degenerative changes, including extravasated erythrocytes, hemosiderin deposition, cystic change, and intravascular thrombi, are also present.

10. **Giant cell angiofibroma,** a slowly growing occasional painful tumor, has a predilection for the eyelids and orbital region of adults, although it has been identified in a number of other anatomic sites. The tumor is usually about 3 cm in greatest dimension, well circumscribed, variably encapsulated, with cystic and/or hemorrhagic areas. Microscopically, cellular areas of round to spindled, cytologically bland cells and multinucleated stromal cells (which often line pseudovascular spaces as is common in giant cell fibroblastoma) are set in a background of myxoid to collagenous stroma with small to medium-sized blood vessels. Both the mononuclear and multinucleated cells are immunoreactive for CD34 and CD99, and occasionally also for BCL2.

11. **Nuchal-type fibroma** and **Gardner-associated fibroma** are virtually identical in terms of the microscopic features of dense, paucicellular collagenous bundles that overgrow and occupy the dermis, subcutis, and deep soft tissues (*Cancer.* 1999;85:156). Recurrent fibromas may have features indistinguishable from a desmoid fibromatosis. The possibility of Gardner syndrome should be raised in the presence of this tumor (*Am J Surg Pathol.* 2007;31:410).

B. **Intermediate (locally aggressive)**

1. **Superficial fibromatoses.** Palmar fibromatosis develops in men >30 years old (with a male to female ratio of 4:1) as asymptomatic, isolated firm nodules that evolve into cord-like bands between nodules involving adjacent fingers. Plantar fibromatosis is seen more often in children and adolescents as painful subcutaneous nodules (*Am J Surg Pathol.* 2005;29:1095).

The microscopic features evolve over time. Greater cellularity is present early on, consisting of bland plump to spindled cells that have a low mitotic rate set in a background of collagen and elongated vessels (**e-Fig. 46.13**). Older lesions are much less cellular and have a stroma that consists of dense, often hyalinized collagen. The extent of surgical excision is the primary determinant of the rate of recurrence.

2. **Desmoid-type fibromatosis** (desmoid tumor, musculoaponeurotic fibromatosis) usually involves the head and neck region in children, and the proximal extremities and abdominal wall in adolescents and older women (*Hematol Oncol Clin North Am.* 2005;19:565). Both soft tissues and mesenteric desmoids may be associated with Gardner syndrome. A circumscribed mass measuring 5 to 10 cm with a firm white trabeculated surface is the typical gross appearance;

the macroscopic circumscription may be deceptive because subtle and extensive infiltration into the interstitium between muscle bundles and along fascial planes is often present microscopically. Although desmoid tumor is classically a proliferation of fibroblasts, a number of patterns are seen, ranging from spindle cells forming bundles and fascicles in a dense collagenous background, to plump fibroblasts in a pale, less fibrotic stroma (e-Fig. 46.14). Small blood vessels may be conspicuous, and when red cell extravasation is present, the lesion can resemble nodular fasciitis. Some mitotic figures may be present, and scattered small lymphoid nodules may be noted at the interface with surrounding normal tissues. If skeletal muscle is involved, it is usually infiltrated with remnants of muscle embedded in the fibrous proliferation (e-Fig. 46.15). SMA expression is common, and 46%–50% of cases have nuclear reactivity for β-catenin (*Am J Surg Pathol.* 2007;31:1299).

3. **Lipofibromatosis** (infantile subcutaneous fibromatosis), another fibrous tumor of childhood, is a slowly growing, painless, ill-defined mass occurring in a variety of sites including the distal extremities (*Am J Surg Pathol.* 2000;24:1491). Grossly, the tumor is an ill-defined white-tan to yellow mass that usually measures <5 cm in greatest dimension. Spindled fibroblastic cells form bands that surround and may separate lobules of fat; the growth pattern resembles fibrous hamartoma but without the nodules of immature mesenchyme. The tumor may express CD34, BCL2, S-100, actin, epithelial membrane antigen (EMA), and CD99, an unusual phenotypic profile for a fibrous tumor.

4. **Infantile digital fibroma–fibromatosis** (inclusion body fibromatosis, recurring digital fibrous tumor of Reye) is seen in the fingers and/or toes (30% of cases are multifocal), excluding the thumb and great toe, as a firm nodule or nodules. The fibrous proliferation resembles a desmoid tumor, with confluent infiltration and replacement of the dermis and deeper soft tissues including the skeletal muscle. Isolated adnexal structures are surrounded by the moderately cellular spindle cell proliferation. Paranuclear bodies consisting of actin microfilaments are one of the unique features of this tumor.

5. **Juvenile nasopharyngeal fibroma** occurs almost exclusively in adolescent males, often presenting with epistaxis. Extensive local growth occurs in the confined spaces of the nasopharynx and into the paranasal sinuses and pterygopalatine fossa. These tumors are firm and have a white-tan cut surface. A diffuse bland fibrous proliferation with a prominent component of small blood vessels is the typical microscopic appearance. This tumor is seen in the setting of familial adenomatous polyposis. The stromal cells may express nuclear β-catenin.

C. **Intermediate (rarely metastasizing)**
   1. **Solitary fibrous tumor** and **hemangiopericytoma** are grouped together as related (if not identical) neoplasms in the current WHO classification.
      a. **Solitary fibrous tumor** is classically found on the pleura, but has been reported in many different locations in a broad age range of patients. Grossly, the tumor is a well circumscribed, nonencapsulated, firm, white mass measuring ≤8 cm, and may show hemorrhage and focal myxoid change. Microscopically, bland plump to spindle-shaped cells with a patternless architecture surround branching blood vessels of the type associated with the hemangiopericytoma (e-Fig. 46.16). The cellularity often varies within individual tumors, and the hypocellular background stroma can have a myxoid fibrous appearance, and can resemble a nerve sheath tumor. The tumor cells are immunoreactive for CD34 and CD99, but a subset of tumors also show reactivity for SMA, BCL2, and EMA and even focal positivity for desmin, cytokeratin, and/or S-100.
         Malignant solitary fibrous tumors have increased mitotic activity (≥4 mitoses per 10 high-power fields), focal necrosis, increased cellularity, marked cytologic atypia in a patchy distribution, and infiltrative margins (*Am J Surg Pathol.* 1998;22:1501), although the clinical behavior of an individual tumor is not always correlated with the histologic features. Some tumors have a solidly cellular fibrosarcoma-like pattern.

b. Hemangiopericytoma. By the current WHO classification scheme, the diagnosis of hemangiopericytoma is limited to soft tissue tumors that morphologically resemble the cellular areas of a solitary fibrous tumor (e-**Fig. 46.17**), and that are composed of cells that have the immunoprofile of the solitary fibrous tumor. By this definition, most cases of hemangiopericytoma occur in the deep soft tissues, primarily in the retroperitoneum of the pelvis, but also in the limb girdles and proximal limbs. Most cases are <15 cm in greatest dimension. Mature adipose tissue is found rarely in hemangiopericytoma (lipomatous type).

2. **Inflammatory myofibroblastic tumor** (inflammatory pseudotumor, inflammatory fibrosarcoma) has a predilection for the mesentery, small intestine (ileocecal region), lung, and bladder, throughout childhood and into young adulthood. In addition to local symptoms related to the mass, 5%–10% of cases have systemic manifestation (fever, anorexia, weight loss, hypochronic microcystic anemia, and/or hypergammaglobulinemia, thrombocytosis) as a manifestation of cytokine production, likely interleukin-6 (IL-6).

   The tumor forms a white to tan, whorled, fleshy to myxoid, circumscribed mass measuring from 1 to 25 cm in diameter that may also show areas of necrosis, hemorrhage, and calcification. Three basic histologic patterns can be found in any one tumor, although one or two patterns may dominate (e-**Fig. 46.18**): dense fascicles of spindle cells with a mixed population of plasma cells, lymphocytes, and eosinophils in the background; loosely cellular foci with a myxoid and edematous background resembling nodular fasciitis; and hypocellular, collagenized foci with minimal inflammation and dystrophic calcifications. Mitotic figures are found among the spindle cells, but they are not atypical. Some tumors have a round cell population. The differential diagnosis includes two unrelated lesions, calcifying fibrous pseudotumor (which has psammomatous calcifications) and inflammatory fibroid tumor (which presents in the stomach or small intestine) (*Int J Surg Pathol.* 2002;10:189 and *Adv Anat Pathol.* 2007; 14:178).

   Immunohistochemically, a subset of tumors [approximately 50%–60%, corresponding to those cases that harbor a rearranged anaplastic lymphoma kinase (*ALK*) gene] shows cytoplasmic staining for the *ALK* gene product (*Am J Surg Pathol.* 2001;25:1364). However, virtually all cases are immunoreactive for vimentin, most show reactivity for SMA and variable reactivity for muscle-specific actin (MSA) and desmin, and 25%–30% are reactive for cytokeratin. ALK-positive tumors may have a more favorable clinical outcome than the ALK-negative tumors (*Am J Surg Pathol.* 2007;31:509).

3. **Congenital–infantile fibrosarcoma** occurs in children ≤2 years old (and can be present at birth) and has a predilection for the superficial or deep soft tissues of the distal extremities, although cases also present in the trunk, head and neck, and intestinal tract. The cut surface of the tumor (which can measure up to 10 to 15 cm in diameter) ranges from white to tan, fleshy to firm, and may show areas of hemorrhage, necrosis, and/or myxoid and cystic degeneration; careful gross examination usually shows that the tumor has an infiltrative irregular margin.

   Congenital–infantile fibrosarcoma has a range of histologic features. Interlacing, broad fascicles of spindle cells resembling the herringbone pattern of the adult type fibrosarcoma or monophasic synovial sarcoma are present in some tumors (e-**Fig. 46.19**). Alternatively, the tumor may be composed of more primitive appearing, shorter spindle cells in a poorly organized pattern. Small foci of palisading necrosis or confluent areas of hemorrhage are other features. Mitotic figures are readily identified. Nuclear pleomorphism, atypical mitoses, and a pale background stroma should raise the possibility of embryonal rhabdomyosarcoma (ERMS). These tumors have the same t(12;15) translocation as cellular mesoblastic nephroma (Table 46.1).

D. Malignant

1. **Adult fibrosarcoma** is a diagnosis of exclusion, rendered only after other types of spindle cell sarcomas (such as dermatofibrosarcoma, congenital–infantile

TABLE 46.4	Differential Immunohistochemical Profile of Adult-Type Fibrosarcoma and Other Spindle Cell Sarcomas					
	FS	**SS**	**LMS**	**MPNST**	**SFT**	**DFSP**
Vim	+	+	+	+	+	+
CK	−	±	−	±	−	−
EMA	−	±	−	±	−	−
SMA	±	−	+	−	−	−
S-100	−	±	±	±	−	−
CD34	−	−	−	−	+	+
CD99	−	+	−	−	−	−

Abbreviations: FS, fibrosarcoma; SS, synovial sarcoma; LMS, leiomyosarcoma; MPNST, malignant peripheral nerve sheath tumor; SFT, solitary fibrous tumor; DFSP, dermatofibrosarcoma protuberans; VIM, vimentin; CK, cytokeratin; EMA, epithelial membrane antigen; SMA, smooth muscle actin; S-100, S-100 protein.

fibrosarcoma, solitary fibrous tumor, monophasic synovial sarcoma, and malignant peripheral nerve sheath tumor [MPNST]) have been ruled out on the basis of immunohistochemistry (Table 46.4). When strictly defined, adult fibrosarcoma is primarily seen between ages 50 and 75 years, and has a predilection for the deep soft tissues of the head and neck, trunk, and extremities.

Fibrosarcoma forms a well-circumscribed mass the cut surface of which has a white to tan appearance and a firm consistency. Sweeping fascicles of compact spindle cells produce the quintessential herringbone pattern (e-**Fig. 46.20**). The background stroma shows a variable collagen content. Immunopositivity is limited to vimentin and, focally, SMA.

2. **Sclerosing epithelioid fibrosarcoma,** a rare variant of fibrosarcoma, occurs over a wide age range, usually in the deep soft tissues of the lower extremities and limb girdles. The tumor produces a well-circumscribed mass measuring up to 20 cm in greatest dimension, and has a firm white cut surface, although cystic and myxoid areas may be present. The rounded or epithelioid cells that compose the mass have minimal eosinophilic to clear cytoplasm, a low mitotic rate, and are arranged in acini, strands, and nests within a dense collagenous matrix. The tumor cells express vimentin but not CD34, HMB-45, and CD45 (*Cancer Genet Cytogenet.* 2000;119:127). A small subset of cases shows focal weak expression of EMA and/or cytokeratin.

3. **Low-grade fibromyxoid sarcoma,** another variant of fibrosarcoma, presents as a painless deep soft tissue mass that has, in some cases, been present for many years. Most tumors present in adults, but the tumor is well recognized in children. Microscopically, a prominent capsule or pseudocapsule surrounds a bland spindle cell proliferation, with alternating and blending fibrogenic and myxoid areas that show variation in cellular density from one area to another (e-**Fig. 46.21**). Mitotic figures are sparse in number. A subset of tumors (approximately 40%) contains poorly formed giant collagen rosettes consisting of a central hyalinized core surrounded by a rim of fibroblasts that usually have epithelioid morphology. Another small subgroup has foci of increased cellularity and cytologic atypia of the type usually found in intermediate grade fibrosarcomas, but the prognostic significance of this finding has yet to be established. Both the t(7;16) and t(11;16) translocations are present in low-grade fibromyxoid sarcoma with or without giant collagen rosettes. Fusion-gene–positive tumors are usually EMA positive, are immunoreactive for CD99 and BCL2, but do not express SMA, S-100, and desmin (*Arch Pathol Lab Med.* 2006;130:1358).

4. **Myxofibrosarcoma** occurs over a wide age range, but has a predilection for patients older than 60 years. Most cases present in the dermis and subcutis; only about one third occur in the deep soft tissue. Myxofibrosarcoma usually

arises in the limb girdles and limbs. The myxoid character on gross examination resembles liposarcoma but is more infiltrative. A multinodular growth pattern, variable cellularity within a myxoid stroma, and incomplete fibrous septa that course through the tumor are consistent microscopic features (*Ultrastruct Pathol.* 2004;28:321). Low-grade tumors are hypocellular and have a prominent myxoid matrix that contains only scattered plump or stellate tumor cells, with very low mitotic activity. High-grade tumors (e-**Fig. 46.22**) show marked cellular pleomorphism, multinucleated giant cells, a high mitotic rate (with easily identified atypical mitotic forms), and areas of solid growth. The tumor cells express vimentin, but otherwise do not have a characteristic immunophenotype.

5. **Acral myxoinflammatory fibroblastic sarcoma** is a neoplasm arising in an articular-juxta-articular location of the hands and feet, although a few examples from other sites have been reported. As the appellation implies, these tumors occur over a broad adult age range, and have an appearance that can be mistaken for an inflammatory process. There is infiltration of surrounding tissues by a mixed cellular infiltrate composed in part of large histiocyte-like cells, some resembling "bizarre" ganglion-like cells and multivacuolated lipoblast-like cells (*Am J Surg Pathol.* 1998;22:911; *Ann Diagn Pathol.* 2002;6:272).

VI. **FIBROHISTIOCYTIC TUMORS.** As the name of this category suggests, these neoplasms are composed of cells that have fibrohistiocytic morphology. However, electron microscopy and immunohistochemistry have firmly established that the cells comprising these tumors (other than the foamy macrophages) are, in fact, not histiocytes but rather primitive mesenchymal cells, fibroblasts, and myofibroblasts.

A. **Benign**

1. **Giant cell tumor of tendon sheath** (GCTTS) (tenosynovial giant cell tumor, nodular tenosynovitis) is a localized tumor that arises from the synovium of joints, bursae, and tendon sheath or adjacent tissues. It is uncertain as to whether this lesion is best classified as a fibrohistiocytic tumor (as in the WHO classification) or as a tumor differentiating toward synovial cells. It is regarded as one of a family of articular and extra-articular neoplasms that includes diffuse-type tenosynovial giant cell tumor and pigmented villonodular synovitis. These tumors share a common translocation (Table 46.1).

   The hand, and less often the wrist, ankle, foot, knee, elbow, and hip, are various sites of the tumor, which clinically presents as a painless mass, mainly in adults. GCTTS forms a firm lobulated yellowish-brown to tan circumscribed mass that measures from 0.5 to 4 cm; erosion into adjacent bone is seen in larger lesions. Mononuclear cells with rounded to plumb-spindled features, foamy macrophages, siderophages, and multinucleate giant cells with a variably prominent hyalinized stroma (e-**Fig. 46.23**) are the elements of this multinodular neoplasm.

2. **Diffuse-type giant cell tumor** (pigmented villonodular tenosynovitis) presents as an intra-articular proliferation predominantly in the knee and hip joint, whereas the extra-articular tumor predominantly involves the periarticular soft tissues in the region of the knee and thigh (some extra-articular tumors have been localized to muscle and subcutis). The tumor has a resemblance to GCTTS, although giant cells are less numerous or absent altogether. Pseudosynovial and blood-filled pseudoalveolar spaces are a common finding in the otherwise monotonous mononuclear proliferation (e-**Fig. 46.24**). Mitotic activity is usually present (in rare cases, >5 mitoses per 10 high-power fields), but atypical mitotic figures are absent. The immunoprofile of CD68, MSA, and desmin expression is the same as for GCTTS.

   Classification of this neoplasm as an intermediate (locally aggressive) tumor is based on the fact that >45% of intra-articular and up to 50% of extra-articular tumors recur. Clearly malignant tumors are associated with the metastasis; this subgroup has a high mitotic rate (>20 mitoses per 10 high-power fields), necrosis, and cellular atypia (*Am J Surg Pathol.* 1997;21:153).

3. **Deep benign fibrous histiocytoma** is a rare tumor of the subcutis, deep soft tissues, and even viscera that occurs over a wide age range, but usually in young

adults. A circumscribed mass, commonly <4 cm in greatest dimension, the tumor is composed of a monomorphic population of bland, plump to spindle cells with indistinct cell borders and storiform profiles. Osteoclast-like giant cells may be present. Stromal myxoid change or hyalinization may also be present.

4. **Fibrohistiocytic lesions** that typically occur in the skin (see Chapter 39) are dermal dendrocytic proliferations like the reticulohistiocytoma and juvenile xanthogranuloma (*Am J Surg Pathol.* 2003;27:579).

B. **Intermediate (rarely metastasizing)**

1. **Plexiform fibrohistiocytic tumor** primarily occurs in the first three decades of life and has a preference for the extremities and head and neck. Grossly, it is a firm, multinodular, and poorly circumscribed mass usually measuring <3 cm in greatest dimension. Microscopically, the architectural pattern is that of nodules or elongated groups of cells with a plexiform arrangement; three cell types are present in the nodules: central multinucleated giant cells, mononuclear histiocyte-like cells, and spindled fibroblast-like cells. Because one of the cell types may dominate, an appreciation of the overall architecture is important for diagnosis. The tumor cells express SMA and vimentin; CD68 reactivity is also present but is confined to the giant cells and mononuclear histiocyte-like cells. Approximately 30%-35% of cases locally recur, and <5% metastasize to regional lymph nodes and beyond (*Arch Pathol Lab Med.* 2007;131:1135; *Am J Dermatopathol.* 2004;26:141).

2. **Giant cell tumor of soft tissue** occurs in the superficial soft tissue of the lower and upper extremities, and occasionally at other sites. It is a circumscribed, nodular mass that has a soft, fleshy, gray to red-brown cut surface. Individual nodules of the mass measure up to 1.5 cm and are separated by fibrous septa that contain hemosiderin-laden macrophages. Admixed mononuclear round to oval cells and multinucleated osteoclast-like giant cells are set in a richly vascular stroma. Mitotic activity can be brisk (up to 30 mitotic figures per 10 high-power fields are often present), but cellular pleomorphism and atypia are absent. Metaplastic bone is noted in up to 50% of cases, and definitive foci of vascular invasion are identified in 30% of cases. The multinucleated giant cells are strongly CD68 immunopositive, whereas the mononuclear cells express SMA and vimentin but show only focal CD68 immunoreactivity.

C. **Malignant**

1. **Pleomorphic malignant fibrous histiocytoma (MFH)/undifferentiated high-grade pleomorphic sarcoma** is the diagnostic term reserved for tumors that, by all current investigational methods, show no evidence of differentiation along a defined cell lineage. Considerable reassessment and revisionism have been directed toward the question of whether MFH represents a specific tumor type or a final common pathway of high-grade sarcomas (*Am J Surg Pathol.* 1992;16:213; *Am J Surg Pathol.* 1996;20:131; and *Am J Surg Pathol.* 2001;25:1030).

The tumor preferentially arises in the extremities and trunk, usually in the deep soft tissue. Individuals older than 40 years present with a rapidly enlarging mass, and about 5% present with metastatic disease, usually in the lung. The tumor may measure in excess of 20 cm and has a white to tan-white, fleshy to fibrous cut surface, with areas of necrosis and hemorrhage. Microscopically, the pattern is often complex (e-**Fig. 46.25**), with field-to-field variation in terms of spindle cells, rounded to ovoid cells, and multinucleated cells. The consistent feature is high nuclear grade with numerous atypical mitotic figures. Extensive necrosis with cystic degeneration and hemorrhage are other common features. Some of these tumors are immunoreactive for SMA and/or desmin, so the differential diagnosis of pleomorphic leiomyosarcoma or myofibrosarcoma must be considered (*Histopathology.* 2001;38:499). The CD68 positivity present in most cases is regarded by some investigators as nonspecific.

2. **Giant cell MFH/undifferentiated pleomorphic sarcoma with giant cells** is a rare neoplasm that is composed of undifferentiated pleomorphic cells with associated stromal osteoclastic giant cells (in contrast to pleomorphic multinucleated tumor cells). Because it is now recognized that a prominent stromal

osteoclastic giant cell reaction is a feature of many poorly differentiated carcinomas as well as sarcomas, putative cases of giant cell MFH should be carefully studied to exclude the presence of an even focal definable line of differentiation indicative of a specific carcinoma or sarcoma type.

3. **Inflammatory MFH/undifferentiated pleomorphic sarcoma with prominent inflammation** is a diagnosis now reserved for an undifferentiated high-grade pleomorphic sarcoma with a prominent neutrophilic infiltrate, in addition to histiocytes, eosinophils, and xanthoma cells. Most cases arise in the retroperitoneum. Some of these tumors may be dedifferentiated liposarcoma (*J Pathol.* 2004;203:822).

VII. SMOOTH MUSCLE TUMORS

A. Benign

1. **Angioleiomyoma** is a deep dermal or subcutaneous neoplasm often associated with pain that in women typically occurs in the lower extremities, but in men more often occurs in the head and upper extremities. These tumors, usually measuring ≤2 cm, consist of three subtypes: a solid subtype of mature smooth muscle cells with virtually no mitotic activity and small slit-like vascular channels; a venous subtype composed of less compact smooth muscle bundles, with venous type vascular channels that blend with the intervascular smooth muscle; and a cavernous subtype with dilated vascular channels with indistinct smooth muscle walls.

B. Leiomyoma of deep soft tissue is a rare neoplasm that, as its name suggests, usually develops in deep subcutis, skeletal muscle, the pelvic retroperitoneum, or the abdominal cavity (typically in the omentum and mesentery). This tumor can measure in excess of 30 cm. It is composed of bland appearing highly differentiated smooth muscle cells that have minimal atypia and a very low mitotic rate (for tumors in the extremities and intra-abdominal tumors in men, the mitotic rate is <1 mitosis per 50 high-power fields; for peritoneal/retroperitoneal tumors in women, the mitotic rate is ≤5 per 50 high-power fields). Although degenerative changes such as fibrosis, myxoid change, hyalinization, or calcification may be present, necrosis is absent. The diagnosis of a deep leiomyoma should be approached with caution from the perspective of no atypia and virtually no mitotic activity (*Adv Anat Pathol.* 2002;9:351 and *Ann Diagn Pathol.* 2003;7:60).

Pilar leiomyoma and uterine smooth muscle tumors are discussed elsewhere (see Chapters 39 and 33, respectively). There is a substantial literature on the cytogenetics of uterine leiomyomas, but considerably less on the extrauterine counterparts (*Cancer Genet Cytogenet.* 2005;158:1).

C. Malignant

1. **Leiomyosarcoma** is typically a sarcoma of mid-life and beyond. There are four clinicopathologic settings: a retroperitoneal tumor, a tumor arising from a large blood vessel with a preference for veins of the lower extremity and inferior vena cava; a subcutaneous or intramuscular tumor of the extremities; and a dermis-based neoplasm. Uterine and intestinal leiomyosarcoma are not considered in this chapter, although the uterus is the most common primary site overall for leiomyosarcoma.

Except for cutaneous leiomyosarcoma, these tumors usually measure in excess of 6 cm and have a trabeculated or smooth, glistening, white-gray cut surface. High-grade tumors are accompanied by necrosis and hemorrhage. Architecturally, the tumors are composed of intersecting bundles of eosinophilic spindle cells with elongated nuclei with blunted ends (**e-Fig. 46.26**). Nuclear pleomorphism and an increased mitotic rate with atypical mitotic forms are characteristic. Poorly differentiated leiomyosarcoma is a pleomorphic high-grade sarcoma the smooth muscle differentiation of which is highlighted by immunoreactivity for SMA, desmin, and h-caldesmon. Focal expression of keratin, EMA, CD34, and S-100 may be present.

A distinct clinicopathologic group of smooth muscle neoplasms is recognized in the immunocompromised setting; these tumors are associated with genomic integration of Epstein–Barr virus (EBV) (*J Clin Pathol.* 2007;60:1358 and *Am J Surg Pathol.* 2006;30:75) and have been described in both visceral and soft tissue sites. Pathologically, these tumors have low-grade spindle cell features to the extent that the traditional criteria for the diagnosis leiomyosarcoma are not met in all cases, and are sometimes therefore designated as EBV-associated smooth muscle tumors.

VIII. PERICYTIC (PERIVASCULAR) TUMORS. Tumors in this category show evidence of myoid/contractile perivascular cell differentiation. Morphologically, they have a tendency to grow in a circumferential perivascular pattern.

A. **Benign**

1. **Glomus tumor** usually occurs in the subungual region of the hand, wrist, and foot, but not to the exclusion of other sites including the viscera. Glomus tumors are <1 cm in most cases, and are painful with minimal tactile stimulation or exposure to cold. Microscopically, these tumors consist of a mixture of glomus cells (characterized as uniform, small, rounded cells with eosinophilic to amphophilic cytoplasm and a central nucleus), smooth muscle cells, and central vascular space (e-Fig. 46.27). Based on the relative proportion of these three elements, there are three subtypes of glomus tumor: solid, composed of nests of glomus cells surrounding capillary-sized vessels; glomangioma, composed of small clusters of glomus cells surrounding dilated vessels; and glomangiomyoma, in which there is a transition from typical round glomus cells to elongated cells that resemble mature smooth muscle.

2. **Myopericytoma,** previously interpreted as a hemangiopericytoma, usually arises in the subcutis of the distal extremities. Less than 2 cm in greatest dimension, this tumor is unencapsulated but well circumscribed. Microscopically, the tumor is composed of a densely cellular population of oval to spindle-shaped cells with eosinophilic to amphophilic cytoplasm arranged in multilayered concentric profiles around compressed blood vessels. Mitotic figures are inconspicuous. There is diffuse immunopositivity for SMA and focal immunopositivity for CD34.

B. **Malignant**

1. **Malignant glomus tumor** (glomangiosarcoma) is rare and seemingly arises from a benign-appearing glomus tumor. The characteristic findings are a visceral or subfascial origin, a size >2 cm, marked nuclear atypia, and atypical mitotic figures. However, a subset of tumors does not have all of these findings; these cases are designated as tumors of uncertain malignant potential (*Am J Surg Pathol.* 2001;25:1). The round cell type is composed of poorly differentiated round cells, so SMA and pericellular type IV collagen are required for diagnosis. A spindle cell variant has features of leiomyosarcoma or fibrosarcoma.

IX. SKELETAL MUSCLE

A. **Non-neoplastic disorders**

1. **Preparation of skeletal muscle biopsies.** Histopathologic examination of skeletal muscle biopsies, whether attained through an open biopsy or through a needle biopsy, continues to have a critical role in the evaluation of patients with suspected myopathy (*Curr Neurol Neurosci Rep.* 2004;4:81). One portion of the biopsy should be formalin fixed and paraffin embedded according to standard laboratory protocols; another should be frozen for enzyme histochemistry studies; and the remainder should be fixed in glutaraldehyde for electron microscopic studies. Although the histopathologic evaluation of skeletal muscle biopsies is a key component in the evaluation of neuromuscular disorders, and can be used to diagnose a variety of inherited, inflammatory, and toxic myopathies, it should only be performed in the context of a thorough history and clinical examination that has included appropriate laboratory studies (including measurement of serum creatine kinase) and electromyography. A number of inflammatory, toxic, and axial myopathies have characteristic histopathologic findings, and immunohistochemical studies can be used to characterize inflammatory infiltrates when present (*Autoimmunity.* 2006;39:161).

2. **Muscular dystrophies** and other congenital myopathies are diagnosed primarily based on clinical and electromyographic features. Increasingly, the

histopathologic evaluation of muscle biopsies in these settings has been supplanted by genetic testing as an increasing number of diseases has been characterized at a genetic level (*Pediatr Dev Pathol.* 2006;9:427 and *Brain Pathol.* 2001;11:206).

3. **Mitochondrial myopathies,** which traditionally have been diagnosed based on the demonstration of so-called ragged-red fibers by Gomori trichrome stain, are increasingly diagnosed based on genetic testing because the genetic abnormalities in mitochondria that underlie these diseases have recently been characterized (*Submicrosc Cytol Pathol.* 2006;38:201 and *Biosci Rep.* 2007;27:23).

B. **Benign tumors**

1. **Rhabdomyoma** by definition shows skeletal muscle differentiation, and includes cardiac rhabdomyoma and extracardiac rhabdomyoma (which has two subtypes: fetal and adult). Both cardiac and fetal rhabdomyomas may be hamartomas rather than true neoplasms; tuberous sclerosis and nevoid basal cell carcinoma syndrome, respectively, accompany these tumors.

   a. **Fetal rhabdomyoma** occurs almost exclusively in children younger than 10 years, with a predilection for the postauricular region and chest wall. The tumor forms a nodule in the subcutis or deeper soft tissues that has a circumscribed noninfiltrative pattern and is composed of bundles of fetal myotubes with interspersed small immature-appearing mesenchymal cells. The classic or myxoid pattern must be differentiated from embryonal rhabdomyosarcoma, the latter of which has a less well-organized pattern, hyperchromatic nuclei, and mitotic figures. The so-called intermediate or cellular pattern (juvenile rhabdomyoma) is characterized by skeletal muscle differentiation beyond the fetal myotube stage.

   b. **Adult rhabdomyoma** is solitary in 75%–80% of cases, but in about 25% of cases is multinodular and even multicentric. Microscopically, lobules of large uniform polygonal cells with abundant granular, vacuolated, or eosinophilic cytoplasm; well-defined cell borders; and round nuclei with a prominent nucleolus are present. Cytoplasmic cross-striations and rod-like inclusions are also present, in addition to abundant glycogen. Complete excision is recommended, because recurrence occurs in >40% of cases that have been incompletely excised.

   c. **Genital rhabdomyoma** presents almost exclusively in the vagina in women between the ages of 35 and 50 years as a solitary 1- to 3-cm polyp that may have been present for several years. Microscopically, bland, interlacing, haphazardly arranged rounded to strap-like cells that have abundant eosinophilic cytoplasm with cross-striations, cytoplasmic glycogen, and a centrally located round nucleus with a prominent nucleolus are present. The tumor cells are embedded in a fibrous stroma with dilated vessels. Local excision is curative.

C. **Malignant tumors**

1. **Embryonal rhabdomyosarcoma** (ERMS) is the most common soft tissue sarcoma of childhood (50%–60% of cases), typically presents before 10 years of age, and accounts for 75%–85% of all rhabdomyosarcomas. The other types of rhabdomyosarcoma, alveolar and pleomorphic rhabdomyosarcomas, comprise 20%–30% and ≤5%, respectively. ERMS has a predilection for the head and neck (25%–35% of cases) and pelvis–genitourinary tract (30%–40% of cases). Unlike alveolar rhabdomyosarcoma (ARMS), a minority of ERMS presents in the peripheral soft tissues. The three basic microscopic patterns of ERMS are botryoid, spindle, and not otherwise specified (NOS), which proportionately account for 5%, 10%, and 85% of cases, respectively. The botryoid and spindle subtypes have a "superior" outcome, whereas the NOS subtype has an "intermediate" to "poor" prognosis (*Pediatr Dev Pathol.* 1998;1:550). Pathologic staging of childhood rhabdomyosarcoma has a number of variables (Table 46.5).

   Because most ERMSs occur at sites that do not lend themselves to primary surgical resection with the prospect of negative tumor margins, biopsies and post-treatment excisions are the two specimen types seen most often in the laboratory. In general, ERMS is a soft, often gelatinous–myxoid mass the shape and size of which accommodate its anatomic site. When the tumor arises in

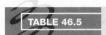

TABLE 46.5	Tumor, Node, Metastasis (TNM) Staging of Childhood Rhabdomyosarcoma[a]				
Stage	**Sites**	**T invasiveness**	**T size**	**Regional nodes**	**Metastases**
I	Orbit	T1 or T2	a or b	N0N1 or NX	M0
	Head and neck[b]	T1 or T2	a or b	N0N1 or NX	M0
	Genitourinary[c]	T1 or T2	a or b	N0N1 or NX	M0
II	Bladder/prostate	T1 or T2	a	N0 or NX	M0
	Extremity	T1 or T2	a	N0 or NX	M0
	Cranial parameningeal	T1 or T2	a	N0 or NX	M0
	Others[d]	T1 or T2	a	N0 or NX	M0
III	Bladder/prostate	T1 or T2	a	N1	M0
	Extremity	T1 or T2	b	N0N1 or NX	M0
	Cranial parameningeal	T1 or T2	b	N0N1 or NX	M0
	Others[d]	T1 or T2	b	N0N1 or NX	M0
IV	All	T1 or T2	a or b	N0 or N1	M1

T1, confined to anatomic site of origin; T2, extension; a, <5 cm in diameter; b, ≥5 cm in diameter; N0, not clinically involved; N1, clinically involved; NX, clinical status unknown; M0, no distant metastasis; M1, distant metastasis present.
[a]TNM pretreatment staging classification for the Intergroup Rhabdomyosarcoma Study-IV.
[b]Excluding parameningeal.
[c]Nonbladder/nonprostate.
[d]Includes trunk, retroperitoneum, and so on.
From *Pediatr Dev Pathol.* 1998;1:550.

a hollow space or viscus like the nasopharynx, common bile duct, bladder, or vagina, it has a polypoid configuration that features the botryoid pattern of small primitive cells concentrated beneath the surface epithelium; interspersed among the small cells, differentiated rhabdomyoblasts may be identified. Otherwise, the tumor (which may measure up to 20 cm in diameter) has a round to ovoid configuration without a delicate capsule or pseudocapsule; the cut surface has a faint multilobular appearance in which hemorrhage is more common than necrosis, with a consistency that reflects the content of the stroma.

It is a mistake to think that ERMS is a "round cell" neoplasm. The morphology of the tumor cells is diverse, ranging from short spindle or round to ovoid cells with or without a delicate cytoplasmic tail, to larger cells with pale vacuolated to eosinophilic cytoplasm (e-**Fig. 46.28**). The intercellular space has a pale mucoid to myxoid appearance. Where there is stroma, the tumor cells are larger, more compact, and more likely to have bright eosinophilic cytoplasm. In many tumors, the fact that no two high-magnification microscopic fields have identical features reflects the polymorphous character of many ERMS. Diffuse and/or lobular growth patterns are seen either as a dominant or mixed feature. Those tumors composed of predominately spindle cells resemble a leiomyosarcoma or fibrosarcoma, but with immature rhabdomyoblasts among the spindle cells.

A difficult assessment is the determination of "viable" tumor in a posttreatment biopsy. By convention, if the biopsy contains tumor cells with features seen in the pretreatment biopsy, residual viable tumor is present. Differentiated rhabdomyoblasts with negative Ki-67 (MIB-1) staining are considered nonproliferative and nonviable.

The immunophenotype correlates with the degree of skeletal muscle differentiation. Primitive ERMS may show only vimentin expression, although myoD1 and/or myogenin nuclear positivity is often present in scattered tumor cells. Differentiating rhabdomyoblasts show desmin and/or MSA expression, whereas differentiated cells also are immunoreactive for myosin.

2. **ARMS** is the quintessential malignant round cell neoplasm of childhood. Most cases are diagnosed in adolescents and young adults, although the tumor also occurs in infants. Primary sites include the extremities, perispinal and perineal regions, and the paranasal sinuses. Microscopically, the tumor has two general patterns: solid sheets of uniform high-grade round cells without extracellular mucin, and the classic alveolar pattern with incomplete fibrovascular septa dividing the loosely arranged cells into nests (e-**Fig. 46.29**). Both patterns can be seen in metastatic ARMS (the initial encounter with the tumor may be in a lymph node or bone metastasis as ARMS may present with disseminated metastatic disease). Most ARMS are strongly immunopositive for desmin and neuron-specific enolase (NSE).

   Regardless of the pathologic stage, ARMS is an "unfavorable" histology neoplasm and managed as such. Approximately 90% of tumors have a balanced *PAX3*- or *PAX7-FKHR* translocation (Table 46.1). The less common t(1;13) is found more often in those tumors in younger children and is correlated with a more favorable outcome (*Curr Oncol Rep.* 2002;4:123).

3. **Pleomorphic rhabdomyosarcoma** is a high-grade sarcoma that presents in the deep soft tissues of the lower extremities. Less than 5% of cases occur in children. It is a poorly differentiated pleomorphic round to spindle cell neoplasm in which the cells have abundant eosinophilic cytoplasm with or without cross-striations. The tumor cells express desmin and MyoD1, and show variable expression of myogenin, SMA, and MSA.

4. **Ectomesenchymoma** is a rare neoplasm that occurs in children for the most part. It may have ERMS- or ARMS-like features, with populations of cells with a range of neural differentiation, from ganglion cells to more primitive neuroectodermal cells that express a variety of neural and myogenic markers.

X. VASCULAR DISEASES

A. **Inflammatory lesions.** Inflammatory disorders of the vessels, including the vasculitides, are covered in more detail in the chapter on the cardiovascular system (see Chapter 9).

B. **Reactive vascular proliferations** include lesions that are generally thought to be reactive and non-neoplastic, although many mimic vascular tumors clinicopathologically.

   1. **Papillary endothelial hyperplasia** (Masson's vegetant hemangioma) is usually subdivided into a primary type (occurring in a vein in the head and neck or fingers) and a secondary type (arising in a pre-existing hemangioma, hemorrhoidal vein, or thrombohematoma). Microscopically, numerous, small, delicate papillae with hyaline cores project into a vascular lumen (e-**Fig. 46.30**). Often there is a transition between an organizing fibrin clot and the papillary endothelial hyperplasia. A single layer of plump endothelial cells without appreciable cytologic atypia differentiates it in part from angiosarcoma, which does not arise from a blood vessel or hematoma. With continued organization of the clot, the papillae fuse and form an anastomosing network of vessels with eventual recanalization.

   2. **Glomeruloid hemangioma** is an uncommon, multifocal, primarily intravascular capillary proliferation that is associated with Castleman disease and the POEMS (*p*olyneuropathy, *o*rganomegaly, *e*ndocrinopathy, *M* protein, and *s*kin changes) syndrome. Glomeruloid capillary proliferations within blood vessels of the dermis, deep soft tissue, or viscera are the microscopic features. Glomeruloid capillary tufts have an outer layer of pericytes but are lined by bland endothelial cells with or without cytoplasmic vacuolation.

   3. **Bacillary angiomatosis** is a reactive vascular proliferation that occurs almost exclusively in immunocompromised patients. It is caused by gram-negative bacilli of the genus *Bartonella*.

   4. **Vascular transformation of lymph nodes** (nodal angiomatosis) occurs as a secondary change in lymph nodes due to lymphatic and/or venous obstruction. Ectatic capillary-sized vessels within the subcapsular space and nodal sinuses are the microscopic features. The differential diagnosis is Kaposi sarcoma.

C. Benign vascular tumors

1. **Hemangioma** is the most common cutaneous and soft tissue tumor of infancy and childhood, and accounts for approximately 7% of benign soft tissue tumors overall. Although most hemangiomas are superficially located, the liver and parotid gland may be involved in infants (*J Pediatr Surg.* 2007;42:62 and *Ann Diagn Pathol.* 2002;6:339). Recently, there has been substantial revision in the classification of vasoformative lesions into vascular neoplasms or malformations based in part on glucose transporter 1 (GLUT-1) immunoreactivity in the majority of vascular neoplasms and its absence in malformations (*Clin Plast Surg.* 2005;32:99 and *Hum Pathol.* 2000;31:11).

   a. Juvenile capillary hemangioma is the most common type of hemangioma, usually diagnosed in infants and children, and has a predilection for the head and neck. Most lesions show complete involution by the time the child is 6 or 7 years old, although a minority persist. Clinically, the tumor is a purple to reddish macule or nodule centered in the skin or subcutaneous tissue. Microscopically, lobules of capillary-sized vessels are supplied by a feeder vessel (e-**Fig. 46.31**). Vascular space formation varies from minimal with cellular lobules and scattered mitotic figures, to those with obvious luminal formation.

   There are several variants of juvenile capillary hemangioma: lobular capillary hemangioma (so-called pyogenic granuloma) in the superficial dermis with or without surface ulceration and associated inflammation; tufted angioma resembling a cellular juvenile capillary hemangioma but with discontinuous capillary lobules; verrucous hemangioma with a mixture of cavernous and capillary vessels immediately beneath a hyperkeratotic, acanthotic epidermis; and cherry angioma as a suspected involuted lobular capillary hemangioma.

   b. Cavernous hemangioma occurs in the same age range and anatomic distribution as juvenile hemangiomas but is less frequent, shows virtually no tendency to regress, and may be locally destructive due to the extrinsic pressure on adjacent structures. A pattern of grouped dilated, thin-walled blood vessels with an inconspicuous endothelial lining is the microscopic appearance. The blue-rubber-bleb nevus syndrome (characterized by cavernous hemangiomas of the skin and gastrointestinal tract) and Maffucci syndrome (cavernous hemangiomas and enchondromas) are two associated syndromes.

   c. Arteriovenous hemangioma, also known as arteriovenous malformation, is a benign vascular malformation associated with arteriovenous shunts. It is found more commonly in the skin than in the deep soft tissue. It is composed of a mixture of arterial vessels and thick-walled veins with variable circumscription, and may have areas of vascular thrombosis and associated dystrophic calcification.

   d. Venous hemangioma (venous malformation) typically presents during adulthood in the deep soft tissue. Ectatic vessels often show thrombosis and dystrophic calcification.

   e. Spindle cell hemangioma occurs in young adults and is found in the skin and subcutis of the distal extremities, especially the hand. Microscopically, thin-walled cavernous vessels lined by bland flattened endothelium are admixed with solid areas composed of plump spindled cells. The tumor involves a large pre-existing vessel in many cases. Recurrences are common (>50% of cases), often with a discontinuous growth pattern.

   f. Synovial hemangioma, as the name implies, arises in synovium-lined spaces, most commonly in the knee in the second decade of life. Microscopically, variably sized thin-walled vascular spaces occupy the stroma of hyperplastic synovium with associated marked hemosiderin deposition. The differential diagnosis includes pigmented villonodular synovitis and trauma-associated hemarthrosis as in hemophilia.

   g. Intramuscular angioma (intramuscular hemangioma, skeletal muscle hemangioma) most frequently arises in the lower extremity, particularly the muscles of the thigh. Microscopically, it is a poorly circumscribed and diffusely infiltrating mass in the muscle composed of variably sized vessels ranging from large thick-walled veins to cavernous vascular spaces, small arteries, and capillaries, and thus has features more in keeping with an arterial-venous malformation. Despite the presence of mitotic activity and intraluminal capillary tufting, freely anastomosing vascular channels are not present.

2. **Epithelioid hemangioma** occurs mainly in women between 20 and 40 years old as a small, dull erythematous plaque in the head and neck. Microscopically, it is a well-circumscribed nodule in the dermis or subcutis, or less frequently in the deep soft tissue, that has a vague lobular pattern of clustered small capillary-sized vessels around a feeder vessel. The endothelial cells are plump and have abundant cytoplasm with impingement on the lumen of the vascular channel (so-called tombstone appearance). When lymphocytes and eosinophils are prominent, the lesion is an example of "angiomatoid hyperplasia with eosinophilia."

3. **Angiomatosis** is, by definition, a poorly circumscribed, diffuse network of vascular structures within a soft tissue site. In virtually all cases it presents during childhood or adolescence as diffuse soft tissue swelling. The GLUT-1 immunonegative vessels are consistent with the interpretation that angiomatosis is a malformation. There are two histologic patterns: mixed-vessel–type lesions resembling an intramuscular angioma, and capillary-predominant–type lesions with a lobular pattern. Mature adipose tissue may be intermixed accounting for an earlier designation as infiltrating angiolipoma.

4. **Lymphangiomas** are cavernous and/or cystic vascular lesions composed of dilated lymphatic channels that occur most commonly in the head and neck of young children (as, e.g., a hygroma). Thin-walled dilated lymphatic vessels of varying size are lined by flattened endothelium, beneath which are lymphoid aggregates (e-Fig. 46.32).

5. **Atypical vascular lesion of the breast** presents as papules, nodules, or erythema several years (average 5 years, range 2 to 20 years) after external radiation for carcinoma of the breast. This lesion is composed of thin-walled vascular spaces resembling lymphatics and is confined to the superficial dermis. An infiltrating, more diffuse pattern into the deeper dermis and atypia of endothelial cells should be viewed with concern (*J Am Acad Dermatol*. 2007;57:126).

D. **Intermediate (locally aggressive) vascular tumors**

1. **Kaposiform hemangioendothelioma,** an uncommon deep soft tissue tumor, occurs primarily in children and teenagers and may be associated with the Kasabach–Merritt syndrome, especially in the presence of a retroperitoneal mass measuring ≥20 cm. The multinodular, poorly circumscribed, infiltrating tumor mass is highly cellular microscopically with an overall lobular architecture. Individual lobules consist of a mixture of capillary-sized vessels that blend with more slit-like spindle vessels, with an absence of mitoses and cytologic atypia (*Am J Surg Pathol*. 2004;28:559). There are overlapping microscopic features with the hemangioma (*J Pediatr*. 1997;130:631). These tumors are lethal in 20% of cases because of the associated coagulopathy.

E. **Intermediate (rarely metastasizing) vascular tumors**

1. **Retiform hemangioendothelioma,** an uncommon neoplasm, arises in the skin of the distal extremities, primarily in young adults, and has a high recurrence rate without wide excision. Grossly, the tumor is a reddish-purple slowly growing plaque centered in the reticular dermis, usually <2 to 3 cm in maximal dimension. The tumor is characterized microscopically by elongated, arborizing, narrow vessels that resemble the rete testis (*Am J Surg Pathol*. 1994;18:115). The endothelial cells are monomorphic with a low mitotic rate, hyperchromatic nuclei, and hobnail morphology. The stroma between the vascular channels is prominent and often shows an abundant lymphocytic infiltrate.

2. **Papillary intralymphatic angioendothelioma** (Dabska tumor) occurs in infants and children with a predilection for the skin, and usually presents as a slowly growing nodule or plaque. On microscopic examination, thin-walled vascular spaces that contain intraluminal papillary tufts of endothelial cells with a hobnail morphology are present.

3. **Kaposi sarcoma** is a low-grade clonal endothelial proliferation that is caused by human herpesvirus 8 (HHV8) infection. The clinicopathologic features of Kaposi sarcoma are discussed in more detail in the chapter on nonmelanocytic tumors of the skin (Chapter 39).

F. **Malignant vascular tumors**

1. **Epithelioid hemangioendothelioma** (intravascular bronchioloalveolar tumor) is a low-grade malignant endothelial neoplasm that occurs in patients of all ages, although it is rare in early childhood. The superficial and deep soft tissues, viscera (liver), and bone are various primary sites. About 10% of patients have multiorgan disease at the time of presentation.

   Grossly, the tumor presents as a poorly circumscribed multilobular infiltrative mass measuring up to 10 cm in greatest dimension, or as multiple lesions. A vascular origin is not apparent. Microscopically, the tumor consists of cords, short strands, solid nests, or individual cells that have rounded to slightly spindled features (e-**Fig. 46.33**). The cells are low grade with a low mitotic rate. Endothelial differentiation is evident by the formation of intracytoplasmic lumina (signet ring–like features), but distinct vascular channels are not prominent. The neoplastic cells are classically embedded within a chondroid-like to hyalinized stroma. Atypical morphologic features—including an increased mitotic rate, increased nuclear pleomorphism, more spindled cytology, and necrosis—correlate with more aggressive behavior. The tumor cells express CD31, CD34, and *Ulex Europaeus* antigen, and variably express Factor XIII–related antigen. Of note, 25%–30% of tumors show focal cytokeratin expression, which can lead to an incorrect diagnosis of metastatic signet ring cell carcinoma.

2. **Angiosarcoma,** a rare malignancy composed of endothelial cells, recapitulates the functional and morphologic features of normal endothelium to a variable degree. The tumor is divided into several groups: cutaneous angiosarcoma (associated and unassociated with lymphedema); angiosarcoma of the breast; radiation-induced angiosarcoma; and angiosarcoma of the deep soft tissue. The malignancy is a poorly circumscribed hemorrhagic mass measuring from 1 to 2 cm to >10 cm, with histologic features that vary from hemangioma-like (but with scattered, enlarged, atypical endothelial cells with occasional mitotic figures and an infiltrating growth pattern) to a high-grade spindle cell sarcoma with a hemorrhagic background (e-**Fig. 46.34**). Intraluminal papillae lined by hyperchromatic cells are sometimes present. Vascular channels with a dissecting pattern of infiltration through the dermis or other surrounding tissues should be viewed with concern (see atypical vascular lesion of breast discussed above).

   Epithelioid angiosarcoma, a well-recognized variant of angiosarcoma in the deep soft tissues, is composed of malignant epithelioid cells with abundant eosinophilic or amphophilic cytoplasm, large vesicular nuclei, and prominent nucleoli (e-**Fig. 46.35**).

XI. **CHONDRO-OSSEOUS TUMORS**

A. **Benign**

1. **Chondroma** occurs over a broad age range usually in the fingers and toes, with a juxta-articular and tendinous predilection. There is a local recurrence rate of 15%–20%. Chondromas are typically composed of lobules of mature hyaline cartilage, but there are variants: chondroblastic chondroma (when the lesion is cellular), fibrochondroma (when there is prominent fibrosis), and osteochondroma (when there is prominent ossification). Chondromyxoid fibroma and chondroblastoma typically arise in bone but have been reported in the soft tissues. If the chondroid tumor is from the base of the skull, chondroid chordoma should be considered.

B. **Malignant**

1. **Mesenchymal chondrosarcoma,** a rare variant of chondrosarcoma, is seen in individuals between 15 and 40 years old and presents in the soft tissues (25%–30%) or bone (70%–75%), with some preference for the head and neck (meninges, orbit), spine, and lower extremities. Microscopically, neoplastic-appearing hyaline cartilage is interspersed in a background of nodules or

sheets of undifferentiated malignant small round cells, with or without a hemangiopericytoma-like appearance. The undifferentiated cells show vimentin and membranous CD99 immunopositivity, and the cartilage expresses S-100.

2. **Extraskeletal osteosarcoma** usually arises in the deep soft tissue, most commonly in the thigh, although the buttock, shoulder girdle, trunk, and retroperitoneum in individuals between 40 and 60 years old. About 10% of patients have a history of prior radiation or trauma to the site. The prognosis is poor with a 5-year survival of 25%.

   Neoplastic bone is usually most prominent in the center of the tumor, whereas more peripheral regions of the neoplasm tend to be more densely cellular (this zonation is the reverse of the pattern present in myositis ossificans and can be a useful feature for differential diagnosis).

XII. PERIPHERAL NERVE TUMORS. The tumors of presumed peripheral nerve or nerve sheath derivation comprise some of the more common soft tissue neoplasms in routine practice.

A. **Benign**

1. **Traumatic neuroma** is a non-neoplastic proliferation in response to nerve injury, often after a surgical procedure. It is a firm, tender nodule measuring <5 cm that is composed of small proliferating nerve fascicles in a haphazard architectural pattern of Schwann cells and fibroblasts in a fibromyxoid stroma (e-**Fig. 46.36**).

2. **Mucosal neuromas** on the lips, mouth, eyelids, and intestines are manifestations of multiple endocrine neoplasia IIB. The irregular nerve bundles in the submucosa have a prominent perineurium; often the immediately adjacent stroma shows myxoid change.

3. **Neurofibromas** are divided into three types based on a growth pattern: localized, diffuse, and plexiform.

   a. **Localized neurofibroma** is sporadic, usually superficial and solitary, and unassociated with a genetic syndrome. The dermis and subcutis are the sites of predilection. Microscopically, the circumscribed nodule is composed of neural bundles with wavy nuclei and strands of collagen in a neurofibrillary background that contains mast cells. The differential diagnosis is a dermal melanocytic nevus with extensive neurotization.

   b. **Plexiform neurofibromas** are manifestations of neurofibromatosis 1 (NF1), as are diffuse neurofibromas (*Lancet Neurol.* 2007;6:340). Plexiform neurofibromas develop in early childhood as superficial soft tissue masses, and vary in size and extent of local involvement. An entire length of nerve can be transformed into the so-called "bag-of-worms" appearance in which multiple nerve bundles characteristically show expansion of the endoneurium by a myxoid stroma, with later extension beyond the perineurium into the adjacent soft tissue (e-**Fig. 46.37**). The interstitium is composed of thickened irregular fibrous bundles with interspersed short to fusiform spindle cells, and a diffuse pattern may accompany the plexiform component in the surrounding soft tissues. Foci of increased cellularity with associated enlarged, hyperchromatic nuclei should be viewed with concern about malignant transformation (e-**Fig. 46.38**).

   c. **Diffuse neurofibroma** has a predilection for the head and neck as a plaque-like elevation of the skin. The dermis and subcutis are effaced by a uniformly cellular proliferation within a fibrillary collagenous matrix containing Schwann cells with short uniform nuclei (e-**Fig. 46.39**) and occasional Meissner body–like formations. Some tumors are associated with other mesenchymal elements including ectatic vessels and mature entrapped adipose tissue.

4. **Schwannoma** (neurilemoma) most often occurs in patients between 20 and 40 years old, but is also seen in children. Most schwannomas present as a solitary mass in the head and neck, on the flexor surfaces of the upper and lower extremities, or in association with spinal and paraspinal sensory nerves. Multiple schwannomas are manifestations of NF2 and schwannomatosis (*Annu*

Rev Pathol. 2007;2:191). Bilateral vestibular schwannomas are one of several diagnostic features of NF2.

The tumors vary in size, but virtually all are invested by a true capsule of the epineurium. The cut surface ranges from white to yellow-white, with or without cystic degeneration. Most tumors are <5 cm in greatest dimension, although those that arise in the paraspinal retroperitoneum can be larger. The characteristic low-power microscopic pattern (e-**Fig. 46.40**) consists of alternating Antoni A areas (consisting of organized spindle cells with [e-**Fig. 46.41**] or without Verocay bodies) and Antoni B areas (consisting of less cellular regions in which the oval to spindled cells are arranged more haphazardly in a loose fibrous matrix). There is considerable histologic variability in schwannomas; despite atypical findings, especially in so-called ancient-type schwannomas, these tumors rarely undergo malignant transformation (characterized by invasion through the capsule, epithelioid or small cell transformation, high-grade nuclear abnormalities, and atypical mitotic figures). It is noteworthy that epithelioid morphology alone is an insufficient criterion for malignancy because there is an epithelioid variant of schwannoma. The tumor cells are diffusely immunopositive for S-100 protein and collagen type IV, with intercellular reactivity reflecting basement membrane-like deposition.

5. **Granular cell tumor** occurs in virtually all age ranges, although more frequently in adults than children. There is a predilection for the skin and sites in the head and neck. One unique type, the congenital epulis of the anterior gingival region in neonates, does not express S-100 protein (non-neural granular cell tumor). Several histologic patterns are seen, including closely apposed nests and ribbons, infiltrating cords, and confluent sheets of uniform polygonal to slightly spindled cells with a central nucleus that is surrounded by abundant uniform granular cytoplasm (e-**Fig. 46.42**). Pseudoepitheliomatous hyperplasia may be present in the overlying epidermis or squamous mucosa. Malignancy is rare, but is well documented (*Am J Surg Pathol.* 1998;22:779). Strong immunoreactivity for S-100, NSE, and CD68 is the usual phenotype of the neural granular cell tumor.

6. **Neurothekeoma** (nerve sheath myxoma), a rare tumor in children and young adults, presents in the head and neck and shoulders. Microscopically, nodules of bland, plump spindle cells are present in a myxoid matrix, separated by fibrous connective tissue (e-**Fig. 46.43**). The cells show little pleomorphism and have a low mitotic rate. Tumors that show increased cellularity, cytologic atypia, increased mitotic figures, extension into adjacent or deep soft tissues, and even vascular invasion are regarded as the atypical variant (*Am J Surg Pathol.* 1998;22:1067).

7. **Perineurioma** is an uncommon neoplasm composed of perineural cells whose expression of EMA is similar to that of meningothelial cells. The two types of perineurioma include those that arise within or external to a nerve (*Arch Pathol Lab Med.* 2007;131:625). The tumor has several histologic patterns, including a lacy and reticulated network of delicate to somewhat more plump fusiform spindle cells, and a more cellular pattern of storiform perivascular spindle cells. The background may be sclerotic or, more typically, myxoid.

B. **Malignant.** All malignant tumors that arise from peripheral nerves are currently classified as malignant peripheral nerve sheath tumors (MPNSTs). A sarcoma can be classified as an MPNST if it has arisen from a peripheral nerve, if it has arisen from a pre-existing benign nerve sheath tumor (in most cases, a neurofibroma), or if it demonstrates histologic and immunophenotype features that reflect Schwannian differentiation.

MPNSTs are large (in excess of 5 cm) fusiform neoplasms and have a fleshy mucoid cut surface with large areas of hemorrhage and necrosis. Microscopically, they are composed of interlacing fascicles or broad sweeping profiles of malignant spindle cells that have wavy or comma-shaped nuclei. The cellular density often varies, producing a "light-cell, dark-cell" appearance (e-**Fig. 46.44**). Nuclear palisading is present in some tumors, as are hyalinized cords and nodules that may resemble large rosettes. The immunophenotype tends toward Schwannian differentiation when S-100 positivity is demonstrated (only in 50% of cases), but is more commonly positive for LEU-7, collagen type IV, and myelin basic protein.

Variant patterns of MPNST include rhabdomyoblastic differentiation (malignant triton tumor in NF), glandular formation, and heterotopic bone and/or cartilage formation.

XIII. TUMORS OF UNCERTAIN DIFFERENTIATION. For many of the tumors in this category, the cell type that produces the tumor, the normal cell type that the tumor is recapitulating, or both is unknown.

A. Benign

1. **Intramuscular myxoma** occurs primarily in adults between 40 and 60 years old as a solitary, painless, slowly growing intramuscular mass arising in the thigh, buttocks, or limb girdle. Most tumors are about 5 cm in maximal dimension, and are well circumscribed with a pale gelatinous or myxoid cut surface. The tumor cells are small, bland, stellate to spindle in shape, have a very low mitotic rate, and are present in an abundant myxoid matrix that contains an inconspicuous vascular network (e-**Fig. 46.45**). The cellular variant of the neoplasm can be a diagnostic challenge.

   Simple excision is followed by a low recurrence rate of <5% of cases. The differential diagnosis of a myxoma includes many other myxoid tumors of the soft tissues (*Histopathology.* 1999;35:291 and *Ann Diagn Pathol.* 2000;4:99). One or more myxomas of the soft tissues with fibrous dysplasia defines Mazabraud syndrome. Multiple cutaneous and mucosal myxomas are features of the Carney complex (*Lancet Oncol.* 2005;6:501).

2. **Juxta-articular myxoma,** as the name suggests, usually arises in the vicinity of a large joint (primarily the knee). The lesion a predilection for men between 20 and 40 years old, and is usually <5 cm in maximal dimension. This tumor is indistinguishable from an intramuscular myxoma, although some cases may have hemorrhage and hemosiderin deposition, chronic inflammation, and fibrosis.

3. **Digital myxoma** (digital mucus cyst) usually occurs on a finger, usually in adult women as a painful nodule <1 cm in diameter. Histologically, it resembles intramuscular myxoma. Cutaneous myxoma (also known as superficial angiomyxoma) is a cutaneous or subcutaneous lesion that occurs primarily in adults between 30 and 50 years of age.

4. **Deep "aggressive" angiomyxoma** is a slowly growing locally infiltrative tumor that usually occurs in the pelviperineal soft tissue of women, but is also seen as a scrotal mass (*Int J Gynecol Pathol.* 2005;24:26 and *Int J Urol.* 2003;10:672). It forms a soft, poorly circumscribed mass measuring 10 to 20 cm in greatest dimension that has a gelatinous cut surface. Small stellate to spindled cells with ill-defined cytoplasm and bland nuclei are set in a myxoid stroma rich in collagen fibers (e-**Fig. 46.46**). Numerous, variably sized, thick- or thin-walled vascular channels are present, from which smooth muscle seems to spin off and merge with the surrounding stroma. The tumor cells express vimentin and desmin, and also usually show nuclear expression of estrogen and progesterone receptors.

   The tumor has the propensity to recur, which is not unexpected given its infiltrative and poorly defined margin. Local control is usually possible without radical surgery, and the tumor does not metastasize.

5. **Pleomorphic hyalinizing angiectatic tumor of soft parts** (hemosiderotic fibrohistiocytic lipomatous lesion), a slowly growing tumor, usually arises in the subcutis of the lower extremity in adults. The tumor is characterized by a background of thin-walled ectatic blood vessels within a stroma that contains large, pleomorphic, plump spindled to round tumor cells that have a low mitotic rate. Although the tumor may recur after excision, aggressively in some cases, its potential for metastatic spread appears limited (*Am J Surg Pathol.* 2004;28:1417).

B. Intermediate (rarely metastasizing)

1. **Angiomatoid fibrous histiocytoma,** a slowly growing tumor usually arising in the lower dermis or subcutis of the limbs, trunk, or head and neck, occurs in children and young adults. The tumor may achieve a size of 12 cm, although most cases are much smaller. Its cut surface is usually multinodular and

hemorrhagic, with blood-filled cystic spaces. The neoplastic population consists of plump to spindled cells, with interspersed pseudoangiomatous or aneurysmal spaces (e-**Fig. 46.47**). Hemorrhage and inflammation are usually present in the background (*Hum Pathol.* 1999;30:1336). The tumor cells express vimentin, desmin, CD57 (Leu-7), and CD68. This neoplasm has a characteristic pattern of cytogenetic abnormalities (Table 46.1).

2. **Ossifying fibromyxoid tumor** is seen in adults as a longstanding painless extremity mass measuring 3 to 5 cm in greatest dimension. Soft tissue, skin, and bone are some of the primary sites of the tumor. Microscopically, lobules of uniform, round to spindled cells are arranged in cords and nests, and are set in a fibromyxoid to collagenous matrix (*Am J Surg Pathol.* 2003;27:421). An incomplete fibrous pseudocapsule or shell of lamellar bone is present around the periphery. Although microscopic features do not reliably predict behavior, increased cellularity and an increased mitotic rate (up to 10 mitotic figures per 10 high-power fields) is associated with a higher rate of recurrence. These tumors have an inconsistent immunophenotype, but can express cytokeratin, S-100 protein, glial fibrillary acidic protein, and CD99.

3. **Mixed tumor, myoepithelioma,** and **parachordoma** are three closely related tumors that display varying proportions of epithelial and/or myoepithelial elements (*Ann Diagn Pathol.* 2007;11:190). All three are typically painless swellings in the subcutis or deep soft tissues of the extremities, and have often been present for several years. The tumors occur primarily in adults, although up to 20% of cases occur in children younger than 10 years (*Am J Surg Pathol.* 1997;21:13).

   These three tumors have some resemblance to a pleomorphic adenoma. The epithelial and myoepithelial elements characteristically form a wide range of architectural patterns, and divergent differentiation is often observed. The tumors usually have a low mitotic rate. Malignant degeneration into either a carcinoma or sarcoma is occasionally observed. However, a subset of histologically benign cases also recurs and metastasizes, so morphologic features cannot be used to reliably predict prognosis. Some have questioned whether the ossifying fibromyxoid tumor is related to these three tumors.

4. **Giant cell fibroblastoma** is the unique morphologic manifestation of dermatofibrosarcoma protuberans that presents in early childhood as a soft tissue mass in the subcutis of the trunk, thigh, or perineum. It is an ill-defined tumor composed of delicate to spindle cells within a fibrous to fibromyxoid to hyalinized stroma, with scattered multinucleated giant cells associated with nonvascularized spaces. Similar cells are found in giant angiofibroma, pleomorphic lipoma, neurofibroma, and collagenoma (*Diagn Pathol.* 2007;2:47 and *Am J Dermatopathol.* 2004;26:141).

5. **Perivascular epithelioid cell tumors** (PEComas) are a family of presumably related neoplasms with morphologic and immunophenotypic similarities (*Histopathology.* 2006;48:75). The archetypes of this category are angiomyolipoma and lymphangiomyomatosis; clear cell "sugar" tumor of the lung and so-called myomelanocytic tumor of the ligamentum teres are additional examples. The characteristic microscopic finding is of a variable proportion of epithelioid and spindle cells with clear to eosinophilic granular cytoplasm and round nuclei, often featuring a perivascular orientation of tumor cells around a thinwalled blood vessel. A vague nesting pattern may also suggest a paraganglioma. Necrosis and vascular invasion are seemingly reliable features of malignancy. Immunohistochemically, the tumor cells are positive for the melanocytic markers HMB-45 and melan-A, positive for SMA, less often positive for desmin, and nonreactive for S-100 and cytokeratin.

C. **Malignant**

1. **Ewing sarcoma/primitive neuroectodermal tumor** (EWS/PNET), one of the several prototypic malignant round cell tumors of children and young adults, presents in the soft tissue, bone, viscera, skin, and other anatomic sites. Although once thought to be an uncommon tumor, EWS/PNET now accounts for about 20% of malignant soft tissue tumors in children, and is recognized throughout

adulthood. Whether in bone or soft tissue, these tumors are usually in excess of 6 cm; larger tumors occur in a "silent" location like the paraspinal or pelvic retroperitoneum.

A biopsy followed by post-treatment resection is the management sequence in most cases (because few of these tumors are candidates for primary resection), and these biopsies offer many diagnostic challenges because of the associated necrosis and compression artifact. Typically, the tumor is composed of uniform round cells with clear to finely vacuolated cytoplasm that surrounds a central nucleus that has fine to slightly coarse chromatin. Mitotic figures are present but are not especially numerous in most cases. Architecturally, broad sheets, lobules, nests, and strands are some of the growth patterns (e-**Fig. 46.48**); other features include Homer–Wright rosettes, condensed small cellular nodules within otherwise monotonous sheets of round cells, some spindling (possibly an artifact), and a pale mucoid background. Clear cytoplasm is usually an indication of abundant diastase-digestible glycogen. Vimentin and CD99 immunostains are diffusely positive with a cytoplasmic and membrane pattern, respectively. Punctate cytokeratin reactivity is seen focally in up to 20%–25% of cases.

Chromosomal translocations that form fusions between the *EWS* gene and a member of the *Ets* family of transcription factors are characteristic of EWS/PNET (Table 46.1). Demonstration of the translocation by molecular techniques is a valuable aid for diagnosis (*Am J Surg Pathol.* 2002;26:965). Secondary structural rearrangements, mainly deletions and trisomy, have been correlated with a poor outcome.

2. **Desmoplastic small round cell tumor** (DSRCT), originally reported as presenting as peritoneal masses in young men in their second or third decade, is now recognized to also occur in soft tissues, various organs, bone, and brain, in a broader age group than initially described. This tumor, like EWS/PNET, is composed of malignant round cells with a nested pattern within a desmoplastic stroma (e-**Fig. 46.49**). Rosette and glandular formations may be seen. A cautionary note is that several other malignant round cell neoplasms also can have desmoplastic stroma: blastemal predominant Wilms tumor, EWS/PNET, and ERMS or ARMS. The immunophenotype of DSRCT is summarized in Table 46.6. This tumor has a characteristic *EWS-WT1* fusion (Table 46.1).

3. **Synovial sarcoma** typically presents in the periarticular soft tissues in patients between the ages of 15 and 40 years. It is now recognized that this tumor can arise in virtually any site or organ. Despite its appellation, no biologic

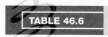

TABLE 46.6 | **Differential Immunohistochemical Phenotypes of Malignant Round Cell Tumors**

	VIM	CK	CD45	DES	CD99	WT-I	CHR	TDT	MPX/CD68
RMS	+	−	−	+	−	−	−	−	−
NB	±	−	−	−	−	−	+	−	+
HLM	+	−	+	−	+*	−	−	+	±**
EWS/PNET	+	±	−	−	+	−	+	−	−
DSRCT	+	+	−	+	±	+	±	−	−
BWT	+	−	−	±	−	+	−	−	−
NEC	−	+	−	−	−	−	+	−	−

Abbreviations: RMS, rhabdomyosarcoma; NB, neuroblastoma; HLM, hematolymphoid malignancy (leukemia, lymphoma, granulocytic sarcoma); EWS/PNET, Ewing sarcoma/primitive neuroectodermal tumor; DSRCT, desmoplastic small round cell tumor; BWT, blastemal Wilms tumor; NEC, neuroendocrine carcinoma; vim, vimentin; CK, cytokeratin; DES, desmin; CHR, chromogranin; TdT, terminal deoxynucleotidyl transferase; MPX, myeloperoxidase.
*CD99 is expressed in lymphoblastic leukemia/lymphoma.
**MPX is expressed in acute myeloid leukemia (M1, M2) and CD68 in acute monocytic leukemia (M5).

or pathologic relationship between synovial sarcoma and synovium has been demonstrated. The frequency of synovial sarcoma varies with age; it constitutes 8%–10% of all soft tissue sarcomas in the first two decades, but is uncommon in older adults.

The two classic histologic subtypes are the monophasic type (which is a spindle cell sarcoma with hemangiopericytoma-like foci) and the biphasic type (which contains epithelial-like glands [e-Fig. 46.50] or nests). A third, poorly differentiated type, has features of a primitive round cell sarcoma. Regardless of subtype, the immunophenotype includes vimentin expression, cytokeratin and/or EMA expression, and CD99 expression. The t(X;18) is characteristic of the tumor.

4. **Clear cell sarcoma** (melanoma of soft parts) occurs in the deep soft tissues of the foot and ankle, commonly in association with tendons and aponeuroses. It is seen in children and young adults. Nests to broad fascicles of plump spindled to polygonal cells with abundant eosinophilic to clear cytoplasm, with vesicular nuclei with a prominent eosinophilic nucleolus, are the histologic features (e-Fig. 46.51). Multinucleated cells may be found. Like the cutaneous melanoma, the immunophenotype includes vimentin, HMB-45, and melan-A (MART-1) positivity.

   Although some of the morphologic and immunophenotypic features overlap with cutaneous melanoma, the two tumors are distinctively different at the molecular genetic level. The balanced translocations characteristic of clear cell sarcoma (Table 46.1) have never been detected in cutaneous melanoma.

5. **Alveolar soft part sarcoma,** most commonly seen in patients between 15 and 35 years of age, has a predilection for the orbit and base of the tongue in children, and the deep soft tissue of the extremities (especially the thigh) in adults. Other than a mass with varying dimension, there is nothing specific about the gross features of the tumor. Microscopically, the findings indicate uniform, large epithelioid or polygonal cells that have abundant eosinophilic granular cytoplasm and are typically arranged in nests separated by delicate fibrous septa and sinusoidal vessels (e-Fig. 46.52). However, the tumor may have a more diffuse, nonalveolar pattern, especially in children. Rod-shaped or rhomboid crystalline inclusions, when present, are highlighted by a periodic acid–Schiff (PAS) stain after diastase digestion. The nonreciprocal der(17)t(X;17) translocation is the characteristic cytogenetic feature of this tumor.

6. **Extraskeletal myxoid chondrosarcoma,** which typically arises in the deep soft tissues of the proximal extremities, is seen in patients between 35 and 60 years of age. Its multilobulated, myxoid gross appearance is reflected in its microscopic composition of small, uniform, round cells with minimal atypia, finely granular eosinophilic cytoplasm, and bland round to oval nuclei that are arranged in clusters, cords, and delicate networks within a prominent myxoid matrix (e-Fig. 46.53). Cartilaginous differentiation is not present despite the appellation.

   The tumor is associated with a limited set of translocations that produce rearrangements of the *CHN* gene (Table 46.1). The same rearrangements are not present in chondrosarcoma of skeletal origin or extraskeletal mesenchymal chondrosarcoma.

7. **Extrarenal malignant rhabdoid tumor** is an extremely aggressive neoplasm of the liver, axial soft tissues, and central nervous system (atypical teratoid–rhabdoid tumor) in children typically younger than 2 years (*Cancer.* 2007;110:2061 and *Pathol Int.* 2006;56:287). This tumor can present in newborns with disseminated disease, including placental involvement, and is in all respects identical to renal malignant rhabdoid tumor. Grossly, it is a poorly circumscribed, highly infiltrative neoplasm that has a soft, grayish tan, and often necrotic cut surface. Various microscopic patterns may be associated with this high-grade malignant round cell neoplasm. Few or many obvious rhabdoid cells that have eccentric vesicular nucleus, prominent nucleolus, and the characteristic eosinophilic filamentous inclusion (which contains vimentin or cytokeratin) may be present. Oftentimes, immunohistochemistry for the latter two

intermediate filaments may demonstrate many more inclusions than are obvious on microscopic examination. The tumor cells also express CD99 in a patchy or focal pattern.

Somatic biallelic inactivation of the *hSNF5/INI1/SNARCB1* gene is the underlying genetic feature that can be demonstrated by an absence of nuclear

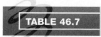

TABLE 46.7	Tumor, Node, Metastasis (TNM) Staging Scheme for Soft Tissue Sarcoma

DEFINITION OF TUMOR, NODE, METASTASIS (TNM)

PRIMARY TUMOR (T)

TX	Primary tumor cannot be assessed
T0	No evidence of primary tumor
T1	Tumor 5 cm or less in greatest dimension
T1a	Superficial tumor[1]
T1b	Deep tumor
T2	Tumor more than 5 cm in greatest dimension
T2a	Superficial tumor[1]
T2b	Deep tumor

REGIONAL LYMPH NODES (N)

NX	Regional lymph nodes cannot be assessed
N0	No regional lymph node metastasis
N1	Regional lymph node metastasis

DISTAL METASTASIS (M)

MX	Distant metastasis cannot be assessed
M0	No distant metastasis
M1	Distant metastasis

HISTOLOGIC GRADE (G)

GX	Grade cannot be assessed
G1	Well differentiated
G2	Moderately differentiated
G3	Poorly differentiated
G4	Poorly differentiated or undifferentiated (four-tiered systems only)

STAGE GROUPINGS

I	T1a	N0	M0	G1–2	G1[2]	Low[3]
	T1b	N0	M0	G1–2	G1	Low
	T2a	N0	M0	G1–2	G1	Low
	T2b	N0	M0	G1–2	G1	Low
II	T1a	N0	M0	G3–4	G2–3	High
	T1b	N0	M0	G3–4	G2–3	High
	T2a	N0	M0	G3–4	G2–3	High
III	T2b	N0	M0	G3–4	G2–3	High
IV	Any T	N1	M0	Any G	Any G	High or Low
IV	Any T	N0	M1	Any G	Any G	High or Low

[1]Depth is evaluated relative to the investing fascia of the extremity and trunk. Superficial is defined as lack of any involvement of the superficial investing muscular fascia in extremity or trunk lesions. All retroperitoneal and visceral lesions are considered deep lesions.

[2]In a three-tiered grading system, G1 is considered "low grade" and G2 and G3 are considered "high grade".

[3]In a two-tiered grading system ("low" versus "high" grade), G1 and G2 are considered "low grade" and G3 and G4 are considered "high grade".

From: Greene FL, Page DL, Fleming ID, Fritz AG, Balch CM, Haller DG, Morrow M, eds. *AJCC Cancer Staging Manual.* 6th edition. New York: Springer; 2002. Used with permission. (A new AJCC TNM staging system is scheduled for release in 2009; after its publication, the new staging scheme will appear on the website for this book.)

reactivity for BAF47. Molecular demonstration of alterations involving this locus can be used to differentiate extrarenal malignant rhabdoid tumor from poorly differentiated carcinomas and sarcomas that have a rhabdoid phenotype as an epiphenomenon.

8. **Epithelioid sarcoma** presents in young adults in their second through fourth decades. The distal type of epithelioid sarcoma involves the fingers, hand, or wrist, or the equivalent sites in the distal lower extremity. The more aggressive proximal type of epithelioid sarcoma involves the pelvis, perineum, and/or genital tract and has clinical and pathologic features of malignant rhabdoid tumor (*Cancer Res.* 2005;65:4012).

In the distal type, arcades and nodules of uniform epithelioid cells with eosinophilic cytoplasm may show a transition into areas of spindled cells, both set in a background of abundant collagen (e-**Fig. 46.54**). The nodules can undergo central necrosis, creating an appearance that resembles a necrobiotic granuloma (with the potential misinterpretation as granuloma annulare because both epithelioid sarcoma and granuloma annulare present in the fingers or toes).

Recurrent epithelioid sarcomas may have features of a high-grade pleomorphic sarcoma with only a remote resemblance to the primary tumor. Epithelioid sarcoma expresses EMA, vimentin, and low- and high-molecular-weight cytokeratins, as well as CD34 in 40%–50% of cases.

9. **Undifferentiated–poorly differentiated sarcoma** is the pathologic diagnosis of last resort. The morphologic scenario usually differs on the basis of age: In children, the problematic tumor is usually a primitive or high-grade round cell neoplasm, whereas in adults it is an equally high-grade pleomorphic neoplasm with anaplasia, bizarre mitoses, and necrosis. In children, the diagnosis of "undifferentiated round cell sarcoma" becomes the diagnosis after the various differentiated malignant round cell neoplasms have been excluded by immunohistochemical and molecular testing (see Table 46.6); "sarcoma of undetermined histogenesis" is an ever shrinking category among sarcomas of children (*J Pediatr Hematol Oncol.* 2001;23:215). In adults, after sarcomatoid carcinoma and melanoma have been excluded on the basis of a thorough immunohistochemical evaluation, "undifferentiated high grade pleomorphic sarcoma" or "pleomorphic malignant fibrous histiocytoma sarcoma" is often the diagnosis.

XIV. **REPORTING.** The surgical pathology report of a soft tissue tumor should include the location of the tumor, the depth of the tumor (see Table 46.7), the surgical procedure, the size of the tumor, the histologic type of tumor, and the biologic potential or managerial category (clinically benign, clinically intermediate, or clinically sarcoma). The extent of tumor necrosis should be noted, as well as the status of the margins. The results of any ancillary studies, including immunohistochemistry, electron microscopy, routine cytogenetic analysis, and/or molecular testing, should also be reported (*Mod Pathol.* 1998;11:1257).

Suggested Readings

Fletcher CDM, Unni KK, Mertens F. *Pathology and Genetics of Tumors of Soft Tissue and Bone. World Health Organization Classification of Tumors.* Lyon, France: IARC Press; 2002.

Kenpson RL, Fletcher CDM, Evans HL, et al. *Tumors of the Soft Tissues. Atlas of Tumor Pathology, 3rd Series, Fascicle 30.* Washington, DC: Armed Forces Institute of Pathology; 2001.

Pfeifer JD. *Molecular Genetic Testing in Surgical Pathology.* Philadelphia, PA: Lippincott, Williams & Wilkins; 2006.

Weiss SW, Goldblum JR. *Soft Tissue Tumors, 5th ed.* St. Louis, MO: Mosby; 2007.

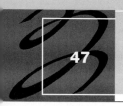

47 BONE NEOPLASMS AND OTHER NON-METABOLIC DISORDERS
Omar Hameed and Michael J. Klein

I. **NORMAL MICROSCOPIC ANATOMY.** The bones are composed of compact bone, which is derived from intramembranous ossification, and coarse cancellous bone, which is the osseous remnant of endochondral ossification. Compact bone makes up the cortices of long bones and constitutes their diaphyses and the surface portion of their metaphyses, as well as the compacta of the flat and irregular bones. Cancellous bone is present in the medullary cavity and is abundant at the ends of the long bones. In bone, form follows function (Wolff's law). In the shafts of bones, most of the forces act upon the surface. Here, the compact bone, which is 90% solid and only 10% space, bears the compression, tension, shear, and torsional forces. The medulla, shielded from forces, contains practically no bone at all. The ends of the bones are supported by the vertical plates and horizontal struts of the cancellous bone, yet cancellous bone is only 25% bone and 75% marrow by volume; here the cortex is very thin.

Bone matrix is classified as woven or lamellar depending on the predominant fiber arrangement of its collagen. In woven bone, the collagen fiber pattern is random. This type of bone is found in the fetal skeleton and in processes in which there is very rapid bone production. In lamellar bone, the bone collagen fibers are arranged in stacks of tightly packed fibers that are parallel in the same stack. In the next layer, the collagen fibers are also parallel to one another, but their direction is different than the collagen in the previous stack so that the bone appears to be layered. Both compact and cancellous bone consists of lamellar bone after the age of 3 years. After this age, woven bone is almost always pathologic, although the etiology is often not discernible without imaging studies (Bullough PG. *Orthopedic Pathology*, 4th ed. St. Louis: CV Mosby; 2004). In compact bone, the lamellae are arranged concentrically around central vascular canals termed Haversian canals; each vascular canal and its associated lamellae are referred to an osteon or Haversian system. In cancellous bone, the lamellae are arranged in linear, parallel plates (**e-Fig. 47.1**).* Adjacent osteons are separated from each other and from interstitial lamellae (see the section on circulatory diseases) and circumferential lamellae (which encircle the inner or outer cortex and are remnants of periosteal intramembranous ossification) by basophilic staining cement lines. Cement lines are sliding planes that are richer in calcium than surrounding bone matrix but the exact composition of which is unknown; they are produced by osteoblasts when bone is synthesized following osteoclast resorption (reversal cement lines) or after a period of inactivity (arrest cement lines). In the former type, the lamellae are discontinuous on either side of the cement line and in the latter the lamellae are continuous on either side (**e-Fig. 47.2**).

II. **SPECIMEN PROCESSING**

A. **Gross handling and selection of sections.** The approach to specimen handling is largely one of common sense. Small biopsy specimens should be submitted for sectioning in their entirety. If there is any doubt about whether they contain bone, they should be fixed, briefly decalcified, and rinsed. Most bone biopsies performed with needles are sufficiently thin for adequate fixation and decalcification, whereas curettings may sometimes need to be sliced into thinner fragments. The amount of curettings to submit for sectioning depends on their volume and whether the curettings are uniform. When it is feasible, all curettings should be submitted. If the lesion curetted is a hyaline cartilage tumor, as much of the histology as possible

---

*All e-figures are available online via the Solution Site Image Bank.

should be reviewed to identify atypical chondrocytes as well as any subtle interface with normal surrounding bone.

Other large specimens such as total joint replacements and bone resections also need to be sliced into thinner fragments. Although this may be accomplished with large band saws or other power-type saws, motorized saws are dangerous and somewhat time consuming to maintain properly, especially in a laboratory that receives a limited number of bone specimens. Vibrating or oscillating saws, which are usually available in autopsy suites, should be avoided if possible, because they do not section uniformly and their oscillating movement creates tension and compression artifacts that often make bone sections impossible to interpret properly. A very easy approach is to hold bone specimens steadily in a tabletop vise or clamp and to cut them with a hacksaw in which two fine-tooth blades are separated by 2- to 3-mm-thick washers. Such an apparatus is easily and cheaply made, although there are commercial instruments available for the same purpose. It is to be emphasized that double-bladed instruments should be scrupulously cleaned between every specimen to avoid tissue cross-contamination between different cases.

The handling and disposition of larger resection specimens depends on the reason for the procedure. For malignant tumors in which patients have not received neoadjuvant (after biopsy but prior to resection) chemotherapy, grading, staging, and adequacy of resection are the major clinical issues. Amputations from these patients should include sections from the soft tissue and vascular margins as well as those from the tumor itself. Tumor sections should be taken in such a way as to document the pertinent tumor histology, whether the tumor involves the medulla and/or cortex, and how far the tumor extends into soft tissues. The specimen should be cut in such a way as to disclose the greatest extent of tumor; review of the imaging studies can guide the selection process. Careful attention should be paid to taking sections from any areas that are grossly disparate from the appearance of the majority of the tumor. Radical resections for malignant tumors that are not amputations need the same sectioning methods, but any area of the resection constituting a margin must be sectioned and appropriately designated. This includes the bone resection margin, overlying soft tissue dissection margins, and the margins of any skin and soft tissue encompassing a prior biopsy site.

Specimens resected from patients who have received neoadjuvant chemotherapy (currently used in osteosarcoma and in Ewing's sarcoma/primitive neuroectodermal tumor [EWS/PNET]) need more extensive sampling to estimate the extent of treatment-associated necrosis. This means that one or more thin slabs should be cut through the entire extent of the bone and tumor, and that the entire slab or slabs should be fixed, decalcified, mapped, and examined not only for tumor stage but for extent of necrosis. The slabs should be photographed so as to produce a section map; if a specimen x-ray machine is available, specimen radiographs can be used both as section maps and as controls for adequate specimen decalcification (e-Fig. 47.3). Additional sections may be taken if there are areas not in the slab selected that appear as though they might be viable; the pathologist's task in this enterprise is to find viable tumor if any is present. It is worthwhile to remember that to extrapolate the degree of necrosis in a single slab into necrosis of the tumor as a whole makes the assumption that what happens in that slab is representative of the entire lesion. In a distal femur, for example, a 3- to 5-mm-thick slab of the bone samples only 7%–10% of the entire bone given the volume ratio of the slab to the entire bone.

B. Decalcification. The main difference between processing of bone specimens and of softer tissues is the requirement for an extra step of decalcification. Removal of calcium insures that bone collagen is no harder than the paraffin in which it is embedded, and that microtomy of bone tissues will approximate that for other types of specimens. Decalcification may be performed in a number of ways. In acid decalcification, hydrogen ions are in effect substituted for calcium ions. Electrolysis in effect accomplishes the same end, but this is done in an electrolyte solution with a weak electrical current; ionic exchange is the slowest of these methods but is the most gentle on the tissue and results in the fewest artifacts. In practice, most histology laboratories rely on weak acid decalcification because this method is the fastest and there is pressure from eager clinicians for rapid turnaround times in diagnosis. In using acid decalcification methods in particular, a few caveats must be kept in mind. First, the tissue must always be fixed adequately prior to decalcification to prevent artifacts that interfere with adequate staining or that can degrade the tissue after sections are prepared. This means that the tissue must be adequately thin (no more than 3- to 4-mm thick) prior to fixation, and that the tissue remains in formalin or some other suitable fixative for an interval adequate to coagulate the proteins for routine staining. In addition, if immunohistochemistry needs to be performed, adequate fixation helps to insure that the decalcification process will less alter tissue antigens. Second, when decalcification is performed with acid solutions, specimens must be rinsed in running water to ensure that the residual pH of the tissue is sufficiently neutral for hematoxylin staining. Failure to neutralize this acid not only results in understaining with hematoxylin, but it will cause stained sections to lose their hematoxylin staining in an accelerated manner. If time is insufficient for adequate specimen rinsing, the specimen should be neutralized in a dilute basic solution such as sodium bicarbonate. Third, if sections are left in dilute acid for a much longer period than necessary for calcium removal, tissue hydrolysis will remove the nucleic acids that cause nuclear hematoxylin staining and nuclei will appear acidophilic. This so-called "overdecalcification" artifact is generally not reversible. Overdecalcification may not interfere with many diagnostic interpretations, but it is important not to mistake this artifact for tissue necrosis, particularly in postchemotherapy specimen interpretation.

Adequate decalcification will vary by the tissue being decalcified. For example, woven bone, even though it tends to have higher calcium concentrations than lamellar bone, will often section adequately with incomplete decalcification because the former has less organization and less cutting resistance. The decision regarding whether the tissue is ready for embedding is often subjective and revolves around whether the tissue is pliable, trims easily, or can be penetrated with a needle. Complete decalcification is best judged either by testing the supernatant fluid with a colorimetric indicator or comparing specimen radiographs prior to and after decalcification. These tests are seldom practical in a very busy general surgical pathology practice.

C. **Approach to the interpretation of bone specimens.** Patient complaints related to the musculoskeletal system constitute nearly one third of physician office visits in the United States, so orthopedic problems are extremely common. While surgical pathologists are often asked to rule out bone tumors as the etiology of a clinical problem, it is useful to keep in mind that fractures alone are about 3,000 to 4,000 times more common than all primary bone tumors combined, and that metastatic tumors to bone are at least 20 times more common than primary bone tumors. The accurate diagnosis of bone diseases requires the correlation of patient demographics along with the clinical history and imaging studies to put the problem in its correct context prior to any histologic examination of tissue. Symptoms and signs are fairly similar in orthopedic diseases; these consist of pain, loss of function, deformities, and (in the case of tumors) sometimes a mass or a sense of fullness. Pain is the most common symptom, and although it may vary considerably, pain severe enough to wake a patient from sleep is the type suspicious for neoplastic diseases.

D. **Importance of radiological findings.** The surgical pathology of orthopedic diseases most often consists of defining the nature of bone lesions that are space occupying on imaging studies, advising the clinician if an infection may be present, and histologically documenting miscellaneous bone diseases that are not diagnosable by imaging studies alone. Because surgical pathologists usually render biopsy diagnoses with the assumption that a biopsy is representative of the pathologic process, it is natural to assume the same parameters in bone biopsies. This is a potentially dangerous assumption, because most orthopedic diseases are invisible without imaging studies. This means that to assure that a biopsy is representative of a process, the smaller the biopsy specimen, the greater is the need to see imaging studies defining that process. Because bones are deep seated, imaging studies are required to grasp the extent and behavior of bone lesions. For a surgical pathologist, correlating imaging studies with histologic findings depends on knowledge of normal bone and joint anatomy, the way this anatomy produces radiographic images, and the rudimentary alterations of these images by pathologic processes. This means not only what a process does to normal bone, but also how normal bone alters the process (*Adv Anat Pathol.* 2005;12:155).

The majority of the radiographic image produced by long bones is due to beam attenuation by cortical bone in the shafts and by cancellous bone in the ends (**e-Fig. 47.4**). The attenuation produced by flat bones is primarily due to cortical bone, and that of irregular bones depends on the proportion of bone elements in any given part of the bone.

Space-occupying lesions within bone usually cause bone destruction, bone production, or some combination of the two. Destructive lesions are not seen in a single radiographic view until at least 40% of the bone in the path of the x-ray beam is destroyed. This means that almost an entire thickness of cortex must be destroyed to see the lesion if an intact and a destroyed cortex are superimposed in one view, or that at least 40% of cancellous bone must be destroyed in a bone end. It is partly for this reason that orthogonal views of bones are taken (e.g., posteroanterior and lateral views) so that destructive lesions may be isolated in routine radiographs. Radiodense lesions superimpose on the extant bone, causing more attenuation and easier visibility on a routine radiograph. In contrast, a lesion that is less dense than bone may fill the entire medullary cavity of a bone, but if it does not destroy the cortex it will be invisible regardless of the view because the dominant attenuator of the x-ray beam is the cortex, not the medullary fat or marrow. It is for these reasons that other imaging studies such as computed tomography (CT) scans and magnetic resonance imaging (MRI) are performed. These studies yield information that is complementary to that derived from routine radiographs. While they may be more sensitive in yielding information, a particular type of imaging modality should be used in concert with routine radiographs to answer a particular clinical question not answered by the radiographs.

III. **DIAGNOSTIC FEATURES OF BONE LESIONS.** There are very few general categories of bone disease (Table 47.1), although there are many individual diseases (McCarthy EF, Frassica FJ. *Pathology of Bone and Joint Disorders with Clinical and Radiographic Correlation.* Philadelphia: WB Saunders; 1998). Most patients can be separated into general diagnostic categories on the basis of their imaging studies. For example, traumatic diseases, which are among the commonest problems, will demonstrate fractures with or without bone displacement or dislocations on routine radiographs. Metabolic bone diseases (discussed in Chapter 48), which characteristically affect the entire skeleton, usually demonstrate generalized radiolucency or osteopenia. Congenital and developmental diseases will usually affect more than one bone, are often symmetrical, and often demonstrate modeling deformities. Infections show a variety of radiographic abnormalities, depending on the type of organism present, the localization of the infection, and its chronicity. Avascular necrosis and idiopathic infarction demonstrate radiodensities in end arterial distributions; they are wedge-shaped at the convex ends of long bones and medullary in their diaphyses. Primary tumors of bone are usually localized defects that vary in their radiographic appearance in accordance with their biologic behavior. Metastatic tumors are usually localized defects that affect more than one bone or more

TABLE 47.1   Bone Diseases by Category

Congenital
Developmental/acquired
Traumatic
Circulatory
Metabolic and Paget disease
Infectious
Iatrogenic
Neoplastic and tumor-like

than one focus in one bone, but they can be mistaken for primary tumors if they are solitary. Joint diseases change the quality or quantity of the space between the bone ends normally seen in radiographs; they may also produce joint erosions or joint deformities. The salient features of some miscellaneous bone diseases that pathologists sometimes encounter are presented in Table 47.2.

A. Congenital and developmental diseases. Very few of these disorders come to the attention of surgical pathologists, for most of them are diagnosed on the basis of their clinical and imaging appearances. Some of them, such as the histiocytoses and storage disorders, may be confirmed histologically, or may be seen incidentally, such as when there is a hip replacement for avascular necrosis associated with Gaucher disease. Many others, such as most of the sclerosing dysplasias exclusive of diseases with specific histologies (e.g., osteopetrosis), demonstrate bone of increased density but are not specific or separable from one another histologically without demonstrating the changes seen in the radiographs (e-**Fig. 47.5**).

B. Traumatic disorders. Fractures are numerically the most frequent bone and joint disorders. They do not usually come to the attention of surgical pathologists because most treatment is closed or does not produce tissue for diagnosis. In contrast, open fractures requiring debridement and acute fractures of the femoral neck undergoing joint replacement are sometimes received in pathology laboratories. Acute fractures usually demonstrate some degree of accompanying hemorrhage, reactive changes such as dilated sinusoids in still viable nearby marrow, and fragmented bone trabeculae. Subacute fractures will also demonstrate devitalization of the bone at the fracture site (empty osteocyte lacunae and necrosis of marrow), although histologic evidence of healing is usually not evident for 7 to 10 days. Fractures that do not heal and fractures that are thought to be pathologic are sometimes sampled to rule out the presence of tumor or infection. It is very important to know that there is a history of trauma when reviewing tissue, or there is some danger of misinterpreting microcallus or reactive changes as matrix production by a tumor. Even if the history is not available, imaging studies will reveal if a tumor is present, and it is worthwhile to remember that primary bone tumors that produce bone matrix are rarely the sites of fracture. There are histologic parameters to separate bone and cartilage formation by tumor from that of trauma, although it takes some experience to recognize them. Bone or osteoid production by tumor matrix is often lacelike and becomes sheet-like as more bone is produced. Bone produced as a repair phenomenon may be focally lacelike, but more often it rapidly acquires a microtrabecular architecture and then becomes trabecular as it matures. In reactive bone there is almost always a zonation of maturity that is dependent on both the area in the lesion sampled and the time from trauma. While bone and cartilage are both common findings in both osteosarcoma and in fracture callus, cartilage tends to disappear as callus matures but it persists in osteosarcoma (e-**Fig. 47.6**). In addition, the progression from bone to cartilage back to bone is orderly in reactive processes but is totally random in bone tumors.

C. Circulatory disturbances

1. Bone necrosis. Osteonecrosis occurs in areas where the bone circulation has an end arterial distribution. The most common sites are near the convex surfaces of joints where epiphyseal arterial branches supply the cancellous bone in the distribution of a cone. When this area of bone is deprived of circulation, avascular or aseptic necrosis of the bone results. The cancellous bone up to the calcified zone of the articular cartilage, deriving its blood supply from nutrient arteries to the epiphysis, undergoes infarction. The overlying articular cartilage, which derives its oxygen and nutrients from the synovial fluid, remains viable. These changes are not immediately visible on routine radiographs because there are no changes in density of the necrotic bone. Radionuclide bone scans do demonstrate early hypervascularity in the zone surrounding the necrotic area, and MRI demonstrates edema and loss of marrow fat because of early adipocyte necrosis. The wedge-shaped area of radiodensity characteristic of late osteonecrosis develops for a variety of reasons, but deposition of calcium salts due to saponification of free fatty acid esters may be of greatest importance (although it is often difficult to recognize calcium salts

TABLE 47.2 Salient Features of Miscellaneous Nonneoplastic Bone Diseases that Pathologists May Occasionally Encounter

Tumor/Lesion	Location	Age	Radiological findings	Pathological findings	Differential diagnosis
Congenital/ Developmental	Diffuse, sometimes localized; usually symmetrical	<10	Modeling abnormality	Disease-dependant	Very broad
Traumatic	Any part of any bone	Any	Fracture lines; dislocations	Hemorrhage; organization; woven bone and chondroid matrix	Osteosarcoma and chondrosarcoma
Circulatory					
Avascular necrosis	Convex ends of LBs	5–40	Wedge-shaped radio-density; crescent sign; collapse of articular cartilage	Necrotic marrow and bone; subarticular plate fracture	None
Idiopathic infarction	Medulla of LBs	>20	Hazy density sometimes resembling smoke	Necrotic marrow and bone; calcification and ossification of marrow fat	Enchondroma*
Paget disease	Any portion of any bone; almost always extending to articular ends	>50	Early: bone resorption in wedge-shaped edge Later: course trabeculation; loss of corticomedullary demarcations	Osteoclastic resorption + increased vascularity and marrow fibrosis; "mosaic" cement lines in middle to late stages	Hyperparathyroidism; myelodysplasia and myelofibrosis; metastatic carcinoma with fibrosis
Infectious					
Hematogenous	Cortex of LBs	2–15	Early: ↑ uptake on bone scan; change of marrow signal on MRI; Later: mixed sclerosis and radiolucency	Marrow fibrosis with osteonecrosis and exudate/mixed inflammatory cell infiltrate	Round cell tumors and Langerhans cell histiocytosis
Direct	Any; open trauma or deep ulcer	Varies	Mixed sclerosis and radiolucency	Marrow fibrosis with osteonecrosis and exudate/mixed inflammatory cell infiltrate	Round cell tumors and Langerhans cell histiocytosis

*Radiological differential diagnosis.
LBs, long bones; MRI, magnetic resonance imaging.

in decalcified sections because they are dissolved by the decalcification process). Clinical symptoms become severe when the necrosis has extended to the articular cartilage with loss of congruency of the usual convex–concave joint surface and destruction of the subarticular plate. It is not uncommon for the articular cartilage and superficial subarticular plate to detach from the underlying cancellous bone. Because dead bone matrix and living bone have the same inherent strength and stiffness, this probably happens because the subarticular bone no longer has the capacity for remodeling in the face of repetitive forces, and accumulated shear stress causes it to detach. When this event occurs, the radiodense subarticular bone attached to the articular cartilage forms a crescentic shadow that may be seen radiographically (e-**Fig. 47.7**).

2. **Bone infarctions.** These are also presumably the result of a disruption in end arterial circulation. In the diaphysis, a bone infarct is largely confined to the medulla. This portion of the bone derives its blood supply from nutrient arteries that penetrate the cortex to supply the sinusoids of the medullary cavity and the inner cortex. The saponified marrow fat resulting from fat necrosis may appear to contain hazy or smoky radiodensities, and biopsies will reveal fat necrosis and a few scant trabeculae with empty osteocyte lacunae (e-**Fig. 47.8**). The outer cortex is supplied mainly by perforating arterioles derived from arteriae comitantes of the periosteum. The cortical portions of this circulation travel longitudinally via Haversian canals and interconnect within the cortex via the Volkmann canals. Because the circulation in the cortex is microscopically collateralized, the cortex of long bones is somewhat more protected against infarction than is the medullary cavity. Within the cortex, there are interstitial lamellae derived from the remnants of old Haversian systems or inner or outer circumferential lamellae that have not fully resorbed but have no active blood supply; because of this, these lamellae are devoid of osteocytes and are physiologically dead (e-**Fig. 47.9**). Because all cortical bone is compact bone, this means that small foci of empty osteocyte lacunae within the cortex do not imply that there is avascular necrosis even though this bone is histologically dead. Ordinarily, it is necessary for both nutrient and periosteal blood supplies to be disrupted to cause a true cortical infarction. This happens most often in conjunction with trauma and with infections.

D. **Paget disease.** This disease has some histologic features in common with high-turnover metabolic bone diseases, but it is not a metabolic disease because it does not diffusely affect the entire skeleton and has no known associated metabolic defect (metabolic bone diseases are covered in Chapter 48). Paget disease is characterized by an imbalance or uncoupling of osteoclastic and osteoblastic activities, with osteoclastic bone resorption predominating early in the disease and osteoblastic activity persisting late in the disease. These histologic manifestations are correlated radiographically with characteristic radiolucency early in the disease, radiodensity in the late stages, and a mixed pattern for most of the interval between (*Skeletal Radiol.* 1995;24:173). Because the bone microarchitecture is altered, there is loss of the normal bone contour radiographically, and there is gradual loss of the normal cortical appearance and an increasingly coarse appearance to the bone trabeculations. A biopsy from an early radiolucent lesion demonstrates large bizarre osteoclasts producing large and irregular resorption pits (Howship's lacunae) on trabecular surfaces. These are often accompanied by paratrabecular fibrosis and dilated marrow sinusoids. As the resorption pits become filled in by osteoblast activity, irregularly shaped cement lines (sometimes likened to grout lines in a mosaic) mark the demarcation between the old and new bone. The bone on either side of these cement lines demonstrates either lamellar bone, in which the layers are discontinuous on either side, or lamellar bone on one side and woven bone on the other side. As the disease progresses and osteoclast activity slows, the bone becomes thicker and more interconnected than normal, but its arrangement and increased irregular cement lines make it more prone to deformities and fractures (e-**Fig. 47.10**).

E. **Infectious disorders.** Infections of bone arise either by direct introduction of organisms into the bone due to open trauma or overlying infections of soft tissue or by secondary hematogenous spread. Most hematogenous osteomyelitis occurs in the first two decades of life. Its usual site in the bone is in the metaphysis adjoining the growth plate of a long bone because the microcirculation is stagnant in this area. Osteomyelitis due to open trauma can occur at any age; osteomyelitis associated with overlying infections is most often associated with peripheral vascular disease and so is seen later in life. Most infections of the bone are bacterial, but infections with fungi and lower virulence organisms may occur in immunocompromised hosts.

The vast majority of hematogenous osteomyelitis is due to coagulase-positive *Staphylococcus aureus*, but many other organisms may infect bones. Histologically, microorganisms are seldom seen in bone biopsies of patients with osteomyelitis because the sheer number of organisms required for the sensitivity of high power or oil-immersion microscopy to detect bacteria is very high. Because of this, bacterial cultures should always be taken when infections of bone are suspected clinically—preferably prior to the institution of antibiotic therapy. A single bacterial culture is on the order of 10 million times more sensitive than histology—even when special stains for organisms are added to the regimen. Infections in bone are often accompanied by necrosis of at least some of the affected bone. The primary reason for this is that edema accompanies inflammation, and edema in the closed confines of the cortex compromises the medullary nutrient arteries and sinusoids due to resulting increased pressure. The innermost cortical circulation may be similarly compromised by increased intramedullary pressure. If the pressurized exudate finds its way into empty Haversian and Volkmann canals, it may push its way through these intracortical spaces and eventually dissect the periosteum with its perforating arteries from the cortex. If the cortex is deprived of its dual circulation, then it in turn becomes necrotic; this necrotic bone is called sequestrum. The combination of necrotic bone sequestrum, marrow fibrosis and/or fat necrosis, and mixed inflammatory infiltrates (usually including neutrophils and plasma cells) provides good histologic corroboration of osteomyelitis, but the demonstration of organisms is the gold standard for the diagnosis of infections (e-Fig. 47.11).

F. Iatrogenic disorders. Treatment-related disorders are seldom a major problem in the pathologic diagnosis of orthopedic disease, provided that an accurate clinical history is communicated to the surgical pathologist. For example, the diagnosis of osteosarcoma would be very unusual in a patient of the sixth decade without prior radiation of the site, or without some other underlying premalignant bone lesion. Administration of various therapeutic regimens may lead to secondary alterations in bones; perhaps the most notable of these is the amyloidosis of bones, tendon sheaths, and ligaments that develops from β-2-microglobulin accumulation in long-term hemodialysis patients. Substances that have been given parenterally but that are not metabolized may also be deposited in bones or joints; without prior knowledge of therapeutic treatment, it may be difficult to make an accurate diagnosis (e-Fig. 47.12).

G. Neoplastic and tumor-like lesions. Primary tumors of bone are quite rare, accounting for only 0.2% of all malignancies, or an incidence of 1 per 100,000 individuals per year (Fletcher, CDM, Unni K, Mertens K, eds. *Tumors of Soft Tissues and Bone*. Lyon, France: IARC Press; 2002). There is a bimodal age distribution, with one peak in adolescence and a smaller one in patients older than 60 years. Among other characteristics, each bone tumor has its own age predilection, which is very useful from a differential diagnostic standpoint. Primary benign bone tumors are probably less common than primary malignant tumors if the very common nonossifying fibroma, osteochondroma, and enchondromas of the hands are excluded. In addition to benign and malignant bone neoplasms, there are a number of nonneoplastic lesions that can present in a manner similar to neoplastic conditions (Table 47.3); all of these lesions are discussed below, and their main features are presented in Tables 47.4 and 47.5. Pathological stage is among the findings that are recommended to be reported for bone tumors (*Hum Pathol.* 2004;35:1173) and the American Joint Committee on Cancer (AJCC) Tumor, Node, Metastasis (TNM) staging scheme (Table 47.6) and/or the simpler Musculoskeletal Tumor Society scheme (Table 47.7) can be used for this purpose.

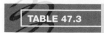

TABLE 47.3	WHO Classification of Bone Tumors

Cartilage tumors	**Ewing sarcoma/primitive**
Osteochondroma	**Neuroectodermal tumor**
Chondroma	Ewing sarcoma
Enchondroma	
Periosteal chondroma	**Hematopoietic tumors**
Multiple chondromatosis	Plasma cell myeloma
Chondroblastoma	Malignant lymphoma, not otherwise specified
Chondromyxoid fibroma	**Cell tumor**
Chondrosarcoma	Giant cell tumor
Central, primary, and secondary	Malignancy in giant cell tumor
Peripheral	**Notochordal tumors**
Dedifferentiated	Chordoma
Mesenchymal	
Clear cell	**Vascular tumors**
	Hemangioma
Osteogenic tumors	Angiosarcoma
Osteoid osteoma	
Osteoblastoma	**Smooth muscle tumors**
Osteosarcoma	Leiomyoma
Conventional	Leiomyosarcoma
Chondroblastic	**Lipogenic tumors**
Fibroblastic	Lipoma
Osteoblastic	Liposarcoma
Telangiectatic	
Small cell	**Neural tumors**
Low-grade central	Neurilemmoma
Secondary	
Parosteal	**Miscellaneous tumors**
Periosteal	Adamantinoma
High-grade surface	Metastatic malignancy
Fibrogenic tumors	**Miscellaneous lesions**
Desmoplastic fibroma	Aneurysmal bone cyst
Fibrosarcoma	Simple cyst
	Fibrous dysplasia
Fibrohistiocytic tumors	Osteofibrous dysplasia
Benign fibrous histiocytoma	Langerhans cell histiocytosis
Malignant fibrous histiocytoma	Erdheim–Chester disease
	Chest wall hamartoma

From: Fletcher CDM, Unni K, Mertens K, eds. *World Health Organization Classification of Tumours. Pathology and Genetics. Tumours of Soft Tissues and Bone.* Lyon: IARC Press; 2002. Used with permission.

1. **Cartilage-forming tumors**
   a. **Osteochondroma.** This is a cartilage-capped bony protrusion (e-**Fig. 47.13**) that arises from the surface of any bone that models or grows by endochondral ossification. On imaging, osteochondromas demonstrate a marrow cavity and a cortex continuous with those of the host bone. Although classified as bone neoplasms, osteochondromas may also result from displacements of the cartilaginous grown plate. This is consistent with their metaphyseal location and the fact that they cease to grow after skeletal maturation. Most osteochondromas are sporadic and solitary; however, multiple lesions are present in osteochondromatosis, which is an autosomal dominant hereditary condition. The presence of *EXT-1* mutations in the germline of these patients has been used as evidence of the classification of osteochondroma as a neoplasm

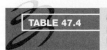

TABLE 47.4	Commonest Location(s), Usual Age Distribution, and Salient Pathological Features of Benign Bone Tumors and Tumor-like Lesions

Tumor/lesion	Location	Age	Salient pathological findings
Cartilaginous			
Osteochondroma	Metaphysis of LBs	10–30	Cartilage-capped bony protrusion
Chondroma	Hands/feet; medulla of LBs	Any	Variably cellular hyaline cartilage
Chondroblastoma	Epiphysis/apophysis of LBs	10–20	Chondroid-like matrix; S-100-positive cells with grooved nuclei
Chondromyxoid fibroma	Metaphysis of LBs	10–30	Hypocellular chondromyxoid lobules surrounded by more cellular spindle-cell areas
Osseous			
Osteoma	Facial bones	Adults	Mineralized compact bone
Osteoid osteoma	Cortex of LBs	10–30	"Nidus" of immature bone surrounded by sclerotic bone
Osteoblastoma	Vertebrae; cortex of LBs	10–30	Identical to osteoid osteoma but larger; often no sclerosis
Fibrous			
Fibrous dysplasia	Ribs; jaw; LBs-medullary	10–30	Irregular woven bone within fibroblastic stroma
Osteofibrous dysplasia	Tibial cortex	<20	Similar to fibrous dysplasia but with appositional osteoblasts
Desmoplastic fibroma	LBs; jaw; pelvis	20–30	Fibromatosis-like proliferation
Nonossifying fibroma	LBs	5–15	Bland spindle cells in storiform pattern + histiocytes + giant cells
Histiocytic			
Benign fibrous histiocytoma	LBs; pelvis	>20	Identical to nonossifying fibroma but variable
Langerhans cell histiocytosis	Skull; jaw; metaphysis and diaphysis of LBs	5–15	Mixed inflammatory cells and eosinophils; S-100/CD1a-positive cells with grooved/multilobated nuclei
Erdheim–Chester disease	LBs	>40	Foamy histiocytes and fibrosis
Giant cell tumor	Epiphysis/metaphysis of LBs	20–45	Evenly placed giant cells among mononuclear cells with identical nuclei; normal serum calcium/phosphate/blood urea nitrogen/creatinine
Others			
Aneurysmal bone cyst	Vertebrae; flat and LBs	10–20	Blood-filled spaces separated by fibrous septae; giant cells
Simple cyst	Metaphysis of LBs	10–20	Fluid-filled "cysts" lined by connective tissue
Hemangioma	Vertebrae; flat and LBs	20–50	Capillary and/or cavernous sized vessels

LBs, long bones.

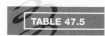

TABLE 47.5	Commonest Location(s), Usual Age Distribution, and Salient Pathological Features of Malignant Bone Tumors		
Tumor/lesion	Location	Age	Salient pathological findings
Cartilagenous			
Chondrosarcoma	Flat bones; metaphysis, and epiphysis of LBs		
Conventional (NOS)	Metaphysis	20–80	Variably cellular hyaline cartilage permeating bone
Dedifferentiated	Metaphysis	>30	Conventional chondrosarcoma + high-grade spindle cell sarcoma
Mesenchymal	Metaphysis	20–50	Undifferentiated small cell tumor + hyaline cartilage
Clear cell	Epiphysis	20–70	Conventional tumor with abundant large clear tumor cells
Osseous			
Osteosarcoma	Metaphysis of LBs; jaw	10–20; >40	
Conventional	Medullary		Osteoid formed directly by malignant cells
Low-grade central	Medullary		Mildly atypical fibroblastic proliferation + thick bone trabeculae
Telangiectatic	Medullary		Blood-filled spaces + fibrous septae + highly malignant osteoid
Parosteal	Cortex outside periosteum		Mildly atypical fibroblastic proliferation + thick bone trabeculae
Periosteal	Cortex inside periosteum		Abundant cartilage matrix with variable malignant osteoid
Fibrous/fibrohistiocytic			
Fibrosarcoma	Metaphysis of LBs; may extend to end of bone	20–60	Malignant spindle cells in a fascicular pattern
Malignant fibrous histiocytoma	Metaphysis of LBs; may extend to end of bone	20–80	Malignant spindle cells in storiform pattern + histiocytic cells (other patterns may be seen)
Hematolymphoid			
Myeloma	Skull; vertebrae; pelvis; LBs	>40	Variably atypical (monoclonal) plasma cells
Lymphoma	Any	Any	Lymphoid proliferations similar to nonbony lesions
Epithelial			
Adamantinoma	Cortex of tibia and/or fibula	25–35	Epithelial cells + fibroblasts + woven or lamellar bone
Metastatic carcinoma	Any	>40	Malignant epithelial cells; morphology/IHC helps confirm origin
Others			
Ewing sarcoma	Diaphysis of LBs	5–20	Small round blue cells ± rosettes; characteristic IHC; translocation
Chordoma	Base of skull; sacrum	>30	Lobules of vacuolated cells embedded in myxoid matrix
Angiosarcoma and hemangioen- dothelioma		20–60	Anastamosing vascular channels lined by highly atypical cells OR vacuolated cells in myxoid background; characteristic IHC

LBs, long bones; NOS, not otherwise specified; IHC, immunohistochemistry.

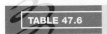

TABLE 47.6	Tumor, Node, Metastasis (TNM) Staging Scheme for Malignant Bone Tumors (Excluding Myeloma and Lymphoma)

HISTOLOGICAL GRADE (G)

GX	Grade cannot be assessed
G1	Well differentiated – low grade
G2	Moderately differentiated – low grade
G3	Poorly differentiated – high grade
G4	Undifferentiated – high grade

PRIMARY TUMOR (T)

TX	Primary tumor cannot be assessed
T0	No evidence of primary tumor
T1	Tumor $\leq$8 cm in greatest dimension
T2	Tumor >8 cm in greatest dimension
T3	Discontinuous tumors in the primary bone site

REGIONAL LYMPH NODES (N)

NX	Regional lymph nodes cannot be assessed
N0	No regional lymph node metastasis
N1	Regional lymph node metastasis

DISTANT METASTASIS (M)

MX	Distant metastasis cannot be assessed
M0	No distant metastasis
M1	Distant metastasis
M1a	Lung
M1b	Other distant sites

American Joint Committee on Cancer (AJCC) Stage Groupings

Stage IA	T1	N0	M0	G1, 2
Stage IB	T2	N0	M0	G1, 2
Stage IIA	T1	N0	M0	G3, 4
Stage IIB	T2	N0	M0	G3, 4
Stage III	T3	N0	M0	Any G
Stage IVA	Any T	N0	M1a	Any G
Stage IVB	Any T	N1	Any M	Any G
	Any T	Any N	M1b	Any G

From: Greene FL, Page DL, Fleming ID, Fritz AG, Balch CM, Haller DG, Morrow M, eds, *AJCC Cancer Staging Mannual.* 6th edition. New York: Springer; 2002. Used with permission. (A new AJCC TNM staging system is scheduled for release in 2009; after its publication, the new staging scheme will appear on the website for this book.)

(*J Clin Invest.* 2001;108:511). While multiple hereditary osteochondromas are associated with an increased incidence of secondary chondrosarcoma, the malignant change also takes place in solitary osteochondromas, most of which do not harbor such mutations.

b. **Chondromas.** These comprise a group of lesions that are composed of variably cellular mature hyaline cartilage (e-**Fig. 47.14**). Enchondromas arise within the medullary cavity and most commonly involve the small bones of the hand and feet or long tubular bones, whereas periosteal chondromas arise on the cortical surface (about half involve the humerus). Most of these lesions are incidental, but some, especially in long bones, can present with pathological fractures. Radiographically, chondromas appear as well-demarcated lucent lesions with variable amounts of stippled mineralization (e-**Fig. 47.15**). Ollier disease is characterized by multiple widespread enchondromas associated with bone deformities that develop early in life, whereas Mafucci's syndrome is characterized by multiple enchondromas with associated soft tissue angiomas. Both of these developmental disorders are associated with a significantly increased incidence of secondary chondrosarcoma, although the incidence is higher in

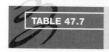

TABLE 47.7	Musculoskeletal Tumor Society Staging Scheme for Malignant Bone Tumors (Excluding Myeloma, Lymphoma and Ewing Sarcoma)		
Grade			
G1	Low-grade		
G2	High-grade		
Site			
T1	Intracompartmental (within the bone)		
T2	Extracompartmental (spread beyond the bone)		
Distant metastasis (M)			
M0	No regional or distant metastasis		
M1	Regional or distant metastasis		
Stage groupings			
Stage IA	G1	T1	M0
Stage IB	G1	T2	M0
Stage IIA	G2	T1	M0
Stage IIB	G2	T2	M0
Stage III	Any	Any	M1

Modified from: Enneking WF. A system of staging musculoskeletal neoplasms. *Clin Orthop Relat Res.* 1986;204:9–24.

patients with Mafucci's syndrome. Enchondromas in these patients tend to be more cellular and myxoid, so the histological appearances alone cannot always be used to diagnose malignant transformation. In such cases, clinical (e.g., rapid growth), radiological (e.g., cortical destruction, soft tissue masses), and/or pathological (e.g., necrosis, permeation of bone trabeculae) findings must be used in combination to arrive at the correct diagnosis.

c. **Chondroblastoma.** This benign neoplasm is characteristically an epiphyseal or apophyseal tumor that often presents with arthritic pain and/or joint stiffness due to its close proximity to joints. Histologically, the tumor is composed of discrete, round mononuclear cells with ovoid, folded, or grooved nuclei (e-**Fig. 47.16**). A pink extracellular material resembling early cartilage is also present, sometimes with "chicken-wire" calcification, but the lesion very seldom produces true hyaline cartilage. Giant cells are often present. If these are abundant, and the matrix is scant, the lesion can be confused with a giant cell tumor. The radiological identification of a sclerotic rim or a demarcated edge with or without calcification (e-**Fig. 47.17**), as well as the fact that almost all patients with this lesion are young and still have open growth plates, help distinguish chondroblastoma from giant cell tumor. In addition, immunohistochemistry demonstrates that the neoplastic chondroblasts are usually S-100 positive.

d. **Chondromyxoid fibroma.** This tumor presents in the metaphyses of growing individuals. It is characteristically well circumscribed, eccentric, and may demonstrate bone expansion (e-**Fig. 47.18**). Histologically, there are lobular aggregates of spindle-shaped to stellate cells arranged within a chondroid to myxoid matrix. Importantly, these lobules are surrounded by zones of hypercellularity in which mononuclear and multinucleated giant cells are evident (e-**Fig. 47.19**). The behavior is benign.

e. **Chondrosarcoma (not otherwise specified).** This is one of the few primary malignant tumors that affects adults with fully mature skeletons. It is classified as primary when there is no pre-existing lesion or secondary when it arises in a pre-existing bone lesion such as osteochondroma or Ollier disease. Chondrosarcoma most commonly involves the flat bones of the trunk and proximal tubular bones of the extremities. Radiographically, it tends to be large and radiolucent, with radiodense stippling, curlicues, and rings due to matrix calcification or ossification. When it is a central (medullary) lesion, there is often cortical destruction and sometimes cortical thickening. When peripheral, the cartilage matrix is usually >3 cm in thickness (e-Fig. 47.20). Histologically, it is composed of mature appearing hyaline cartilage except that the chondrocytes have varying degrees of increased cellularity, nuclear atypia, or even mitotic activity. Chondrosarcoma can show variable degrees of differentiation, ranging from minimally hypercellular tumors resembling enchondromas with scattered enlarged hyperchromatic tumor cell nuclei that are sometimes binucleate (grade I), to unequivocally malignant tumors with markedly atypical cells and easily identifiable mitotic figures (grade III). Grade II tumors have features intermediate between the two (e-Fig. 47.21). Regardless of their grade, chondrosarcomas (when sampled adequately) invariably show permeation of existing marrow spaces between bony trabeculae (e-Fig. 47.22). This is very helpful in distinguishing low-grade tumors from enchondromas, especially in the small bones of the hands and feet where enchondromas may show a degree of hypercellularity and/or binucleation quite reminiscent of that seen in low-grade chondrosarcomas of larger, more proximal bones. The presence of tumor cell necrosis can also point to a diagnosis of chondrosarcoma. Nevertheless, there are cartilaginous tumors that remain difficult to accurately categorize, especially when the radiological features of malignancy are not clearly evident. Occasionally, complementary imaging studies such as CT scans may help to identify true bone destruction in a central cartilage tumor, or MRI will demonstrate the extent of a cartilage cap in a peripheral cartilage tumor; these criteria, in turn, can help to identify the true biological nature of the lesion when a small biopsy cannot (e-Fig. 47.23). The prognosis of chondrosarcoma is mostly dependant on grade and completeness of resection (as no other modality of treatment is effective), with 5-year survival rates ranging from 90% for low-grade tumors to 53% in higher grade tumors.

  f. Dedifferentiated chondrosarcoma. In addition to areas of classic chondrosarcoma (usually low grade), this tumor is characterized by the presence of a distinct, second, clearly defined, high grade, noncartilaginous sarcomatous component (e-Fig. 47.24). The later is most frequently represented by a malignant fibrous histiocytoma-like component, but osteosarcoma, fibrosarcoma, and rhabdomyosarcoma have also been reported. This tumor is associated with a very poor prognosis.

  g. Mesenchymal chondrosarcoma. This rare tumor is also characterized by a dimorphic pattern and is composed of a highly undifferentiated small round cell component that is often arranged in a hemangiopericytomatous pattern, intermixed with a variable number of islands of hyaline cartilage (e-Fig. 47.25). Although it may occur at any age, the peak age incidence of patients with this tumor (2nd and 3rd decades) is earlier than that seen in patients with other chondrosarcomas. Mesenchymal chondrosarcoma has a high incidence of local recurrence and distant metastasis, although the latter may not occur for 5 to 10 years.

  h. Clear cell chondrosarcoma. Another rare type of chondrosarcoma, this tumor shows a predilection for the ends of long bones after the growth plates have closed (e-Fig. 47.26). It is characterized histologically by the presence of abundant large round clear cells with well-defined cell borders, intermixed with areas of conventional low-grade chondrosarcoma (e-Fig. 47.27). The clear cells contain large amounts of intracellular glycogen and stain strongly for S-100 protein. The prognosis is similar to that of low-grade chondrosarcoma. Metastases occur in about 20% of patients, and may behave indolently or aggressively. Clear cell chondrosarcoma has a high predilection for metastasis to other bones.

2. Bone-forming tumors

  a. Osteoma. This is a well-circumscribed, radiodense, benign lesion that most frequently arises in the jaws and paranasal sinuses (e-Fig. 47.28), but can also be seen in long bones. Some cases are sporadic, whereas others arise in association with familial polyposis coli (see Chapter 14). Histologically, osteomas are composed of mineralized compact bone matrix with a variable admixture of mature and immature bone and no cellular stroma (e-**Fig. 47.28**).

b. **Osteoid osteoma.** This benign, self-limited tumor usually presents with pain that often wakes patients from sleep but is relieved by aspirin. Although it usually involves the cortices of long bones, osteoid osteoma has been reported in almost every skeletal site. Radiographically, there is a central area of radiolucency surrounded by dense reactive sclerosis (e-**Fig. 47.29**). The quantity of sclerosis varies by location in the bone. If the lesion is cortical, the reactive sclerosis may obscure the lesion such that it can only be seen by thin-cut CT scans. In the medullary cavity, there may be little or no sclerosis. Histologically, the radiolucent area, termed the "nidus," is composed of vascularized fibroconnective tissue in which immature new bone is being formed. This new bone is usually arranged in microtrabecular arrays lined by plump appositional osteoblasts that lack nuclear pleomorphism (e-**Fig. 47.30**). Simple excision or curettage of the nidus of an osteoid osteoma is curative.

c. **Osteoblastoma.** This tumor is virtually identical histologically to osteoid osteoma but, unlike the latter, is not limited in growth potential. When diagnosed, osteoblastomas are usually larger than 2 cm in diameter. Radiographically, they may resemble large osteoid osteomas, they may be expansile like aneurysmal bone cysts (ABCs), and they may even appear as aggressive as malignant tumors. There is also a predilection to involve the axial skeleton, especially the vertebral pedicles and arches. Occasionally, osteoblastomas may be very cellular, and their osteoblasts may be several times the size of usual osteoblasts. Tumors having predominant areas of this histologic feature have been termed "aggressive osteoblastoma" or "epithelioid osteoblastoma" (e-**Fig. 47.31**). The prognosis of osteoblastomas is excellent if amenable to excision.

d. **Osteosarcoma.** This is the most common nonhematopoietic primary malignant neoplasm of bone. The peak incidence of this tumor is late childhood and adolescence; however, there is a second peak in patients older than 40 years, most cases of which develop secondarily in pre-existing bone lesions (e.g., Paget disease) or following irradiation. The metaphyses of long bones (femur, tibia, humerus) are the most common sites of involvement; isolated diaphyseal involvement is rare, and involvement of the epiphyses of long bones or small bones of the hands and feet is exceptionally rare. Other sites of involvement include the jaws, skull, and axial skeleton. Most cases of osteosarcoma present with pain (often dull and unremitting) with or without a palpable mass. Radiologically, there is almost always evidence of a destructive bony lesion, often with evidence of new bone formation. There may also be an interrupted periosteal reaction and soft tissue involvement (e-**Fig. 47.32**). The histological hallmark of osteosarcoma is the presence of osteoid or bone formation directly by tumor cells. Osteoid appears as dense, pink, amorphous material (resembling collagen or amyloid) that has a lacelike or sheet-like appearance (e-**Fig. 47.33**). Intermixed within, and often in direct contact with this osteoid matrix, are the neoplastic tumor cells, which can be quite variable in appearance, including polyhedral cells, spindle cells with variable nuclear atypia, small blue cells (resembling EWS, see below), and large, markedly atypical cells. The predominant matrix produced by the tumor can be bone or osteoid, cartilaginous, or fibrous. Historically, osteosarcomas have been subclassified based on the predominant matrix production (osteoblastic, chondroblastic, or fibroblastic), but this classification has no prognostic importance. Instead, as described below, osteosarcomas are best classified based on radiological and/or pathological features that have been shown to have distinct prognostic implications (*Am J Clin Pathol.* 2006;125:555).

i. **Central osteosarcomas.** These arise within the medullary cavity and include:

(a) **Conventional intramedullary osteosarcoma.** This is the prototypical osteosarcoma, for which most of the above information refers. Neoplastic tumor cells in conventional osteosarcoma are often polyhedral or spindle-shaped with unequivocally malignant features. Given that preoperative chemotherapy for these tumors is the current standard of care (which has significantly improved the 5-year survival rate of this tumor from 20% to >80%), it is important to carefully "map" the tumor in the resection specimen (as discussed earlier) to determine the extent of tumor necrosis compared to the volume of viable plus nonviable tumor, because a good long-term outcome is associated with >90% tumor necrosis. Additional chemotherapy is often offered to patients with less necrosis as a second-line attempt to further improve their survival.

(b) **Low-grade central osteosarcoma.** This rare type of osteosarcoma (1%–2%) is composed of a variably cellular spindle cell/fibroblastic proliferation that lacks the degree of cytological atypia seen in conventional osteosarcoma. In addition, bone production is usually evident as irregular, somewhat thick, anastamosing, or branching bony trabeculae. These trabeculae simulate the woven bone of fibrous dysplasia or the longitudinal seams of bone seen in parosteal osteosarcoma (see below), and are separated by a spindle-cell stroma. Review of the radiological findings often reveals subtle signs of malignancy that are useful in making the diagnosis (e-**Fig. 47.34**). This tumor has a much more indolent course compared to conventional osteosarcoma; however, there is still a high recurrence rate if the tumor is inadequately excised, often with grade progression.

(c) **Telangiectatic osteosarcoma.** This tumor is characterized by large, blood-filled spaces separated by highly cellular fibrous septae that contain markedly pleomorphic cells with a variable amount of osteoid production (e-**Fig. 47.35**). Radiologically, this tumor is radiolucent and expansile, and resembles ABC. Compared to other osteosarcomas, it is more likely to present with a pathological fracture. Although not necessarily associated with improved survival, this aggressive osteosarcoma is very sensitive to chemotherapy.

(d) **Small cell osteosarcoma.** This tumor is composed of small round blue cells and histologically resembles EWS, except that there is histologic evidence for osteoid formation (although it is often scant). It is usually entirely radiolucent. It has a capricious clinical behavior, often but not always resistant to usual osteosarcoma chemotherapy. Although the usual reciprocal chromosomal translocation described in EWS (see below) has not been generally observed, this lesion has been shown to have membrane positivity for CD-99, which has led some authors to theorize that it is a variant of EWS with divergent differentiation.

ii. **Surface osteosarcomas.** About 1 in 20 osteosarcomas occurs in association with the bone surface rather than in the medullary cavity. The vast majority of these are low-grade tumors showing radiodensity and osseous differentiation. They include:

(a) **Parosteal osteosarcoma.** Parosteal osteosarcoma accounts for approximately 4% of osteosarcomas and the majority of surface osteosarcomas. It characteristically involves the posterior distal femur, is associated with the outer fibrous layer of the periosteum, and tends to wrap around the bone. Histologically, it consists of well-formed bony trabeculae, often arranged in parallel streamers separated by a hypocellular spindle stroma as seen in low-grade central osteosarcoma (e-**Fig. 47.36**). Cartilaginous differentiation is also common, often seen as a cartilage cap and sometimes causing confusion with osteochondroma. Radiographically, however, there is no continuity of the interior of this lesion and the medullary cavity, the adjacent bony cortex is not continuous with the outside of parosteal osteosarcoma (e-**Fig. 47.37**), and the intertrabecular spaces do not contain fatty or hematopoietic marrow. The prognosis of parosteal osteosarcoma is similar to that of low-grade intramedullary osteosarcoma. If inaccurately diagnosed as benign, or if inadequately excised, these lesions will recur. Recurrences may be low grade, but they may also be high grade; low-grade parosteal sarcoma undergoing high-grade transformation is termed *dedifferentiated parosteal osteosarcoma* and has a prognosis similar to conventional osteosarcoma.

(b) Periosteal osteosarcoma. This tumor arises between the cortex and overlying periosteum most commonly in the tibial or femoral diaphysis, and is characterized by abundant cartilaginous matrix and a somewhat greater degree of cytological atypia than is seen in parosteal osteosarcoma.

(c) High-grade surface osteosarcoma. This tumor is histologically identical to conventional intramedullary osteosarcoma, except that it arises on the bone surface. The prognosis is similar to that of conventional intramedullary osteosarcoma.

3. Fibrous tumors and tumor-like conditions

a. Fibrous dysplasia. This space-occupying lesion has been classified variously as developmental, tumorous, or tumor-like. It usually presents as a solitary lesion, although it may affect multiple bones in a single limb bud distribution or multiple bones without limb bud distribution. The polyostotic form is one of the manifestations of the McCune–Albright syndrome, which includes pigmented skin lesions and endocrinopathies. Fibrous dysplasia may be asymptomatic, but deformities, secondary fractures, and even pain may be the presenting manifestation. Radiographically, the lesion is almost always intramedullary, and it tends to affect those portions of bone formed by endochondral ossification. While secondary cortical atrophy may take place because of intramedullary expansion of the lesion, fibrous dysplasia usually does not involve the cortex. Fibrous dysplasia is often expansile and results in modeling deformities of the host bone. It is well circumscribed and radiolucent, but less radiolucent than the underlying bone that it has replaced; radiologists often refer to its appearance as having a "ground glass" quality (e-Fig. 47.38).

Histologically, fibrous dysplasia consists of various combinations of any tissue produced by bones, so fibrous tissue, bone, cartilage, and vascular tissues are produced in various combinations. The usual microscopic pattern, however, consists of loosely arranged, vascularized fibrous tissue in which disconnected, curved, microtrabeculae of bone are disposed. These trabeculae are not only woven in their collagen fiber pattern, but when a section is examined under polarized light, the fabric of their collagenous background forms a continuum with the fabric of the fibrous tissue (e-Fig. 47.39). Cartilage formation is not unusual, and occasionally cartilage is formed in such excess that lesions may be mistaken radiographically and histologically for cartilaginous neoplasms. Activating G-protein mutations have been identified in fibrous dysplasia, raising the possibility that it represents a true neoplasm (*J Pediatr.* 1993;123:509). Treatment is usually focused on relief of deformities or other morbid symptomatology. The prognosis is usually excellent.

b. Osteofibrous dysplasia. This fibro-osseous lesion is self-limited and is invariably seen in the tibia, fibula, or both. Its peak incidence is in the first two decades of life. Radiographically, the lesion is radiolucent and usually based in the anterior cortex; it may extend to the medullary cavity. The lesion may be unilocular or multilocular; while it tends to be circumscribed, it may also diffusely involve the diaphysis and cause secondary bowing deformities (e-Fig. 47.40). Histologically, osteofibrous dysplasia resembles fibrous dysplasia except that the microtrabeculae of bone tend to be rimmed by appositional osteoblasts even at their very earliest synthesis (e-Fig. 47.41). The fibrous stroma tends to be more cellular than in fibrous dysplasia, and is less contiguous with the trabeculae in polarized light. The bone tends to mature at the periphery with the surrounding normal bone. The lesion tends to undergo spontaneous involution with time, although sometimes it behaves more aggressively.

c. Nonossifying fibroma (fibrous cortical defect). This is the commonest space-occupying lesion of bone, estimated to affect one in four individuals.

Even though it is thought to be developmental, in rare cases the lesion behaves as a tumor of limited biologic potential. Unless it fractures, patients are generally without symptoms; the lesions are typically discovered incidentally during the course of evaluation for some other condition. The routine radiographs are virtually diagnostic. The lesion is a well-circumscribed radiolucent defect in the metaphyseal cortex with scalloped sclerotic borders, and it is almost always longer in the cephalocaudal than axial direction (e-**Fig. 47.42**). Histologically, the lesion consists of spindle cells arranged in a distinctly storiform pattern. There may be a fair number of multinucleated giant cells, histiocytic cells with foamy cytoplasm, and histiocytes containing hemosiderin pigment (e-**Fig. 47.43**). While bone formation is not observed (hence the name), lesions that have fractures or microscopic infarctions are admixed with reactive bone. Because this lesion may be focally cellular, it is important to review the radiographs to avoid misdiagnosis. Most nonossifying fibromas are self-healing and do not require clinical intervention.

   d. Desmoplastic fibroma. This rare tumor occurs in adolescents and young adults, with the mandible being the most commonly affected site. Radiologically, it often expands the involved bone, is entirely radiolucent, and is usually well circumscribed. Histologically, it is composed of bland fibroblastic or myofibroblastic cells in a background of collagen identical to that found in desmoid tumors and/or soft tissue fibromatosis (e-**Fig. 47.44**). Although it is benign, it behaves similarly to fibromatosis of soft tissue in that there is a high recurrence rate when not completely excised.

   e. Fibrosarcoma. This tumor constitutes approximately 5% of all primary malignant bone tumors with a relatively uniform age distribution between the 2nd and 6th decades. It usually involves the metaphyses of long bones resulting in pain, swelling, and a destructive radiological lesion without radiographically detectable matrix. Histologically, fibrosarcomas are usually quite cellular with malignant spindle cells arranged in a fascicular or herringbone pattern (e-**Fig. 47.45**). The differential diagnosis includes other malignant spindle-cell tumors such as fibroblastic osteosarcoma, leiomyosarcoma, malignant fibrous histiocytoma, as well as desmoplastic fibroma.

4. **Histiocytic and fibrohistiocytic tumors**
   a. Benign fibrous histiocytoma. This rare bone lesion is histologically similar to its soft tissue counterpart. There is a wide age distribution, with more than half of the cases developing in patients older than 20 years. The tumor most commonly involves either the epiphysis or diaphysis of long bones, or the pelvis. Radiographically, the lesion is well defined and radiolucent, and may expand the bone. Similar to benign fibrous histiocytoma elsewhere, the lesion is composed of spindle-shaped fibroblasts, at least focally arranged in a whorled or storiform pattern, intermixed with histiocytes and giant cells (e-**Fig. 47.46**). Mitoses may be evident. The main differential diagnosis is a secondary fibrohistiocytic reaction within another primary bone lesion, such as giant cell tumor or nonossifying fibroma.

   b. Malignant fibrous histiocytoma. This tumor is also similar to its soft-tissue counterpart, with most cases developing in patients older than 40 years. It can also complicate Paget disease, irradiation, and infarction. Most cases involve the long bones of the extremities or the pelvis. Histologically, there is a mixed population of spindle cells, histiocytic cells, and giant cells. Pleomorphic tumor cells, abnormal mitotic figures, and the characteristic storiform pattern of growth are also evident (e-**Fig. 47.47**). Almost all of the histological subtypes described in soft tissue have also been described in bone. The management and prognosis of this tumor most closely resemble osteosarcoma; the focal identification of osteoid or bone matrix is sometimes the only histologic difference between these two tumors, although most osteosarcomas arising in this age group are secondary to a prior disease or treatment.

   c. Langerhans cell histiocytosis. This comprises a group of neoplastic Langerhans cell proliferations that can be unifocal (solitary eosinophilic granuloma), multifocal (Hand–Schuller–Christian disease), or disseminated (Letterer–Siwe disease). All of these can produce bone lesions that tend to present early in multifocal and disseminated forms. Langerhans cell histiocytosis most frequently involves the craniofacial bones, but other bones such as the femur, pelvis, and ribs may also be involved. Radiographically, the lesions appear radiolucent and rapidly destructive, sometimes with associated exuberant periosteal new bone formation when they occur in long bones (e-**Fig. 47.48**). Histologically, there is a mixed inflammatory infiltrate including neutrophils, eosinophils, lymphocytes, and histiocytes (with or without giant cells) in which Langerhans cells are identified. Langerhans cells have eosinophilic to clear cytoplasm and contain oval, grooved, or multilobated nuclei (e-**Fig. 47.49**); immunohistochemically, they characteristically express S-100 and CD1a. Because there is a histologic similarity to chronic osteomyelitis, lesions thought to be Langerhans cell histiocytosis should be cultured, and the culture results should be known prior to formulating a final diagnosis. Langerhans cell histiocytosis has a very good prognosis except in the disseminated form, which is associated with a poor outcome (*Pediatr Blood Cancer.* 2005;45:37).

d. **Erdheim–Chester disease.** This rare disorder of unknown etiology is characterized by the presence of skeletal and extraskeletal foamy histiocytic infiltrates with associated fibrosis (e-**Fig. 47.50**). Most patients are older than 40 years, and there is usually bilateral symmetric or patchy sclerosis of the medullary cavity of the involved bones (most frequently the long bones of the extremity). Given the frequent and progressive infiltration of vital organs (such as the kidney, heart, or lung), most patients succumb within a few years.

e. **Giant cell tumor.** This tumor comprises around 4%–5% of all primary bone tumors and has a peak incidence between 20 and 45 years of age; it is rarely seen in skeletally immature individuals or in patients older than 50 years. Although there is some controversy as to its exact origin, it is placed in the histiocytic category because its giant cells are modified histiocytes and at least some of its stromal cells also express histiocytic markers. Giant cell tumor typically affects the ends of long bones and extends to the articular or apophyseal portions of the bone. The pelvis or small bones of the hand or feet are more rarely affected. Given the often juxta-articular location of the tumor, joint swelling and limitation of movement are common presenting symptoms. Radiologically, the tumor is radiolucent and eccentric, may expand the bone, and is well demarcated (e-**Fig. 47.51**). There is almost never a periosteal reaction associated with the tumor.

The histological hallmark of the tumor is the presence of sheets of round, oval, or elongated mononuclear cells with an open chromatin pattern evenly intermixed with numerous osteoclast-like giant cells with nuclei similar to the mononuclear cells (e-**Fig. 47.52**). The cell borders are often indistinct, so that on low power the lesion appears as a syncytium. Mitoses are variable in number; atypical mitoses are occasionally seen and do not necessarily predict malignant behavior. The presence of the characteristic mononuclear cells and the even interposition of the giant cells are essential for the diagnosis, as giant cells can be a component of many bone lesions. Other histological features occasionally seen in giant cell tumors include a focal storiform pattern, which, when abundant foam cells are present, can easily be confused with benign fibrous histiocytoma. There also may be areas of fibrosis, as well as secondary cystic areas resembling ABC (see below). The most important differential diagnosis is the so-called "brown tumor" of hyperparathyroidism (see Chapter 48); the lack of radiological or biochemical evidence of hyperparathyroidism, as well as the absence of additional bone lesions, can be very helpful in this regard. Another important differential diagnosis is so-called "giant-cell reparative granuloma" that characteristically involves the mandible and is composed of granuloma-like aggregates of giant cells in a fibrovascular stroma, but which lacks the mononuclear cells characteristic of giant cell tumor (e-**Fig. 47.53**).

Most cases of giant cell tumor behave in a benign fashion; some, however, are associated with local aggressiveness and occasionally (~ 2%) with distant metastasis. Most of these metastases are slow growing and rarely lethal. Except for the rare, so-called "malignant giant cell tumor," there are no reliable histological features that can predict a malignant outcome.

Malignant giant cell tumor is defined as a sarcomatous lesion arising within a giant cell tumor, or as a sarcoma that appears in the same area in which a bona fide giant cell tumor was treated (e-Fig. 47.54). The former instance is sometimes referred to as a primary malignant giant cell tumor; the latter as a secondary malignant giant cell tumor. The prognosis is related to the histology, size, and grade of the malignant component.

5. Hematolymphoid tumors

a. Solitary plasmacytoma and multiple myeloma. These tumors are malignant proliferations of plasma cells that account for the majority of tumors arising primarily in bone. The presentation of myeloma is quite variable (see Chapter 44), but involvement of the skeletal system is usually manifested by bone pain and/or pathological fractures. Radiologically, plasmacytoma and the lesions of multiple myeloma are lytic, well demarcated, and without a rim of sclerotic bone; however, multiple myeloma may also present with "generalized osteoporosis" without any detectable foci of discrete bone destruction. Histologically, the tumors are composed of plasma cells and their precursors at various stages of development (e-Fig. 47.55). The main differential diagnosis is often other hematolymphoid tumors; however, myeloma cells are occasionally quite anaplastic and can resemble carcinoma or high-grade sarcoma. Accordingly, immunohistochemical reactivity for CD138 or CD38 (among other markers; see Chapter 44) may be very useful to confirm the diagnosis.

b. Lymphoma. Most bone lymphomas are secondary to disease elsewhere, but primary bone lymphomas may also occur. In general, lymphomas presenting in bone are classified as primary provided no lymph node involvement is present both at the time of presentation and for a long interval afterward (the length of this interval varies according to different authors). Most primary lymphomas of bone represent examples of diffuse large B-cell lymphoma or other high-grade tumor, because most lower grade lymphomas and leukemias present with diffuse marrow involvement rather than as a tumorous mass. Primary Hodgkin's lymphoma of bone is exceedingly rare. Radiologically, lymphomas usually present as radiolucent lesions, sometimes disproportionately destructive when compared with the patient's clinical symptoms (e-Fig. 47.56). In about 20% of cases, the lesions present as radiodensities. The histological findings recapitulate those seen in extraskeletal sites. The prognosis is dependent on the type of lymphoma and stage.

6. Vascular tumors

a. Hemangioma. Although incidental hemangiomas are relatively common, clinically symptomatic tumors account for <1% of primary bone tumors and tend to present in late adulthood. Hemangioma is most frequently seen in the vertebrae, followed by the craniofacial skeleton and metaphyses of long bones. It appears as a radiolucent, often expansive lesion in long bones but as a vertically striate "corduroy pattern" lesion in intact vertebrae. Histologically, it is composed of capillary sized or cavernous vessels that permeate the marrow and are lined by bland endothelial cells (e-Fig. 47.57). As the name indicates, this tumor, as well as the closely related lymphangioma, is benign with low rates of recurrence following excision.

b. Angiosarcoma and hemangioendothelioma. This group accounts for <1% of bone tumors and may present at any age group, although the peak incidence is in young adulthood. It constitutes a spectrum of lesions ranging from locally destructive but indolent tumors with a good response to surgery or local radiation, to poorly differentiated malignant tumors with a high metastatic rate. Most tumors are radiolucent with poor margination; however, a sclerotic rim is occasionally identified.

While angiosarcomas are often solitary, hemangioendotheliomas tend to present as multifocal lesions in the same bone or in the same limb bud distribution and may be mistaken for skeletal metastases (e-**Fig. 47.58**). Angiosarcomas are usually characterized, at least focally, by the presence of irregularly anastamosing vascular channels that are lined by highly atypical endothelial cells, but they may largely consist of solid, patternless aggregates of polyhedral or spindle cells (e-**Fig. 47.59**). Poorly differentiated angiosarcomas may fail to express vascular markers. It should be noted that angiosarcomas are known to express cytokeratins, which is an important consideration when metastatic carcinoma is in the differential diagnosis. Most angiosarcomas are associated with a poor outcome.

Epithelioid hemangioendothelioma is composed of cords, nests, or sheets of plump cells that, in their attempt to form vessels, are often vacuolated, and some of the vacuoles may contain erythrocytes. An extracellular myxoid or hyalinized stroma is characteristic, although not always identified. Immunohistochemical reactivity with vascular markers such as CD31, CD34, and Factor VIII–related antigen can be used to confirm endothelial differentiation, and may help to exclude a diagnosis of metastatic signet-ring adenocarcinoma. Epithelioid hemangioendothelioma may have an indolent course.

7. Epithelial tumors

   a. Adamantinoma. This tumor comprises <1% of malignant bone tumors. There is a wide age distribution, with the median age of patients between 25 and 35 years. The tibia is most frequently involved, followed by the fibula, or both sites synchronously. Radiologically, an intracortical radiolucent lesion is evident, which may involve the medullary cavity (e-**Fig. 47.60**). Histologically, classic adamantinoma is composed of epithelial cells having a basaloid, tubular, or squamoid appearance; a predominantly spindle cell pattern; as well as mixtures of the above (e-**Fig. 47.61**). A storiform fibroblastic proliferation that contains variable amounts of woven or lamellar bone may also be present. Rarely, the tumor is predominantly composed of the latter component, with only rare scattered epithelial cells (single or in small nests, sometimes only detected by immunohistochemistry). Such tumors have been termed as having an "osteofibrous dysplasia-like pattern" or as "differentiated adamantinomas," and usually present in patients younger than 20 years. Adamantinomas are invariably immunopositive for various keratins and epithelial membrane antigen, and often also for vimentin. Classic adamantinomas are indolent tumors with a high local recurrence rate and metastasis in about 20% of patients; differentiated adamantinomas almost never metastasize.

   b. Metastatic carcinomas. These are the most common tumors affecting the skeleton, which is the third most common site to be involved by metastatic tumor after the lungs and liver. Primary carcinomas of the breast, lung, prostate, kidney, and thyroid gland compose >80% of all bone metastases. Radiologically, metastatic deposits can be radiolucent or radiodense or can display a mixed pattern (e-**Fig. 47.62**). Given their high incidence, metastatic carcinoma should always be in the differential diagnosis of solitary or multiple bone lesions in patients older than 40 years. The histology usually resembles that of the primary carcinoma, if it is known; it should be noted that a fibroblastic, osteoblastic, or vascular response to the secondary tumor may occasionally be quite prominent and overshadow the tumor cells, which may only be focally evident (e-**Fig. 47.63**). Consequently, immunohistochemistry may reveal isolated subtle tumor cells that are not obvious in small biopsy specimens.

8. Miscellaneous neoplasms

   a. EWS/PNET. In addition to its classic presentation in the diaphyses of long bones, EWS can involve axial bones such as the pelvis and ribs, as well as soft tissues (see Chapter 46) and other organs. EWS/PNET has been described at various ages, but most patients are younger than 20 years. Although patients usually have pain and a mass, they may also present with fever and leukocytosis suggestive of an infectious process. Radiologically, a destructive, permeative lesion is usually evident, often with an overlying multilayered but discontinuous "onion-skin" periosteal reaction (e-**Fig. 47.64**). Occasionally, there is a large soft-tissue mass with no obvious bone destruction on the routine radiographs, but the intraosseous component becomes evident on a CT scan or MRI. Histologically, EWS/PNET is the prototype for "small blue round cell tumors" as it is composed of sheets of such cells, often with glycogen-containing clear cytoplasm (e-**Fig. 47.65**). Evidence of neuroectodermal differentiation may be manifested by extracellular eosinophilic neuropil-like structures or Homer–Wright rosettes (composed of groups of tumor cells that surround a central core of eosinophilic extracellular material). Immunohistochemically, EWS/PNET shows characteristic strong immunoreactivity for CD99, negativity for CD45, and variable reactivity for neural markers such as neuron-specific enolase, synaptophysin, CD57, neurofilament, and S-100 protein. Cytokeratins may also be positive.

A characteristic feature of this tumor is the presence of a recurrent balanced reciprocal translocation involving the *EWS* gene on chromosome 22 and a member of the *Ets* family of genes, the most common of which (85% of cases) is the *FLI1* gene on chromosome 11 (*Br J Cancer.* 1994;70:908). Immunohistochemistry, polymerase chain reaction, and fluorescent in situ hybridization have all been used to confirm the diagnosis by detecting expressed *FLI1*, the fusion transcript, or the translocation itself, respectively. The prognosis of EWS has greatly improved with multimodality treatment, and 5-year survival rates are now approaching 70%.

   b. **Chordomas.** These are derived from notochordal remnants and account for approximately 4% of malignant bone tumors. Most tumors present after 30 years of age with a peak incidence between 50 and 60 years of age. The midline of the axial skeleton, particularly the sacrum and the base of the skull, is usually affected. Radiologically, a lucent lesion is seen with scattered calcifications; there is often a large associated soft-tissue component (e-**Fig. 47.66**). Histologically, chordomas are composed of lobules of tumor in which sheets, cords, or nests of vacuolated, eosinophilic to clear cells are embedded in myxoid matrix (e-**Fig. 47.67**). Chordomas express cytokeratins, epithelial membrane antigen, and S-100 protein, an immunohistochemical profile that is helpful in distinguishing this tumor from chondrosarcoma (which is cytokeratin and epithelial membrane antigen negative). Chordomas are aggressive tumors that are most notable for local recurrence when incompletely excised, but also have a metastatic potential. A controversial entity, "chondroid" chordoma, characterized by areas of mimicking hyaline cartilage, appears to have a better prognosis, whereas "dedifferentiated" chordoma, with its high-grade sarcomatous component, is associated with a very poor outcome.

9. **Cystic/cyst-like lesions**
   a. **Simple bone cyst.** This is an intraosseous space-occupying lesion consisting of an accumulation of fluid. The lesion is usually lined by a thin membrane composed of flattened cells of unknown type that may be involved in the production of the fluid, which usually appears serous. The base of the lesion is usually situated at an active growth plate, and the cyst is more or less maintained by continuous modeling of the bone around the area of fluid pressure. The lesion is circumscribed and radiolucent and usually involves the proximal humeral, femoral, or tibial region (e-**Fig. 47.68**). It does not expand the bone or cause deformity unless there has been a fracture with displacement prior to healing, and it tends to be symmetric. While fluid may not be obvious radiographically, the contents are demonstrable by MRI. Histologically, the diagnosis is one of exclusion and depends upon correlation of the imaging, operative findings, and lack of any other diagnostic tissue. Because most simple cysts are treated conservatively by injection of steroids or other sclerosing agents, it is unusual to see the lining of a simple cyst histologically unless there has been repeated fracture.

b. **Intraosseous ganglion.** This is a subarticular defect in the cancellous bone filled with mucoid fluid. The bone surrounding the defect is remodeled and sometimes sclerotic (e-**Fig. 47.69**). The defect is histologically similar to the subarticular cysts associated with overlying osteoarthritis (geodes) except that the subarticular plate and articular cartilage are radiographically intact in patients with intraosseous ganglia. The lesion is presumed to arise from a microscopic continuity of the subarticular plate with the joint space that either cannot be detected by imaging studies or that has healed; this etiology would allow pressurized synovial fluid to come in contact with the intertrabecular medullary space. There are no diagnostic features histologically as the concentrated fluid is practically acellular and resembles the contents of tenosynovial ganglia.

c. **Aneurysmal bone cyst.** This peculiar lesion derives its name from its expansile character. It is not a true cyst, but rather a collection of blood-filled spaces that are separated by fibro-osseous tissue septa containing a varying amount of multinucleated giant cells and immature bone. Most ABCs occur prior to 20 years of age. The lesion usually arises as an eccentric radiolucent lesion in metaphyses of long bones (e-**Fig. 47.70**). When it is central and symmetric it can often be distinguished from a simple cyst because it causes the bone to become wider than the growth plate. The bone destruction associated with ABC is perhaps the most rapidly associated with any osseous lesion. While its internal edge tends to be well marginated radiographically, ABC sometimes extends across adjacent bones, particularly if it arises in the spine. Complementary imaging studies, particularly MRI, reveal peculiar fluid–fluid levels on T2-weighted axial and sagittal views (e-**Fig. 47.71**); these levels are caused by the signal differences in erythrocytes and plasma, reflect erythrocyte sedimentation, and demonstrate that blood in intact ABC is both unclotted and stagnant or slow moving.

Histologically, there are vascular spaces that progress from very small capillary spaces to very large sinusoids separated by fibrous septae and sometimes by bone (e-**Fig. 47.72**). Within the septae are fibroblasts, scattered multinucleated giant cells, and osteoblasts associated with the bone production. Rarely, the lesion is almost entirely solid, although sometimes the solid variant may demonstrate fluid levels on imaging. In about half the cases, there is some other lesion associated with the cyst and admixed with curetted fragments; this has been termed secondary ABC. The associated lesion is usually benign, although malignant tumors have also been described in association with ABC. Gene rearrangements in chromosome 17 have been described in ABC, raising the possibility that the lesion is truly neoplastic. The genetic abnormalities thus far seem to apply mainly to the primary variety of this lesion, and have also been found in the solid variant (*Am J Pathol.* 2004;165:1773).

10. **Other rare primary bone neoplasms.** There are other benign and malignant soft-tissue neoplasms that can primarily arise in bone, including leiomyoma, leiomyosarcoma, lipoma, liposarcoma, and Schwannoma. All of these are histologically similar to their soft-tissue counterparts (see Chapter 46).

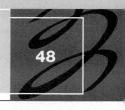
METABOLIC DISEASES OF BONE
Deborah Novack

I. NORMAL ANATOMY. Because of its accessibility and composition of both cortical and trabecular (cancellous) bone, the iliac crest is the site of choice for evaluation of systemic metabolic bone diseases. Cortex forms the external layer of all bones, comprises approximately 80% of bone mass, and supports most of the tissue's mechanical function. Trabecular bone, the meshwork surrounded by marrow or fat, is much more metabolically active than cortex. To support both its mechanical and metabolic functions, bone is dynamically regulated, and the skeleton is replaced completely every 10 years. The process of replacement, known as remodeling or turnover, is accomplished by the coordinated action of bone-forming osteoblasts and bone-resorbing osteoclasts, and is regulated by a variety of systemic factors including calcium, phosphorus, and parathyroid hormone (PTH). The goal of iliac crest trochar biopsy is to assess this process.

In either the cortex or trabeculum, remodeling begins when mononuclear osteoclast precursors (derived from hematopoietic progenitors) arrive at a bone surface, fuse, and differentiate into functional polykaryons (Fig. 48.1). Mature osteoclasts polarize and secrete acid and proteases onto an isolated microenvironment of the bone surface, excavating a pit known as Howship's lacuna. This resorption phase ends with the osteoclasts' apoptosis, and a reversal phase follows, characterized by activation of osteoblasts (of mesenchymal origin) to replace the excavated bone; the activity of osteoclasts and osteoblasts is normally tightly coupled, and the amount of bone synthesized matches the amount resorbed. Newly secreted matrix called osteoid becomes mineralized to form mature bone. The remodeling cycle ends when new bone formation is complete, and the osteoblasts are either incorporated into the new bone matrix as osteocytes, or become quiescent surface bone lining cells. The net result of each cycle is the formation of a new osteon, a packet of bone delineated by a "cement line" in which the collagen fibers are aligned. These lamellae of bone are easily seen when decalcified hematoxylin and eosin (H&E)-stained sections are examined under polarized light (e-Fig. 48.1).*

Osteoclasts can be identified by their characteristic appearance as multinucleated cells on the bone surface, with discrete nuclei (in contrast to megakaryocytes, which have fused nuclei). The most sensitive method of identifying osteoclasts histologically is expression of tartrate-resistant acid phosphatase (TRAP), which stains osteoclasts bright red (e-Fig. 48.2), although this is not usually necessary for diagnosis. Osteoblasts appear as cuboidal cells on the bone surface, often in rows, with abundant cytoplasm and an eccentric nucleus (e-Fig. 48.3). However, the strength of the undecalcified biopsy is in the evaluation of the function of these cells rather than their morphology.

Osteoblasts secrete matrix proteins onto the bone surface, but several days are required for mineral deposition. Therefore, the extent of bone surface covered by osteoid (osteoid surface) is one indicator of osteoblast activity. The thickness of the osteoid seams reflects the rate of mineral apposition, because mineralization converts osteoid to bone. Decalcification required for standard paraffin processing removes the distinction between newly synthesized osteoid and mature calcified bone. In contrast, undecalcified plastic sections can be stained in several ways to demonstrate osteoid. The vonKossa stain, a silver-based stain used

---

*All e-figures are available online via the Solution Site Image Bank.

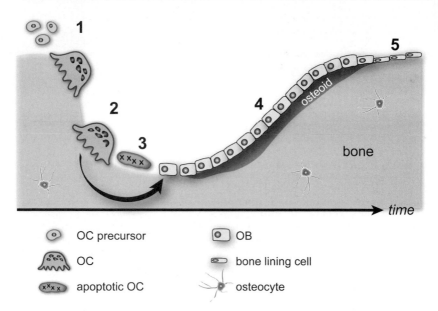

Figure 48.1. The bone remodeling cycle. 1. Osteoclast (OC) precursors are recruited to the bone surface, where they fuse and differentiate into mature polykaryons. 2. The osteoclasts resorb both organic and inorganic matrix of bone. 3. The resorption phase ends with osteoclast apoptosis. 4. During the reversal phase, osteoblasts (OB) differentiate from mesenchymal precursors, under the influence of factors from osteoclasts (*curved arrow*), and secrete new bone matrix known as osteoid. 5. At the end of the remodeling cycle, some osteoblasts have been incorporated into the bone and become osteocytes, whereas others remain on the surface as synthetically quiescent bone-lining cells.

with a basic fuchsin counterstain, shows calcified bone matrix as dark brown or black, whereas the unmineralized matrix (osteoid) appears pink-red (e-**Fig. 48.4A**). A trichrome stain, either Gomori or modified Masson, also distinguishes mineralized bone from osteoid (e-**Fig. 48.4B**). These latter stains allow easier interpretation of cellular morphology than the vonKossa, and also highlight peritrabecular or marrow fibrosis.

A second critical marker of osteoblast function is tetracycline labeling. Tetracycline family antibiotics are calcium-chelating fluorochromes that bind to actively mineralizing bone surfaces, can be taken orally, and are well-tolerated. They are given in 2 courses, separated by 2 weeks. If bone formation is active during both intervals, examination of unstained sections by fluorescence microscopy demonstrates two bright bands of labeling (a double label) (e-**Fig. 48.5**, *arrows*). Similarly, active bone formation during only one of the labeling periods yields a single tetracycline label (e-**Fig. 48.5**, *arrowheads*). Combination of the extent of labeled trabecular bone surface and the distance between labels provides the mineral apposition rate and bone formation rate. In a normal subject, most surfaces with osteoid, as seen on trichrome or vonKossa stains, have double labels.

During normal endochondral bone development, cartilage formed at the growth plate is replaced by bone in the primary spongiosa through the action of osteoclasts. Toluidine blue stains cartilage purple, and cartilage may be found within trabeculae near the growth plate in children (e-**Fig. 48.6**). However, a finding of entrapped cartilage in an iliac crest bone biopsy in an adult, or >1 cm from the growth plate in a child, is indicative of osteoclast dysfunction such as in osteopetrosis.

II. INDICATIONS FOR BIOPSY, TISSUE SAMPLING, AND PREPARATION

A. Indications for biopsy. The most common indications for metabolic bone biopsy are end-stage renal disease (ESRD) and unexplained hypercalemia or hyperphosphatemia, osteoporosis unresponsive to therapy, or suspected osteomalacia. Patients who have multiple or unexplained fractures (particularly if they are failing to heal), unexplained bone pain, or an elevation in serum alkaline phosphatase may also be candidates.

B. Biopsy procedure. A critical component of evaluation of metabolic bone biopsies is in vivo fluorochrome labeling of bone. Use a regimen of tetracycline (250 mg orally four times a day [PO qid]) for 3 days, followed by a 14-day interval, then 3 more days of therapy (250 mg PO qid). Biopsy is performed on the third day after the last dose. Biopsy interpretation may be confounded by recent antibiotic use of drugs in the tetracycline family. Inadequate labeling can be caused by malabsorption syndromes or by taking tetracycline with meals, dairy products, iron-containing medications, antacids, or calcium supplements.

Biopsy is performed as an outpatient procedure. The most accessible site for biopsy is the anterior iliac crest, a biopsy of which can be taken using a vertical or horizontal approach. A small incision is made to expose the periosteum, the trephine is inserted and advanced with steady pressure, and the specimen is extracted. When obtained, the specimen should be placed directly in 70% ethanol. The biopsy site is packed with surgicel. Patients typically return to full activity within 24 hours.

C. Sample preparation. The specimen should be fixed in 70% ethanol for at least 48 hours, and this solution is suitable for shipping and long-term storage at room temperature. Following dehydration with xylene, the specimen is mounted in methyl methacrylate in a process that requires 7 to 10 days. The tissue core is sectioned parallel to its long axis at 5 to 7 μm using a tungsten blade. Undecalcified sections are stained with vonKossa, Gomori, or modified Masson trichrome, and toluidine blue. One section is decalcified and stained with H&E. Thicker 10-μm sections are coverslipped without staining for examination under fluorescence.

D. Quantitative versus qualitative evaluation. The American Society for Bone and Mineral Research has described a nomenclature for a basic set of structural and kinetic features identified by nondecalcified bone biopsy (*J Bone Miner Res* 1987;2:595), and there are two commercially available systems that allow quantitative analysis based on these standards (OsteoMeasure, OsteoMetrics, Inc. and Bioquant Osteo II, BIOQUANT Image Analysis Corporation). Reference values, based on somewhat limited populations, have been published (*J Bone Miner Res* 1988;3:133, *J Bone Miner Res* 2004;19:1628, *Bone* 2000;26:103, *Engl J Med* 1988;319:1698). Although some laboratories perform quantitative analysis on all specimens, qualitative assessments are often adequate for diagnosis of individual patients. Quantitative analysis is most useful in the setting of research studies.

III. DIAGNOSTIC FEATURES OF METABOLIC BONE DISORDERS

A. Osteoporosis. In the setting of osteoporosis or osteopenia, biopsy establishes rate of bone remodeling (turnover), degree of mineralization, architectural integrity, and effects of treatment. Iliac crest bone biopsy is a poor indicator of bone mass, as bone volume/tissue volume (BV/TV) is variable within this region. Trabecular connectivity, which describes the intactness of the trabecular meshwork, correlates with bone mass. In osteoporosis/osteopenia, trabeculae are very small and often appear as isolated islands (low connectivity), rather than as an interconnected grid (good connectivity) (e-**Fig. 48.7**). In high-turnover osteoporosis, osteoid surface is enhanced (e-**Fig. 48.8A**), with normal or increased numbers of osteoclasts and osteoblasts. The extent of double tetracycline-labeled trabecular bone surface is also increased, although the distance between the double labels is usually normal (e-**Fig. 48.8B**). In low-turnover osteoporosis or osteopenia, there is little osteoid, few osteoclasts or osteoblasts, and rare or absent trabecular double tetracycline labels (e-**Fig. 48.9**). Even in low-turnover states, double labeling in the cortex is usually present, and is a good positive control for adequate tetracycline dosing and specimen processing.

Many patients with osteoporosis have been treated with bisphosphonates, often for several years. Although biopsy studies have shown that normal turnover is intact in most patients (*JAMA* 2006;296:2927), some cases of severely suppressed bone turnover have been reported and are associated with increased fractures (*J Clin Endocrinol Metab* 2005;90:1294, *N Engl J Med* 2006;355:2048). Bisphosphonates target the osteoclast, decreasing resorption and enhancing apoptosis, producing changes that can be seen on sections, with osteoclasts appearing either hyperchromatic with pyknotic nuclei (e-**Fig. 48.10A**) or round and unpolarized (e-**Fig. 48.10B**).

B. **Osteomalacia.** In osteomalacia, newly formed organic bone matrix fails to mineralize normally, and the result is wide osteoid seams, often greatly increased in extent along the trabecular bone surface (e-**Fig. 48.11A**). Some osteoid may be completely unlabeled by tetracycline (e-**Fig. 48.11B**), whereas other surfaces may show irregular and diffuse fluorescence (e-**Fig. 48.11C**); double tetracycline labels are rare. Florid osteomalacia due to nutritional rickets is now rare, but milder cases may be found unexpectedly, and bone biopsy is the only definitive diagnostic tool. In these cases, poor tetracycline labeling of osteoid-covered surfaces is necessary to diagnose osteomalacia.

C. **Renal osteodystrophy.** Patients with ESRD have a wide array of metabolic abnormalities that may affect bone and are known collectively as renal osteodystrophy. Three predominant patterns have been described: high bone turnover with osteitis fibrosa (hyperparathyroid bone disease), low bone turnover (including low-turnover osteomalacia and adynamic bone disease), and mixed uremic osteodystrophy. The most important role of biopsy is in the setting of hypercalcemia, in which a finding of PTH-driven high turnover indicates a need for parathyroidectomy, whereas a finding of low turnover is a contraindication for this surgery.

In high-turnover renal osteodystrophy, elevated PTH levels drive bone resorption by many osteoclasts; peritrabecular fibrosis, also known as osteitis fibrosa, may also be present (e-**Fig. 48.12A**). Bone formation is accelerated, often with formation of disorganized woven bone (seen on polarization; e-**Fig. 48.12B**) and increased tetracycline double labels (e-**Fig. 48.12C**). Trabeculae may be irregular in shape, and the cortex may be porous due to increased resorption.

In either form of low-turnover osteodystrophy, trabecular surfaces appear quiescent, with few osteoblasts or osteoclasts. Trabecular connectivity may also be decreased, and this parameter is more useful than the overall BV/TV (as mentioned in the discussion of osteoporosis). In the osteomalacic form of renal osteodystrophy, mineralization is delayed and wide osteoid seams identified by vonKossa or trichrome staining (e-**Fig. 48.13A**) are not tetracycline labeled (e-**Fig. 48.13B**). In a dynamic bone disease, both osteoid (e-**Fig. 48.13C**) and tetracycline labels (e-**Fig. 48.13D**) are minimal or absent.

As the name implies, mixed uremic osteodystrophy shows features of increased PTH and defective mineralization. Additionally, the appearance may vary considerably within the specimen (e-**Fig. 48.14A**), with areas of increased turnover adjacent to more quiescent regions with poor mineralization. Some areas may show abundant osteoid and robust tetracycline double labels (e-**Fig. 48.14B** and C) adjacent to broad single labels or unlabeled osteoid (e-**Fig. 48.14D**).

D. **Glucocorticoid-induced osteoporosis.** Because long-term glucocorticoid therapy is widely used in chronic inflammatory disease and in organ transplantation, there is a high prevalence of glucocorticoid-induced bone disease. Early in treatment, glucocorticoids increase bone resorption, but more prolonged therapy eventuates in adynamic bone. The number of osteoclasts and osteoblasts is decreased, as is tetracycline double labeling.

E. Most cases of primary hyperparathyroidism are now diagnosed based on elevated serum calcium and PTH levels. However, in normocalcemic patients with variable or borderline PTH levels, bone biopsy can be useful in making the diagnosis of primary hyperparathyroidism because histologic findings represent the net effect of PTH over time. As in secondary hyperparathyroidism (such as in high-turnover renal osteodystrophy), sections typically show increased osteoid surfaces, some with woven bone, increased tetracycline labeling, and elevated numbers of osteoclasts and osteoblasts. Osteitis fibrosa cystica, the formation of cystic bone loss due to elevated osteoclast activity associated with marrow fibrosis, is found only in severe cases and, due to routine testing of serum calcium, is rarely seen. However, peritrabecular fibrosis may be present. Another effect of PTH is to increase the porosity of the cortex, which may be difficult to distinguish from the trabecular bone.

Suggested Readings

Monier-Faugere MC, Langub MC, et al. Bone biopsies: a modern approach. In: Avioli LV, Krane SM, eds. *Metabolic Bone Disease and Clinically Related Disorders*. San Diego, CA: Academic Press; 1998:237–273.

Recker RR, Barger-Lux MJ. Bone biopsy and histomorphometry in clinical practice. In: Favus M, ed. *Primer on the Metabolic Bone diseases and Disorders of Mineral Metabolism*. Washington, DC: American Society for Bone and Mineral Research; 2006:161–169.

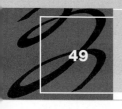

49

JOINTS AND SYNOVIUM

Peter A. Humphrey

I. NORMAL ANATOMY. Joints are composed of the ends of contiguous bones, and the associated soft tissue elements, including cartilage, ligaments, tendons, and synovium (Bullough PG in SE Mills ed., *Histology for Pathologists,* 2nd ed. Philadelphia: Lippincott Williams & Wilkins; 2007:97–121). Diarthrodial movable joints, which are the most common type, are usually covered by hyalin cartilage. Histologically, this articular cartilage is hypocellular, with a glassy extracellular matrix, composed mainly of collagen, proteoglycan, and water. Embedded within the matrix are chondrocytes within surrounding spaces (lacunae). There are four zones in articular cartilage—superficial, intermediate, deep, and calcified (e-**Fig. 49.1**)*—and chondrocytes have a different appearance depending on their location. Those near the surface of the articular cartilage are small and flattened; in the middle zones, the chondrocytes are more rounded and arranged in columns. The deep and calcified layers of articular cartilage are separated by a thin, basophilic line known as the tidemark, which represents the mineralized front. The calcified cartilage base interdigitates with underlying subchondral bone.

Ligaments, which join two adjacent bones, are formed mainly of collagen. At the insertion site onto bone the ligamentous tissue is calcified. Tendons are connective tissue structures connecting muscle to bone. Microscopically, scant fibroblasts are found within parallel collagen bundles.

Synovium is a glistening white membrane with delicate villous projections that lines the inner surface of the joint capsule (*Am J Clin Pathol* 2000;14:773)(e-**Fig. 49.2**). The inner lining surface is created by synovial cells, including fibroblastlike cells and histiocytes, which are arranged as a thin 2- to 3-cell layer of closely-packed synoviocytes with elliptical nuclei and abundant cytoplasm. A fibrous or fibroadipose supporting layer lies beneath the synovial cell layer. Synovium also lines the flexor tendons of the hand and bursae (subcutaneous and subtendinous sacs).

II. GROSS EXAMINATION AND TISSUE SAMPLING. Joint or synovial soft tissue may be received as needle core tissue, as fragments from arthroscopic or open synovectomy, as fragments from revised total joint arthroplasty, or as excisions of soft tissue tendon sheath or extra-articular masses. If fragments are received, the number, color, shape, and aggregate size of the fragments should be recorded. If meniscus tissue is submitted, fibrillations or tears should be noted. If chalky white deposits are identified, some of the tissue should be placed into absolute (100%) alcohol to preserve the crystals. Decalcification may be required for calcified cartilage, bone, or soft tissue. Fragments that appear different from normal should be selected for embedding, along with representative unremarkable-appearing fragments.

    A. Revision arthroplasties. The presence or absence of necrosis, purulent exudate, and foreign material should be recorded. The explanted prosthesis should be described, including any identification numbers or defects.

    B. Soft tissue tumors. For excised soft tissue tendon sheath or juxta-articular masses size, color, consistency, shape, and nodularity (single vs. more) should be provided. The outer surface of the specimen should then be inked, and cut sections should be characterized as to color, presence or absence of hemorrhage and necrosis, and distance of tumor to inked margin. One section per centimeter of tumor is a useful

---

*All e-figures are available online via the Solution Site Image Bank.

guide for section submission. Demonstration of tumor in relation to the closest inked margin(s) and to any recognizable normal tissue is important.

C. **Joint replacement surgeries.** Joint tissue may also be removed along with bone in orthopedic joint replacement surgeries, such as knee and total hip replacement procedures, which are most often performed for osteoarthritis. In such cases, where there is identifiable bone and attached articular cartilage, gross examination is particularly important. The overall dimensions and shape of the submitted bone and soft tissue should be recorded. Articular cartilage presence or absence, color, thickness, and abnormalities such as loss, cleft or tuft formation, crystalline deposits, and bony and cartilaginous overgrowths (osteophytes or exostosis) should be documented. Synovium color, thickness, and consistency and any nodules or villous projections should be described. One or several sections of synovium should be submitted for formalin fixation. Any associated gross bone defects, such as subchondral cyst formation and superficial bony necrosis, should be noted. Again, if chalky white deposits are identified, tissue should be placed into absolute (100%) alcohol to preserve the crystals. Sections of macroscopically abnormal areas should be submitted for histologic examination as follows. The bone and overlying cartilage should be fixed overnight in formalin, decalcified, and sectioned into 3- to 5-mm slices. One or two sections are usually sufficient to document cartilaginous and associated bone abnormalities. Junctions of normal and abnormal cartilage with underlying bone should be demonstrated with the sections.

D. **Synovial fluid.** Examination can be extremely useful in the diagnosis of different types of arthritis, especially infectious arthritis.

III. **DIAGNOSTIC FEATURES OF COMMON DISEASES OF JOINTS AND SYNOVIUM**

A. **Osteoarthritis** (also known as degenerative joint disease) is defined by the American College of Rheumatology as a "heterogeneous group of conditions that leads to joint symptoms and signs which are associated with defective integrity of articular cartilage, in addition to related changes in the underlying bone at the joint margins." (*Semin Arthritis Rheum* 2005;35(1):1). It is the most common disease of the joints, with a prevalence after the age of 65 years of about 60% in men and 70% in women. The etiology of osteoarthritis is multifactorial, with inflammatory, metabolic, and mechanical causes. Major trauma, repetitive joint use, chronic inflammatory arthritis, and congenital malformations are major risk factors. The diagnosis is usually based on clinical and radiographic features. Pathologically, although the name osteoarthritis indicates an inflammatory condition, disruption of the articular cartilage is the fundamental finding. The joints most commonly affected are the distal and proximal interphalangeal joints of the hands, the hips and knees, and the cervical and lumbar spine.

Grossly, cartilaginous thinning, disruption, and fibrillation can be seen. In areas of complete cartilage loss, the underlying bone is exposed; this bone has a dense polished appearance like marble (known as eburnation). Microscopically, vertical clefts in the cartilage are characteristic (e-**Fig. 49.3**). There may be associated villous hyperplasia and mild chronic inflammation of the synovium (which should not be confused with rheumatoid arthritis). Papillary masses of metaplastic cartilage, bone, or adipose tissue may form in the synovial membrane; detachment of the masses results in intra-articular loose bodies (known as rice bodies). In eburnated areas, the bone may show sclerotic thickened bony trabeculae, cysts with fluid and fibromyxoid tissue, and superficial bony necrosis (Bullough PG, Silverberg SG. *Surgical Pathology and Cytopathology*, 4th ed. Philadelphia: Elsevier; 2006:678–699). It should be noted that in the vast majority of cases, the pathologic findings are confirmatory of the clinical diagnosis, so it has been suggested that routine pathologic examination in uncomplicated total hip and total knee arthroplasties may not be necessary. In only a small percentage of cases is the pathologic diagnosis different from the clinical impression; in discrepant cases, the pathological diagnosis in most cases is avascular necrosis, rheumatoid arthritis, pseudogout, or pigmented villonodular synovitis (*J Arthroplasty* 2000;15:69, *Bone Joint Surg Am* 2000;82:1531). Because of these rare cases with unexpected findings, microscopic examination is warranted.

B. Rheumatoid arthritis is a chronic multisystem disease of unknown cause. The hallmark of rheumatoid arthritis is a persistent inflammatory synovitis, typically involving the peripheral joints in a symmetric distribution. Clinically, the synovial inflammation causes swelling, tenderness, and limitation of motion. Histologically, the main attribute is joint destruction. There is hypertrophy and hyperplasia of the synovium, along with a lymphoplasmacytic infiltrate, generating a papillary/polypoid chronic synovitis (e-**Fig. 49.4**). Lymphoid follicles and acute fibrinous surface exudate (e-**Fig. 49.5**) can also be seen. Synovial giant cells and bone and cartilage fragments may be present in the synovium. This overall histologic picture is not specific for rheumatoid arthritis, and similar changes may be seen in other arthridites such as systemic lupus erythematosus and psoriasis (Bullough PG, Silverberg SG. *Surgical Pathology and Cytopathology,* 4ᵗʰ ed. Philadelphia: Elsevier; 2006:678–699). Destruction of cartilage and joint fusion (ankylosis) can occur due to pannus (inflamed synovium and granulation tissue) formation over the surface of the articular cartilage, with invasion into cartilage and even bone and joint capsule.

Extra-articular manifestations of rheumatoid arthritis, which usually occur in patients with high titers of rheumatoid factor, include rheumatoid nodules, vasculitis, pleuropulmonary involvement (such as fibrosis and serositis), and splenomegaly with neutropenia in Felty's syndrome. Rheumatoid nodules develop in about 25% of patients with rheumatoid arthritis. Although common locations include olecranon bursa, the proximal ulna, and Achilles tendon, they can also be found in the heart, lung, pleura, kidney, and meninges. Histologically, there is a central zone of fibrinoid necrosis surrounded by palisading histiocytes (e-**Fig. 49.6**).

C. Synovitis associated with loose large joint arthroplasty can be seen when there is failure of a total joint replacement, and can be related to a foreign body-type inflammatory response or infection. The foreign material can be metal, plastic/polyethylene, and/or methyl methacrylate cement. Microscopically, 1- to 3-mm metallic particles may be found within macrophages. Needle-shaped, polarizable fragments of polyethylene plastic can be found in foreign body giant cells. Because the methyl methacrylate cement is lost upon processing, only empty spaces within foreign body-type giant cells are present in histologic sections after routine processing. These different types of foreign material can also elicit an exuberant fibrohistiocytic response (e-**Fig. 49.7**).

When neutrophils are seen, particularly numerous neutrophils, the possibility of infection should be considered. Frozen section of the inflamed tissue from a failed joint replacement may be requested, and the number of neutrophils per high-power field (HPF) should be reported. At least 5 HPFs on at least two sections should be examined. Observation of ≤5 neutrophils per HPF in tissue (not fibrin) is associated with high specificity (of about 95%) in identification of the absence of infection, whereas the presence of >5 neutrophils per HPF has a sensitivity of up to 69% in identification of the presence of infection (*Mod Pathol* 1998;11:427).

D. In crystal-induced synovitis, deposition of microcrystals in joints and periarticular tissues results in gout (urate crystals), pseudogout (also known as chondrocalcinosis—calcium pyrophosphate dihydrate crystals), and apatite disease (hydroxyapatite crystals) (*Am J Clin Pathol* 2000;14:773). Gout and pseudogout are definitively diagnosed by light microscopic detection of crystals in joint fluid. Gouty tophi are formed when urate crystals are deposited in subcutaneous soft tissue, synovium, bone, or bursae, with a granulomatous response dominated by histiocytes and foreign body giant cells (e-**Fig. 49.8**); fixation of the tissue in alcohol is necessary to preserve the crystals. A deGalantha histochemical stain can be used to highlight the crystals.

E. Infectious arthritis is diagnosed by clinical history and joint fluid examination, including Gram stain of a centrifuged cell pellet and microbiologic culture.

F. Hemosiderotic synovitis follows chronic intra-articular hemorrhage, which can occur in patients with hemophilia and synovial hemangioma. Microscopically, there are fine villous projections early in the disease course. Hemosiderin is present within synoviocytes and macrophages (e-**Fig. 49.9**). Osteoarthritis usually ensues.

G. Baker's cyst, which can be found in osteoarthritis and rheumatoid arthritis, is a synovial-lined cyst in the popliteal space that is formed by herniation. In contrast, ganglia (ganglion cysts), located near a joint capsule or tendon sheath, are not synovial-lined cysts and do not communicate with the joint cavity.

H. Tissue from a **torn meniscus** from the knee may be submitted as tissue shavings or as a fibrocartilaginous loose body. Histologically, there is little to be observed in this avascular, collagenized tissue, because reparative fibrosis and neovascularization are uncommon.

I. Each **intervertebral disc** is a type of joint (amphiarthrodial), and tissue fragments from a prolapsed disc may be submitted. Microscopically, fibrous tissue, fibrocartilage, and cartilaginous tissue can be seen. Chondrocyte necrosis and/or groups of proliferating chondrocytes may be found. The presence of neovascularization indicates herniation (*Hum Pathol* 1988;19:406).

J. **Synovial tumors** are uncommon and can arise from synovium of the tendon sheaths, bursae, and joint spaces (Unni KK, Inwards CT, Bridge JA, Kindblom L-G, Wold LE. In: *Tumors of the Bones and Joints*, AFIP Atlas of Tumor Pathology, Series 4, Washington, DC: American Registry of Pathology; 2005:383–391, Weiss SW, Goldblum JR. In: *Soft Tissue Tumors*, 5th ed., St. Louis, MO: Mosby:, 2008:769–788).

1. **Tenosynovial giant cell tumor, localized type (nodular tenosynovitis)** is the most common benign tumor of the tendon sheath and synovium. It appears to be a neoplasm rather than a reactive process. These giant cell tumors are usually found in adults on the fingers, and uncommonly on the ankle and knee (*Cancer* 1986;57:875). Grossly, they are circumscribed lobulated masses a few centimeters in diameter, with mottled pink-gray cut surfaces that often show flecks of yellow or brown (representing lipid and hemosiderin, respectively). Microscopically, there is a vague nodularity at low magnification; at higher powers of magnification, rounded mononuclear cells, giant cells, foam cells, and collagen are seen in varying proportions (e-**Fig. 49.10**). Hemosiderin deposition may be present. Mitotic figures are uncommon and when they exceed 2 figures per 10 HPFs, the likelihood of recurrence is greater. Immunohistochemistry and electron microscopy have demonstrated macrophage and synovial cell features (and osteoclast attributes in the giant cells), but are not required for the diagnosis. Cytogenetic studies have demonstrated clonal abnormalities (especially involving 1p11–13) but are not needed for diagnosis.

   Tenosynovial giant cell tumors are benign, with a recurrence rate of about 10% to 20%, related to mitotic activity (as noted above), cellularity, and incomplete excision (Weiss SW, and Goldblum JR. In: *Soft Tissue Tumors*, 5th ed., St. Louis, MO: Mosby; 2008:769–788). Accordingly, margin status and a high mitotic rate should be reported.

2. **Tenosynovial giant cell tumor, diffuse type,** is also known as extra-articular pigmented villonodular synovitis. It is much less common than intra-articular pigmented villonodular synovitis. The knee, ankle, and foot are predominant sites of occurrence. Grossly, the tumor is a large, multinodular, white to yellow-brown mass, without villous projections. Microscopically, there are sheets of rounded to polygonal mononuclear cells, with the formation of clefts and pseudoglandular spaces. Giant cells are fewer in number compared to the localized giant cell tumor. Xanthoma cells, spindle cells, and chronic inflammatory cells are present. Scant data exist on outcome for these patients, although recurrence rates appear high, at 40% to 50% (Weiss SW, and Goldblum JR. In: *Soft Tissue Tumors*, 5th ed., St. Louis, MO: Mosby; 2008:769–788).

3. **Pigmented villonodular synovitis** typically involves the joint space of the knee of young adults, although ankle, hip, and shoulder involvement have also been reported. Localized and diffuse forms are recognized. The localized form is characterized by focal involvement of the synovium, with either nodular or pedunculated masses; the more common diffuse form affects virtually the entire synovium. Grossly, tissue from the diffuse form removed by open synovectomy is spongy,

diffusely thickened, and brownish-yellow. Microscopically, subsynovial fibrohistiocytic cells with uniform round to oval nuclei are seen. Foam cells and iron pigment are always present, and giant cells are common and tend to be arranged in groups. Aside from the villous structures, the overall appearance is similar to tenosynovial giant cell tumor (e-**Fig. 49.11**).

The gene expression profile of the neoplasm resembles that of activated macrophages (*Arthritis Rheum* 2006;54:1009), and structural rearrangements of 1p11-12 have been reported in the lesion; however, these special studies are not needed to establish the diagnosis. The localized form has an excellent prognosis and a low recurrence rate when managed surgically, whereas the diffuse form has a reported recurrence rate of up to 46%. Radiation treatment has shown mixed results. Combined surgical and nonsurgical approaches may be necessary, and in some patients, total joint arthroplasty may be the only effective treatment (*J Am Acad Orthop Surg* 2006;14:376).

4. **Malignant giant cell tumor of tendon sheath/pigmented villonodular synovitis** is rare type of sarcoma, and can be diagnosed when histologically benign giant cell tumor of tendon sheath/pigmented villonodular synovitis is admixed with overtly malignant areas, or when malignancy is seen in a recurrence of the benign tumor. Histological indicators of malignancy include diffuse infiltrative growth, scant giant cells, cytological atypia, necrosis, and a mitotic count of >10 per 10 HPFs.

5. **Synovial chondromatosis** is defined as "a benign nodular cartilaginous proliferation arising in the synovium of joints, bursae, or tendon sheaths" (Miller MV, King AR, Mertens F; In: Fletcher CDM, Unni KK, Mertens F, eds. *Pathology and Genetics of Tumours of Soft Tissue and Bone*. Lyon, France: IARC Press; 2002:246). It is usually monoarticular in distribution, involving the knee or hip in adults. Grossly, there are multiple osteocartilaginous nodules, each measuring <1 mm to several millimeters in diameter, which may be embedded within synovium and/or mobile as loose bodies (note that loose bodies can also be seen in epiphyseal osteonecrosis, osteochondral fracture, and osteochondritis dissecans, so their presence is not diagnostic). Microscopically, the nodules of hyaline cartilage show clusters of chondrocytes that can show nuclear atypia with nuclear enlargement, hyperchromasia, and binucleation (e-**Fig. 49.12**), findings that should not be viewed as evidence of malignancy. Clonal chromosomal abnormalities have been cited as evidence for a neoplastic process, but cytogenetics is not used for diagnosis. Local recurrence after excision occurs in about 15% of cases. Rare cases of chondrosarcoma arising in synovial chondromatosis have been reported.

6. **Synovial chondrosarcoma** is extremely rare and may be classified as primary or secondary to synovial chondromatosis. Histologic features of malignancy include loss of the "clustering" growth pattern typical of synovial chondromatosis (e-**Fig. 49.13**), with a sheetlike arrangement of chondrocytes, myxoid change in the matrix, areas of necrosis, and spindling at the periphery of chondroid lobules (*Cancer* 1991;67:155). The prognosis is poor.

7. **Synovial hemangioma** is very rare and usually found in the knee of young adults. Microscopically, most are cavernous hemangiomas; some are capillary or arteriovenous hemangiomas (e-**Fig. 49.14**).

8. **Synovial lipoma** is rare. Grossly, the synovium is yellow, thickened, and exhibits excrescences (lipoma arborescens). Microscopically, the synovium is infiltrated by mature adipose tissue (e-**Fig. 49.15**). Recurrence is unusual.

9. Case reports of synovial tumors include intra-articular hemangiopericytoma, intracapsular chondroma, synovial sarcoma, epithelioid sarcoma, malignant fibrous histiocytoma, and lymphoma.

GENERAL PRINCIPLES OF EXFOLIATIVE AND FINE NEEDLE ASPIRATION BIOPSY

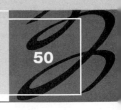

50

Rosa M. Dávila and Lourdes R. Ylagan

I. NONGYNECOLOGIC EXFLOLIATIVE CYTOLOGY

A. Specimen types

1. Body fluids (including urine, cerebrospinal fluid, and sputum) from various sources, including peritoneum and pleural and pericardial cavities.

2. Scrapings, washings, or brushings from various sites, including peritoneal washings, bronchial washings, bronchial brushings, bile duct brushings, and esophageal brushings.

B. Specimen transport and preservation.
Samples without preservative can be submitted to the laboratory only if they are going to be processed immediately. When delays are anticipated, samples should be refrigerated until processing is available. Some specimens, such as urine specimens, undergo cellular degeneration even when refrigerated, so addition of commercially available preservatives may be useful.

C. Specimen processing.
Body fluid specimens and washings can be processed in different ways, and different laboratories have different preferences. Available options include cytocentrifugation with air drying or ethanol fixation of the sample; liquid-based processing using commercially available reagents such as ThinPrep (Cytyc, a Hologic company) and SurePath (BD Diagnostics-TriPath); and production of a paraffin-embedded cell block after formalin fixation.

Scrapings and brushings are performed at the patient's bedside so the samples can be air dried or ethanol fixed. In general, the Papanicolaou stain is applied to ethanol fixed slides, and a Romanowski stain is applied to air-dried slides. Other histochemical stains such as Gomori methenamine silver, mucicarmine, and acid-fast stains, can also be used if needed.

D. Ancillary testing

1. **Immunocytochemistry.** Special stains are commonly applied to cytologic samples, often to confirm the morphologic diagnosis, to help in determining possible primary sites of a tumor, or to determine the presence of specific markers. In general, cell block sections are usually preferred for immunocytochemical staining because most laboratories have experience processing the formalin-fixed, paraffin-embedded tissue sections that are generated from cell blocks.

2. **Flow cytometry.** In the presence of a lymphocyte-rich sample, the possibility of a lymphoproliferative process may need to be addressed by flow cytometry. Body fluids, particularly effusions, are amenable to this type of analysis.

3. **Molecular genetic methods.** Cytological preparations, including body fluid specimens as well as scrapings, washings, and brushings, are suitable substrates for molecular analysis. Regardless of the method used to process samples clinically (whether air dried, ethanol fixed, or used to produce a cell block), it is possible to extract nucleic acids that can be analyzed by a wide variety of genetic assays, including polymerase chain reaction, DNA sequence analysis, gene expression analysis, and fluorescence in situ hybridization.

II. FINE NEEDLE ASPIRATION BIOPSY

A. Fine needle aspiration (FNA) biopsies
are performed by physicians from different specialties.

1. Radiologists usually use 22-gauge needles up to 10 inches in length to reach masses in the lung, liver, retroperitoneum, kidney, and pelvis. Ultrasound guidance or computed tomography is often used to localize the lesion.

2. **Cytopathologists** use 25- to 22-gauge needles, 1 to 3 inches in length, to perform FNA of palpable masses in the salivary glands, lymph nodes, breast, thyroid, and subcutaneous soft tissue.
3. **Other clinicians**
   a. Gastroenterologists use an endoscopic ultrasound-guided needle to perform FNA biopsy of the gastrointestinal tract, mediastinum, pancreas, liver, or accessible retroperitoneal lymph nodes.
   b. Endocrinologists use 25- to 22-gauge needles 1 to 3 inches in length to perform FNA biopsy of the thyroid.
   c. Surgeons use 25- to 22-gauge needles to perform FNA biopsy of the salivary glands, lymph nodes, or breast.
4. When the FNA biopsy is performed by a physician other than a pathologist, it is helpful to send a cytotechnologist to prepare the slides.

B. **Advantages of FNA biopsy** include the following:
   1. The technique is relatively painless.
   2. A diagnosis may be available within 1 hour.
   3. The procedure is relatively inexpensive.
   4. The method provides useful information for the preoperative or pretreatment investigation of pathological processes.
   5. It is not technically demanding.
   6. Complications from the procedure are relatively rare.

C. **Limitations of FNA biopsy** include the facts that the sample may not be technically adequate (e-Fig. 50.1),* the sample may not be representative of the lesion, and specific diagnostic conclusions may not always be possible despite adequate sampling (for example, a diagnosis of follicular carcinoma of the thyroid is based on finding capsular/vascular invasion by the neoplastic cells, which obviously cannot be evaluated by FNA biopsy).

D. **Materials required for FNA biopsy.** Materials used for the performance of FNA include a 25- to 22-gauge needle (0.6- to 1.0-mm external diameter), a syringe pistol handle, (e.g., Cameco, Inrad) (e-Fig. 50.2), syringe with Luer lock tip, 5-mL covered tubes containing RPMI tissue culture media, alcohol prep sponges, antiseptic solution, sterile gauze pads, Coplin jars containing 95% ethanol, Coplin jars with ethanol and 1% HCL (to lyse erythrocytes), a Diff-Quik and Papanicolaou staining set, and a light microscope.

E. **FNA biopsy procedure**
   1. Medical history is reviewed.
   2. Informed consent is obtained; the patient must be informed of the reasons for the procedure, what the procedure entails, and possible complications (such as infection or bleeding). Any history of bleeding or current anticoagulation therapy must be evaluated. In most cases, discontinuation of anticoagulant therapy and International Normalized Ratio testing are required before performing the FNA.
   3. The FNA biopsy area is draped and cleaned with antiseptic solution. Local anesthesia is administered if necessary. Topical anesthetics are rarely used.
   4. At least three samples are obtained from each lesion.
   5. If there is suspicion of an infectious process, additional material for cultures is collected separately and sent for microbiologic work-up.
   6. The biopsy site is tamponaded to prevent bleeding, and then covered with a sterile dressing.

F. **Staining procedure.** After aspiration, the slides are taken to the laboratory for both Papanicolaou and Diff-Quik staining. The needle rinse material is placed into RPMI medium (which provides material for a lymphoma work-up, conventional cytogenetic analysis, or molecular genetic analysis, if needed). All stains must be filtered before staining, and after processing any specimen known to contain malignant cells. Slides for Papanicolaou staining must be fixed in 95% ethanol, 95% ethanol with 1% HCL, or an alcohol-based spray fixative for 5 minutes before staining. Slides used for

---

*All e-figures are available online via the Solution Site Image Bank.

Diff-Quik staining must be air-dried before staining. A 3% glutaraldehyde solution can be used to fix tissue if the need for electron microscopy is anticipated.

G. Cytologic features of cells prepared by different staining procedures

    1. The relative size of a cell when paraffin embedded and stained with hematoxylin and eosin resembles that of a hard-boiled egg. The cell maintains the size at which it would be seen in a routinely processed tissue biopsy (e-**Fig. 50.3**).

    2. The relative size of an ethanol-fixed, Papanicolaou-stained cell resembles that of a poached egg. The nuclear size of paraffin-embedded cells and ethanol-fixed cells is very similar; however, the ethanol-fixed cell has a larger cytoplasmic diameter.

    3. The relative size of a cell that is air dried and Diff-Quik stained is similar to that of a fried egg. Both the nuclear and cytoplasmic diameters are larger than those obtained by the other processing methods.

H. Preliminary diagnosis. The cytopathologist can render a preliminary diagnosis within an hour after the procedure, if requested. The preliminary diagnosis can help ensure that an adequate specimen is obtained and identify the need for ancillary testing.

    1. Negative for malignancy. This diagnosis is rendered when only benign cellular components are obtained. If there is suspicion that the targeted lesion was missed, the clinical setting will direct additional biopsy approaches on an individual basis. If a false-negative result can be excluded, the patient is followed.

    2. Atypical cytology. This terminology is used to communicate the presence of abnormal but inconclusive findings. The report should include a comment as to the reason underlying the atypical cytology designation.

    3. Suspicious for malignancy. This diagnosis is rendered when the cytologic findings are worrisome but lack some features usually seen in malignant neoplasms such as abundant neoplastic cells or significant nuclear abnormalities.

    4. Positive for malignancy. This terminology is used when both the quality and quantity of the malignant cells are unequivocal for a definitive diagnosis of malignancy.

I. The formal screening. This process includes examination of the slides by a cytotechnologist and a cytopathologist. A report is usually generated within 24 hours.

J. Reporting. The report of FNA biopsy results should include the following:

    1. Organ, side, FNA procedure

        a. General category of result (Negative, Atypical Cytology, Suspicious, or Positive for Malignancy)

        b. Specific pathologic diagnoses

    2. Comment section. If a definitive diagnosis cannot be rendered, an explanation should be provided. The comment field can also be used to provide a differential diagnosis and to report the results of additional testing such as flow cytometry or immunohistochemistry.

K. Sources of error in FNA biopsies include the following:

    1. Inadequate sampling due to poor localization of the target lesion, scant cellularity due to poor technique or fibrosis of the lesion, and dilution by blood or fluid.

    2. Inadequate processing due to air-drying artifact, blood-clotting of aspirated material, or failure to smear the aspirate as a monolayer.

    3. Lack of identification of abnormal cells.

    4. Erroneous interpretation of abnormal cells.

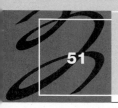

51

FROZEN SECTIONS AND OTHER INTRAOPERATIVE CONSULTATIONS
Michael E. Hull, Peter A. Humphrey, and John D. Pfeifer

I. **INTRODUCTION.** Intraoperative consultations fall into two general categories. Microscopic consultations, known as frozen sections, are performed to establish a tissue diagnosis, determine the nature of a lesion that may require ancillary testing, establish that sufficient diagnostic tissue has been obtained, identify metastatic disease, and assess surgical margins or extent of disease. Nonmicroscopic consultations are performed for evaluation of tissue margins, for specimen orientation, and to triage tissue for ancillary studies, tissue banking, and research.

II. **FROZEN SECTIONS.** High-quality frozen sections can be performed with remarkable speed if equipment is kept in optimum working condition and if the operator is well versed in the technique. In experienced hands, the entire consultation can often be performed in 10 to 15 minutes from the time of the arrival of the specimen in the frozen section room to the notification of the surgeon of the diagnosis. For larger tissue specimens, proper interpretation requires a complete gross examination of the tissue prior to sectioning and a well-trained, experienced pathologist. Informative interactive communication with the surgeon and an adequate clinical history are also absolutely essential for optimization of this process.

    A. **Indications.** Frozen sections are indicated to establish a tissue diagnosis (such as the presence of malignancy, which will guide intraoperative patient management and extent of surgery); for tissue identification (e.g., to confirm the presence of parathyroid tissue in a parathyroidectomy specimen); to determine the nature of a lesion that may require ancillary testing that requires special fixative or medium (e.g., RPMI for flow cytometry, glutaraldehyde for electron microscopy); to establish that sufficient diagnostic tissue has been obtained; to identify metastatic disease; and to assess surgical margins or extent of disease.

        Frozen sections should not be used merely to satisfy a surgeon's curiosity, to compensate for inadequate preoperative evaluation, or as a mechanism to communicate information more quickly to the patient or patient's family.

    B. **The frozen section procedure.** Frozen sections are performed by freezing the tissue in a block of specialized embedding medium, followed by cutting thin (usually 5 micron) sections from the block using a cryostat (refrigerated microtome). The sections are adhered to glass slides, fixed in ethanol, and stained with hematoxylin and eosin (H&E). Small specimens may be completely used for frozen section slide preparation, but if possible, a portion of the tissue should be preserved for routine handling to avoid freezing artifacts that can compromise interpretation of the permanent sections. For larger tissue samples, judgment must be exercised in gross sampling so that the area most likely to be of highest diagnostic yield is selected for frozen section. Cytological imprints from tissues can be an important adjunct in diagnosis, especially for hematolymphoid abnormalities and thyroid lesions (see Part II.G below.)

    C. **The interpretation of frozen sections** requires integration of the histologic morphology in the H&E-stained sections; the gross features of the specimen; and information from the surgeon regarding the origin of the tissue, the indication for the consultation (including the clinical history, radiological findings, and intraoperative observations), and the ways in which the frozen section diagnosis will affect the operative strategy. In difficult cases, deferral of a definitive diagnosis pending

TABLE 51.1 Examples of Frozen Section Evaluation

Tissue	Concordance with permanent section diagnosis	False negative	Comments on utility
Breast	—	—	Limited (see text)
Cervix	73% for evaluation of dysplasia	—	Poor for evaluation of dysplasia
Gallbladder	95% when used to evaluate a mural lesion	—	Useful in the rare instances in which it is required
Liver	—	—	Diagnostic dilemmas that generate deferrals: 1. Hamartoma vs cholangiocarcinoma 2. Regenerative nodule vs hepatocellular carcinoma 3. Adenoma vs hepatocellular carcinoma
Lung	99%	—	Useful; deferral rate of only 3% to 4%
Axillary sentinel lymph nodes for metastatic breast cancer	90%[1] to 96%[2]	15%[1] to 37%[2]	Possibly useful (see text)
Lymph nodes for staging	~100%[3]	20% to 40%[3]	Limited and dependent upon the lymph node location (see text)
Ovary	92%	5%	Useful; errors are disproportionately represented among mucinous tumors

(Continued)

TABLE 51.1 Examples of Frozen Section Evaluation (*Continued*)

Tissue	Concordance with permanent section diagnosis	False negative	Comments on utility
Pancreas	98% when used for diagnosis of primary lesion; almost 100% for margins	1%	Atypical ductal structures, especially in the setting of pancreatitis, may mimic carcinoma; deferral rate of 6% to 7%
Parathyroid	99% (for parathyroid vs nonparathyroid tissue)	—	Useful for distinction of parathyroid vs. nonparathyroid tissue; inadequate for diagnosis of parathyroid carcinoma, or for differentiating adenoma from hyperplasia
Melanoma	—	Up to 50%	Strongly discouraged (see text)
Nonmelanoma	—	About 2%, based on recurrence rates following Mohs' microsurgery[4]	Useful for the evaluation of margins in the resection of tumors with infiltrating borders
Thyroid	98%	10%	Inadequate for follicular lesions, as the sampling required is not practical (see text); better for lesions with papillary architecture; deferral rate is 6%

[1]When nodes with submicrometastases (<0.2 mm) are considered "positive"
[2]When nodes with submicrometastases are considered "negative"
[3]Staging pelvic lymph nodes at prostatectomy
[4]Data on correlation with permanent sections is sparse, as follow-up permanent sections are not performed
— Sparse data or performance of frozen section is variable depending on the indication for the procedure.

examination of formalin-fixed paraffin-embedded sections is an acceptable option. In some difficult cases, it may be necessary to request additional tissue for frozen section analysis.

D. Communication of findings. Clear communication of a concise diagnosis to the surgeon is the last step of the intraoperative consultation. The frozen section diagnosis should be rendered so that the clinical request for the frozen section is directly addressed. The pathologist should transmit the diagnosis by first identifying the patient by two independent identifiers (for example, name and birth date), and then record the exact diagnosis rendered, the identity of the person receiving the information in the operating room, the time of the communication, and the pathologist(s) whose opinion the diagnosis represents. The operating room staff member taking the diagnosis should repeat it back to the pathologist to confirm accurate communication. The results of the frozen section should also be reported in the final surgical pathology report.

E. Accuracy of frozen sections. The efficacy of the frozen section technique will vary from institution to institution based on the types of surgical cases evaluated and the experience of the involved pathologists. Table 51.1 highlights the fact that the accuracy of frozen section diagnosis is dependent on the anatomic site. Regular self-audits of the frozen section service are desirable so that surgeons and pathologists are aware of the performance characteristics of the modality in their own hands. Such audits of single institutions, and pooled data across hundreds of institutions, show that accurate diagnoses are made overall in >95% of cases, whereas discordance with the final diagnosis occurs in 1% to 2% of cases. Deferral of the diagnosis until permanent section diagnosis occurs in 1% to 4% of cases.

F. Sources of error in frozen sections. Errors can be divided into errors of interpretation and errors of sampling; both usually result in false-negative diagnoses. False-positive diagnoses are more rare, likely because experienced pathologists tend to defer to permanent section rather than make a diagnosis of malignancy on substandard material.

Misinterpretation accounts for about one third of errors. Interpretations of frozen sections are more prone to this error than interpretation of permanent sections due to the presence of artifacts that are not encountered in routinely fixed, paraffin-embedded sections. Also, some tissues are more difficult to cut when frozen, especially fatty tissue and lymph nodes with abundant adipose tissue.

Sampling errors occur in two ways. Diagnostic tissue may be present in the frozen block, but the block may not be faced sufficiently for the lesion to be present in the actual frozen section slides; the diagnostic material may then be found in routine permanent sections of the frozen block, a scenario that accounts for another one third of errors. The remaining one third of errors is encountered when the diagnostic tissue is not in the portion of the specimen sampled by the frozen section; good gross pathology skills will minimize, but never eliminate, this problem. Furthermore, it is not feasible to completely sample larger lesions by frozen section, so sampling errors will always exist for large lesions with heterogeneous composition.

Discrepancies between a frozen section and final (permanent section) diagnosis should be documented in the final surgical pathology report, along with the reason for the discrepancy. If the discrepancy is of clinical significance, the attending pathologist should immediately call the attending surgeon to alert the surgeon to the change in diagnosis.

G. Anatomic sites deserving special mention. The anatomic sites with the most discrepancies between frozen section and permanent section are skin, breast, lymph nodes for metastatic disease, the female genital tract (particularly cervix), and thyroid. Frozen sections do have a role in the surgical management of disease in these sites (with the probable exception of melanocytic lesions), but because loss of diagnostic material during the performance of frozen sections is unavoidable, each case must be critically evaluated as to whether the frozen section diagnosis will add enough value to warrant this loss.

    1. Skin. Most authors agree that the intraoperative primary diagnosis of pigmented lesions is contraindicated. Assignment of prognosis and subsequent management in the treatment of melanoma requires accurate assessment of Breslow thickness, and frozen artifact may cause so much specimen distortion as to make a depth of invasion assessment meaningless in both permanent and frozen sections. Freezing artifact, compounded by the actinic damage so frequent in patients with pigmented lesions, conspires to obscure histology. Subtle changes, such as intraepidermal spread by single melanocytes, are very difficult to appreciate in frozen sections, making the method a poor choice for margin assessment as well. For example, the false-negative rate for lentiginous spread of melanoma by frozen section evaluation may be as high as 50%.

2. **Breast.** The initial diagnosis of breast tumors is very rarely made during surgery, owing to the common clinical practice of preoperative fine needle aspiration (FNA) and needle core biopsy. The high fat content of breast tissue makes frozen specimens technically difficult to section and prone to freezing artifact. Evaluation of margins by imprint cytology is an alternative to frozen section, but will miss many positive margins, unless the margins are grossly involved, in which case the examination is redundant.

3. **Lymph nodes for metastatic disease.** Although current diagnostic modalities have reduced the need for breast frozen sections, requests for frozen sections of breast sentinel lymph nodes have increased (e-**Fig. 51.1, A and B**).* Unfortunately, frozen sections of sentinel nodes consume considerable tissue that is then not available for subsequent evaluation by permanent sections; if no metastases are identified, further evaluation of the node has therefore been significantly hampered (e-**Fig. 51.2**).

   Numerous studies have indicated that the sensitivity of frozen section evaluation of sentinel nodes is about 60%, although the specificity is near 100%. It has been argued that the metastases that are typically missed by frozen section are submicroscopic (<0.2 mm in greatest dimension) or are detected by cytokeratin immunohistochemistry alone, and that because the significance of these classes of metastases is not yet clear, the low sensitivity of the approach underestimates it clinical utility. A sensible middle ground seems to be to perform frozen sections when the clinical history and gross examination of the node give a high degree of suspicion for metastasis.

4. **Thyroid.** The widespread use of FNA has altered the approach to frozen section evaluation of the thyroid. Frozen section evaluation of thyroid excision specimens is best performed in conjunction with imprint cytology, the latter of which is more sensitive for the nuclear grooves, inclusions, and chromatin-clearing characteristic of papillary carcinoma. Because the distinction between follicular adenoma and carcinoma by frozen section would require thorough sampling of the tumor and capsule for invasion and angioinvasion, frozen section is poorly suited to this application (e-**Fig. 51.3**).

5. **Female genital tract.** Of all the neoplastic processes of the female genital tract, ovarian neoplasms are probably the best suited to intraoperative frozen section diagnosis. However, the diagnosis of cervical dysplasia is fraught with difficulties due to frozen section artifact and low concordance with permanent section diagnosis.

III. **OTHER INTRAOPERATIVE CONSULTATIONS.** Intraoperative nonmicroscopic consultations are often required even though no frozen section is needed. Indications include gross diagnosis (such as benign simple ovarian cyst or leiomyoma of uterus); gross confirmation of the presence of a lesion or mass; identification of a margin or region of interest that requires special sampling for permanent sections; specimen orientation; triage of tissue for ancillary testing modalities that require special processing or fixatives (in which case good judgment is required to ensure a balance between the need for tissue for routine histopathologic evaluation and the need for tissue for specialized testing); and collection of tissue for tumor-banking or research studies.

   A. **Opening of a viscus organ** for gross examination and fixation. Gastrointestinal specimens commonly require opening in the operating room so that the surgeon can

---

*All e-figures are available online via the Solution Site Image Bank.

see whether lesional tissue has been excised. In partial intestinal excisions for inflammatory disease, in which the risk for malignancy is increased, a careful intraoperative examination may inform the surgeon of a previously undetected tumor that may have implications for additional surgical therapy.

Similarly, gross examination and opening of the adnexa and/or uterus can aid in determining the extent of surgery that is required. Such gross examination often leads to frozen sections when ovarian surface papillary excrescences are identified, or when solid or complex architecture features are discovered in ovarian cysts.

B. **Tissue banking.** Tumor for banking must be chosen so that the remaining lesional tissue material will still be suitable for a complete diagnostic evaluation. The banked tissue should not include a surgical margin or have an important relationship to an anatomic structure that would impact staging or the need for adjuvant therapy. In cases of small specimens, it may be necessary to defer banking for the sake of a thorough diagnostic evaluation.

Suggested Readings

Cetin B, Aslan S, Hatiboglu C, Babacan B, Onder A. Frozen section in thyroid surgery: is it a necessity? *Can J Surg*. 2004;47:29–33.

Cioc AM, Ellison C, Proca DM, Lucas JG, Frankel WL. Frozen section diagnosis of pancreatic lesions. *Arch Pathol Lab Med*. 2002;126:1169–1173.

Coffey D, Kaplan AL, Ramzy I. Intraoperative consultation in gynecologic pathology. *Arch Pathol Lab Med*. 2005;129:1544–1557.

Gephardt GN, Zarbo RJ. Interinstitutional comparison of frozen section consultations. A College of American Pathologists Q-Probes study of 90,538 cases in 461 institutions. *Arch Pathol Lab Med*. 1996;120:804–809.

Laucirica R. Intraoperative assessment of the breast. *Arch Pathol Lab Med*. 2005;129:1565–1574.

Lechago J. Frozen section examination of liver, gallbladder, and pancreas. *Arch Pathol Lab Med*. 2005;129:1610–1618.

Marchevsky AM, Changsri C, Gupta I, Fuller C, Houck W, McKenna RJ. Frozen section diagnoses of small pulmonary nodules: accuracy and clinical implications. *Ann Thorac Surg*. 2004;78:1755–1759.

Medeiros LR, Rosa DD, Edelweiss MI, et al. Accuracy of frozen-section analysis in the diagnosis of ovarian tumors: a systematic quantitative review. *Int J Gynecol Cancer*. 2005;15:192–202.

Mitchell ML. Frozen section diagnosis for axillary sentinel lymph nodes: the first six years. *Mod Pathol*. 2005;18:58–61.

Smith-Zagone MJ, Schwartz MR. Frozen section of skin specimens. *Arch Pathol Lab Med*. 2005;129:1536–1543.

Young MP, Kirby RS, O'Donoghue EP, Parkinson MC. Accuracy and cost of intraoperative lymph node frozen sections at radical prostatectomy. *J Clin Pathol*. 1999;52:925–927.

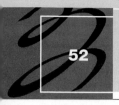

52 ELECTRON MICROSCOPY
Frances V. White

I. INTRODUCTION. Transmission electron microscopy (EM) has been used by surgical pathologists over the past 50 years for the diagnosis of a wide range of diseases in various organ systems (Table 52.1). This method allows for the visualization of subcellular morphology, with appreciation of disease processes and structural abnormalities that cannot be resolved by light microscopy. EM is an essential part of the work-up of medical renal biopsies, peripheral nerve biopsies, and muscle biopsies. It is also useful in evaluating metabolic and inherited diseases, providing an initial differential diagnosis, or ruling in or out a specific disease process. The role of EM in the diagnosis of neoplasms has decreased since the advent of immunohistochemical and molecular techniques, but it is still an ancillary tool for the evaluation of atypical tumors or when other techniques yield indeterminate results. Although not usually needed, EM is occasionally used to demonstrate infectious agents or evidence of drug toxicity.

In recent years, EM has been combined with immunohistochemical and in situ hybridization methods, allowing antigen detection and localization at the subcellular level. These combined methods require special fixation and processing protocols. Although immunoelectron microscopy is currently used primarily in research laboratories, the method is now considered to be a promising diagnostic technique in oncological surgical pathology, in particular for the identification and localization of targets for gene therapy.

II. METHODOLOGY. Tissue for EM must be immediately fixed. A thin slice of tissue should be immersed in a cold fixative such as buffered 2%–4% glutaraldehyde, or buffered glutaraldehyde plus paraformaldehyde, and then diced into 1-mm cubes using a sharp, clean scalpel. Specimens are usually postfixed in osmium tetroxide, dehydrated in ethanol, and then embedded in an epoxy resin or plastic. Semithin (1-μm-thick) sections are cut from the blocks and stained with toluidine blue or methylene blue, and light microscopic examination of the semithin sections is used to select the blocks from which thin sections are cut and placed on grids. The thin sections are usually stained with uranyl acetate and lead citrate; however, other stains may be selected to enhance electron contrast of specific particles or structures, depending on the tissue type and diagnostic question. Tissue processing typically takes a couple of days, but with microwave techniques, grids can be ready within 5 hours postfixation.

For some disease processes, if glutaraldehyde-fixed tissue is not available, EM can be performed on formalin-fixed wet tissue or paraffin-embedded tissue. Wet tissue is preferable to paraffin-embedded tissue, but previous prompt fixation in formalin is essential. Autopsy material, whether fixed in glutaraldehyde or formalin, is usually unsatisfactory due to the prolonged postmortem interval prior to fixation.

A focused differential diagnosis based on integration of clinical history and light microscopic findings is essential for the correct interpretation of ultrastructural findings. Except for the most routine specimens, the case pathologist should personally review the semithin sections by light microscopy and select the blocks for further processing. In addition, the case pathologist should communicate his differential diagnosis to the electron microscopist and specify the cell type and subcellular structures of interest. Obviously, sampling error is minimized and the most information is obtained when the case pathologist is directly involved in scanning the tissue grids.

Subcellular Feature	Cell/Tissue Type	Use
Peroxisomes	Liver	Increased number in alcoholic liver disease, chronic passive congestion, oral contraceptives, various hepatitides
Siderosomes	Mitochondria	Sideroblastic anemia
Genetic diseases		
Cilia	Epithelial cells	Primary ciliary dyskinesia
Lysosomes	Neurons	Identification of lipoidosis and several types of mucopolysaccharidoses
Peroxisomes	Hepatocytes	Identification of several types of mucopolysaccharidoses
	Liver and kidney	Absence in Zellweger syndrome and neonatal adrenoleukodystrophy
Neoplasmas		
Intercellular junctions	Epithelial cells; selected mesenchymal nonlymphoid tumors	Distinction between lymphoma and carcinoma
Intracellular or intercellular lumina	Glandular epithelium	Identification of adenocarcinomas
Microvillous core rootlets	Glandular epithelium of alimentary tract	Identification of gastrointestinal origin of metastatic carcinomas
Cytoplasmic tonofibrils	Squamous epithelium	Identification of squamous differentiation in epithelial tumors
Premelanosomes and melanosomes	Melanocytic cells	Identification of melanomas
Neurosecretory granules	Neuroendocrine and neuroectodermal cells	Identification of neuroendocrine and neuroectodermal neoplasms
Birbeck granules	Langerhans cells	Identification of Langerhans proliferations such as Langerhans cell histiocytosis
Other		
Viruses and parasites	Solid tissues, fecal specimens, body fluids	Identification of infectious agent
Electron-dense deposits and/or other basement alterations	Glomeruli	Identification and classification of glomerular diseases
	Adjacent to vascular smooth muscle	CADASIL syndrome

CADASIL, cerebral autosomal dominant arteriopathy with subcortical infarcts and leukoencephalopathy.

III. KIDNEY. EM, in conjunction with routine histology and immunofluorescence, is an essential part of the work-up of medical renal biopsies to diagnose glomerular disease. It is also performed on renal allograft biopsies when recurrent or de novo glomerular disease is suspected. The protocol for triaging renal biopsies is presented in detail elsewhere in this manual (see Chapters 19 and 55). Because EM makes it possible to visualize the individual components of the glomerular capillary wall, including endothelium, glomerular basement membrane, and visceral epithelial cells, it is used for identification and localization of discrete electron-dense deposits in glomeruli, either of immunoglobulins or amyloid and amyloid-like proteins. The glomerular basement membrane can also be evaluated for abnormal thickening, thinning, and/or splitting and for the presence of electron lucent, granular, or other deposits. Tubular basement membranes, arterioles, and the interstitium can also be evaluated by EM for pathogenic changes, for example, nonimmune deposits such as amyloid, light chain dense deposits, and cryoglobulins. Chapter 19 describes in detail the ultrastructural findings in specific renal diseases.

IV. NEOPLASMS. The role of EM in the diagnosis of neoplasms has decreased since the advent of immunohistochemical and molecular markers. EM, however, is still a useful ancillary method in selected cases and for poorly differentiated tumors for which immunohistochemical and molecular studies are inconclusive. In general, a differential diagnosis is first developed based on light microscopic findings, and EM is then used to look for evidence of cellular differentiation toward tumors in the differential diagnosis. For example, desmosomes, tonofilaments, melanosomes, and premelanosomes may be sought in the differential diagnosis of carcinoma versus melanoma. EM does not differentiate reactive, benign, neoplastic, and malignant processes.

V. INHERITED METABOLIC DISEASES. Initial studies in the work-up of inherited metabolic diseases often include a biopsy of affected organs (such as liver, muscle or peripheral nerve). For select diseases, EM findings may be pathognomonic. In most cases, however, light microscopy and EM findings are useful in narrowing the differential diagnosis and providing direction for further laboratory studies. Definitive diagnosis typically requires enzyme studies of fibroblast cultures and/or molecular studies.

A. Prenatal studies. EM can be performed on amniotic cells and chorionic villous tissue obtained for prenatal diagnosis. Ultrastructural studies on noncultured amniotic cells can yield a rapid diagnosis or differential for certain metabolic diseases, including type 2 glycogen storage disease, lysosomal storage diseases, and peroxisomal disorders.

B. Liver. Inherited metabolic diseases often result in hepatocellular dysfunction, either as part of a systemic disorder or as part of disease limited to the liver. In the work-up of hepatitis and cholestatic liver disease in infancy and childhood, a portion of the liver biopsy is routinely placed in glutaraldehyde for possible ultrastructural studies. In cases where obstruction and infection have been ruled out, EM is performed to look for evidence of primary metabolic disease. Certain metabolic diseases have pathognomonic or near-pathognomonic findings, such as type 2 and 4 glycogen storage diseases and Wilson disease. Various abnormalities in the number and structure of mitochondria and peroxisomes are characteristic of specific diseases, as are lysosomal inclusions. Ultrastructural findings are always interpreted in conjunction with light microscopic findings, clinical history, biochemical assays, and other laboratory studies.

C. Lung. The protocol for lung biopsy in the work-up of interstitial lung disease in infancy includes placing a portion of tissue in EM fixative on hold. Based on light microscopic findings, the tissue may be further processed for ultrastructural analysis. Diseases that have characteristic ultrastructural findings include pulmonary interstitial glycogenosis, surfactant processing abnormalities (surfactant protein B [SPB] deficiency and adenosine 5'-triphosphate [ATP]-binding cassette transporter A3 [ABCA3] abnormalities), and certain lysosomal storage disorders.

D. Heart. Glycogen storage disease type 2 (Pompe disease) can be diagnosed based on ultrastructural findings in cardiac biopsies. Adriamycin toxicity involving the heart results in characteristic cytoplasmic changes that can be seen by light microscopy in semithin sections prepared for EM.

VI. NEUROPATHOLOGY SPECIMENS. EM is critical for the evaluation of peripheral nerve biopsies and muscle biopsies (*Can J Vet Res.* 1990;54:1) and is also useful in the evaluation of selected neuro-oncologic specimens (*J Neuropathol Exp Neurol.* 2002;61:1027). EM examination of skin and conjunctival biopsies is used in the diagnosis of neuronal ceroid lipofuscinosis, infantile neuroaxonal dystrophy, and cerebral autosomal dominant arteriopathy with subcortical infarcts and leukoencephalopathy (CADASIL).

VII. PRIMARY CILIARY DYSKINESIA. At present, EM is the method of choice for the diagnosis of primary ciliary dyskinesia (*Acta Otorhinolaryngol Belg.* 2000;54:309 and *Nat Rev Mol Cell Biol.* 2007;8:880). Ciliary biopsies and brushings are obtained from the nasal mucosa and lower airway. The most frequent ultrastructural abnormalities are decreased numbers or absence of outer and/or inner dynein arms, some of which are associated with specific genetic abnormalities with an autosomal recessive inheritance pattern (*Respiration.* 2007;74:252). Ultrastructural abnormalities in other ciliary components have also been reported, but not in a consistent manner. Difficulties in interpretation result from significant overlap of EM findings in chronic inflammatory processes and from an inherent difficulty in the visualization of inner dynein arms.

VIII. MICROVILLUS INCLUSION DISEASE. Microvillus inclusion disease presents as intractable secretory diarrhea in the neonate. Characteristic light microscopic findings include villous atrophy and loss of the brush border; however, EM is required for diagnosis. Pathognomonic ultrastructural findings include absent or decreased numbers of stubby microvilli on the apical cytoplasmic membrane of enterocytes, along with cytoplasmic membrane–bound inclusions with microvillus projections. Morphologic variants have been reported.

Suggested Readings

D'Agati VD, Jennette JC, Silva FG. *Non-neoplastic Kidney Disease. Atlas of Nontumor Pathology* (First series, Fascicle 4). Washington DC: American Registry of Pathology Press; 2005.

Iancu TC. The ultrastructural spectrum of lysosomal storage diseases. *Ultrastruct Pathol.* 1992;16:231–244.

Sherman PM, Mitchell DJ, Cutz E. Neonatal enteropathies: defining the causes of protracted diarrhea of infancy. *J Pediatr Gastroenterol Nutr.* 2004;38:16–26.

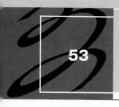

53 HISTOLOGY AND HISTOCHEMICAL STAINS
Kevin D. Selle

I. RECEIPT, ACCESSIONING, AND GROSS DISSECTION. Most, if not all, biopsies and large tissue specimens are routed to the pathology laboratory. Under normal circumstances the specimens are received in 10% neutral buffered formalin (formalin begins the fixation process and prevents autolysis and decomposition). The specimen is first logged into the surgical pathology computer system and given a unique identifying number, referred to as an accession number or case number. After being accessioned, the specimen is taken to the gross dissection room; depending on the practice setting, residents, fellows, pathologist assistants, and/or trained technicians are responsible for gross processing of the specimen under the supervision of an attending pathologist. Gross processing entails describing the specimen by its size, shape, color, and overall general appearance, followed by placing samples of the tissue in processing cassettes (for biopsies, the entire tissue specimen is placed in a cassette; for larger specimens, regions of tissue are sampled according to established protocols). Each cassette is labeled with the accession number as well as a part designator and number; this numbering scheme is designed to allow the location of a particular section of tissue within the context of the whole specimen.

II. PROCESSING. The loaded cassettes are stored in 10% neutral buffered formalin until automated tissue processing. The normal processing cycle is approximately 8 hours long and, in general, is designed to remove the water from the specimen and replace it with paraffin. Automated, closed-system tissue processors use agitation, vacuum, and increased temperature to optimize the process. In general terms, the process is as follows. First, the tissue is subjected to 10% neutral buffered formalin to assure complete fixation. Complete fixation aids in the dehydration steps, and prevents tissue shrinkage and other artifacts caused by excessive or rapid dehydration; chemically, formalin fixation produces methylene cross-links between nucleic acids and/or proteins. Once the tissue is well fixed it is subjected to several changes of graduated alcohols in a gradient starting at 70% and ending at 100%, a process that removes water from the tissue at a slow controlled rate designed to prevent excessive shrinkage and disruption of the architecture and cellular components. When complete dehydration of the tissue has been accomplished, a clearing agent is used to remove the alcohol and allow tissue infiltration by paraffin; this clearing agent must therefore be miscible in both alcohol and paraffin. Xylene is most often used for this purpose, although commercial xylene substitutes are available. In the next step of processing, heated paraffin infiltrates into the tissue. Paraffin is a solid at room temperature but has a relatively low melting point, and so is a good choice as an infiltration and embedding medium. While pure paraffin wax was used in the past, current commercially available paraffins are formulated with various plastic polymers to allow better infiltration and a more rigid crystalline structure, both of which aid subsequent microtomy.

III. EMBEDDING. Properly fixed and processed tissue sections are embedded in molds to prepare them for microtomy. The tissue is removed from the cassette and oriented in the base of a mold that is of a size to allow paraffin to surround the tissue section. During embedding, the tissue is oriented with the understanding that the surface placed down in the mold will become the face of the tissue block, and will thus be the surface cut into first by the microtome blade. Attention must be given to tissues requiring specific orientation such as tubular structures requiring complete cross-sections (e.g., ureteral margins). Orientation is critical to proper tissue representation on the finished slide and leads to proper pathologic diagnosis, so the importance of proper embedding cannot be overstated. After proper orientation, the mold and tissue are touched to a cold plate to begin to solidify the paraffin so that the tissue is held in place as the mold is filled with paraffin. The empty cassette is placed on top of the mold so that it becomes the back of the tissue block, conveniently retaining the identification of that tissue sample. Finally, the mold is allowed to cool so that the paraffin block containing the oriented tissue can be easily removed.

IV. MICROTOMY. Proper microtomy requires a well trained and highly skilled microtomist, usually a trained histotechnician or histotechnologist. The microtome instrument is designed to hold the paraffin tissue block firmly in place as it is cyclically presented to a stationary microtome blade. Each turn of the microtome handle (each cycle) advances the tissue block a set distance, so microtomes must be kept clean and in good working order. Most tissues are sectioned at 4–5 microns thick; however, some tissues are cut thinner at 3 microns (e.g., kidney biopsies and lymph node biopsies), and others thicker at 5–6 microns (e.g., bone and brain).

In practice, the paraffin block is first "faced in" to reach a level within the tissue where there is a representative tissue section plane; the block is then cooled on wet ice to further harden the paraffin and aid microtomy. If proper care is taken, individual sections come off of the microtome blade connected to each other, a string of tissue sections called a "ribbon." The tissue ribbon is then floated on a warm water bath at a temperature 6°–8° below the melting point of the paraffin to make the paraffin very pliable, which aids in mounting the sections on a glass microscope slide labeled with the corresponding accession number and part identifier for that particular block (in addition, the convection currents formed in the water bath help to gently stretch the tissue sections, removing any wrinkles).

V. HEMATOXYLIN AND EOSIN STAINING. Slides that have been sectioned are stained to reveal their histologic detail. The primary stain used for pathologic diagnosis is the hematoxylin and eosin stain. Hematoxylin is derived from the log wood tree, and has long been in use in the pathology laboratory. By itself it is not a dye, but after it is oxidized to hematein and combined with a metallic mordant it acquires a strong affinity for nuclear chromatin. Eosin is a dye that, at a pH of approximately 4.6–5.0, is a strong anion and thus has an affinity for positively charged, cationic, tissue protein groups. At the proper pH, eosin combines at different rates to tissue proteins and thus produces a graduation of three distinct shades from light pink to pinkish red.

There are several methods for performing the hematoxylin and eosin stain that can be used to achieve slight variations in the end stain to match the preference of the pathologist. The two general variations of hematoxylin and eosin staining in common use are regressive methods and progressive methods. Progressive methods involve staining slides for a designated period of time, then stopping the reaction as soon as optimal staining has occurred; every tissue stains slightly differently with hematoxylin based on its type, fixation, and prior decalcification; therefore, the length of time in hematoxylin is critical using the progressive method. Regressive methods overstain the tissue sections with hematoxylin then differentiate the hematoxylin using acid alcohol; by overstaining and then differentiating the hematoxylin by the regressive method, a darker, crisper stain can be achieved with the assurance that all hematoxylin-positive elements are represented.

The routine regressive staining protocol for the hematoxylin and eosin stain is as follows. The tissue sections are dried completely in an oven because water left on or under the tissue sections can allow the sections to fall off of the slide during the staining process. The slides are then deparaffinized by soaking in xylene, the xylene is removed by alcohol, and the slides are rehydrated by 95% alcohol and then water before staining with hematoxylin. Excess hematoxylin is then removed with a water rinse; the slides are differentiated using acid alcohol, then rinsed; and the hematoxylin is "blued" by immersion in a weak ammonia water solution. The slides are rinsed again, placed in 80% alcohol, and stained with eosin. Excess eosin is removed by alcohol rinses, and the slide is prepared for mounting with a coverslip and resinous medium by removal of the alcohol using xylene rinses.

VI. OTHER FREQUENTLY USED HISTOCHEMICAL STAINS. Tissue stains range from very simple to complex in methodology, and can be used to demonstrate most major tissue elements relevant to pathologic diagnosis. They are based on the chemistry of various dyes and metals, and most were developed prior to the advent of immunohistochemistry. In general, a histochemical stain consists of the main chemical reaction that demonstrates the specific tissue element of interest, followed by chemical reactions that provide staining of the background uninvolved tissue elements, often including nuclear detail. Histochemical stains are usually grouped by the tissue element they stain.

A. Carbohydrates. In humans, carbohydrates exist as various sugars and polymers linked to proteins. Simple sugars cannot be detected by standard histochemical procedures because they are water soluble; however, polymers such as glycogen can be detected. Naturally occurring polysaccharides can be classified into four groups based on their histochemical staining differences: neutral polysaccharides (Group I), acid mucopolysaccharides (Group II), glycoproteins (Group III), and glycolipids (Group IV). Amyloid must also be included because, even though it is not a carbohydrate, its histochemical staining properties are similar to those of polysaccharides. The histochemical stains most often used to detect carbohydrates, and to differentiate one type of carbohydrate from another, are mucicarmine, Alcian blue, colloidal iron, Congo red, thioflavin T, and the periodic acid–Schiff (PAS) reaction.

1. Mucicarmine. The mucicarmine method is used to detect tissue mucins and uses the tissue dye carmine. When carmine is reacted with aluminum it forms a compound that has a net positive charge and is attracted to the negative acid groups of epithelial mucins. Metanil yellow and Weigert's Hematoxylin are used as counterstains and produce yellow staining of the background tissue elements and blueblack nuclear staining (e-Fig. 53.1).*

2. Alcian blue. Alcian blue, a phthalocyanine basic dye, forms salt bridges with the acid groups in mucopolysaccharides. Staining tissue sections in an Alcian blue solution at pH 1.0 produces staining of only sulfated mucopolysaccharides, whereas staining at pH 2.5 produces staining of all mucopolysaccharides. These two methods make it possible to differentiate sulfated from carboxylated mucopolysaccharides; further differentiation between mucosubstances of connective tissue origin versus mucosubstances of epithelial origin can be achieved by the addition of hyaluronidase digestion (e-Fig. 53.2).

3. Colloidal iron. The colloidal iron stain is based on the chemical principle that at low pH colloidal ferric ions can be absorbed by both carboxylated and sulfated mucopolysaccharides, as well as by other glycoproteins. The absorbed ferric ions are detected by use of the Prussian blue reaction (see below).

4. Congo red. Congo red reacts with cellulose and amyloid. The dye is a linear molecule that attaches to amyloid in a sheetlike fashion resulting in so-called "apple green" birefringence when subjected to polarized light. This "apple green" birefringence is considered specific for amyloid in Congo red–stained tissue sections (e-Fig. 53.3).

5. Thioflavin T. Thioflavin T is a fluorescent tissue dye that has an affinity for amyloid. Thioflavin T fluoresces yellow to yellow-green when the tissue section is viewed by fluorescence microscopy, but the dye is not as specific for amyloid as is Congo red.

6. PAS reaction. The PAS reaction is invaluable in histochemistry because of its versatility. In this reaction, the glycol groups of polysaccharides, mucosubstances, and basement membranes are subjected to oxidation by a solution of periodic acid. The oxidation of the glycols results in the formation of dialdehydes. The dialdehydes are then reacted with Schiff's reagent, a colorless solution created by reducing basic fuchsin in the presence of sulfurous acid. When reacted with the previously oxidized tissue, Schiff's reagent is bound to the dialdehyde groups and gains a red color (e-Fig. 53.4).

The differentiation of glycogen from other mucosubstances can be achieved using the PAS stain as follows. Two identical tissue sections are cut. The first section is treated (or digested) with either amylase or diastase to remove any glycogen in the tissue, and then both sections are stained following the PAS procedure. If

---

*All e-figures are available online via the Solution Site Image Bank.

the substance in question is glycogen, it will be present in the undigested section but not in the digested one (e-Fig. 53.5).

B. **Connective tissues.** Connective tissue is made up of three elements in varying amounts, cells, a variety of protein fibers, and so-called ground substance. The commonly used connective tissue stains are used to demonstrate cells and various protein fibers, and include the reticulin stain, trichrome stain, Jones' methenamine silver (JMS) stain, phosphotungstic acid hematoxylin (PTAH) stain, Verhoeff–Van Gieson (VVG) stain, and Oil red O stain. Each of these stains has many different modifications, based on the preferences of the lab and pathologists involved. Because ground substance is principally composed of mucopolysaccharides, it can be demonstrated by the carbohydrate stains mentioned previously.

1. **Reticulin.** The reticulin stain is similar to the PAS stain in that glycols are first reduced to dialdehydes by the use of an acid. The tissue is next sensitized to accept metallic silver ions with an ammoniacal silver solution, and the silver ions that are attached on and around the dialdehyde groups are then reduced to metallic silver. Finally, the tissue sections are toned from brown to black by replacing the metallic silver with metallic gold; sodium thiosulfate is used to remove any remaining unreacted silver in the tissue to prevent darkening of the slide over time. The end result is that reticulin fibers are stained black against a clear background (e-Fig. 53.6).

2. **JMS.** The JMS stain uses methenamine to form a complex with silver, which is then reacted with dialdehyde groups formed by the reduction of glycol units in the basement membrane in a process similar to that of the reticulin stain (e-Fig. 53.7).

3. **Trichrome.** There are a number of variations of the trichrome stain; in general, they all use three dyes with affinities for different connective tissue elements. The first step in the trichrome stain involves mordanting the tissue with a heavy metal fixative such as Bouin's fixative. The tissue is then dyed with a nuclear stain, most often an iron hematoxylin. Next, an acidic dye such as acid fuchsin or Biebrich scarlet is used to stain the cytoplasm of cells, collagen, and muscle; either phosphotungstic acid or phosphomolybdic acid is then used to remove the acid dye from the collagen (because the cytoplasm of cells is less permeable than collagen, with proper timing the dye can be removed from collagen without complete removal from other tissue elements). Finally, collagen is stained using aniline blue. As the name suggests, the method produces tissue sections that are stained in three colors: black cell nuclei, red cell cytoplasm and muscle, and blue collagen and mucus (e-Fig. 53.8).

4. **VVG.** The VVG is another compound stain. The tissue section is first overstained with an iron hematoxylin solution, and the hematoxylin is then differentiated by removal with ferric chloride; because elastic fibers have the greatest affinity for iron hematoxylin, they are the last to decolorize, so it is possible to halt the differentiation at the point when the elastic fibers are the only tissue elements still stained. The tissue section is then treated with Van Gieson's solution, which contains the dye acid fuchsin; in a very strong acid solution the dye selectively stains only collagen. Picric acid, used to maintain the proper pH during staining, stains the rest of the tissue elements yellow. The VVG stain demonstrates red stained collagen, black elastic fibers, and a yellow background (e-Fig. 53.9).

5. **PTAH.** The PTAH stain requires mordanting of the tissue section in Zenker's fixative prior to staining. Because phosphotungstic acid is present in the staining solution in excess over hematoxylin, all of the hematoxylin is bound into a tungsten–hematein lake, which selectively binds to cell nuclei, fibrin, and cross-striations in muscle fibers. The excess unreacted phosphotungstic acid stains the remaining tissue elements red to red–brown.

6. **Pentachrome.** The pentachrome stain is a compound stain that essentially combines the elastic fiber staining of a modified VVG stain with a modified trichrome stain. Alcian blue is first used to stain mucosubstances, then iron hematoxylin is used to stain elastic fibers. Following the differentiation of the iron hematoxylin, a combined Crocein scarlet and acid fuchsin solution is used to stain muscle, cellular cytoplasm, amorphous ground substance, and collagen red. Phosphotungstic

acid in solution is then used to decolorize the collagen and amorphous ground substance, which is then subsequently stained yellow using a saturated alcoholic Safran solution.

7. **Oil red O.** This stain is used to demonstrate fat in tissue sections or lipid droplets in cell cytoplasm. The dye Oil red O is highly soluble in lipids and, when used in solution with isopropanol, is actually more soluble in fat than in the alcohol.

This stain requires the use of frozen section tissues because the alcohol and xylene steps in standard paraffin processing remove virtually all lipids from the tissue. The staining itself is fairly straightforward: Frozen tissue sections are cut, fixed with formaldehyde, and then stained in the Oil red O solution. The sections are next rinsed free from any excess stain and then counterstained using hematoxylin. The stain results in blue cell nuclei with fat droplets that are stained bright red.

C. **Microorganisms.** There are many different stains that can be used to demonstrate microorganisms, specifically bacteria and fungi, in tissue sections. The most commonly used stains are the Gram stain, the acid-fast bacilli (AFB)n, Fite's modification of the AFB, Grocott's Methenamine Silver (GMS), Warthin–Starry, and PAS.

1. **Gram stain.** The tissue Gram stain is not much different from the standard Gram stain performed in the microbiology lab. In the tissue Gram stain, however, after the use of crystal violet to demonstrate Gram-positive bacteria by a blue color, basic fuchsin (a red dye) is used to demonstrate Gram-negative organisms as well as cell nuclei. Differentiation of Gram-positive and Gram-negative bacteria is still a critical step; overdifferentiation is a common staining error. The final step in the Brown–Hopps Gram stain involves treating the tissue with a picric acid solution that renders the background yellow. In addition to identification of bacteria, some cases of *Actinomyces, Nocardia,* coccidioidomycosis, blastomycosis, cryptococcosis, aspergillosis, rhinosporidiosis, and amebiasis can stain (e-**Fig. 53.10**).

2. **AFB stain.** The tissue AFB stain is simply a modification of the standard Ziehl–Neelsen and Kinyoun stains that are based on the fact that carbol-fuchsin, a solution created by reacting basic fuchsin with phenol in alcohol, is soluble in lipids. Tissue sections are first treated with the carbol-fuchsin solution and then differentiated using acid alcohol; bacteria that have waxy, lipid-containing cell walls resist decolorization with acid alcohol and are said to be "acid fast." A methylene blue counterstain is used to highlight other tissue elements and provide a background to highlight the red microorganisms (e-**Fig. 53.11**). A slight modification of this procedure can be used to specifically stain for *Nocardia* species in tissue sections. Another modification of this stain, known as Fite's AFB stain, is used when *Mycobacterium leprae* is suspected (e-**Fig. 53.12**).

3. **GMS.** This stain uses most of the same chemical reactions and principles as the JMS stain. In the GMS stain, however, a stronger oxidizer, chromic acid, is used instead of the weaker periodic acid. Because the cellular walls of fungi are very thick and contain much more carbohydrate than basement membranes and reticulin fibers of the surrounding tissue, the stronger oxidizer allows for creation of dialdehyde groups from the carbohydrates of the fungi cell walls with overoxidation and subsequent destruction of these groups in subsequent basement membranes and other carbohydrate structures in the tissue section. The GMS stain uses a light green counterstain, resulting in fungus cell walls that are various shades of black to taupe in a light green background (e-**Fig. 53.13**).

4. **Warthin–Starry.** The Warthin–Starry method is used primarily for the demonstration of spirochetes, but other bacteria are also stained. The procedure is based on the principle that bacteria in general (and spirochetes in particular) have the ability to bind silver ions.

The staining procedure therefore involves impregnation of the spirochetes in the tissue with silver ions, with subsequent reduction of these ions to metallic silver using a developer containing hydroquinone. The stain demonstrates black spirochetes against a yellow to pale brown background. The spiral morphology of this form of bacteria can be fully appreciated by the use of this method (e-**Figs. 53.14 and 53.15**).

5. PAS. This stain is often used for the demonstration of fungi in tissue, but is most helpful when a counterstain of light green is applied. The method used in stains for microorganisms is no different than when used for carbohydrates.

D. Nervous system. Most of the stains used on tissues from the nervous system are for demonstration of either nerve fibers or the myelin sheath. Two commonly used stains for central nervous system tissues are the Bielschowsky and the Luxol Fast Blue.

   1. Bielschowsky. The Bielschowsky and all of its modifications are silver stains that follow the principles and general steps of the reticulin stain. In the Bielschowsky technique, the tissue sections are impregnated with a 20% silver nitrate solution and then treated with an ammoniacal silver solution to which formaldehyde has been added. Nerve endings, neurofibrils, neurofibrillary tangles, and neuritic plaques are all stained black.

   2. Luxol fast blue. Luxol fast blue, a phthalocyanine dye that is soluble in alcohol, is attracted to bases found in the lipoproteins of the myelin sheath. For this stain, tissue sections are treated with Luxol fast blue over an extended period of time (usually overnight) and then differentiated with a lithium carbonate solution. Because Luxol fast blue has a strong affinity for the lipoproteins of the myelin sheath, it remains bound to these lipoproteins even after removal from other tissue elements. The myelin sheath is stained blue against a colorless background.

E. Pigments and minerals. Pigments are substances deposited in the interstitium of tissues, or as inclusions or granules in the cytoplasm of cells. Pigments can be derived from minerals such as iron and calcium, or can be endogenous such as melanin. The following staining techniques are used for the demonstration of the most commonly encountered pigments.

   1. Iron. The Prussian blue reaction is the most common staining technique for the demonstration of iron in tissue sections. Prussian blue stains only weakly bound iron. Strongly bound iron, such as iron in hemoglobin, will not stain. The principle of this stain is simple: When treated with potassium ferrocyanide in an acidic solution, ferrous ions in tissue react to form an insoluble blue pigment. A nuclear fast red counterstain is usually applied to demonstrate the background tissue morphology (c-**Fig. 53.16**).

   2. Urates. A modified GMS stain can be used to demonstrate uric acid crystals. No oxidation of the tissue sections is performed; instead, the sections are reacted in the methenamine solution for an extended period at an elevated temperature. Silver ions deposit on the uric acid crystals, which in turn reduce the silver ions to metallic silver, so no toning is necessary. A light green counterstain is usually applied, and the resulting stained section demonstrates black uric acid crystals in a green background. This stain requires the use of alcohol-fixed tissues because uric acid is soluble in water.

   3. Calcium (von Kossa method). The von Kossa method to stain for calcium is very simple. Tissue sections are incubated in a 5% silver nitrate solution under a very strong light source. The silver ions deposit on the calcium and are reduced to metallic silver by the strong light, in much the same process as occurs in photographic film. The stained section is rinsed free of any unreacted silver ions by a sodium thiosulfate wash, and then counterstained with nuclear fast red to highlight the background tissue morphology (e-**Fig. 53.17**).

   4. Copper (rhodanine method). Copper can be demonstrated in tissues using several methods, but the most sensitive method uses rhodanine. Tissue sections are subjected to a saturated solution of 5-(p-dimethylaminobenzylidine) rhodanine in aqueous solution. The rhodanine reacts with proteins that have bound copper rather than directly with the copper itself. The excess stain is rinsed from the sections, and the sections are counterstained with Mayer's hematoxylin, an aqueous hematoxylin that will not overstain the rhodanine reaction. This tissue stain demonstrates bound copper as a granular red pigment with pale blue cell nuclei (e-**Fig. 53.18**).

   5. Argyrophil staining. Argyrophil substances within a cell bind silver ions. They are "silver loving" but do not reduce silver to its visible metallic form. There are

TABLE 53.1 Common Histochemical Stains

Stain	Tissue element demonstrated	Result
Alcian blue pH 2.5	All acidic mucopolysaccharides	Blue
Alcian blue pH 1.0	Only sulfated acid mucopolysaccharides	Blue
Colloidal iron	Both carboxylated and sulfated mucopoly-saccharides and all glycoproteins	Blue
Mucicarmine	Epithelial mucins; cryptococcus capsule	Red
PAS	Neutral mucopolysaccharides, glycogen, basement membranes, and fungi	Rose-red
Congo red	Amyloid	Apple-green
Thioflavin T	Amyloid	Yellow
Reticulin	Reticulin fibers	Black
Trichrome	Nuclei, collagen, muscle	Black, Blue, Red
JMS	Basement membranes	Black
PTAH	Fibrin, muscle striations	Deep purple
Pentachrome	Nuclei, collagen, muscle, elastic fibers Fibrin, muscle, mucin	Black, Yellow, Red, Black, Red, Blue
Oil red O	Fat	Red
VVG	Elastic fibers	Black
AFB	Acid-fast bacilli	Red
Fite's AFB	*Mycobacterium leprae*	Red
Gram	Differentiating gram-positive from Gram-negative bacilli	Gram positive bacteria blue; Gram negative bacilli red
GMS	Fungi	Taupe to black
Warthin–Starry	Spirochetes	Black
Steiner	Bacteria, particularly *Helicobacter pylori*	Black
Dieterle	Spirochetes and legionella	Black
Giemsa	Bacteria, primarily H. pylori	Blue
Bielschowsky	Nerve endings, neuron fibrils, tangles and plaques	Black
Luxol fast blue	Myelin	Blue
Iron (Prussian blue)	Iron	Blue
Copper (rhodanine)	Copper	Red to red-orange
Calcium (von Kossa)	Calcium	Black
Calcium (Alizarin red S)	Calcium	Red
Uric acid (Gomori's)	Urate crystals	Black
(Fontana-Masson)	Argentaffin granules Melanin	Black
Bile pigments (Hall's bile)	Bile pigments	Emerald green
Churukian–Schenk	Argyrophil granules	Black
Leder	Cells of myeloid lineage	Red

Abbreviation: PAS = Periodic acid-Schiff; JMS = Jones' methenamine silver; PTAH = phosphotungstic acid hematoxylin; VVG = Verhoeff–Van Gieson; AFB = acid-fast bacilli; GMS = Grocott's Methenamine Silver.

several different techniques for the demonstration of argyrophil substances, all of which are chemically similar to the Warthin–Starry technique. A solution of silver nitrate is used to impregnate the argyrophilic substances in the tissue, and a reducing solution containing hydroquinone is then used to reduce the bound silver ions to metallic silver. Nuclear fast red is often used as a counterstain. By this approach, argyrophilic substances are stained black.

6. **Argentaffin staining (Fontana–Masson method).** Argentaffin substances not only bind silver ions like argyrophilic substances, but also reduce bound ionic silver to metallic silver without the use of a developer or other reducing agent. This property of argentaffin substances, which include melanin, underlies the Fontana-Masson stain. An ammoniacal silver solution is used to treat tissue sections, and the argentaffin substances within the tissue not only bind the silver ions in the solution but reduce them to metallic silver. Gold chloride is used as in the reticulin stain to tone the metallic silver from brown to black. Nuclear fast red is the counterstain of choice for this stain (e-Fig. **53.19**).

7. **Bile pigments.** Bile pigment stains are used on liver sections to distinguish bile pigments from lipofuchsin. Fouchet's reaction demonstrates biliverdin, bilirubin, and most other bile pigments. The tissue sections are treated with an aqueous solution of trichloroacetic acid and ferric chloride, which renders an emerald green precipitate, and van Gieson's solution is used as a counterstain (as in the VVG procedure). Stained tissue sections show bile pigments as emerald green, collagen as red, and other tissue elements as yellow.

F. **Enzymes.** Most enzyme stains require the use of frozen section tissues because formalin fixation and paraffin processing tend to inactivate cellular enzymes. The vast majority of enzyme stains are used in the evaluation of diseases that affect skeletal muscle.

The only enzyme stain performed on routinely processed tissue is the Leder stain, which demonstrates the presence of chloroacetate esterase in cells of myeloid lineage (chloroacetate esterase is an enzyme that can survive the rigors of formalin fixation and paraffin processing but not acid decalcification, so application of the stain to bone marrow specimens requires the use of nonacid decalcification). In the Leder method, tissue is treated with a solution of naphthol-chloroacetate and pararosaniline, and reaction with the cellular chloroacetate esterase forms a red precipitate. Hematoxylin is used as the counterstain to demonstrate nuclear detail (e-Fig. **53.20**).

G. **Staining table.** Table 53.1 presents tissue stains listed by their most common name, the tissue element that they demonstrate, and the resulting coloration or specific result.

Suggested Readings

Bancroft JD, Gamble M, eds. *Theory and Practice of Histological Techniques*, 5th ed. Edinburgh, United Kingdom: Churchill Livingston; 2002.

Carson FL. *Histotechnology: A Self-Instructional Text*, 2nd ed. Chicago, IL: ASCP Press; 1997.

Sheehan DC, Hrapchak BB, eds. *Theory and Practice of Histotechnology*, 2nd ed. Columbus, OH: Battelle Press; 1980.

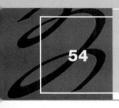

54 IMMUNOHISTOCHEMISTRY
Peter A. Humphrey

I. INTRODUCTION. Immunohistochemistry is one of the most powerful and widely-used ancillary methods in surgical pathology. The technique makes it possible to simultaneously visualize cell type and differentiation markers in standard tissue sections by light microscopy, and has revolutionized diagnostic surgical pathology.

Antigens in tissue sections were first detected using antibodies via immunofluorescence performed on frozen sections (*Proc Soc Exp Biol Med.* 1941;47:200). Although immunofluorescence is still used in the evaluation of medical kidney biopsies (see Chapter 19), currently the most common approach for diagnostic detection of antigens uses formalin-fixed paraffin-embedded (FFPE) tissue sections and immunoperoxidase methodology. This enzymatic labeling technique has evolved from simple direct peroxidase conjugation of the primary antibody, to the use of multi-step peroxidase–antiperoxidase avidin–biotin (and related) conjugate methods which, along with amplification techniques such as tyramide and polymer-based labeling, allow for much greater sensitivity in antigen detection (Taylor CR, Shi S-R, Barr NJ, Wu N. Techniques of immunohistochemistry: Principles, pitfalls, and standardization. In: Dabbs D, ed. *Diagnostic Immunohistochemistry.* Philadelphia: Elsevier; 2006: 1–42).

The laboratory utilization of immunohistochemistry (also known as immunohistology and immunostaining) requires appropriate test selection, specimen acquisition and management, methodology, validation, reporting, and interpretation (Taylor CR, Cote RJ, eds. *Immunomicroscopy. A Diagnostic Tool for the Surgical Pathologist,* 3rd ed. Philadelphia: Elsevier; 2006). This chapter provides a concise overview of these elements.

II. TEST SELECTION (PRE-ANALYTICAL PHASE). Immunohistochemical stains are usually ordered after examination of hematoxylin and eosin (H&E)-stained sections. Common indications for immunohistochemistry are the diagnosis and characterization of neoplasms, but there are others as well, such as detection of infectious organisms and evaluation of prognostic and/or predictive factors.

The use of specific immunostains is driven by the clinical and morphological context of each individual case. Panels of antibodies are often used, and these panels should be devised based on the anticipated value added to the clinical, radiographic, and pathological differential diagnosis. Panels of antibodies should thus be directed toward a specific question. Various approaches have been used to help construct appropriate immunostain panels, including algorithmic approaches and tabular approaches. Web sites with information on the specificity and sensitivity of various immunostains, and on construction of immunostain panels based on differential diagnosis of specific neoplasms, also exist (see below).

III. SPECIMEN TYPE AND TISSUE MANAGEMENT. Immunostains can be performed on cytological specimens (Barr NJ, Wu NC-Y. Cytopathology/FNA. In: Taylor CR, Cote RJ, eds. *Immunomicroscopy. A Diagnostic Tool for the Surgical Pathologist,* 3rd ed. Philadelphia: Elsevier; 2006), although they are usually performed on standard histological tissue sections. Whereas the use of FFPE tissue sections offers obvious logistical advantages, some antigens require the use of fresh tissue or tissue preserved with ethanol-based fixatives. The discussion here focuses on tissues fixed in 10% neutral buffered formalin, because this is the tissue type most commonly available for analysis in routine clinical practice.

Immediate fixation in neutral pH formalin for 12 to 48 hours at room temperature is desirable. Formalin induces cross-links that may mask some epitopes, resulting in loss of immunoreactivity. Acid decalcification of bone samples can also cause loss of immunoreactivity. "Unmasking" of some epitopes from FFPE tissue (and tissue treated with acid decalcification) can be accomplished by antigen retrieval techniques. Enzyme digestion was used in the past, but now simple heat treatment (heat-induced antigen retrieval) is the most commonly used approach to optimize antigen detection. (For details on specimen fixation, processing, and antigen retrieval see Chapter 2 of Taylor CR, Cote RJ, eds. *Immunomicroscopy. A Diagnostic Tool for the Surgical Pathologist*, 3rd ed. Philadelphia: Elsevier; 2006). Unstained tissue sections cut onto charged slides or poly-L-lysine (or gelatin or albumin)-coated slides are typically used for immunohistochemistry, but it is possible to perform immunostains on sections that have already been stained with H&E (*Am J Clin Pathol.* 2005;124:708); because success with such restaining protocols is variable, unstained tissue sections remain the best resource for immunostains. Immunostaining should be performed on freshly cut sections from the paraffin block, because unstained sections exposed to air may lose antigen immunoreactivity over the course of days to weeks.

IV. **METHODOLOGY**

   A. **The primary antibody** is an immunoglobulin molecule that binds to the target antigen in tissue sections. The primary antibody may be either a monoclonal antibody derived via the hybridoma technique or a polyclonal antibody from an antiserum. In general, polyclonal antibodies tend to be more sensitive but less specific than monoclonal antibodies. Unlike monoclonal antibodies, polyclonal antibodies are not reliable reagents of unlimited supply; different batches of antisera may result in polyclonal antibody heterogeneity.

      Each antibody, whether polyclonal or monoclonal in origin, needs to be tested for sensitivity and specificity in target antigen detection, and the reaction conditions for its use need to be optimized. Titration experiments must be performed to achieve a working dilution of the primary antibody that yields the greatest contrast between specific staining and nonspecific staining. If prediluted reagents and kits are used, it is recommended that the manufacturer protocol be followed because validation was performed with those reaction conditions.

   B. **Background staining** results from nonspecific antibody binding and from endogenous enzymes that nonspecifically interact with the chromogenic substrate. Nonspecific antibody binding is more likely to occur with polyclonal antibodies. Endogenous enzymes that cause background staining are found in normal cells including erythrocytes, neutrophils, eosinophils, hepatocytes, and neoplastic cells; their activity can often be blocked (e.g., endogenous peroxidase can be blocked by incubation with hydrogen peroxide).

   C. **Detection systems**

      1. **Direct conjugate-labeled antibody method.** In this method, the label—such as peroxidase or fluorescein—is directly chemically linked to the primary antibody. Disadvantages to this approach include a requirement for a large amount of primary antibody for labeling and a lack of signal amplification.

      2. **Indirect or sandwich method.** The primary antibody is unlabeled, and a secondary antibody, reactive against the primary antibody, carries the label.

      3. **Unlabeled antibody method.** Also known as the peroxidase–antiperoxidase (PAP) method, this procedure uses an unlabeled primary antibody, an unlabeled bridge antibody, and a complex of an antiperoxidase antibody and the peroxidase molecule itself. The bridge antibody, directed against both the primary antibody and the antiperoxidase antibody, links the primary antibody–tissue antigen reaction to the signal generated by the peroxidase. This approach has largely been replaced by the more sensitive approaches below.

      4. **Avidin–biotin or streptavidin–biotin conjugate method.** A biotinylated secondary antibody is used to recognize the primary antibody; avidin or streptavidin complexed with biotinylated peroxidase is then bound to the secondary antibody (both avidin and streptavidin have extremely high affinity for biotin). These reactions deliver several peroxidase molecules to the primary antibody

binding site and so boost sensitivity. Streptavidin has several advantages over avidin, including decreased background staining.

5. **Tyramine amplification (catalyzed signal amplification [CSA]) methods.** With these methods, there is increased sensitivity due to greater accumulation of biotin at the antigen–primary antibody reaction site as a result of the catalytic activity of peroxidase on biotinylated tyramine.

6. **Polymer-based labels.** This approach uses dextran chain polymers to localize numerous enzyme molecules to the antigen site by linking multiple antibody and enzyme molecules together along the polymer chain (Fig. 54.1). This method avoids problems with endogenous biotin.

7. **Alkaline phosphatase** can be used instead of peroxidase when the target antigen is in tissues rich in myeloid cells that contain high levels of endogenous peroxidases, such as bone marrow.

8. **Chromogens** are the color-producing reactants in the detection system. The methods using peroxidase, diaminobenzidine (DAB, produces a brown color), and 3-amino-9-ethyl carbazole (AEC, produces a red color) are commonly used.

9. **Counterstaining** is most often accomplished using the nuclear stain hematoxylin. Care must be taken not to overstain the tissue sections, especially when the target antigen is located in the nucleus.

10. **Antibody cocktails** can be used to detect two or more antigens at the same time. Single color (*Am J Surg Pathol.* 2005;29:579) or two color (*Am J Clin Pathol.* 2005;123:231) approaches can be used.

11. **Automation.** Automated immunostaining devices are in routine use in many laboratories and can improve standardization, throughput, and reproducibility of immunohistochemical procedures.

12. **Quantitative immunohistochemistry.** In the past, immunohistochemical reactions have been manually scored in a semiquantitative manner by pathologists, via analysis of the grade of staining intensity and estimates of the percentage of cells stained in the area of interest. Such scoring has been particularly important for a few markers, for example, detection of HER2/*neu* immunoreactivity in breast carcinoma to determine the eligibility of breast cancer patients for trastazumab (Herceptin) therapy (*J Clin Oncol.* 2007;25:118). Because image analysis improves the consistency of quantitative immunohistochemical scoring, it is likely that digital microscopy (see Chapter 62) with image analysis will be increasingly used in this context in the future.

V. VALIDATION. Positive and negative controls should be included in every sample run and reviewed along with the test immunohistochemical reaction. A positive tissue or cell control known to express the antigen under investigation should be used, and should be subjected to the same reaction conditions in the same analytical run as the test tissues or cells. Some laboratories place a positive control tissue section on the same slide as the test tissue section; for some immunostains there may be an internal positive control in the test tissue. A negative control can be generated using a tissue known to lack the antigen of interest or by replacing the primary antibody with an irrelevant nonimmune antibody or antiserum; a search should also be made in the test tissues for negative internal controls.

VI. REPORTING. Immunohistochemical stain reports should include specific content elements (Table 54.1).

VII. INTERPRETATION. Interpretation of immunostains, including significance, should be integrated with the interpretation of the clinical, radiographic, gross, and histopathological findings of the case, as well as the results of any additional ancillary tests (such as molecular genetic tests). After evaluation of positive and negative controls, the test tissue sections should be assessed for presence of the area(s) of interest, localization of immunohistochemical signal, intensity of signal, and number of immunoreactive cells or foci. In some cases, especially for limited and small tissue samples, the area of interest may not be present in the additional sections used for immunohistochemistry. Specific attention should be directed toward background staining, and artifacts such as localization of signal along tissue edges (edge artifact) or in areas of necrosis.

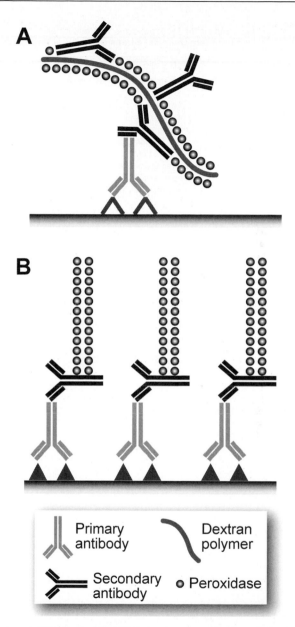

Figure 54.1. Immunohistochemical detection using the polymer method. This technique allows linkage of numerous molecules of enzyme (either peroxidase or alkaline phosphatase) to one **(B)** or more **(A)** molecules of secondary antibody. Delivery of a large number of enzyme molecules to the antigen–primary antibody reaction site yields high sensitivity. Modified from Taylor CR, Cote RJ, eds. *Immunomicroscopy. A Diagnostic Tool for the Surgical Pathologist*, 3rd ed. Philadelphia: Elsevier, 2006.

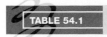

TABLE 54.1	Guidelines for Incorporation of Results of Immunohistochemical Stains in Surgical Pathology Reports*

1. All immunostain results should be reported, whether positive, negative, or noncontributory
2. A differential diagnosis justifying immunostain selection should be given
3. The report should also include
    - the nature of the specimen tested: frozen section, paraffin section, cytoprep, etc.
    - the paraffin block number used to obtain sections for immunostaining
    - the antibodies used, including where appropriate, the clone number
    - the result of staining for each antibody, including cellular localization when relevant
4. An interpretation of the findings in the context of the diagnosis, with reference to the associated surgical pathology report if immunohistochemical results are reported separately
5. Exact protocols, antigen retrieval methods, and reaction conditions need not be part of the report but must be available in laboratory manuals and records.

*Modified from Taylor CR, Cote RJ, eds. *Immunomicroscopy. A Diagnostic Tool for the Surgical Pathologist*, 3rd ed. Philadelphia: Elsevier; 2006:41, Table 1.8.

Appropriate location of the signal—for example, cytoplasm versus nucleus—should be noted.

Immunostain results can profoundly influence a diagnosis or can be noncontributory, so the role of immunostains in arriving at the final diagnosis should be specified. For example, a comment in the report should indicate that immunostains were used to establish, confirm, or support a diagnosis, or that they were noncontributory. For predictive markers such as HER2/*neu*, guidelines for reporting should be followed (*J Clin Oncol.* 2007;25:118).

VIII. **SOURCES OF DATA ON ANTIBODIES AND ANTIGENS, INCLUDING CONSTRUCTION OF MARKER PANELS.** The chapters in this book provide information on the most useful immunostains for the evaluation of diseases of each organ system and/or tissue type. Other sources for detailed information on useful marker panels include books (Common panels for immunohistochemical studies: Tables 7.3 to 7.30 in Lester SC, ed. *Manual of Surgical Pathology*, 2nd ed. Philadelphia: Elsevier; 2006:76–146) as well as internet sites (one helpful commercial site is my.statdxpathiq.com).

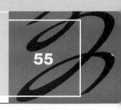

IMMUNOFLUORESCENCE
Anne C. Lind and Rosa M. Dávila

55

I. INTRODUCTION/OVERVIEW. These ancillary studies are used to support fixed tissue diagnoses and to provide additional diagnostic and prognostic information as it relates to autoimmune diseases, vesiculobullous diseases, transplantation, and glomerular disease. Fresh tissue submitted in a preservative, nonfixative, transport medium such as Michel's medium or fresh frozen tissue is required. Transport medium can be held at room temperature. Temperature extremes should be avoided. Currently, immunofluorescence studies cannot be performed on formalin-fixed, paraffin-embedded tissue. A specialized microscope and a room where the majority of ambient light can be extinguished are required for either direct or indirect immunofluorescence examination.

II. DIRECT IMMUNOFLUORESCENCE

A. Skin/mucosa. Cutaneous/mucosal biopsies for immunofluorescence are stained with fluorescein-labeled antibodies to immunoglobulins (IgG, IgA, IgM), complement (C'3), and collagen IV. The patterns of staining that correlate with specific diseases are discussed in more detail with the corresponding diagnoses in the chapter on inflammatory disorders of the skin (Chapter 38).

    1. Bullous pemphigoid. A biopsy of perilesional tissue to include the edge of a blister is optimal. Some studies have reported a high false-negative rate for tissue from the lower extremity; if possible, tissue for direct immunofluorescence should be obtained from above the knee. Direct immunofluorescence is positive in approximately 85% to 90% of cases of bullous pemphigoid.

    2. Pemphigus vulgaris. A biopsy of perilesional tissue, without including the edge of a blister, is optimal. Direct immunofluorescence is positive in approximately 90% to 95% of cases of pemphigus vulgaris.

    3. Dermatitis herpetiformis. A biopsy of perilesional tissue, avoiding excoriated areas, is optimal. Direct immunofluorescence is positive in approximately 80% of cases of dermatitis herpetiformis.

    4. Vasculitis. A biopsy of lesional tissue is required. Sources vary on recommendations regarding age of lesion; however, the majority favor a lesion that has been present for <48 hours.

    5. Lupus. A biopsy of an established lesion that has been present for at least 8 weeks, preferably 12, is required to detect immunofluorescence positivity in discoid lupus. In the past, prognostic information regarding disease activity was associated with immunofluorescence positivity in sun-protected, nonlesional skin in systemic lupus.

B. Kidney. What constitutes an adequate renal biopsy is not well defined. However, it is generally suggested that two tissue cores be obtained and that the tissue should be distributed for light microscopy, immunofluorescence, and electron microscopic analysis (*Mod Pathol* 2004;17:1555). Renal biopsies are usually performed under ultrasound guidance, and the tissue cores are evaluated in the ultrasound suite with a dissecting microscope. It is important to avoid air drying of the tissue; therefore, the tissue is placed in a Petri dish with a balanced salt solution while it is examined with the dissecting microscope. Because glomerular diseases are a common indication for renal biopsy, the tissue is distributed in such a way that approximately two or more glomeruli are examined by electron microscopy, two or more by immunofluorescence, and 10 or more by light microscopy. The tissue assigned to electron microscopy is placed in glutaraldehyde. Tissue for immunofluorescence is frozen, and tissue for

689

light microscopy is placed in formalin. When a biopsy needs to be transported to the laboratory from a remote site, it should be placed in a container with transport medium such as Michel's medium.

Light microscopic evaluation of the renal biopsy is performed using hematoxylin and eosin, periodic acid Schiff (PAS), trichrome, and methenamine silver stained sections. The PAS and silver stains facilitate examination of the basement membranes, and the trichrome stain highlights areas of interstitial fibrosis. Evaluation with antibodies against IgG, IgM, IgA, C'3, C1q, fibrinogen, albumin, κ, and λ are performed by direct immunofluorescence. Transplant kidney biopsies are also stained for C4d to assess the presence of humoral rejection, usually seen as immunopositivity of the peritubular capillaries.

C. Pulmonary transplantation. In the event of suspected humoral rejection after pulmonary transplantation, biopsy of pulmonary parenchymal tissue acquired via transbronchial biopsy can be submitted in Michel's medium for evaluation of complement (C4d) by direct immunofluorescence. It is worth noting that evaluation for the presence of C4d can also be accomplished using an immunoperoxidase method on formalin-fixed tissue.

III. INDIRECT IMMUNOFLUORESCENCE. Blood (5 to 10 mL) drawn into a tube without anticoagulant is required for all indirect immunofluorescence studies. The serum is removed and is applied to an epithelial substrate. The substrate varies with the clinical diagnosis, and the clinical diagnosis should guide the decision to pursue the appropriate indirect immunofluorescence study. For indirect immunofluorescence, serial dilutions (1:10 to 1:1280) of serum are inoculated onto the tissue substrate together with fluorescein-labeled IgG.

A. Pemphigus vulgaris. The primary utility for indirect immunofluorescence is for the diagnosis of pemphigus vulgaris and to follow response to therapy. Serial dilutions are performed and documentation of the end-point of positivity of intercellular IgG is reported. Commercially prepared slides using guinea pig or monkey esophagus are used. As in other serologic tests, it is possible to get a prozone effect in patients with pemphigus vulgaris, so additional dilutions may be required to avoid a false-negative result.

B. Paraneoplastic pemphigus. The substrate for evaluation of paraneoplastic pemphigus is murine/rat bladder epithelium. Because this test is not commonly ordered, it is usually only performed at reference laboratories.

C. Bullous and/or cicatricial pemphigoid. Circulating antibodies are detected in fewer than half of the patients with documented pemphigoid, making ancillary testing by indirect immunofluorescence minimally useful for this disease process.

D. Dermatitis herpetiformis. Circulating antibodies are not detectable in the serum of patients with dermatitis herpetiformis; therefore, indirect immunofluorescence is not indicated.

E. Reference laboratories. Reference laboratories are a useful resource for indirect immunofluorescence testing for rare diseases. Evaluation of epidermolysis bullosa is performed by Beutner Laboratories (Buffalo, NY). Testing for paraneoplastic pemphigus is performed by Mayo Clinical Laboratories (Rochester, MN). Some research laboratories also perform specialized testing for rare vesiculobullous dermatoses, however testing in this setting may not be approved for clinical use.

FLOW CYTOMETRY
Friederike Kreisel

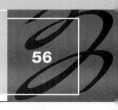

56

I. BASIC PRINCIPLE. Flow cytometry simultaneously measures and analyzes multiple physical and/or chemical characteristics of single particles, usually cells, as they flow in a fluid stream through a beam of light. With this technique any suspended microparticle, ranging in size from 0.2 to 150 μm can be analyzed. Many protocols for the preparation of cell suspensions exist. Peripheral blood or bone marrow aspirate specimens already represent a suspension of single cells but they must be prevented from clotting by using collection tubes containing disodium EDTA, sodium citrate, or heparin. Enrichment of leukocytes can be achieved by lysis of accompanying red blood cells with ammonium chloride buffer or use of density-gradient separation (*Flow Cytometry in Clinical Diagnosis,* 3rd ed. Chicago: ASCP Press; 2001:31–65). Solid tissue should be collected in RPMI medium, and the tissue should be minced into small pieces and passed through a fine mesh.

II. FLOW CYTOMETER is composed of three main systems (*Basic Principles in Clinical Diagnosis,* 3rd ed. Chicago: ASP; 2001:31–65) (Fig. 56.1).

    A. The flow system. The sample is injected into a stream of sheath fluid within the flow chamber. Through the principle of hydrodynamic focusing, the particles are forced into the center of the stream and transported to the laser beam for analysis. Only one particle or cell should move through the laser beam at a given moment. The sample pressure is always greater than the sheath fluid pressure; increasing the sample pressure increases the flow rate of the sample by increasing the width of the sample core, allowing more cells to enter the stream at a given moment. A higher flow rate is generally used for the immunophenotyping of cells. A lower flow rate is important in applications where greater resolution is needed, such as DNA analysis.

    B. The optical system. Lasers illuminate the particles in the sample stream and optical mirrors and filters that route the different wavelengths of the generated light scatter and fluorescent signals to the appropriate photodetectors.

        1. Light scatter. Light scattering occurs when a particle or cell deflects laser light. Forward-scattered light (FSC) is in line with the laser light beam and represents a measurement of the cell surface size. Side-scattered light (SSC) is collected perpendicular to the laser light beam and analyses the granularity or internal complexity of a cell. Leukocytes can be separated into different subpopulations using FSC and SSC. For example, lymphocytes will show both a low forward scatter and a low side scatter due to the small size and lack of cytoplasmic granulation. In contrast, neutrophils are larger in size and show granular cytoplasm as well as a complex nucleus, and therefore will show both a high forward and side scatter (e-Fig. 56.1).*

        2. Fluorescence. Another way to identify particular subpopulations is to conjugate fluorescent dyes to monoclonal antibodies directed toward antigens on a particular cell subset. These fluorescent dyes absorb light energy over a range of wavelengths that is characteristic for that compound. With the absorption of light energy, an electron in the fluorescent dye is raised to a higher energy level. Subsequently, the excited electron will return to its ground state, thereby emitting the excess energy as a photon of light. The light that is given off is called fluorescence; its wavelength is then captured by a detector.

---

*All e-figures are available online via the Solution Site Image Bank.

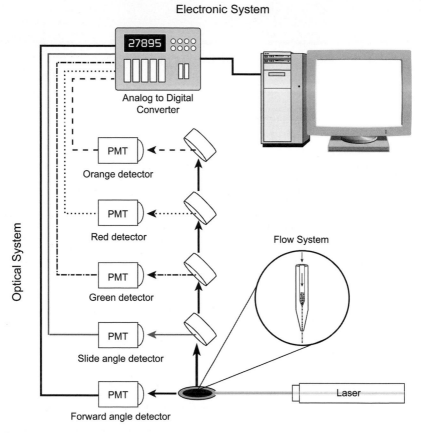

Figure 56.1. The flow cytometer is composed the flow system, optical system, and electronic system. The flow system transports cells in a stream to the laser beam for analysis. The optical system consists of lasers to illuminate the cells in the sample stream and optical filters to direct the resulting light signals to the appropriate detectors. The electronic system converts light signals into electronic signals that are processed by the computer.

The staining procedure can be carried out in a direct or indirect staining process (*Flow Cytometry, First Principles*. New York: Wiley-Liss; 1992;75–102). The direct staining procedure involves a single staining incubation, followed by several washes to remove nonspecifically bound antibodies. The indirect staining procedure involves the incubation of cells with a nonfluorescent monoclonal antibody directed toward the specific antigen. After washing nonspecifically bound antibody, there is a second incubation with a fluorescent antibody that will react with the monoclonal antibody. Although more time consuming, the indirect staining procedure is less expensive.

Argon ion lasers are the most common lasers used in flow cytometry because the 488-nm light emitted can be absorbed by more than one fluorochrome. Examples of fluorochromes that are conjugated to antibodies are fluorescein isothiocyanate (FITC) and phycoerythrin (PE) (*Flow Cytometry*, 3rd ed. Oxford: Oxford University Press; 2005:23–33). FITC absorbs light in the range of 460 to 510 nm and then fluoresces in the range of 510 to 560 nm, with a peak at ~525 nm, giving a green fluorescent color. PE absorbs light in the range of 480 to 565 nm and fluoresces at ~570 nm, creating a red fluorescent color. Although both fluorochromes absorb light at ~488 nm, the resulting peak emission wavelengths differ in such a way that they can be detected by different detectors. This enables different fluorochromes to be used simultaneously in one sample. Combined with the FSC and SSC data, the staining pattern of each subpopulation will aide in delineating which cells are present in a sample and in what percentage they are present (e-**Fig. 56.2**).

C. Electronic system. Photodetectors convert the generated FSC, SSC, and fluorescent light signals into electrical impulses.

1. Photodetectors. Generally, two types of photodetectors are used in flow cytometry: photomultiplier tubes (PMTs) and photodiodes (*Flow Cytometry, First Principles.* New York: Wiley-Liss; 1992;15–40). PMTs have voltages applied to them to amplify the electrical current generated from the light signals. These are mostly used to detect weaker signals generated by SSC and fluorescence. Photodiodes are less sensitive to light signals and are used to detect stronger FSC. Amplification of a signal detected by a photodetector can also be achieved by increasing the amplification, by means of log amplification or linear amplification. Log amplifiers are usually used to separate negative from dim positive signals and are commonly used to analyze fluorescence signals in cells stained with fluorochrome-labeled antibodies because these cells often exhibit a great range of fluorescence intensities. Linear amplifiers are generally used to analyze forward and side scatter signals.

2. Conversion into a digital value. The intensity of the electronic impulses derived from the photodetectors is assigned a digital value by means of an analog to digital converter (ADC). The role of the ADC is to analyze a continuous distribution of signals falling into a channel of a certain light intensity range and to organize these signals into a data plot. An electronic threshold is used to limit the number of events to the population of interest. For example, the threshold can be set on FSC to eliminate events that represent debris is smaller than the threshold channel number. After the acquired data are saved, cell populations can be displayed as different data plots. A single parameter, such as FSC or FITC (FL1) can be displayed as a single-parameter histogram, on which the horizontal axis represents the signal intensity expressed as the parameter's signal value in channel numbers and the vertical axis represents the number of events per channel (e-**Fig. 56.3**). Signals with identical intensities accumulate in the same channel. Two parameters, such as FITC (FL1) and PE (FL2) can be displayed simultaneously in a dot plot (e-**Fig. 56.4**). One parameter is displayed on the *x* axis and the other parameter is displayed on the *y* axis.

A subset of data can be defined through a gate. Based on FSC and SSC, a gate can be set on a selected population of interest and analysis restricted to only that subset.

D. Uses

1. Cell markers. Flow cytometry has become a valuable ancillary study methodology for classifying acute leukemias and lymphomas. Monoclonal antibody technology has provided flow cytometry with a large variety of antibodies specific to nuclear, cytoplasmic, and surface antigens characteristic of particular cell subsets. These are organized as clusters of differentiation (CD) antigens, which help differentiate cells into the different subpopulations of the hematopoietic and lymphoid system. Selected CD markers that are used in the diagnosis of acute leukemias and lymphomas are discussed in Chapters 42 and 43. Flow cytometric scattergrams of an example of precursor B-lymphoblastic leukemia are outlined in e-**Fig. 56.5**. Typical flow cytometric findings of chronic lymphocytic leukemia are shown in e-**Figs 56.6** and **56.7**. Antibodies form a strong bond with corresponding antigens and are "visualized" by attaching a fluorochrome, such as FITC or PE.

2. DNA content. Besides analyzing surface or cytoplasmic properties of a cell, flow cytometry can also be used to analyze DNA contents of a cell (*Flow Cytometry in Clinical Diagnosis*, 3rd ed. Chicago: ASCP Press; 2001:641–662). Several types of fluorescent stains are available depending on which DNA bases within the helix are targeted. Most of these require the use of laser with significant ultraviolet output

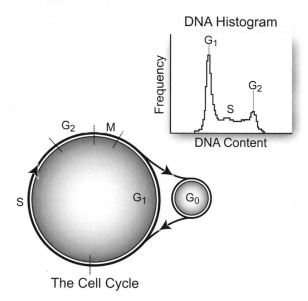

Figure 56.2. Histogram of DNA distribution from a cycling population of cells. The eukaryotic cell cycle is divided into several successive phases: G_0, G_1, S, G_2, and M. The DNA flow histogram correlates to the distribution of different kinds of nuclei present at a particular moment.

to be specific. For example, HOECHST 33342 or 4′,6-diamidino-2-phenylindole (DAPI) are specific for the adenosine/thymine base pairs, whereas mithramycin and chromomycin A3 preferentially target the guanine/cytosine base pairs. Propidium iodide is not very specific because it stains all double-stranded nucleic acids, but it can be included as a DNA stain in conventional cytometers with low-power argon lasers because it absorbs light at 488 nm.

DNA staining is generally performed to assess the amount of DNA in the nucleus of a cell or to analyze cell division. Because most normal cells contain the same amount of DNA (diploid or euploid amount of DNA), measurement of DNA content of a cell will differentiate normal cells from aneuploid malignant cells. The histograms from malignant tumors will show abnormal peaks corresponding to more (hyperdiploid) or less (hypodiploid) DNA than normal cells.

3. **Cell cycle analysis.** The cell cycle is composed of four phases. Cells in G1 are recovering from division or are preparing for division; cells in S phase are in the process of synthesizing new DNA. Cells in G2 phase have finished DNA synthesis and therefore have double the normal amount of DNA (tetraploid), and the M phase is the division into two similar daughter cells. Cells in G0 phase are not cycling at all. The cell cycle can be plotted as a histogram with number of cells per channel on the y axis and the fluorescence intensity of cells stained for DNA content on the x axis (Fig. 56.2).

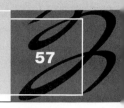

CYTOGENETICS

57

Shashikant Kulkarni and John D. Pfeifer

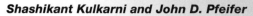

I. **INTRODUCTION.** The three significant milestones in the history of clinical cytogenetics are the preparation of chromosome spreads from peripheral blood cultures (*Exp Cell Res* 1960;20:613), the development of hypotonic methods to obtain enhanced chromosome spreads (*Cancer Res* 1960;20:462), and the discovery that fluorescent quinacrine compounds could be used to demonstrate a unique banding pattern for each human chromosome pair (*Hereditas* 1971;67:89). The remarkable advancement of the field of human cytogenetics is emphasized by the fact that it has been only 50 years since the correct number of human chromosomes was established. The various banding methods in current use not only permit identification of each chromosome, but also make it possible to detect specific alterations associated with hereditary syndromes and neoplasms.

II. **TRADITIONAL CYTOGENETIC ANALYSIS.** Although cytogenetic analysis is commonly used in the evaluation of congenital disorders (specifically, to diagnose syndromes associated with abnormalities of chromosomal number or structure, to establish the chromosomal sex in cases of sexual ambiguity, and to screen for karyotypic abnormalities in patients with multiple birth defects) and for prenatal diagnosis, the technique's primary application in surgical pathology is in the evaluation of neoplastic disorders. The utility of the technique in surgical pathology rests on the fact that specific cytogenetic abnormalities have been recognized that are closely, and sometimes uniquely, associated with morphologically and clinically distinct subsets of lymphoma and leukemia, or with soft tissue neoplasms.

A. **Advantages.** The power of conventional cytogenetics lies in its ability to provide simultaneous analysis of the entire genome without any foreknowledge of the chromosomal regions involved in the disease process. In most cases, the type and location of an identified chromosomal abnormality is either directly diagnostic or can be used to direct additional testing. Contrary to some predictions, the advent of technologies such as array comparative genomic hybridization has not diminished the importance of traditional cytogenetics; in fact, these novel molecular techniques achieve some of their greatest utility when they are used in conjunction with traditional clinical cytogenetics.

B. **Limitations.** The clinical utility of traditional cytogenetic analysis is restricted by two general features of the method. From a technical standpoint, analysis can only be performed on viable tissue specimens that contain proliferating cells (see section on culture initiation below). From a sensitivity standpoint, analysis has resolution of only about 3 to 4 Mb at an 850-band level, and only about 7 to 8 Mb at a 400-band level. Traditional cytogenetic analysis is therefore only suited for detection of numerical abnormalities and gross structural rearrangements. The method does not have the sensitivity to detect mutations such as small deletions and amplifications and single base pair substitutions.

C. **Basic laboratory procedures.** Chromosomes that can be individually distinguished by light microscopy can only be obtained during cell division, so the fundamental requirement for traditional cytogenetic analysis is a tissue specimen that contains actively proliferating cells or cells that can be induced to proliferate in vitro. The basic method for the production of metaphase chromosomes for cytogenetic analysis is shown in Figure 57.1.

1. **Culture initiation.** Different specimen types have different sample and handing requirements (Table 57.1). Inappropriate handling, as well as delay between

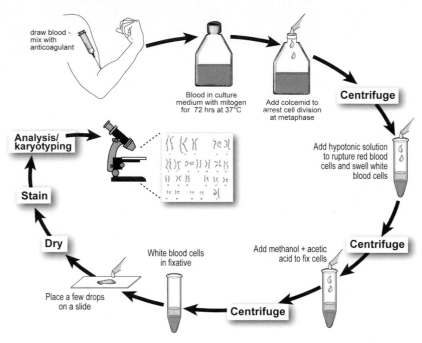

Figure 57.1. Overall scheme for the production of metaphase chromosomes for traditional cytogenetic analysis.

specimen collection and culture initiation, can markedly decrease the likelihood that the sample will grow in vitro, so communication and coordination with the cytogenetics laboratory are essential.

In vitro culture relies on a sterile microenvironment, so specimens should be collected under sterile conditions. In practice, sterility is most difficult to achieve when sampling solid tissues; in this setting, clean instruments and a clean cutting surface, together with transport of the specimen in medium supplemented with broad-spectrum antibiotics, can be used to minimize contamination.

TABLE 57.1	**Specimen Requirements**
Tissue type	**Sample collection**
Peripheral blood	Preservative-free sodium heparin; transport refrigerated or at room temperature
Bone marrow aspirate	Preservative-free sodium heparin; the first several milliliters of the aspirate usually contain the greatest proportion of cells, so is the optimal sample for cytogenetic analysis; transport at room temperature
Solid tissue	Collect and transport in sterile culture medium containing broad-spectrum antibiotics; carefully select maximally viable tumor for analysis; transport on ice to minimize autolysis and microbial overgrowth

Bone marrow and solid tissue neoplasms consist of cell types that proliferate spontaneously in culture, although often at a low rate. Lymph nodes are composed of cells that have a low intrinsic proliferative rate but that can be induced to divide much more rapidly by the addition of mitogens. Phytohemagglutinin stimulates proliferation of T lymphocytes. Lipopolysaccharide, protein A, 12-O-tetradecanoly-phorbol-13-acetate, Epstein–Barr virus, and pokeweed mitogen induce proliferation of B lymphocytes, and are also required for successful culture of some leukemias and lymphomas of B-cell origin.

2. **Culture maintenance.** The length of in vitro culture depends on cell type. Because bone marrow cultures contain spontaneously proliferating cells, they can be harvested after only a 24- to 48-hour culture interval, if not directly after specimen collection. Peripheral blood cultures usually require a 72-hour culture interval. The growth rate of solid tissue specimens is difficult to predict; some solid tumors require culture periods of 2 weeks or longer.

3. **Cell harvest.** Colcemid, a synthetic analogue of colchicine (an alkaloid from the bulb of the Mediterranean plant *Colchicum*) prevents separation of sister chromatids and is used to block the proliferating cells in metaphase, thus allowing an accumulation of cells at metaphase stage. A hypotonic solution is then used to swell the cells so that, after fixation, the chromosomes are adequately spread for microscopic analysis.

Because cells in culture do not proceed through the cell cycle in synchrony, chemical synchronization of cell division is often required to obtain an acceptable mitotic index. A common chemical approach involves addition of excess thymidine, which stalls cells at the S phase of the cell cycle by decreasing the amount of 2′ deoxycytidine 5′-triphosphate (dCTP) available for DNA synthesis. When the excess thymidine is removed (or the effect of excess thymidine is eliminated by the addition of deoxycytidine), normal DNA replication resumes, and the collective release of the cells from S phase produces a transiently high mitotic index. Alternatively, 5-fluorodeoxyuridine (which inhibits the enzyme thymidylate synthetase) can be used to stall cells at the G1/S boundary; in this method, addition of thymidine releases the block.

4. **Banding.** The different techniques that can be used to stain metaphase chromosomes can be divided into two general categories: methods that produce specific alternating white and dark regions (bands) along the length of each chromosome, and methods that stain only a defined region of specific chromosomes (Table 57.2). The dark bands are gene-poor, adenine-thymine (AT)-rich regions, whereas the light bands are gene-rich, guanine-cytosine (GC)-rich regions. The quality of staining depends on several technical factors, including sufficient separation of the chromosomes in the metaphase spread to allow clear visualization. Although there are no internationally accepted standards for banding resolution, ideograms are used as reference points (e-**Fig. 57.1**).* Many countries, including the United States, Canada, United Kingdom, France, Japan, and Australia, have established standards that specify the minimum requirements for the number and quality of cells that must be processed for chromosome analysis depending on sample type, although many cases require more detailed analysis.

5. **Microscopic analysis.** The method used to stain the chromosomes dictates whether bright field microscopy or fluorescence microscopy is used to visualize the chromosomes. Conventional photography has traditionally been used to produce high-resolution prints of the stained chromosomes, but electronic imaging systems are rapidly replacing conventional photographic processes. The final step in cytogenetic analysis is the production of a karyotype, which consists of the chromosomal complement of the cell displayed in a standard sequence on the basis of size, centromere location, and banding pattern (e-**Fig. 57.2**).

D. **Assay failure.** Many of the common causes of failure to obtain a cytogenetic result (Table 57.3) can be avoided by careful selection of viable tissue with prompt specimen transport in the appropriate medium to the cytogenetics laboratory. Nonetheless,

---

*All e-figures are available online via the Solution Site Image Bank.

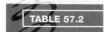

TABLE 57.2	Major Chromosome Staining and Banding Techniques

Method	Staining pattern
Techniques that produce specific alternating bands along each chromosome	
Giemsa banding (G-banding)	Dark bands are AT rich; light bands are CG rich
Quinacrine banding (Q-banding)	Bright regions are AT rich
Reverse banding (R-banding)	AT-rich regions stain lightly (have dull fluorescence), CG-rich regions staining darkly (have bright fluorescence)
4,6-Diamidino-2-phenylindole staining (DAPI staining)	DAPI binds AT-rich regions; produces a pattern similar to Q-banding
Techniques that stain selective chromosome regions	
Constitutive heterochromatin banding (C-banding)	Stains heterochromatin (α-satellite DNA) around the centromeres; can also be used to demonstrate some inherited polymorphisms
Telomere banding (T-banding)	Technical variation of R-banding used to stain telomeres
Silver staining for nucleolar organizer regions (NOR staining)	Stains the NORs (which contain active ribosomal RNA genes) on the satellite stalks of acrocentric chromosomes
Fluorescence in situ hybridization (FISH)	Staining pattern is dependent on the probe

several causes of assay failure are inherent to in vitro culture and cannot be eliminated by even the most meticulous laboratory technique.

Cytogenetic analysis of solid tumors highlights a number of these intrinsic technical limitations. First, because benign solid tumors contain few mitotic cells, cultures are susceptible to overgrowth by nonneoplastic cells. Second, even high-grade malignant solid tumors often grow poorly in vitro, especially if grown without the appropriate culture medium and growth factor supplementation. Third, the number of neoplastic cells in a solid tumor sample can be difficult to determine based on gross examination, and the material submitted to the cytogenetics laboratory may consist primarily of stromal cells and inflammatory cells. Fourth, the viability of the neoplastic cells is often uncertain; even tumor samples that are not grossly necrotic may contain predominantly nonviable tumor cells. Fifth, in vitro culture selects for subclones within the neoplastic population that have a growth advantage, so the karyotype may not be representative of the entire neoplasm. Sixth, contamination is often unavoidable for samples collected in the frozen section area or gross room,

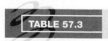

TABLE 57.3	Common Reasons for Failure of Traditional Cytogenetic Analysis

Culture Failure
No viable cells present in the sample (necrotic tumor sample or improper specimen handling)
Inappropriate sample (peripheral blood without blasts is submitted instead of bone marrow)
Overgrowth by nonneoplastic cells
Overgrowth by a nonrepresentative clone of tumor cells
Microbial overgrowth

Post Culture Failure
Technical errors involving cell harvest, slide preparation, or staining
Misdiagnosis (an abnormality is overlooked, or an abnormality is incorrectly interpreted)

or from specimens arising from anatomic sites normally colonized by bacteria, such as the oral cavity, gastrointestinal tract, or skin.The overall failure rate of conventional cytogenetic analysis is difficult to quantify for many tissue types, neoplasms, and diseases, so it is difficult to provide objective statements regarding the utility of analysis in routine surgical pathology. In studies that specifically address this issue for hematolymphoid neoplasms, cytogenetic analysis has a success rate for detecting characteristic chromosomal aberrations that varies from 33% to 100%, depending on the specific diagnosis, but is about 70% overall (*Am J Clin Pathol* 2004;121:826). For solid tumors, the success rate of analysis is less certain; reports describing cytogenetic abnormalities of many solid tumors often do not provide data on failed analyses or negative cases. Objective measures (including, e.g., sensitivity, specificity, and predictive value of a positive or negative result) of traditional cytogenetic analysis as an ancillary testing methodology in routine clinical practice are therefore often unknown.

III. METAPHASE FLUORESCENCE IN SITU HYBRIDIZATION. Virtually all metaphase chromosome in situ hybridization analysis is performed using probes that are directly or indirectly labeled with fluorescent labels. Guidelines for the use of metaphase fluorescence in situ hybridization (FISH) in clinical laboratory testing have been developed by the American College of Medical Genetics (http://www.acmg.net/Pages/ACMG_Activities/stds-2002/e.htm), and standardized nomenclature for reporting results has been developed (discussed in more detail below).

Metaphase FISH is essentially a modified Southern blot in which the target DNA consists of chromosomes rather than membrane-bound DNA. Technically, the method has four steps: the probe and metaphase target are denatured by a high temperature and formamide, the probe is hybridized to the chromosomal target, unbound probe is removed by posthybridization washes, and, finally, the bound probe is detected by fluorescence microscopy. A fluorochrome-based counterstain is virtually always used to help detect the chromosomes during microscopic examination; the use of 4,6-diamidino-2-phenylindole (DAPI) as a counterstain makes it possible to localize the position of the bound probe to specific chromosomal bands.

A variety of fluorophores can be incorporated into metaphase FISH probes either directly or indirectly. The choice of labels is largely governed by practical issues, such as the excitation and emission filters on the microscope that will be used to view the chromosome spreads.

A few probe kits have been approved by the U. S. Food and Drug Administration (FDA) for in vitro diagnostic testing, although many probes for metaphase FISH are classified as analyte-specific reagents (ASRs) so are exempt from FDA approval. Standards and guidelines for clinical use of ASRs have been established by the American College of Medical Genetics, as have recommendations for interpretation of a metaphase FISH result (http://www.acmg.net/Pages/ACMG_Activities/stds-2002/e.htm).

A. Repetitive sequence probes. The most widely used repetitive sequence probes bind to a-satellite sequences of centromeres; these probes produce strong signals because a-satellite sequences are present in hundreds of thousands of copies. Chromosome-specific centromere-specific probes have been developed for most human chromosomes based on differences in a-satellite sequences, and are particularly useful for demonstrating aneuploidy. These FISH probes can be used on both metaphase and interphase preparations, and simultaneous analysis of more than one locus is possible when a cocktail of differentially labeled probes is used in the same hybridization. Other repetitive sequence probes include probes that recognize β-satellite sequences (located on the short arms of acrocentric chromosomes) and probes that recognize the telomeric repeat sequence TTAGGG.

B. Unique sequence probes. Probes of this type are used to detect sequences that are present only once in the genome. They are usually derived from genomic clones, but can also be produced from complementary DNA or by polymerase chain reaction (PCR). Different cloning vectors are used to produce unique sequence probes of different length, including plasmids for probes 1 to 10 kb long, bacteriophage λ for probes up to 25 kb long, bacterial artificial chromosomes (BACs) for probes up to about 300 kb long, and yeast artificial chromosomes (YACs) for probes from 100 kb to 2 Mb long. The availability of mapped BAC libraries, originally developed as part of the Human Genome Project, has greatly simplified the production of probes for any locus under study (http://genome.ucsc.edu/cgi-bin/hgGateway and http://bacpac.chori.org/).

Unique sequence probes (also known as locus-specific identifier probes, or LSI probes) are used primarily to detect changes in the copy number of a specific locus, to confirm the presence of rearrangements involving a specific locus, or to detect so-called cryptic rearrangements that cannot be identified by examination of chromosomes stained by routine banding methods (e-**Fig. 57.3**). The advantages and disadvantages of metaphase FISH analysis using unique sequence probes directly parallel those of interphase FISH (as discussed in Chapter 58).

C. **Whole chromosome probes** (WCPs), also known as chromosome painting probes or chromosome libraries, consist of thousands of overlapping probes that recognize unique and moderately repetitive sequences along the entire length of individual chromosomes. They are isolated through flow sorting of specific chromosomes, microdissection of specific chromosomes accompanied by PCR amplification, or via production of somatic cell hybrids. WCPs are used to identify rearrangements that are not evident by routine banding methods, to confirm the interpretation of aberrations identified by routine banding methods, or to establish the chromosomal origin of rearrangements that are difficult to evaluate by other approaches. These probes are designed for use with metaphase chromosome preparations because hybridization to the decondensed chromatin in interphase nuclei gives a splotchy, undefined hybridization pattern. WCPs for each human chromosome are commercially available.

IV. MULTIPLEX METAPHASE FISH (also known as multicolor FISH) and spectral karyotyping (SKY) are related techniques in which metaphase chromosome spreads are hybridized with a combination of probes labeled with different fluorophores. Because N different fluorophores can produce $(2^N - 1)$ different color combinations, five different fluorophores yield sufficient different color combinations to uniquely label WCPs so that all 24 different human chromosomes can be identified in one hybridization.

For both multiplex FISH and SKY, a cocktail consisting of labeled probes for each of the 24 chromosomes is hybridized to metaphase chromosome spreads, and the fluorescent emissions are measured by computerized imaging systems. Specialized software is used to determine the combination of fluorophores present along the length of each chromosome, which makes it possible to assemble a karyotype.

A. Advantages. Multiplex FISH and SKY are used to detect aneuploidy, detect interchromosomal rearrangements, and identify marker chromosomes (extrachromosomal material of unknown origin). In many cases, multiplex-FISH or SKY makes it possible to establish the chromosomal origin of rearrangements that cannot be defined based on routine cytogenetic analysis. A Web-based database has been developed to facilitate identification of chromosomal aberrations detected by multiplex FISH (http://www.ncbi.nlm.nih.gov/sky/), a database that contains links to other Web sites that can be used to integrate the cytogenetic map with physical and sequence maps.

B. Disadvantages. The lower limit of the size of individual DNA chromosomal fragments that can be visualized by either technique is in the range of 1 to 2 Mb, although neither technique provides direct information on the involved chromosomal bands. Similarly, multiplex FISH and SKY will only reveal intrachromosomal deletions and duplications that are large enough to result in a change in size of the affected chromosome; neither technique is designed to detect interchromosomal rearrangements such as inversions, and neither is informative in regions of repetitive DNA.

C. Modifications of multiplex FISH and SKY. Mixtures of so-called partial chromosome paints, each of which hybridizes to only a band or subband of an individual chromosome, can be used to produce a pseudocolor-banded karyotype at a resolution of about 550 bands (*Cytogenet Cell Genet* 1999;84:156). The use of partial chromosome paints makes it possible to use multiplex FISH and SKY methodology to identify translocation breakpoint and to detect intrachromosomal rearrangements.

V. COMPARATIVE GENOMIC HYBRIDIZATION. Although comparative genomic hybridization (CGH) often has a higher sensitivity than conventional cytogenetic analysis, of even greater significance is the fact that CGH can be performed using DNA extracted from fixed as well as fresh tumor samples. The technique therefore makes it possible to perform a genome-wide scan for structural alterations even on those cases for which conventional cytogenetic analysis is not feasible or is unsuccessful. CGH essentially opens the entire formalin-fixed tissue archive to at least limited cytogenetic analysis.

For a typical CGH test, genomic DNA from a tumor sample is labeled with a green fluorophore, and genomic DNA from a paired normal tissue sample is labeled with a red fluorophore. The green and red probes are mixed and used in a single hybridization.

A. Metaphase CGH. This technique is basically a variation of metaphase FISH used to survey the entire genome for chromosomal deletions and amplifications (*Science* 1992;258:818, *Trends Genet* 1997;13:405). The labeled probe mixture is used in a hybridization to metaphase chromosomes prepared from normal cells, and the ratio of the green to red fluorescent signals is measured along the length of each chromosome. Areas where the ratio deviates significantly from the expected one-to-one relationship indicate a change in DNA copy number in the tumor; areas where the green to red ratio is significantly greater than one are areas of chromosomal gain (usually amplifications), and areas where the green to red ratio is significantly lower than one are areas of chromosomal loss (deletions). The smallest chromosomal alterations that can be reproducibly detected are about 3 Mb long.

B. Array CGH. This approach uses a microarray consisting of an ordered arrangement of DNA molecules (features) linked to a solid matrix support. The labeled probe mixture is hybridized to the microarray, and the ratio of the green to red fluorescent

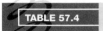

TABLE 57.4	Common Symbols and Abbreviations Used in Karyotype Designations
Abbreviation or symbol	**Description**
add	Additional material of unknown origin
square brackets [ ]	Number of cells in each clone
cen	Centromere
single colon (:)	Break
double colon (: :)	Break and reunion
comma (,)	Separates chromosome number, sex chromosomes, and abnormalities
del	Deletion
der	Derivative chromosome
dmin	Double minute(s)
dup	Duplication
i	Isochromosome
idem	Identical abnormalities as in prior clone
inv	Inversion
ins	Insertion
mar	Marker chromosome
minus sign (−)	Loss
multiplication sign (×)	Multiple copies, also designates copy number with ish
plus sign (+)	Gain
question mark (?)	Uncertainty of chromosome identification or abnormality
r	Ring chromosome
rcp	Reciprocal
slash (/)	Separates cell lines or clones
semicolon (;)	Separates chromosomes and breakpoints in rearrangements involving more than one chromosome
t	Translocation

signals is measured for each feature. Because each DNA feature has been mapped to a specific region of the genome, the ratio of the green to red fluorescent signals for each feature provides information on the gain or loss of the corresponding chromosomal region. The resolution of array CGH is in theory limited only by the number of features in the array; commercially available arrays currently provide a resolution of <10 Kb.

VI. **HUMAN CHROMOSOME NOMENCLATURE.** Technical advancements, together with an ever more complete understanding of human chromosomal structure, necessitate periodic revision of nomenclature guidelines. The document in current use is the *International System for Human Cytogenetic Nomenclature* from 2005, abbreviated ISCN 2005, which includes ideograms for all of the chromosomes that serve as useful reference points because of their universal acceptance and availability.

A. **Chromosome region and band designations.** The centromere divides each chromosome into a short (or p) arm and a long (or q) arm. Each chromosome arm ends in a terminus, designated pter and qter for the short and long arms, respectively. A list of the more frequent symbols and abbreviations used to describe human karyotypes is shown in Table 57.4.

Chromosome arms are divided into regions based on landmarks, defined as consistent and distinct morphologic areas that aid in the identification of that chromosome. The regions adjacent to the centromere of the short arm and long arm are designated as p1 and q1, respectively, the next distal as p2 and q2, and so on. Chromosome regions are divided into bands, and the bands are divided into subbands, both of which are numbered sequentially. The terminal band on the long arm of chromosome 11 is therefore written as 11q25, indicating chromosome 11, long arm, region 2, band 5, and is referred to as "eleven q two-five."

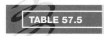

TABLE 57.5   **Examples of Human Chromosome Nomenclature**

Designation	Description
Description of karyotypes	
Constitutional sex chromosome aneuploidies	
45,X	Turner Syndrome
47,XXY	Klinefelter Syndrome
Autosomal chromosome aneuploidies	
47,XY,+21	Male with trisomy 21 (Down syndrome)
48,XY,+21c,+21	Male with trisomy 21, with gain of an additional chromosome 21 in his tumor cells
Abnormalities in neoplasms	
47,XX,+10,t(11;22)(q24;q12)	Female whose tumor cells have two cytogenetic abnormalities: an additional chromosome 10, and a reciprocal translocation between the long arm (q) of chromosome 11 at region 2, band 4, and the long arm (q) of chromosome 22 at region 1, band 2
Description of metaphase FISH results	
47,XY,+mar.ish der(3)(wcp3+)	In this tumor, traditional cytogenetic analysis shows a marker chromosome; metaphase FISH using a whole chromosome paint for chromosome 3 shows that the marker is derived from chromosome 3

Abbreviation: FISH, fluorescence in situ hybridization.

B. Description of karyotypes. ISCN nomenclature provides rules for karyotype designations. The first item of the designation is the total number of chromosomes (including the sex chromosomes) followed by the sex chromosomes. Chromosomal abnormalities follow the sex chromosome designations using established symbols and abbreviations. For each chromosome described, numerical changes are listed before structural aberrations. Table 57.5 provides examples of the karyotypic designation of numerical and structural abnormalities detected by traditional cytogenetic analysis. The rules for designating the karyotype of constitutional abnormalities are also used for designating the abnormalities associated with neoplasms, although the biology of tumors requires additional definitions and guidelines.

C. Description of FISH results. ISCN 2005 also includes rules for designating cytogenetic findings derived from various in situ hybridization techniques (a summary of the more common symbols and abbreviations is shown in Table 57.5). For metaphase chromosome in situ hybridization, the results of conventional cytogenetic analysis (if performed) are listed first, followed by the results of in situ hybridization analysis. Ideally, loci are designated according to Genome Data Base (GDB) nomenclature (http://gdbwww.gdb.org/); when GDB designations are unavailable, probe names are used.

Suggested Readings

Gersen SL, Keagle MB, eds. *The Principles of Clinical Cytogenetics*, 2nd ed. Totowa, NJ: Humana Press; 2005.

Rooney DE, ed. *Human Cytogenetics: Constitutional Analysis: A Practical Approach*, 3rd ed. Oxford: Oxford University Press; 2001.

Shaffer LG, Tommerup N, eds. *ISCN 2005: An International System for Human Cytogenetic Nomenclature*. Basel, Switzerland: Karger AG; 2005.

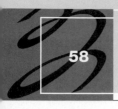

FLUORESCENCE IN SITU HYBRIDIZATION

58

Anjum Hassan and Arie Perry

I. INTRODUCTION. Florescence in situ hybridization (FISH) uses tagged probes that bind to chromosome-specific DNA sequences of interest, thereby allowing for the identification of both structural and numeric aberrations that specify certain hematopoietic and nonhematopoietic malignancies. Although FISH can be performed on dividing (metaphase) cells, it has several major advantages over conventional cytogenetics in that it can be applied in many clinical settings (Table 58.1), can be performed on nondividing (interphase) cells, can be performed on air-dried or formalin-fixed specimens, can facilitate detection of molecular abnormalities in neoplasms with low proliferation rates such as multiple myeloma, and can facilitate detection of numeric abnormalities. In surgical pathology, the technique is used primarily to detect somatic cancer-associated alterations with known diagnostic, prognostic, or therapeutic implications.

FISH provides insight into intranuclear target DNA localization and copy number. Therefore, using locus-specific probes (with the exception of XY sex chromosome determinations in males), two signals per nucleus are expected, so four common alterations are readily detectable: aneusomy (gain or loss of a chromosome), gene deletion, gene amplification, and translocation (e-Figs. 58.1 through 58.4).* Sex chromosome determinations can be useful in patients with sex-mismatched bone marrow or organ transplants (e-Fig. 58.5) to monitor engraftment success or failure.

II. ADVANTAGES AND LIMITATIONS OF FISH

A. Specimens, retained morphology, and combined FISH/immunohisto-chemistry. FISH is applicable to a variety of specimen types, including fresh or frozen tissue, cytologic preparations, and formalin-fixed paraffin-embedded (FFPE) tissue (Table 58.2). The latter provides a particularly rich source of archival material.

In clinical diagnostic testing, morphologic preservation is one of the principal advantages of FISH, particularly for studies on heterogeneous tissue samples, in that it eliminates the need for microdissection (e-Fig. 58.6). An extension of this morphologic advantage comes from the possibility of combining FISH with immunohistochemistry, wherein separate assessments can be rendered in immunopositive and negative cellular populations.

B. FISH versus other cytogenetic and molecular techniques. When compared with metaphase cytogenetics (see Chapter 57), interphase FISH has several clear advantages. One advantage is the lack of a requirement for mitotically active cells through cell cultures, which removes potential artifacts due to in vitro growth selection biases such as overgrowth of nonneoplastic stromal elements. In contrast, FISH is not a genomic screening tool; it provides a targeted approach for alterations that have been initially identified by more global molecular techniques, such as classic cytogenetics, loss of heterozygosity screening, comparative genomic hybridization (CGH), array CGH (aCGH), array single nucleotide polymorphism analysis, and gene expression profiling.

In terms of resolution, FISH is more sensitive than conventional karyotypic analysis and CGH (limited to alterations of several Mb in size) but less sensitive than polymerase chain reaction (PCR)-based assays for detecting small alterations (which can be designed to detect even single base pair mutations). Because FISH probes are typically at least 20 kb long, and most average 100 to 200 kb long, alterations need

---

*All e-figures are available online via the Solution Site Image Bank.

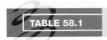

TABLE 58.1	Examples of Diagnostic Tests by Fluorescence in Situ Hybridization (FISH)

Prenatal testing
  Trisomy 13, 18, 21
  XY aneusomies
Microdeletion syndromes
  Cri-du-chat (5p)
  Prader-Willi/Angelman (15q)
  Di George syndrome (22q)
Transplant pathology
  XY FISH on sex-mismatched organ transplant
  Disease relapse using known genetic alterations in primary tumor
Oncology (diagnostic, prognostic, and/or predictive markers)
  Chromosomal aneusomies
  Gene/Locus deletions
  Gene amplifications
  Translocations

to be fairly large for reliable detection by FISH; consequently, FISH cannot detect small intragenic mutations, deletions, or insertions.

Minimal residual disease or early recurrences are better detected by PCR of blood or fresh tissue specimens rather than FISH. This usually involves detection of abnormal fusion transcripts resulting from chromosomal translocations, picking up as few as one abnormal per million normal cells, a level of sensitivity that cannot be attained by FISH techniques to date. In contrast, FISH is more sensitive than PCR at identifying gene deletions or amplifications from samples of mixed cellularity, such as neoplasms with clonal heterogeneity or contaminating nonneoplastic elements (*J Neuropathol Exp Neurol* 1997;56:999); in this setting, FISH can typically detect gains, translocations, or amplifications in as few as 5% and deletions in 15% to 30% of the cells within a sample.

C. Tissue microarray-FISH. This technology takes advantage of multispecimen paraffin blocks (tissue microarrays, or TMAs) constructed from hundreds of 0.6- to 2.0-mm neoplastic, nonneoplastic, and control tissue cores of interest. TMA-FISH markedly increases efficiency by reducing data acquisition time, as well as probe, reagent, and storage space requirements. TMA studies have shown excellent morphologic, antigenic, and genomic concordance compared to the traditional whole slide approaches (*Adv Anat Pathol* 2001;8:14), and although complications due to tumor heterogeneity can be problematic, adequate sampling can be optimized by

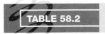

TABLE 58.2	Examples of Specimen Types Applicable to Fluorescence in Situ Hybridization (FISH)

Fresh/frozen tissue
Cytology specimens
  Body fluids (e.g., urine)
  Intraoperative smears
  Cell culture preparations
Formalin-fixed paraffin-embedded (FFPE) tissue
  Thin sections (4 to 6 microns)
  Disaggregated nuclei
  Archived unstained sections
  Previously stained sections (e.g., negative immunohistochemistry controls)

incorporating multiple cores from each specimen. TMA-FISH is an excellent method for new probe validation, proficiency testing, interlaboratory comparisons, and quality assurance/quality control (*J Histochem Cytochem* 2004;52:501).

D. Disadvantages and pitfalls of FISH. Although recent technical advances have greatly enhanced the clinical applicability of FISH, a number of limitations remain. Signal fading is one of the main disadvantages. Clinical labs typically circumvent this pitfall by capturing digital images as a permanent record of each case; a permanent record is not otherwise possible unless chromogenic in situ hybridization (CISH) is used. Unfortunately, multicolor CISH is not as simple as multicolor FISH; currently available chromogens lack the spectral versatility, sensitivity, and spatial resolution attainable with fluorochromes. Some commercial CISH applications bypass this problem by providing the test and reference probes separately, so that in place of one dual-color FISH assay, two single-color CISH experiments are performed. Recently developed photostable quantum dots offer a potential alternative for permanent fluorescent signals (*J Histochem Cytochem* 2003;51:981). Other limitations include a variety of artifacts, particularly common in paraffin sections, that make correct interpretation of FISH results dependent on significant experience.

1. **Truncation artifact.** This artifact is due to the underestimation of copy number because of an incomplete DNA complement within transected nuclei. It is therefore important to assess controls cut at the same thickness.

2. **Artifacts due to aneuploidy and polyploidy** can result in confusing signal counts, and are a particularly common finding in malignant and even some benign neoplasms. Although the simplest approach is to interpret absolute losses (<2 copies) and gains (>2 copies), "relative" losses and gains can also be delineated based on a reference ploidy, obtained either by flow cytometry or the assessment of multiple chromosomes by FISH. For example, cells with 4 chromosome 9 centromeres and 2 copies of the *p16* gene region on 9p21 would be interpreted as having polysomy 9 and a hemizygous p16 deletion (**e-Fig. 58.7A**); a similar tumor with no p16 signals would be interpreted as polysomy 9 with homozygous p16 deletion (**e-Fig. 58.7B**).

3. **Autofluorescence.** This is a particularly common problem in FFPE tissue sections. Although autofluorescent tissue fragments are usually larger and more irregular than true signals, some fragments have just the right size to mimic true nuclear signals. The use of multiple filters is helpful, because autofluorescence will often appear at several wavelengths of light, whereas true signals only fluoresce at one wavelength.

4. **Partial hybridization failure.** This issue is most problematic when combining a highly robust probe (e.g., centromere) with a comparatively weak probe (e.g., small locus-specific probe). This artifact can be minimized by counting only in regions where the majority of cells have discernable signals. Signals from both probes should be seen in normal cells (e.g., endothelial cells) within the region for the counts to be considered reliable.

E. Additional technical considerations. Many different FISH protocols are available; they vary depending on individual preferences and specimen type. Simple protocols are generally better, requiring less "hands on" time, fewer opportunities for error, and fewer troubleshooting requirements. Automated instruments are now available to minimize hands on time, although they are expensive. In general, the basic steps of the protocols are similar to those of immunohistochemistry and include deparaffinization, pretreatment/target retrieval, probe and target DNA denaturation, hybridization (a few hours to overnight), posthybridization washes, detection, and microscopic interpretation/imaging. FISH is therefore typically a 2-day assay, although same-day assays are possible if the probes are particularly robust (e.g., centromere probes).

Similar to immunohistochemistry, microwave- or heat-induced target retrieval often enhances hybridization more effectively than do chemical forms of pretreatment (*Anal Cell Pathol* 1994;6:319). Nonetheless, optimal pretreatment and digestion vary from specimen to specimen and depend on a number of variables, including method of fixation and processing. Some hybridization buffers are also significantly more efficient and may lower probe concentration requirements considerably, which can be particularly beneficial with expensive commercial probes. Lastly, a variety of amplification steps are available for enhancing weak signals, although such steps are rarely necessary with good probes. One exciting advancement made possible by high-level signal amplification techniques is the potential use of smaller probes, down to the level of 1 kb or less (*Biotechniques* 27:608, 1999).

III. **FISH PROBES AND PROBE DEVELOPMENT.** Several basic probe types are used for FISH. Centromere-enumerating probes (CEPs) were among the first to be developed and remain ideal for detecting whole chromosome gains and losses, such as monosomy, trisomy, and other polysomies. CEPs target highly repetitive 171-bp sequences of α-satellite DNA, so are associated with excellent hybridization efficiencies and typically produce large, bright signals. Unfortunately, sequence similarities in some pericentromeric regions result in cross-hybridization artifacts with the potential for overestimating signal counts. Another artifact is caused by the interesting phenomenon observed in nonneoplastic brain specimens in which certain chromosomes in interphase nuclei are packaged such that paired centromeres are in close proximity, a process known as somatic pairing (*Hum Genet* 1989;83:231, *Cytogenet Cell Genet* 1991;56:214); because of the close proximity, FISH yields an unexpected fraction of cells harboring a single large signal rather than two smaller ones, potentially leading to overinterpretation of monosomy. Despite these technical limitations, CEPs remain extremely useful for detecting aneusomies and are still among the best FISH probes available. The presence of repetitive DNA sequences in subtelomeric regions has led to the development of commercially available probes for each chromosomal arm as well.

A whole chromosome paint (WCP) probe consists of a cocktail of DNA fragments that targets all the nonrepetitive DNA sequences of an entire chromosome. Because a WCP covers such a large region, it produces a diffuse signal in interphase nuclei (although some of the smaller acrocentric chromosomes yield sufficiently discrete signals for enumeration, even in interphase nuclei). For this reason, WCPs are not often used in interphase FISH, but instead are primarily used in advanced cytogenetic applications (see Chapter 57).

Currently, the most versatile FISH probes are locus-specific identifier probes (also known as LSI, or gene-specific, probes). These probes target distinct chromosomal regions of interest and use single copy rather than repetitive DNA sequences. To yield signals of sufficient size in interphase FFPE nuclei, the probe typically needs to be at least 20 kb long; the largest LSI probes are >1 Mb long, although most fall into the 100- to 300-kb range. The assortment of LSI probes available commercially has expanded greatly over the last few years. Additionally, cloning vectors, such as cosmids, bacterial artificial chromosomes (BACs), P1 artificial chromosomes (PACs), and yeast artificial chromosomes (YACs), are excellent sources for developing homemade FISH probes. In the past, development of LSIs required a rather lengthy and tedious process of screening vector libraries, but the BAC libraries generated as part of the Human Genome Project have made it possible to rapidly identify vectors that contain sequences of interest, gene names, or physical maps of individual chromosomes (http://www.genome.ucsc.edu). Similarly, mapped BAC clones spread throughout the human genome at 1-Mb intervals have also become available (http://mp.invitrogen.com). However, regardless of how a probe is obtained, it is important to verify its identity, either by screening for the DNA sequence of interest by PCR or by performing metaphase FISH to determine that the probe localizes to the appropriate cytogenetic band (e-Fig. 58.8).

IV. **CLINICAL APPLICATIONS.** FISH testing is clinically useful when a cytogenetic alteration (deletion, gain, amplification, translocation) is sensitive and specific for a single tumor type, either as a diagnostic biomarker (as in many hematopoietic malignancies) or as a prognostic biomarker helping to predict which tumors will be aggressive or indolent (Her-2/*neu* amplification testing in breast cancer). Some translocation and deletions detected by FISH are also helpful in predicting response to a specific therapy; examples include detection of t(11;18) in a subset of mucosa-associated lymphoid tissue (MALT) lymphomas (which tend to be resistant to conventional therapy) or detection of del(13q) and/or t(4;14) in a subset of cases of multiple myeloma (which tend to have a worse prognosis). The most common clinical applications of FISH testing currently include

HER-2 neu amplification testing for breast cancer, UroVysion testing in urine cytology specimens, 1p/19q deletion testing in gliomas, and testing for signature translocations associated with specific hematologic, soft tissue, and/or pediatric malignancies. Clinically relevant examples for each alteration type detectable by FISH are summarized in Table 58.3.

A. Aneusomies and deletions. Aneusomies represent gains and losses of whole chromosomes. Deletions are losses of distinct chromosomal regions, varying in size from loss of a specific gene or portion of a gene to an entire chromosomal arm. Aneusomies and deletions are among the most common alterations detected in neoplasms by FISH (Table 58.3), although it is sometimes difficult to distinguish specific tumor-associated polysomies and monosomies from nonspecific gains and losses that are secondary changes due to the genomic instability that is characteristic of many malignancies. The use of reference probes helps to distinguish such chromosomal gains or high-level polysomies from true gene amplification (e-**Fig. 58.3**).

One of the most common FISH applications is testing for deletions of 1p and 19q in diffuse gliomas. The presence of 1p and 19q codeletion (typically one entire arm from each) has diagnostic, prognostic, and predictive value in that this genetic signature (e-**Fig. 58.2, A** and **B**) is associated predominantly with pure oligodendrogliomas with enhanced therapeutic responsiveness and overall survival time (*J Neuropathol Exp Neurol* 2003;62:111). There is no current consensus for the optimal way to enumerate signals for chromosomal losses and gains, although in clinical cases a common approach is to use two individuals who count signals in 100 cells each; when the counts are concordant, they are simply added for a total enumeration of 200 cells, but when there is a discrepancy or the counts are borderline for an alteration, then either the same individuals count additional cells or a third enumerator is used. Despite the clinical utility of 1p and 19q testing, the precise gene targets on these chromosomes remain unclear.

In other tumor types, a specific tumor suppressor is known to be targeted by various chromosomal deletions (Table 58.3). Notable examples include the *INI1/hSNF5* gene on 22q11.2 in malignant rhabdoid tumors and atypical teratoid/rhabdoid tumors, the *NF2* gene at 22q12 in meningiomas, the *RB1* gene at 13q14, the *TP53* gene at 17p13.1 in multiple myeloma, and the *NF1* gene at 17q11.2 in malignant peripheral nerve sheath tumors.

In terms of tumor-specific chromosomal gains and losses, Vysis (http://www.vysis.com) has recently marketed a number of multicolor probe cocktails for clinical and translational studies, each with different recommendations for minimum number of nuclei counted and cutoffs for alterations. For example, the UroVysion (e-**Fig. 58.9**) and LAVysion probe sets have been shown to increase diagnostic sensitivities in body fluid cytology specimens for urothelial carcinoma (*J Urol* 2003;169:2101) and lung carcinoma (*Am J Clin Pathol* 2005;123:516), respectively. Similarly, the chronic lymphocytic leukemia (CLL) and ProVysion FISH assays have been shown to identify prognostically relevant subsets of CLL (*Cancer Gen Cytogenet* 2005;158:88) and prostatic adenocarcinoma (*Genes Chrom Cancer* 2002;34:363) patients, respectively. Likewise, the detection of specific aneusomies and deletions by FISH has been clinically useful in identifying diagnostically challenging cases of glioblastoma (particularly the small cell variant), medulloblastoma (especially the anaplastic/large cell variant), and prognostically relevant subsets of leukemia/myelodysplastic syndrome.

B. Gene amplifications. High-level gene amplifications typically occur in one of two patterns. If the amplified gene is present on small extrachromosomal segments known as double minutes, FISH will show numerous individual signals (e-**Fig. 58.3, A** and **C**). If the gene amplification consists of contiguously arranged gene copies within a single chromosomal region manifested as a homogenously stained region on chromosomal banding, FISH will show regions of hybridization so close together that they coalesce into abnormally large linear or globular signals (e-**Fig. 58.3B**); rough estimates are made regarding how many signals are contained within the coalescent signals based on their overall size. In both settings, CEP probes are often used as references for chromosome number to distinguish polysomies (i.e., gains of the entire chromosome; e-**Fig. 58.3D**) from true gene amplification.

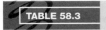

	Cancer-Associated Alterations Commonly Detected by
TABLE 58.3	**Fluorescence in Situ Hybridization (FISH)**

Type	Tumor type (references)	Alterations/Probes	Association
Aneusomies/ Deletions	Oligodendroglioma	1p– with 19q–	Diagnostic, prognostic, predictive
	Urothelial carcinoma	+3, 7, or 17; 9p–	Diagnostic
	Lung carcinoma	+7p, 8q, 5p, or 6	Diagnostic
	CLL	13q–, 11q–, 17q–	Diagnostic, prognostic
	GBM	+7, –10	Diagnostic
	Prostatic carcinoma	8p–, 8q+	Prognostic
	Medulloblastoma	17p–, 17q+; (i17q)	Diagnostic
	Leukemias/MDS	+8, +12; –5, –7	Diagnostic, prognostic
	MRT, AT/RT	*INI1/hSNF5* (22q–)	Diagnostic
	Meningioma	*NF2* (22q–)	Diagnostic
	Multiple myeloma	*RB1* (13q–), *TP53* (17p–)	Prognostic
	MPNST	*NF1* (17q–)	Diagnostic
Amplifications	Breast carcinoma	*HER-2/neu*	Prognostic, predictive
	Neuroblastoma	*N-myc*	Diagnostic, prognostic
	GBM	*EGFR*	Diagnostic
	Medulloblastoma	*MYCN, c-myc*	Diagnostic, prognostic
Translocations	EWS/PNET	*EWS-FLI1*, EWS-BA	Diagnostic
	Synovial sarcoma	*SYT-SSX*, SYT-BA	Diagnostic
	Alveolar RMS	*PAX3-FKHR*, FKHR-BA	Diagnostic
	DSRCT	*EWS-WT1*, EWS-BA	Diagnostic
	M/RC liposarcoma	CHOP-BA	Diagnostic
	Clear cell sarcoma	*EWS-ATF1*, EWS-BA	Diagnostic
	IMT	*ALK-TPM3, ALK-TPM4, ALK-CARS*, ALK BA	Diagnostic, prognostic
	Burkitt lymphoma	*MYC-IGH*, MYC-BA	Diagnostic
	MALT lymphoma	*API2-MALT1, IGH-MALT1,* MALT1-BA	Diagnostic
	Follicular lymphoma	*IGH-BCL2*	Diagnostic
	ALCL	ALK-BA	Diagnostic
	Mantle cell lymphoma	*IGH-CCND1*	Diagnostic
	Multiple myeloma	*IGH-CCND1, IGH-FGFR3,* IGH-BA	Prognostic
	CML	*BCR-ABL*	Diagnostic, MRD
	AML	*AML1-ETO*, CBFB-BA, *PML-RARA*, RARA-BA, MLL-BA, *BCR-ABL*	Diagnostic, prognostic, predictive
	ALL	*TEL-AML1, BCR-ABL,* MLL-BA	Diagnostic, prognostic, predictive

CLL, chronic lymphocytic leukemia; GBM, glioblastoma; MDS, myelodysplastic syndrome; MRT, malignant rhabdoid tumor; AT/RT, atypical teratoid/rhabdoid tumor; MPNST, malignant peripheral nerve sheath tumor; EWS, Ewing sarcoma; PNET, primitive neuroectodermal tumor; RMS, rhabdomyosarcoma; DSRCT, desmoplastic small round cell tumor; M/RC, myxoid/round cell; IMT, inflammatory myofibroblastic tumor; MALT, mucosa-associated lymphoid tissue; ALCL, anaplastic large cell lymphoma; CML, chronic myelogenous leukemia; AML, acute myelogenous leukemia; ALL, acute lymphoblastic leukemia; BA, break-apart probe set; MRD, minimal residual disease assessment.

Of the current clinical applications of FISH in surgical pathology, the assessment of *HER-2/neu* amplification status in breast cancer is one of the most common, but controversial (*Cancer* 2003;98:2547). There is agreement that *HER-2/neu* assessment provides clinically useful information, however, the optimal diagnostic approach is still debated. *HER-2/neu* gene amplification is present in 20% to 35% of breast carcinomas (e-Fig. 58.3C) and provides both prognostic and predictive information with the following associations for positive tumors: reduced patient survival, especially in lymph node–positive cases; increased responsiveness to adriamycin-based therapeutic regimens; increased responsiveness to Herceptin (trastuzumab), which specifically targets the overexpressed surface protein; and decreased responsiveness to radiation therapy, cyclophosphamide, methotrexate, 5-fluorouracil, hormonal therapy, and Taxol (paclitaxel). Additionally, due to the significant risk of cardiotoxicity with combined Adriamycin (doxorubicin) and Herceptin therapy, testing is justified to identify patients with a low probability of response.

In pediatric pathology, testing of neuroblastomas for *MYCN* amplification has similarly become standard of care, with positive cases typically showing an aggressive biology (*J Pathol* 2002;198:83). A similar pattern is encountered in a subset of the central nervous system counterpart, medulloblastoma; *MYCN* and *c-myc* amplifications are particularly common in the highly aggressive anaplastic/large cell variant.

EGFR amplification, often in combination with monosomy 10 or chromosome 10q deletion, helps to distinguish the clinically aggressive and therapeutically refractory small cell variant of glioblastoma from the more biologically favorable and chemotherapeutically responsive lookalike, anaplastic oligodendroglioma.

C. Translocations. The list of known tumor-associated chromosomal translocations is already impressive and continues to grow. Translocation analysis by FISH is particularly useful as an ancillary diagnostic aid in primitive-appearing hematopoietic and soft tissue malignancies (Table 58.3). Chromosomal translocations are unique among the FISH assays in that interpretation relies on the spatial relationships of the signals rather than on their number. For optimal probe design, detailed knowledge of the breakpoints is needed, although reliable probes are commercially available for most of the common translocations.

1. Fusion FISH. Also known as FISH-F, this strategy uses two locus-specific probes with different fluors (color tags), targeting two different partners in a translocation (e.g., *BCR* on 22q and *ABL* on 9q). Separated or "split" signals (e.g., two green, two red signals; e-Fig. 58.4A) are therefore present in translocation-negative cells, but "fusion" yellow or red-green signals are present in translocation-positive cells due to the juxtaposition of the target loci by the translocation (e.g., one fusion, one green, one red signal; e-Fig. 58.4B). FISH-F results must be scored carefully to avoid overinterpreting small cellular populations in which green and red signals overlap purely by chance. Based on signal proximities in normal controls, typical conservative cutoffs require the presence of fused signals in >30% cells for FISH-F (*Mod Pathol* 2006;19:1).

2. Break-apart FISH. Also known as FISH-BA, this strategy uses two probes localizing just proximal and distal to one of the two breakpoints of interest. The two probes are therefore in close proximity in normal cells, resulting in fusion signals (e.g., two fusion signals; e-Fig. 58.4C). Cells harboring the translocation will contain at least one pair of split signals (e.g., one fusion, one green, one red signal; e-Fig. 58.4D). The advantages of FISH-BA are that split signals do not occur purely by chance, the test yields a positive result even when the translocation can involve multiple partner genes (e.g., C-MYC at chromosome 8, band 24 can fuse with multiple partner genes in Burkitt lymphomas including immunoglobulin H at 14q32, or less commonly, light chain loci on 2q11 or 22q11), and commercial break-apart probes yield large, easily interpretable signals. Disadvantages of FISH-BA include that it provides no information regarding the identity of the fusion partner. Based on signal proximities in normal controls, typical conservative cutoffs for positive test results require the presence of split signals in >15% of cells for FISH-BA (*Mod Pathol* 2006;19:1).

3. Other approaches. A strategy that has been used to increase the sensitivity of FISH-F is to include one particularly large FISH probe that spans a breakpoint region. In the presence of a translocation, the large DNA probe is split, leading to an extra signal (hence the name FISH-ES) smaller than the remaining nonsplit, nonfused signals (e.g., one fusion, one normal green, one normal red, and one ES red signal). Because it is unlikely that individual cells will contain both a fusion signal and an extra signal, smaller populations of tumor cells can be confidently identified in heterogeneous specimens (e.g., minimal residual disease in chronic myelogenous leukemia).

An even more reliable method to increase the sensitivity of FISH-F is to use two large probes that span both breakpoint regions. By this approach, a tumor harboring the target translocation will harbor two fusion or "double fusion" signals marking the two derivative chromosomes (hence the name D-FISH). However, if a positive tumor additionally has superimposed changes (such as, e.g., polyploidy, the deletion of one of the derivative chromosomes, an unbalanced translocation), the FISH pattern becomes considerably more complex and difficult to interpret with certainty.

V. DEVELOPMENT OF A FISH TEST FOR CLINICAL USE. The clinical utility of FISH, together with the ease of assay development, makes the methodology an ideal basis for development of new molecular genetic tests. The basic format for developing a new FISH test is outlined in Table 58.4.

The first critical step is the identification of distinct molecular cytogenetic alterations known to be associated with a particular tumor type or genetic syndrome; these data typically come from genomic screening studies. Next, DNA probe availability must be addressed; acquisition is simple if a probe is commercially available, but if not, homemade probes can be developed as described above. For deletions, regional chromosomal gains, or gene amplifications, the CEP from the same chromosome is often used as the reference probe; alternatively, a marker on the opposite chromosomal arm as the locus under study can serve as a copy number reference. Depending on the frequencies of

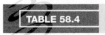 **Development of New Fluorescence In Situ Hybridization (FISH) Tests**

TABLE 58.4

Identify a cytogenetic biomarker
Chromosomal gain/loss
Gene/locus deletion
Gene amplification
Translocation
Obtain test and reference DNA probes
Commercial
Homemade (e.g., bacterial artificial chromosomes [BAC] clones)
Assess potential clinical relevance
Diagnostic aid
Prognostic aid
Predicts response or lack of response to patient therapy
Determine appropriate specimen cohort to test and clinical endpoints needed
Archival paraffin-embedded tissue vs. fresh/frozen vs. cytology
Retrospective vs. prospective
Morphologically overlapping tumor entities to assess specificity
Times to disease progression, metastasis, and/or patient death
Patient age or other demographically relevant prognosticators
Extent of resection/surgical margin status
Types of adjuvant therapy administered
Biostatistics needed to answer study questions?
Statistical power analysis: Number of specimens needed for statistical significance

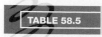

TABLE 58.5	Examples of Symbols and Abbreviations Used in Interphase Fluorescence in Situ Hybridization (FISH) Nomenclature

Abbreviation or symbol	Description
Plus sign (+)	Present on a specific chromosome
Minus sign (−)	Absent on a specific chromosome
++	Duplication on a specific chromosome
Period (.)	Separates cytogenetic results from ish results
con	Connected or adjacent signals
ish	When used by itself, refers to hybridization to chromosomes
nuc ish	Nuclear or interphase in situ hybridization
pcp	Partial chromosome paint
sep	Separated signals (which are usually adjacent in normal cells)
wcp	Whole chromosome paint

various translocations, breakpoint inconsistencies, and variant translocations, FISH-F, FISH-BA, FISH-ES, D-FISH, or a combination strategy can be designed.

Once the appropriate DNA probes are obtained, diagnostic accuracy is evaluated using tumor types with overlapping morphologic features. If prognostic value is the issue, there must be sufficient clinical follow-up to accurately determine statistical

TABLE 58.6	Examples of Nomenclature Used for Neoplasms Evaluated by Interphase Fluorescence in Situ Hybridization (FISH)*

Designation	Description
nuc ish 11p13(WT1×2), 22q12(EWS×2), (WT1 con EWS×1)	Interphase FISH of a tumor cell using single-fusion probes. A probe for WT1 at 11p13 shows two signals, as does a probe for EWS at 22q12. However, one WT1 and one EWS signal are juxtaposed (or connected), suggesting that they lie on the same chromosome, consistent with a t(11;22)(p13;q12) translocation.
nuc ish 22q12(EWSR1×2) (5′EWSR1sep 3′EWSR1×1)	Interphase FISH of a tumor cell using a break-apart probe set for the EWS locus at 22q12. Two sets of EWS signals are present, but on one copy of chromosome 22, the probes are separated (most likely as a result of a rearrangement of the EWS locus).
nuc ish 22q12(5′EWS,3′EWS con 5′EWS,3′EWS)× 2[169/200]	Interphase FISH using the same break-apart probe set as in the above example. However, in this tumor, the two probes remain juxtaposed on both copies of chromosome 22 (which provides no evidence of a rearrangement of the EWS locus). The indicated results are present in 169 of 200 nuclei evaluated.
nuc ish 8q24(MYC×2) (5′MYC sep 3′MYC×1) [119/200]	Interphase FISH using a breakapart probe set. In this tumor, a split of red and green signals was detected. This is consistent with a c-myc-containing chromosomal rearrangement in 119 of 200 nuclei evaluated.
nuc ish 8q24(5′MYC,3′MYC con 5′MYC,3′MYC)× 2[174/200]	Interphase FISH was performed using a commercial c-myc (8q24) break-apart probe set. In this particular case, a split of red and green signals was not detected in 174 of 200 nuclei evaluated.

* The assistance of Diane Robirds, CLSp(CG) in the preparation of this table is gratefully acknowledged.

associations to patient outcomes, such as time to tumor recurrence, presence or absence of metastases, and patient death. If responsiveness to a specific form of therapy is being tested, patients must be treated uniformly, and data on times to recurrence, parameters of response versus progression, and/or survival times must be collected; confounding variables that often affect prognosis should also be considered (e.g., patient age, demographics, extent of surgery, and forms of adjuvant therapy). Depending on the clinical setting, biostatistical support may be required to determine the sample numbers required to provide sufficient statistical power.

VI. FISH NOMENCLATURE. Technical advancements, together with an ever more complete understanding of human chromosomal structure, necessitate periodic revision of nomenclature guidelines. The document in current use is the *International System for Human Cytogenetic Nomenclature* from 2005, abbreviated ISCN 2005, which includes rules for designating cytogenetic findings derived from various in situ hybridization techniques, including interphase FISH. A summary of the more common symbols and abbreviations is shown in Table 58.5.

If interphase in situ hybridization is performed, results are presented in the following order: The abbreviation nuc ish is listed first, followed by the chromosome band to which the probe maps, followed by the locus designation, a multiplication sign, and the number of signals present (Table 58.6). If both conventional cytogenetic analysis and metaphase in situ hybridization are performed, the results of the conventional cytogenetic analysis is listed first, followed by a period, followed by the abbreviation ish, followed by the in situ hybridization results presented in the same order as described above. If conventional cytogenetic analysis is performed in conjunction with interphase in situ hybridization, the results are described on separate lines of nomenclature. Ideally, loci are designated according to Genome Data Base (GDB) nomenclature (http://gdbwww.gdb.org); when GDB designations are unavailable, probe names are used. If two or more probes for the same or different loci are used, they are separated by commas.

By these guidelines, simultaneous analysis by FISH-F using probes on different chromosomes expected to produce separate signals in normal cells, but juxtaposed signals in cells harboring the target rearrangement, uses the abbreviation con (for connected) to indicate juxtaposed signals; this finding suggests that the target loci are present on the same chromosome (Table 58.6). Similarly, analysis by FISH-BA using probes that are juxtaposed in normal cells, but that become separated in cells that harbor the target chromosomal rearrangement, uses the abbreviation sep to indicate separated signals; this finding suggests that a rearrangement of the target region is present.

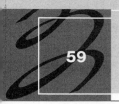

59 PCR-BASED METHODS FOR MOLECULAR GENETIC TESTING
Barbara A. Zehnbauer and John D. Pfeifer

I. INTRODUCTION. Clinical molecular diagnostic methods have been integrated into many laboratory disciplines, and guidelines and recommendations from both professional societies and regulatory agencies have been developed to assist in the development and performance of clinical molecular pathology testing (Table 59.1). Most molecular tests performed in surgical pathology focus on somatic or acquired DNA variations in the cells of the disease process that provide information that aids in diagnosis, identifies prognostic indicators, stratifies patients into effective treatment options, helps monitor treatment response, and identifies patients at increased risk of disease. Because polymerase chain reaction (PCR)-based approaches are quick, reliable, and sensitive, PCR has become a central technology for much of clinical molecular genetic testing.

II. SPECIMEN REQUIREMENTS, HANDLING, AND PROCESSING. Clinical PCR-based molecular testing in the setting of surgical pathology requires the same attention to detail regarding efficient specimen collection, identification, preparation, and routing as any other pathology test.

Specimen requirements are dictated by the disease process, including the type of tissue, amount of tissue, type of sample (e.g., fresh or frozen tissue, formalin-fixed paraffin-embedded (FFPE) tissue, cytology specimen), and the extent of the disease in the sample. The amount of tissue required for PCR-based testing is relatively small, which contributes to the clinical utility of the technique.

Regardless of specimen type, two general features of the tissue sample influence molecular assays. First, there must be a sufficient quantity of the specific target cell (and therefore target DNA or RNA) in the sample. Second, the size or integrity of the nucleic acid molecules after isolation from the tissue can dramatically affect the sensitivity of the detection of specific alterations, thus nucleic acid degradation (whether due to enzymatic, heat, pH, or mechanical forces) can reduce the sensitivity of testing.

A. Tissue type. Fresh peripheral blood, bone marrow, solid tissue biopsies, enriched cell populations (for example, from flow cytometry), and FFPE tissue sections are all sources of nucleic acids for molecular analysis. Specimens should be collected and transported to the molecular pathology laboratory using aseptic techniques, if possible. Transport on ice reduces cell lysis, minimizes nuclease activity, and reduces nucleic acid degradation.

B. Tissue quality. Prompt preservation of solid tissue samples by freezing or fixation minimizes nuclei acid degradation. Hematologic specimens (peripheral blood, bone marrow) should be collected in the presence of an anticoagulant, preferably ethylenediamine tetraacetic acid (EDTA) or acid-citrate dextrose (ACD); heparin should be avoided because heparin carryover after nucleic acid isolation may inhibit subsequent PCR steps. Freezing of hematologic specimens presents distinct obstacles to the preparation of good quality nucleic acid and should generally be avoided.

Sections of FFPE tissue are suitable substrates for PCR-based molecular analysis. Fixed tissue has several advantages as a test substrate; fixation suspends the degradation of nucleic acids, and fixed specimens can be easily stored and transported. However, a significant limitation of fixed tissue is that the quality of the extracted nucleic acids is extremely variable due to the fact that all fixatives, including formalin, chemically degrade nucleic acids to some extent.

C. Tissue quantity. Minimum sample requirements are determined by the assay methodology and extent of target cell involvement in the tissue. Although

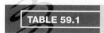

TABLE 59.1	Selected Resources for Clinical Molecular Pathology Laboratory Operational Guidelines	

Entity	Site	Tool(s)
Clinical Laboratory Improvement Amendments 1988	http://www.cms.hhs.gov/clia/	Clinical laboratory accreditation requirements and compliance lists
College of American Pathologists (CAP)	http://www.cap.org	Laboratory accreditation Molecular pathology laboratory inspection checklist Proficiency surveys • Molecular oncology (MO) • Medical genetics (MGL) • Pharmacogenetics (PGX) • Monitoring engraftment (ME) • Molecular microbiology (HIV, HCV, infectious diseases [ID]) • Microsatellite instability (MSI) • Sarcoma translocation (SARC) • Nucleic acid testing (viral; NAT)
Clinical and Laboratory Standards Institute	http://www.nccls.org	Molecular methods guidelines • Genetic diseases • IgH and TCR gene rearrangements • Nucleic acid amplification • Nucleic acid sequencing • Collection and handling of specimens • Proficiency testing
American College of Medical Genetics (ACMG)	http://www.acmg.net	Standards and guidelines for clinical genetics laboratories Policy statements for molecular testing of genetic diseases
US Food and Drug Administration (FDA)	http://www.fda.gov	Medical devices 21CFR809.30 In vitro diagnostic products for human Use • Analyte specific reagents (ASRs)
Association for Molecular Pathology (AMP)	http://www.amp.org	Molecular pathology professional organization (including genetics, hematopathology, infectious disease, solid tumors) CHAMP listserve for AMP members Test directories • Solid tumors • Hematopathology • Infectious diseases

Abbreviations: HIV, human immunodeficiency virus; HCV, hepatitis C virus; IgH, immunoglobulin heavy chain; TCR, T cell receptor.

conventional genomic Southern hybridization requires approximately 10 μg of DNA (approximately 10^6 cells) per enzymatic digest for detection of single copy genomic DNA targets, PCR-based assays have significantly lower DNA requirements. A typical PCR-based assay requires only 20 to 200 ng of DNA (about 10^3 to 10^4 cells), although multiplexed PCR may require a bit more DNA to equally represent all targets. The sensitivity of PCR for detection of a few target molecules in a large

TABLE 59.2	Nomenclature When Bayes' Theorem for One Variate Is Applied in Laboratory Testing	
	Number of subjects with positive test result	Number of subjects with negative test result
Number of subjects with disease	TP	FN
Number of subjects without disease	FP	TN

Definitions:
TP = True positives *or* number of diseased patients correctly classified by the test.
FP = False positives *or* number of patients without the disease misclassified by the test.
FN = False negatives *or* number of diseased patients misclassified by the test.
TN = True negatives *or* number of patients without the disease correctly classified by the test.
Diagnostic sensitivity = TP / (TP + FN)
Diagnostic specificity = TN / (FP + TN)
Predictive value of positive test = TP / (TP + FP)
Predictive value of negative test = TN / (TN + FN)
Efficiency of the test *or* number fraction of patients correctly classified = (TP + TN) / (TP + FP + FN + TN)
Youden Index = [(sensitivity + specificity) − 1]

background of unaltered DNA molecules (1 in 10^5) is one of the principle strengths of the methodology.

III. **ANALYTIC/TECHNICAL VERSUS DIAGNOSTIC AND OPERATIONAL ASPECTS OF TESTING.** The familiar probabilistic model used to define the likelihood that a particular patient is correctly classified based on a test result (Table 59.2) can be applied to molecular genetic tests as with any other laboratory test. However, it is important to recognize that the quantitative performance of a lab test can be evaluated at four different levels (Table 59.3), and that test performance at one of the four levels does not necessarily predict performance at the other levels. Differences between these four levels of analysis are often overlooked even though they account for many of the confusing or seemingly conflicting results regarding the utility of molecular genetic testing in surgical pathology.

IV. **BASIC PCR METHODOLOGY**

A. **Amplification.** Selective amplification of the target sequence is achieved through the use of oligonucleotide primers that hybridize to the 5′ and 3′ ends of the DNA target sequence (Fig. 59.1). In addition to the two primers and input (template) DNA, the reaction mixture also includes the four deoxynucleotide triphosphates (dATP, dCTP, dGTP, dTTP) and a heat-stable (thermostable) DNA polymerase. The first step of the PCR itself involves heating the mixture to a high temperature to denature the target DNA. In the second step, the reaction is cooled to allow the primers to anneal to

TABLE 59.3	Four Levels at Which a Laboratory Test Can Be Evaluated
Level	**Measures**
Analytic/technical	Technical sensitivity, technical specificity, precision, accuracy, proficiency
Diagnostic	Diagnostic sensitivity, diagnostic specificity, Youden Index
Operational	Predictive value of a positive result, predictive value of a negative result, efficiency
Medical decision-making	Cost-benefit analysis, stratification to optimal treatment regimen, stratification to gene-targeted treatment regimen

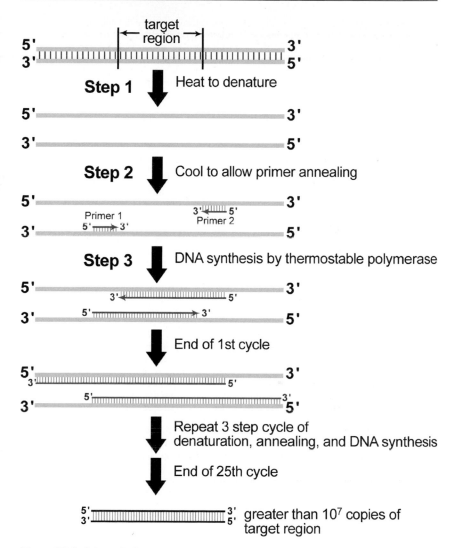

Figure 59.1. Schematic diagram of polymerase chain reaction (PCR). Each cycle consists of three steps: The reaction mix is heated to denature the double-stranded DNA template, the reaction mix is cooled to permit annealing of oligonucleotide primers to sequences that flank the target region, and then the reaction mix is warmed to permit the thermostable polymerase to synthesize new DNA strands. Each newly synthesized DNA strand then acts as a template in subsequent three-step cycles of denaturation, annealing, and DNA synthesis, producing exponential amplification of the target region.

their complementary sequence in the target DNA, and in the third step the reaction is heated to the temperature at which the thermostable DNA polymerase has optimal activity. As a result of this three-step denaturation, annealing, and polymerization cycle, the two primers will initiate synthesis of new DNA molecules from opposite strands of the input DNA heteroduplex. With each repetition of the three-step cycle, the newly synthesized DNA strands will also act as templates for further DNA synthesis, so DNA duplexes in which both strands have the fixed length of the target sequence (so-called amplicons) accumulate exponentially.

PCR makes it possible to selectively amplify a specific DNA target sequence within a background of heterogeneous DNA sequences, such as total genomic DNA or complementary DNA (cDNA) derived from unfractionated cellular RNA. However, each of the components in a PCR, including the input DNA, the oligonucleotide primers, the thermostable polymerase, the buffer, and the cycle parameters, has an effect on the sensitivity, specificity, and fidelity of the reaction.

B. **Factors that affect PCR testing on an analytic/technical level**
   1. **Advantages of PCR**
      a. **PCR is simple, quick, and inexpensive.** A single PCR cycle of melting, annealing, and extension is usually completed within 3 minutes, and consequently an entire PCR amplification of 25 to 35 cycles can be performed in only a few hours. Because of the high level of amplification achieved by PCR, the product DNA can be visualized after simple gel electrophoresis, avoiding the hazards and expense of radiolabeling methods.
      b. **PCR has high sensitivity and specificity.** When optimized, PCR can detect one abnormal cell in a background of 10^5 normal cells, and can even be used to analyze single copy genes from individual cells (*Methods Enzymol* 2002;356:295,334). PCR can also be used to detect a broad range of genetic abnormalities ranging from gross structural alterations, such as translocations and deletions, to single base pair changes.
      c. **PCR products are easily labeled for detection.** For primer-mediated labeling, a labeled chemical group (usually a fluorophore) is attached to the 5′ end of either or both oligonucleotide primers. Alternatively, the PCR product can be directly labeled by including one or more modified nucleotide precursors into the PCR mix.
      d. **Phenotype–genotype correlations are possible.** When performed on tissue sections, PCR provides only an indirect correlation of morphology and genetic abnormalities. Microdissection—in which the region of interest is carved out of the FFPE tissue block, scraped from tissue sections or cytology slides, or collected more precisely with a micromanipulator apparatus—provides some enrichment for morphologic–genetic correlations. More precise phenotypic-genotypic analysis is achieved by collecting individual cells by laser capture microdissection, by flow cytometry, or even by using immunomagnetic methods. In situ PCR performed on histologic tissue sections themselves is perhaps the ultimate method of providing morphologic localization of genotypic expression.
   2. **Limitations of PCR**
      a. **PCR analyzes only the target region.** Testing provides information on only the target segment amplified by the specific primer set used.
      b. **PCR amplifies only intact target regions.** Mutations that damage a primer-binding site (including insertions, deletions, and even point mutations) preclude amplification of the target region by PCR and can easily lead to errors in test interpretation. Similarly, mutations that alter the structure of the target region itself (e.g., large insertions, deletions, inversions, or translocations) may also preclude amplification.
      c. **Amplification bias.** PCR bias refers to the fact that some DNA templates are preferentially amplified versus other templates within the same reaction. PCR bias can be caused by differences in template length, random variations in template number (especially with very low target abundance, producing an artifact known as allele dropout), and random variations in PCR efficiency with each cycle. Amplification bias can even result from differences in the target sequence itself as small as a single base substitution. PCR bias can cause 10- to 30-fold differences in amplification efficiency in some settings, a difference that can influence quantitative PCR (Q-PCR) test results and loss of heterozygosity analysis. PCR bias can be a particularly troublesome problem in multiplex PCR.

d. Technical factors. There are several technical factors that can lower the sensitivity and specificity of PCR in routine clinical practice below that obtained in optimized research settings. Nonspecific inhibitors of PCR are sometimes present in patient samples, including heparin and uncharacterized components of cerebrospinal fluid, urine, and sputum. With the extreme sensitivity of PCR, strict attention to the physical organization and methodologies of the laboratory are required to avoid cross-contamination of specimens.

However, the most important technical limitations are introduced when fixed rather than fresh tissue specimens are used for testing, due to the degradation of DNA and messenger RNA (mRNA) that occurs prior to and during fixation, as noted above. Nucleic acid degradation compromises test sensitivity and specificity when it makes it necessary to amplify shorter target sequences or use a nested PCR approach, both of which increase the risk of amplification of nonspecific sequences and cross-contamination (*Am J Surg Pathol* 2002;26:965).

C. Factors that affect testing on a diagnostic level. The intrinsic biologic variability of disease has the greatest impact on the diagnostic sensitivity and specificity of molecular testing. Because only a subset of patients with a specific disease harbors a characteristic mutation, more than one genetic variant may characterize a specific disease, the same mutation may be characteristic of more than one disease, a mutation characteristic of disease may be present in healthy individuals (reduced penetrance), and so on; even a molecular genetic method with perfect analytic performance will have a lower sensitivity and specificity when used for diagnostic testing of patient samples.

Another diagnostic limitation of the use of PCR in routine clinical testing is a result of the fact that the technique is so sensitive that it amplifies target DNA and RNA sequences from cellular debris as well as from viable cells (*Cancer* 1997;80:1393). Consequently, in the absence of histologic confirmation of the presence of live tumor cells, the significance of PCR-based detection of tumor-derived nucleic acids in lymph nodes or even peripheral blood is uncertain.

D. Factors that affect testing on an operational level. Purely operational factors can introduce uncertainty into the interpretation of results when testing is performed prospectively in routine clinical practice. If the probability that a case is subjected to additional analysis depends on the initial test result itself, clinical variables, or both, selection bias (also called verification bias, posttest referral bias, and work-up bias) is introduced into the test. Discrepant analysis (also known as discordant analysis) can also introduce uncertainty in the interpretation of test results. Finally, even mundane factors such as differences in disease prevalence can have a marked effect on the predictive value of positive and negative test results.

E. Implications for clinical testing. Taken together, the analytic/technical features of molecular genetic assays, biologic variability, variation in assay design, and differences in distribution of disease in patient populations have many implications for testing applied in routine clinical practice.

  1. Characteristics of tests with clinical utility. In most aspects, the criteria used to evaluate the clinical utility of other hospital laboratory tests should also be applied when considering the role of the molecular pathology laboratory in patient care (Table 59.4).

  a. The relative merit of the molecular testing should focus on the ability of the test findings to improve patient care rather than on the presence of the technical capacity to perform the test. For clinical utility, the molecular diagnostic test must be an improvement in the standard of patient care by providing new or refined information with the potential for clinical stratification of disease subtypes, prognostic categories, treatment regimens, gene-targeted therapies, survival statistics, or disease progression. The test results should complement the findings of established tests, such as cytogenetics, immunohistochemistry, and cell surface marker analysis. In the context of surgical pathology, the test results must be correlated with the histopathologic features of the case.

  b. Routine clinical use of molecular tests must consider practical aspects of clinical prevalence (the disease should represent a significant health problem or

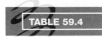

TABLE 59.4	Characteristics of Molecular Tests with Clinical Utility

Criterion	Utility
The disorder must be a significant health problem.	Disease prevalence and adverse effect on affected individuals are measurable and serious.
Treatment alternatives are available to alter disease course.	The genotype does affect the patient's clinical outcome.
A reliable molecular test is available to distinguish true-positive and false-positive results.	Focus on molecular changes known to be associated with disease pathology
Pretest and posttest counseling resources are available.	Interpretation of molecular findings with the data from the clinical presentation and other pathology tests
The test is cost-effective and /or cost-beneficial.	More costly or invasive disease monitoring methods are unnecessary. Specific treatment options and / or prognostic outcomes are indicated by the molecular results.
Referring clinicians accept the test as worthwhile to aid their decision-making.	Diagnosis, treatment, and / or clinical outcome are enhanced by the addition of the molecular pathology results to other medical tests.

diagnostic dilemma), test run frequency, clinically relevant turnaround-time, sensitivity, and specificity. Testing for diseases that are common in many populations (e.g., cancer, microbial infections, genetic predispositions) and have well-defined molecular markers will be performed in many laboratories. Molecular genetic testing for rare disorders will be routinely available only at selected laboratories with specific clinical programs or areas of institutional focus and expertise.

c. Testing must include steps to validate the result, and will include positive and negative assay controls, definition of the details and limits of interpretation of test results, and provisions for proficiency testing of the analytic method, competency of the technologists, and interpretive expertise of the laboratory director.

d. Results must be reported in a context that explains the molecular assay data and integrates the findings with other pathology results to avoid seemingly contradictory reports in comparison with other laboratory tests that possess different levels of resolution or detection.

e. Biosafety, legal, ethical, and privacy issues must consistently be observed.

2. **Discordant cases.** Cases will arise in which there is a lack of concordance between the diagnosis suggested by the molecular test results and the morphologic diagnosis. The debate over the best approach to resolve the ambiguity presented by these cases reflects the fundamental impact of molecular genetics on the classification of disease as well as the status of morphology as the historical standard of diagnosis by which new methods are measured. Rather than arbitrarily assuming that genetic testing or morphology is superior in all cases, the most reasonable way to handle discordant cases is to acknowledge the presence of the discrepancy, and then reappraise the clinical data, pathological findings, and therapeutic implications of all the test results.

For those cases in which the diagnosis suggested by morphology and genetic testing are different, prospective clinical trials are required to assess whether stage, prognosis, and response to treatment are more accurately predicted by the molecular test results than by the morphologic findings on which current staging and treatment protocols are based. Although it is often assumed that molecular genetic tests provide a more objective basis for diagnosis or therapy in cases in which there is a disagreement with traditional morphology, it is important to recognize that no formal prospective, randomized studies have demonstrated that this is true. Epidemiologically, there is a distinction between diagnostic testing and prognostic testing, with different study designs required to assess the performance of tests in these different settings (*J Clin Epidemiol* 2002;55:1178, *Ann Intern Med* 2003;139:950).

V. VARIATIONS OF PCR

A. Nested PCR. In this technique, two consecutive PCRs are performed on the same DNA sample; an initial amplification of a longer target sequence followed by a second amplification of a shorter sequence contained within the first amplicon. The second PCR may involve two internal primers (fully nested) or one internal primer and one of the original primers (seminested). Performance of nested reactions provides a marked increase in sensitivity compared with traditional PCR, and is desired in situations when the target sequence is present at an extremely low copy number, such as when the mutation is present in only a small subset of the cell population under study, when the nucleic acids have been degraded as a result of tissue fixation, or, for reverse transcriptase–PCR (RT–PCR) as discussed below, when the target mRNA is expressed at an extremely low level. Because the increased sensitivity carries an increased risk of cross-contamination, reproducible nested PCR results therefore require strict attention to laboratory technique, rigorous use of controls, and confirmation of product identity.

B. RT–PCR makes it possible to amplify RNA extracted from a tissue sample; a cDNA strand is synthesized from the RNA template using the enzyme reverse transcriptase, and the cDNA is then amplified by conventional PCR. Fresh (or fresh frozen) tissue is the preferred source of RNA for RT–PCR. RNA from fixed tissue is an acceptable substrate for testing (e-**Fig. 59.1**),* although it always suffers some degree of degradation depending on the prefixation interval, the type of fixative, the length of fixation, and the method used to isolate the RNA.

1. Advantages of RT–PCR. RT–PCR permits direct amplification of multiexon sequences by eliminating the intervening introns, and thus greatly simplifies mutation scanning methods. Similarly, RT–PCR makes it much simpler to demonstrate the presence of translocations that create fusion genes by making it possible to directly detect the fusion transcripts encoded by the translocations. RT–PCR can also be used to detect changes in mRNA structure that result from alternative splicing, to demonstrate aberrant splicing due to mutations, and to evaluate the level of gene expression through the quantitative methods discussed below.

2. Limitations of RT–PCR. RNA is a more technically demanding substrate with less stability than DNA. Tissue samples must be processed rapidly to avoid mRNA degradation, especially because many mutations render transcripts more susceptible to cellular mechanisms that clear abnormal transcripts from the cell and result in unstable mRNA. A nested PCR approach is often necessary when the target RNA is present at very low levels, but RT–PCR carries an increased risk of contamination and amplification of nonspecific sequences, because the transfer of the first PCR product to a separate tube for the nested PCR entails transmission of a highly amplified DNA preparation.

C. Quantitative-PCR. An ideal PCR would generate a perfect 2-fold increase in the number of copies of the amplicon in each cycle of the reaction. In reality, inhibitors of the reaction, accumulation of pyrophosphate molecules, decreasing polymerase activity, and reagent consumption all contribute to a plateau phase in the later stages of the reaction during which the amplicon is no longer accumulating at an exponential rate (*Clin Chem Lab Med* 2000;38:833). Reliable quantitation of PCR therefore involves more than simple measurement of the amount of product DNA present at the end of 30 to 40 cycles of the reaction. Quantitative-PCR (Q-PCR), also referred to as real-time PCR, uses real-time measurements of DNA accumulation (usually via fluorescence-based approaches) during the early exponential phases of PCR progress to provide precise estimates of the initial concentration of the target sequence(s).

---

*All e-figures are available online via the Solution Site Image Bank.

A wide variety of different chemistries for Q-PCR are in routine use, including the so-called *Taq*Man (also known as 5' exonuclease or hydrolysis real-time PCR), molecular beacon (which can be designed to distinguish targets differing by only a single nucleotide), scorpion (also known as self-probing amplicons), hybridization probe, and intercalating dye methods. Regardless of the chemistry, changes in fluorescence that result from target amplification are measured by a detector for each cycle of the reaction and are calculated by a computer to construct an amplification plot of fluorescence versus the cycle number to quantify the concentration of the input target DNA sequence.

1. **Advantages of Q-PCR.** The method can be applied to fresh as well as FFPE tissue, and phenotype–genotype correlations are possible through analysis of specific cell populations collected, e.g., via microdissection or laser capture microdissection. Quantitative reverse transcriptase-PCR (Q-RT-PCR) is also a robust analytic approach.

2. **Disadvantages of Q-PCR.** Even for optimized assays, testing can be complicated by amplification bias, which in the context of Q-PCR has two major sources; PCR drift due to random fluctuations in amplification efficiency in the early cycles of the reaction when the templates are present at very low concentration, and PCR selection due to mechanisms that systematically favor amplification of some particular target(s). For Q-RT-PCR, a lack of completion of the reverse transcription reaction can introduce additional variables into the analysis.

3. **Use of Q-PCR in nonquantitative settings.** Because the probes used in Q-PCR (and Q-RT-PCR) have specificity for the target amplicon, the amplification plot not only confirms the presence of the DNA product, but also confirms its identity. Intercalating dyes can also provide confirmation of both the presence and identity of the DNA product when coupled with subsequent melting curve analysis. Because Q-PCR eliminates the need for gel electrophoresis to demonstrate successful amplification while simultaneously confirming product identity, Q-PCR is often used as a 'one-step' alternative to conventional PCR or RT-PCR even when quantitation is not required.

D. **Multiplex PCR.** Multiplex PCR is the simultaneous amplification of multiple target sequences in a single reaction through the simultaneous use of multiple primer pairs. The technique saves time and money, is ideal for conserving templates that are in short supply, and has been successfully applied to many amplification approaches, including nested PCR and Q-PCR. However, even in optimized reactions, multiplex PCR may be complicated by amplification bias due to PCR drift and PCR selection. Rigorous optimization of primer design and careful titration of the relative primer concentration among separate primer pairs are essential for robust, reproducible multiplex PCR performance.

E. **Methylation-specific PCR.** Methylation of CpG sites in human DNA has been associated with transcriptional inactivation of imprinted genes, is important for X chromosome inactivation, and is an important mechanism for developmentally regulated and tissue-specific gene regulation. An altered pattern of methylation is also characteristic of many human diseases. Changes in the CpG methylation pattern in some malignancies have been associated with differences in response to specific chemotherapeutic agents and overall survival.

Recently developed methylation-specific PCR techniques exploit the sequence differences produced when methylated CpG and unmethylated CpG are treated with sodium bisulfite (*Proc Natl Acad Sci U S A* 1996;93:9821). This chemical modification will not alter methyl cytosine but will depurinate cytosine to produce a transversion and replacement with thymidine in subsequent DNA synthesis during PCR. Because the two strands of genomic DNA are no longer complementary after sodium bisulfite treatment, PCR with appropriately designed primers makes it possible to infer the methylation status of the original untreated DNA. Methylation-specific PCR can be applied to DNA extracted from fresh tissue, FFPE tissue, and even archival cytology specimens.

F. **Telomerase repeat amplification protocol (TRAP).** The hexanucleotide TTAGGG repeat sequence of human telomeres is essential for the maintenance of chromosome stability and integrity, and abnormalities of telomere length have been associated with a number of developmental abnormalities and malignancies. The PCR-based TRAP assay is a simple, sensitive, and reproducible method for measurement of telomerase activity as an adjunct in early diagnosis, for prognostic testing, or as a means to identify drugs that inhibit telomerase function.

The technique has limitations: The protein extract used for testing can only be prepared from fresh cells or tissue samples, false-negative and false-positive reactions are commonly encountered, and heterogeneity within a tumor can lead to significant variability in the test result. Although early studies suggested that altered telomerase activity is a characteristic finding in a variety of neoplasms, a growing body of evidence suggests that telomerase activity demonstrated by the TRAP assay is neither a consistent feature of malignancy nor specific for a malignant phenotype (*Hum Pathol* 2004;35:393). Attempts to correlate a malignant phenotype with telomerase activity measured by other techniques (such as RT–PCR-based measurement of the level of expression of mRNA encoding the human telomerase reverse transcriptase [hTERT] catalytic subunit of telomerase, or immunohistochemical analysis of hTERT) have likewise produced mixed results.

VI. APPLICATIONS OF PCR

A. Direct DNA sequence analysis. The dye terminator cycle sequencing method for direct DNA sequencing is currently used for virtually all routine DNA sequence analyses. This technique (e-**Fig. 59.**2) uses synthetic oligonucleotide primers complementary to a known sequence of the template strand to be analyzed, and is greatly simplified by the use of fluorescently labeled, chain-terminating dideoxynucleotide triphosphates. As initially described, enzymatic extension of the primer was performed only once per sequencing reaction, but the utility of the method is greatly increased by the modification known as cycle sequencing (or linear amplification sequencing). Cycle sequencing is similar to conventional PCR in that it uses a thermostable DNA polymerase and a temperature cycling format for DNA denaturation, annealing, and enzymatic DNA synthesis, but only one primer (the sequencing primer) is added to the reaction mixture. Automated DNA sequencing uses nucleotides or primers that are labeled by fluorophores, and is the method of choice in most clinical labs.

B. Indirect DNA sequence analysis. Identification of normal and mutant alleles at a specific locus that correlate with presence of disease often provides indirect DNA sequence information of clinical utility without detection of specific nucleotide sequences. Virtually all of the indirect methods are based on PCR and can be applied to a broad range of clinical specimens. Examples of indirect methods include the following.

1. Allelic discrimination by size. Alleles that vary by small insertions or deletions can be distinguished based on the size of the PCR product after gel electrophoresis, perhaps the most straightforward method for indirect DNA sequence analysis.

2. Allelic discrimination based on susceptibility to a restriction enzyme. Using the technique known as restriction fragment length polymorphism (RFLP) analysis, mutations that either create or destroy a restriction endonuclease site can easily be distinguished by a two-step process that involves DNA digestion with the restriction endonuclease followed by gel electrophoresis to size fractionate the digested DNA. Virtually all RFLP analysis is performed on PCR product DNA.

3. Allele-specific PCR. Allele-specific PCR (also known as the amplification refractory mutation system, or ARMS) uses oligonucleotide primers designed to discriminate between normal and mutant target DNA sequences that may differ by a single base (*J Mol Diagn* 2007;9:272). Simultaneous analysis of multiple loci via a multiplex PCR format is possible if the amplicons from the different loci are different sizes. PCR conditions must be optimized with sufficient stringency so that amplification only occurs when complete DNA sequence complementarity exists between primer and target molecules.

4. Single-strand conformational polymorphism (SSCP) analysis is one of the most simple and widely used techniques employed as a physical mutation scanning system. Single-stranded DNA molecules fold into complex three-dimensional structures that are stabilized primarily by intrastrand base-pairing hydrogen bond formation that alters the mobility of the molecule during nondenaturing gel electrophoresis. SSCP has limited resolution of DNA fragment sizes (100 to 400 bp long is optimal). Although a base sequence may be indicated by the altered mobility, SSCP does not provide information about either the location of the base change within the DNA fragment or the chemical identity of the base change. Subsequent direct DNA sequence is required for this resolution. In practice, the DNA fragments evaluated by SSCP are generated by PCR.

5. **Melting curve analysis.** PCR amplification of a locus from a heterozygous individual actually yields four different types of duplexes: two homoduplexes and two heteroduplexes. Each duplex has a characteristic melting temperature, and although small, the differences in melting temperature between the duplexes can be reliably detected by high-resolution melting analysis. Differences in the melting transition of PCR products can therefore be used to infer sequence variations such as single nucleotide polymorphisms, small deletions, and small insertions. The most straightforward methods melt unlabeled PCR products in the presence of DNA-binding dyes such as SYBR Green that differentiate double-stranded from single-stranded DNA by changes in fluorescence intensity (*Nat Protoc* 2007;2:59).

C. **Clonality assays.** Demonstration that the cells in a lesion share a common genetic alteration can be used to support classification as a neoplasm rather than as a polyclonal reactive process, although it is important to emphasize that clonal neoplasms are not necessarily malignant.

1. **Assays based on immunoglobulin and T-cell receptor genes.** Most PCR clonality assays performed clinically are used to assess lymphoid infiltrates based on evaluation of immunoglobulin gene or T-cell receptor gene rearrangements. PCR primer design is an important component of these assays; because generation of immunoglobulin and T-cell receptors involves deletions, template-independent nucleotide additions, and single base-pair changes, consensus primers are designed to bind to conserved sequence regions, and multiple sets of primers are used to insure that a broad range of rearrangements can be detected. Demonstration of a monoclonal or oligoclonal population of cells within an infiltrate is very often, but not always, indicative of malignancy. These specific gene rearrangements are also lineage specific for these lymphoid populations. Rare oligoclonal or monoclonal gene rearrangements may characterize reactive lymphoid proliferations.

2. **Clonality assays based on specific gene mutations.** This class of assays focuses on detection of specific mutations in individual genes, including single-base-pair changes and larger scale structural changes (such as deletions, or insertions of viral genomes). This type of analysis can be useful when attempting to show that two neoplasms represent independent synchronous or metachronous tumors rather than one tumor with metastases.

D. **Microsatellite instability assays.** Defects in the DNA mismatch repair system produce a characteristic pattern of mutations known as microsatellite instability (MSI). Direct analysis of the genes responsible for mismatch repair is not desirable in routine clinical practice because it requires complete DNA sequencing of two to five causative genes, there are no specific mutation "hot spots," and the genes may be inactive as a result of epigenetic silencing rather than mutation. PCR-based analysis offers a more efficient, though indirect, method to identify defects in the DNA mismatch repair system via detection of the short increases or decreases in the length of the short tandem repeat (STR, or microsatellite) sequences that are the characteristic feature of MSI. Mutations in the genes that normally monitor the fidelity of DNA replication of these repeated sequences is defective and allows for the generation of the variable lengths of repeats in the tumor cells.

Laboratory testing regimens for MSI are not yet standardized in terms of the number and identity of microsatellite loci that must be analyzed for a particular tumor type, or in terms of the number of loci that need to show length alterations to be considered indicative of MSI. These issues have only been formally addressed in the context of colorectal cancer (*Cancer Res* 1998;58:5248).

DNA derived from either fresh tissue or FFPE tissue can be analyzed in the MSI assay. Comparison of the size of the PCR products from the target STR loci in the neoplasm versus normal tissue is used to detect changes in the length of the microsatellite sequences indicative of MSI. In most cases, the profile of PCR-amplified sequences permits straightforward classification as indicative of MSI or not; however, there are no uniform criteria for interpretation of marginal test results, although standards have been proposed (*Mutat Res* 2001;461:249). Sources of variation in MSI analysis include the presence of contaminating nonneoplastic tissue (which can limit test reliability because demonstration of MSI in even the most sensitive testing regimens requires that neoplastic cells comprise at least 10% of the total population), the identity of the microsatellite markers used in the analysis (the susceptibility of a given microsatellite to instability is highly dependent on both the number of repeats and the length of the repeat units), and the potential for biased amplification of some alleles.

E. Infectious disease testing. PCR-based molecular genetic approaches frequently have higher sensitivity than do standard special stains, and can often provide information not typically available from special stains, such as species-specific identification and drug sensitivity. Molecular methods are also a useful way to detect organisms that cannot be cultured (for example, human papillomavirus [HPV]) or that are notorious for their slow growth in culture (for example, *Mycobacterium tuberculosis*).

1. Bacteria

a. Mycobacteria. In most studies, PCR designed to detect mycobacteria targets the highly conserved gene that encodes the 65 kd heat shock protein, but other target loci include the genes encoding 16S ribosomal RNA (rRNA) or the repetitive insertion element IS6110. PCR testing has been successfully applied to FFPE tissue from a wide variety of sites, including the respiratory tract, gastrointestinal tract, genitourinary tract, skin, bone, liver, and lymph nodes, and also to cytology specimens. Alternative isothermal amplification approaches originally developed for use in the clinical microbiology laboratory have also been adapted for use with processed tissue specimens (*Expert Rev Mol Diagn* 2004;4:251).

b. Helicobacter pylori. Although the genome of *H. pylori* is remarkable for the polymorphism between different clinical isolates, PCR-based methods have nonetheless been developed that permit successful detection of virtually all reported forms of *H. pylori* by PCR from either fresh or FFPE tissue, including the nonculturable coccoid form of the organism. The most common target loci in PCR assays include the 16S rRNA gene, urease gene, or arbitrarily chosen regions of the *H. pylori* genome. Recently developed Q-RT-PCR methods that target the 23S rRNA gene permit simultaneous detection of *H. pylori* and antibiotic resistant testing.

c. Other bacterial pathogens. PCR has been used to detect *Bacillus anthracis* organisms in patient specimens associated with bioterrorism or accidental environmental release from bioweapons facilities (*J Clin Microbiol* 2002;40:4360).

2. Fungi. Most PCR assays target sequences within the fungal rRNA genes. PCR can be performed using universal primers that bind to highly conserved sequences in the region, followed by direct or indirect DNA sequence analysis of the PCR product to identify the specific fungal pathogen. Alternatively, sequence differences in the 18S rRNA gene can be used to design primers that are specific for individual fungal pathogens. Sequence polymorphisms of the mitochondrial large subunit rRNA gene have also been used as a target in PCR tests to identify fungal pathogens in tissue specimens, and Q-PCR methods have also been developed for detection of fungal pathogens in tissue specimens.

3. Viruses

a. HPV. Most PCR protocols for HPV testing make use of consensus primers targeted to the viral L1 gene that are potentially capable of detecting all HPV types that affect the anogenital region. Following amplification using consensus primers, the HPV type can be determined by either DNA sequence analysis or membrane hybridization with type-specific probes. However, both approaches are labor intensive and difficult to automate, which makes them poorly suited for screening a large volume of patient specimens.

b. **Hepatitis C virus.** RT–PCR methods used to detect hepatitis C virus (HCV) in liver biopsy specimens focus on the 5' noncoding region of the virus that is highly conserved between the (at least) 6 genotypes and >90 subtypes of HCV that have been described worldwide. Maximal RT–PCR test sensitivity can only be achieved via a nested RT–PCR approach, or when the PCR products are evaluated by Southern blot hybridization.

c. **Epstein–Barr virus.** A Q-PCR methodology has been described that targets five highly conserved segments of the Epstein–Barr virus genome (*J Mol Diagn* 2004;6:378). The method can be applied to FFPE tissue, but maximum test sensitivity is obtained only when analysis involves all five marker loci.

d. **Respiratory viruses.** Although PCR assays have been developed for many individual viruses, a multiplex RT–PCR assay for seven common respiratory viruses (specifically, adenovirus, influenza virus types A and B, respiratory syncytial virus, and parainfluenza virus types 1, 2, and 3) is one of the most efficient molecular approaches thus far described (*J Mol Diagn* 2004;6:125). The multiplex assay not only has a specificity of 100% for each viral pathogen, but also has sensitivity for each virus that is superior to either direct immunofluorescence antibody staining alone or antibody staining combined with viral culture.

A nested RT–PCR assay has been described for detection of the coronavirus responsible for severe acute respiratory syndrome (SARS) (*Am J Clin Pathol* 2004;121:574). The method can be applied to FFPE tissue from both open lung biopsies as well as autopsy specimens, a feature of the assay that is important given the virulence of the pathogen. The rapidity and simplicity of the approach make it ideally suited for diagnosis given the epidemiology of SARS outbreaks.

4. **Protozoans**

a. **Toxoplasmosis.** Several different PCR-based assays (for use with either fresh or FFPE tissue) have been developed for detection of *Toxoplasma gondii,* the etiologic agent of toxoplasmosis. The assays have clinical utility because serologic diagnosis of active infection is unreliable because immunoglobulin M levels do not correlate with recent infection, and because reactivation of disease is not always accompanied by changes in antibody levels.

b. **Leishmaniasis.** A number of different loci serve as targets in PCR-based tests for leishmaniasis, including repetitive nuclear DNA sequences, genes encoding rRNA, and kinetoplast DNA. In fact, PCR using primers that amplify a 120-bp fragment of kinetoplast DNA has a higher sensitivity than all other diagnostic methods that have been evaluated, including serologic testing, microbiologic culture, routine histopathologic evaluation, and immunohistochemical staining.

c. **Intestinal parasites.** A nested PCR that targets the gene encoding the small subunit rRNA gene of microsporidia has been described that can be used with fresh tissue for species-specific detection of four different pathogenic microsporidia; because different pathogenic microsporidia can have different sensitivities to antimicrobial agents, testing provides an opportunity to establish the diagnosis as well as direct therapy. PCR targeted to genes encoding 18S rRNA or oocyst wall proteins can be used to document infection with *Cryptosporidium.*

F. **Identity determination.** Although the advantages of DNA-based identification analysis have been most widely publicized in forensics and parentage studies, this testing also has a role in the routine practice of surgical pathology, including resolution of specimen identity issues, differentiation of synchronous and metachronous tumors from metastases, evaluation of tumors in transplant recipients, evaluation of bone marrow engraftment, diagnosis of hydatidiform moles (e-**Fig. 59.3**), and demonstration of natural chimerism.

PCR-based approaches for DNA typing have greatly expanded the range of testing because they require such small amounts of DNA and can be performed on fresh, fixed, or even partially degraded specimens. Virtually all DNA typing is currently performed using a set of 13 core short tandem repeat (STR) loci (also known as microsatellite loci) chosen by the Federal Bureau of Investigation of the United States for use in a national database of convicted felons known as the Combined DNA Index System (CODIS). Commercial kits for either monoplex or multiplex PCR amplification of CODIS loci have greatly simplified STR typing and made the method accessible to most molecular genetics laboratories.

Suggested Readings

Pfeifer JD. *Molecular Genetic Testing in Surgical Pathology*. Philadelphia: Lippincott Williams & Wilkins; 2006.

Rudin N, Inman K, eds. *An Introduction to Forensic DNA Analysis*, 2nd ed. Boca Raton, FL: CRC Press Publishers; 2002.

Strachan T, Read AP. *Human Molecular Genetics*, 3rd ed. London: Garland Science; 2004.

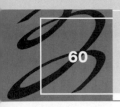

60 MICROARRAYS
Mark A. Watson

I. **INTRODUCTION.** Nucleic acid microarrays are an ordered arrangement of DNA molecules (*probes* or *features*) on a solid surface. A sample of DNA or RNA derived from cells or tissue (*target*) is then hybridized to the array to quantify the level of nucleic acid corresponding to each probe. Microarrays can be utilized for a number of different experimental and clinical applications (Fig. 60.1).*

  A. **Array comparative genomic hybridization (aCGH).** This microarray-based assay is used to compare genome copy numbers between biospecimens. Often, a patient tumor DNA sample is directly compared to a corresponding nonmalignant or germline DNA sample from the same individual to assess quantitative changes in a tumor genome. This approach is rapidly becoming a higher-resolution complement to more traditional cytogenetic and fluorescent in situ hybridization (FISH) assays.

  B. **Genotyping.** Microarray technology can be used to assay single nucleotide polymorphism (SNP) genotypes or copy number variation across 1 to 2 million genomic loci in a single DNA sample. This approach is useful in identifying correlations between phenotype and genotype in familial linkage or genome-wide association (population-based) studies.

  C. **Sequencing by hybridization** uses microarray technology to determine the complete nucleotide sequence of a DNA target, usually 100 to 300 kilobases in length. Unlike conventional sequencing chemistry using capillary gel electrophoresis, the target sequence need not be a contiguous stretch of DNA, but may consist of a set of regions of diagnostic relevance distributed throughout the genome.

  D. **Genome tiling.** Very high density microarray designs contain nucleotide probes with 10 to 35 nucleotide spacing across the entire genome. These high-resolution probe arrays allow for identification of methylation and DNA-protein binding patterns at the single nucleotide level.

  E. **Gene expression.** By hybridizing cellular RNA to microarrays with probes directed to messenger RNA (mRNA) targets, it is possible to perform qualitative (i.e., detection of alternative splicing) and quantitative gene expression analysis simultaneously on 30,000 to 50,000 genes from a single RNA specimen. Measurement of transcript abundance (i.e., *gene expression profiling*) has been the most common use of microarray technology in investigative and diagnostic pathology.

II. **MICROARRAY TECHNOLOGY.** Nucleic acid microarrays are fabricated using several different technologies and probe types, depending on the intended application (Fig. 60.1).

  A. **Bacterial artificial chromosome (BAC) arrays.** BAC cloned DNA is deposited onto a solid surface (usually a glass microscope slide) by a robotic, mechanical spotting device. Each BAC clone represents a large stretch of genomic DNA from a specific chromosomal region, usually several hundred kilobases in length. BAC arrays have been particularly useful in assessing genome-wide DNA copy number changes in tumor specimens and have enhanced the resolution of traditional cytogenetic studies using aCGH. Validated BAC arrays are used in a number of clinical laboratories. However, compared with newer, oligonucleotide-based platforms, they suffer from poor resolution and require a sufficient laboratory infrastructure to grow and maintain BAC libraries that are used to generate the DNA probes.

---

*All e-figures are available online via the Solution Site Image Bank.

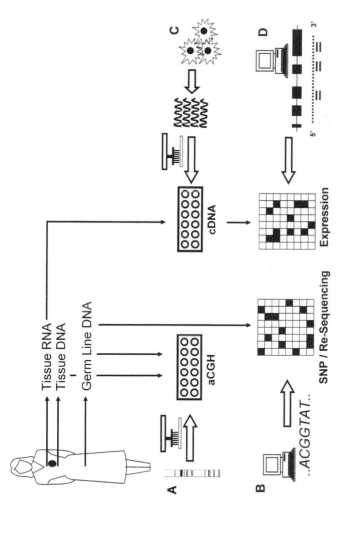

Figure 60.1. Microarray applications and technology. Microarray technology can be used for many different applications, depending on the nucleic acid composition of the array (probes) and the test material (target) that is hybridized to it. **A:** For array comparative genomic hybridization (aCGH) assays, fragments of genomic DNA (i.e., bacterial artificial chromosomes) are spotted as probes onto the microarray surface. Genomic DNA from the patient's tissue and germline are then cohybridized to the array to identify regions of chromosomal gain or loss. **B:** Alternatively, genomic DNA sequence can be used to computationally design oligonucleotide probes that detect specific alterations in DNA samples (either germline or tissue) for either single nucleotide polymorphism (SNP) genotyping or DNA resequencing studies. **C:** Complementary DNA (cDNA) clones generated from cellular RNA also can be spotted as probes onto the microarray and patient tissue RNA subsequently hybridized to quantify relative messenger RNA (mRNA) transcript abundance for gene expression profiling experiments. **D:** Similarly, oligonucleotides can be designed based on known gene exon structure and spotted on the array surface to perform quantitative or qualitative assessment of mRNA expression.

B. **Complementary DNA (cDNA) microarrays.** Some of the earliest microarray designs used cDNA probes. Messenger RNA from a defined tissue or cell source is converted into a double-stranded cDNA plasmid clone library. Plasmid DNA from each clone is then spotted onto the microarray surface. Genome sequence information is not necessarily required for microarray design, a particular advantage for studying experimental organisms for which genome sequence information is not available. However, because cDNA probes correspond to relatively long stretches of transcribed mRNA, cross-hybridization and lack of specificity can often limit the accuracy of cDNA microarray results. Like BAC arrays, the effort and infrastructure necessary to store, grow, purify, monitor quality control, and track individual cDNA clones is considerable and not easily standardized. This last constraint has and will continue to limit the use of cDNA microarrays as clinical diagnostic tools.

C. **Oligonucleotide microarrays.** A completely sequenced and annotated human genome, coupled with improved synthesis chemistries, has shifted the fabrication of nucleic acid microarrays toward the use of synthetic oligonucleotide probes, usually 60 to 75 nucleotides in length. Probe sequences may be customized for specific genes, gene transcripts, or gene transcript segments using defined nucleic acid sequences. Sophisticated bioinformatics programs can select optimized oligonucleotide sequences for any gene or transcript of interest while minimizing cross-reactivity with other sequences and standardizing hybridization properties such as melting temperature and G/C sequence content. "Use of oligonucleotide probes" has provided a new level of standardization and flexibility to the design of sequence content on nucleic acid microarrays which is aptly suited for clinical diagnostic assays.

D. **In situ synthesized microarrays.** Another strategy for microarray design involves simultaneously synthesizing specific oligonucleotide probes in situ using combinatorial photochemistry. Affymetrix GeneChip microarrays use a series of micron-scale "masks" to direct light to specific locations on the microarray surface. Photoreactive nucleotides (A, C, G, T) are sequentially passed over the array surface in the presence of each mask. Depending on the mask pattern, a specific nucleotide is added to the growing chain of oligonucleotides at a specific position. In this combinatorial method, the use of 25 different masks sets (A, C, G, T) in 100 sequential nucleotide addition steps can result in 4^{25} (1×10^{15}) different sequences that are simultaneously created on the array surface. Alternate methods use a "maskless" approach for in situ probe synthesis. A sheet composed of micron-scale electronic mirrors can be programmed to direct light to specific areas of the microarray during sequential steps of photochemical oligonucleotide synthesis. The method is similar to GeneChip fabrication, but does not rely on the creation of fixed lithographic masks and therefore allows for flexible design on a single array basis.

E. **Bead arrays.** One of the newer and perhaps most innovative approaches to microarray design involves the use of a beaded microarray. In this approach, micron-sized beads, each containing a unique oligonucleotide gene sequence in tandem with a unique nucleotide address sequence, are allowed to randomly assemble onto a solid surface. By repeated interrogation of each bead address sequence, the identity of each bead at each position is deduced. The "decoded" array can then be used for its intended hybridization assay.

III. **MICROARRAY ASSAYS.** Microarray assays are complex (e-**Fig. 60.1**), because of both the amount of data generated and the exacting specimen requirements that are necessary to produce high-quality data.

A. **Study design.** To date, most microarray-based studies have been designed as biomarker discovery experiments, with the aim of defining a panel of multiple biomarkers that can then be transitioned into a more conventional clinical assay. Microarray experiments generally fall into several classes (*Science.* 1999;286: 531).

1. **Class discovery.** In such studies, experimental specimens are classified based solely on their microarray data values, and the results of the classification are reviewed to identify new, previously unappreciated clinical or pathological classifications. Perhaps the most elegant illustration of this approach has been the

reclassification of breast adenocarcinoma based on microarray-generated gene expression profiles (*Clin Cancer Res.* 2005;11:5678).

2. **Class distinction.** In this type of study designed to identify novel predictive biomarkers, patterns of gene expression, copy number, or sequence variation are sought that demonstrate a correlation to an already known parameter such as clinical outcome or treatment response.

3. **Single sample classification.** Ultimately, to achieve clinical utility, it is necessary to create a robust molecular signature that can be prospectively applied to individual patient specimens and accurately predict clinical phenotype. In this approach, a specific subset of probes on the microarray (sometimes a customized array designed for a specific diagnostic purpose) is examined and a weighted discriminate index is calculated. The resulting index provides a probability measure that a given specimen falls into a specific, predefined diagnostic category. Studies that independently validate a previously identified signature are relatively rare to date, but are obviously a critical step in transitioning any assay into routine clinical use.

B. **Statistical considerations.** In principle, microarray data analysis is no different than evaluating whether a single biomarker demonstrates a statistically significant difference between defined sample classes using traditional statistics. By definition, a traditional significance threshold of $p = .05$ allows for a 5% false-positive (false discovery) rate. Therefore, when analyzing 50,000 to 2,000,000 independent biomarker values obtained by a microarray assay, as many as 100,000 values will appear to be 'significant' by chance alone. To contend with this problem of multiple testing, several methods have been applied to calculate a true significance threshold when analyzing thousands of variables in relatively few numbers of samples (*Genome Biol.* 2003;4:210). Although these approaches minimize the number of false-positive results for a given sample set, they can in no way substitute for data validation using multiple, independent sets of samples across different technology platforms and laboratories.

C. **Specimen requirements.** Because of the inherent complexity of microarray-based assays, specimen quality assurance is essential.

1. **Specimen collection.** Careful consideration must be given to specimen collection for microarray studies. Although DNA and DNA methylation patterns are relatively stable and probably less sensitive to environmental conditions, the same is not true for mRNA that is the target of microarray-based gene expression profile assays. Global changes in gene expression may occur in tissue biospecimens as a result of tissue warm ischemia time (*Am J Pathol.* 2002;161:1743), creating artificial differences in gene expression patterns based on collection procedures rather than important clinical differences. For peripheral blood and bone marrow specimens, the method in which a specimen is collected and processed can also influence gene expression signatures (*Physiol Genomics.* 2004;19:247). Finally, most tissue specimens are inherently heterogeneous collections of many cell types. Variable cellular composition between tissue specimens may lead to differences in genomic and transcriptional profiles generated from microarray assays. For example, two prostate tumor samples, the first of which contains 5% neoplastic cellularity and the second of which contains 70% neoplastic cellularity, may demonstrate two different gene expression signatures based simply on the content of neoplastic epithelial cells present in the tissue. Similarly, measurement of a tumor-associated change in DNA copy number will vary considerably depending on the content of neoplastic cells. For this reason, many investigators use techniques such as laser microdissection to isolate more homogeneous cell populations for both gene expression and DNA copy number microarray analysis (see Chapter 61).

2. **Specimen processing.** Generally, diagnostic surgical pathology tissue specimens are subjected to formalin fixation and paraffin embedding. This process results in chemical cross-linking and degradation of nucleic acid. DNA extracted from formalin-fixed, paraffin-embedded (FFPE) tissue may be suitable for microarray-based DNA analysis. However, most investigators have found that RNA derived

from FFPE tissue is unsuitable for traditional gene expression microarray-based assays. Freshly procured, snap-frozen biospecimens remain the "gold standard" for microarray analysis, particularly for RNA-based gene expression assays. Many clinical centers do not have access to resources needed for the processing and storage of frozen samples; in the context of research studies, a number of solutions have been proposed to circumvent the limited availability of fresh-frozen biospecimens for microarray analysis (see Chapter 61). Such advances should enable routine prospective analysis of clinical specimens for RNA- or DNA-based microarray assays in the future.

D. **Target preparation.** To prepare samples for microarray assays, RNA or DNA derived from a tissue or cell specimen is converted into a synthetic target in the presence of labeled deoxynucleotides. To analyze clinical specimens containing small amounts of cellular material, such as diagnostic core or needle aspiration biopsies, most protocols for microarray target synthesis use some method of molecular amplification including polymerase chain reaction (PCR), isothermal DNA polymerization, or in vitro transcription (*J Cancer.* 2004;90:1111).

IV. **DATA ANALYSIS** is by far the most complicated aspect of any microarray study (*Nat Rev Genet* 2001;2:418 and *BMC Bioinformatics.* 2005;6:115). Principal steps in microarray data analysis involve the following.

A. **Image analysis.** Current microarray technology allows for laser scanning of several square centimeters of microarray surface at the resolution of micron-sized image elements. The result is a primary image data file that can be hundreds of megabytes in size. Although a number of software solutions and data repositories have been developed to hold and distribute experimental microarray data, regulatory issues related to storage and transfer of data in a clinical setting have yet to be addressed.

The first step in microarray analysis involves the conversion of these raw, pixilated images into numerical values that relate to hybridization signal intensity at each feature (probe). For two-color arrays, the fluorescence intensity must be sequentially captured and analyzed for each emission spectrum. In other microarray platforms such as the Affymetrix GeneChip, multiple probes are used to assay for a single transcript or genomic locus. For this reason, the signal from multiple different probes must be integrated to create a single, averaged intensity value. Due to the widespread use of the Affymetrix platform, several different algorithms have been developed to translate raw hybridization data into gene expression values. Using standardized data sets, the sensitivity and specificity of each of these algorithms to detect known changes in copy number between samples has been evaluated at length.

B. **Normalization.** After image data have been converted into numerical values for each probe or probe set represented on the array, the composite set of data is usually normalized to a reference point to allow for comparison between sets of array data (e-**Fig. 60.2**). For example, inter-array normalization algorithms compensate for global differences in the signal intensity between arrays. Inter-gene normalization algorithms are useful for identifying common patterns of gene expression between study samples, even when absolute gene expression values are considerably different. Other types of data transformation techniques, such as log transformation of two-color signal ratios, may also be appropriate, depending on the nature of the primary microarray data set.

C. **Visualization and data reduction.** After normalization, data must be visualized and statistically analyzed to address a specific research question (e-**Fig. 60.2**). There are a number of relatively standard methods in which voluminous and multidimensional microarray data may visualized.

1. **Hierarchical clustering.** Samples (targets) are organized based on their similarity in gene marker values and, genes (probes) based on their similarity across samples. Several different measures of similarity can be used and several different algorithms can be applied to perform the clustering. However, no particular algorithm can be considered more 'correct.' In fact, although hierarchical clustering is a useful tool to provide a manageable view of immense data sets, it does not necessarily impart any underlying 'truth' to microarray data.

2. **Heat maps** are colorimetric representations of numerical data, usually presented in combination with hierarchical clustering. These visualization schemes provide a convenient method to identify patterns or blocks of similarity between gene markers and/or samples.
3. **k-Means** clustering and **principal components analysis (PCA).** These data reduction methods are particularly useful for reducing the level of microarray data complexity. A large number of variables (i.e., microarray probe values) are placed into a finite number of 'bins' based on their similarity of values across a much smaller number of observations (i.e., target samples). The number of bins created (the 'k' in k-means) can be adjusted to create a much smaller set of similar, collective values, which can then be used as the basis for further analysis.

    In PCA, samples are plotted in 'gene marker space,' where the distance between samples is related to their similarity based on gene marker values. However, for a 47,000-element microarray, gene marker space is represented in 47,000 different dimensions. Therefore, the goal of PCA is to reduce 47,000 dimensions into two to three principle components. Then, relatedness between samples can be plotted.

D. **Annotation.** A final significant challenge in data analysis is to determine how patterns of gene expression can be related to biologically meaningful results. As annotation and our understanding of the human genome continue to improve, investigators have been able to classify a large number of human genes into ontologies based on function, cellular location, and structural determinants. Several software programs are available that can map lists of biomarkers to these ontologies, which often result in a clearer view of altered biological processes associated with differential gene expression. For single cellular and simple multicellular organisms, this approach has led to sophisticated models for cell signaling and transcriptional regulatory networks, whereas for other mammalian species this type of analysis is still evolving.

E. **Validation.** Like any other diagnostic test, the results of any microarray assay must be validated through independent testing. Validation of microarray assays is particularly problematic for many reasons. First, microarray assays are relatively expensive ($200 to $800 per sample), which creates financial constraints on the number of samples that can be analyzed. Second, given the stringent specimen requirements needed to perform most microarray assays, availability of suitable specimens is often limiting. Finally, as discussed above, the large number of variables associated with a microarray data set requires that a relatively large number of observations (e.g., samples) are analyzed to create any degree of statistical confidence. To perform data validation for microarray results in the face of these limitations, investigators have devised a number of approaches (*Expert Rev Mol Diagn.* 2003;3:587).

    1. **Cross-validation.** One of the most popular approaches for data validation is sequential sampling or 'leave-one-out' cross-validation analysis in a single sample set. In an analysis of N study samples, $N - 1$ samples are used for the initial statistical analysis to identify groups of signature genes. The ability of these genes to correctly classify the Nth sample is then calculated and the gene list modified, discarding biomarkers that perform poorly and solidifying those with the best performance This process is repeated, removing all N samples, one at a time, until a list of genes with the best class prediction score is created. The advantage of this method is that no additional data or experimentation is needed for validation. However, because the cross-validation is still applied to a single set of samples (i.e., the 'test' and 'validation' sets are one in the same), the ability to generalize conclusions to independent or larger sample sets may still be limited.
    2. **Sample set splitting.** If an initial microarray sample set is large enough, it is also possible to divide the experiment into independent sets of test data and validation data. In this scheme, patterns of 'significant' gene expression are identified using the first set of samples, and patterns are validated in a second set of arrays. Although this approach uses two truly independent data sets, it necessarily limits the number of independent samples available for the discovery phase and validation phase. The desire to split a limited number of samples into test and validation sets raises the question of sample size requirement for performing microarray analyses

with sufficient statistical power (*Physiol Genomics.* 2003;16:24). Although multiple methods have been proposed to calculate required sample sizes, the number of samples required will ultimately depend on the expected biological effect. For example, relatively few study samples may be necessary to identify fundamental genomic differences between acute myelogenous leukemia and acute lymphocytic leukemia, as these tumor cell types are biologically very distinct. In contrast, a considerably larger study set may be required to identify reliable differences in molecular signatures associated with clinical outcome within acute lymphocytic leukemia patients, if the intrinsic biological basis for patient outcome is more subtle.

3. **Meta-analyses.** Microarray data results may be validated using multiple, independent study data sets. As an increasing number of microarray studies are published and corresponding data sets are made publicly available in microarray data repositories, it has become increasingly possible to validate patterns of gene expression identified in one experiment using other microarray experiments in the published literature. In fact, meta-analyses of microarray data are becoming more frequent, and although some studies demonstrate that significant patterns of gene expression can be validated in experiments conducted by independent investigators (*N Engl J Med.* 2006;355:560), other such analyses have demonstrated clear differences between studies (*J Natl Cancer Inst.* 2005;97:927).

V. **CLINICAL APPLICATIONS.** To date, microarray technology has been used primarily for basic science studies that involve whole genome analyses to identify novel biomarkers or elucidate biological signaling pathways. However, as this technology continues to mature, nucleic acid microarrays are now being used as a clinical diagnostic platform.

A. **Gene expression profiling as an ancillary diagnostic tool for the pathologist.** Perhaps one of the most useful applications of gene expression microarray technology has been its use in the diagnosis of histologically ambiguous tumor specimens. Gene expression profiles can molecularly define the cell lineage of metastases of unknown origin (particularly adenocarcinoma) with 80–90% accuracy based on thorough retrospective analysis of clinical data (*Cancer Res.* 2005;65:4031). Gene expression data can also be used to discriminate histological 'look-alikes' with distinct cell origins, such as small round blue cell tumors (*Nat Med.* 2001;7:673). Of greater interest are results demonstrating that molecular profiling can subclassify histologically indistinguishable tumors into biologically relevant subtypes. The first study to define this principle was conducted in diffuse large B-cell lymphoma, where gene expression patterns clearly segregate tumors with aggressive and indolent molecular profiles that also have significance for patient survival (*Curr Opin Hematol.* 2002;9:333). Gene expression profiles of invasive ductal breast carcinoma can also clearly define 'basal-cell' and 'luminal cell' tumor types (among others) that have unique biological characteristics and therapeutic response profiles (*Clin Cancer Res.* 2005;11:5678). An even more intriguing application of microarray-based molecular profiling involves complete tumor reclassification based not on anatomic site or histopathological features, but by patterns or modules of gene expression (*Nat Genet.* 2004;36:1090). Given that the phenotypic behavior of tumor cells and their response to molecular therapies may be more dependent on molecular profiles than organ site of origin, this approach has the potential to significantly modify the role of pathology and the practice of clinical oncology.

B. **Predicting disease behavior.** Gene expression profiles of primary tumor samples have been used to develop predictive signatures of local and distant metastasis, both for specific tumor types and more globally (*Nat Genet.* 2003;33:49). Further clinical validation of such signatures could, for example, define a new diagnostic category of "lymph node potential positive" tumors, which might play an equal if not more important role than traditional histopathology for staging cancer patients and therapeutic decision making.

C. **Predicting survival.** Several large clinical studies have identified gene expression signatures that predict patient survival in breast cancer, lung cancer, leukemia, lymphoma, and many other tumor types. Results from these studies are usually individually validated using statistical methodology or through independent training and test patient populations. However, an increasingly worrisome finding is that clinically predictive gene expression signatures are not reproducible across multiple studies of the same tumor type (*J Natl Cancer Inst.* 2005;97:927). Proposed explanations for these discordant findings include the use of differing and nonstandardized microarray platforms, the examination of patient cohorts that are not matched for clinical and treatment parameters, and the relatively complex phenotype of survival, which is dependent on many variables in addition to tumor molecular signatures.

D. Predicting therapeutic response. In the context of neoadjuvant chemotherapy trials, gene expression microarray analyses of pretreatment tumor biopsy specimens have been used to develop predictive signatures of treatment response (*Nat Med.* 2006;12:1294). To date, these studies have been small and retrospective. However, the ability to use tumor gene expression data to prospectively manage patient treatment will be an important step toward the concept of personalized medicine.

E. Non-tumor pathology. Microarray technology has been applied to biomarker discovery in other fields of pathology and clinical medicine such as neuropathology (Alzheimer's Parkinson's epilepsy, schizophrenia), immunopathology (systemic lupus, multiple sclerosis), organ transplantation, reproductive endocrinology, trauma and sepsis, and cardiovascular disease. However, in multiorgan disease processes, the appropriate target cell population for study is often either (a) not obvious or (b) difficult to obtain from a large number of relevant fresh-frozen biospecimens from patients. Therefore, many microarray studies focusing on noncancer disease processes have been limited to very small sample sizes. Known and unknown variability within these disease processes and between patients make establishing definitive patterns of gene expression associated with disease phenotype difficult.

F. Genotyping. DNA sequence alterations, either SNPs present in germline DNA or somatic point mutations which occur in tumor cells, are important diagnostic markers for disease predisposition, diagnosis, and treatment. Microarray technology is a high-throughput method for genotyping individuals at as many as 1 million loci across the genome, and is beginning to have enormous implications for clinical genetics. For example, familial linkage studies designed to identify inherited disease genes associated with tumor syndromes have greatly benefited from this technology. Microarray-based genotyping has also been used in genetic association studies to define loci associated with disease predisposition and clinical phenotype. Although most applications of genotyping microarrays have been used to discover a single disease locus of interest, it is likely that complex, multigenic diseases may eventually require genotyping at multiple loci to accurate classify a genetic phenotype.

G. Genome copy number. Another major application of microarray technology involves assessment of genome copy number (*Hum Mol Genet.* 2003;12 Spec No 2:R145). Tumor cells experience a wide variety of chromosomal gains and losses, and although these events have been traditionally measured using cytogenetic techniques, microarrays are becoming an increasingly useful method to correlate gene copy number changes with clinical and pathological features of tumors. Microarray-based gene copy number assessment has been used to define critical regions or even single genes whose gain or loss had previously been measured only on the scale of chromosome arm losses or gains. This has led to the rapid identification of new oncogenes and tumor suppressor genes which are subsequent targets of future biomarker and therapeutic studies. Microarray analysis of gene copy number has also identified genomic alterations that are characteristic of particular tumor types and that can be associated with clinical outcome.

Microarray analysis of gene copy number has also identified genomic alterations that are characteristic of particular tumor types and which can be associated with clinical outcome. Germline genomes of normal populations contain a large number of copy number polymorphisms as well (20). This normal variability in locus copy number is likely to have enormous significance for disease predisposition and pharmacogenomics, making the use of copy number based microarray analysis a likely tool for future patient management.

H. Methylation. Methylation of CpG dinucleotides occurs frequently in tumor genomes and is associated with transcriptional silencing of key tumor suppressor genes.

Microarray technology has allowed for whole-genome methylation profiling to distinguish subtypes of leukemia and to identify patterns of methylation associated with treatment response, among many other evolving applications.

I. **DNA resquencing.** A final, but perhaps most promising application of microarrays involves their use in gene resequencing. Oligonucleotide microarrays can be constructed to interrogate individual bases of DNA sequence, thus providing a method for sequencing clinical samples by hybridization. Microarrays have been designed to sequence the genomes of the severe acute respiratory syndrome and human immunodeficiency virus, for the purposes of strain classification and predicting response to antiviral agents, respectively. In other applications, investigators have developed a "MitoChip," a microarray designed to sequence the entire mitochondrial genome, because specific mitochondrial mutations occur frequently in human cancer cells and therefore have become intriguing candidates for tumor biomarkers. A microarray designed to resequence the entire p53 tumor suppressor gene has been used to predict clinical outcome and therapeutic response in patients based on the spectrum of somatic p53 sequence alterations in their primary tumors; the sensitivity of this approach is >90% and, with the exception of detecting nucleotide insertions and deletions, is comparable to that of traditional dideoxy sequencing (*Cancer Res.* 2000;60:2716).

Only recently has the sequence of the cancer genome been explored to any degree of detail. However, there is already compelling evidence that specific gene sequence alterations in tumors will predict vulnerability and resistance to specific therapies such as the epidermal growth factor receptor inhibitor, gefitinib (*N Engl J Med.* 2004;350:2129). As more and more clinically relevant somatic sequence alterations are identified in viruses, tumor cells, and other pathologic specimens, the ability to perform rapid resequencing of multiple genetic loci on a single clinical specimen will be incredibly important. In this respect, as compared to traditional sequencing methodologies, microarrays and the sequencing by hybridization approach should become routine clinical molecular diagnostic tools that will supplement many traditional histopathological and immunohistochemical approaches currently used to evaluate pathology specimens.

VI. **USE OF MICROARRAYS IN THE CLINICAL LABORATORY.** Although nucleic acid microarrays have been used for numerous research studies with potential clinical significance, the routine use of this technology platform in the clinical laboratory will still require several significant advancements.

A. **Array content.** Because the microarray format is well suited to measure multiple markers from a single sample, it is ideal for the clinical laboratory that performs prospective analysis on single clinical specimens. For discovery experiments, thousands of individual genetic markers may be simultaneously assayed, but in doing this, each marker is optimized for neither sensitivity nor specificity. In clinical testing, this may be problematic for measuring low levels or subtle alterations of gene expression, or for detecting genomic alterations that may be present in only a subset of cell populations. By designing disease-specific marker sets, optimizing hybridization conditions for each marker, and placing redundant probes for each marker on the same array, it may be possible to increase the sensitivity and precision of microarray assays, although this has only recently become a design consideration. A microarray used for discovery purposes may assay 10,000 genes using a single set of probes; a similar sized array could also assay 100 genes using 100 different probe measurements. The ability to create large numbers of redundant probe sets and control sequences should provide a level of precision not currently available from most research-based microarrays.

B. **Automation and standardization.** Another potential advantage of microarray technology is that it can be highly automated and regulated, attributes that are critical for any clinical laboratory test. Newer sample (target) preparation methods use single tube, 'hands-off' chemistries that will facilitate routine use in the clinical laboratory. Self-contained microarray cassettes, such as those manufactured by Affymetrix and other vendors, provide an acceptable format for regulated clinical tests. Finally, as diagnostic biomarkers become more established, microarray platforms will need to evolve into clinical diagnostic tools that meet all regulatory requirements of standard clinical tests. Regulatory requirements will require additional standardization and inter-laboratory assay validation, which only recently has received appropriate attention (*Nat Biotechnol.* 2006;24:1151). Already several assays have been validated and are being adapted to an in vitro diagnostic platform for use in clinical laboratories (*Mol Diagn.* 2005;9:119). As additional biomarker targets are validated, these assays should become more and more prevalent in clinical laboratories, and microarray technology will become integrated within the standard practice of diagnostic pathology.

C. Assay complexity. Microarrays are indisputably high-complexity assays, and although streamlined protocols, automation, and standardized array manufacturing can mitigate some inherent technical complexity, microarray assays may still remain in the domain of specialized clinical laboratories. Like most hybridization-based assays, the time required to perform microarray analysis even in its most automated format may still require 3 to 4 days. Assay turnaround time could be problematic when assay results are needed to guide immediate therapy. Finally, because microarray assays are based on signal detection by hybridization, there is an inherent limit to sensitivity as compared to amplification-based PCR detection assays.

D. Sample requirements. Another technical limitation of microarray assays is their requirement for high sample quality. Although exact specimen requirements depend on the analyte measured (mRNA, genomic DNA, methylated DNA), the use of formalin-fixed tissue or other specimens that have been collected under routine hospital conditions currently limits the use of microarray technology in a number of clinical settings. Methods are available for amplifying and labeling nanogram quantities of nucleic acids samples (both DNA and RNA), so the ability to use small numbers of cells obtained from minimally invasive procedures such as fine needle aspiration, swabs, or lavages will allow microarray-based assays to be used for diagnostics in a number of different clinical scenarios. Refinements in the use of routine pathology tissue specimens that have been fixed and embedded in paraffin will allow full integration of this technology into routine histopathological assessment.

E. Clinical relevance. The biggest challenge for implementing microarray technology in the clinical laboratory, however, is not array technology itself but rather the clinical validity of the array biomarker content. To date, the majority of microarray platforms have been designed as whole genome discovery tools. Studies have used a relatively small number of observations (patients) and a large number of variables (genes), an approach which has consistently led to high false-positive rates that are unacceptable for clinical assay validation. Most microarray data generated and reported in the literature (particularly gene expression data) have not been reproducible (*J Natl Cancer Inst.* 2005;97:927). Therefore, while microarray technology itself holds great promise for use in a clinical laboratory, there is still a need for many larger, prospective correlative studies to support the use of microarray-based biomarker panels in routine diagnostic pathology.

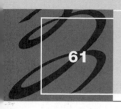

61

BIOSPECIMEN BANKING
Mark A. Watson

I. SIGNIFICANCE TO PATHOLOGY AND TRANSLATIONAL RESEARCH. National initiatives such as The Cancer Genome Atlas (http://cancergenome.nih.gov) and Genome-Wide Association Studies (http://grants.nih.gov/grants/gwas), together with a completely sequenced and highly annotated human genome, have greatly enhanced the resources available to better understand the molecular and genetic basis of human disease. Technologies such gene expression profiling, methylation scanning, comparative genome hybridization, and high-throughput resequencing have also made it possible to harness genomic information to identify disease-specific molecular alterations that occur in human tissues. However, to ultimately understand the significance of basic biological findings toward the improved diagnosis and treatment of human disease, primary human biospecimens (for tissue and body fluids) must be available for clinicogenomic correlative studies. Six important principles embody the rationale for a well-run biospecimen bank.

   A. **Availability of large biospecimen cohorts.** The number of specimens available for study must be relatively large to generate statistically significant findings. For example, because of the large number of variables (e.g., gene expression values) generated from DNA microarray experiments compared to the much smaller number of observations (patients), traditional statistical approaches generate a large number of false-positive results; that is, genes whose expression appears to classify subpopulations of patients, but only does so by mere chance. Validating findings from such whole-genome approaches requires large numbers of patient specimens for study.

   B. **Accurately diagnosed biospecimens.** Several anecdotal examples have illustrated how gene expression profiling can correctly classify specimens that were histologically misidentified by routine clinical pathology (*Am J Pathol.* 2001;159:1231). However, initial diagnostic mislabeling can seriously impede supervised learning approaches to identify new biomarkers. In addition to issues of diagnostic accuracy, knowledge of the precise cellular makeup of specimens (particularly for heterogeneous tissues) is important to properly interpret both gene expression profile and DNA sequencing data. Techniques such as laser capture microdissection can be used to isolate homogeneous cell populations (*Acta Histochem.* 2007;109:171), but requires considerable technical expertise. An added level of complexity in longitudinal studies is that multiple specimens collected from the same patient need to be accurately coded and tracked to ensure that the intended specimen (e.g., initial presentation vs. relapse) is used for downstream analyses.

   C. **Availability of specimens with high molecular integrity.** Although genomic DNA is relatively stable and unaffected by variables in clinical specimen processing and storage, the same is not true for cellular RNA and protein. Cellular RNA and protein may be degraded in cells ex vivo if clinical specimens are not rapidly and properly processed and stored (*J Mol Diagn.* 2000;2:60). More insidiously, the messenger RNA and protein complement of cells may rapidly change as a function of processing time and methodology (*J Surg Res.* 2001;99:222).

   D. **Maximal utilization of diverse biospecimens.** Because of the number and diversity of potential biomarkers that can be discovered as a result of basic scientific studies, patient specimen repositories should contain a wide variety of specimens in a format that can be distributed to as many investigators as possible. For example, preoperative serum from cancer patients may be useful for identifying tumor-associated serum markers for early detection, while nucleated cell fractions from bone marrow, peripheral blood, or cavity washings from the same patient may be used to evaluate potential markers for tumor metastasis detection (Fig. 61.1). Collected specimens may be rare or small in size, so strategies to efficiently consolidate specimen resources (such as tissue microarrays [TMAs]) or to molecularly amplify limiting amounts of genomic material from needle biopsies, tissue touch preps, or washings are critical to providing a useful specimen resource to the research community.

E. Biospecimen annotation. Given the cost and effort associated with whole-genome analyses of clinical specimens, molecular data associated with human biospecimens are equally, if not more valuable than the specimen itself. A data system that can accurately track individual samples within large clinical specimen sets and that allows for accurate integration and correlation of sequence, expression, biomarker, and clinical data is obviously crucial. A large and viable specimen resource is only useful if it is linked to complete and accurate clinical data that can be used to substantiate or refute clinical hypotheses. At the same time, increasing concerns for medical record privacy and, in particular, genetic data privacy require proper measures to protect patient confidentiality.

F. Biospecimen custodianship. There have been increasing concerns regarding ownership of tissue specimens (*JAMA.* 2004;292:2500) and the intellectual property that is generated from their use. There is also a continuing need to appropriately honor the intent and privacy of patient donors. These considerations require the establishment of an unbiased agent who can judiciously administer and regulate the collection and distribution of specimens for research purposes.

The biospecimen bank has become such an integral part of modern translational research that several national and international agencies, such as the National Cancer Institute, have created dedicated offices and guidelines for bank operation (http://biospecimens.cancer.gov). The principles of biospecimen banking obviously relate to the general practice of pathology; therefore, it is almost exclusively the pathologist and the pathology department that have sufficient expertise to govern these activities. The development and maintenance of a biospecimen resource involves many policies and processes that are outlined in Figure 61.2, summarized in this chapter, and described in more detail elsewhere (*Br J Cancer.* 2004;90:1115 and *Mol Diagn.* 2000;5:287).

II. BIOSPECIMEN COLLECTION. The types of biospecimens collected and the methods used to process and store them will depend greatly on their projected use. In establishing a biospecimen bank, however, the intended use is often unknown. Therefore, a wide variety of biospecimens may be collected and archived for study. Because the cost associated with biospecimen procurement and storage is not insignificant ($20 to $150 per specimen), careful consideration should be given to the scope and focus of the biospecimen bank's operation.

A. Defining the scope of operation. The type and number of participants from whom biospecimens will be collected will depend on the stated mission and available resources of the biospecimen bank. In some cases, small banks may collect only defined specimens from participants enrolled in specific clinical trials. In other cases, the bank may be diseased-based and seek to generically collect all available tissue specimens for a given disease type. When resources or institutional boundaries do not permit the creation of a large centralized facility, several small banks may elect to create a federated system where each bank operates independently but is linked by a common informatics network (*Adv Exp Med Biol.* 2006;587:65). A biospecimen bank need not be a 'bank' at all, but may simply serve to collect, process, de-identify, and immediately distribute biospecimens to investigators; the Cooperative Human Tissue Network frequently operates as such a tissue broker (*Cancer.* 1993;71:1391). A biospecimen bank may also simply exist as a more formal representation of diagnostic paraffin block specimens already available in the pathology department.

B. Regulatory requirements. Unlike other aspects of pathology practice, biospecimen banking is considered a research activity and therefore must conform to regulatory requirements that are different than those for a clinical laboratory.

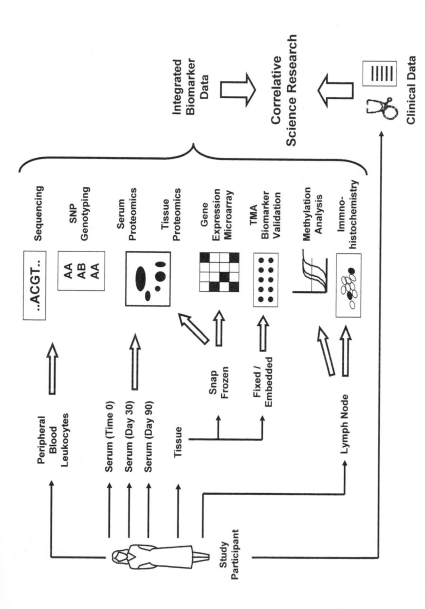

Figure 61.1. From a single participant, a biospecimen resource may collect multiple specimen types and corresponding data to enable a wide variety of translational research projects. A corresponding informatics system is often required to track and maintain these data. SNP, single nucleotide polymorphism; TMA, tissue microarray.

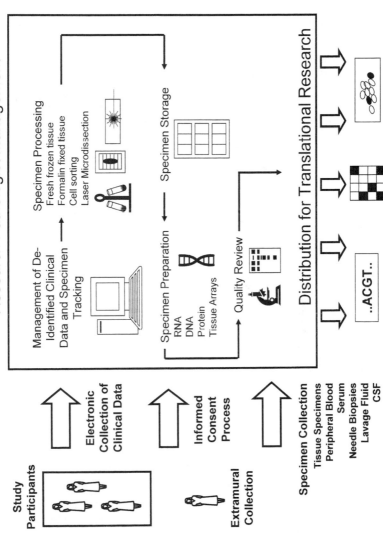

Figure 61.2. Flow diagram of the many processes and resources required to operate a typical full service biospecimen resource. CSF, cerebrospinal fluid;

Policies have evolved significantly at the national level over the past 5 years, and also vary greatly between states and institutions. Generally, the following points need to be considered with regard to biospecimen-based human subjects research.

1. **Institutional review board (IRB) review.** The intended purpose, scope, and policies of the biospecimen bank must be reviewed by the IRB. In some cases, a Certificate of Confidentiality, a document that asserts the right of the tissue bank director (or honest broker) to protect the confidentiality of biospecimen data even under court order, may be required (*Genet Test.* 2004;8:209).

2. **Participant consent.** In most cases of prospective biospecimen collection, some form of informed participant consent is required. Explicit informed consent may be waived if it is impossible or impractical to obtain and the risk to the participant is minimal. Some institutions have ruled that generic language present in a hospital admissions document or surgical consent form provides sufficient consent for biospecimen collection, assuming that the specimens are distributed and used in a de-identified or anonymous manner. Generally, however, explicit written consent for biospecimen banking should be obtained from the participant. Many generic templates for the language used in such a document are available (*J Lab Clin Med.* 2004;144:229). Because the main risk to an individual participating in a biospecimen banking program is loss of confidentiality, measures used to protect such confidentiality and the risks associated with this loss are the main risks to convey to the participant. However, when human biospecimens are being used for genomic and disease-predisposition studies, and when research results from biospecimen use generate patentable biomarker inventions, properly documented more specific informed participant consent may be critical.

3. **Investigator agreements.** In addition to IRB requirements that must be satisfied by the biospecimen bank for the initial collection, coding, and storage of biospecimens, any investigator seeking to use biospecimens from the bank may need to meet additional regulatory requirements. For example, approval of an independent IRB protocol may be required. In addition, the investigator may be expected to sign a Data Use Agreement or other investigator agreement that establishes what the investigator will or will not do with distributed biospecimens. If specimens are to be distributed to an investigator outside of the bank's institution, a material transfer agreement (MTA) may also be necessary.

C. **Specimen types**

1. **Tissues.** Collected tissues may be snap-frozen or fixed in a variety of cross-linking or precipitating fixatives. Snap-frozen tissue provides the highest quality protein and nucleic acid derivatives, and is often required for genomic or proteomic studies. However, the logistics of frozen tissue collection are difficult, and proper storage is relatively expensive. Formalin-fixed, paraffin embedded (FFPE) tissue blocks are easy to obtain, easy to store, and very familiar to any pathology service. However, the quality of molecular derivatives from such tissues is vastly inferior and rarely amenable to array-based or proteomic studies (*Lab Invest.* 2007;87:383). Fixation of tissue in precipitating fixatives such as ethanol, acetone, and others (*Arch Pathol Lab Med.* 1994;118:298 and *Mod Pathol.* 2001;14:116), followed by embedding in low-melting-point paraffin or acrylic (*J Mod Diagn.* 1999;1:17), provides tissue with excellent histological detail and molecular material that is superior to that of traditional FFPE tissue (e-**Fig. 61.1**).* However, RNA and protein quality still do not match that of material derived from frozen tissue.

2. **Blood components.** Serum and plasma (often from multiple time points throughout a patient's clinical course) are often banked. They are the preferred biospecimen for proteomic analysis, but when properly aliquoted from multiple patients from multiple time points, they can often occupy a large amount of storage space. Peripheral blood leukocytes are the ideal source for germline DNA for genetic and genomic studies, and can be stored or processed without the need for additional cell-separation protocols such as mononuclear cell isolation. Bone marrow may also be banked.

---

*All e-figures are available online via the Solution Site Image Bank.

3. **Other body fluids.** Urine, sputum, cavity lavages, and effusions may also be collected and stored as they serve as useful analytes to discover disease-associated proteins or cellular biomarkers. However, large fluid volume specimens (such as urine) may be difficult and expensive to process and store for long periods of time, particularly for a future unknown use. Furthermore, analysis of such biospecimens may require only a small amount of material per assay, which then necessitates that collections be excessively aliquoted to prevent multiple freeze–thaw cycles of the same specimen. As an alternative, the cellular component of these fluids may be isolated by centrifugation and stored as cell pellets.

D. **Collection methods.** Depending on the biospecimen type and its intended application, there are a number of important considerations involved in collecting specimens for a biospecimen bank.

1. **Specimen acquisition.** For most general tissue bank activities, tissue specimens are collected in the course of routine treatment, such as a surgical resection of a solid tumor, a therapeutic needle aspiration to remove joint or body cavity fluid, or a diagnostic bone marrow biopsy. In these cases, it is important that biospecimen collection for research purposes not compromise the diagnostic utility of the specimen. In many cases, such as the resection of a small breast tumor or malignant prostate gland, it is important that biospecimen procurement occur under the direct guidance of a pathologist who can supervise and assure that diagnostic integrity (e.g., an intact tumor margin) is not compromised. In these cases, the procedure and resulting biospecimen should be minimally invasive and limited in size or quantity (e.g. a needle core biopsy). Such small specimens may be perfectly suitable for their intended downstream analyses, but may required careful attention to processing and storage, as discussed below. Other protocols may allow for redundant tissue sampling at the time of a diagnostic procedure; for example, for a patient with a suspicious liver mass, standard of care may dictate that two specimens from a computed tomography–guided needle biopsy be submitted for diagnostic evaluation, while two additional needle cores may be taken for the research tissue bank. In certain cases, the research bank may receive tissue samples that harbor clinically relevant diagnostic findings that are not present in the routinely processed tissue samples; for this reason, the institutional pathology department should develop policies regarding clinical versus research specimen collection, which may include holding all research specimens in escrow until a final clinical diagnosis is rendered. Finally, an IRB-approved study protocol may require the collection of biospecimens above and beyond what is needed for routine standard of care. For example, a tissue biopsy or peripheral blood specimen collected before and at multiple time points after a course of therapy.

2. **Biospecimen preservation.** For molecular and genomic analyses, proper tissue preservation is critical. A specimen's molecular profile (i.e., gene expression, protein phosphorylation) can rapidly change from the time it is first collected until the time when it is ultimately preserved by freezing or fixation (*J Surg Res.* 2001;99:222) due to 'warm ischemia time.' Although few evidence-based guidelines exist, warm ischemia time should be limited and at least documented so as not to introduce additional preanalytical variability into biospecimen-based studies. Although snap-frozen tissue is the preferred substrate for many studies, several commercial and 'home-brew' tissue preservatives are available that provide acceptable biospecimen preservation (*BMC Genomics.* 2004;5:88). Delays in blood processing can affect proteomic biomarker profiles (*Expert Rev Proteomics.* 2006;3:409); unlike tissue, whole blood cannot be immediately snap-frozen, but must be centrifuged to remove the specific plasma or serum component, which then, in turn, must be aliquoted and rapidly frozen. As with tissue, a number of commercial products are available to preserve blood cell components at ambient temperature without freezing, although these products are relatively expensive and require specialized downstream isolation procedures (*Cytometry A.* 2004;59:191 and *Physiol Genomics.* 2004;19:247).

3. **Remote site collection.** For multi-institutional research protocols, it may be necessary to collect biospecimens from remote sites, often from health centers or

medical offices that have little experience in dealing with intricate biospecimen requirements such as snap-frozen tissue. Proper and efficient collection of biospecimens from such sites may require preassembled specimen procurement kits (e-Fig. 61.2) and personnel training to ensure the uniform collection of biospecimens from all sites.

4. **Specimen quantity.** New molecular amplification strategies such as polymerase chain reaction, whole-genome amplification, and transcript amplification allow investigators to use nanogram quantities of DNA and RNA for analysis. Instrumentation for proteomic analysis has also become considerably more advanced and, although it is not possible to amplify protein analytes from biospecimens, tissue requirements have been minimized even for these technologies. Therefore, even limited size biospecimens such as needle aspirates, tissue touch preps, and core biopsies are valuable and frequently amenable to molecular analyses. Obviously, however, such specimens must be judiciously distributed to maximize their research potential. Conversely, the collection of large tissue specimens is not necessarily desirable; for example, large resected carcinoma specimens are often not properly preserved when fixed or frozen in their entirety. For such cases, tissue specimens should be divided into samples no greater than 1 cm^3 for fixation and/or freezing.

5. **Associated data collection.** Clinical and pathologic data corresponding to the participant and specimen are as important as the specimen itself. Without these associated data, it is impossible to perform correlative studies. The scope of the data that are collected and stored with the biospecimen will depend on the mission of the biospecimen bank. It is usually impractical to gather detailed clinical information represented as written notes in a clinical chart or report; instead, it may be more efficient to rely on electronic sources of data. Although data is usually represented in text format, surgical pathology reports provide an accurate and detailed source of pathology information about tissue specimens that are collected and diagnosed as part of routine clinical care. In some centers, an electronic medical record may provide access to basic patient demographics and clinical diagnostic data. For cancer patients and their specimens, the hospital tumor registry is often a reasonably detailed and standardized source for cancer-related clinical and pathology data. Except for specific studies, it is generally advisable to collect a limited but standardized data set corresponding to each collected case, rather than an exhaustive (and inevitably incomplete) data set for every specimen.

E. **Biospecimen data management.** As depicted in Figure 61.1, biospecimen banks may house a complex array of specimens and associated data. It is critical that specimens be accurately tracked and annotated if they are to be useful. Although smaller banks may rely on written log books and electronic spreadsheets to track specimen information, these methods will become rapidly constraining as the bank becomes larger and more diversified. Basic data types that may be required in a biospecimen bank information system include the following:

1. **Receipt, study association, and consent tracking.** An accurate record must be maintained of when and from where biospecimens were received, and for what protocol they are intended. The consent with which the specimens were collected is also important to regulate how the specimens can be used.

2. **Inventory and storage.** It is important to accurately maintain the availability and storage location of each specimen so that it can be rapidly retrieved on demand.

3. **Quality assurance.** Quality assurance measures such as tissue histology review, warm ischemia time, details of specimen processing, and nucleic acid quality should be maintained for each specimen.

4. **Clinical annotation.** As discussed above, a minimal set of clinical and pathology annotation data should be associated with each specimen.

5. **Distribution and utilization.** The efficacy of a biospecimen bank is judged almost entirely on its distribution of biospecimens for productive translational research. Therefore, detailed data concerning specimen distribution to investigators and utilization for specific research studies are essential in justifying the activity and operation of the bank.

A small number of commercial software packages are available to assist in the management of biospecimen banks. More frequently, individual centers develop their own data systems, often developing rather arbitrary and custom data schemes and data definitions. Although such applications may serve the immediate needs of the bank, they present a significant obstacle to collaboration among different biospecimen resource centers. To address this challenge, the NCI's Cancer Biomedical Informatics Grid program has fostered a group of pathologists, biologists, and informatics specialists working to develop data standards and tools for pathology and biospecimen resources (https://cabig.nci.nih.gov/workspaces/TBPT). Among these tools is the caTissue software application, a freely available web-based tool for managing biospecimen inventory (https://cabig.nci.nih.gov/tools/catissuecore).

III. **BIOSPECIMEN PROCESSING.** Many of the same principles of specimen processing used in the clinical laboratory apply to biospecimens banked for research purposes. However, because specimens collected for research purposes may be used for experimental studies that are not a part of traditional diagnostic histopathology, special specimen processing needs must be considered.

A. **Frozen tissue.** Although the histological quality of frozen tissue is inferior to that of traditionally fixed, paraffin-embedded material, most molecular studies require high-grade DNA, RNA, and protein that can be obtained only from frozen specimens. Tissue may be frozen in liquid nitrogen, an isopentane cryobath (such as is available in most pathology frozen section rooms), or a make-shift dry ice–ethanol bath. Tissue specimens should be no larger than 1 cm^3 to ensure rapid and consistent freezing throughout the specimen. If the specimen is to be used for histological sectioning for quality review or laser microdissection, it may first be embedded in freezing media such as optimal cutting temperature (OCT) compound. Because OCT material does not interfere with nucleic acid isolation, but may have an effect on proteomic studies, it may be advisable to freeze both embedded and non-embedded tissue for the widest range of downstream uses. After being frozen, tissue may be stored in cassettes in $-80°C$ ultralow freezers or liquid nitrogen (LN_2) vapor inventory systems. Although the latter are more expensive and difficult to maintain, specimens stored in LN_2 are immune to the power failures and mechanical breakdowns that can occur with electric freezers. Any frozen storage system should be equipped with a temperature-recording device to document appropriate storage conditions and a remote alarm system that can contact the laboratory supervisor in the event of a machine failure or power loss.

B. **Fixed tissue.** FFPE tissue specimens are not as well-suited for molecular and genomic analyses. However, the quality of fixed tissue specimens intended for research can be improved using several quality control measures.

1. **Control and document fixation and processing times.** By minimizing the time for which tissues are fixed, overfixation (which leads to excessive antigen cross-linking and molecular degradation) can be avoided. Documentation of processing times for each specimen can remove this preanalytical variable in studies that use tissue specimens collected over different time periods or from different locations.

2. **Use of 'molecularly friendly' fixatives.** Several commercially available and 'home brew' precipitating fixatives preserve tissue and tissue histology while minimizing the damaging effects to protein antigens and nucleic acids caused by cross-linking fixatives such as formalin (*Arch Pathol Lab Med*. 1994;118:298 and *Mod Pathol*. 2001;14:116).

3. **Vacuum storage.** Although there are no convincing data to suggest an added benefit, many biospecimen repositories recommend that paraffin tissue blocks and, more importantly, cut unstained sections, be vacuumed sealed and stored at 4°C. The premise of this storage approach is that antigenicity and nucleic acids are protected from further degradation by both removal of oxygen and reduced temperature.

C. **Blood components.** For the storage of serum and plasma, whole blood must be immediately spun to remove the appropriate liquid component from cellular material. The isolated serum or plasma must then be immediately aliquoted and frozen.

Processing must be performed rapidly before cell lysis and protein degradation occurs. Consortia of proteomics investigators have published recommendations on blood processing for proteomic studies (*Expert Rev Proteomics.* 2006;3:409) and although some of these guidelines are evidenced based, robust guidelines have not been firmly established. Many investigators freeze whole blood at the site of collection as a convenient way to store blood for future genomic DNA isolation; however, freezing blood in glass Vacutainer tubes presents a safety hazard, requires considerably more freezer space to store, and inevitably causes cell lysis, which results in DNA that is frequently lower in yield, degraded, and contaminated with heme products that can effect downstream assays. Although more labor intensive for the collection site, immediate spinning of whole blood followed by selective removal, washing, aliquoting, and freezing of the buffy coat creates a high-quality specimen that is easy to store and results in higher DNA yield and quality. In some cases it may be desirable to isolate the peripheral blood mononuclear cell (PBMC) fraction and preserve these cells; this approach has the advantage of removing peripheral blood granulocytes and preserving the monocyte fraction that can be manipulated for future uses such as flow cytometry and cell immortalization. However, viable preservation of PBMC is expensive, requires additional expertise, and is seldom necessary for simple DNA isolation. When PBMC isolation is not a consideration, whole blood may be stored at 4°C for as long as 72 hours with little loss in PBMC viability (*Ann Epidemiol.* 2000;10:538).

D. Laser microdissection. For some investigations involving genomic analysis, it may be desirable to have material derived from homogeneous cell populations. Laser microdissection is a method that allows an investigator to visualize tissue microscopically and to use a laser to either 'capture' or cut the desired cells away from surrounding tissue (e-Fig. 61.3). The isolated cells may then be used for DNA, RNA, or protein isolation for molecular analysis (*Acta Histochem.* 2007;109:171 and *Methods Mol Biol.* 2005;293:187). Although laser microdissection instrumentation is expensive and the technique requires expertise, it has become routine in many biospecimen banks.

E. TMAs provide another format to maximize utilization of limiting tissue specimens (*Methods Mod Med.* 2005;103:89). They are constructed by sampling one to three 0.8-mm (up to as large as 3 mm) tissue cores from a donor paraffin tissue block and assembling them into an array of as many as 300 cores in a recipient block (e-Fig. 61.4). The resulting recipient block can then be sectioned as a traditional tissue block, making it possible to perform immunohistochemistry or fluorescence in situ hybridization on each of the 300 cores on a single slide. TMAs allow researchers to easily validate patterns of biomarker expression in a large sample series using relatively inexpensive technology. Few special reagents are required, and basic TMA instrumentation is relatively inexpensive, but expert reading and informatics tracking of the 300 cores per slide is required. A recognized disadvantage of the TMA format is that it is prone to sampling error as only a small sample from each block is incorporated into the array.

F. Nucleic acid. Genomic technologies have shifted research requirements from fixed tissue sections to derivative nucleic acids, so many biospecimen banks now produce DNA and RNA for research investigators. Nucleic acid can be effectively derived from frozen and fixed tissue using several standard protocols, although the quality from the latter is inferior as discussed above. In some cases, it may be desirable to isolate nucleic acid directly from collected specimens, such as DNA from peripheral blood. Nucleic acids (RNA and DNA) are more stable when isolated and can be more conveniently stored as compared to the parent tissue or fluid. However, the initial cost and effort to generate DNA and/or RNA from every banked specimen as it is received is great, so prospective preparation of nucleic acids should be considered only when material will be of immediate use.

IV. QUALITY ASSURANCE. A biospecimen resource should provide material only to investigators with appropriate quality control. In fact, one of the main reasons for a pathologist-supervised biospecimen resource is that it is pathologists who best understand the approach to and importance of clinical specimen quality control.

A. Specimen identification. Just as in any clinical laboratory, proper specimen labeling and identification are critical; because a bank may store biospecimens for prolonged periods of time, maintenance of proper specimen identification is important. Most biospecimen banks are not subject to the regulatory review of clinical laboratories, but even as a purely research effort, biospecimen banks should implement standard clinical laboratory practices to prevent sample mislabeling. These practices may include use of preprinted barcode labels, double data entry, and routine data auditing.

B. Representative tissue sampling. In most cases, biospecimens that are submitted for clinical diagnosis and those that are submitted to a bank for research purposes are not identical. They may be collected at slightly different times or locations, or may involve sampling bias. For example, in a heterogeneous prostate tumor, a tissue biopsy banked for research may contain no neoplastic cells although the routinely processed tissue for diagnosis shows adenocarcinoma; distribution of the banked specimen under the assumption that it truly reflects the diagnostic material may result in a compromised research study. Consequently, it is important that individual biospecimens received by the bank undergo individual diagnostic review either prospectively or prior to distribution for a research study. Such a review of tissue or cellular samples may involve confirmation of a histopathological diagnosis as well as notation of general cellular features such as histological preservation, tissue cellularity, and necrosis. A special circumstance arises when a novel finding or diagnosis is observed in a banked research specimen that was not reported from the material for diagnosis; resolution of such a problematic circumstance will depend on the policies of both the IRB and pathology service, but should be documented as part of the bank's standard operating procedures.

C. Tissue preservation and molecular integrity. When the bank will be responsible for generating and distributing nucleic acids (DNA and RNA) for correlative science research, it is important that molecular integrity is verified. As discussed above, the quality of nucleic acid is directly related to the manner in which the biospecimen was collected and preserved. Fixation and delays in specimen processing (warm ischemia time) can compromise nucleic acid quality as can repeated freeze–thaw cycles (e-Fig. 61.5). Inherent necrosis and tissue cellularity in the specimen can also affect the quality of nucleic acids. Documentation of molecular specimen quality can be accomplished by readily available (albeit often expensive) instrumentation designed for quality review of small amounts of nucleic acid, including fiberoptic spectrophotometers and capillary microelectrophoresis systems. Metrics have been developed which relate quantitative results from these instruments to expected performance in downstream applications and assays (*BMC Mol Biol.* 2007;22:8).

V. BIOSPECIMEN UTILIZATION. The success of any biospecimen bank is measured by the utilization of collected biospecimens for productive translational research. Distribution of biospecimens for funded research projects is also an important revenue source to support the larger biospecimen-banking effort. Although there is often a 3- to 5-year lag time before a new biospecimen bank is routinely used, while the bank is developing and maturing its collection, a fundamental principle of biospecimen banking is that the collection should be biased in favor of those biospecimens that will be used for funded research projects. Measures that can help promote the productive utilization of a biospecimen resource include the following:

A. Advertisement of available resources is best accomplished through a Web-based catalog of available sources.

B. Streamlined administrative processes. Often, investigators are unfamiliar with procedures for requesting specimens, obtaining appropriate IRB approval, and creating necessary MTAs. Having a standardized and facilitated process for dealing with regulatory steps necessary for biospecimen distribution will greatly enhance utilization of a biospecimen resource.

C. High-quality annotated specimens. Translational research can be accelerated only when biospecimens distributed to the investigator are properly quality controlled and "assay ready." Minimal but sufficient clinical and/or pathology data should be supplied with each specimen to easily enable the correlative analysis.

D. Facilitated and judicious distribution. The process of case selection, specimen retrieval and processing, specimen annotation, and distribution can be time consuming and expensive. As a biospecimen bank matures, an increasing number of requests from investigators may overtax the bank's available resources and can result in significant delays in providing specimens for research. Competing interests for a limited number of biospecimens may also become problematic as bank utilization increases. Therefore, a biospecimen bank should establish a utilization review committee so that the finite effort and physical resources of the bank can be allocated fairly to the research community. This committee should be an unbiased representation of pathologists and scientists, with allocation decisions based on scientific merit of proposed projects, investigator track record with previous requests, funding status, and likelihood that distributed biospecimens will meaningfully contribute to grant or scientific publication development.

VI. SUPPORT. Unlike the clinical pathology laboratory, a research biospecimen bank must find its own means of financial support. Frequent sources of support include the following:

A. Institutional support. Academic institutions or departments often support the initial development and operation of a biospecimen bank, which is not surprising considering the central importance of the bank in the mission of translational research. In return, the institution expects a return on its investment in terms of the number of biospecimen-based projects, publications, and research grants that can be enabled through such a resource.

B. Extramural funding. Unlike traditional, hypothesis-based research grants, there are few extramural (non-institutional) funding mechanisms to specifically support biospecimen banks. A bank or tissue procurement shared resource facility may, however, be a key funded component of larger initiatives such as National Institutes of Health program project grants, center grants, or disease-focused programs (e.g., Specialized Programs of Research Excellence, or SPOREs). As the importance of biospecimen banking becomes increasingly evident, special funding opportunities may become available.

C. Investigator fees. A viable specimen resource will need to develop investigator fees for the services it provides, including biospecimen collection, storage, and processing. These fees should be calculated realistically and take into account all operations and resources that are required from the initial collection of a biospecimen to its final distribution to an investigator. Such fees should be structured to also allow for bank growth and further development. At the same time, fees should not be so burdensome as to deter the conduct of sound research, particularly for pilot translational studies for which investigator funding may be limited, or where a unique opportunity exists to collect biospecimens (perhaps in the context of a clinical trial), store them, and use them at a later date when additional research funding is obtained. Obviously, the greater a bank's participation in funded research, the easier it will be to maintain long-term support for the operation and the more likely it will be that the bank will significantly contribute to translational research.

Suggested Readings

Eiseman E, Haga SB. *Handbook of Human Tissue Source: A National Resource of Human Tissue Samples.* Santa Monica, CA. Rano corporation, 2004.

International Society for Biological and Environmental Repositories (http://www.isber.org/)

National Cancer Institute (NCI) Office of Biorepositories and Biospecimen Research (http://biospecimens.cancer.gov)

NCI Specimen Resource Locator (http://pluto3.nci.nih.gov/tissue/expediter.cfm)

IMAGING TECHNOLOGIES IN SURGICAL PATHOLOGY: VIRTUAL MICROSCOPY AND TELEPATHOLOGY

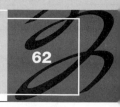

62

Jochen K. M. Lennerz, Peter A. Humphrey, and Erika C. Crouch

I. **CONVENTIONAL LIGHT MICROSCOPY** is the core tool in diagnostic surgical pathology (*Lab Invest.* 2007;87:403). The future of pathologic diagnosis will, however, include the electronic mode of image presentation, with diagnoses rendered after viewing the cells or tissue on a computer screen rather than with an optical microscope. Digital cameras have replaced 35-mm film cameras (*Adv Anat Pathol.* 2003;10:88), and these static gross and microscopic digital images are now the standard for surgical pathology teaching and research. The next phase of imaging in pathology will be to incorporate new imaging technologies into the routine practice of diagnostic pathology.

To evaluate new imaging technologies, it is essential to separate knowledge of histopathology from the skill of using a microscope. Histopathological diagnosis depends far more on the professional competence and skill of the pathologist rendering the diagnosis than on the "technology" or the "microscope" used. For the foreseeable future, using an optical microscope to examine tissue sections on glass slides will remain the standard for the practice of diagnostic histopathology. However, pathologists will increasingly view these sections on computer monitors rather than through conventional optical microscopes because digitized glass slides permit electronic consultations, digital morphometry, and stable image storage that go beyond the capabilities of current microscopy-based diagnostic pathology. These capabilities will increase the amount of clinically useful information obtained from a given pathologic specimen.

II. **VIRTUAL MICROSCOPY** is a technique whereby glass slides are scanned and converted to digital data files or "virtual slides," with viewing of the digital images on a computer screen (whole slide imaging). The visual characteristics, in terms of resolution and range of magnification, are primarily determined by the optical features of the scanning system and are overall comparable with those of glass slide microscopy (*BMC Clin Pathol* 2006;6:4). In contrast to a conventional light microscope on which the magnification, focus, and condenser can be adjusted at any time, a decision of the so-called 'scanning depth' has to be made prior to digital scanning. The scanning depth includes the selection of the region of interest, as well as decisions regarding the scanning power and the number of horizontal levels to be obtained in the plane of the tissue section (so-called z-stacking). Scanning power includes the physical magnification (e.g., 20×) and resolution (e.g., 2048 × 4800 pixels), while z-stacking is dependent on the section thickness and enables virtual focusing up and down through the thickness of the tissue and cells. Depth of focus presents particular problems for the interpretation of 3-dimensional cytological specimens that rely on a 3-dimensional assessment of cellular morphology (*Cancer Cytopathol.* 2007;111:203).

Average scanning time for a single horizontal level (non–z-stacked) is about 2 to 3 minutes and generates a file that is enormous (range from ~200 MB to 1.5 GB). While radiology follows the DICOM (Digital Imaging and Communications in Medicine) standard, no uniform (open source) virtual-slide file format is currently available. However, some interfaces are able to convert the different virtual-slide file formats. The controversial issue of an image standard for pathology is beyond the scope of this chapter (*J Telemed Telecare.* 2005;11:109); however, a variety of file types (jpeg, tiff) can exist side by side. New open-source formats (bigtiff.org) enable versatile retrieval of files with sizes beyond current standards.

Each virtual file consists of multiple parts, called file segments, which include an identification tag, a scanned barcode linked to the laboratory information system (LIS), a low-power overview, and the images at selected power. Image acquisition methods vary (linear, meander, array), and at this time all available systems produce tiled images, that is, small images that are retrieved and stitched together to form the final image on screen at the selected power. The individual image files are typically open source (jpeg, jpeg2000, tiff), and most interfaces allow electronic zooming or additional magnification beyond the scanned power.

Resolution and functionality have recently achieved levels that are comparable with conventional light microscopes. Scanning time, in contrast, is not yet optimal (a reasonable goal is about 20 seconds, including z-stacks). This scanning time is mainly dependent on optical physics, determined by the objective, the image acquisition, the processor, and computational speed. The image acquisition device or CCD (charged coupled device) consists of several hundred thousand individual picture elements (pixels) and transforms the physical into a virtual image (pixel values). Whole slide images can therefore be acquired via single optical lenses moving in a linear fashion over the slide. Some scanners improve scanning time by using a meander-shaped scanning pattern to acquire images, but both the linear and meander methods have inherent physical limitations that become most apparent when acquiring multiple images within each plane of section. In contrast, 'lens array microscopy,' which uses arrays of detectors (miniaturized lenses) to simultaneously capture information from larger areas of the tissue section, may soon be able to meet the high standards of diagnostic pathology (*Hum Pathol.* 2004;35:1303).

A. Implementation of virtual microscopy in the surgical pathology laboratory requires an electronic and organizational infrastructure, and purchase of a slide scanning instrument, which are still quite expensive. Infrastructure and workflow has to be planned and maintained, which requires an efficient interaction of all involved parties, including information technology (IT), laboratory, and LIS personnel. Dedicated and trained technical personnel (image technologists) are required to load and maintain the scanning instrument, perform initial screening (and rescanning if necessary), monitor scan quality, and distribute the virtual files in a manner that can be conveniently viewed by the pathologist. A file server with the necessary storage (upgradeable tera- to petabyte range or beyond), databases for the virtual files (linked and updated to the LIS), and the necessary maintenance and updates have to be organized by a knowledgeable IT person. Protocols for backup copies and deletion of files have to be established. The pathologist needs high-quality LCD monitors of sufficient size (>21 inches) for peripheral vision (*Hum Pathol.* 2006;37:1543) with extended desktop functionality to be able to simultaneously see the LIS, Final report, gross description, images of the specimen, and the slide viewer with histologic images displayed at suitable resolutions.

B. Diagnostic applications of virtual microscopy include consultations, scanning/storage of selected cases for future needs, routine diagnosis, and quality assurance control.

   1. Consultation is one of the greatest immediate strengths of virtual slide microscopy. The introduction of a second opinion, expert opinion, and even 'peer-review diagnosis' via electronic (e-) consultations have begun. In addition to convenience (no packing or mailing), there are several advantages to e-consultations. Electronic distribution is almost instantaneous and allows consulting pathologists to review the virtual slide(s) nearly any time and anywhere. Online, real-time conferencing and simultaneous viewing by two or more pathologists is easily achieved. In addition, there are no risks of losing the primary data (i.e., tissue blocks or slides).

   2. Slides selected for scanning may include controls, original frozen section, representative diagnostic slides and consultation cases where glass slides must be returned to the original referring hospital. Storage of virtual slides creates a permanent copy of the slide(s) and permits review when the patient undergoes another biopsy or resection, in legal cases and/or when the case is presented at a hospital conference.

   3. Routine virtual microscopic diagnosis of all slides should soon be technically feasible. However, it is not yet clear whether digitizing all slides will result in cost and time savings. With existing technology it can take up to 8 minutes to scan a single slide, which can be a rate-limiting factor.

4. **Quality assurance programs** may be enhanced by review of virtual slides from cases with diagnostic discrepancies. Files can be flagged for subsequent review, and trends in diagnostic errors easily identified.

C. **Education.** Virtual microscopy is already an indispensable tool for medical education in pathology, including medical student teaching, teaching of pathology residents and fellows, and continuing medical education for practicing pathologists. At Washington University School of Medicine, virtual slides have been used for several years in the first- and second-year medical school courses (e.g., http://128.252.124.67/). Many national pathology conferences and slide seminars now post virtual slides on a Web site before the meeting, and some Web sites are also building a collection of teaching cases (see, e.g., the United States and Canadian Academy of Pathology [USCAP] Virtual Slide Box at www.uscap.org). Other examples of teaching via virtual slides include teaching of histology to medical students (*Anat Rec.* 2005;285B:19), a tutorial on Gleason grading of prostatic adenocarcinoma (*Hum Pathol.* 2005;36:381), didactic presentations using a combination of PowerPoint and virtual microscopy (*Ann Diagn Pathol.* 2003;7:67), and online virtual atlases (e.g., breast at www.webmicroscope.net). Education and experience with interpretation of virtual slides is critical for pathology residents and fellows; at the very least, it prepares trainees for the American Board of Pathology virtual microscopy practice examination (http://www.abpath.org/VMInstr.htm).

D. **Research applications** for virtual microscopy in surgical pathology include quantitative image analysis and images of tissue microarrays used to study patterns of gene and protein expression. Virtual images can provide documentation for specimens or tissue microarrays retained in tissue banks (*Eur J Cancer.* 2006;42:3110) or for patients enrolled in clinical trials. As for diagnostic pathology, virtual slides make it possible to easily share specimens among investigators at different sites, anytime. Virtual slides also allow for the electronic publication of whole slides rather than selected fields, facilitating the transfer of new information to practicing pathologists.

Image analysis can be performed on any of the above-mentioned files, as for example, quantification of immunohistochemistry signals in breast pathology, which has recently been approved by the U.S. Food and Drug Administration (FDA). Widely accepted freeware and a variety of morphometric small and typically customized subprograms ("plugins") are available; the most versatile solution for image processing and analysis is the NIH freeware ImageJ (*Biophot Int.* 2004;11:36), available at http://rsb.info.nih.gov/ij/. The versatility of this program derives from an open architecture that allows users to implement plugins. Over the years many plugins (mostly research-derived) have been developed; for example, 'Image J for microscopy' (http://www.macbiophotonics.ca/imagej) includes numerous tools, such as intensity and time analysis, particle analysis, colocalization analysis, intensity processing, color processing, stack-slice manipulation, z-functions, t-functions, deconvolution, and annotation. Other image analysis solutions are available (see Resources).

III. **TELEPATHOLOGY** is the practice whereby pathologists render diagnoses from a distance by viewing electronically transmitted images. The transmission medium can include an ordinary telephone line, high-speed digital line, satellite, or the Internet. With some overlap, three systems are currently available: dynamic, static, and virtual telepathology.

A. **Dynamic telepathology systems.** In these systems, pathologists view images in real time by electronic control of a distant robotic microscope with motorized optics and stage. Dynamic robotic telepathology has been primarily used to provide intraoperative frozen section diagnoses to hospitals without on-site pathologists (*Hum Pathol.* 2007;38:1330). Typically, in less than a minute a digital overview of the slide is created. Linked computers enable the pathologist to remotely control the movement of the slide on the microscope. Reported diagnostic accuracy has been high, comparable to conventional light microscopy. A variation of the dynamic method is the submission of a live ("streaming") image from a remotely located microscope without direct (robotic) control; instructions are given via telephone. One important disadvantage of either method is the extra time (factor 2–4) needed to review remotely controlled slides when compared to standard glass slide review. Moreover, robotic and streaming systems are not able to store the whole slide, making reassessment difficult and limiting diagnostic documentation to selected fields. Perhaps even more significant are organizational and logistical issues. In one study (*J Neuropathol Exp Neurol.* 2007;66:750) the lack of an on-site presence affected every stage of the intraoperative consultation including the gathering of patient information, gross specimen examination and handling, frozen section and smear preparation, communication between various parties involved, and documentation of the consultation process. Thus, implementation of telepathology requires substantial planning, communication, and training of both pathologists and support personnel. Indeed, prior to implementation of any of the imaging technologies into routine practice, the laboratory must establish and follow multiple steps including design, verification, validation, and implementation of assurance/quality control (e.g., documented diagnostic accuracy testing).

B. Static telepathology systems. Use images that have been selected, stored, and forwarded to the pathologist. Static systems are mainly used to obtain second opinions on difficult cases. Overall, the diagnostic accuracy approaches that of conventional glass slide optical microscopy. Problems leading to discordance include field selection and poor image quality (*Hum Pathol.* 2003;34:1228). For large or complex specimens, the handicaps of preselected images are more pronounced.

C. Virtual slide telepathology. The use of whole slide imaging in the telepathology setting, has begun to replace other setups. This also includes time-sensitive settings (e.g. intraoperative frozen section diagnosis) where scanning time is currently a limiting factor in all setups. The quicker control of a virtual slide and the advantages of file retrieval outweigh the benefits of robotic control or 'streaming' microscopy. While solutions for the large files are available (e.g. bigtiff.org), image archiving will need to be addressed.

IV. EMERGING IMAGING-RELATED TECHNOLOGIES include spectral imaging (*Cytometry A.* 2006;69[8]:735, 748) and nonconventional optical techniques, computer-aided detection (e.g., visual field tracking, pattern recognition, image segmentation), and the application of artificial intelligence to image analysis. These techniques remain to be tested in routine surgical pathology.

V. FUTURE. Significant issues must be addressed to allow the routine implementation of virtual microscopy and telepathology in diagnostic pathology. There are unresolved regulatory issues concerning pathology practice from a distance, including mechanisms of reimbursement. There is also a debate as to whether virtual microscopy instrumentation is subject to governmental approval, and whether users must be certified prior to rendering diagnoses using these technologies. The validation (*J Biomed Opt.* 2007;12:051801) and incorporation of digital pathology images into the electronic medical record and the integration of digital surgical pathology and radiologic data are largely unexplored. Despite these uncertainties, there is little question that recent advances in imaging technologies provide the unique opportunity to improve patient care.

Resources

apill.upmc.edu (Advancing Practice, Instruction and Innovation Through Informatics Conference)

cap.org (College of American Pathologists: Futurescape conference Series)

Giszczynski y D. Telepathology: revolution or evolution? *Medical Laboratory Observer.* September, 2007.

Gu J, Ogilvie RW. *Virtual Microscopy and Virtual Slides in Teaching, Diagnosis, and Research (Advances in Pathology, Microscopy, and Molecular Morphology).* Boca Raton, FL: CRC Press; 2005.

pathologyinformatics.org (Pathology informatics, the overall field and fellowships)

pathology.wustl.edu/virtualpathology

webmicroscope.net (European Virtual Microscopy network, lab quality, seminars)

Page numbers followed by f indicate figures; page numbers followed by t indicate tabular material.